95.00

Rotherham Health Care Library

B013112

D1582210

This book is due for return on or before the last date shown below.

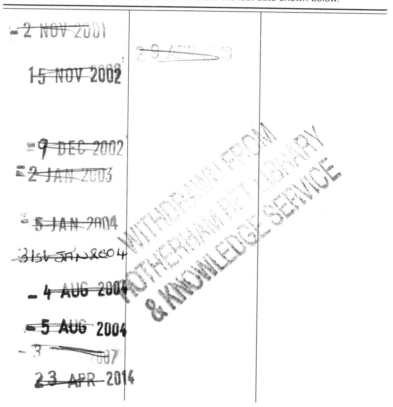

- 2 NOV 2001

15 NOV 2002

2 9 APR

- 9 DEC 2002

- 2 JAN 2003

- 5 JAN 2004

31st JAN 2004

- 4 AUG 2004

- 5 AUG 2004

- 3   007

23 APR 2014

WITHDRAWN FROM
ROTHERHAM HEALTH LIBRARY
& KNOWLEDGE SERVICE

Don Gresswell Ltd., London, N21   Cat. No. 1207

DG 02242/71

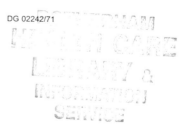

ROTHERHAM
HEALTH CARE
LIBRARY &
INFORMATION
SERVICE

13112

Diagnosis and Treatment of
LUNG CANCER

An Evidence-Based Guide for the
Practicing Clinician

Diagnosis and Treatment of
LUNG CANCER

An Evidence-Based Guide for the Practicing Clinician

FRANK C. DETTERBECK, M.D.
Division of Cardiothoracic Surgery
Department of Surgery
The University of North Carolina at Chapel Hill
Chapel Hill, North Carolina

MARK A. SOCINSKI, M.D.
Division of Hematology and Oncology
Department of Medicine
The University of North Carolina at Chapel Hill
Chapel Hill, North Carolina

M. PATRICIA RIVERA, M.D.
Division of Pulmonary Diseases and Critical Care
School of Medicine
The University of North Carolina at Chapel Hill
Chapel Hill, North Carolina

JULIAN G. ROSENMAN, M.D., PH.D.
Department of Radiation Oncology
School of Medicine
The University of North Carolina at Chapel Hill
Chapel Hill, North Carolina

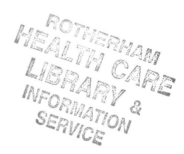

W.B. SAUNDERS COMPANY
A Harcourt Health Sciences Company
Philadelphia • London • New York • St. Louis • Sydney • Toronto

W.B. SAUNDERS COMPANY
A Harcourt Health Sciences Company

The Curtis Center
Independence Square West
Philadelphia, Pennsylvania 19106

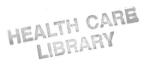

Library of Congress Cataloging-in-Publication Data

Diagnosis and treatment of lung cancer / [edited by] Frank C. Detterbeck . . . [et al.].
—1st ed.

p.   cm.

ISBN 0–7216–9192–7

1. Lungs—Cancer.   I. Detterbeck, Frank C.
  [DNLM: 1. Lung Neoplasms—diagnosis.   2. Lung Neoplasms—therapy.
  WF 658D536 2001]

RC280.L8 D53 2001   616.99′424—dc21

00–030059

Acquisitions Editor: Marc Strauss
Project Manager: Amy Cannon
Production Manager: Norm Stellander
Illustration Specialist: Walt Verbitski
Book Designer: Matt Andrews

DIAGNOSIS AND TREATMENT OF LUNG CANCER: An Evidence-Based
Guide for the Practicing Clinician

ISBN 0–7216–9192–7

Copyright © 2001 by W.B. Saunders Company

All rights reserved. No part of this publication may be reproduced or transmitted in any form or by any
means, electronic or mechanical, including photocopy, recording, or any information storage and retrieval
system, without permission in writing from the publisher.

Printed in the United States of America

Last digit is the print number: 9   8   7   6   5   4   3   2   1

A project such as this book cannot be accomplished without a great deal of sacrifice. There is no doubt that the brunt of this was borne by my family. This book is dedicated to my children, Roland and Sabine, and to my wife, Judit, for their constant patience and willingness to allow me the endless hours needed for this undertaking.

FRANK C. DETTERBECK

To my husband, Ben, for his love, support, and patience, which helps me stay focused, and to my children, Benjamin, Alejandro, and Sofia, for their love, support, and impatience, which helps me maintain balance!

M. PATRICIA RIVERA

To my wife, Kimberly, children, Audra, Greg, and Alex, and my parents, John and Janet. Without them, this book would not have been possible. They are the ones I truly work for.

MARK A. SOCINSKI

I would like to dedicate this book to my wife, Maryanne, to my children, Dan, Alex, and James, and to the Radiation Oncology Department. Without their support, my contribution would not be possible.

JULIAN G. ROSENMAN

CONTRIBUTORS

MARK S. BLEIWEIS, M.D.
Assistant Professor, Division of Cardiothoracic Surgery, UNC School of Medicine, Chapel Hill, North Carolina
Surgical Treatment for Stage IV Non–Small Cell Lung Cancer

JAY A. CLARK, M.D.
Clinical Assistant Professor, Department of Radiation Oncology, UNC School of Medicine, Chapel Hill, North Carolina
Radiotherapy Alone for Stage IIIA,B Non–Small Cell Lung Cancer

FRANK C. DETTERBECK, M.D.
Associate Professor, Division of Cardiothoracic Surgery, and Director, Multidisciplinary Thoracic Oncology Program, UNC School of Medicine, Chapel Hill, North Carolina
Objectives and Methods; Epidemiology and Classification of Lung Cancer; Clinical Presentation and Diagnosis; Intrathoracic Staging; Extrathoracic Staging; General Aspects of Surgical Treatment; Surgery for Stage I Non–Small Cell Lung Cancer; Surgery for Stage II Non–Small Cell Lung Cancer; Adjuvant Therapy of Resected Non–Small Cell Lung Cancer; T3 Non–Small Cell Lung Cancer (Stage IIB–IIIA); Pancoast Tumors; Surgical Treatment of Stage IIIA(N2) Non–Small Cell Lung Cancer; Radiotherapy Alone for Stage IIIA,B Non–Small Cell Lung Cancer; Induction Therapy and Surgery for I–IIIA,B Non–Small Cell Lung Cancer; Surgery for Stage IIIB Non–Small Cell Lung Cancer; Surgical Treatment of Stage IV Non–Small Cell Lung Cancer; Limited Stage Small Cell Lung Cancer; Carcinoid and Mucoepidermoid Tumors; Bronchioloalveolar Carcinoma; Tracheal Cancers; Palliative Treatment of Lung Cancer; Satellite Nodules and Multiple Primary Cancers; Pulmonary Metastases from Extrapulmonary Cancer

THOMAS M. EGAN, M.D., M.Sc.
Professor and Associate Division Chief for Thoracic Surgery, Division of Cardiothoracic Surgery, UNC School of Medicine, Chapel Hill, North Carolina
Surgery for Stage II Non–Small Cell Lung Cancer

MATTHEW G. EWEND, M.D.
Kay and Van Weatherspoon Assistant Professor, Chief, Section of Neuro-oncology, Division of Neurosurgery, UNC School of Medicine, Chapel Hill, North Carolina
Surgical Treatment of Stage IV Non–Small Cell Lung Cancer

ANN FISH-STEAGALL, B.S.W., B.S.N.
Nurse Coordinator, Multidisciplinary Thoracic Oncology Program, UNC School of Medicine, Chapel Hill, North Carolina
Clinical Research

WILLIAM K. FUNKHOUSER, JR., M.D., Ph.D.
Assistant Professor, Department of Pathology and Laboratory Medicine, UNC School of Medicine, Chapel Hill, North Carolina
Bronchioloalveolar Carcinoma; Satellite Nodules and Multiple Primary Cancers

HEIDI H. GILLENWATER, M.D.
Assistant Professor, Division of Hematology/Oncology, University of Virginia, Charlottesville, Virginia
Extensive Stage Small Cell Lung Cancer

JAN S. HALLE, M.D.
Assistant Professor, Department of Radiation Oncology, and Co-Director, Multidisciplinary Thoracic Oncology Program, UNC School of Medicine, Chapel Hill, North Carolina
Radiotherapy for Stage I,II Non–Small Cell Lung Cancer; Chemoradiotherapy for Stage IIIA,B Non–Small Cell Lung Cancer

THOMAS A. HENSING, M.D.
Clinical Instructor, Division of Hematology/Oncology, UNC School of Medicine, Chapel Hill, North Carolina
Chemoradiotherapy for Stage IIIA,B Non–Small Cell Lung Cancer

HAROLD JOHNSON, M.D.
Resident, Department of Radiation Oncology, UNC School of Medicine, Chapel Hill, North Carolina
Radiotherapy for Stage I,II Non–Small Cell Lung Cancer

DAVID R. JONES, M.D.
Assistant Professor, Division of Thoracic and Cardiovascular Surgery, University of Virginia, Charlottesville, Virginia
Intrathoracic Staging; Extrathoracic Staging; Surgery for Stage I Non–Small Cell Lung Cancer; Pancoast Tumors; Surgical Treatment of Stage IIIA(N2) Non–Small Cell Lung Cancer; Surgery for Stage III Non–Small Cell Lung Cancer; Bronchioloalveolar Carcinoma; Tracheal Cancers; Palliative Treatment of Lung Cancer; Satellite Nodules and Multiple Primary Cancers

ARNOLD D. KALUZNY, Ph.D.
Professor, Department of Health Policy and Administration, and Director, Public Health Leadership Program, UNC School of Public Health, Chapel Hill, North Carolina
Clinical Research

BARBARA A. KALUZNY, B.S.
Outreach Clinical Trials Coordinator, Multidisciplinary Thoracic Oncology Program, UNC School of Medicine, Chapel Hill, North Carolina
Clinical Research

ANDY C. KISER, M.D.
Cardiothoracic Surgery, Pinehurst Surgical Clinic, Pinehurst, North Carolina
General Aspects of Surgical Treatment; T3 Non–Small Cell Lung Cancer (Stage IIB–IIIA); Carcinoid and Mucoepidermoid Tumors

DANA P. LOOMIS, Ph.D.
Associate Professor, Department of Epidemiology, UNC School of Public Health, Chapel Hill, North Carolina
Epidemiology and Classification of Lung Cancer

KEVIN MARTINOLICH, M.D.
Pulmonary Medicine, Knoxville Pulmonary Group, Knoxville, Tennessee
Pulmonary Assessment and Treatment

PAUL L. MOLINA, M.D.
Associate Professor, Department of Radiology, UNC School of Medicine, Chapel Hill, North Carolina
Extrathoracic Staging

DAVID E. MORRIS, M.D.
Assistant Professor, Department of Radiation Oncology, UNC School of Medicine, Chapel Hill, North Carolina; and Clinical Affiliate, Department of Radiation Oncology, Wake Forest University School of Medicine, Winston-Salem, North Carolina
Limited Stage Small Cell Lung Cancer; Tracheal Cancers; Palliative Treatment of Lung Cancer

L. ALDEN PARKER, M.D.
Associate Professor and Chief, Section of Thoracic Radiology, Department of Radiology, UNC School of Medicine, Chapel Hill, North Carolina
Intrathoracic Staging

M. PATRICIA RIVERA, M.D.
Assistant Professor, Division of Pulmonary Diseases and Critical Care, and Co-Director, Multidisciplinary Thoracic Oncology Program, UNC School of Medicine, Chapel Hill, North Carolina
Epidemiology and Classification of Lung Cancer; Clinical Presentation and Diagnosis; Pulmonary Assessment and Treatment

JULIAN G. ROSENMAN, M.D., Ph.D.
Professor, Department of Radiation Oncology, UNC School of Medicine, and Adjunct Professor, UNC Computer Science Department, Chapel Hill, North Carolina
General Aspects of Radiotherapy for Lung Cancer; Adjuvant Therapy of Resected Non–Small Cell Lung Cancer; Pancoast Tumors; Radiotherapy Alone for Stage IIIA,B Non–Small Cell Lung Cancer

SUZANNE M. RUSSO, M.D.
Fellow, Department of Radiation Oncology, UNC School of Medicine, Chapel Hill, North Carolina
General Aspects of Radiotherapy for Lung Cancer

JOHN D. SADOFF, M.D.
Fellow, Division of Cardiothoracic Surgery, UNC School of Medicine, Chapel Hill, North Carolina
Pulmonary Metastases from Extrapulmonary Cancer

MARK A. SOCINSKI, M.D.
Assistant Professor, Division of Hematology/Oncology, and Co-Director, Multidisciplinary Thoracic Oncology Program, UNC School of Medicine, Chapel Hill, North Carolina
General Aspects of Chemotherapy; Adjuvant Therapy of Resected Non–Small Cell Lung Cancer; Induction Therapy and Surgery for I–IIIA,B Non–Small Cell Lung Cancer; Chemoradiotherapy for Stage IIIA,B Non–Small Cell Lung Cancer; Chemotherapy for Stage IV Non–Small Cell Lung Cancer; Limited Stage Small Cell Lung Cancer; Extensive Stage Small Cell Lung Cancer

WILLIAM A. SOLLECITO, Dr.P.H.
Research Professor and Associate Director of the Public Health Leadership Program, UNC School of Public Health, Chapel Hill, North Carolina
Objectives and Methods; Clinical Research

THOMAS E. STINCHCOMBE, M.D.
Fellow, Division of Hematology/Oncology, UNC School of Medicine, Chapel Hill, North Carolina
General Aspects of Chemotherapy

PREFACE

Medicine is both an art and a science. Because medicine involves caring for individual patients, there will always be an art to the practice of medicine. Each patient presents a number of medical conditions, values, and biases, as well as practical issues that influence which intervention is chosen as the best treatment for a particular disease. The art of medicine involves judgment in weighing these various considerations in order to select the treatment that is best for the individual.

However, the practice of medicine cannot be guided only by a series of individualized approaches for particular patients. Clearly, there is a need to incorporate clinical science into the practice of medicine. Clinical science, which is grounded on reproducible results for defined clinical situations, allows generalized truths to be defined. Unfortunately, clinical science is continually evolving and is rarely refined enough to clearly define the "truth." Thus, it is important not only to know the conclusions that have been drawn from clinical research, but also to be able to weigh the strength of the data supporting one approach over another when clinical science is incorporated into actual practice.

Lung cancer is by far the most frequent cause of death from cancer. Much information has been accumulated by scientific studies that point the way to better therapeutic approaches to patients with lung cancer. Unfortunately, the complexity and sheer volume of information is overwhelming, and the approach to the diagnosis and treatment of lung cancer is often determined by dogma and biases instead of scientific data. The purpose of this book is to present a concise overview of the data regarding lung cancer in a way that can be applied to clinical practice. This requires that the available data be concisely summarized, but with enough detail so that the strength of the data can be assessed. The ability to weigh the strength of the data allows the clinician to combine both the art and the science of medicine in order to select the best approach for each individual patient.

This book is written for clinicians who are involved in the care of patients with lung cancer. This includes pulmonologists, thoracic surgeons, medical oncologists, radiation oncologists, primary care physicians, nurses, and others who desire insight into currently available data about the diagnosis and treatment of lung cancer. The focus of this book is on the practical issues that such clinicians face in their daily practice. In order to achieve this goal, the contributing authors chosen for this book were selected from a group of clinicians who are actively involved in caring for patients with lung cancer. In addition, all the authors are part of a multidisciplinary team that has worked together closely and grappled with clinical issues involving patients with lung cancer on a daily basis over the course of several years. We hope that this book is a useful and unbiased source of information that will contribute to improving the treatment of patients with lung cancer.

FRANK C. DETTERBECK
M. PATRICIA RIVERA
MARK A. SOCINSKI
JULIAN G. ROSENMAN

NOTICE

Medicine is an ever-changing field. Standard safety precautions must be followed, but as new research and clinical experience broaden our knowledge, changes in treatment and drug therapy become necessary or appropriate. Readers are advised to check the product information currently provided by the manufacturer of each drug to be administered to verify the recommended dose, the method and duration of administration, and the contraindications. It is the responsibility of the treating physician, relying on experience and knowledge of the patient, to determine dosages and the best treatment for the patient. Neither the publisher nor the editor assumes any responsibility for any injury and/or damage to persons or property.

THE PUBLISHER

This book would not have been possible without the extensive contributions of Betsy Mann. Her work as an Editorial Assistant was superb, and her thoroughness and attention to detail are reflected throughout the book. More importantly, her support and dedication was crucial in bringing this project to completion. We also thank Kimberly Flynn for her contributions in preparing the figures.

CONTENTS

Diagnosis and Treatment of
LUNG CANCER

An Evidence-Based Guide for the
Practicing Clinician

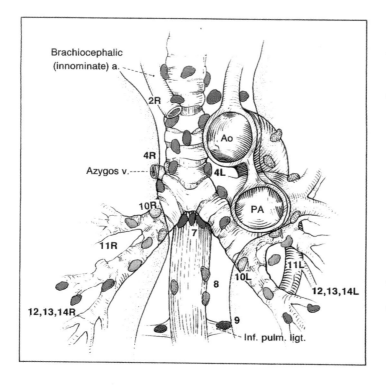

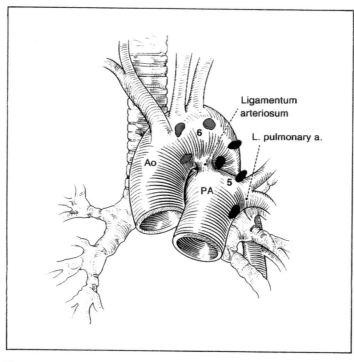

N₂ NODES
SUPERIOR MEDIASTINAL NODES

- **1** Highest Mediastinal
- **2** Upper Paratracheal
- **3** Pre- and Retrotracheal
- **4** Lower Paratracheal (including Azygos Nodes)

AORTIC NODES

- **5** Subaortic (A-P window)
- **6** Para-aortic (ascending aorta or phrenic)

INFERIOR MEDIASTINAL NODES

- **7** Subcarinal
- **8** Paraesophageal (below carina)
- **9** Pulmonary Ligament

N₁ NODES

- **10** Hilar
- **11** Interlobar
- **12** Lobar
- **13** Segmental
- **14** Subsegmental

Figure 5–4. Regional lymph node stations for lung cancer staging. A-P, anteroposterior. (Adapted from Mountain CF, Dresler CM. Regional lymph node classification for lung cancer staging. Chest. 1997; 111:1718–1723.).

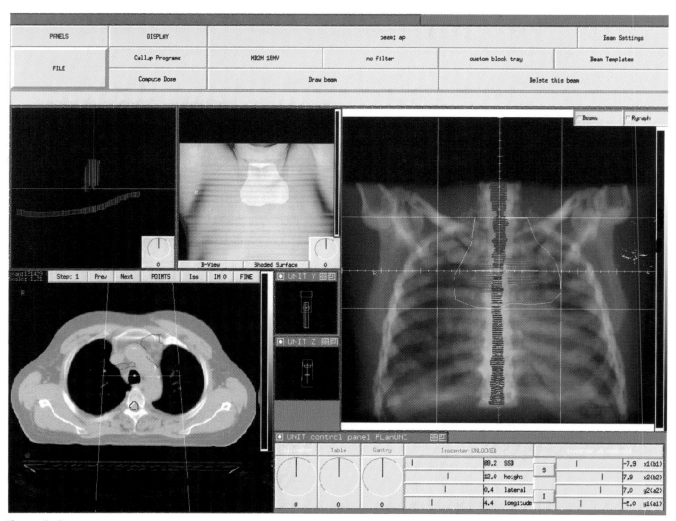

Figure 9–3. A typical "screen shot" from the 3D treatment planning system used at the University of North Carolina.

PART 1

OBJECTIVES, METHODS, AND CLINICAL RESEARCH

1

OBJECTIVES AND METHODS

Frank C. Detterbeck and William A. Sollecito

Books generally do not include a section on objectives and methods. However, one of the major goals of this book is to provide a careful, scientific review of existing data about lung cancer. Like any other scientific endeavor, a clear understanding of the objectives and careful attention to the methods used makes achievement of the goals more likely. Indeed, a fair amount of research and analysis has been done regarding what constitutes a high quality review.[1-6] Adherence to the principles set forth by these and other authors minimizes the effects of biases and enhances the validity of a review. Unfortunately, most review articles do not measure up to these standards,[5, 7] probably because the principles of writing a scientific review are not widely appreciated.[4] Therefore, in order to create a valid review and analysis of data pertaining to lung cancer, we carefully defined our objectives and methods before writing this book. These are outlined in the following pages.

OBJECTIVES

This book has two overriding objectives. First, it is written to be *useful to practicing clinicians* who care for patients with lung cancer. Second, it is based on a *review of existing data* on this subject, rather than a repetition of widely accepted dogma. Secondary goals are to be *thorough* in reviewing data, yet to present it in a *concise format*. Finally, this book aims to provide a *multidisciplinary viewpoint;* we tried to put aside "turf battles" and single-discipline viewpoints.

Clinical Relevance

This book is written for clinicians who treat patients with lung cancer. This includes pulmonologists, thoracic surgeons, medical and radiation oncologists, as well as primary care physicians who wish to have in-depth knowledge of this disease. The book deals with clinical questions that are faced in daily practice and is written from the viewpoint of a clinician who is facing an individual patient. For example, although sensitivity and specificity may be useful measures to assess the value of a test, use of these measures is an awkward way to answer the questions of an individual patient faced with a positive (or negative) clinical finding or test. In this situation, knowledge of the false positive rate (or false negative rate) of that particular finding is more useful.

In order to be useful to a busy clinician, the data presented not only must be relevant but also must be able to be quickly and easily reviewed. Therefore, we divided the material into many separate chapters to allow the desired data to be found more quickly. We also made extensive use of tables to summarize the data. In addition, at various points, we provided a series of summary statements or *take home messages* of the available data, indicated by highlighted boxes. In order that these statements be given the appropriate weight and not be viewed as dogma, we developed a data rating system to concisely rate the data upon which each statement is based. This system will be explained in detail later. Finally, because not everything can be expressed in terms of data tables and summary statements, we provided—at the risk of appearing dogmatic—a brief collection of the editors' comments on the topic of each chapter. Although much of this section is rooted in the data, it also provides a place to state policies that are based on relatively arbitrary decisions in areas in which no data is available as a guide.

A Guide Based on the Evidence

A tremendous amount of data about lung cancer exists. Unfortunately, much of the data that is available has not filtered into many areas of clinical practice, probably in part due to the sheer volume and complexity of the material.[8,9] Furthermore, the quality of the reports is uneven, and the myriad of smaller studies involving nonhomogeneous patient populations has resulted in few clearly defined standards of care. However, the frequent lament that no definite conclusions can be reached because the ideal studies (randomized, blinded, and so on) have not been conducted is of no use to the practicing clinician. We must still look at the data that is available and try to make the best decisions possible for the patients we are confronted with today. Therefore, this book examines the available data that addresses the clinical issues in lung cancer. The methods used to retrieve, analyze, and summarize the data are explained in the following pages.

Multidisciplinary Perspective

This book has been written by a single team of clinicians representing a variety of disciplines. We are all part of a multidisciplinary thoracic oncology program in which the team discusses each patient's workup and treatment and develops a consensus treatment plan. As a result, all of the authors and editors of this book, working closely with one another, have grappled with clinical issues in the field of lung cancer on a daily basis for several years. In order to provide a more balanced perspective, most chapters have been written by two or three authors. More important, we sought the input of all of the editors for each of the chapters, representing the disciplines of pulmonary medicine, thoracic surgery, medical oncology, and radiation oncology, in order to present a multidisciplinary view.

METHODS

Data Retrieval

The authors conducted Medline computer searches for each of the topics discussed, using both main words and related topics. Because it has been shown that such searches may miss 30% to 40% of the desired data,[1, 10, 11] we also carefully reviewed the table of contents of a number of medical journals for pertinent articles published from 1994 to 2000. These journals are listed in Table 1–1 and represent the 10 most common sources of clinical articles on lung cancer. In our initial library of 1000 articles accumulated over 5 years, approximately 75% of the clinical articles on lung cancer were published in one of these journals. In addition, we reviewed all articles from the authors' and editors' files and from the reference lists in other articles. This search has yielded a library of more than 3000 clinical articles related to lung cancer. Each of these articles was carefully read and analyzed, with the goal of including all pertinent high quality data.

We occasionally wrote to authors of published or presented studies requesting clarification, more details, or updated material, but we did not make any attempt to address the issue of publication bias by requesting information from unpublished studies. We found this simply to be beyond the scope of what we were able to do. However, we made use of available meta-analyses and summary statements from the Ontario Cancer Treatment and Research Foundation, which attempted to address the issue of publication bias. The latter group has issued treatment recommendations in a number of areas in which many randomized studies concerning lung cancer have been carried out, which is the type of situation in which publication bias is likely to be greatest.

In general, we included only articles published in English, from 1980 through April 2000. Many changes that affect data concerning lung cancer occurred around 1980, including the consistent separation of small cell and non–small cell cancer types, the more widespread use of mediastinoscopy, the availability of computed tomography scanning, the use of actuarial survival curves, the advent of cisplatin-based chemotherapy, and the development of better radiation therapy equipment. In the case of rare tumors or unusual aspects of lung cancer, we did include earlier literature, and we also included references to older historical controls, where appropriate.

Although the emphasis was on modern data, the authors made every effort to be comprehensive. Our aim was to be inclusive, rather than exclusive. We included data from both articles and abstracts whenever the publication provided enough detail to allow interpretation. If two reports were published from the same institution based on the same patient population, we excluded the earlier report unless it contained information not found in the later report. In those instances in which a large amount of data was available (eg, more than 10 studies), we chose criteria to limit the papers included, and these are noted in the appropriate tables. Most often, this involved deciding on a minimum number of patients. In some instances, only randomized trials were selected.

Validity Assessment

Each study included in this book was scrutinized for flaws in methodology or design. However, it is rare that a study was excluded on these grounds. Assessing validity and quality is a matter of degree, not meeting an arbitrary setpoint. In those instances in which sufficient high quality (eg, prospective, randomized) data was available, the papers of lesser validity (eg, nonrandomized) were not included. Nevertheless, in a review such as this, in which many clinical questions are addressed for which only a limited amount of data exists, we found it necessary in many instances to accept most pieces of data available. Rather than exclude many studies, we found it more appropriate to accept papers with the recognition that flaws exist. We analyzed and discussed these shortcomings and noted them in the text and footnotes. Furthermore, throughout

TABLE 1–1. TEN MOST COMMON SOURCES OF CLINICAL ARTICLES ON LUNG CANCER

Annals of Thoracic Surgery
Cancer
Chest
International Journal of Radiation Oncology, Biology, Physics
Journal of Clinical Oncology
Journal of Thoracic and Cardiovascular Surgery
Lung Cancer
Radiology
Seminars in Oncology
Thorax

the book we scored the quality of the data using the instrument described in a later section of this chapter.

Methods of Data Presentation

The authors made a concerted effort to collate the data from different studies, which often reported results in slightly different ways. We endeavored to glean as much data as possible from each report. In doing so, we had to make some assumptions, such as whether a definition used by one set of authors was similar to that used by other authors. Sometimes patient populations were similar but not completely the same. Our goal was to overlook small inconsistencies in the spirit of having a larger "reasonable" database to use for analysis. The "rough edges," where assumptions were made or patient populations differed, are indicated in the text and in footnotes. When variability regarding the results of different studies was encountered, we sought inherent differences in the studies that would explain it. We categorized the individual studies according to such differences in many of the tables to try to explain this variability.

Analysis of how studies are similar or different requires some judgment. For this reason, we specifically involved at least two authors in each chapter and asked each of them to independently evaluate the data. Thereafter, agreement was reached among the authors of the chapter and the editors so that the book would represent a consensus rather than arbitrary decisions. In addition, we noted the assumptions in footnotes so that readers can decide for themselves whether our judgments are valid.

In order to present an objective summary of available studies, we explicitly defined the criteria used to include or exclude studies from the tables and figures. Although we attempted to adhere rigidly to these criteria, undoubtedly some studies have been overlooked. Such omissions are not due to any author bias but simply represent human error. We welcome any information from readers concerning studies that were missed.

Statistical Analysis

Statistical analysis is clearly an important tool to assist in the understanding of data. However, such analysis is useful and valid only if the assumptions about the underlying data are valid. Comparison of the data from many authors has required making some assumptions and acceptance of comparisons between very similar, but not necessarily identical, patient populations or treatments. Therefore, a detailed statistical analysis, such as a formal meta-analysis, was not carried out. We felt this would be inappropriate and would create the false impression that the trials are completely homogeneous. We believe that a careful study of the data presented in the tables provides the reader with a better opportunity to judge the validity of the comparisons than a statistical analysis would offer.

Summary Statements

In an attempt to draw conclusions about the clinical issues from the available data, we presented summary statements in highlighted boxes at several points in each chapter. We tried to keep these statements brief. In addition, we provided a coded synopsis of the data upon which each statement is based to prevent the statements from being viewed as dogma. In order to code the data, we developed a data rating system based on the amount of data available, the quality of the data, and the consistency of the findings. Three types of data are identified: purely descriptive data (indicated in plain text), comparisons based on nonrandomized studies (indicated in italics), and comparisons based on randomized studies (indicated in bold).

An explanation of the definitions used in this data rating system is provided in the last section of this chapter. An understanding of these details is not absolutely necessary for every reader, although use of these definitions makes the system more objective and the ratings consistent among different reviewers. An example of this data rating system in use is shown in the box below.

ASSESSMENT OF LEVELS OF EVIDENCE

Other Evidence-Rating Systems

In order to address the needs of clinicians practicing the art of medicine, a method of summarizing the strength of

DATA SUMMARY: PANCOAST TUMORS			
	AMOUNT	QUALITY	CONSISTENCY
FNA has a >90% success rate in achieving diagnosis	High	High	High
Curative radiotherapy in "good risk" patients has a 5-year survival of 15%–20%	High	High	High
Radiotherapy and surgery results in a 5-year survival of 30% (20%–40%)	High	High	Moderate
Lobectomy may result in better survival than limited resection	*Mod*	*Mod*	*Poor*

Type of data rated:
Plain text: descriptive statement   *Italics: controlled comparison*   **Bold: randomized comparison**

conclusions is needed. The clinician must weigh a variety of considerations in guiding a patient to a decision, such as the patient's biases and fears, the local availability of a particular treatment, and how convincingly a benefit to a treatment has been demonstrated. Dogmatic statements can be either accepted or rejected, but not weighed. The same shortcoming applies to more recently published clinical guidelines, which have generally used the format of algorithms.[12] Furthermore, such clinical guidelines, which do not allow room for clinical judgment, can really be issued only for situations in which a clear answer for the majority of patients is available.[13] A method of summarizing the strength of a conclusion in a concise way that is more generally applicable is what is needed to help guide the decisions of individual patients.

There are many aspects of study design, implementation, and reporting that determine the quality and validity of a study. Rating systems were designed to categorize the strength of conclusions by assigning the studies to a level of evidence category.[3,14] Although these systems were useful in developing evidence-based clinical practice guidelines for specific interventions, they were designed primarily for situations in which a lot of high quality (eg, randomized, blinded) data exists. For the majority of clinical questions, however, such data does not exist. Therefore, we found the previously published rating systems not well suited to this book, which aims to provide a review of data on the entire spectrum of clinically relevant issues in lung cancer.

Types of Data

Before discussing a system of rating studies, it is important to note that there are different types of data that are useful to clinicians. The simplest type is purely *descriptive*, such as the incidence of non–small cell lung cancer or the natural history of non–small cell lung cancer. To answer such questions, single-cohort studies are perfectly adequate; in fact, it would make no sense to demand a randomized, two-cohort study.

Sometimes patients with a certain given characteristic are compared relative to others without this characteristic. An example would be the survival of patients with poor performance status compared with those with good performance status. However, there is no ability to add this characteristic to or remove it from a patient or to make this characteristic independent of other parameters of the cohort population (eg, weight loss). Randomization of patients to have or not have this characteristic cannot be done (although this characteristic could be used to stratify patients in a randomization regarding an active intervention).

Because such data describes a fact (eg, survival of stage I patients) about a group of patients, we found it most appropriate to group such data with the descriptive type of data. Such a comparison of one group with another (eg, stage I versus stage II) raises the questions of what type of controls are used (historical versus contemporary, from different institutions or studies versus from the same institution) and whether such data should be grouped with the comparative type of data. There are several arguments against this.

First, the fact that the characteristic cannot be added to or removed from a patient makes it inherently different from studies investigating the effect of an active treatment. Such given characteristics define a group of patients. This is opposed to an active intervention, in which the composition of the patient groups and their similarity is very much the question.

Second, it turns out that comparisons of patients with given characteristics most often involve concurrent groups from the same institution; therefore, the study quality is usually fairly good.

Third, the importance of such data is more similar to descriptive data than to active interventions. This does not mean it is not important to know such data, for example, the survival of patients with good performance status or poor performance status. However, because this characteristic cannot be changed, it does not carry the same significance as whether a particular treatment that can be either chosen or not chosen results in a measurable benefit. Therefore, we rated data about given characteristics in the same way as for descriptive studies, even though a comparison to another group is generally made.

The most important clinical questions involve assessing an active intervention (eg, the benefits of surgery or a new chemotherapy regimen). This involves *comparative data,* in which the results in the active intervention group are compared with those in a nonintervention, or control, group. Even though such data may come from a single-cohort study, the data cannot stand alone; by necessity, such data must be compared with another cohort. The ability to actively control the intervention allows the investigator to manipulate the groups, such as by randomization.

For comparative questions, randomized studies are clearly the ideal.[15] Nonrandomized trials using historical controls have been shown to seriously overestimate treatment effects, even when adjusted for known prognostic factors.[15] Randomized trials, on the other hand, probably underestimate treatment effects and are prone to false negative results.[15, 16] An analysis of the literature regarding treatment questions for which both randomized and nonrandomized studies existed consistently found that 80% of the nonrandomized studies showed a benefit to the treatment, whereas 80% of the randomized studies showed *no benefit to the same treatment.*[15] These caveats for both nonrandomized and randomized studies must be kept in mind.

Although the amount of effort necessary to carry out a randomized study raises the expectation of high quality, this is not always the case. In fact, it is surprising how often major flaws are present, such as too small a sample size to allow an adequate power of detection or an imbalance between the groups with regard to a known prognostic factor.[16] For most comparative clinical questions, however, randomized studies are not available. Data from nonrandomized studies certainly can be used and, in many instances, provide a convincing answer to a clinical question, keeping in mind the caveats just noted. This is especially true in epidemiologic investigations that do not use randomization but instead offer other methods (eg, matching) to improve the validity of comparisons among cohorts. Although the questions addressed by such comparative randomized and nonrandomized studies are the same, the differences in the data from these two types of studies warrant considering them separately.

Thus we find it most appropriate to recognize three types of data: descriptive data, comparative data addressed by nonrandomized studies, and comparative data addressed by randomized clinical trials. These groups are inherently different; therefore, the standards to which the data are held must be defined differently.

DATA RATING SYSTEM

We developed a data scoring system that is more generally applicable, and this is used throughout this book. The strength of a conclusion is based on three things: the *amount* of data available that pertains to it, the *quality* of that data, and the *consistency* of the conclusions reached by the studies. For example, even if only two studies addressing a question are available, the conclusion might be quite strong if they are high quality studies with very consistent results. On the contrary, even a large number of studies of reasonable quality will not be convincing if the conclusions reached by the studies are at odds with one another.

Some people argue that the value of a conclusion is also influenced by the clinical importance of the conclusion. However, no methods are available to measure clinical importance. Furthermore, the clinical importance does not affect the strength of a conclusion based on the data, but only how this is valued. Therefore, we left it to the reader to judge the clinical importance, rather than attempting to rate this in any manner.

Our scoring system ranks the available data as high, moderate, or poor in each of these three categories. Very small studies, such as series involving fewer than 20 patients, are generally of questionable validity, especially in regard to generalization of results. Therefore, such studies are usually not counted in determining the amount (number of studies), the quality, or the consistency of available data. The quality ranking is based on the quality of the majority of the studies, recognizing that a fair amount of variation exists in most instances. Assessment of consistency is possible only if at least two studies exist. Although 100% consistency between only two studies may not yield as strong a conclusion as if this were true for 10 studies, this is really a matter of the amount of data available rather than the consistency. We generally omitted any conclusions in which the data was rated poor in at least two of the three categories. We included such statements primarily when they are widely cited, in order to point out that very little supportive data exists.

Each of the types of data—descriptive, comparative via nonrandomized studies, and comparative via randomized trials—is assessed in a similar way, although the definitions used vary slightly. It is quite intuitive that the strength of the conclusions is also a reflection of the type of data available. For example, a series of high quality, randomized studies is more convincing than a series of nonrandomized studies. We addressed this by indicating descriptive data assessments in plain text, nonrandomized comparative data in italics, and randomized comparative data in bold.

Amount Rating

The data rating system is shown in Table 1–2. As mentioned earlier, the data is ranked as high, moderate, or poor

TABLE 1–2. DATA RATING SYSTEM

	DESCRIPTIVE	COMPARATIVE NONRANDOMIZED	COMPARATIVE RANDOMIZED
Amount			
High	4–5 studies	4–5 cohorts[a]	4–5 trials
Mod	2–3 studies	2–3 cohorts[a]	2–3 trials
Poor	1[b]	1 cohort[b]	1 trial[b]
Quality			
High	Consecutive patients, well-defined population and treatment	Concurrent, well defined Well matched patient groups	Well defined; $P < 0.05$ Power $\geq 80\%$
Mod	Consecutive patients, moderately well defined	Moderately well controlled Contemporary controls, different institutions, but well-defined, similar patient population Historical controls, same institution, no known change in treatment	Minor flaws; $P < 0.1$ Power $\geq 60\%$ Some details missing Some stratification imbalance
Poor	Selected patients Ambiguous population	Poorly controlled Historical controls and different institutions Population or treatment probably different	Major flaws Power $<60\%$ Major details missing Significant stratification imbalance
Consistency			
High	$\geq 80\%$ agreement (and $\pm \leq 10\%$ for quantitative data)	$\geq 80\%$ agreement and $\pm \leq 10\%$[c] (and $\geq 30\%$ difference between groups[d] or $P < 0.05$ if high quality study[e])	$\geq 80\%$ agreement
Mod	$\geq 60\%$ agreement (and $\pm \leq 20\%$)	$\geq 60\%$ agreement and $\pm \leq 20\%$[c]	$\geq 60\%$ agreement and $\geq 30\%$ difference between groups[d]
Poor	No clear pattern	Much overlap between results	No clear pattern

[a]Cohorts for the smallest of the two groups being compared.
[b]Or any number of studies with <20 patients.
[c]Among the patient cohorts representing each group.
[d]Or $<30\%$ difference between groups if claiming a negative (no difference) result.
[e]If high quality study (concurrent, well stratified), then high consistency if $P < 0.05$.

in each of the three categories: the amount of data, the quality of the data, and the consistency of the data. Similar definitions are used for ranking each of the three types of data (descriptive, comparative nonrandomized, and comparative randomized). However, the different nature of these three types of data demands slightly different definitions. For example, descriptive data involves a single group of patients per study; the amount of data is based on the number of studies. Comparative data involves two groups. In randomized data, each trial contains two groups; the amount of data is based on the number of trials. For nonrandomized, comparative data, however, a trial may involve only one group, the comparison being made to a historical control or a control population at another institution. In assessing multiple nonrandomized, comparative data, the number of patient cohorts included in one group may not be the same as the number of patient cohorts included in the other group with which it is being compared. The number of patient cohorts in the smaller of the two groups being compared (either the experimental or the control group) determines the amount rating for nonrandomized, comparative data. Thus, the different types of data have very similar ratings for amount (4–5, 2–3, or 1), differing only by slight differences in the definitions (number of studies, number of cohorts in the smaller of the two groups, or number of trials).

Quality Rating

The quality ratings for the three types of data are also similar in principle, although it is in this category that the greatest differences exist in the detailed definitions for each category. This is because what constitutes a high quality study of one type (eg, descriptive) is quite different from that of another (eg, randomized trial).

For descriptive data, a high quality trial would be one involving a well-defined population of consecutive patients.

For comparative, nonrandomized data to be rated as high quality, the groups should be well matched according to prognostic factors and involve concurrent controls from the same institution.

A high quality randomized trial should have a P value of < 0.05 if a positive study, have a power of detection of at least 80%, and involve a carefully defined, well-matched patient population stratified for recognized prognostic factors. If moderate doubts exist about the homogeneity of the patient populations, the trials would be classified as being of moderate quality. For example, this might involve randomized trials with a power of detection $\leq 80\%$ (but $>60\%$) or demonstrating a strong trend but not a P value of <0.05. (It has been suggested that randomized controlled trials use a P value of 0.1 to minimize their tendency to show false negative results.[15])

For nonrandomized, comparative data, a moderate quality study might involve controls from a different era or institution but contain sufficient detail to indicate that there was no discernible difference in the patient population or treatment. Poor quality studies would be those with major flaws or ambiguity that were below the standards of moderate quality.

The overall quality rating of a series of studies ad-

TABLE 1–3. ABBREVIATED DATA RATING SYSTEM

Amount

High	4–5 studies/*cohorts*/**trials**
Mod	2–3 studies/*cohorts*/**trials**
Poor	1 study/*cohort*/**trial**

Quality

High	Well defined
	consecutive patients, clear inclusion criteria
	concurrent controls
	power ≥80%, P < 0.05
Mod	Moderately well defined
	consecutive patients, vague inclusion criteria
	matched historical controls
	power ≥60%, P < 0.1
Poor	Ambiguously defined
	selected patients
	unmatched controls
	major flaws/imbalances

Consistency

High	≥80% agreement
	and ± 10% of quantitative result
Mod	>60% agreement
	and ± ≤20% of quantitative result
Poor	No clear pattern

Different types of data are indicated as follows:
Plain text: descriptive data
Italics: Comparative data from nonrandomized studies
Bold: Comparative data from randomized studies

dressing a particular topic should reflect the highest quality of the preponderance of the data. This would represent the majority of studies in most instances, but might represent the largest number of patients in others. For example, two large studies of high quality would overshadow three poor quality studies involving only small numbers of patients.

Consistency Rating

Data that shows high consistency should exhibit agreement in at least 80% of the studies (eg, four of five). Furthermore, if the data involved is quantitative, as opposed to a simple qualitative difference between the arms, the numerical values should be within 20% of one another (or ± 10% from the average) in at least four of five studies. For example, if five of six studies (>80%) showed that a treatment was beneficial *and* the survival rates for the treatment population were within 20% of one another, a consistency rating of high would be given. The requirement of ≤20% difference in quantitative results is similar to the definition of minimal heterogeneity between studies proposed by others.[14] The use of a standard deviation rather than an arbitrary 20% might be more accurate but would make the scoring system too unwieldy and complex.

For comparative nonrandomized data, this 20% variation would apply to at least 80% of the studies for a particular cohort (investigational or control). Furthermore, the difference between cohorts should be large enough to confidently detect a difference. A requirement of $P < 0.05$ or a somewhat arbitrary 30% difference in quantitative results was chosen. A rating of moderate consistency would involve agreement among at least 60% of studies (eg, 3 of 5 or 2 of 3) and no more than 40% variation for these 60% of studies.

SUMMARY

Use of this data rating system has been quite straightforward, although at first glance the definitions may seem complex. A look at the highlighted example shown (Data Summary: Pancoast Tumors) is self-explanatory in conveying the strength of the conclusion statements, even without knowing the definitions used. These definitions, however, allowed us to be relatively objective in assigning a data rating. A simplified, abbreviated version of the data rating system is shown in Table 1–3. This system has provided a simple, objective, and concise way to rate the strength of the data supporting conclusions covering a wide spectrum of issues in lung cancer.

References

1. Oxman AD, Guyatt GH. Guidelines for reading literature reviews. Can Med Assoc J. 1988;138:697–703.
2. L'Abbé KA, Detsky AS, O'Rourke K. Meta-analysis in clinical research. Ann Intern Med. 1987;107:224–233.
3. Cook DJ, Guyatt GH, Laupacis A, et al. Rules of evidence and clinical recommendations on the use of antithrombotic agents. Chest. 1992;102:305S–311S.
4. Squires BP. Biomedical review articles: what editors want from authors and peer reviewers. Can Med Assoc J. 1989;141:195–197.
5. Mulrow CD. The medical review article: state of the science. Ann Intern Med. 1987;106:485–488.
6. Evans WK, Will BP, Berthelot J-M, et al. Cost of combined modality interventions for stage III non–small-cell lung cancer. J Clin Oncol. 1997;15:3038–3048.
7. Oxman AD, Guyatt GH, Singer J, et al. Agreement among reviewers of review articles. J Clin Epidemiol. 1991;44:91–98.
8. Evans WK, Newman T, Graham I, et al. Lung cancer practice guidelines: lessons learned and issues addressed by the Ontario Lung Cancer Disease Site Group. J Clin Oncol. 1997;15:3049–3059.
9. Haynes RB, McKibbon KA, Fitzgerald D, et al. How to keep up with the medical literature, I: why try to keep up and how to get started. Ann Intern Med. 1986;105:149–153.
10. Poynard T, Conn HO. The retrieval of randomized clinical trials in liver disease from the medical literature: a comparison of MEDLARS and manual methods. Control Clin Trials. 1985;6:271–279.
11. Dickersin K, Hewitt P, Mutch L, et al. Perusing the literature: comparison of MEDLINE searching with a perinatal trials database. Control Clin Trials. 1985;6:306–317.
12. Ettinger DS, Cox JD, Ginsberg RJ, et al. NCCN non–small-cell lung cancer practice guidelines. Oncology. 1996;10(suppl):81–111.
13. Eddy DM. Designing a practice policy: standards, guidelines, and options. JAMA. 1990;263:3077–3084.
14. Guyatt GH, Sackett DL, Sinclair JC, et al. Users' guides to the medical literature, IX: a method for grading health care recommendations. JAMA. 1995;274:1800–1804.
15. Sacks H, Chalmers TC, Smith H Jr. Randomized versus historical controls for clinical trials. Am J Med. 1982;72:233–240.
16. Freiman JA, Chalmers TC, Smith H Jr, et al. The importance of beta, the type II error and sample size in the design and interpretation of the randomized control trial: survey of 71 "negative" trials. N Engl J Med. 1978;299:690–694.

2

CLINICAL RESEARCH

*Ann Fish-Steagall, William A. Sollecito, Barbara A. Kaluzny,
and Arnold D. Kaluzny*

THE IMPORTANCE OF CLINICAL RESEARCH

The focus on *outcomes* and *evidence-based medicine* has placed a premium on the role of clinical trials in the practice of medicine. Specifically, within the world of oncology, clinical trials represent the means by which to improve clinical practice.[1] Whether sponsored by pharmaceutical or biotechnology companies or by the National Cancer Institute (NCI), clinical trials represent a dynamic process that has a profound impact on the practice of oncology. It is crucial for physicians and patients to realize the stake that we all have in clinical research if we are interested in improving the outcome for patients with lung cancer. Clinical trials offer the potential benefit of new treatments or methods of disease prevention to trial participants. Unfortunately, only an estimated 2% to 3% of adult patients enroll in clinical trials.[2] Without clinical research, no progress will be made.

The objective of this chapter is to provide the practicing clinician with sufficient understanding of the design of clinical trials to have a solid basis for interpreting the validity of the results. It is important that all people involved be able to recognize the virtues and flaws of reported studies in order to prevent erroneous conclusions, which can be more damaging than a total lack of data. In addition, this chapter provides an understanding of how clinical trials are organized, funded, and conducted. It is hoped that such an understanding will help garner the

support of physicians for the process of clinical research. Although the process may at times be unwieldy, cumbersome, and painstakingly slow, support is needed because there is no other way to make progress in the clinical care of patients. A number of developments are underway that are likely to affect provider and patient participation in such trials in the years ahead. Nonetheless, a more widespread understanding and involvement is still the best way to improve the process of clinical research.

DEFINITION AND TYPES OF CLINICAL TRIALS

Definition of a Clinical Trial

A *clinical trial* involves dealing with patients in a controlled fashion with a treatment that is carefully selected, is medically and ethically justified, and has the potential to yield the desired results. The difference between a clinical trial and ad hoc, off study treatment is that clinical trials seek to apply the scientific method to the practice of medicine in order to objectively evaluate whether the anticipated effects are actually realized. This requires that the patient groups are well defined and homogeneous, the treatment administered is reasonably consistent, and the data is carefully collected so that results can be evaluated. Because of the extensive deliberation involved in choosing a treatment to be evaluated and the careful collection of outcomes data, *any arm* of a clinical trial usually represents better treatment than a traditional approach or a less rigorously devised "individualized" treatment plan.

There are several types of clinical trials because there are different types of treatment questions to be answered. However, all clinical trials have several standard components, including clearly defined study objectives, patient eligibility criteria to ensure that the treatment is used in an appropriate context, and defined endpoints to be measured. In order to make participation in the trial appealing to physicians and patients, the trial protocol should provide an explanation of the rationale and background data describing why this is a promising treatment question to study. The trial protocol should also include an estimate of the expected outcome so that the ability of the trial to actually provide an answer to the question can be assessed. In many cases, the planning process requires the help of a statistician. A report of the trial results should include mention of each of these components (background, objectives, eligibility, criteria, endpoints, statistical design) so that the results can be interpreted appropriately.

Clinical trials are typically categorized into one of four classes, usually called phases I through IV, and each of these is described next.

Phase I

A new drug or new treatment that appears promising in preclinical studies is first brought into limited patient use in the context of a phase I trial, usually involving 10 to 20 patients. The patients who are suitable for this type of trial have no other treatment options, and it is hoped that they might benefit from the new approach. However, the focus is on ensuring that the drug is used safely, rather than on defining efficacy. Phase I studies can be conducted only at centers designated by the NCI and are subject to careful surveillance. Typically, the dose of drug given is gradually increased in a limited number of patients (usually three to six) to define the maximum safe therapeutic dose, which is then confirmed by adding an additional limited cohort of patients. Although some data about beneficial effects are collected, a phase I trial is not designed to permit an assessment of treatment efficacy.

Phase II

A drug, drug combination, or a new treatment that appears safe as demonstrated by a phase I study is further evaluated in a phase II trial in a larger cohort of patients, usually 20 to 100. The objective is to gather further data about toxicity patterns and pharmacokinetics and to provide preliminary data on the efficacy of the drug or treatment strategy being studied. Phase II trials are generally not randomized and usually do not include enough patients to allow reliable comparison of the new treatment with other treatment approaches. The goal of phase II trials is to confirm the safety of the drug or treatment and to determine whether sufficient therapeutic merit is suggested by the data to warrant a randomized trial comparing the new treatment with standard therapy. The Food and Drug Administration (FDA)

requires adequate safety data from phase II studies before a drug is allowed to be sold commercially.

Phase III

The primary goal of a phase III trial is to provide an unbiased comparison of two or more treatment regimens. To achieve this goal, the classic study design is a randomized trial, which may sometimes be blinded (to the patient) or double blinded (to both the patient and the physician) in order to minimize the chance that subjective bias will be reflected in the data. At least one of the treatment arms typically involves the current standard of care. Phase III trials must involve large numbers of patients (usually 200–1000) in order to prove or disprove superiority of a new treatment with sufficient power (typically 80%) at an accepted level of statistical significance (usually $P < 0.05$). (See Trial Size for an explanation of *power*.) The number of patients needed also depends on the expected survival (or other endpoint) of the control arm, as will be discussed later. A phase III trial must demonstrate efficacy before the FDA will approve the use of a drug for a specific clinical condition.

Phase IV

Phase IV studies are designed to evaluate the long-term effects, cost-effectiveness, and therapeutic merit of a drug or treatment in large populations. In these studies, the patient population is not carefully defined, and there is often variability in the way the drug is used or the treatment is administered. This is appropriate for drugs or treatment approaches that have become standard therapy either because of the results of phase III studies or simply by widespread convention without supporting data (which is more often the case). Such studies are important because they can identify rare treatment effects that were not apparent during the conduct of phase I, II, or III trials of the drug or treatment. The pharmaceutical industry sometimes employs phase IV studies as part of marketing rather than research and development.

TRIAL DESIGN

The design of clinical trials is a complex subject that spans several areas of expertise, including clinical medicine as well as quantitative sciences such as biostatistics and epidemiology. The design used in a specific trial depends on a variety of factors, including the phase (I, II, III, or IV), the number of treatments being compared, whether the trial involves one investigative site or multiple investigative (multicenter) sites, whether the treatment is curative or palliative, duration of treatment, and—one of the most important— whether it is ethical to include a placebo-treated group in the study. It is difficult to cover this wide range of study design issues here; other books are available that address this subject in detail.[3] The rest of this section primarily addresses issues that pertain to phase II and phase

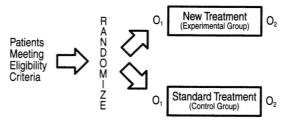

FIGURE 2–1. A schematic illustration of the basic design of a randomized parallel group trial. O_1, pretreatment baseline observations; O_2, posttreatment observations. (Modified from Gillings DB, Douglass CW. BIOSTATS: A Primer for Healthcare Professionals. Chapel Hill, NC: CAVCO Publications; 1985:262–265.)[5]

III studies in order to provide a basis for critical assessment of the quality of a study and the validity of the results.

Randomized Parallel Group Trial

The workhorse of assessment of treatment efficacy is the randomized parallel group design, shown in Figure 2–1. This design is also known as a randomized pretest-posttest control group design.[4] The most important features of this design are the use of randomization to assign patients to experimental and control groups and the inclusion of pretreatment or baseline measures (O_1). These features control for confounding variables, or biases, that threaten the interpretation of the clinical trial results. For example, individual biologic differences among patients are controlled by the randomization procedure, which is a uniquely unbiased mechanism for assigning patients to treatments. Changes from baseline (O_1-O_2) eliminate external effects that may occur differentially in both treatment groups and have the additional advantage of providing indications of differential rates of improvement in disease outcomes between the experimental and control groups. This design can be easily extended to include three or more treatments. In some trials, both a standard treatment and placebo are included as control groups to give a three-treatment, randomized, parallel group design. Further improvements are accomplished through the inclusion of multiple posttreatment measures to establish evidence regarding efficacy and safety over time.

Randomized Crossover Trial

The second commonly used design in clinical trials is the randomized crossover trial. This design applies only to diseases or physical conditions for which the treatment is palliative rather than curative and that, therefore, recur when medication or treatment is withheld. For example, this design may be applicable in an oncology population to test the efficacy of an antiemetic treatment administered during chemotherapy. The key feature of a crossover design is that each patient is assigned to a sequence consisting of all treatments. For example, for a two-treatment crossover trial, each patient is randomly assigned to alternative sequence groups: one sequence consisting of the new treatment followed by the standard treatment and the other consisting of the standard treatment followed by the new treatment.

The crossover trial has the same benefits of randomization that the parallel group trial possesses. In addition, this design has the advantage of providing more precise comparisons of treatments by using each patient as his or her own control; this feature reduces between-patient variability and generally results in a need for fewer patients to be studied than would be required in a parallel group trial. The fact that each patient receives both treatments is often viewed as a benefit for ethical reasons as well, because no patient is denied the new therapy or procedure. One important caution with the use of crossover trials is that a *wash-out period* is needed after the first treatment has been stopped in order to allow each patient's physiologic condition to return to its baseline levels. This wash-out period should be long enough to prevent the therapeutic effect of the first treatment from carrying over into the time period of the second treatment. If this precaution is not taken, a carryover effect may distort the result of the study. Further discussion of crossover trials is presented by Pocock[3] and Gillings and Douglass.[5]

Trial Size

Carrying out a clinical trial involves selection of a sample of patients who are thought to be representative of a larger population of patients who have the condition that the new drug is designed to treat or cure. The most important consideration in choosing patients for a given clinical trial is that they be truly representative of patients who would benefit from the treatment or drug being tested; to guarantee this requires a careful choice of investigators and, in turn, a careful choice of patients, with strict adherence to study inclusion and exclusion criteria listed in the study protocols.

The inclusion of an adequate number of patients—that is, a large enough sample size to be able to make a correct decision about whether or not the study treatment yields a significant improvement in the disease condition being studied—is also critical to ensure that inferences can be made from the study sample to the larger patient population. In a comparative trial, adequate sample size is needed to determine whether the difference between the new therapy (experimental group) and the standard treatment (control group) is statistically significant, that is, whether one can conclude that a true difference in outcome exists in the population of patients to be treated with a new therapy.

Historically, many clinical trials that have failed to show statistical significance have had an inadequate sample size.[3] Therefore, it is critical that sample size computations be carried out during the design of a clinical trial in order to ensure that the true value of a clinical investigation can be ascertained. The determination of adequate sample size in a clinical trial depends on several key components that need to be estimated in advance. It is sometimes difficult to know the value of these components before conducting a study. However, every effort should be made to determine these components as precisely as possible in order to maximize the ability to make a correct decision about the efficacy of treatments being tested.

One consideration related to sample size is the phase of a study. In general, both phase II and phase III trials require careful sample size calculation, but because phase II trials are carried out earlier in the clinical testing process, it is sometimes more difficult to obtain adequate information to estimate components of sample size. As a result, phase II sample sizes may sometimes be based on the number of available patients, and they generally have much smaller numbers of patients than phase III trials. However, whenever phase II studies are comparative trials, they should undergo the same rigorous standards for determining sample size that are applied to phase III studies.

Some studies are designed properly but still have insufficient sample size owing to dropouts or accrual difficulties, resulting in an inability to identify a sufficient number of appropriate patients. Adjustments for dropouts and nonevaluable cases should be factored into the sample size computation. Occasionally, the planned sample size is limited because of a desire to obtain study results more quickly. The practicality of choosing fewer patients must be balanced against the risk of having insufficient power to make a correct decision.

Power is the primary component of sample size determination in a comparative clinical trial. It is a mathematical concept describing the likelihood of finding a statistically significant difference between experimental and control groups in the sample of patients included in a clinical trial when a true difference exists in the population being studied. In other words, power determines our ability to detect a difference that really exists between experimental and control groups. Insufficient power can cause the difference between the experimental and control groups in key efficacy measures not to reach statistical significance even though the treatments truly are different. Power can be represented as a percentage; as noted by Pocock,[3] adequate power is usually defined as being 80% or higher. This means that the trial has a 20% chance of not detecting a significant difference that is really present (ie, a 20% risk of a type II error). Sample size computations require a computational factor to be included, based on the level of power chosen.

A second important component in the determination of sample size in a comparative clinical trial is the size of the expected difference between experimental and control groups in key efficacy measures. For treatments that are thought to be major breakthroughs, a large difference would be expected in key endpoints. However, in oncology and other disease conditions for which few adequate treatments are available, even small differences, such as an increase of 5% to 10% in 5-year survival, are desirable. In these situations, it becomes important to be able to reliably detect a small difference by demonstrating statistical significance.

The smaller the difference to be detected, the larger the sample size that is needed. The expected size of difference (often referred to as *delta*) is chosen in advance by the investigator. This is sometimes an iterative process in which alternative levels of delta are specified and sample sizes for each are reviewed to determine their feasibility.

The next component in determining sample size is the level of statistical significance to be used (also referred to as the *type I error rate*). For example, when a significance level of .05 is chosen, 95% of the time $(1.00-0.05)$ a correct decision will be made about not finding a significant

difference when the treatment is not efficacious, and 5% of the time an erroneous conclusion will be made that there is a difference when there actually is not (ie, there is a 5% chance of committing a type I error).

The final component in determining sample size is the variance of the measures to be used to determine efficacy. Both in regard to estimating variance and in specifying delta, the most important issue is that in most clinical trials there are several key outcome measures. The recommended approach is to choose the two or three most important measures and compute sample size based on each, and whenever possible choose the largest sample size. All other components being equal, the larger the variance of a measure, the larger the sample size needed.

In choosing key efficacy measures to compute sample size, it is often feasible to choose a categorical measure of outcome such as the proportion of patients showing clinical improvement in some key study criteria. In such cases, the variance is computed directly from the proportion; thus, using the value of the proportion, the variance does not need to be computed directly. (The size of variance increases as proportions get closer to 50%.)

Table 2–1 illustrates how the factors discussed earlier affect the necessary sample size in a clinical study. This table lists the sample size needed in each treatment group (experimental and control) in order to show a statistically significant difference $(P < 0.05)$ with 80% power (80% chance of detecting a difference that is actually there) according to the percentage of the control group achieving a categorical endpoint measure (eg, proportion of patients surviving 5 years) and according to the expected difference between the experimental group (P_E) and control group (P_C) ($P_E - P_C = 5\%$, 10%, 15%, and 20%). The sample size estimates in Table 2–1 apply only to categorical outcome measures; other tables must be used to compare differences in a continuous measure such as median survival time.

As an example of how to use Table 2–1, let us consider a study in which the endpoint is an improvement in the proportion of patients surviving 5 years. If it is expected

TABLE 2–1. NUMBER OF PATIENTS NEEDED (PER GROUP) TO SHOW A STATISTICALLY SIGNIFICANT DIFFERENCE* WITH 80% POWER OF DETECTION

PERCENTAGE OF CONTROL GROUP ACHIEVING ENDPOINT	DIFFERENCE IN PERCENTAGE ACHIEVING ENDPOINT: EXPERIMENTAL VERSUS CONTROL GROUP ($P_E - P_C$)			
	5%	10%	15%	20%
5	420	130	69	44
10	680	195	96	59
15	910	250	120	71
20	1090	290	135	80
25	1250	330	150	88
30	1380	360	160	93
40	1530	390	175	97
50	1560	390	170	93

It is assumed that the lower outcome rate is obtained in the control group.
*$P = 0.05$, two-sided test.
P_C, control group; P_E, experimental group.
Data from Lee E. Statistical Methods for Survival Analysis. Belmont, Calif: Lifetime Learning Publications, 1980, p 386.[27]

that there would be a 5-year survival rate of 15% in the control group and 25% in the experimental group, then the expected difference between the two groups would be 10% ($P_E - P_C$). Reading across the third row ($P_C = 15\%$) to the second column ($P_E - P_C = 10\%$), it can be noted that achieving statistical significance would require at least 250 patients in each group. If a larger difference had been expected, such as $P_E - P_C = 20\%$, then only 71 patients would be needed in each group to achieve statistical significance. Thus the expected difference in the endpoint measures ($P_E - P_C$) has a profound impact on the sample size needed to show a difference. It is all too easy to be tempted to use an unrealistically optimistic estimate of the expected difference between the treatment and control groups in designing a trial, in order to accommodate the practical limitation of being able to accrue a large number of patients to a clinical trial. It can also be seen how miscalculations in the baseline outcome of the control group can have a major effect on whether the sample size accrued was large enough to show a statistically significant difference. One way to improve on the accuracy of this estimate is to conduct a thorough literature review as part of the design of a trial.

PITFALLS IN STUDY INTERPRETATION

A randomized controlled trial, often conducted as a multi-institutional venture, is usually expected to be of good quality and to yield reliable results. Unfortunately, this is not always the case. Several frequently overlooked but common sources of erroneous conclusions are outlined below.

Interpretation of Nonsignificant Studies

When the effectiveness of the test treatment is substantial, the interpretation of statistically significant findings in a comparative clinical trial is well understood and clinical interpretation is usually fairly straightforward. When statistical comparisons in a controlled clinical trial are not statistically significant (eg, $P \geq 0.05$) the clinical meaning requires a careful review because the lack of significance may be due to factors other than ineffectiveness of the test treatment. In order to review these factors in a logical manner, it is important to ask a series of questions such as those described in Table 2–2. The rationale behind these questions is discussed next.

A first step in determining the importance of a finding that is not statistically significant is to review its clinical significance based on the observed difference between the experimental and control groups at some critical time point, such as a 5-year survival rate, or in a categorical response measure at study endpoint. This preliminary test helps us to assess the benefit of a treatment before addressing the statistical issues surrounding the test result. If an observed difference that was found not to be statistically significant is too small to be clinically important, then little will be gained from further analysis of the issue.

TABLE 2–2. QUESTIONS TO REVIEW WHEN ASSESSING A STUDY THAT IS NOT STATISTICALLY SIGNIFICANT

1. Is there an observed difference between the experimental and control groups that is clinically important?
2. Are the experimental and control groups homogeneous at baseline?
3. Are there equal numbers of patients in the experimental and control groups?
4. Is the sample size sufficient to achieve statistical significance?

Next, one should always review the actual P value computed, rather than simply determining whether it is statistically significant or not. In the absence of other confounding factors (such as multiple comparisons), P values that approach the predetermined target significance level, such as 0.05 or 0.10, may be strongly indicative of a clinically important trend. Those P values that are much larger than the predetermined significance level (eg, ≥ 0.20) indicate very definitive evidence of a lack of treatment efficacy, regardless of other factors. Clinically significant differences that yield P values approaching statistical significance may be evidence of an important treatment effect; the lack of a significant P value may be the direct result of a lack of power of the statistical test, which can be due to larger-than-expected variability in the data, insufficient sample size (number of patients in each treatment group), or both.

Variability that is larger than expected may be due to heterogeneity of background or disease status characteristics in the study group leading to a wider-than-expected range of response to the treatment. In reviewing journal articles, this is a difficult issue to examine unless a complete description of each patient or a listing of each patient's response measures is presented. However, a reasonable assessment of homogeneity can be gained from a baseline (before treatment) comparison of study and control groups relative to demographics, background characteristics, and key prognostic factors. Significant differences at baseline may indicate heterogeneity, which may influence variability in response. However, even when treatment groups are homogeneous at baseline, there may be various factors related to patient characteristics that cause variations in response to treatment.

The more common and more easily detected cause of lack of statistical power in a clinical trial is insufficient sample size. This may be due to the selection of a small sample to begin with or to patients excluded during the course of the trial because of protocol violations or other non–treatment-related issues. To guard against this latter problem, most statistical procedures in survival studies account to some degree for dropouts and losses to follow-up. Another potential cause of loss of power in a comparative trial is imbalance across treatment groups because maximum power is achieved through enrollment of equal numbers of patients in each treatment group. However, for ethical or other reasons, different numbers of patients may be randomized to various treatment groups in oncology trials. In this case, the effect on power should be assessed.

One method for determining whether the power of a clinical trial is insufficient because of the sample size is to use a table such as Table 2–1 to assess the sample size needed to achieve statistical significance for a difference that is clinically important. If the sample size in the nonsignificant study being reviewed is less than indicated in the table, the lack of statistical significance may be due to failure to include enough patients in the trial (ie, insufficient power). To prevent this problem, researchers should follow procedures such as those described under Trial Size. If a clinical study detects a clinically important difference but the statistical comparison yields a nonsignificant result, then a review of such a table can help to explain this finding. In fact, it may provide evidence of the clinical importance of this treatment despite the inability of the trial to achieve statistical significance because a likely explanation for the lack of statistical significance can be provided. However, before concluding definitely that such a treatment is clinically valuable, additional study is needed using the appropriate sample size to determine definitive evidence of success or failure.

Balance and Stratification

In a randomized trial, it is important that the two treatment arms be comparable in every respect except for the difference in the treatment given. In most situations, a number of prognostic factors have been identified for the patient cohort being studied. Although it is anticipated that the randomization process will evenly distribute prognostic factors (including unrecognized factors) between the two arms, this is not necessarily always the case. Unless the two arms are well balanced with respect to all the major prognostic factors, the strength of the conclusion will be diminished. A report of a clinical trial should include such an analysis of *baseline homogeneity* between the trial groups. Studies frequently report how well the two groups are matched with respect to a number of factors, including some that are not of prognostic significance but unfortunately omit mention of others that are of prognostic importance.

In order to ensure that the groups are well matched, patients are sometimes stratified with respect to several major prognostic factors. Stratification is unnecessary in most large randomized trials because increasing sample size can help to ensure an adequate balance of prognostic factors in all treatment groups. However, in smaller studies or in cases in which a specific prognostic factor is rare and may be unevenly distributed across treatments, the use of stratification helps to guarantee balance by ensuring that a fixed number of patients with each level of a prognostic factor is assigned to each treatment.[3]

When stratification is used, analyses are somewhat more complicated because within-stratum treatment comparisons are carried out and then averaged across strata to provide an overall estimate of treatment effect. Likewise, when imbalance in prognostic factors exists at baseline, a more complex analysis is required using multivariable analysis methods. (See the following discussion.)

Subset Analysis

As described earlier in this chapter, it is critical to have a sufficient sample size in order to achieve the power neces-sary to make a correct inference about treatment effectiveness. It is for this reason that comparisons between experimental and control groups based on subsets of patients should be interpreted cautiously. Generally, subgroup analyses will not have adequate power to demonstrate statistical significance for an observed difference. Thus, subgroup analysis results can be misleading.

A second caution regarding subgroup analysis has to do with the statistical concept of multiple comparisons. Simply stated, if one makes a large number of unplanned statistical comparisons in a clinical study, some will yield statistical significance due to random chance. In fact, the type I error rate (1 in 20 if $P<0.05$ is chosen) becomes larger the greater the number of separate analyses that are performed. Thus one may incorrectly conclude that a difference between experimental and control groups is real when it is not.

In general, subset analyses should be avoided unless they are preplanned, that is, stated as being of interest in the study protocol. When unplanned subgroup analyses are carried out, they should be based on a sound clinical rationale in order to avoid the implication that they are "fishing expeditions." In all cases, they should be assessed with caution. In some cases, with proper caution, subgroup analyses can be informative and can be viewed as hypothesis-generating exercises, which are useful for planning further studies. This can be especially valuable when primary hypotheses based on the entire sample of patients fail to yield statistical significance, and a subgroup of patients yields a clinically important trend that merits further study. In such cases, a new trial that focuses on the subgroups of interest may be designed with adequate sample size to provide valid conclusions.

Multivariable Analysis

The advent of advanced software packages has made it easy to carry out very complex multivariable analyses (ie, those analyses in which one outcome measure is analyzed as a function of multiple explanatory variables and prognostic factors). Examples of these methods include general linear models based on least squares regression for continuous measures, logistic regression models for categorical outcome measures, and Cox proportional hazards regression models for survival measures. Although multivariable analysis greatly facilitates analysis of complex clinical findings, this type of analysis can lead to erroneous conclusions in several ways. Although none of these pitfalls should deter one from using multivariable models for assessing clinical studies, they do point out the need to be cautious in making conclusions that are based solely on complex multivariable analyses.

First, all such complex modeling approaches are based on assumptions underlying the modeling procedure. Although these assumptions are rarely defined in publications, they may have implications for the validity of conclusions from such models. Also important, especially for logistic regression, is the goodness of fit of the model, which has a direct impact on the validity of conclusions. Unfortunately, this is rarely reported in publications involving regression analyses. Another area of caution when many variables have been included in a multivariable analysis model is the pattern of missing values in the explanatory variables. When several patients have different missing values, the effective sample size for the specific analysis being carried out may be dramatically reduced, and this may have a direct impact on the ability to achieve statistical significance.

Meta-Analysis

As noted by Pocock, "for most diseases, it is unrealistic to expect that any single trial can totally resolve a therapeutic issue. . . . Replication of a clinical trial in different circumstances is a valuable step in checking the original [trial's] validity."[3(p 242)] This is good advice, and much has been written about the use of meta-analysis as a technique for formalizing the process of combining evidence from multiple studies by providing a single statistic to summarize the results of a set of similar studies.

The first step in carrying out a meta-analysis is to define a set of similar studies to provide information about a treatment's efficacy or, in epidemiology, to provide a single-risk estimate. The use of a careful literature review is the first step in this process; failure to conduct such a review is the first pitfall to consider in reviewing a meta-analysis. It is critical to consider the possibility of publication bias, which refers to a concern that positive studies are more likely to be published. When this occurs, estimates of the magnitude of a treatment effect may be biased upward in meta-analyses of published literature. Although this is a pitfall that must be considered, Hunter and Schmidt[6] pointed out that this is a general problem with all published study findings and is not limited to meta-analyses.

A more serious consideration in reviewing meta-analyses is whether it is legitimate to pool the results of various studies in light of the risk of possible diversity of treatments and trial designs. The homogeneity of studies included in a meta-analysis can be assessed to some degree by reviewing the characteristics of each study, such as the study population characteristics (demographics, prognostic factors, and inclusion and exclusion criteria), the number and types of treatment arms, and the duration of the trial. The goal is to avoid combining apples with oranges. Other issues related to the homogeneity of trials can be adjusted for through proper (study-specific) weighting in a meta-analysis. These include size of sample and size of variance of estimates from each study. Variability in the quality of studies being combined is another critical element to consider in reviewing meta-analyses, although it is often difficult to assess this unless considerable background information is provided.

In addition to a careful review of published design factors, various methods are available for assessing the consistency and strength of results from a meta-analysis. These include formal sensitivity and influence analyses—methods by which analyses are repeated after excluding controversial or other specific studies in order to assess robustness of the overall result. In reviewing meta-analyses, care should be taken to check for the presence and results of these types of analyses.

In general, the broader the disease indication, the more

pitfalls one must take into account when reviewing meta-analyses. However, valuable information can be obtained through the proper use of this powerful technique. For further information about the use and limitations of meta-analyses, see Hunter and Schmidt[6]; and information compiled by Bullock and Svyantek.[7]

DEVELOPMENT AND CONDUCT OF CLINICAL TRIALS

Often, there is wide agreement about whether it is important to study a particular issue, but a surprising amount of disagreement about details related to the design and conduct (eg, drug dosage) of a clinical trial. An understanding of how trials are developed and conducted is useful to gain insight into how the details of clinical trials are chosen. Traditionally, most phase II and phase III clinical trials have been developed through one of the cooperative oncology groups supported by the NCI.

Alternatively, some trials are sponsored by the pharmaceutical or biotechnology industry. In the past, these mainly involved studies that were conceived within a particular company, which then contracted with individual sites or with a commercial research organization to carry out the trial. More recently, investigator-initiated trials that are supported through industry have become much more common. In this case, the trial is conceived and conducted by an independent investigator, but financial support for the cost of conducting the trial is provided by a pharmaceutical company.

A major change is taking place in the organization of clinical research by the NCI, as is discussed later in this chapter. One of the goals is to broaden the base of investigators who are able to develop a clinical trial. In this scenario, any investigator can submit a proposal to the appropriate Disease-Specific Concept Review Committee of the NCI. If the concept is meritorious, the new NCI infrastructure will provide financial and organizational support to see that the study is carried out, regardless of whether or not the investigator is affiliated with a particular oncology group or institution. This system is under development and is being piloted in lung cancer, as well as several other types of cancer. How well this will work in practice remains to be seen, but it is hoped that this structure will result in more widespread investment of physicians in clinical research.

Cooperative Group Trials

The development of a local (single-institution) clinical trial is the easiest to understand. Such a trial is initiated by a clinician or group of clinicians who propose a treatment plan for a particular group of patients. Ideally, the objectives and the treatment plan should be spelled out in detail, as well as the eligibility requirements for patient inclusion. Unfortunately, sometimes the treatment plan and inclusion criteria are defined only vaguely. With most prospective trials, ethical approval must be obtained from the institutional review board (IRB), and the patients must sign a consent form to be part of the trial. Such single-institution trials, which often involve comparisons with historical groups of patients as controls, lack statistical power to evaluate treatment effectiveness but can be useful in assessing toxicity and response (phase I and II questions).

Larger trials, such as those needed to answer phase III questions, usually involve the collaboration of multiple institutions and are usually conducted under the auspices of one of the cooperative oncology groups. A trial that is developed within one of the larger cooperative oncology groups is first proposed as a concept within the appropriate committee of the cooperative group. If the concept meets approval, a formal protocol is written. The protocol is then subjected to criticism and debate within the initiating committee and other committees within the group, as well as the group's executive committee, which must give approval. The trial must then meet the approval of the Cancer Therapy Evaluation Program (CTEP) of the NCI in order to be eligible for NCI (and cooperative group) funding. Once all of these hurdles are overcome, the trial is activated, but before accrual can begin, the trial must be approved by the IRB of each institution that would like to participate.

Any changes to the protocol (due to ambiguities or because new data has become available) must be made through a formal amendment. The principal investigator must monitor the safety of the treatment and the quality of the data accumulated. Any major safety issues must be communicated immediately to the appropriate committee of the cooperative group and the NCI. Data is collected by local protocol nurses and data managers and collated by the statistical center of the cooperative group. Following completion of the study period and after sufficient time has elapsed for the results to be sufficiently mature statistically to warrant an assessment, the data is reviewed by the data monitoring committee of the group and released for publication.

In order to increase patient accrual, a trial initiated by one group may allow participation by other cooperative groups through the intergroup mechanism. A formal arrangement and agreement to participate must be reached before this can begin. Sometimes there is a substantial amount of negotiation about details of the trial, but the initiating group retains the power to decide which changes it is willing to make in order to get broader participation.

Industry-Sponsored Trials

The development of an industry-sponsored trial is usually more rapid and does not involve as many people and steps as in the development of a cooperative group trial. A concept is proposed by a company or by an independent investigator. Scientific review is obtained from as many people as is deemed necessary. The safety issues and regulations that apply to these trials are the same as those for cooperative group trials. Before a decision is made to support a trial, the company involved assesses the scientific validity of the trial as well as practical issues related to completion of the trial. A number of study sites are selected on the basis of demonstrated interest, the ability to accrue patients, and the ability to collect reliable data. The sponsoring company provides financial support for the data

collection. The local IRB at each site must approve the study before any patients can be enrolled.

In investigator-initiated, industry-supported trials, the data is usually analyzed and published by the investigator. In industry-initiated trials, the data is evaluated and released by the company involved, which introduces a potential for bias. However, data that is biased is of no value either to a pharmaceutical company or to the medical community. Pharmaceutical companies are interested in providing data that will stand up to careful scrutiny and be accepted by the scientific community. Often, sponsoring companies require that the data be reviewed by an external, independent organization to prevent bias.

INFRASTRUCTURE FOR CLINICAL TRIALS

National Cancer Institute–Funded Infrastructure

Since the 1950s, the NCI has been the world's largest sponsor of clinical trials of cancer, supporting a broad range of treatment studies of new drugs and procedures, both surgical and radiotherapeutic. Developmental work for new treatments (phase I and II trials) has traditionally been carried out in a limited number of institutions, whereas definitive studies comparing new treatments to the standard of care (phase III trials) have required multicenter collaborations (J. Abrams. Background of pilot projects: report of the National Cancer Institute Clinical Trials Program Review Group. Attachment 1, memorandum to BSA Subcommittee and Expert Panel Members. Bethesda, Md: National Cancer Institute; February 26, 1998).

Cooperative Oncology Groups

The NCI supports multiple sites and investigators in North America to collaborate in several clinical trials cooperative groups. Table 2–3 lists the seven cooperative groups actively involved in clinical research in lung cancer. Each of these groups maintains the necessary infrastructure (scientific committees, statisticians, data managers, quality control monitors) to perform large, randomized clinical trials. Collectively, the cooperative groups accrue about 20 000 new patients to treatment trials each year. Group activities take place at thousands of sites nationwide, including university hospitals, cancer treatment centers, community hospitals, and outpatient offices and clinics.

Although most trials are conducted by the respective

TABLE 2–3. COOPERATIVE GROUPS ACTIVELY INVOLVED IN CLINICAL RESEARCH IN LUNG CANCER

American College of Surgeons Oncology Group (ACoSOG)
Cancer and Leukemia Group B (CALGB)
Eastern Cooperative Oncology Group (ECOG)
National Cancer Institute of Canada (NCIC)
North Central Cancer Treatment Group (NCCTG)
Radiation Therapy Oncology Group (RTOG)
Southwest Oncology Group (SWOG)

cooperative groups and thus only members of that group are eligible to accrue patients to that protocol, the NCI has increasingly made selected trials available to various NCI cooperative groups in order to speed accrual to large phase III and IV trials. These are known as *intergroup studies*. These studies are developed, designed, opened, and analyzed by one group, but members of other groups have access to the study and are able to accrue patients. Each cooperating group agrees to collect data for members of that group and forward it to the group initiating the study. Periodic intergroup meetings are also held to coordinate studies that are under development within each of the individual groups.

Community Clinical Oncology Program

The NCI has long recognized that cutting edge treatment and clinical research should not remain confined to academic centers. This belief led to the development in 1983 of the Community Clinical Oncology Program (CCOP), with the goal of providing community oncologists with state-of-the-art protocols as well as achieving the participation of many more patients in studies so that progress could be made more quickly. The infrastructure created by CCOP provided a mechanism for awarding cooperative agreements to community-based consortia of physicians and hospitals, designated as CCOP research bases, to support enrolling patients in clinical trials.[8]

NCI cooperative groups and selected NCI-funded cancer centers are designated as research bases responsible for designing the protocols for the clinical trials, collecting and analyzing study data, and monitoring data quality and patient accrual. Each CCOP must affiliate with at least one and not more than five NCI-supported research bases. CCOPs are the working groups of physicians, support staff, and hospitals that conduct cancer research at the community level. The number of patients that a CCOP enrolls on research-based protocols serves as the primary measure of CCOP performance.

National Cancer Institute Pilot Organization

Whether conducted under the sponsorship of the NCI or various pharmaceutical or biotechnology companies, clinical trials occur within an ever larger and changing health service industry.[9] Many changes in the structure and conduct of clinical research are taking place. At the core of these changes is movement away from episodic treatment by an autonomous provider and toward care provided by clinicians who are part of a larger delivery system involved with some form of a managed care arrangement. These changes have resulted in significant alterations in the manner in which the NCI is conducting phase III treatment trials. These changes involve the major components of the process, including the generation of trial ideas, the information infrastructure, the organizational structure of the trial, and the network of investigators performing the trials. Major elements of the change are outlined in the following paragraph.[10]

- *State-of-the-science meetings.* These involve a review of a particular treatment issue in order to stimulate ideas for multicenter (phase III) trials. These meetings include not only investigators from the NCI's clinical trials cooperative groups (the traditional source of ideas) but also clinical and basic scientists from academia and industry, patient advocates, and others. The first state-of-the-science meeting took place in mid-1999.

- *Disease-Specific Concept Review Committees.* These are bodies that approve or disapprove proposals for phase III trials. Any researcher, regardless of affiliation, may submit an idea. Unlike in the previous review procedure, one-third of each committee's members are from the NCI, one-third from the cooperative groups, and one-third from the advocacy community and investigators outside the groups. Previously, review was centralized largely within the NCI. The first such committees, in the areas of genitourinary and lung cancers, met in the spring of 1999.

- *National network of physicians.* This network is designed to allow patients to be enrolled in any trial approved by the Concept Review Committees. This is in contrast to the previous system, in which investigators were limited to their own group's trials. Development of this network is being piloted in the areas of lung, breast, gastrointestinal, and genitourinary cancers as well as adult leukemia. Initially, only members of cooperative groups will belong to the network, but as the new system becomes established, others will be able to join.

- *Cancer Trials Support Unit (CTSU).* The CTSU provides a uniform system of patient registration and data collection for all network trials. A CTSU contract is awarded through open competition to an organization equipped to provide state-of-the-art clinical trials communications and data management.

- *Common informatics system.* This links network physicians with the NCI and CTSU. The online system includes common forms, common data elements, and electronic interfaces among data centers and sponsors for easy updating and reporting.

Infrastructure for Industry-Sponsored Trials

Industry-sponsored research often requires investigators to contract directly with pharmaceutical or biotechnology companies to carry out trial-related duties. It has also become common for industrial sponsors to delegate the management of clinical trials to intermediaries such as clinical contract research organizations (CROs) and site management organizations (SMOs). The role of CROs has expanded, and often the CRO carries out a variety of activities ranging from study design to submission of new drug applications (NDAs) to the FDA. SMOs that have been formed to coordinate the activities of investigator sites require some formal membership or partnership by the investigative site with the SMO.

The same responsibilities for quality and safety apply regardless of whether trials are contracted directly by industry, through intermediaries such as CROs or SMOs, or through federal agencies such as the NCI. The role and responsibility of sponsors, CROs, SMOs, and investigators are clearly defined by regulations of the FDA and have been detailed by laws described in the Code of Federal Regulations.[11] Sponsors are responsible for selecting and monitoring each clinical study site to validate study data and ensure patient safety. These tasks are accomplished through periodic site visits by the sponsor or its agents (eg, CROs).

Investigators are responsible for obtaining IRB approval and written informed consent from all patients who enroll in a trial, maintaining clearly documented dispensing records of study drugs and notifying the sponsor of the occurrence of any adverse reactions that are thought to be causally related to the study drug. Investigators must record individual patient data and keep this data for 2 years following the marketing approval of the new drug or the discontinuation of the Investigational New Drug status by the FDA.

ISSUES IN TRIAL PARTICIPATION

Clinical research is a difficult undertaking. As with any scientific endeavor, the requirement that as many variables as possible be controlled other than the one being tested means that careful preparation is necessary. In addition, data must be carefully recorded. The number of possible variables and the ability to control them in a clinical setting is more difficult than in research conducted in a laboratory. The fact that clinical research must be conducted by many different physicians and protocol nurses, who are often in different institutions across the country, compounds the problem. Furthermore, a place for clinical research must be created in the context of clinical medical care, which is affected by a myriad of financial and societal pressures. Finally, the necessity in our modern society for clinical research to be not only ethically sound but also able to stand up to media and legal scrutiny creates an additional layer of organization and regulations. Some of these issues are discussed briefly in the remaining pages of this chapter.

Patient Issues

Previous research has found that between 19% and 33% of patients who are offered clinical trial therapy refuse it.[12, 13] Reasons for refusal include the perceived cost and risk versus the perceived benefit, distrust of experimentation, and lack of receptivity to information.[14, 15] In one of the few studies assessing the effect of protocol characteristics on patient enrollment, an analysis of 23 phase III breast cancer protocols, revealed that patients were less likely to be enrolled if the protocol included an assessment of drug toxicity as a study endpoint and if the protocol included a number of treatment modalities to which the patient could be assigned.[2]

Research into how patients weigh potential treatment benefits against toxicity has generally shown that patients have a much lower threshold to want treatment than medical staff.[16, 17] A survey of patients who had received chemotherapy found that on average, a survival benefit of 4 months was considered sufficient for patients to view a treatment as worthwhile if the toxicity was mild or moderate.[18] Although these studies do not specifically address participation in clinical trials, they do suggest that patients' views of the ratio between treatment benefits and toxicity

are probably not a major factor preventing trial participation. Logistic issues may play a greater role in a patient's reluctance to participate in clinical trials. The realities of time lost from the job during treatment and difficulties in obtaining access to medical facilities for appropriate follow-up tests are factors contributing to the patient's reluctance to get involved.

The naive fear of experimentation can usually be allayed if the patient is made aware of the amount of scientific and ethical discussion and consensus that is behind a protocol that has come through the development process to the point of activation. A patient's fear of experimentation may also be related to misunderstandings. For example, a patient may attribute every death that occurs on a protocol as being *due to the treatment*, ignoring the effects of the disease that is being treated. The patient's receptivity to information and the physician's communication skills are important factors. A physician may fail to present the advantages of a trial or the patient may not understand the process described and feel too confused and uncertain to participate, despite a good presentation. Some patients will decline the trial because they are in a state of denial about their cancer diagnosis. However, a patient's fear of experimentation may also be related to mistrust of the individual provider or the institution. For example, a patient may distrust the participating institution because of a previous experience resulting in unresolved complaints, temporary or long-standing problems with the reputation of the institution, or a perceived conflict between a physician-recommended "best" therapy and the trial therapy.

A particularly critical issue facing patient participation in clinical trials is whether treatment will be reimbursed. The use of investigational drugs presents major problems for patients seeking reimbursement from their insurance carrier. Moreover, as increasing portions of the population are enrolled in managed care plans, the challenges are likely to become more acute as managed care companies implement strict cost-containment measures. The popular press has provided extensive coverage of various insurance payment denials because of experimental treatment, and the increasing complexity of health services delivery has presented both challenges and opportunities to the clinical research community.[9]

Nonetheless, serious efforts are presently underway to develop a working relationship between various managed care providers and the National Institutes of Health (NIH) and NCI clinical trial program.[19] These efforts include federal funding of a large cooperative research project involving the NCI and 10 of the largest health maintenance organizations (HMOs) in the country[20] and a cooperative agreement between the NCI and the Department of Defense to involve Civilian Health and Medical Program of Uniformed Services (CHAMPUS) patients in NCI-approved clinical trials.[21] Moreover, significant progress is being made to systematically assess the cost of clinical trials in order to factor the cost into various reimbursement policies.[22]

Physician Issues

Good clinical research requires a commitment from participating physicians. From a larger perspective, commitment to the welfare of patients and improvement in outcomes for patients should make participation in clinical research automatic. However, from a practical standpoint, a significant investment of time is necessary because clinical research cannot be done only when time permits. One must be organized enough to have selected protocols for participation, understand the trial background and design, and have obtained approval by the IRB before an eligible patient is encountered.

Discussion of the trial with the patient requires a substantial time investment. The physician must be able to make the patient understand the value of trial participation and the safety of the trial and must maintain equipoise in the case of a randomized study. The fact that no credit or reimbursement is given for the extra time required to carry out these tasks is a significant impediment to finding room for clinical research in a busy clinical practice. Much material is available to assist physicians and other clinical personnel in approaching the patient about clinical trials in order to increase the likelihood of patient acceptance. The way in which the trial is presented to the patients and their families is critical. Various brochures and videotapes are available and useful, but personal contact—particularly by the treating physician and the nurse oncologist—is important. Other support material usually available as part of patient resource libraries includes materials and computer information on drug treatment, resources to assist in pain management, dietary information, and information on personal issues (eg, wigs and cosmetics). In addition, support groups provide an important resource to help recently diagnosed patients meet the challenges of their illness and their involvement in clinical trials.

The character of the doctor-patient relationship is a major reason for physicians to decide not to offer trial enrollment to their patients.[23] Issues of trust and clinical judgment influence the decision process, and often physicians may choose not to select otherwise eligible patients for trial enrollment because of characteristics not specified in the protocol. Advanced age has been shown to be a significant factor in the exclusion of patients from clinical trials.[12] Other reasons include the strength of the patient's support system, the patient's home situation, the cost to the patient, and anticipated poor compliance with the protocol treatment.[24]

A significant problem is the fact that most physicians harbor particular biases about treatment that may be influenced by anecdotal experiences, practical issues such as availability of particular treatment options, and political or personality issues within the local community. Physicians may have a bias against specific trials because of the particular drugs used or concerns about the protocol design.[12] Physician bias can be reflected in the very protocols that are submitted to an IRB for review. For example, in a study of 23 phase III breast cancer protocols, protocols that reduced cost or had no cost to patients for one or more treatment drugs had a positive and significant relationship to protocol adoption, as measured by referral to an IRB.[2] Most often, however, their bias is based on a more general sense that there is literature demonstrating the value of a particular approach, when in fact there is not. Unless a great deal of time is taken to critically review most of the literature, one is susceptible to overemphasizing small and incomplete pieces of information that appear to support a particular approach. It is hoped that this book will permit the available data to be accessed quickly and will help foster an honest examination of whether statements that are commonly touted are based on data or conjecture and dogma.

As cancer treatment becomes more and more complex, often involving several treatment modalities, there is an even greater potential for strong biases because the number of people participating in the treatment is larger. Furthermore, there is great potential for miscommunication, which can greatly erode a patient's confidence in the treatment. A forum in which all the involved parties meet to discuss patient and protocol issues on a regular basis is extremely useful in this regard. Although 1 to 2 hours a week may need to be set aside for this purpose, much time is saved by reducing confusion and promoting communication in a timely fashion.

Cost Issues

Underlying the various patient and physician issues is the question of cost; namely, is the cost of caring for patients on clinical trials substantially greater than for those who receive standard care? Although cost has always been a factor in clinical trials, the advent of managed care has forced the issue, and its resolution will shape the perspective of managed care toward clinical trial reimbursement.

Two studies have concluded that the cost of caring for patients on clinical trials is not significantly higher than for patients receiving standard care.[25, 26] In a study comparing the cost of standard care with the cost of care for 61 patients enrolled in NCI phase II or phase III cancer chemotherapy clinical trials at the Mayo Clinic from 1988 to 1994, analysis revealed that the cost for clinical trial patients was slightly higher, but the differences were not statistically significant[25] (Fig. 2–2). Patients were matched

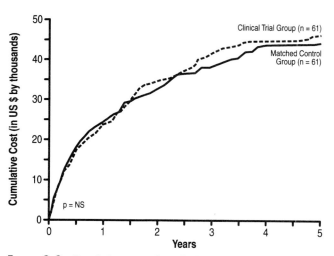

FIGURE 2–2. Cumulative cost of medical care of patients treated on phase II or III clinical cancer trials versus matched patients treated for cancer within the same geographical area and period of time. (From Wagner J, Alberts S, Sloan J, et al. Incremental cost of enrolling cancer patients in clinical trials: a population based study. J Natl Cancer Inst. 1999; 91:847–853.[25])

with respect to age, gender, site of primary cancer, stage of cancer, date of diagnosis, and clinical trials eligibility.[25] A similar finding was reported in a retrospective study of 135 Kaiser Permanente (Northern California) patients in clinical trials compared with a matched group of patients receiving standard care.[26]

Data Quality Issues

There can be no doubt that prospective data is much better than retrospective data. Prospective data provides the opportunity to collect data in a manner consistent with the study design rather than trying to retrofit the data to the design. Furthermore, the requirement that most clinical research be controlled and conducted according to a defined protocol means that a consistent focus on the study requirements and data collection is necessary. This fact is clearly recognized by the NCI and industry through funding for research nurse positions. However, the current climate in health care is having a negative impact on such positions. The trend toward minimizing costs by promoting *multitasking*— requiring people to do many different jobs as time permits—is not conducive to the kind of focused attention to detail that is required to collect accurate data. Furthermore, the approval of minute details of patient care demanded by insurance carriers makes clinical research more difficult.

CLINICAL RESEARCH PERSONNEL

In order to ensure adequate and good quality data, clinical research must be conducted by a team approach. The clinical research team consists of the principal investigator, co-investigator, research nurse, data manager, investigational pharmacist, statistician, and clinical nursing staff. The role of each is briefly described below.

The principal investigator (PI) has primary responsibility for the scientific integrity of the study. The principal investigator is usually the individual who has developed the protocol or, in the event of a multi-institutional protocol, has taken the responsibility of serving as the local study representative. The principal investigator is responsible for initiating the regulatory process, presenting the trial to various review boards, and writing the consent form. The principal investigator also is responsible for implementing the study.

The research nurse plays a key role in providing information to the patient and family, treating the patient, and ensuring that the details of the study are carried out appropriately. In addition, the research nurse usually participates in screening potential patients and in recruiting for the study. The nurse is involved in the informed consent process together with the physician and is available to the patient for answering questions and triaging problems. The research nurse must educate patients, family members, and home health nurses regarding the nature of the treatment and potential toxicities. The research nurse implements the physician's orders as outlined by the study. The nurse observes responses and toxicities to the treatment and documents them for data collection.

The data manager collects all the information regarding the patient's treatment, toxicity, and responses and records it for statistical analysis. The data manager usually uses standardized forms prepared by the sponsor or cooperative group for data collection. The data manager must pay attention to detail in order to ensure accurate data entry. The accuracy with which data is entered will be reflected in the final statistical analysis.

Phase I and phase II clinical trials may involve investigational drugs. When investigational drugs are used in a clinical trial, an investigational pharmacist should be involved. The investigational pharmacist is primarily responsible for drug inventory, drug dispensing, and record keeping for drugs used during the study.

The statistician is responsible for many aspects of clinical trials. The statistician is usually involved during the development of a trial to help determine the sample size needed and to help evaluate the study design. The statistician evaluates data during the trial and reports the final analysis when the trial is complete. The statistician is extremely important to the integrity of the study.

The clinical nursing staff is responsible for administering protocol therapy. The staff should be well versed in the immediate and long-term toxicity profile of the treatment. The nursing staff should also be aware of the risks and benefits of the particular therapy involved. The patients may ask questions of the nursing staff during their treatment time; therefore, it is important that the clinical staff be educated about the clinical trials. It is also the responsibility of the clinical nurse to immediately report any toxicity noted during a patient's treatment. The clinical nurse should be aware of the need for intermittent laboratory or radiologic studies. The clinical nurse should also note when the patient should return to the clinic and should reinforce these orders with the patient.

Institutional Review Board

A critical component of the clinical trial process is the protection of human subjects. The central issue is that patients are informed and that there is assurance that the benefits outweigh the risks. To achieve this, institutions wishing to participate in NIH-funded clinical trials are required to have an IRB or to affiliate with an institution with an IRB that is approved by the NIH Office for the Protection of Research Risk (OPRR) and to have all protocols and consent forms approved by the IRB before a patient is entered on trial. The designated IRB must meet specific OPRR criteria in terms of membership and function. The IRB must also monitor and review, on a regular basis, all NIH-funded trials conducted within the institution. The IRB must be kept abreast of amendments or toxic events as they relate to individual study, and protocols and consent forms must be reviewed at least once a year. Documentation of toxic events must be reported to the IRB and, under certain conditions, to the NCI. Large institutions generally have an IRB in place. Physicians within the community must affiliate with one of these institutions to open and accrue patients to clinical trials.

EDITORS' COMMENTS

Clinical research lies at the heart of all advances that have been achieved in the treatment of lung cancer. Major strides have occurred in the field of clinical research since 1980, from the widespread use of actuarial survival to the sophisticated design of multi-institutional clinical trials. Often, much of this is taken for granted. However, without this methodology, only gross differences in outcomes can be detected.

The treatment of lung cancer now has clearly moved beyond the obvious gross conclusions that can be reached from anecdotal studies or simple retrospective reviews of undefined patient groups. Elucidation of further details in order to achieve clinically important advances, such as increases in survival time by 5%, 10%, or 20%, requires good quality clinical research. This requires carefully planned studies and often involves cooperation among many institutions.

There is much opportunity for further progress in the treatment of lung cancer. Achievement of this goal requires an investment in the process of clinical research. It is disappointing that currently only 2% of patients with lung cancer are treated in the context of a clinical trial. Much can be done to make the process of participation easier, but the fact remains that physicians must be willing to invest some time and effort and must not allow personal biases to stand in the way of carefully planned trials that are based on a thorough review of the literature.

Further progress in the treatment of lung cancer will also require some insight into the science of clinical research. Many advances have occurred in the field of clinical research, and it is important that there be a more widespread appreciation of some of the basic principles and limitations. This is important not only so that future trials will be designed and conducted in an optimal fashion but, more important, so that the results of published trials can be critically evaluated and erroneous conclusions can be avoided. Unfortunately, most practicing physicians have had little training in the science of clinical research. It is hoped that this chapter has provided some useful insight into the process and principles involved in clinical research.

References

1. Ford L, Kaluzny A, Sondik E. Diffusion and adoption of state-of-the-art therapy. Semin Oncol. 1990; 17:485–494.
2. Barnsley J, Hynes D, Warnecke RB. Ensuring access to quality care. In: Kaluzny AD, Warnecke RB, eds. Managing a Health Care Alliance: Improving Community Cancer Care. San Francisco, Calif: Jossey Bass; 1996:59–82.
3. Pocock SJ. Clinical Trials: Practical Approach. New York: John Wiley & Sons; 1993.
4. Campbell DT, Stanley JC. Experimental and Quasi-Experimental Designs for Research. Chicago, Ill: Rand McNally College Publishing; 1963.
5. Gillings DB, Douglass CW. BIOSTATS: A Primer for Healthcare Professionals. Chapel Hill, NC: CAVCO Publications; 1985:262–265.
6. Hunter JE, Schmidt FL. Methods of Meta-Analysis. London: Sage Publications, 1990.
7. Bullock RJ, Svyantek DJ. Analyzing meta-analysis: potential problems, an unsuccessful replication, and evaluation criteria. J Appl Psychol. 1985; 70:108–115.
8. Warnecke RB, Kaluzny AD. The challenge of improving cancer care. In: Kaluzny AD, Warnecke RB, eds. Managing a Health Care Alliance: Improving Community Cancer Care. San Francisco, Calif: Jossey Bass; 1996:3–30.
9. Kaluzny AD, Warnecke RB. Working within a changing health care system. In: Kaluzny AD, Warnecke RB, eds. Managing a Health Care Alliance: Improving Community Cancer Care. San Francisco, Calif: Jossey Bass; 1996:171–187.
10. NCI overhauls clinical trials system. J Natl Cancer Inst. 1999; 91:312.
11. Miller L, Millstein LG. The FDA and the regulatory oversight of the clinical research process in drug development. In: Blidt B, Montagne M, eds. Clinical Research in Pharmaceutical Development. New York: Marcel Dekker; 1996:80–108.
12. Hunter CP, Frelick RW, Feldman AR, et al. Selection factors in clinical trials: results from the Community Clinical Oncology Program Physician's Patient Log. Cancer Treat Rep. 1987; 71:559–565.
13. Begg C, Zelen M, Carbone PP, et al. Cooperative groups and community hospitals: measurement of impact in the community hospitals. Cancer. 1983; 52:1760–1767.
14. Win RJ. Obstacles to the accrual of patients to clinical trials in the community setting. Semin Oncol. 1994; 21:112–117.
15. McCabe MS, Varricchio CG, Padberg RM. Efforts to recruit the economically disadvantaged to national clinical trials. Semin Oncol Nurs. 1994; 10:123–129.
16. Slevin ML, Stubbs L, Plant HJ, et al. Attitudes to chemotherapy: comparing views of patients with cancer with those of doctors, nurses, and general public. BMJ. 1990; 300:1458–1460.
17. Brundage MD, Davidson JR, Mackillop WJ. Trading treatment toxicity for survival in locally advanced non–small cell lung cancer. J Clin Oncol. 1997; 15:330–340.
18. Silvestri G, Pritchard R, Welch HG. Preferences for chemotherapy in patients with advanced non–small cell lung cancer: descriptive study based on scripted interviews. BMJ. 1998; 317:771–775.
19. Winslow R. Managed-care trade group approves plan to spur clinical-trial involvement. Wall Street Journal. July 1, 1997:B6.
20. Wagner E. Increasing Effectiveness of Cancer Control Interventions. Bethesda, Md: National Cancer Institute; 1998.
21. NCI Med News. TRICARE beneficiaries can enter cancer treatment clinical trials. Available at: http://imsdd.meb.uni-bonn.de/cancernet/600113.html. Accessed March 7, 2000.
22. Brown M. Cancer patient care in clinical trials sponsored by the National Cancer Institute: what does it cost? J Natl Cancer Inst. 1999; 91:818–819.
23. Taylor KM. The doctor's dilemma: physician participation in randomized clinical trials. Cancer Treat Rep. 1985; 69:1095–1100.
24. Kotwall C, Mahoney LJ, Myers RE, et al. Reasons for non-entry in randomized clinical trials for breast cancer: a single institutional study. J Surg Oncol. 1992; 50:125–129.
25. Wagner J, Alberts S, Sloan J, et al. Incremental cost of enrolling cancer patients in clinical trials: a population based study. J Natl Cancer Inst. 1999; 91:847–853.
26. Fehrenbacher L, Fireman B, Gruskin L, et al. The cost of care in cancer clinical trials: a matched, controlled analysis of participation in selected National Cooperative Group Trials. Available at: http://asco.infostreet.com/prof/me/html/99abstracts/har/m_1610.htm. Accessed May 18, 2000.
27. Lee E. Statistical Methods for Survival Analysis. Belmont, Calif: Lifetime Learning Publications, 1980.

PART 2

GENERAL ASPECTS OF LUNG CANCER

EPIDEMIOLOGY AND CLASSIFICATION OF LUNG CANCER

M. Patricia Rivera, Frank C. Detterbeck, and Dana P. Loomis

INCIDENCE OF LUNG CANCER

Lung cancer is one of the most lethal cancers known to humankind because of the high incidence of the disease and the high case fatality rate (ratio of mortality to incidence).[1] In the United States, lung cancer constitutes 13% of all malignant tumors, but it accounts for 28% of all cancer deaths each year (31% in men and 25% in women) (Fig. 3–1).[1] A downturn in the incidence of lung cancer in men began in the late 1980s, and from 1990 to 1995 incidence rates decreased by 2.3% per year (Fig. 3–2A). Whereas the incidence of lung cancer appears to have leveled off in men, a sharp rise in the incidence has occurred in women (from 6 per 100 000 in 1960 to >40 per 100 000 in 1990) (Fig. 3–2B). It appears, however, that the incidence rates of lung cancer among women may be stabilizing. An estimated 164 100 new cases of lung cancer (89 500 in men and 74 600 in women) will be diagnosed in the United States in 2000.[1] Approximately 80% of lung cancers are non–small cell lung cancer (NSCLC). The majority of cases occur in current or former cigarette smokers.

Worldwide, lung cancer is the leading type of cancer (1.04 million new cases; 12.8% of all cancers worldwide) and the leading cause of mortality from cancer (921 000 deaths; 17.8% of all cancer deaths worldwide).[2] The global incidence of lung cancer is increasing at a rate of 0.5% per year.[3,4] The majority (58%) of new lung cancer cases occur in developed countries. It is by far the most common cancer among men, with the highest rates occurring in North America and Europe. Moderately high rates also occur in South America and Australia.[2] The worldwide incidence of lung cancer is lower in women than in men (10.8 versus 37.5 per 10⁵). As in men, the highest rates in women occur in North America and Northern Europe.[2]

LUNG CANCER MORTALITY

Lung cancer is the leading cause of cancer death in both men and women in the United States.[1] In fact, lung cancer accounts for as many cancer deaths annually as the next four leading causes of cancer deaths combined in this country (Fig. 3–1). The number of deaths due to lung cancer in men in the United States appears to be leveling off and may even be beginning to decline (Fig. 3–3A). Mortality from lung cancer among men decreased by an average of 1.6% per year from 1990 to 1995.[1] However, a frightening increase in lung cancer mortality in women has occurred from 1950 to 2000 in the United States and other developed countries.[5] Between 1969 and 1989, deaths from

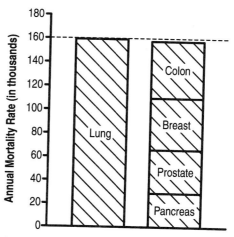

FIGURE 3–1. Mortality of lung cancer compared with next four leading causes of cancer deaths. (Data from Landis SH, Murray T, Bolden S, et al. Cancer statistics 1999. CA Cancer J Clin. 1999;49:8–31.[8])

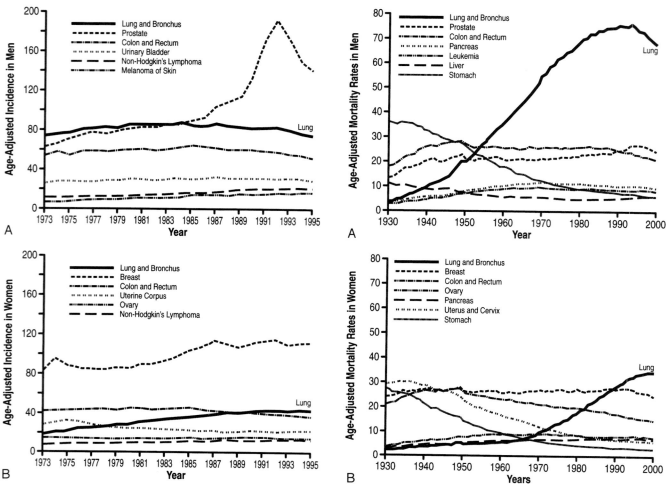

Figure 3–2. Incidence of lung cancer in the United States: *A*, Incidence in men *B*, Incidence in women. (From Landis SH, Murray T, Bolden S, et al. Cancer statistics 1999. CA Cancer J Clin. 1999;49:8–31.[8])

Figure 3–3. Mortality of lung cancer in the United States over time. *A*, Mortality in men. *B*, Mortality in women. (From Greenlee RT, Murray T, Bolden S, et al. Cancer statistics 2000. CA Cancer J Clin. 2000; 50:7–33.[1])

lung cancer among women increased by more than 200% in Japan, Australia, New Zealand, Denmark, Norway, Poland, and Great Britain, and increased by more than 300% in Canada and the United States.[6,7] In 1986, lung cancer surpassed breast cancer as the leading cause of cancer death among women in the United States (Fig. 3–3*B*) and is expected to account for 25% of all cancer deaths in women in 2000.[1]

The close relationship between lung cancer incidence (new cases per year) and mortality (deaths per year) is a result of the low median 5-year survival rate. Although mortality due to some solid tumors, such as stomach cancer and cervical cancer, has been declining in the United States, the number of deaths from lung cancer has continued to rise.[1] Although the survival rate of patients with lung cancer has shown some improvement (Fig. 3–4), lung cancer remains a disease with a high fatality rate (5-year survival rate of 15% in 1989–1994).[8] It is estimated that 156 900 individuals (89 300 men and 67 600 women) in the United States will die of lung cancer in 2000.[1] Furthermore, although 5-year survival is only 15% in the United States,

the average survival in Europe and in developing nations is an even more grim 8%.[2]

Because of the long latency period between exposure to carcinogens and the development of lung cancer, interventions made in the 1990s to prevent lung cancer are not expected to affect overall mortality until decades later.[9] As projected by Brown and Kessler,[10] reductions in lung cancer mortality in this century will depend on the success of current smoking prevention efforts. Figure 3–5 shows projections of age-adjusted death rates from lung cancer with and without projected reductions in the incidence of smoking. Unfortunately, data indicates that the rate of active smoking among high school students is increasing; in 1997, 38% of students had smoked within 1 month and 18% had smoked at least one pack of cigarettes within 1 month.[11] Although lung cancer mortality in men decreased an average of 1.6% per year from 1990 to 2000 and will probably continue to decrease,[1] lung cancer mortality in women is not expected to decline until after 2010.[10] Thus, it is clear that lung cancer will remain a major health problem for at least the next 30 to 40 years, even if there

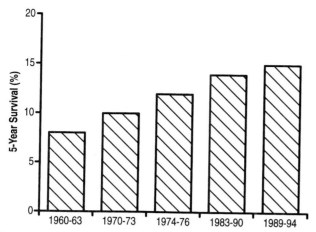

FIGURE 3–4. Lethality rate of lung cancer in the United States over time. (Data from Wingo PA, Tong T, Bolden S. Cancer statistics 1995. CA Cancer J Clin. 1995;45:8–30[5] and Landis SH, Murray T, Bolden S, et al. Cancer statistics 1999. CA Cancer J Clin. 1999;49:8–31.[8])

is a decline in incidence as a result of smoking cessation interventions.[10,11]

RISK FACTORS

Although approximately 85% to 90% of all patients with lung cancer have a history of direct exposure to tobacco, it is likely that the cause of lung cancer is multifactorial and involves more than a simple association with smoking. Table 3–1 lists factors that have been reported to increase the risk of lung cancer. Several of the more important risk factors are discussed next.

Tobacco

That lung cancer might be caused by tobacco was first suggested by Rottman in 1898.[12] Over the next 40 years,

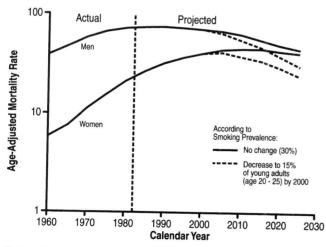

FIGURE 3–5. Projected lung cancer mortality over time. (From Brown CC, Kessler LG. Projections of lung cancer mortality in the United States: 1985-2025. J Natl Cancer Inst. 1988;80:43–51, by permission of Oxford University Press, Oxford, England.[10])

TABLE 3–1. RISK FACTORS FOR LUNG CANCER

Tobacco exposure	Gender
Environmental tobacco smoke	Diet
Occupational exposure	Chronic lung disease
Genetic factors	Prior tobacco-related cancer

Inclusion criterion: Widely accepted risk factors for lung cancer, according to the authors' judgment.

physicians referred to the association between tobacco exposure and lung cancer, but no evidence was available in human beings until Muller[13] reported substantial differences between the smoking habits of people with and without the disease. It was not until 1950, when several more case-control studies were reported, that the relationship between cigarette smoking and the development of lung cancer received serious attention.[14–16] In 1964, cigarette smoking was declared to be the major cause of lung cancer among American men.[17] In the 30 years following the initial warning by the U.S. Surgeon General, a vast amount of epidemiologic evidence incriminated cigarette smoking as the main cause of the increased incidence of and mortality from lung cancer.[18–25] The risk is higher than most people think. For a 35-year-old male smoker, the chance of dying of lung cancer before age 75 is estimated to be 13% and the chance of dying of any smoking-related disease is 28%.[26] One of every six deaths in the United States (from any cause) is caused by smoking.[27]

Cigarette smoke is a complex aerosol classified as either mainstream smoke or sidestream smoke. Mainstream smoke is produced at a high temperature (up to 950°C) as air is drawn through the column of tobacco in the cigarette. It is the predominant source of smoke for the active smoker. The particle size of cigarette smoke (0.1-1.0 μm) is in the range that will lead to deposition in the airways and alveoli of the lung.[28] Tobacco smoke contains irritants, oxidants, free radicals, and more than 40 carcinogenic agents.[29] The irritant agents in smoke lead to acute and chronic changes in the lung that may result in increased retention of carcinogens and increased vulnerability of the lung to the effects of these carcinogens.[21] N-nitrosamines and polycyclic aromatic hydrocarbons (eg benzopyrene and dimethylbenzanthracene) are the two major classes of tobacco-related inhaled carcinogens. N-nitrosamines are formed during tobacco processing and pyrosynthesis and originate from nicotine and arecoline.[30] The polycyclic aromatic hydrocarbons and N-nitrosamines exert their mutagenic/carcinogenic action through the formation of DNA adducts.[31]

Three major prospective studies demonstrated a clearcut dose-response relationship between the development of lung cancer and the degree of exposure to cigarette smoke, as measured by the total number of cigarettes smoked per day, the age at which smoking began, and the duration of smoking.[19,24,25] Many other case-control studies have demonstrated similar findings.[20,22,32–34] Figure 3–6 shows the effect of the number of cigarettes smoked, the duration of smoking, and the age at which smoking began, as reported in some of these studies. The age-adjusted relative risk of developing lung cancer in people who smoke >20 cigarettes per day is approximately 20 (a 2000% increased

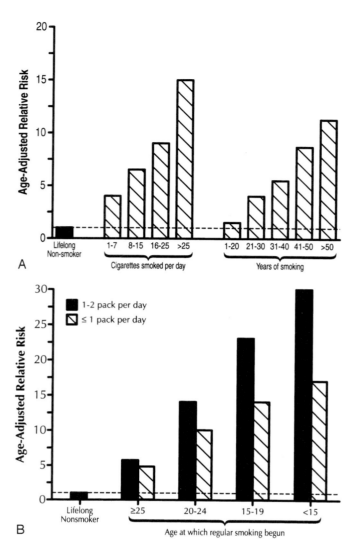

FIGURE 3–6. *A*, Effect of dose and duration of smoking on the incidence of lung cancer compared with lifelong nonsmokers. *B*, Relative risk of lung cancer in smokers at a uniform age (55-64 years) according to age at which regular smoking began, compared with lifelong nonsmokers. (*A*, Data from Damber LA, Larsson L-G. Smoking and lung cancer with special regard to type of smoking and type of cancer: a case-control study in north Sweden. Br J Cancer. 1986;53:673–681.[20] *B*, Data from Peto R. Influence of dose and duration on lung cancer rates. In: Zaridge D, Peto R, eds. Tobacco: A Major International Health Hazard. Lyon, France. International Agency for Research on Cancer. 1986:23–33.[23])

risk).[19,24,32] There is some debate about whether the increase is linear or exponential.[35] The duration of smoking is also strongly correlated with the risk of lung cancer,[20,35] and there is evidence that smoking one pack of cigarettes per day for 40 years is associated with a higher risk of lung cancer than smoking two packs per day for 20 years.[23]

The pattern and intensity of smoking, as well as the composition of the cigarette, are important determinants of the dose of carcinogens delivered to the smoker's lungs. Several prospective studies have shown higher risk of lung cancer among smokers who reported inhaling deeply or frequently.[19,22,36,37] High tar cigarettes are associated with an increased risk for the development of lung cancer.[37,38] Between 1950 and 1990, the percentage of filter tip cigarettes sold in the United States increased from 56% to

97%.[37] The use of filters likely reduces the exposure to carcinogens, thus reducing the risk of lung cancer.[37–40] However, lowering the tar and nicotine content by using filters leads the smoker to inhale more deeply and to smoke more intensely (ie, increase the puff volume, increase the number of cigarettes smoked per day, or both).[41–44] In addition, the tobacco in filtered cigarettes is richer in nitrates than that in the nonfiltered cigarettes manufactured during past decades.[45] More intense smoking, deeper inhalation of tobacco smoke, and higher delivery of carcinogens (nitrogen oxides, nitrosated compounds) to the periphery of the lung may explain the increasing incidence of adenocarcinomas in smokers.[46,47]

Smoking is associated most strongly with squamous cell and small cell lung cancer (SCLC).[36,48] Although the predominant cell type in nonsmokers is adenocarcinoma,[49,50] most of the patients who develop this type of lung cancer have a history of smoking. Numerous studies have demonstrated that the risk of adenocarcinoma increases with exposure to tobacco smoke in a linear fashion, although the rate of increase is less than for squamous cell and SCLC.[51] Thus, smoking is clearly associated with each of the four major histologic types of lung cancer (squamous cell, adenocarcinoma, large cell, and small cell).[51]

Initially, epidemiologic studies of lung cancer and smoking emphasized men, who began smoking earlier and consumed greater quantities of tobacco than did women in almost all countries. However, the percentage of white men who are current smokers has been decreasing since the first Surgeon General's report linking cigarette smoking to lung cancer. On the other hand, since 1980, the prevalence of smoking among women has increased significantly in many countries, including the United States. Changes in smoking practices have been accompanied by increasing relative and attributable risks for lung cancer in women.[52,53]

Nearly half of cases of lung cancer now involve patients who have quit smoking, often many years earlier.[54] Several large studies have demonstrated that the risk of lung cancer diminishes over time after cessation of smoking.[18,24,36,55–57] However, even after 15 to 20 years, the relative risk has consistently been found to be two to three times higher for a former smoker than for someone who never smoked, and even after 30 years, the relative risk remains higher for a former smoker than for a lifelong nonsmoker.[18,24,36,56,57] A graphic presentation of the relative risk determined by one of these studies is shown in Figure 3–7A.[18] This study involved over 1.2 million people (43% men) from all 50 states from 1982 to 1986 and is known as the Cancer Prevention Study II (CPS II) of the American Cancer Society.[18] The increased relative risk that is consistently seen in the first 1 to 2 years after smoking cessation compared with that of current smokers is commonly attributed to subtle symptoms of cancer that prompt the individual to quit smoking.[18,55]

Although the relative risk of developing lung cancer decreases according to the number of years since smoking cessation, the risk is linked to the person's age at the time of quitting. The risk of lung cancer increases with age, however, in both smokers and nonsmokers. In fact, the relative risk of lung cancer after smoking cessation decreases at about the same rate that the relative risk of lung cancer increases as people age, so that the absolute risk of

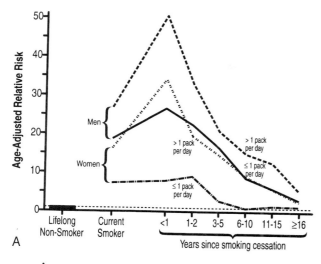

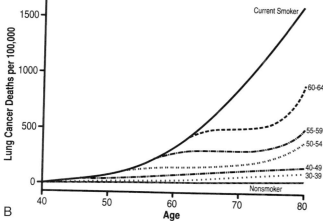

FIGURE 3–7. *A,* Effect of smoking cessation on the age-adjusted relative risk of lung cancer for men and women compared with lifelong nonsmokers, from the CPS II study. *B,* Effect of smoking cessation on the absolute risk of lung cancer in men, by age at the time of quitting smoking, from the CPS II study. (*A,* Data from Centers for Disease Control, Public Health Service, US Department of Health and Human Services. The Health Benefits of Smoking Cessation. Washington, DC: US Govt Printing Office; 1990.[18] *B,* From Halpern MT, Gillespie BW, Warner KE. Patterns of absolute risk of lung cancer mortality in former smokers. J Natl Cancer Inst. 1993;85:457–464, by permission of Oxford University Press, Oxford, England.[55])

lung cancer remains approximately the same over time as it was when the person quit smoking.[23,55] This is shown in Figure 3–7*B*, in which data from the CPS II study is expressed as absolute risk. Of course, because people who have quit smoking do not exhibit an increased risk of lung cancer as they age, their *age-adjusted relative risk* does decrease over time after smoking cessation.

Environmental Tobacco Smoke

Environmental tobacco smoke (ETS), or sidestream smoke, is produced at a lower temperature (350°C) than mainstream smoke[58] and is comprised of smoke released during the smoldering of the cigarette between puffs and the mainstream smoke exhaled by the smoker. Inhalation of sidestream smoke (diluted by ambient air) by a nonsmoker is referred to as *passive smoking*. Studies have shown that

sidestream smoke actually has higher concentrations of some *N*-nitrosamines than mainstream smoke.[59] ETS is predominantly an indoor problem, and the exposure levels depend on the intensity of the smoking, room size, and air exchange.

Pooling the data reveals that the relative risk of developing lung cancer in nonsmokers exposed to ETS is 1.2 times greater than the risk in unexposed nonsmokers.[60] There is strong evidence that the risk is proportional to the level and duration of exposure, with 10 of 14 large studies showing a statistically significant association between level of exposure and risk.[61] At the highest level of exposure, the relative risk is approximately 1.75, with all of 17 large studies showing a statistically significant association.[61,62] Approximately 2% to 3% of lung cancers diagnosed each year can be attributed to ETS.[63]

Occupational Exposure

Table 3–2 lists the occupational agents classified as known carcinogens for lung cancer (group 1) by the International Agency for Research on Cancer.[64–67] Sufficient evidence implicating these agents exists in animal studies as well as human studies. Table 3–3 presents the occupational agents listed as probable carcinogens (group 2A) and possible carcinogens (group 2B) by the same agency. For most of the agents in the last two groups, animal evidence suggests an effect, but there is limited data in human beings to confirm this. Epidemiologic studies indicate that the relative risk of lung cancer from exposure to most of the agents listed in Table 3–2 at the levels typically encountered is approximately 1.3 to 1.6, although it is 3 to 4 for people exposed to asbestos, arsenic, or chromium.[64] To put this in

TABLE 3–2. OCCUPATIONAL AGENTS ASSOCIATED WITH LUNG CANCER: KNOWN CARCINOGENS (GROUP 1)

AGENT	EPIDEMIOLOGY
Arsenic	Byproduct of copper, lead, zinc, and tin ore smelting. Synergistic action with cigarette smoking.
Asbestos	Mining, milling, textile, insulation, shipyards, and auto mechanics. Synergistic association with cigarette smoking.
Beryllium	Exposure in mining, manufacture of ceramics and electronic equipment.
Bis(chloromethyl) ether	Used in manufacture of ion exchange resins, polymers, and plastics.
Cadmium	Electroplating, batteries, plastics, and pigments.
Chromium	Metal alloys, electroplating, paint pigments, cement, rubber, photoengraving, and composition floor coverings.
Nickel	Electroplating, manufacturing of steel and other alloys, ceramics, storage batteries, electric circuits, and petroleum refining.
Polycyclic aromatic hydrocarbons	Smelting of nickel-containing ores, aluminum, iron, steel and coke production, untreated mineral oils, soots from combustion and diesel engine exhausts
Radon	Underground mining.
Vinyl chloride	Production of plastics, packaging materials, and vinyl floor tiles.

Based on the International Agency for Research on Cancer (IARC) classification.[65–67]

TABLE 3–3. OCCUPATIONAL AGENTS ASSOCIATED WITH LUNG CANCER: PROBABLE AND POSSIBLE CARCINOGENS

PROBABLE CARCINOGENS (GROUP 2A)	POSSIBLE CARCINOGENS (GROUP 2B)
Acrylonitrile	Acetaldehyde
Formaldehyde	Silica
Diesel exhaust	Welding fumes

Based on the International Agency for Research on Cancer (IARC) classification.[65-67]

perspective, the relative risk associated with smoking more than one pack of cigarettes per day is approximately 15 to 25.[19,20,24] However, many occupational studies have been based on rather crude indicators of actual exposure, such as having been employed in an industry in which the suspected agent was used. Estimates based on such gross measures of exposure tend to understate the risk.

An excellent review of occupational lung carcinogens was published in 1996.[64] Based on the relative risk ratios and the number of individuals exposed to carcinogens in various occupations, it is estimated that approximately 9% of lung cancers in men and 2% in women are caused by occupational exposures. Over half of the occupational cases of lung cancers are caused by asbestos. However, the data concerning relative risk of lung cancer due to occupational exposure is based on populations with a much higher level of exposure than what is currently encountered in the United States. Therefore, the proportion of occupationally related lung cancers is likely to diminish with the passage of time.[64] A few of the more commonly encountered occupational and environmental factors associated with lung cancer are discussed briefly in the following sections.

Asbestos

Asbestos is a class of naturally occurring fibrous minerals (silicates of magnesium and iron) that have been used extensively because of their unique physical and chemical properties, including tensile strength, resistance to acid, and ability to insulate against heat and electricity. More than 3000 products containing asbestos in some form have been identified, including fire-resistant cloth, cement, wicks, electrical appliances, water pipes, floor and roofing tiles, and brake linings. Asbestos fibers consist of two subgroups: serpentine fibers (which includes chrysotile asbestos) and amphibole fibers (which includes amosite, crocidolite, and tremolite asbestos).[68]

The association between asbestos and lung cancer is complex, and to discuss it is beyond the scope of this chapter. In brief, asbestos is a well recognized carcinogen that most likely acts as a tumor promoter and is the most frequent occupational cause of human lung cancers.[68] (Asbestos is also associated with the development of mesothelioma, but that is a separate issue.) A dose-response relationship between the degree of asbestos exposure and the development of lung cancer has been demonstrated.[69] Exposure to all types of asbestos fibers is associated with a significantly increased risk of lung cancer.[69] The relative risk of lung cancer in asbestos workers in general is approximately 2 (95% confidence interval [CI] 1.9-2.11), whereas it is 6 in individuals who develop an interstitial

and pleural fibrosis known as *asbestosis* (95% CI 4.98-7.0), as compared with the general population (when corrected for smoking).[64] When smoking is combined with asbestos exposure, the relative risk of lung cancer is multiplicative and has been reported to increase to 50.[70] Most of the data regarding the risk of lung cancer comes from people with a high degree of exposure, and there is little risk associated with the levels of exposure encountered today in countries such as the United States, which regulate asbestos exposure.[64]

Beginning with the earliest reports of increased lung cancer risk among asbestos workers, there has been interest in determining whether the development of asbestosis is a necessary step in the development of asbestos-related lung cancer. It has been suggested that asbestosis, rather than asbestos per se, accounts for the increased risk of lung cancer in former asbestos workers.[71] Asbestos-related lung cancers occur predominantly in the lower lobes,[71] which is also where asbestosis most often develops, in contrast to the upper lobe predominance of cigarette-related lung cancers.[72] Assessing the hypothesis that lung cancer due to exposure to asbestos occurs only in the presence of asbestosis has been difficult because few studies have adequate data about all of the necessary variables (ie, degree of asbestos exposure, radiographic changes, and smoking).[71] Several studies with data regarding these three variables provide some evidence that only those patients with radiographic evidence of fibrosis (asbestosis) develop lung cancer.[73-75] Both asbestos and lung cancer are so strongly associated with asbestos exposure, however, that a rigorous test of the hypothesis requires exceptionally precise adjustment for the amount of exposure.

Radon

Radon is a decay product of naturally occurring uranium in the earth. Although radon gas is inert, radon decay products, also called *radon daughters,* are radioactive metals that adhere to particles suspended in the air. They may cause bronchogenic carcinoma when they are inhaled into the respiratory system and interact directly with pulmonary epithelial and other cells. Underground miners who are occupationally exposed to radon and its decay products experience a markedly increased risk of lung cancer, on the order of that associated with smoking.[64] Radon also accumulates in indoor air, so that exposures can occur in homes and other buildings. The risk associated with these exposures has been difficult to define, however. The average concentration of radon in outdoor air is about 0.2 picocurie per liter (pCi/L), whereas the average concentration in buildings is 1.5 pCi/L.[64,76] The concentration in homes and buildings varies widely, and the level is difficult to predict without actual measurements, although higher concentrations are associated with poor ventilation.

Indoor radon exposure accounts for an average of 50% to 80% of the total radiation received in the United States.[76] Although normal lifetime environmental exposure is only a small percentage of that of uranium mine workers, there is reasonable evidence that the risk of lung cancer from radon is a linear phenomenon without a risk threshold.[64] As a result, there is probably a low risk of lung cancer from residential radon exposure, similar on average to the risk associated with exposure to sidestream tobacco smoke (relative risk, approximately 1.2).[64,76]

Diesel Engine Exhaust

Exposure to diesel exhaust in the workplace or in the ambient environment is widespread. Although animal studies have shown this agent to be carcinogenic, it is classified as a probable carcinogen because epidemiologic studies that document exposure levels have been difficult to conduct. A review of studies demonstrates an average relative risk of 1.3 for workers whose jobs involve exposure to diesel exhaust compared with individuals who are not exposed (95% CI, 1.13-1.44).[64] Most of these studies have corrected for the effect of smoking, but accurate information about individual exposures has generally not been available.[64]

Silica

Silica exposure occurs in mining and sandblasting, as well as in masonry, concrete, gypsum, and pottery industries. As a result, many people are exposed to silica. A review of 15 studies found an average relative risk of lung cancer of 2.8 (95% CI, 2.5-3.15) in individuals with silicosis (an interstitial fibrosis of the lung caused by silica exposure).[64] Studies that excluded confounding exposures reported an average relative risk of 1.3 in workers exposed to silica (95% CI, 1.21-1.45), but the results are not entirely consistent, and silica is currently classified as a probable carcinogen.[64]

Genetic Factors

An inherited host susceptibility to cancer may partly explain why only a fraction of individuals who smoke and only a portion of individuals exposed to occupational carcinogens develop lung cancer. Family clusters of lung cancer have been well documented.[77,78] First degree relatives of lung cancer patients have been found to have a 2-fold to 6-fold increase in the risk of developing lung cancer, independent of tobacco exposure,[79-82] especially as the number of affected family members increases.[83,84] Family

studies have repeatedly shown a 2-fold to 4-fold increase in the risk of lung cancer in *nonsmokers* who are relatives of lung cancer patients compared with nonsmokers who have no family history of lung cancer.[82-86] Several studies have reported that the increased risk (2-fold to 3-fold) of developing lung cancer is particularly apparent in *young* adults who have a first degree relative with a history of lung cancer (in both smokers and nonsmokers).[82,87] Although these studies have corrected for age and smoking, they have usually not corrected for ETS exposure. A 30% increased risk of lung cancer was found in lifetime non-smokers who had a first degree relative (parent or sibling) with lung cancer in a large multicenter study in the United States, which adjusted for exposure to environmental tobacco smoke (646 female lung cancer patients and 1252 population controls).[88] This study also found that having a female relative (mother or sister) with lung cancer increased the risk of developing lung cancer 3-fold.[88]

The data regarding the risk of lung cancer in relation to age, family history, and smoking status has been found to fit a model of genetic predisposition, inherited in an autosomal codominant or dominant fashion, if it is assumed that such a gene would lead to an earlier onset of lung cancer.[86,89] This model would predict that 15% of the population are carriers, that approximately 60% are exposed to environmental factors that place them at risk, that carriers will develop lung cancer 20 to 25 years earlier than noncarriers, and that almost all cases of lung cancer will be seen in carriers of this putative gene.[86,89,90] Whether such a genetic predisposition really exists remains to be demonstrated. A large study of twins did not suggest that inheritance played a significant role in the development of lung cancer.[91] However, this study excluded women and patients who were diagnosed with lung cancer before age 50—two groups in which a genetic factor may play a large role, based on the data just presented.

Because the metabolites of carcinogens, not the carcinogens themselves, usually initiate cancer,[92] individual susceptibility to tobacco and environmental carcinogens may de-

DATA SUMMARY: SMOKING AND OCCUPATIONAL RISK FACTORS FOR LUNG CANCER			
	AMOUNT	QUALITY	CONSISTENCY
The risk of lung cancer increases with tobacco exposure in a dose- and time-dependent manner (approximate average adjusted relative risk of 20)	*High*	*High*	*High*
The adjusted relative risk of lung cancer decreases after smoking cessation but remains 2 to 3 times that of a lifelong nonsmoker 20 years after cessation in most individuals	*High*	*High*	*High*
The adjusted relative risk of lung cancer from exposure to environmental tobacco smoke is approximately 1.2	*High*	*High*	*High*
The adjusted relative risk of lung cancer from exposure to asbestos is approximately 2 (in patients who may or may not have evidence of asbestosis)	*High*	*High*	*Mod*
The excess risk of lung cancer due to asbestos is seen primarily in individuals with asbestos-related fibrosis	*Mod*	*Mod*	*High*
The adjusted relative risk of lung cancer from exposure to most occupational and environmental factors is approximately 1.5 (radon, beryllium, cadmium, nickel, silica)	*High*	*High*	*High*

Type of data reported: Plain text: descriptive statement   *Italics: controlled comparison*   **Bold: randomized comparison**

pend on competitive gene-enzyme interactions that affect activation or detoxification of these metabolites[76] Genes of the cytochrome P-450 system control the oxidative metabolism of some environmental carcinogens, and it has been suggested that individuals with increased oxidative activity may be at risk for developing cancer because of a higher level of activated carcinogens.[93–95] Furthermore, increased metabolism of the antihypertensive drug debrisoquine has been associated with an increased risk of lung cancer.[96]

Gender

Many reports suggest that women who smoke are more susceptible to developing lung cancer than their male counterparts.[40,97–100] The rate of increase in the incidence of lung cancer among women in the United States is rising more rapidly than what would be expected based on changing trends in smoking rates alone. Moreover, because of a slower decline in the prevalence of smoking among women than among men, the exposure of women to tobacco carcinogens has gradually approached—and is likely to surpass—that of men. Thus, if current trends continue, the incidence of lung cancer in women is expected to surpass that in men by 2030. Zang and Wynder[97] conducted a hospital-based case-control study of 1889 case subjects who had lung cancer and 2070 control subjects who had diseases unrelated to smoking. The study revealed that women start smoking at a later age, smoke fewer cigarettes, smoke brands containing less tar, and inhale less deeply than men. Despite this, women demonstrated a 1.2-fold to 1.7-fold higher odds ratio of developing lung cancer that was seen consistently for each of the major cell types (adenocarcinoma, small cell, large cell, and squamous cell) and at every level of exposure to cigarette smoke. This finding was not altered by adjustments for weight, height, or body mass index (Fig. 3–8). Furthermore, a higher proportion of women than men with lung cancer were never smokers, suggesting that women may have a higher baseline susceptibility to lung cancer in addition to a higher risk for a given amount of tobacco exposure.[97] Other investigators have also found greater susceptibility to lung carcinogens in women smokers.[36,40,98–101] The few studies that have not found a higher relative risk in women have usually not adjusted for dose or duration of exposure,[24,56] although one large study found no difference in gender susceptibility despite a detailed correction for the amount of smoking.[102]

Potential biologic explanations for gender differences in lung cancer risk include (1) gender differences in nicotine metabolism, (2) male-female variations in cytochrome P-450 enzymes, and (3) the effect of hormones on the development of lung cancer.[97] It has been shown that nicotine can be a precursor for tobacco-specific carcinogens[103]; therefore, gender differences in nicotine metabolism may be a plausible reason for a higher susceptibility to tobacco carcinogens in women. It has also been reported that the total plasma clearance of nicotine, normalized for body weight, is lower in women than in men.[104,105]

Evidence has been accumulating that cytochrome P-450 in liver microsomes plays a central role as a drug-metabolizing enzyme and that there are gender-dependent differences in the properties of this enzyme.[106] Data also shows that some cytochrome P-450 enzymes (1A1, 1A2, 2E1) in human liver are involved in bioactivation of toxic components in cigarette smoke condensate, including polycyclic aromatic hydrocarbons and certain nitrosamines.[107] Moreover, Ryberg et al[108] found that DNA adduct levels were higher in female than in male lung cancer patients after adjusting for smoking dose.[108] In addition, the patients with higher DNA adduct levels generally had a shorter duration of smoking before the clinical onset of lung cancer. The authors concluded that their observations suggest that women are exposed to higher levels of nicotine and thus may have a higher relative risk for tobacco-induced lung cancer.[108]

An increased risk of lung cancer in women who received estrogen replacement therapy was noted in a large scale epidemiologic cohort study, but no adjustment was made for the amount of smoking.[109] Another study found a statistically significant synergy between estrogen replacement therapy and cigarette smoking as well as an elevated risk of adenocarcinoma of the lung in women associated with hormone replacement (odds ratio, 1.7; 95% CI, 1.0-2.5).[110] Furthermore, Zang and Wynder[97] found that women 55 years or older with lung cancer, particularly adenocarcinoma, were nearly twice as likely never to have smoked than were younger women with lung cancer, whereas no comparable age-related difference in smoking was found either among male lung cancer case subjects or among female control subjects.[97] Finally, an increased risk of developing lung cancer was found in several studies of women who have a personal history[40,111–113] or a family history[114] of a female reproductive organ cancer, implying that a hormonal factor may increase the risk of both types of cancer.

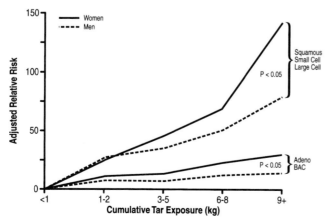

FIGURE 3–8. Gender-specific relative risk of lung cancer adjusted for age and body weight, by cumulative exposure to tar from cigarette smoking. (From Zang EA, Wynder EL. Differences in lung cancer risk between men and women: examination of the evidence. J Natl Cancer Inst. 1996;88:183–192, by permission of Oxford University Press, Oxford, England.[97]) Adeno, adenocarcinoma; BAC, bronchioloalveolar carcinoma.

Diet

Diet was not suspected of playing any role in the development of lung cancer until 1975, when Bjelke[115] reported that the risk of lung cancer in a Norwegian cohort varied with an index of vitamin A consumption, irrespective of the amount smoked. Since then, many epidemiologic studies have indicated that increased consumption of fruits and vegetables is associated with a reduced lung cancer risk in smokers, ex-smokers, and those who have never smoked (relative risk, ~0.5).[34,116–121] In a comprehensive review of this subject in 1992, 30 of 32 studies found a decreased risk of lung cancer with an increased consumption of fruits and vegetables (most of these studies corrected for the influence of smoking).[122] Furthermore, 24 of 25 studies that calculated statistical significance and included at least 20 patients who developed lung cancer found a statistically significant effect, with a median risk of 0.45 for those with the highest levels of fruit and vegetable consumption compared with the lowest levels (usually divided into quartiles).[122] Such data, together with strongly positive data for almost every cancer site studied,[122] has led the National Research Council to recommend consumption of five servings of fruits and vegetables per day to reduce the risk of cancer.[123]

Several studies have also found an association between higher serum β-carotene levels and a lower risk of lung cancer, as noted in a review in 1993.[9] These observations are further supported by the results of laboratory studies in animals and cell cultures.[124,125] The dietary factors best studied to date are the retinoids, in the form of either preformed vitamin A (retinol) or precursors known as *carotenoids*.[126,127] Vitamin A is necessary both to maintain proper differentiation of epithelial cells and to inhibit the proliferation of neoplastic cells after transformation.[128]

Based on results obtained from epidemiologic and laboratory studies, several large clinical studies have been conducted to investigate the role of vitamins in the prevention of lung cancer. A randomized, double-blind, placebo-controlled trial evaluated whether daily α-tocopherol (vitamin E), β-carotene, or both would reduce the incidence of lung cancer in 29 133 male Finnish smokers.[129] An unexpected *higher* incidence of lung cancer (relative risk 1.18; $P = 0.01$) was found in the group of subjects who received supplemental β-carotene (which increased the serum β-carotene levels 10-fold). However, in the placebo group, an apparent protective effect on lung cancer incidence was found in the group of subjects with higher *baseline* serum levels of both α-tocopherol and β-carotene. A second multicenter, randomized, double-blind, placebo-controlled trial involving 18 314 smokers, ex-smokers, and asbestos exposed workers was closed early after investigators also found a higher relative risk (1.28; $P = 0.02$) of lung cancer in the group treated with a combination of β-carotene and vitamin A.[130] However, a third randomized trial involving 21 071 male physicians (50% of whom never smoked) found no effect of β-carotene in combination with low-dose vitamin A on the risk of lung cancer.[131] Thus, whether supplementation with these vitamins is harmful has not been proven conclusively; however, it must be concluded that such supplementation is unlikely to be of benefit.

Many authors have suggested that a diet with a high proportion of fat is associated with an increased risk of lung cancer, with an average risk of 1.6 in a detailed review (range, 0.8-6.1).[119] This has not been studied as extensively as the benefit of a high intake of fruits and vegetables. Although the studies have adjusted for smoking status, possible confounding due to the amount or duration of smoking or the intake of fruits and vegetables has not been well studied.[119] The available data suggests that the dietary intakes of fat and of fruits and vegetables are not correlated

and that the risk associated with increased fat intake remains when corrections for fruit and vegetable intake are made.[119,120] The component, or components, of dietary fat responsible for the increased risk has not been clearly identified.[119] Other factors, such as increased use of processed foods and adoption of the lifestyle associated with more developed countries, may also be confounding factors.[132] Therefore, although the majority of the data does suggest an increased risk of lung cancer associated with a high dietary fat intake, it is difficult at this point to come to a clear conclusion because of the variability of the results and the incomplete study of confounding factors.

Chronic Obstructive Pulmonary Disease

In the early 1960s, Passey[133] suggested that the irritating properties of tobacco smoke, resulting in chronic inflammation and destruction of lung tissue, were of pathogenic significance in the development of lung cancer, rather than a direct action by tobacco carcinogens. Several years later, after noting that bronchial inflammation was accompanied by squamous cell metaplasia and dysplasia, Kuschner[134] suggested that chronic inflammation provided a cocarcinogenic mechanism for neoplastic cell transformation on exposure to polycyclic aromatic hydrocarbons. Subsequently, several prospective studies have reported that chronic obstructive pulmonary disease (COPD) is an independent predictor of lung cancer risk.[135–139] The number of patients in these studies ranged from 226 to >14 000 (total of 35 103 patients), with an average follow-up period ranging from 1.7 years to >10 years.

A relative risk of approximately 4 (range, 2.7-5) in patients with substantial COPD has been reported consistently in these studies, compared with controls without pulmonary impairment[135,137–139] or with baseline population controls.[136] Substantial COPD was defined as a forced expiratory volume in 1 second (FEV_1) of <40%,[139] as an FEV_1 of <60% or 70% of predicted value,[135,137,138] or on clinical grounds (average FEV_1 of 1.1 L).[136] Several of these studies demonstrated that the risk increased linearly as the FEV_1 decreased.[135,137–139] Most of these studies were able to adjust for the influence of smoking[137–139] and demonstrated a statistically significant predictive value of the FEV_1 by multivariate analysis when multiple confounding factors were considered.[137–139]

The presence of chronic sputum production has also been associated with a higher relative risk of lung cancer, although to a lesser degree.[137–140] The relative risk reported in several studies is approximately 1.5 (range, 1.3-2.1).[137–140] In some studies chronic sputum production has been found to be a statistically significant predictor of lung cancer by multivariate analysis.[138,139] The definition of chronic sputum production (most commonly defined as sputum production for >3 months per year) and the reliability of patients' assessment of this condition may account for some variability in the results.[139] There appears to be no association of lung cancer with asthma.[138]

NATURAL HISTORY

Lung cancer is a rapidly lethal disease if left untreated once a diagnosis of lung cancer has been made or sus-

DATA SUMMARY: FAMILIAL, DIETARY, AND OTHER RISK FACTORS FOR LUNG CANCER

	AMOUNT	QUALITY	CONSISTENCY
A family history of lung cancer is associated with an increased adjusted relative risk (approximately 3)	*High*	*High*	*Mod*
Female gender is associated with an increased adjusted relative risk of lung cancer (approximately 1.5)	*High*	*High*	*Mod*
Increased consumption of fruits and vegetables is associated with a reduced risk of lung cancer	*High*	*Mod*	*High*
Increased consumption of dietary fat is associated with an increased risk of lung cancer	*High*	*Mod*	*Mod*
Randomized trials of supplemental β-carotene have shown an increased risk of lung cancer	**Mod**	**Mod**	**Mod**
The presence of chronic obstructive pulmonary disease is associated with an increased risk of lung cancer (approximately 4-fold)	*High*	*Mod*	*High*

Type of data reported: Plain text: descriptive statement   *Italics: controlled comparison*   **Bold: randomized comparison**

pected. Overholt et al[141] reported in 1975 that 95% of 1960 lung cancer patients who were untreated were dead within 1 year. A more contemporary study of 130 untreated patients with NSCLC is shown in Figure 3–9. These results have been corroborated by several other authors, as shown in Table 3–4. The median survival for patients with stage I-III NSCLC is approximately 5 months, and the 1-year survival is approximately 15%. *All* patients (including patients with stage I disease) were dead within 3 years without treatment. Similar results were reported by Flehinger et al[142] in an analysis of 45 patients with clinical stage I cancer, found as a result of two large screening trials, who did not undergo resection. Even though 44% of these patients did receive some treatment (radiation), only two patients in the entire group survived 5 years.[142] The median survival for patients with SCLC has been reported to be 12 weeks for limited stage disease and 5 weeks for extensive stage disease (see Chapter 24).[143]

Estimates of the natural history of lung cancer have also been made using serial chest radiograph (CXR) measurements. Such estimates have been found to be consistent with the repeated tumor doubling (exponential growth) model of cancer growth,[144] although slowing of growth is often seen as the tumor mass enlarges (see Chapter 10). The doubling time is estimated to be approximately 100 days for NSCLC (squamous cell, 90 days; adenocarcinoma, 160 days; large cell, 90 days) and 30 days for SCLC, based on an analysis of 228 patients for whom such data was available.[144] The time from malignant change to death is approximately 40 tumor doublings, with the diagnosis usually being made after 35 doublings when the tumor has reached 3 cm. This results in an estimated time from malignant change to diagnosis of about 10 years and, following diagnosis, an average time to death of about 18 months for NSCLC.[144] In patients with SCLC, the estimated time from malignant change to death is approximately 3 years.

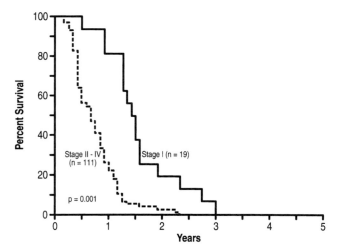

Figure 3–9. Survival of untreated patients with NSCLC. Stage I patients had cT2N0M0 tumors; patients with stage II-IV tumors are combined, because individual survival curves were similar. (From Vrdoljak E, Mise K, Sapuner D, et al. Survival analysis of untreated patients with non–small cell lung cancer. Chest. 1994;106:1797–1800.[189])

TABLE 3–4. NATURAL HISTORY OF UNTREATED NON–SMALL CELL LUNG CANCER

STUDY	N	STAGE	SURVIVAL MST (mo)	1 y %	2 y %
Vrdoljak et al[189]	50	cI, II	13	56	8
Hyde et al[190a]	293	cI-IIIb	—	—	4
Roswit et al[191a]	246	cI-III	5	16	0
Zelen[143]	193	cIII	4[b]	14[b]	—
Reinfuss et al[192]	162	cIII	4	9	0
Wellons et al[193]	139	cI-IV	3	12	3
Leung et al[194]	57	cIII	9	30	4
Paul et al[195]	50	pIIIa,b	5	12	0
Vrdoljak et al[189]	17	cIIIa	9	24	0
Hyde et al[190a]	775	cIV	—	—	1
Zelen[143]	522	cIV	2[b]	<10[b]	—

Inclusion criteria: Studies of ≥100 total patients reporting the natural history of untreated patients with non–small cell lung cancer.
[a]Includes small cell lung cancer.
[b]Average of squamous cell, adenocarcinoma, and large cell.
MST, median survival time (in months).

More complex estimates of the natural history of lung cancer have been made using data from two large studies of screening CXRs involving approximately 10 000 patients each.[145,146] From these studies, it is estimated that the average duration of a detectable, although asymptomatic, stage is approximately 4 years. However, the ability to detect the cancer during that time is <20% per screening examination. Furthermore, the ability to cure cancer during an early stage is approximately 50%.[145,146] Similar estimates were obtained independently from another screening study in Czechoslovakia.[147] The estimates from these studies are surprisingly consistent with each other and consistent with clinial observations.

A number of studies have shown that once a diagnosis of lung cancer has been made, an abnormality can often be discerned in retrospect on previous chest radiographs, even though it was not noted at the time the film was taken.[148–151] In fact, evidence of the cancer could be found 2 years earlier in retrospect in an average of 41% of patients in studies reporting such data (range, 20%–58%).[148–150] The fact that an abnormality can be seen in retrospect to have been present, often for years, cannot be used to argue that the natural history of untreated lung cancer *once a diagnosis has been made* is much longer than the 1 to 2 years indicated by the data just cited. Instead, it points out the limited ability of CXRs to *prospectively* identify small lung cancers. An interval increase in the stage was found to have occurred in 43% of patients in whom a lesion had been missed.[151] The *retrospective* ability to find a lesion on a previous CXR is of little practical use.

Spontaneous remission of cancer has been reported in a wide variety of tumor types but is extremely rare in lung cancer. A review in 1997 reported 15 well documented cases, which were usually diagnosed by a surgical biopsy.[152] These cases involved each of the major histologic types and had clear documentation of the pathologic findings, often with independent pathologic review. Although four patients underwent a partial resection (R$_2$), no additional treatment directed against the tumor was given to any of the patients. Two-thirds of the patients had stage III disease, and most of the remainder had stage IV. The follow-up period averaged 9 years (range, 3.5-19 years).[152]

HISTOLOGIC CLASSIFICATION

Lung cancer is divided broadly into two main categories: small cell and non–small cell. SCLCs grow rapidly, metastasize widely, and are treated primarily by chemotherapy.[153] Different histologic subtypes of SCLC have been described and various classification schemes proposed. However, only the distinction between pure small cell tumors and tumors that have both small cell and non–small cell components has any clinical and prognostic significance. Therefore, classification of SCLC subtypes according to this scheme, as proposed by the International Association for the Study of Lung Cancer (IASLC) in 1988,[154] has the greatest practical value (Table 3–5).

NSCLCs are divided into squamous cell cancers, adenocarcinomas, and large cell (undifferentiated) carcinomas. Further classification of subtypes, as proposed by the World

TABLE 3–5. HISTOLOGIC CLASSIFICATION OF LUNG CANCER

HISTOLOGIC TYPE	AGE-ADJUSTED INCIDENCE RATE[a]
Dysplasia/carcinoma in situ	—
Small Cell	
Pure small cell	9.4
Mixed (small cell and large cell)	8.8[b]
Combined (small cell and squamous cell	0.5[b]
or adenocarcinoma)	0.1[b]
Non–Small Cell	
Large cell	9.6
Large cell/undifferentiated	9.4
Giant cell	0.2
Clear cell	0.0
Squamous cell carcinoma	15.3
Epidermoid carcinoma	—
Spindle cell variant	—
Adenocarcinoma	15.3
Acinar adenocarcinoma	13.6[c]
Papillary adenocarcinoma	0.3
Bronchioloalveolar carcinoma	1.4
Solid carcinoma with mucus formation	—[c]
Adenosquamous carcinoma	0.8
Bronchial gland carcinoma	0.6
Adenoid cystic carcinoma	0.2[b]
Mucoepidermoid tumor (MET)	0.4[b]
Carcinoid tumor	0.5
Typical	0.37[b]
Atypical	0.13[b]
Sarcoma	0.1
Sarcoma	0.06[b]
Carcinosarcoma	0.04[b]

Based on the World Health Organization classification system[155] and on the International Association for the Study of Lung Cancer classification for small cell lung cancer.[154]

[a]Age-adjusted incidence rates per 100,000 population according to SEER registry statistics 1983–1987. Data from Travis.[156]
[b]Estimated from proportion of types in this category.
[c]Includes all adenocarcinomas not classified as papillary or bronchioloalveolar.

Health Organization (WHO),[155] is shown in Table 3–5, although other classification schemes are in use.[156,157] The classification system used is not of major importance because the different types of NSCLC generally behave similarly to one another, as shown in Figure 3–10. However, a few subtypes of NSCLC exhibit sufficiently distinct clinical characteristics to make it appropriate to consider them separately. Carcinoid tumors, mucoepidermoid tumors, and adenoid cystic carcinomas are often classified with adenocarcinomas. These tumors grow more slowly than other types of NSCLC and exhibit distinct epidemiologic and biologic characteristics; therefore, they should be considered separately, regardless of the pathologic grouping (see Chapters 27 and 28). Bronchioloalveolar carcinomas are also classified as adenocarcinomas, although these tumors have a somewhat better prognosis and demonstrate a clinical presentation and pattern of spread that warrant separate analysis (see Chapter 26). Patients with large cell cancers with neuroendocrine granules have been reported to have poorer survival.[158–161] Finally, primary sarcomas and carcinosarcomas of the lung are seen rarely (0.1% and 0.07% of lung cancers), carry an intermediate prognosis (5-year

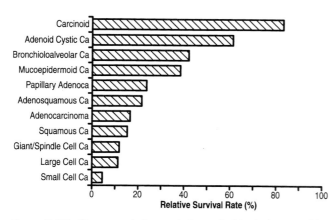

FIGURE 3–10. Five-year relative survival rates by histologic type, taking into account the mortality of the general population. (From Cancer. Vol 75, No. 1 suppl 1995, 191–202.[156] Copyright © 1995 American Cancer Society. Reprinted by permission of Wiley-Liss Inc., a subsidiary of John Wiley & Sons, Inc.)

survival of 30% and 21%), and are not discussed further in this book.

The incidence of the various histologic types of lung cancer from several large population-based series is shown in Table 3–6. Small cell cancers account for approximately 20% of lung cancers. Squamous cell carcinomas are the largest single group at 35% and are the most common major cell type in all except one of the series. Adenocarcinoma accounts for approximately 25%, with large cell and other types constituting the remainder.

Smoking has been shown to be a risk factor for all of the major cell types, but the association is strongest for squamous cell and small cell cancers and less pronounced for adenocarcinoma.[20,33,36,40,97,162–164] Adenocarcinoma is the most common cell type in nonsmokers[49,50,165] and is also the most common cell type in women in most series.[166–173] Although the risk of adenocarcinoma as a result of smoking is less than the risk of squamous cell or small cell cancer, it is estimated that 86% of adenocarcinomas are caused by smoking.[100]

Many studies have reported that the proportion of adenocarcinomas among lung cancers has been increasing.[166,170–174]

A review of Table 3–6 does not suggest an obvious trend over time, but the study periods included are broad. However, incidence rates over time show a disproportionate increase for adenocarcinoma, especially in women (Fig. 3–11A, B). Better pathologic methods of typing cancers have resulted in a decrease in the number of cancers classified as undifferentiated or "other," and the WHO definitions have resulted in many tumors formerly classified as large cell being reclassified as adenocarcinoma.[170–175] However, an increase in the proportion of adenocarcinomas remains that is beyond what can be explained by these factors.[170,174,176–178] This trend is seen for both men and women.[166,167,171,172,174,178] The increase in the proportion of adenocarcinomas is accompanied by a slight decrease in the proportion of squamous cell and, to a lesser extent, small cell cancers.[166,167,173,178]

The reason for the shift in the proportions of the various histologic types of lung cancer has not been clearly identified. However, circumstantial evidence points to changes in smoking habits as a plausible explanation.[45,166] Smoke from nonfiltered cigarettes contains large particles, which are deposited primarily in the more central airways, whereas filtered smoke is associated with peripheral cancers.[45,162] The greater use of filtered cigarettes since the 1960s could explain a reduced risk of squamous cell and small cell cancers, which are generally located more centrally, and an increased risk of adenocarcinomas, which are more often peripheral. Indeed, a large case-control study found that switching to filtered cigarettes diminishes the risk of developing a squamous cell or small cell cancer but has no effect on the risk of developing an adenocarcinoma.[40] Furthermore, research in smoking habits has shown that when women switch to filtered cigarettes, they are much more likely than men to substantially increase the number of cigarettes smoked and the depth of inhalation in order to compensate for the lower yield of these cigarettes.[98] This could explain why a more pronounced increase in adenocarcinoma has been seen in women. Women have been found to be more likely to smoke filtered cigarettes exclusively, although a higher incidence of adenocarcinoma among those smoking only filtered cigarettes could not be documented in this study.[163] Furthermore, changes in the type of cigarettes smoked (eg, presence and type of

TABLE 3–6. INCIDENCE OF MAJOR HISTOLOGIC TYPES OF LUNG CANCER FROM SEVERAL LARGE POPULATION-BASED SERIES IN CHRONOLOGIC ORDER

STUDY	YEARS INCLUDED	N	PERCENTAGE				
			Small	Squamous	Adeno	Large	Other
Greenberg et al[169]	1973–1976	1580	22	48	20	8	3
Vincent et al[170]	1962–1975	1682	19	38	24	9	9
Beard et al[167]	1935–1984	591	19	30	34	16	1
Dodds et al[173]	1974–1981	8897	17	30	29	7	17
Travis et al[156]	1973–1987	147 637	17	31	29	7	10
Auerbach and Garfinkel[176]	1973–1989	505	12	38	27	12	10
Barbone et al[196] a	1979–1986	755	29	35	21	12	3
Humphrey et al[165]	1987	18 983	20	36	32	10	2
Fry et al[197]	1992	73 898	16	28	27	10	20
Average			**19**	**35**	**27**	**10**	**8**

Inclusion criteria: Population-based series of lung cancer reporting histologic types in ≥500 patients.

aMen only.

Adeno, adenocarcinoma.

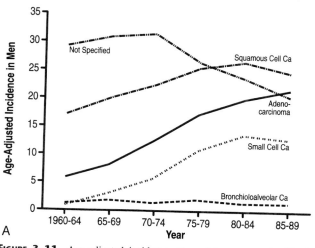
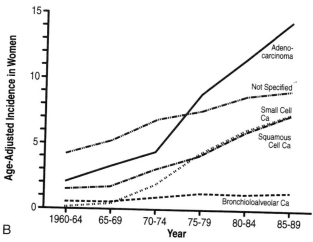

Figure 3–11. Age-adjusted incidence rates of lung cancer by histologic type in the state of Connecticut during 1960 to 1989. *A*, Incidence per 100 000 men. *B*, Incidence per 100 000 women. (From Cancer. Vol 74, No. 5, 1994, 1556–1567.[166] Copyright © 1994. American Cancer Society. Reprinted by permission of Wiley-Liss, Inc., a subsidiary of John Wiley & Sons, Inc.)

filter, type of tobacco) have led to an increase in the amount of NNK (a tobacco-specific *N*-nitrosamine) in smoke, although the tar and nicotine contents have been reduced.[45] NNK is a strong inducer of lung adenocarcinoma in laboratory studies.[45]

CLASSIFICATION BY STAGE

Development of a Staging System

The purpose of a staging system is to define homogeneous groups of patients that are distinct from one another in order to provide a common language for communication about patients with cancer. This is necessary in order to compare treatment results and to be able to assess whether the results of a particular approach are likely to be applicable to individual patients prospectively. Thus, treatment results and the definition of homogeneous groups are major factors underlying a staging system. However, patient outcomes can be expected to change over time as improvements in treatment are made, and this may affect the homogeneity of stage groups. Furthermore, as the amount of knowledge increases, nuances are likely to be defined, promoting separation of an increasing number of distinct groups.

Initially, a simple staging system was used that separated

patients into two groups: *limited stage* (meaning any patient with tumor confined to the chest) and *extensive stage* (meaning any patient with systemic metastases). This system was refined somewhat by considering the applicability of radiotherapy (RT), so that limited stage was defined as disease localized to the chest that could be encompassed in a "reasonable" RT port. This simple staging system is still in use today for patients with SCLC.

A more detailed staging system was officially defined by the American Joint Commission for Cancer (AJCC) in 1976. This system was revised in 1986[179] and again in 1997[180] to the system that is used currently. The separation of different groups in the current system is based primarily on a retrospective review of the cancer-specific survival of 5319 patients with lung cancer during the years 1975 to 1988. Eighty percent of these were consecutive patients seen at the M.D. Anderson Cancer Center, and 20% were from a surgical registry (the Lung Cancer Study Group). Except for a brief period (1975-1980), patients with SCLC were excluded from the M.D. Anderson registry, with the result that only about 20% of the entire series involved patients of both histologic types.[180] Various treatments were used during this period, but undoubtedly the most effective was surgery for those with early stage tumors. This data, as well as published reports from other large series, was taken into consideration by the committees of the AJCC and the UICC (Union Internationale Contre le Cancer),

DATA SUMMARY: NATURAL HISTORY AND HISTOLOGIC CLASSIFICATION			
	AMOUNT	**QUALITY**	**CONSISTENCY**
The natural history of untreated stage I-III non–small cell lung cancer is a median survival of 6 months and a 1-year survival of 15%	High	High	High
Small cell lung cancer accounts for 20% of lung cancers	High	High	High
Squamous cell carcinomas account for 35% of lung cancers	High	High	High
The proportion of adenocarcinoma among patients diagnosed with lung cancer is increasing	High	High	High

Type of data rated: Plain text: descriptive statement   *Italics: controlled comparison*   **Bold: randomized comparison**

and TNM classes were grouped together based on similar survival results. Most of the data for patients with early stage disease probably represents pathologic stage (determined after resection); however, the TNM classes that are grouped together exhibit similar survival rates when defined by clinical (pretreatment) stage as well as by pathologic stage.[180]

As improvements in treatment are made, the prognosis for various stage subgroups may change. Furthermore, as the sensitivity of diagnostic tests improves, patients who would previously have been assigned to a lower stage will be classified with a higher stage, although the survival of these patients has not changed. This phenomenon, known as *stage migration,* results in better survival of all stages involved simply by changing the way patients are classified, even though the survival of the individual patients has not changed.[181] Thus, comparisons of patients classified in the same stage group but from a different time period will be fraught with error despite a detailed stage classification.

The TNM staging system is based on definition of the anatomic extent of disease. This seems to work fairly well for patients with early stage disease but does not succeed well in separating patients with extensive locally advanced or metastatic disease into prognostically homogeneous groups. Other factors, such as performance status, have a major impact on the length of survival of these patients. Alternative staging systems, which have included a clinical symptom assessment in the stage classification, have been proposed but not adopted, perhaps because of their complexity.[182,183] Perhaps a simplified hybrid system, including performance status (PS) only in patients with more advanced stage disease, would have some value, but this has not been studied.

Staging based on anatomic extent of disease is appealing because intuitively it would be expected to correlate with the need for local therapy (eg, surgery or RT) versus systemic treatment (eg, chemotherapy). However, as our understanding of cancer biology and the ability of cancer cells to metastasize becomes more sophisticated, this approach of using a description of gross disease to guide treatment strategy seems increasingly simplistic and inappropriate. The guiding principle underlying a staging system, therefore, should be to distinguish patients who are similar with respect to tumor biology. Such groups will be more likely to continue to exhibit similar prognoses (although the survival may improve over time) and respond to similar treatment strategies (although these are subject to change). This suggests that markers of biologic behavior, such as the expression of oncogenes, may play a role in the future in a more sophisticated stage classification system based on tumor biology rather than on gross anatomy. At present, however, the ability to predict tumor biology is rudimentary, and anatomic stage classification remains the only practical and widely accepted approach.

The TNM Staging System for Lung Cancer

The staging system for lung cancer is based on the TNM classification. The T factor is used to describe the extent of the primary tumor, the N factor the extent of regional

TABLE 3–7. THE TNM SYSTEM FOR STAGING LUNG CANCER

T	CONCEPT	DEFINITION
T1	Small	≤3 cm
T2	Larger	>3 cm
	More peripheral	Visceral pleural involvement
	More central	Tumor in lobar bronchus (atelectasis to hilum)
T3	More peripheral	Involving: ribs, diaphragm, mediastinal pleura, pericardium, phrenic nerve
	More central	In mainstem bronchus (<2 cm from carina)
T4	Extension to major adjacent structures or organs	Involving: trachea, carina, esophagus, heart, superior vena cava, aorta, vertebral body, recurrent laryngeal nerve
	More diffuse	Malignant pleural effusion

N	CONCEPT	DEFINITION
N0	No nodal involvement	No nodal involvement
N1	Nodes within lung	Involvement of nodal stations 10–14
N2	Ipsilateral mediastinal	Involvement of nodal stations 1–9 (ipsilateral or midline)
N3	Contralateral mediastinal	Involvement of contralateral nodal stations 2, 4
	Supraclavicular	Involvement of supraclavicular nodes

M	CONCEPT	DEFINITION
M0	Locoregional disease	No evidence of distant metastases
M1	Disseminated disease	Distant metastases present

SPECIAL SITUATIONS

Focus of in situ cancer	*Tis*
Small primary tumor confined to the wall of the trachea or mainstem bronchus	T1
Tumor with a satellite nodule *in the same lobe*	T4
T, N, or M status not able to be assessed	TX/NX/MX

Based on the 1997 American Joint Commission for Cancer and the Union Internationale Centre le Cancer (UICC) staging system.[180,198]

lymph node involvement, and the M factor the presence of distant metastases. Table 3–7 provides a description of the different T, N, and M categories. Increasing T stage denotes primary tumors that are larger, more peripheral, or more central. Further progression of T stage denotes involvement of major extraparenchymal structures (eg, heart, esophagus). Nodal staging also proceeds in a logical fashion from parenchymal lymph nodes to mediastinal lymph nodes. What is important is not the *number* of nodes, but the *location* of involved nodes: N1—within the lung parenchyma, N2—ipsilateral mediastinal, and N3—contralateral mediastinal.

Using current methods of treatment, survival in patients with lung cancer is influenced primarily by the extent of nodal disease and the presence of distant metastases, as shown in Figure 3–12. Recognition of this fact has led to stage grouping, as shown in Table 3–8. It can be seen that stage grouping is essentially defined by nodal status. The T1,2 status plays a minor role. The T3 and T4 status is also used to determine stage grouping, but patients with T3 or T4 tumors who do not have the nodal involvement otherwise characteristic of the stage grouping are uncommon and may present different biologic issues than patients

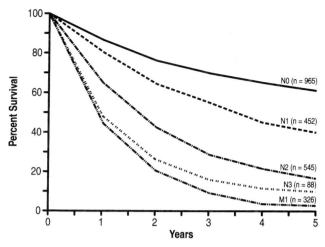

FIGURE 3–12. Influence of lymph node metastases on survival after lung resection in 2377 patients with NSCLC. (From Naruke T. Significance of lymph node metastases in lung cancer. Semin Thorac Cardiovasc Surg. 1993;5:210–218.[202])

having tumors with N2 or N3 nodal involvement. Therefore, these subgroups (T3N0, T3N1, and T4N0,1) should probably be viewed as special situations and included in their respective stage groups with caution.

From a treatment standpoint, it is intuitive to view tumors in the lung parenchyma (T1,2N0,1) as being easily resectable, tumors with a slight extension beyond this (T3 or N2) as being potentially resectable, and more extensive tumors (T4 or N3) as being unresectable unless additional incisions are made (eg, bilateral thoracotomy) or major reconstruction is done. However, this view is simplistic and may not be appropriate as the understanding of tumor biology improves and new treatment options become available. The anatomic definition of gross tumor has less relevance for the use of RT and is not relevant for treatment with chemotherapy alone.

Additional Staging Nomenclature

The method of staging and the time at which the stage is assessed have a major impact on the prognostic implications of the stage classification. For example, the 5-year survival of a patient who is staged clinically to have a

TABLE 3–8. LUNG CANCER STAGE GROUPING

STAGE	T	N	M	ADDITIONAL GROUPS
Ia	T1	N0	M0	
Ib	T2	N0	M0	
IIa	T1	N1	M0	
IIa	T2	N1	M0	T3N0
IIIa	T1-3	N2	M0	T3N1
IIIb	T1-3	N3	M0	T4N0-2
IV	Any	Any	M1	

Based on the 1997 AJCC/UICC staging system.[180, 198]

TABLE 3–9. TYPES OF STAGING ASSESSMENTS

PREFIX	CONCEPT	DEFINITION
c	Clinical	Prior to initiation of any treatment, using any and all information available (including mediastinoscopy)
p	Pathologic	After resection, based on pathologic assessment
y	Restaging	After part or all of the treatment has been given
r	Recurrence	Stage at time of a recurrence
a	Autopsy	Stage as determined by autopsy

Based on AJCC/UICC nomenclature.[198]

T1N1M0 tumor is approximately 34%, whereas that of a patient who is staged as T1N1M0 after resection, when the final pathologic examination has been completed, is approximately 52% (see Tables 12–1 and 12–2). The two types of stage assessment that are encountered most commonly are clinical staging, meaning the stage determined using all information (including the results of mediastinoscopy) available *prior to any treatment,* and pathologic staging, which is determined by the pathologist *after a resection* has been carried out. In order to avoid confusion, the prefix "c" is conventionally used (eg, cN0) when clinical staging has been done, and "p" is conventionally used (eg, pN0) when pathologic (surgical) staging has been carried out. The AJCC also recognizes other situations in which the stage assessment has distinct prognostic implications and has assigned various prefixes, as shown in Table 3–9. Reassessment of stage after treatment is begun (eg, after induction chemotherapy, before a resection is undertaken) is becoming more important and is denoted by the prefix "y."

The AJCC also defines a classification system for the presence or absence of residual tumor after treatment, as shown in Table 3–10. Usually this is used to describe the completeness of a surgical resection. It is obvious that an incomplete resection, in which gross tumor is left behind (R_2), cannot necessarily be compared with a complete resection, in which the margins are microscopically negative and no residual disease remains (R_0). Unfortunately, this data is not provided in many surgical series. As the knowledge about the treatment of lung cancer becomes more sophisticated, it is becoming more important to use such a classification system so that nuances of treatment differences can be understood.

PERFORMANCE STATUS

After tumor stage, PS is the most important determinant of prognosis in patients with solid tumor malignancies. This

TABLE 3–10. RESIDUAL TUMOR AFTER TREATMENT

SYMBOL	CONCEPT	DEFINITION
R_0	No residual	No identifiable tumor remaining, negative surgical margins
R_1	Microscopic residual	No gross tumor remaining, but microscopically positive margins
R_2	Gross residual	Gross (visible or palpable) tumor remaining

Based on AJCC/UICC nomenclature.[198]

is certainly true for SCLC and for NSCLC as well. In two large reviews, the importance of performance status was substantiated in virtually every study of lung cancer that analyzed prognostic factors.[184,185] Two classification schemes are used with equal frequency[186] to describe PS—the Karnofsky and the Zubrod scales. These are named after the authors who proposed them and are shown in Table 3–11 as they were originally defined. The Eastern Cooperative Oncology Group (ECOG) or the WHO scales represent minor modifications of the Zubrod scale.

The definitions used in the Zubrod and Karnofsky classification schemes are slightly different, which hampers conversion from one scale to another. The comparison of the scales shown in Table 3–11 was found by two independent studies to result in the best correlation.[186,187] The breakpoint in the scales that has the greatest clinical importance is between patients who are still ambulatory and those who spend a significant amount of time in bed. This corresponds to a Karnofsky PS of 80 to 100 and a Zubrod PS of 0 or 1 versus patients with poorer PS scores. In these categories, conversion from one scale to another using the comparison shown in Table 3–11 results in the correct classification of > 90% of patients.[186,187] This is useful in comparing the patient selection of different studies with one another.

The largest analysis of prognostic factors has been carried out by Stanley,[188] who analyzed 5138 patients from 1968 to 1978 as part of the Veterans Administration Lung Group protocols. This analysis involved patients with inoperable lung cancer who generally had at least stage III disease, and included patients with both SCLC and NSCLC.[188] PS emerged as the most important prognostic factor. In fact, in this study population (patients with stage III and IV disease), it was even more important than extent of disease (limited versus extensive stage). The prognostic significance of PS with regard to specific stages and types of lung cancer is discussed in more detail in other chapters.

TABLE 3–11. COMPARISON OF KARNOFSKY AND ZUBROD SCALES OF PERFORMANCE STATUS

ZUBROD SCALE[a]	KARNOFSKY SCALE
0 Asymptomatic	100 Asymptomatic
1 Symptomatic, but ambulatory (able to work)	90 Normal activity, minor symptoms 80 Normal activity, some symptoms
2 In bed <50% of day (unable to work, but able to live at home with some assistance)	70 Unable to work, care for self 60 Occasional assistance with needs
3 In bed >50% of day (unable to care for self)	50 Considerable assistance 40 Disabled, full assistance needed
4 Bedridden	30 Needs some active supportive care 20 Very sick, hospitalization needed
	10 Moribund 0 Dead

[a]Descriptions in parentheses are not part of the original definition.
Based on Zubrod and Karnofsky performance status scales.[188, 199–201]

EDITORS' COMMENTS

There is no question that lung cancer is a major health problem, accounting for more cancer deaths than the next four leading causes of cancer mortality *combined*. Although the rate of rise of deaths from lung cancer has decreased, this should not be confused with resolution of the problem. Lung cancer will be the leading cause of cancer mortality until at least 2040. The high current rate of smoking in adolescents underscores the fact that this will remain a major health problem. Perhaps the more recent efforts in the United States to discourage adolescents from smoking will pay off in the future. However, it is likely that such efforts will not occur in developing countries for many years to come.

Lung cancer has not received attention commensurate with its importance as a cause of mortality. Efforts at prevention and treatment of this disease have lagged behind those directed toward other cancers (eg, breast cancer). Undoubtedly, this is largely because most lung cancers are caused by smoking, which is a factor that people can control. This results in less sympathy for victims of lung cancer and makes it difficult for prominent individuals afflicted with this disease to be spokespersons. It is important to realize, however, that most lung cancers currently occur in individuals who have quit smoking many years earlier. Furthermore, stopping smoking is not easy, and the pressures adolescents are subjected to regarding whether or not they begin smoking are complex and cannot be dismissed simply with "it's their own choice."

Smoking remains the major risk factor for the development of lung cancer. In the past, occupational exposure accounted for a small minority of cancers, but substantial efforts have been made to alter the exposure levels, at least in the United States. As a result, the number of lung cancers attributable to occupational exposure in the future will be small.

One could easily think that the major insights in the epidemiology of lung cancer have already been achieved. In reality, many exciting developments are currently taking place in this field. We are just beginning to understand some of the genetic factors that predispose patients to lung cancer. Furthermore, associations of lung cancer with specific aspects of gender, family history, and the development of chronic obstructive pulmonary disease represent a very important advance in our understanding of the epidemiology of lung cancer. Such insights have important implications for screening and early diagnosis of lung cancer. The development of effective screening tools and the ability to diagnose lung cancer at an earlier stage would have a huge impact on the mortality associated with this disease.

Classification systems are crucial because they provide a language with which to communicate accurately about lung cancer. It is important that everyone understands the system and makes an effort to use it to describe not only the gross characteristics but also the details of patients included in a series, even when it is not apparent how these details are important. This is necessary if we are to ferret out the nuances of different results, realizing that progress is made in a series of small steps.

It is important to accept that no classification system

will meet all needs equally. Furthermore, we must realize that classification systems are not static, allowing classification "once and for all." As our knowledge and our treatment approaches change, the results change, and, even more importantly, the issues change. The best system would reflect the biology of the tumor, because patients grouped by tumor behavior characteristics will probably continue to have similarities with one another, even as treatment approaches and results change.

References

1. Greenlee RT, Murray T, Bolden S, et al. Cancer statistics, 2000. CA Cancer J Clin. 2000;50:7–33.
2. Parkin DM, Pisani P, Ferlay J. Global cancer statistics. CA Cancer J Clin. 1999;49:33–64.
3. Magrath I, Litvak J. Cancer in developing countries: opportunity and challenge. J Natl Cancer Inst. 1993;85:862–868.
4. Kurihara M, Aoki K, Hisamichi S. Cancer Mortality Statistics in the World, 1950-1985. Nagoya, Japan: Nagoya University Press;1989.
5. Wingo PA, Tong T, Bolden S. Cancer statistics, 1995. CA Cancer J Clin. 1995;45:8–30.
6. Stanley K, Stjersward J. Lung cancer: a worldwide health problem. Chest. 1989;96:1S–5S.
7. Lopez-Abente G, Pollan M, de la Iglesia P, et al. Characterization of the lung cancer epidemic in the European Union (1970-1990). Cancer Epidemiol Biomarkers Prev. 1995;4:813–820.
8. Landis SH, Murray T, Bolden S, et al. Cancer statistics 1999. CA Cancer J Clin. 1999;49:8–31.
9. Beckett WS. Epidemiology and etiology of lung cancer. Clin Chest Med. 1993;14:1–15.
10. Brown CC, Kessler LG. Projections of lung cancer mortality in the United States: 1985-2025. J Natl Cancer Inst. 1988;80:43–51.
11. US Dept. of Health and Human Services. Cigarette smoking among high school students—11 states, 1991-1997. Morbid Mortal Weekly Rep. 1998;48:686–692.
12. Rottman H. Über Primäre Lungencarzinome [inaugural dissertation]. Universität Würzburg; Würzburg, Germany, 1898.
13. Müller FH. Tabakmissbrauch und Lungencarzinome. Z Krebsforsch. 1939;49:57–85.
14. Scjrenk R, Baker LA, Ballard GP, et al. Tobacco smoking as an etiologic factor in disease: cancer. Cancer Res. 1950;10:49–58.
15. Mills CA, Porter MM. Tobacco smoking habits and cancer of the mouth and respiratory system. Cancer Res. 1950;10:49–58.
16. Levin ML, Goldstein H, Gerhardt PR. Cancer and tobacco smoking. JAMA. 1950;143:336–338.
17. Public Health Service, US Department of Health, Education, and Welfare. A report of the Advisory Committee to the Surgeon General of the Public Health Service. Washington, DC: US Gov Printing Office; 1964.
18. Centers for Disease Control, Public Health Service, US Department of Health and Human Services. The health benefits of smoking cessation. Washington, DC: US Gov Printing Office; 1990.
19. Hammond EC. Smoking in relation to the death of one million men and women. Natl Cancer Inst Monogr. 1966;19:127–204.
20. Damber LA, Larsson L-G. Smoking and lung cancer with special regard to type of smoking and type of cancer: a case-control study in north Sweden. Br J Cancer. 1986;53:673–681.
21. Burns DM. Tobacco smoking. In: Samet JM, ed. Epidemiology of Lung Cancer. New York, NY: Marcel Dekker; 1994:15–49.
22. Cederlof R, Frberg L, Hrubec Z, et al. The relationship of smoking and smoke: social Covariables to mortality and cancer morbidity—a ten year follow-up in probability sample of 55000 Swedish subjects Age 18 to 69 (Part 1 and 2). Stockholm, Sweden: Department of Environmental Hygiene, The Karolinska Institute; 1975.
23. Peto R. Influence of dose and duration of smoking on lung cancer rates. In: Zaridge D, Peto R, ed. Tobacco: A Major International Health Hazard. Lyon, France: International Agency for Research on Cancer; 1986:23–33.
24. Doll R, Peto R. Mortality in relation to smoking: 20 years' observations on male British doctors. BMJ. 1976;2:1525–1536.
25. Rogot E, Murray JL. Smoking and causes of death among U.S. veterans: 16 years of observation. Public Health Rep. 1980:213–222.
26. Mattson ME, Pollack ES, Cullen JW. What are the odds that smoking will kill you? Am J Public Health. 1987;77:425–431.
27. United States Surgeon General. Reducing the health consequences of smoking: twenty-five years of progress. Rockville, Md: Department of Health and Human Services; 1989. USPHS Pub No (CDC) 89-8411.
28. Ingebrethsem BJ. Aerosol studies of cigarette smoke. Rec Adv Tobacco Sci. 1986;12:54–142.
29. International Agency for Research on Cancer. Tobacco: A Major International Health Hazard. Lyon, France: International Agency for Research on Cancer; 1986.
30. Hoffmann D, Health S. Nicotine derived N-nitrosamines and tobacco related cancer: current status and future directions. Cancer Res. 1985;45:935–944.
31. Phillips DH, Herver D, Martin CN, et al. Correlation of DNA adduct levels in human lung with cigarette smoking. Nature. 1988;336:790–797.
32. Samet JM, Wiggins CL, Humble CG, et al. Cigarette smoking and lung cancer in New Mexico. Am Rev Respir Dis. 1988;137:1110–1113.
33. Weiss W, Boucot KR, Seidman H, et al. Risk of lung cancer according to histologic type and cigarette dosage. JAMA. 1972;222:799–801.
34. Rylander R, Axelsson G, Andersson L, et al. Lung cancer, smoking, and diet among Swedish men. Lung Cancer. 1996;14:S75–S83.
35. Doll R, Peto R. Cigarette smoking and bronchial carcinoma: dose and time relationships among regular smokers and life-long non-smokers. J Epidemiol Commun Health. 1978;32:303–313.
36. Lubin JH, Blot WJ. Assessment of lung cancer risk factors by histologic category. J Natl Cancer Inst. 1984;73:383–389.
37. Stellman SD. Cigarette yield and cancer risk: evidence from case-control and prospective studies. In: Zaridze DG, Peto R, eds. Tobacco: A Major International Health Hazard. Lyon, France: International Agency for Research on Cancer; 1986:197–209.
38. Benhamou D, Benhamou E, Auquier A, et al. High tar cigarettes are associated with a higher risk for the development of lung cancer. Int J Epidemiol. 1994;23:437–443.
39. Wynder EL, Kabat GC. The effect of low tar cigarette smoking on lung cancer risk. Cancer. 1988;62:1223–1230.
40. Kabat GC. Aspects of the epidemiology of lung cancer in smokers and nonsmokers in the United States. Lung Cancer. 1996;15:1–20.
41. Lubin JH, Blot WJ, Berrino F, et al. Patterns of lung cancer risk according to type of cigarette smoked. Int J Cancer. 1984;33:569–576.
42. Wilcox HB, Schoenberg JB, Mason TJ, et al. Smoking and lung cancer: risk as a function of cigarette tar content. Prevent Med. 1988;17:263–272.
43. Augustine A, Harris RE, Wynder EL. Compensation as a risk factor to the development of lung cancer in smokers who switch from nonfilter to filter cigarettes. Am J Public Health. 1989;79:188–191.
44. Herning RI, Jones RT, Bachman J, et al. Puff volume increases when low-nicotine cigarettes are smoked. BMJ. 1981;283:187–189.
45. Wynder EL, Hoffmann D. Smoking and lung cancer: scientific challenges and opportunities. Cancer Res. 1994;54:5284–5295.
46. Hoffman D, Rivenson A, Hecht SS. The biological significance of tobacco-specific N-nitrosamines, smoking and adenocarcinoma of the lung. Crit Rev Toxicol. 1996;26:199–211.
47. Wynder EL, Muscat JE. The changing epidemiology of smoking and lung cancer histology. Environ Health Perspec. 1995;103:143–148.
48. Holmes EC. Lung cancer. In: Simmons DH, ed. Current Pulmonology. Boston, Mass: Houghton Mifflin; 1979:239–250.
49. Hirayama S, Taminato T, Kitano N, et al. Non-smoking wives of heavy smokers have a higher risk of lung cancer: a study from Japan. BMJ. 1981;282:183–185.
50. Capewell S, Sankaran R, Lamb D, et al. Lung cancer in lifelong non-smokers. Thorax. 1991;46:565–568.
51. Jinot J. Hazard information. I. Lung cancer in active smokers, long-term animal bioassays, and genotoxicity studies. In: Respiratory Health Effects of Passive Smoking: Lung Cancer and Other Disorders. Washington, DC: US Environmental Protection Agency. 1992.
52. Harris JE. Cigarette smoking among successive birth cohorts of men and women in the United States during 1900-1980. J Natl Cancer Inst. 1983;71:473–479.

53. Fiore MC, Novotny TE, Pierce JP, et al. Smoking in the United States: the changing influence of gender and race. JAMA. 1989;261:49–55.

54. Tong L, Spitz MR, Fueger JJ, et al. Lung carcinoma in former smokers. Cancer. 1996;78:1004–1010.

55. Halpern MT, Gillespie BW, Warner KE. Patterns of absolute risk of lung cancer mortality in former smokers. J Natl Cancer Inst. 1993;85:457–464.

56. Doll R, Gray R, Hafner B, et al. Mortality in relation to smoking: 22 years' observations on female British doctors. BMJ. 1980;280:967–971.

57. Higgins ITT, Mahan CM, Wynder EL. Lung cancer among cigar and pipe smokers. Prev Med. 1988;17:116–128.

58. Baker RR, The effects of ventilation of cigarette combustion mechanisms. Rec Adv Tobacco Sci. 1984;10:88–150.

59. Sandler DP, Everson RB, Wilcox AJ. Passive smoking in adulthood and cancer risk. Am J Epidemiol. 1985;121:37–48.

60. Pershagen G. Passive smoking and lung cancer. In: Samet JM, ed. Epidemiology of Lung Cancer. New York, NY: Marcel Dekker; 1994:109–130.

61. Bayard SP. Summary and conclusion. In: Respiratory Health Effects of Passive Smoking: Lung Cancer and Other Disorders. Washington, DC: US Environmental Protection Agency. 1992.

62. Fontham ETH, Correa P, Reynolds P, et al. Environmental tobacco smoke and lung cancer in nonsmoking women: a multicenter study. JAMA. 1994;271:1752–1759.

63. National Research Council. Environmental Tobacco Smoke. Washington, DC: National Academy Press; 1986.

64. Steenland K, Loomis D, Shy C, et al. Review of occupational lung carcinogens. Am J Ind Med. 1996;29:474–490.

65. International Agency for Research on Cancer. Overall evaluations of carcinogenicity: an updating of IARC Monographs 1–42, Supplement 7. Lyon, France: International Agency for Research on Cancer; 1987.

66. International Agency for Research on Cancer. Diesel and gasoline engine exhausts and some nitroarenes, Monograph 46. Lyon, France: International Agency for Research on Cancer; 1989.

67. International Agency for Research on Cancer. Beryllium, cadmium, mercury and exposures in the glass manufacturing industry, Monograph 58. Lyon, France: International Agency for Research on Cancer; 1993.

68. Hughes JM, Weill H. Asbestos and man-made fibers. In: Samet JM, ed. Epidemiology of Lung Cancer. New York, NY: Marcel Dekker, 1994:185–205.

69. Davis L, Beckett S, Bolton R, et al. Mass and numbers of fibers in the pathogenesis of asbestos-related lung disease in rats. Br J Cancer. 1978;37:673–688.

70. Steenland K, Thun M. Interaction between tobacco smoking and occupational exposures in the causation of lung cancer. J Occup Med. 1986;28:110–118.

71. Browne K. Is asbestos or asbestosis the cause of the increased risk of lung cancer in asbestos workers? [editorial]. Br J Industr Med. 1986;43:145–149.

72. Byers TE, Vena JE, Rzepka TF. Predilection of lung cancer for the upper lobes: an epidemiologic inquiry. J Natl Cancer Inst. 1984;72:1271–1275.

73. Hughes J, Weill H. Asbestosis as a precursor of asbestos related cancer: results of a prospective study. Br J Industr Med. 1991;48:229–233.

74. Liddell F, McDonald J. Radiological findings as predictors of mortality in Quebec asbestos workers. Br J Industr Med. 1980;37:257–267.

75. Sluis-Cremer GK, Bezuidenhout BN. Letter to the editor. Br J Industr Med. 1990;47:215–216.

76. Schottenfeld D. Epidemiology of lung cancer. In: Pass HI, Mitchell JB, Johnson DH, et al, eds. Lung Cancer: Principles and Practice. Philadelphia, Pa: Lippincott-Raven; 1996:305–321.

77. Ogawa H, Kato I, Tominaga S. Family history of cancer among cancer patients. Jpn J Cancer Res. 1985;76:113–118.

78. Lynch HT, Kimberling WJ, Markvicka SE, et al. Genetics and smoking-associated cancers: a study of 485 families. Cancer. 1986;57:1640–1646.

79. Ooi WL, Elston R, Chen VW, et al. Increased familial risk for lung cancer. J Natl Cancer Inst. 1986;76:217–222.

80. Horwitz RI, Smaldone LF, Viscoli CM. An ecogenetic hypothesis for lung cancer in women. Arch Intern Med. 1988;148:2609–2612.

81. Samet J, Humble C, Pathak D. Personal and family history of respiratory disease and lung cancer risk. Am Rev Respir Dis. 1986;134:466–470.

82. Schwartz AG, Yang P, Swanson GM. Familial risk of lung cancer among nonsmokers and their relatives. Am J Epidemiol. 1996;144:554–562.

83. Brownson RC, Alavanja MCR, Caporaso N, et al. Family history of cancer and risk of lung cancer in lifetime non-smokers and long-term ex-smokers. Int J Epidemiol. 1997;26:256–263.

84. Shaw GL, Falk RT, Pickle LW, et al. Lung cancer risk associated with cancer in relatives. J Clin Epidemiol. 1991;44:429–437.

85. Tokuhata GK, Lilienfeld AM. Familial aggregation of lung cancer in humans. J Natl Cancer Inst. 1963;30:289–312.

86. Sellers TA, Bailey-Wilson JE, Elston RC, et al. Evidence for Mendelian inheritance in the pathogenesis of lung cancer. J Natl Cancer Inst. 1990;82:1272–1279.

87. Kreuzer M, Kreienbrock L, Gerken M, et al. Risk factors for lung cancer in young adults. Am J Epidemiol. 1998;147:1028–1037.

88. Wu AH, Fontham ETH, Reynolds P, et al. Family history of cancer and risk of lung cancer among lifetime nonsmoking women in the United States. Am J Epidemiol. 1996;143:535–542.

89. Sellers TA, Potter JD, Bailey-Wilson JE, et al. Lung cancer detection and prevention: evidence for an interaction between smoking and genetic predisposition. Cancer Res. 1992;52(suppl):2694s–2697s.

90. Sellers TA, Chen P-L, Potter JD, et al. Segregation analysis of smoking-associated malignancies: evidence for Mendelian inheritance. Am J Med Genet. 1994;52:308–314.

91. Braun MM, Caporaso NE, Page WF, et al. Genetic component of lung cancer: cohort study of twins. Lancet. 1994;344:440–443.

92. Neber DW. Possible clinical importance of genetic differences in drug metabolism. BMJ. 1981;283:537–542.

93. Economou P, Lechner JF, Samet JM. Familial and genetic factors in the pathogenesis of lung cancer. In: Samet JM, ed. Epidemiology of Lung Cancer. New York, NY: Marcel Dekker; 1994:353–396.

94. Nakachi K, Imai K, Hayashi S, et al. Genetic susceptibility to squamous cell carcinoma of the lung in relation to cigarette smoking dose. Cancer Res. 1991;51:5177–5180.

95. Jacquet M, Lambert V, Baudoux E, et al. Correlation between P450 CYP1A1 inducibility, MspI genotype and lung cancer incidence. Eur J Cancer. 1996;32A:1701–1706.

96. Caporaso NE, Tucker MA, Hoover RN, et al. Lung cancer and the debrisoquine metabolic phenotype. J Natl Cancer Inst. 1990;82:1264–1272.

97. Zang EA, Wynder EL. Differences in lung cancer risk between men and women: examination of the evidence. J Natl Cancer Inst. 1996;88:183–192.

98. Risch HA, Howe GR, Jain M, et al. Are female smokers at higher risk for lung cancer than male smokers? A case-control analysis by histologic type. Am J Epidemiol. 1993;138:281–291.

99. Harris RE, Zang EA, Anderson JI, et al. Race and sex differences in lung cancer risk associated with cigarette smoking. Int J Epidemiol. 1993;22:592–599.

100. Brownson RC, Chang JC, Davis JR. Gender and histologic type variations in smoking-related risk of lung cancer. Epidemiology. 1992;3:61–64.

101. Osann KE, Anton-Culver H, Kuroaski T, et al. Sex differences in lung cancer risk associated with cigarette smoking. Int J Cancer. 1993;54:44–48.

102. Prescott E, Osler M, Hein HO, et al. Gender and smoking-related risk of lung cancer. Epidemiology. 1998;9:79–83.

103. Hecht SS, Hoffmann D. The relevance of tobacco-specific nitrosamines in human cancer. Cancer Surv. 1989;8:273–294.

104. Beckett AH, Gorrod JW, Jenner P. The effect of smoking on nicotine metabolism. J Pharm Pharmacol. 1971;23(suppl):62S–67S.

105. Benowitz NL, Jacob PI. Daily intake of nicotine during cigarette smoking. Clin Pharmacol Ther. 1984;35:499–504.

106. Piekoszewski W, Brandys J, Lipniak M. Studies on sex related differences in elimination of theophylline in the rat after pretreatment with phenobarbital, chrysene or lindane. Acta Pharmacol. 1991;48:9–12.

107. Guengerich FP, Shimada T. Oxidation of toxic and carcinogenic chemicals by human cytochrome P-450 emzymes. Chem Res Toxicol. 1991;4:391–407.

108. Ryberg D, Hewer A, Phillips DH, et al. Different susceptibility to smoking-induced DNA damage among male and female lung cancer patients. Cancer Res. 1994;54:5801–5803.

109. Adami HO, Persson I, Hoover R, et al. Risk of cancer in women receiving hormone replacement therapy. Int J Cancer. 1989;44:833–839.

110. Taioli E, Wynder EL. Endocrine factors and adenocarcinoma of the lung in women. J Natl Cancer Inst. 1994;86:869–870.

111. Annegers JF, Malkasian GD. Patterns of other neoplasia in patients with endometrial carcinoma. Cancer. 1981;48:856–859.

112. Harvey EB, Brinton LA. Second cancer following cancers of the breast in Connecticut, 1935-82. Natl Cancer Inst Monogr. 1985;68:99–112.

113. Curtis RE, Hoover RN, Kleinerman RA, et al. Second cancer following cancer of the female genital system in Connecticut, 1935-82. Natl Cancer Inst Monogr. 1985;68:113–137.

114. Sellers TA, Potter JD, Folsom AR. Association of incident lung cancer with family history of female reproductive cancers: the Iowa Women's Health Study. Genetic Epidemiol. 1991;8:199–208.

115. Bjelke E. Dietary vitamin A and human lung cancer. Int J Cancer. 1975;15:561–565.

116. Fraser GE, Beeson WL, Phillips RL. Diet and lung cancer in Seventh-Day Adventists. Am J Epidemiol. 1991;133:683–693.

117. Mayne ST, Janerich DT, Greenwald P, et al. Dietary beta carotene and lung cancer risk in U.S. nonsmokers. J Natl Cancer Inst. 1994;86:33–38.

118. LeMarchand L, Hankin JH, Bach F, et al. An ecological study of diet and lung cancer in the South Pacific. Int J Cancer. 1995;63:18–23.

119. Ziegler RG, Mayne ST, Swanson CA. Nutrition and lung cancer. Cancer Cases Control. 1996;7:157–177.

120. Wynder EL, Hebert JR, Kabat GC. Association of dietary fat and lung cancer. J Natl Cancer Inst. 1987;79:631–637.

121. Shekelle RB, Lepper M, Liu S, et al. Dietary vitamin A and risk of cancer in the Western Electric Study. Lancet. 1981;2:1185–1189.

122. Block G, Patterson B, Subar A. Fruit, vegetables, and cancer prevention: a review of the epidemiological evidence. Nutr Cancer. 1992;18:1–29.

123. National Research Council, Committee on Diet and Health, Food and Nutrition Board, and Commission on Life Sciences. Diet and Health: Implications for Reducing Chronic Disease Risk. Washington, DC: National Academy Press; 1990.

124. Wald N, Idle M, Boreham J, et al. Low serum vitamin A and subsequent risk of cancer. Lancet. 1980;2:813–815.

125. Chung FL, Morse MA, Eklind KI, et al. Inhibition of tobacco-specific nitrosamine-induced tumorigenesis by compounds derived from cruciferous vegetables and green tea. Ann NY Acad Sci. 1993;686:186–202.

126. Ziegler R. A review of epidemiologic evidence that the carotenoids reduce the risk of cancer. J Nutr. 1989;119:116–122.

127. Willet W. Vitamin A and lung cancer. Nutr Rev. 1990;48:201–211.

128. Byers T. Diet as a factor in the etiology and prevention of lung cancer. In: Sammet JM, ed. Epidemiology of Lung Cancer. New York, NY: Marcel Dekker; 1994:335–352.

129. The Alpha-Tocopherol, Beta Carotene Cancer Prevention Study Group. The effect of vitamin E and beta carotene on the incidence of lung cancer and other cancers in male smokers. N Engl J Med. 1994;330:1029–1035.

130. Omenn GS, Goodman GE, Thornquist MD, et al. Effects of a combination of beta carotene and vitamin A on lung cancer and cardiovascular disease. N Engl J Med. 1996;334:1150–1155.

131. Hennekens CH, Buring JE, Manson JE, et al. Lack of effect of long-term supplementation with beta carotene on the incidence of malignant neoplasms and cardiovascular disease. N Engl J Med. 1996;334:1145–1149.

132. Wakai K, Ohno Y, Genka K, et al. Risk modification in lung cancer by a dietary intake of preserved foods and soyfoods: findings from a case-control study in Okinawa, Japan. Lung Cancer. 1999;25:147–159.

133. Passey RD. Some problems of lung cancer. Lancet. 1962;2:107–109.

134. Kuschner M. The J. Burns Amberson lecture: the causes of lung cancer. Am Rev Respir Dis. 1968;98:573–590.

135. Skillrud DM, Offord KP, Miller RD. Higher risk of lung cancer in chronic obstructive pulmonary disease: a prospective, matched, controlled study. Ann Intern Med. 1986;105:503–507.

136. Davis AL. Bronchogenic carcinoma in chronic obstructive pulmonary disease. JAMA. 1976;235:621–622.

137. Tockman MS, et al, and The Johns Hopkins Lung Project for the Early Detection of Lung Cancer. Airways obstruction and the risk for lung cancer. Ann Intern Med. 1987;106:512–518.

138. Kuller LH, Ockne J, Meilahn E, et al. Relation of forced expiratory volume in one second (FEV_1) to lung cancer mortality in the Multiple Risk Factor Intervention Trial (MRFIT). Am J Epidemiol. 1990;132:265–274.

139. Lange P, Nyboe J, Appleyard M, et al. Ventilatory function and chronic mucus hypersecretion as predictors of death from lung cancer. Am Rev Respir Dis. 1990;141:613–617.

140. Peto R, Speizer FE, Cochrane AL, et al. The relevance in adults of air-flow obstruction, but not of mucus hypersecretion, to mortality from chronic lung disease. Am Rev Respir Dis. 1983;128:491–500.

141. Overholt RH, Neptune WB, Ashraf MM. Primary cancer of the lung: a 42-year experience. Ann Thorac Surg. 1975;20:511–519.

142. Flehinger BJ, Kimmel M, Melamed MR. The effect of surgical treatment on survival from early lung cancer: implications for screening. Chest. 1992;101:1013–1018.

143. Zelen M. Keynote address on biostatistics and data retrieval. Cancer Chemother Rep. 1973;4:31–42.

144. Geddes DM. The natural history of lung cancer: a review based on rates of tumour growth. Br J Dis Chest. 1979;73:1–17.

145. Flehinger BJ, Kimmel M, Melamed MR. Natural history of adenocarcinoma-large cell carcinoma of the lung: conclusions from screening programs in New York and Baltimore. J Natl Cancer Inst. 1988;80:337–344.

146. Flehinger BJ, Kimmel M. The natural history of lung cancer in a periodically screened population. Biometrics. 1987;43:127–144.

147. Walter SD, Kubik A, Parkin DM, et al. The natural history of lung cancer estimated from the results of a randomized trial of screening. Cancer Causes Control. 1992;3:115–123.

148. Soda H, Tomita H, Kohno S, et al. Limitation of annual screening chest radiography for the diagnosis of lung cancer: a retrospective study. Cancer. 1993;72:2341–2346.

149. Heelan RT, Flehinger BJ, Melamed MR, et al. Non–small-cell lung cancer: results of the New York Screening Program. Radiology. 1984;151:289–293.

150. Muhm JR, Miller WE, Fontana RS, et al. Lung cancer detected during a screening program using four-month chest radiographs. Radiology. 1983;148:609–615.

151. Quekel LGBA, Kessels AGH, Goei R, et al. Miss rate of lung cancer on the chest radiograph in clinical practice. Chest. 1999;115:720–724.

152. Kappauf H, Gallmeier WM, Wünsch PH, et al. Complete spontaneous remission in a patient with metastatic non–small-cell lung cancer. Ann Oncol. 1997;8:1031–1039.

153. Cohen MH, Matthews MJ. Small cell bronchogenic carcinoma: a distinct clinicopathologic entity. Semin Oncol. 1978;5:234–243.

154. Hirsch FR, Matthews MJ, Aisner S, et al. Histopathologic classification of small-cell lung cancer: changing concepts and terminology. Cancer. 1988;62:973–977.

155. World Health Organization. The World Health Organization histological typing of lung tumours, 2nd ed. Am J Clin Pathol. 1982;77:123–136.

156. Travis WD, Travis LB, Devesa SS. Lung cancer. Cancer. 1995;75:191–202.

157. World Health Organization. International Classification of Diseases for Oncology, 1976. Geneva, Switzerland: WHO; 1976.

158. Jiang S-X, Kameya T, Shoji M, et al. Large cell neuroendocrine carcinoma of the lung: a histologic and immunohistochemical study of 22 cases. Am J Surg Pathol. 1998;22:526–537.

159. Warren WH, Faber LP, Gould VE. Neuroendocrine neoplasms of the lung. J Thorac Cardiovasc Surg. 1989;98:321–332.

160. Rusch VW, Klimstra DS, Venkatraman ES. Molecular markers help characterize neuroendocrine lung tumors. Ann Thorac Surg. 1996;62:798–810.

161. Dresler CM, Ritter JH, Patterson GA, et al. Clinical-pathologic analysis of 40 patients with large cell neuroendocrine carcinoma of the lung. Ann Thorac Surg. 1997;63:180–185.

162. Yang CP, Gallagher RP, Weiss NS, et al. Differences in incidence rates of cancers of the respiratory tract by anatomic subsite and histologic type: an etiologic implication. J Natl Cancer Inst. 1989;81:1828–1831.

163. Morabia A, Wynder EL. Cigarette smoking and lung cancer cell types. Cancer. 1991;68:2074–2078.

164. Wynder EL, Covey LS. Epidemiologic patterns in lung cancer by histologic type. Int J Cancer Clin Oncol. 1987;23:1491–1496.

165. Humphrey EW, Smart CR, Winchester DP, et al. National survey of

the pattern of care for carcinoma of the lung. J Thorac Cardiovasc Surg. 1990;100:837–843.

166. Zheng T, Holford TR, Boyle P, et al. Time trend and the age-period-cohort effect on the incidence of histologic types of lung cancer in Connecticut, 1960-1989. Cancer. 1994;74:1556–1567.

167. Beard CM, Jedd MB, Woolner LB, et al. Fifty-year trend in incidence rates of bronchogenic carcinoma by cell type in Olmsted County, Minnesota. J Natl Cancer Inst. 1988;80:1404–1407.

168. Osann KE. Lung cancer in women: the importance of smoking, family history of cancer, and medical history of respiratory disease. Cancer Res. 1991;51:4893–4897.

169. Greenberg ER, Korson R, Baker J, et al. Incidence of lung cancer by cell type: a population-based study in New Hampshire and Vermont. J Natl Cancer Inst. 1984;72:599–603.

170. Vincent RG, Pickren JW, Lane WW, et al. The changing histopathology of lung cancer: a review of 1682 cases. Cancer. 1977;39:1647–1655.

171. Ikeda T, Kurita Y, Inutsuka S, et al. The changing pattern of lung cancer by histological type—a review of 1151 cases from a university hospital in Japan, 1970-1989. Lung Cancer. 1991;7:157–164.

172. Wu AH, Henderson BE, Thomas DC, et al. Secular trends in histologic types of lung cancer. J Natl Cancer Inst. 1986;77:53–56.

173. Dodds L, Davis S, Polissar L. A population-based study of lung cancer incidence trends by histologic type, 1974-81. J Natl Cancer Inst. 1986;76:21–29.

174. Valaitis J, Warren S, Gamble D. Increasing incidence of adenocarcinoma of the lung. Cancer. 1981;47:1042–1046.

175. Kung ITM, So KF, Lam TH. Lung cancer in Hong Kong Chinese: mortality and histological types, 1973-1982. Br J Cancer. 1984;50:381–388.

176. Auerbach O, Garfinkel L. The changing pattern of lung carcinoma. Cancer. 1991;68:1973–1977.

177. Barsky SH, Cameron R, Osann KE, et al. Rising incidence of bronchioloalveolar lung carcinoma and its unique clinicopathologic features. Cancer. 1994;73:1163–1170.

178. Charloux A, Quoix E, Wolkove N, et al. The increasing incidence of lung adenocarcinoma: reality or artefact? A review of the epidemiology of lung adenocarcinoma. Int J Epidemiol. 1997;26:14–23.

179. Mountain CF. A new international staging system for lung cancer. Chest. 1986;89(suppl):225S–233S.

180. Mountain CF. Revisions in the International System for Staging Lung Cancer. Chest. 1997;111:1710–1717.

181. Feinstein AR, Sosin DM, Wells CK. The Will Rogers phenomenon: stage migration and new diagnostic techniques as a source of misleading statistics for survival in cancer. N Engl J Med. 1985;312:1604–1608.

182. Feinstein AR, Wells CK. A clinical-severity staging system for patients with lung cancer. Medicine. 1990;69:1–33.

183. Pfister DG, Wells CK, Chan CK, et al. Classifying clinical severity to help solve problems of stage migration in nonconcurrent comparisons of lung cancer therapy. Cancer Res. 1990;50:4664–4669.

184. Buccheri G, Ferrigno D. Prognostic factors in lung cancer: tables and comments. Eur Respir J. 1994;7:1350–1364.

185. Sorensen JB, Badsberg JH, Olsen J. Prognostic factors in inoperable adenocarcinoma of the lung: a multivariate regression analysis of 259 patients. Cancer Res. 1989;49:5748–5754.

186. Verger E, Salamero M, Conill C. Can Karnofsky performance status be transformed to the Eastern Cooperative Oncology Group scoring scale and vice versa? Eur J Cancer. 1992;28A:1328–1330.

187. Buccheri G, Ferrigno D, Tamburini M. Karnofsky and ECOG performance status scoring in lung cancer: a prospective, longitudinal study of 536 patients from a single institution. Eur J Cancer. 1996;32A:1135–1141.

188. Stanley KE. Prognostic factors for survival in patients with inoperable lung cancer. J Nat Cancer Inst. 1980;65:25–32.

189. Vrdoljak E, Mise K, Sapunar D, et al. Survival analysis of untreated patients with non-small-cell lung cancer. Chest. 1994;106:1797–1800.

190. Hyde L, Wolf J, McCracken S, et al. Natural course of inoperable lung cancer. Chest. 1973;64:309–312.

191. Roswit B, Patno ME, Rapp R, et al. The survival of patients with inoperable lung cancer: a large-scale randomized study of radiation therapy versus placebo. Radiology. 1968;90:688–697.

192. Reinfuss M, Skolyszewski J, Kowalska T, et al. Palliative radiotherapy in asymptomatic patients with locally advanced, unresectable, non–small cell lung cancer. Strahlenther Onkol. 1993;169:709–715.

193. Wellons HA Jr, Johnson G Jr, Benson WR, et al. Prognostic factors in malignant tumors of the lung: an analysis of 582 cases. Ann Thorac Surg. 1968;5:228–235.

194. Leung WT, Shiu WCT, Pang JCK, et al. Combined chemotherapy and radiotherapy versus best supportive care in the treatment of inoperable non-small-cell lung cancer. Oncology. 1992;49:321–326.

195. Paul A, Marelli D, Wilson JAS, et al. Does the surgical trauma of "exploratory thoractomy" affect survival of patients with bronchogenic carcinoma? Can J Surg. 1989;32:322–327.

196. Barbone F, Bovenzi M, Cavallieri F, et al. Cigarette smoking and histologic type of lung cancer in men. Chest. 1997;112:1474–1479.

197. Fry WA, Menck HR, Winchester DP. The National Cancer Data Base report on lung cancer. Cancer. 1996;77:1947–1955.

198. American Joint Commission for Cancer. AJCC Cancer Staging Handbook. 5th ed. Philadelphia, Pa: Lippincott-Raven; 1998.

199. Zubrod CG, Schneiderman M, Frei E III, et al. Appraisal of methods for the study of chemotherapy of cancer in man: comparative therapeutic trial of nitrogen mustard and triethylene thiophosphoramide. J Chron Dis. 1960;11:7–33.

200. Karnofsky DA, Bruchenal JH. The clinical evaluation of chemotherapeutic agents in cancer. In: Macleod CM, ed. Evaluation of Chemotherapeutic Agents. New York, NY: Columbia University Press; 1949:199–205.

201. Donehower RC, Abeloff MD, Perry MC. Chemotherapy. In: Abeloff MD, Armitage JO, Lichter AS, et al, eds. Clinical Oncology. New York, NY: Churchill Livingstone; 1995:201–218.

202. Naruke T. Significance of lymph node metastases in lung cancer. Semin Thorac Cardiovasc Surg. 1993;5:210–218.

CLINICAL PRESENTATION AND DIAGNOSIS

Frank C. Detterbeck and M. Patricia Rivera

PATIENT CHARACTERISTICS
  Stage at Presentation
  Age
  Comorbid Illness
  Performance Status
  Care Received

CLINICAL PRESENTATION
  Symptoms
  Radiographic Presentation

DIFFERENTIAL DIAGNOSIS

GENERAL APPROACH TO DIAGNOSIS

DIAGNOSIS OF PRIMARY TUMOR
  Solitary Pulmonary Nodule
  Growth Rate
  Sputum Cytology
  Bronchoscopy
  Transthoracic Needle Aspiration
  Positron-Emission Tomography
    Scanning

  Thoracoscopy

CELL TYPE ACCURACY

SCREENING AND EARLY DETECTION
  Sputum and Chest Radiograph
  Screening With Chest Computed
    Tomography
  Fluorescence Bronchoscopy
  Detection of Genetic Changes

EDITORS' COMMENTS

PATIENT CHARACTERISTICS

Stage at Presentation

At the time of presentation, it is most useful to consider the *clinical* stage, because a pathologic stage is not yet available. The only large population-based series reporting such data for patients with non–small cell lung cancer (NSCLC) comes from a prospective study of 3937 patients registered in Germany from 1984 to 1990.[1] Approximately one third of patients with NSCLC presented with stage IV disease, and nearly half (44%) presented with stage III tumors, as shown in Figure 4–1.[1] This study used the 1986 staging system, which did not divide stages I and II into a and b subsets. This data was corroborated by a large study from the United States involving 55% of all new cases of lung cancer reported to the National Cancer Data Base (NCDB) in 1992. In this study, 38% were found to be stage IV; 31% stage IIIa,b; 7% stage II; and 24% stage I (using the 1986 staging system) among the 62 392 NSCLC patients for whom stage data was available.[2] However, it must be noted that for approximately 20% of the NSCLC cases registered, no stage data was available, and that this study used a combination of pathologic and clinical stage. Data from 3973 patients from Japan has also shown similar results: stage IV, 39%; stage III, 36%; stage II, 5%; and stage I, 20% (based on the 1978 International Union Against Cancer [UICC] staging system).[3]

Small cell lung cancer (SCLC) accounts for approximately 20% of all lung cancers (see Table 3–6). Fifty-seven percent of 11 506 patients with SCLC were found to have stage IV disease (which is extensive stage by defini-

tion) in the large 1992 series of patients reported to the NCDB mentioned earlier.[2] This series reported results by TNM stage even for patients with SCLC and used the 1986 staging system. Stage I tumors were seen in 7%, stage II in 4%, and stage III in 30%. However, in 22% of the 14 722 reported cases of SCLC, data on the TNM stage was not provided. These results are similar to results from several other series of SCLC patients, in which approximately 40% were found to have limited stage and 60% extensive stage disease (see Table 6–1).

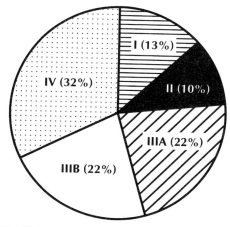

FIGURE 4–1. Clinical stage at presentation of 3823 non–small cell lung cancer patients. (Data from Bülzebruck H, Bopp R, Drings P, et al. New aspects in the staging of lung cancer: prospective validation of the International Union Against Cancer TNM classification. Cancer. 1992;70:1102–1110.[1])

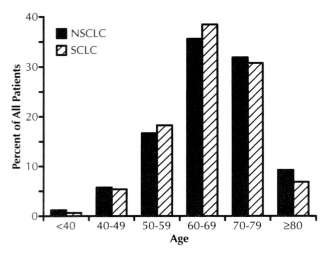

FIGURE 4–2. Age of 92 182 patients at the time of diagnosis of non–small cell and small cell lung cancer from the National Cancer Data Base in 1992. (Data from Fry WA, Menck HR, Winchester DP. The National Cancer Data Base report on lung cancer. Cancer. 1996;77:1947–1955.[2])

Age

The average age of all patients with lung cancer in current population-based series is consistently reported to be 66 or 67.[2,4,5] The reported average age in studies focusing on treated patients is slightly lower, being reported as 61 to 64 in several large series.[5–11] A graph of the age distribution of patients from the largest series is shown in Figure 4–2. However, it is important to remember that the incidence of lung cancer rises linearly with age (see Fig. 3–7B). The reason that fewer patients with lung cancer are seen in the older age groups (>80 years) is that the number of people who reach these age groups diminishes markedly. There is no difference between the ages of patients with NSCLC and those with SCLC.

Comorbid Illness

Little data has been published on the incidence of comorbid illnesses in patients with newly diagnosed lung cancer. The

true assessment of comorbid conditions must come from population-based studies because it is likely that sicker patients will not be referred to centers for diagnosis and possible treatment. One population-based study prospectively collected such data on 3864 patients in the Netherlands who were diagnosed with lung cancer in 1993–1995.[5] This study included an internal audit of data accuracy, which resulted in some modifications of the data and the collection methods. Approximately two-thirds of patients had at least one comorbid condition (60% if <70 years old, 76% if ≥70 years old), as shown in Table 4–1. Cardiovascular conditions were less common in women, and the incidence of specific comorbid conditions was slightly higher in patients >70 years of age. No striking differences were found in the incidence of comorbidities among patients with different histologic types of lung cancer.

The issue, of course, is the frequency of other medical illnesses that would alter the treatment of the lung cancer. Conditions that would likely affect treatment choices include poor functional status, a stroke resulting in a major impairment, lifestyle-limiting chronic obstructive pulmonary disease (COPD), significantly impaired cardiac function or evidence of significant myocardial ischemia, and poor hepatic or renal function. Unfortunately, the incidence of such factors cannot be readily discerned from the data in Table 4–1 because no definition of some conditions (eg, COPD) was provided, and other groups of comorbidities included conditions that would be unlikely to affect the patient's suitability for treatment provided he or she was stable (eg, an abdominal aneurysm or claudication).

Performance Status

A patient's performance status (PS) has been found to be a major prognostic factor, ranking second only to disease stage in patients with lung cancer, as discussed in Chapter 3. This is logical because a declining PS appears to correlate with the extent of cancer that is present.[12] Furthermore, most of the comorbid conditions that are severe enough to affect a patient's suitability for a particular treatment could be expected to affect the PS as well. As a result, the PS may serve as an overall marker of illness severity due to

TABLE 4–1. INCIDENCE OF COMORBID CONDITIONS IN A POPULATION-BASED REGISTRY OF PATIENTS WITH LUNG CANCER (%)

	AGE <70 y			AGE >70 y			ALL PATIENTS
	Male	Female	All	Male	Female	All	
No comorbidity	36	44	**37**	22	25	**23**	31
Cardiovascular	21	9	**19**	31	22	**29**	23
Chronic obstructive pulmonary disease	19	17	**19**	29	19	**27**	22
Cerebrovascular accident (stroke)	3	2	**3**	7	5	**7**	5
Other cancer	11	17	**12**	18	14	**17**	14
Hypertension	10	11	**10**	12	21	**14**	12
Diabetes mellitus	6	5	**6**	8	15	**9**	7
Other	7	5	**7**	10	10	**10**	8
Unknown	9	7	**9**	7	6	**7**	8

Inclusion criterion: Only published population-based study of comorbid conditions in patients with lung cancer.

Data from Janssen-Heijnen MLG, Schipper RM, Razenberg PPA, et al. Prevalence of co-morbidity in lung cancer patients and its relationship with treatment: a population-based study. Lung Cancer. 1998;21:105–113.[4]

TABLE 4–2. PERFORMANCE STATUS AT THE TIME OF DIAGNOSIS OF PATIENTS WITH LUNG CANCER

STUDY	STAGE	YEARS OF STUDY	N	KARNOFSKY PERFORMANCE STATUS (% OF PATIENTS)					WEIGHT LOSS	
				100	80–90	60–70	40–50	≤50	>5%	>10%
Pater and Loeb[208] [a]	All[b]	1965–74	651	8	———71———		———21———		34[c]	13[c]
Chute et al[12]	Extensive	1973–76	943	———80———			———20———		—	—
Lanzotti et al[209]	Extensive	1972	187	0.5	62	21	10	6	48	29
Chute et al[12]	Limited	1973–76	537	———92———			———8———		—	—
Lanzotti et al[209]	Limited	1972	129	5	86	9	—	—	39	20

Inclusion criteria: Population-based or regional tumor registry studies that prospectively recorded performance status data in >250 patients. All studies involved both small cell and non–small cell lung cancer.
[a]Zubrod scale.
[b]Stage distribution: 32% stage I, 32% stage II,III, 36% stage IV.
[c]Recorded as absolute weight loss of >10 or >20 lb.

either the lung cancer itself or to the effect of comorbid conditions.

Data from tumor registries that prospectively recorded PS is shown in Table 4–2. In studies involving patients with extensive stage disease, approximately 60% are PS 0 or 1, 20% are PS 2, and 20% are PS 3,4. Among patients with limited disease, approximately 80% are PS 0 or 1, 10% are PS 2, and 10% are PS 3,4. Approximately 40% of patients of all stages have lost more than 5% of their body weight, and 20% have lost more than 10%. The data from a large series of patients who were placed on chemotherapy treatment protocols (80% stage IV) shows a similar distribution of PS and weight loss, although slightly fewer patients with PS 3,4 were included in the more recent series.[13–16]

Care Received

The condition of patients with lung cancer with respect to suitability for treatment can be estimated by examining the therapy they receive. The largest amount of data from a population-based series comes from the analysis of 92 182 cases of lung cancer in the United States in 1992, as reported to the NCDB.[2] This data is shown in Table 4–3 and represents 55% of all cases of lung cancer occurring in the United States during that year. Based on data presented in this book and published clinical guidelines,[17,18] it can be argued that optimal treatment of NSCLC should include surgery for stages I and II, chemotherapy and radiotherapy (RT) for stage III (except in a subset for whom surgery may be appropriate), and chemotherapy for stage IV. Optimal treatment for patients with both limited and extensive stage SCLC should include chemotherapy. Application of this reasoning to the data in Table 4–3 suggests that 34% to 73% of patients with NSCLC and 21% to 32% of patients with SCLC received suboptimal treatment.[2]

Estimates from data regarding patients' conditions at presentation are crude at best. For example, the reported data is not detailed enough to allow differentiation of definitive radiation of a primary tumor versus palliation of a metastasis that appeared 6 months after diagnosis of a stage III NSCLC. Furthermore, because no data was col-

TABLE 4–3. TREATMENT OF NON–SMALL CELL AND SMALL CELL LUNG CANCER BY STAGE (%)[a]

STAGE	N	SURG	SURG +RT	RT	CHEMO +RT	CHEMO	OTHER	NONE	SUBOPTIMAL[b]
NSCLC									
I	14 717	62	4	(19)	(2)	(1)	(2)	(10)	34
II	4 368	36	24	(20)	(4)	(2)	(6)	(9)	40
III	19 404	8	9	(42)	15	(7)	(5)	(15)	68
IV	23 598	3	(5)	(41)	16	11	(3)	(22)	73
SCLC									
I	996	(6)	—	(5)	35	33	(9)	(12)	32
II	433	(4)	—	(5)	37	31	(12)	(11)	32
III	3497	(1)	—	(6)	45	35	(3)	(11)	21
IV	6552	(1)	—	(8)	29	44	(3)	(16)	28

Inclusion criterion: Largest study of cancer treatment by stage.
[a]Numbers given are the percentage of patients in a particular stage given the treatments listed. Data taken from the National Cancer Data Base report of 92 182 new cases of lung cancer in 1992 (comprising 55% of newly diagnosed cases of lung cancer in the United States in 1992). Stage 0 and cases with unknown staging are excluded.
[b]Suboptimal, suboptimal treatment. Suboptimal treatments are indicated by italics in parentheses. The total percentage of suboptimal treatment is listed in this column.
Chemo, chemotherapy; NSCLC, non–small cell lung cancer; RT, radiotherapy; SCLC, small cell lung cancer; Surg, surgery.
Data from Fry WA, Menck HR, Winchester DP. The National Cancer Data Base report on lung cancer. Cancer. 1996;77:1947–1955.[2]

TABLE 4–4. PREVALENCE OF SYMPTOMS AT PRESENTATION IN 446 PATIENTS WITH NON–SMALL CELL LUNG CANCER

SYMPTOM	%
Cough	46
Weight loss	32
Dyspnea	30
Chest pain	30
Hemoptysis	27
Fever	28
Asymptomatic	15

Inclusion criterion: Selected study of symptoms at presentation.
From Huhti E, Sutinen S, Reinilä A, et al. Lung cancer in a defined geographical area: history and histological types. Thorax. 1980;35:660–667.[24]

lected on PS or comorbid illnesses, it is unclear how often so-called "suboptimal" treatment may have been appropriate because of the patient's condition and how often this treatment was a reflection of nihilism or poor access to optimal care. However, the data regarding the incidence of a poor PS, discussed earlier, suggests that this factor alone cannot account for the number of patients receiving so-called "suboptimal" treatment. The presence of comorbid conditions also does not appear to justify the rate of suboptimal treatment. In the study from the Netherlands, the presence of comorbid conditions was found to correlate with less surgical resection in localized NSCLC but to have little influence on the selection of therapy in nonlocalized NSCLC or in SCLC.[4]

Several studies have suggested that attitudes and experience as well as social and financial factors play a major role in differences in the care patients receive.[2,19–23] The 1992 NCDB analysis found that less aggressive care correlated with treatment at a smaller hospital, treatment at a non–academic or non–cancer center institution, lower economic class, minority ethnicity, and increasing age (by decade >50 years).[2] These factors, some of which may be interrelated, were associated primarily with less aggressive treatment of patients with NSCLC (less surgery, chemotherapy, or chemoradiotherapy).[2] Several other studies have

indicated that access to centers that provide specialized care for patients with lung cancer[19–21] and socioeconomic status[22] are major factors in the care received and the eventual outcome. The study from the Netherlands found that increasing patient age (>70 years) was the only factor found by multivariate analysis to be associated with less aggressive treatment of nonlocalized NSCLC and SCLC (and not with comorbid illness).[4] Other studies have also suggested that age is a major factor associated with less aggressive treatment of patients with lung cancer.[19,23] Taken together, this data suggests that suboptimal treatment is more often a reflection of a nonaggressive approach on the part of the physicians involved as well as age and socioeconomic factors and is less often due to the presence of true markers of poor patient condition.

CLINICAL PRESENTATION

Symptoms

The number of patients with NSCLC who have no symptoms at the time of presentation varies from 2% to 15%.[12,24,25] Common symptoms from a contemporary series are shown in Table 4–4. Between one-third and one-half of the patients have local symptoms related to intrathoracic tumor (cough, dyspnea, chest pain, hemoptysis, hoarseness).[12,24,25] Approximately one-third of patients have symptoms related to metastatic disease at the time of presentation.[12,24,25] This is consistent with the finding that 30% to 40% of patients with NSCLC have stage IV disease and 30% to 40% have stage III tumors. A similar frequency of symptoms of local and metastatic disease has been observed in patients with SCLC.[12] The onset of symptoms occurred approximately 1 year before death in two older studies involving 230 patients from the 1940s[26] and 415 patients from the 1950s.[27]

Radiographic Presentation

An evaluation for a possible lung cancer is usually triggered by an abnormal chest radiograph (CXR), which may

TABLE 4–5. FINDINGS ON CHEST RADIOGRAPH AT PRESENTATION IN 345 PATIENTS WITH LUNG CANCER[a]

FINDING	% OF TOTAL	DISTRIBUTION OF HISTOLOGIC TYPES (%)				
		SCLC	Squam	Adeno	Large Cell	NSCLC[b]
Normal	2	(0)[c]	(57)[c]	(43)[c]	(0)[c]	(100)[c]
Peripheral primary	43	21	28	41	10	79
Central mass	52	31	31	34	4	69
Mediastinal mass	38	41	19	35	5	59
Central mass only	14	22	35	37	6	78
Other findings						
Obstruction	37	34	33	28	5	66
Pleural effusion	22	34	30	32	4	66
Central and other[d]	57	34	31	31	4	66

Inclusion criterion: Only contemporary study of radiographic findings at presentation.
[a]Data from 345 patients registered in a Wisconsin tumor registry in 1990–1992.
[b]Includes squamous cell cancer, adenocarcinoma, and large cell cancer combined.
[c]<10 patients with this finding.
[d]Central mass in addition to a peripheral mass, a pleural effusion, or an obstruction.
Adeno, adenocarcinoma; NSCLC, non–small cell lung cancer; SCLC, small cell lung cancer; Squam, squamous cell.
Data from Quinn D, Gianlupi A, Broste S. The changing radiographic presentation of bronchogenic carcinoma with reference to cell types. Chest. 1996;110:1474–1479.[29]

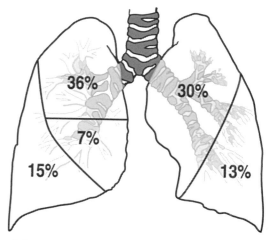

FIGURE 4–3. Lobar distribution of lung cancer among 23 730 cases reported to the SEER registries, 1973–1977. (Data from Byers TE, Vena JE, Rzepka TF. Predilection of lung cancer for the upper lobes: an epidemiologic inquiry. J Natl Cancer Inst. 1984;72:1271–1275.[31])

have been obtained because of particular symptoms. Surprisingly little has been published on the radiographic findings at presentation in cases of lung cancer since a 1969 report of 600 patients seen at the Mayo Clinic between 1954 and 1957.[28] Table 4–5 presents data from a contemporary study of the radiographic findings of 345 patients who were recorded in a tumor registry in Wisconsin from 1990 to 1992.[29] Similar findings were noted in another contemporary series of 396 patients in the Netherlands.[30] A pleural effusion was seen in one-fifth of patients in these series, which included all patients, regardless of cancer stage or cell type. Peripheral masses were seen in 43% of the patients in the Wisconsin study,[29] whereas they were seen in only one-third of patients in the earlier Mayo Clinic study.[28] Analysis of the distribution of histologic types of cancer reveals that the cell types were relatively evenly represented among central and peripheral tumors. In the earlier Mayo Clinic study,[28] most (76%) of the central tumors were either squamous or small cell tumors, and most (75%) adenocarcinomas presented as peripheral tu-

mors. The contemporary series[29] reveals that more central adenocarcinomas are now encountered, and, in fact, only 49% of adenocarcinomas involve a peripheral mass.

Approximately two-thirds of primary lung cancers occur in the upper lobes, as illustrated in Figure 4–3. In this large series involving 23 730 patients, the predominance of upper lobe involvement was seen to an equal degree among SCLCs, squamous cell cancers, and adenocarcinomas.[31] The upper lobe predominance was more marked in younger patients: right upper lobe (RUL) and left upper lobe (LUL) involvement decreased progressively from 49% and 27% for patients age 30 to 39 years of age to 32% and 27% for patients 80 years of age or older, whereas right lower lobe (RLL) and left lower lobe (LLL) involvement increased progressively from 7% and 8% for patients age 30 to 39 years of age to 17% and 16% for patients 80 years of age or older.[31] No difference in the lobar distribution patterns was seen between men and women or between whites and blacks.[31]

DIFFERENTIAL DIAGNOSIS

A pulmonary parenchymal mass may represent a variety of different disease processes, as noted in Table 4–6. A previous CXR is helpful in identifying a chronic benign condition, and the past medical history and number of nodules are useful in identifying metastatic lesions, as discussed in Chapter 31. An acute benign condition is often strongly suggested by the recent clinical history.

A detailed discussion of the differential diagnosis of a parenchymal mass or abnormality is beyond the scope of this book. Let it suffice to say that a review of the recent clinical history and of the medical and radiographic history, together with a review of the radiographic findings by an experienced radiologist, will often strongly suggest a particular diagnosis other than a primary lung cancer, which should then be pursued accordingly. The considerations in this chapter—regarding the likelihood of cancer or the usefulness of particular diagnostic tests, for example—apply to the remaining group of patients, in whom lung cancer is considered a likely possibility.

DATA SUMMARY: PATIENT CHARACTERISTICS AND CLINICAL PRESENTATION

	AMOUNT	QUALITY	CONSISTENCY
35% of patients with NSCLC present with stage IV, 40% with stage III, and 25% with stage I,II disease	Mod	Mod	High
60% of patients with SCLC have extensive stage disease at presentation	High	Mod	High
90% of patients with limited disease have a good performance status (Zubrod 0,1 or Karnofsky ≥80)	Mod	High	High
20% to 30% of patients with lung cancer have >10% weight loss at presentation	Mod	Mod	High
Approximately one-third of patients with lung cancer have symptoms suggestive of metastatic disease at presentation	Mod	Mod	High
Approximately two-thirds of primary lung cancers occur in the upper lobes	Mod	High	High

Type of data rated: Plain text: descriptive statement   *Italics: controlled comparison*   **Bold: randomized comparison**

TABLE 4–6. DIFFERENTIAL DIAGNOSIS OF A PULMONARY MASS OR ABNORMALITY

DIAGNOSTIC CATEGORY	HELPFUL CLINICAL FACTORS
Primary lung cancer	Age, risk factors
Metastatic cancer	Medical history, number of lesions
Chronic benign lesion	
Granuloma/scar	Prior CXR, diffuse calcification
Hamartoma	Prior CRX, fat on fine cut CT
Acute benign lesion	
Rounded atelectasis	Radiographic appearance, resolution
Pseudotumor (fluid in fissure)	Radiographic appearance, resolution
Foreign body/obstruction	Clinical history
Lung abcess	Clinical history
Bacterial pneumonia	Clinical history
Tuberculosis/atypical AFB	Clinical history, ppd skin test
Fungal infection	Clinical history
Pulmonary embolus	Clinical history, resolution
Vasculitis	Clinical history

Inclusion criteria: Major classes of conditions causing pulmonary abnormalities, according to the authors' judgment.

AFB, acid-fast bacillus; CT, computed tomography; CXR, chest radiographs; ppd, purified protein derivative.

GENERAL APPROACH TO DIAGNOSIS

Lung cancer is usually suspected initially on the basis of a CXR, although most patients have symptoms caused by either local or systemic effects of the tumor. Although in theory it makes sense to obtain a diagnosis before detailed staging is carried out, in reality the clinical presentation usually allows a presumptive diagnosis of lung cancer to be made with a fairly high degree of accuracy. This does not obviate the need to make a definite diagnosis. However, achieving a diagnosis and staging are usually done in concert because the most efficient way to make a diagnosis is often dictated by the stage of the cancer. The best sequence of studies and interventions in a particular patient involves careful judgment and weighing of the probable accuracy of a number of presumptive diagnostic issues.

The radiographic presentation usually raises a strong suspicion of lung cancer and, in addition, usually allows a presumptive differentiation between SCLC and NSCLC to be made. No data is available, however, to quantify how often a clinical assessment of SCLC versus NSCLC is correct. If SCLC is suspected, histologic or cytologic confirmation of the diagnosis is best achieved by whatever means is easiest (eg, sputum analysis, supraclavicular node aspiration, bronchoscopy). The distinction between limited or extensive disease is then made radiographically.

In patients suspected of having NSCLC, the method of achieving a diagnosis is usually dictated by the presumed stage of the disease. Patients with stage IV disease usually present with either constitutional symptoms (fatigue, anorexia, weight loss) or organ-specific symptoms suggestive of distant metastases (neurologic symptoms, bone pain). Often, a needle biopsy of a site of metastasis represents the most efficient way both to make a diagnosis and to confirm the stage (especially in the case of a solitary metastatic site). However, sometimes an extrathoracic metastatic site is technically difficult to biopsy. If the patient can be predicted with a high degree of accuracy, on the basis of the radiographic appearance, to have metastatic disease (eg, multiple metastatic sites), it may be more efficient to achieve a diagnosis via transthoracic needle aspiration or bronchoscopy of the primary lesion. This decision must be made by weighing the technical considerations involved in each approach as well as the reliability of diagnosing an extrathoracic lesion as a site of metastasis based on radiographic appearances alone. Such a decision is best made jointly by a radiologist and a pulmonologist, along with a medical or radiation oncologist.

Many other patients present with locally advanced disease involving the mediastinum. In such patients, a search for distant metastases should be undertaken, even in the absence of symptoms (see Chapter 6). If no distant metastases are found, diagnosis and staging are usually accomplished most efficiently by mediastinoscopy. Histologic confirmation of malignant involvement of the mediastinal nodes is necessary because radiographic enlargement carries a 40% false positive (FP) rate* (see Table 5–7). Occasionally, transthoracic or transbronchial needle aspiration is a useful alternative to confirm malignant involvement of an enlarged mediastinal lymph node.

A fourth group of patients presents with a primary tumor in the lung parenchyma with no obvious mediastinal involvement and no symptoms of distant metastases. In many of these patients, mediastinoscopy should be performed, despite radiographically normal mediastinal lymph nodes. For example, in patients with central tumors and adenocarcinomas, the false negative (FN) rate* for CT is approximately 20% to 25% (see Fig. 5–7). Bronchoscopy can be performed at the time of mediastinal node evaluation to diagnose the primary tumor.

In patients who have small peripheral tumors but no symptoms of distant metastases and no radiographic evidence of mediastinal involvement, one can be comfortable that the tumor is localized—if it is indeed a lung cancer. Although transthoracic needle aspiration can be performed to confirm the diagnosis, this does not alter management unless the clinical picture strongly suggests a specific benign diagnosis that is to be confirmed. When a lung cancer is suspected clinically, it is more efficient to forgo a needle biopsy and proceed directly to thoracoscopic biopsy—and subsequent lobectomy if the lesion is found to be a lung cancer.

DIAGNOSIS OF PRIMARY TUMOR

Solitary Pulmonary Nodule

A substantial number of patients present with an asymptomatic solitary pulmonary nodule (SPN) noted on a CXR.

---

*False positive rate is the number of false positive results divided by the total number of positive results (false positive results plus true positive results). False negative rate is the number of false negative results divided by the total number of negative results (false negatives plus true negatives). See Chapter 5 for detailed definitions.

This is usually defined as a lesion up to 3 cm that is surrounded by lung parenchyma. The issue presented by this situation is deciding when the risk that the nodule may represent a lung cancer is low enough that a biopsy is not necessary because even a moderate suspicion of cancer leads to a surgical intervention in most instances. Many factors are involved in making this judgment, including the patient's age, risk factors, size of the lesion, and radiographic characteristics of the lesion. The majority of SPNs are found to be malignant.[32-35] An analysis of 360 U.S. veterans suggested that the incidence of malignancy increased from approximately 60% in 1980 to >90% in the 1990s.[32] Comparison of other series of SPNs, reported over many years, confirms this trend.[33-37] This may be a result of the increased incidence of lung cancer, a decreased incidence of granulomatous disease, or simply a reflection of more selective patient referral. In a recent series, 53% of the benign lesions were granulomas and 11% hamartomas, with the remainder involving a variety of other conditions.[32]

The incidence of malignancy in SPN clearly increases with age, as demonstrated by the data from the most recent series in Figure 4–4A. Earlier series confirm this trend, albeit with slightly lower percentages (20%-30% malignant for age <40 years and 60% for age 50-60 years).[33,38] All series from 1980 to 2000 found that even in patients <40 years, a substantial number of SPNs (20%-30%) are malignant.[32,33,38] The proportion of malignant nodules also increases as the size of the SPN increases, as can be seen in Figure 4–4B. This is also a consistent finding among studies of SPNs. However, even nodules ≤1 cm have been found to be malignant in 30% to 40% of patients.[32,33,38] The majority of the malignant nodules in these studies were primary lung cancers (84%; range, 77%-92%), but metastases were also included.[32-36,38]

Calcification is often seen in chronic benign lesions, but foci of calcification are seen in 5% to 15% of malignant lesions as well.[35,39] The pattern of calcification in malignant nodules is usually eccentric, but occasionally stippled. Four patterns of calcification are often cited as being reliable indicators of benign lesions: diffuse calcification, concen-

tric laminar calcification, dense central calcification (all signs of granulomatous disease), and a "popcorn" pattern of calcification (which is associated with a hamartoma).[40] However, only diffuse calcification is seen with a reasonable frequency, and none of the latter types occurred in a study of 634 SPNs.[35] Diffusely calcified nodules were found to be benign in 100% of 153 patients in a prospective series as confirmed either histologically or by no radiographic change with a minimum follow-up of 2 years in all cases.[35] Unfortunately, no actual data about the reliability of the other three types of benign calcification has been reported in the last 30 years. The frequent citation of laminated and popcorn patterns of calcification as signs of benign disease can be traced back to a study of 207 SPNs published in 1957.[41] Although these patterns of calcification were found to be benign in all 40 of the cases in which they were noted, this was based on the findings of a *radiograph of the resected specimen* and not a preoperative CXR.

The use of computed tomography (CT) to assess the density of nodules has been studied extensively[34,35,38] but has not been widely adopted. Because of differences between scanners, CT densitometry requires construction and rescanning of a phantom to achieve reproducible values. Furthermore, it is not indicated in spiculated lesions or nodules >2 cm, and it fails to provide more information than standard CT in the majority of cases.[34,35] Thin section CT can be used to demonstrate the presence of fat in approximately 50% of hamartomas. This finding has been reported to be 100% accurate in one series of 28 patients with histologic confirmation or follow-up of more than 2 years.[42] More recently, the degree of contrast enhancement (>20 Hounsfield units early difference between contrasted and noncontrasted scan) has shown some promise in predicting malignancy (sensitivity, 93%-100%; FP, 5%-10%; FN, 0%) in two studies with a total of 195 patients.[43,44]

The contours of an SPN have some predictive value, as shown in Table 4–7. Spiculated lesions have a 75% to 85% likelihood of being a primary lung cancer. Nodules with smooth borders are more likely to be benign, but they still carry a rate of malignancy that is too high to ignore.

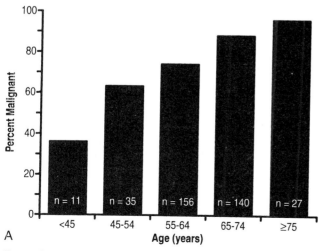

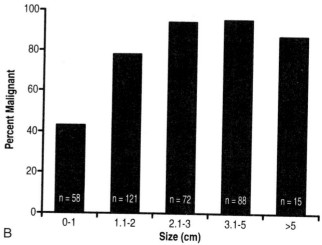

FIGURE 4–4. Incidence of malignancy in solitary pulmonary nodules by age in 360 U.S. veterans *(A)* by age and *(B)* by size. (Data from Rubins JB, Rubins HB. Temporal trends in the prevalence of malignancy in resected solitary pulmonary lesions. Chest. 1996;109:100–103.[32])

TABLE 4–7. PREDICTIVE VALUE OF CHARACTERISTICS OF THE BORDER OF SOLITARY PULMONARY NODULES

STUDY	TYPE OF BORDER	N	% BENIGN	% METASTASIS	% PRIMARY LUNG CANCER
Siegelman et al[35]	Spiculated	218	12	4	84
Zerhouni et al[34]	Spiculated	91	12	4	84
Swensen et al[43]	Spiculated	39	23	———77———	
Average			**16**	**84**	
Siegelman et al[35]	Lobulated	350	58	16	26
Zerhouni et al[34]	Lobulated	48	42	10	48
Swensen et al[43]	Lobulated	41	29	———71———	
Average			**43**	**57**	
Zerhouni et al[34]	Smooth	130	61	22	17
Swensen et al[43]	Smooth	73	58	———42———	
Siegelman et al[35]	Smooth	66	79	9	12
Average			**66**	**34**	
Swensen et al[48]	Shaggy	229	72	———28———	
Average			**72**	**28**	

Inclusion criteria: Studies of ≥100 patients with a prevalence of malignancy of 20%–80%, providing data of the characteristics of the border of solitary pulmonary nodules.

Cavitary lesions may be either malignant or infectious. In two studies (126 patients total) that analyzed the wall thickness at the thickest point on a CXR, 94% of thin-walled cavities (maximal thickness, <5 mm) were reported to be benign, whereas 90% of thick-walled cavities (maximal thickness, >15 mm) were malignant.[45,46] However, these thresholds classified nearly half of all cavitary lesions as indeterminate.

A number of authors have developed mathematical models to predict the risk of malignancy.[47–51] Many of these studies used Bayesian analysis, in which the likelihood ratio for each individual factor is multiplied to estimate the composite likelihood of malignancy.[47,49] However, a prerequisite for the Bayesian approach is that all the factors are independent of one another, which is probably not the case with SPNs. A more recent analysis used logistic regression to evaluate the role of 8 clinical and 11 radiographic factors in 419 patients, with validation of the model in an additional 210 patients.[48] This study involved patients with SPNs 0.4 to 3 cm in diameter and excluded patients with benign patterns of calcification or a history of cancer within 5 years. In 88% of the patients, a definite diagnosis was reached by histology or follow-up of ≥2 years. The significant predictors of malignancy by multivariate analysis were a large-sized lesion, the presence of spiculation, a history of smoking, and (to a lesser extent) older age, location in an upper lobe, and a remote history of malignancy (>5 years ago).[48] Although such mathematical models can be helpful, they are somewhat complex and cumbersome to use.

In summary, several studies have shown that overall, at least 50% of patients age >50 with an SPN will have a malignancy.[32–36,52] Several radiographic features, clinical factors, and the presence of risk factors affect the likelihood of malignancy in an SPN. There is good evidence that, in many circumstances, clinical judgment can predict the likelihood of lung cancer with a high degree of accuracy

(>80%) and allow an appropriate diagnostic and therapeutic plan to be initiated even before a firm diagnosis has been achieved. The converse is more problematic, however. Unless a nodule is diffusely calcified or perhaps has evidence of fat on a fine-cut CT, there are no distinguishing characteristics that predict a benign lesion accurately enough to obviate the need for further investigation. For those patients with an intermediate risk, what is really needed is a test that can *reliably rule out* malignancy. It is likely that most physicians and most patients would be uncomfortable simply following a nodule if the risk of malignancy is >10% or if the FN rate of a test to rule out cancer is over 10%.

Growth Rate

A characteristic feature of malignancies is progressive growth, which is commonly assessed using the doubling time. On average, SCLC exhibits a doubling time of 30 days and NSCLC 100 days (about 3 months), although there is a great deal of variability in individual cases.[53] Consistent with this, Nathan et al[54] observed that <1% of 177 malignant nodules exhibited a doubling time of <7 days or >465 days. In contrast, 70% of 41 benign nodules exhibited a doubling time of <7 days or >465 days. Thus, rapid growth or stability over time (commonly defined as a 2-year period) can be used to rule out cancer, but there are many practical difficulties in the actual application of this method. Evaluation of rapidly growing nodules is complicated by the fact that the life expectancy of a patient with untreated SCLC is approximately 5 weeks (see Chapters 24 and 25). Evaluation of slow growing or stable lesions is difficult because they must be observed for a long period, during which spread of tumor may occur if a cancer is indeed present, or an assessment must be based on small changes in tumor size.

Small changes in the size of nodules are difficult to detect by standard radiographic studies. A 10% variability has been noted between different observers in estimates of nodule diameter on a CXR.[55,56] Furthermore, 5% of malignant nodules were observed to decrease in size for a period of time, as seen on serial CXRs during observation.[56] Assessment of nodule size is undoubtedly more accurate using CT scanning, but issues of exact positioning of the nodule relative to the level of the CT plane, respiratory variation, and differences in slice thickness complicate comparisons made using conventional CT. These issues are very real, particularly in the case of small nodules, because the volume of a sphere is doubled with an increase in the diameter of only 28%. This means that growth typical of an NSCLC (doubling in 100 days) has occurred if a 0.5-cm nodule increases in size by 1 mm in 3 months or a 1-cm nodule has increased to 1.2 cm. These differences are not dramatic and can be easily obscured by technical factors.

One study provided exciting preliminary data that a thin section spiral CT (1-mm collimation; pitch, 1:1) *repeated after 28 days* is sufficiently sensitive to detect interval growth consistent with a cancer.[57] Even with a doubling time of 180 days, the growth of a 1-cm nodule would be detectable at 28 days, as assessed by CT measurements of phantom rods of incrementally increasing size. Growth of a 0.5-cm nodule would be detectable at 28 days if the doubling time was <120 days. This technique was then applied retrospectively to 15 patients with nodules ranging from 4 to 10 mm. All 9 malignant nodules were correctly identified by interval growth consistent with doubling times of 50 to 120 days, whereas all 6 benign nodules showed no growth or a decrease in size (diagnosis proven by resection or stability on follow-up of >2 years in all cases).[57] If this data is confirmed, early repeat thin section CT may come to play a major role in evaluation of pulmonary nodules.

Sputum Cytology

Sputum cytology is the least invasive means of obtaining a specific diagnosis in a patient who is suspected of having lung cancer. The diagnostic accuracy of sputum cytology is dependent on rigorous specimen sampling and preservation techniques. Sputum samples should be collected either after a deep spontaneous cough or after induction with aerosolized hypertonic saline. Where possible, the specimens should be collected fresh and initially examined unfixed.[58] However, good cell conservation at 4°F has been reported for up to 48 hours.[59] At least three sputum samples should be submitted because many studies have consistently shown that, of those cases in which cancer is eventually diagnosed by sputum cytology, the diagnosis is made in only about 60% after one sample is examined but in about 90% after three samples (Fig. 4–5).[59-64] The studies that reported on the efficacy of sputum cytology for diagnosis that are discussed in the following paragraphs all involved multiple carefully collected samples, and this data cannot necessarily be extrapolated to other settings. Furthermore, it must be kept in mind that most of the studies of sputum

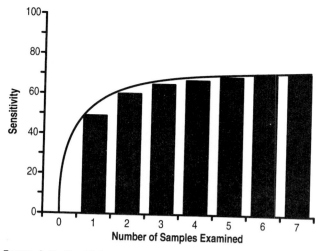

FIGURE 4–5. Sensitivity of sputum cytology in 381 patients with lung cancer, according to the number of specimens examined. (From Rosa UW, Prolla JC, Gastal E da S. Cytology in diagnosis of cancer affecting the lung: results in 1000 consecutive patients. Chest. 1973;63:203–207.[59])

cytology involved patients seen in the 1970s, when central tumors were more prevalent than they are today.

In many patients, the clinical presentation and radiographic appearance predict the presence of cancer with a high likelihood, and the role of sputum cytology is to confirm this. In this situation, the best measure of the value of sputum analysis is the sensitivity, which measures the chance that the diagnosis of cancer will be achieved when cancer is, in fact, present. The average reported sensitivity of sputum cytology for the diagnosis of lung cancer is 64% (range, 52%-92%) in the 10 studies published from 1970 to 2000 and involving >250 patients with lung cancer.[59,62-70] In addition, an average of approximately 10% of patients with cancer have cytology specimens labeled *suspicious,* and approximately 10% of sputum samples are considered inadequate. The average FP rate of sputum cytology is 2% (range, 0%-10%).[59,64,65,67,70-72]

The location and the size of the tumor can also affect the diagnostic yield of sputum cytology. As one would expect, centrally located tumors have a higher positive yield than peripheral tumors (average sensitivity, 71% versus 48% in studies of >250 patients with lung cancer).[59,62-64] A 1997 review of 21 studies confirmed this (sensitivity, 71% versus 46%).[73] Larger tumors also have a higher diagnostic yield, with the sensitivity reported to be about 80% for tumors measuring 2 to 5 cm in diameter but only 40% for tumors measuring <3 cm in diameter.[60,62] A diagnosis could be achieved in ~30% of peripheral tumors <2 cm in diameter.[62] Slight differences exist in the sensitivity among the major histologic types, but this is of little practical value in approaching patients because the histologic type is not known before diagnosis (average sensitivity for squamous cell, 70%; adenocarcinoma, 52%; large cell, 51%; and small cell carcinoma, 62% in studies of >250 patients with lung cancer).[59,62,63,65,75]

Approximately 50% of patients with an inconclusive cytologic result are subsequently found to have cancer. The studies that have addressed this have involved patients with at least three adequate sputum samples available for analysis and have followed the patients for 2 to 8 years.[76,77] The most frequent inconclusive diagnoses made on sputum cytology are either *atypical squamous metaplasia* or *atypical cells suspicious for malignancy*.[76] Follow-up of 70 patients with a diagnosis of atypical metaplasia revealed that 40% had cancer, and 68% of 135 patients with atypical cells suspicious for malignancy were found to have cancer.[76] The patients who did not have a malignancy had a variety of pulmonary conditions, the most common being pneumonia and COPD.[76] In a study of 49 patients with severe dysplasia on sputum cytology, 46% were subsequently found to have cancer.[77]

Data regarding the FN rate of sputum cytology that can be used prospectively is not available because of a lack of definition of the patient population. In several studies that have tabulated negative results, the FN rate was 8% to 27%.[59,64,65,67,70] However, the prevalence of lung cancer was relatively low in many of these studies, which presumably included sputum samples from many patients in whom the suspicion of lung cancer was low. The FN rate *in patients in whom lung cancer is strongly suspected clinically* has not been defined, but the low sensitivity of sputum analysis suggests that a negative cytology report does not exclude carcinoma in such patients. Proposed explanations for an FN diagnosis include bronchial obstruction with concomitant distal atelectasis, necrotic or degenerative cells exfoliated by advanced bulky tumors (due to poorer blood supply), and secondary bronchial inflammation associated with the tumor.[78]

Bronchoscopy

Almost all diagnostic bronchoscopy is currently done with a flexible fiberoptic bronchoscope because it permits visualization of the tracheobronchial tree down to the subsegmental branches. Various techniques can be used in conjunction with a fiberoptic bronchoscope to obtain adequate specimens for cytologic and histologic analysis, including endobronchial biopsy, brushings, washings, bronchoalveolar lavage, transbronchial biopsy, and transbronchial needle aspiration. Assessment of the value of each of these techniques is complex and depends on many anatomic and technical factors, such as whether the lesion is directly visible, the lesion's size and location, the ability to localize nonvisible lesions using fluoroscopy, and the number of samples obtained. Furthermore, preparation and handling of the cytologic specimens is important and should be done in a systematic fashion in collaboration with a cytopathologist. The value of bronchoscopy is discussed according to the location of the primary tumor because this can be estimated from the CXR when the decision is made whether to pursue a diagnostic bronchoscopy. Most studies have defined *central* as being visible in a main or lobar airway, and *peripheral* includes nonvisible lesions as well as lesions in segmental or subsegmental bronchi. The use of bronchoscopy as a tool for mediastinal staging is discussed in Chapter 5 (see Table 5–11).

The average overall sensitivity of bronchoscopy is 82% in studies involving >100 patients from 1970 to 2000.[75,79-84] However, the results are variable, ranging from 67% to 97%, and probably primarily reflect differences in the proportion of patients included with central and peripheral lesions. Recognizing this, most studies have reported results separately for central and peripheral tumors. Those studies reporting such data on ≥100 patients from 1970 to 2000 are shown in Table 4–8. The FP rate for a bronchoscopic diagnosis of cancer has been reported to be 1%.[85,86]

TABLE 4–8. SENSITIVITY OF BRONCHOSCOPY IN DIAGNOSING LUNG CANCER

| STUDY | N[a] | LOCATION | % SENSITIVITY (AMONG PATIENTS BIOPSIED, BY TECHNIQUE) | | | | | |
			All[b]	Biopsy	Brushing	Washing	TBNA	BAL
Buccheri et al[79]	708	Central	—	80	35	31	—	—
Oswald et al[64]	434	Central	61	—	—	—	—	—
Lam et al[210]	329	Central	94	82	74	76	—	—
Pilotti et al[81]	286	Central	78	—	—	—	—	—
Sing et al[73]	214[c]	Central	—	—	64	—	—	—
Zavala[82]	193	Central	94	97	93	—	—	—
Bilaçeroğlu et al[91]	151	Central	—	78	66	40	91	—
Mak et al[89] [d]	125	Central	87	76	52	49	—	—
Average			**83**	**83**	**64**	**48**		
Oswald et al[64]	435	Peripheral	28	—	—	—	—	—
Buccheri et al[79] [e]	337	Peripheral	—	75	44	33	—	—
Sing et al[73]	214[c]	Peripheral	—	—	31	—	—	—
Hattori et al[86]	208	Peripheral	83	—	83	—	—	—
Lam et al[210]	155	Peripheral	86	61	52	52	—	—
Pirozynski[101]	145	Peripheral	—	33	30	—	58	65
Zavala[82]	137	Peripheral	71	69	70	—	—	—
McDougall and Cortese[96]	130	Peripheral	62	49	36	36	—	—
Reichenberger et al[95]	103	Peripheral	66	39	36	28	47	—
Average			**66**	**60**	**48**	**37**		

Inclusion criteria: Studies of ≥100 patients from 1970 to 2000.
[a]Number of patients with lung cancer undergoing bronchoscopy.
[b]Among all patients undergoing bronchoscopy.
[c]Both central and peripheral combined.
[d]Study restricted to patients undergoing three biopsy techniques (biopsy, brushing, washing).
[e]Unclear whether fluoroscopy was used in all patients.
BAL, bronchoalveolar lavage; TBNA, transbronchial needle aspiration.

A diagnosis can be achieved by bronchoscopy in 75% to 100% of patients with central lung cancers (see Table 4–8). Direct forceps biopsy of visible central lesions is the technique used most frequently in most series, and the sensitivity of this test by itself is high. Generally, at least three forceps biopsies of visible lesions are recommended, although two studies have indicated that the diagnosis is made with the first biopsy sample in 90% of patients in whom a bronchoscopic diagnosis is achieved.[87,88] The yield from brushings and washings in central tumors is somewhat lower by itself, but these tests are often combined with biopsy. Transbronchial needle aspiration is used much less frequently but has demonstrated excellent sensitivity in central tumors as well. A comparison of biopsy techniques is problematic because patient selection, technical factors, the number of biopsies taken, and institutional experience with particular techniques vary considerably. Furthermore, brushings, washings, and transbronchial needle aspiration are often done when a forceps biopsy is technically not feasible, and in actual practice several biopsy techniques are usually performed in each patient. A comparison of forceps biopsy, brushing, and washing in 125 patients with central lesions who underwent all three procedures found that a diagnosis was made by brushing alone in only 5% and by washing alone in only 2% of central lesions.[89]

Central lesions can present as an exophytic endobronchial mass, a submucosal spread (often appearing as mucosal edema), or a peribronchial tumor (causing extrinsic compression).[90] The term *infiltrating* is also often used but should be avoided because it leads to confusion; some authors use the term to mean submucosal spread,[79] whereas others use the term to mean extrinsic tumor.[83] As one would expect, the yield is highest for exophytic central lesions and is lower for peribronchial tumors, but even in the latter case, the yield is reported to be 60% to 90% (with forceps biopsy).[79,83,91] For submucosal and necrotic

lesions, the diagnostic yield is reported to be 75% to 80% (with forceps biopsy).[79,83] Therefore, although it may be difficult to tell before the procedure which type of central lesion is present, this is of little consequence when deciding whether to pursue bronchoscopy for diagnosis because the reported diagnostic yield is good for each type, at least if multiple biopsy techniques are employed. The choice of biopsy technique for the different types of central lesions should be guided by technical anatomic factors and institutional experience because the data does not indicate a consistent superiority of one technique over another for different types of central lesions.

Peripheral lesions are defined in most studies as lesions that are not visible in the main or lobar airways, and it is not surprising that the yield of diagnosing cancer is lower than is the case for central lesions. Nevertheless, the average reported sensitivity of bronchoscopy is 70% (see Table 4–8). A few points must be noted in order to interpret these results appropriately. First, these series of peripheral cancers included lesions that were visible in segmental or subsegmental bronchi. Second, all of the studies in Table 4–8 used fluoroscopy routinely for peripheral lesions. The average reported sensitivity of bronchoscopy *without* fluoroscopy for peripheral lesions is 38% (range, 28%-56%).[81,84,85,89] The number of biopsies taken is important, with a sensitivity of 45% for one sample and 70% for six samples being reported in one study.[88] Third, few of the patients included in the reported series have had small lesions. The size of the lesion is critical, with a diagnosis of cancer being achieved in 0 to 33% of lesions <2 cm in most studies,[62,74,92–99] although one study reported a yield of 69% in lesions <2 cm using fluoroscopy and brushes.[86] The yield is reported to be higher if CT shows a bronchus extending to the lesion (~60% versus ~25%), but this is probably also associated with larger sized lesions.[98,99]

The optimal choice of bronchoscopic biopsy procedure

DATA SUMMARY: DIAGNOSIS OF PRIMARY TUMOR BY RADIOGRAPHIC APPEARANCE, SPUTUM CYTOLOGY, OR BRONCHOSCOPY

	AMOUNT	QUALITY	CONSISTENCY
The majority of solitary pulmonary nodules (SPNs) are malignant	High	High	High
Diffuse calcification of an SPN confirms a nodule as benign	Poor	High	—
A spiculated lesion has an 85% chance of being malignant	Mod	High	High
A lesion with a smooth border has a 35% chance of being malignant	Mod	High	Mod
The sensitivity of sputum cytology for diagnosing central lung cancer is 70% when careful handling and analysis of multiple samples are done	High	High	Mod
The sensitivity of sputum cytology for the diagnosis of peripheral cancer is 45% under optimal conditions	High	High	Mod
The sensitivity of bronchoscopy for central lesions is approximately 85%	High	High	Mod
The sensitivity of bronchoscopy for larger peripheral lesions is approximately 70% under optimal conditions (eg, fluoroscopy, multiple samples)	High	High	Mod
The sensitivity of bronchoscopy for small (≤2 cm) peripheral lesions is low (<33%)	High	High	High

Type of data rated: Plain text: descriptive statement   *Italics: controlled comparison*   **Bold: randomized comparison**

for peripheral lesions is not clear. In studies comparing different techniques, each of the techniques contributes appreciably to the number of patients in whom a diagnosis is achieved by bronchoscopy.[82,85,89,100] The results reported for individual techniques vary widely (eg, 33%-75% for transbronchial biopsy and 30%-83% for brushing). The variability appears to be related to institutional differences in expertise and how aggressively various techniques are pursued in peripheral lesions. Proponents of each of the different techniques report good results with their favored technique and worse results with others.[86,95,100,101] The value of postbronchoscopy sputum samples has also been controversial, with some authors reporting good diagnostic yield (58%)[102] and others reporting poor results (16%)[85,96] in peripheral lesions. A comparison of prebronchoscopy and postbronchoscopy sputum in 146 patients with lung cancer revealed no difference in the diagnostic yield,[103] suggesting that if sputum is to be added, it may be better to do it first with the potential of sparing some patients a bronchoscopy.

In summary, bronchoscopy has a high sensitivity for the diagnosis of lung cancer in the case of endoscopically visible lesions. Such lesions can probably be predicted fairly well on the basis of a CXR or CT scan, although it should be noted that the diagnostic yield for nonvisible lesions that are close to the hilum is poor, possibly due to difficulties in angulation of biopsy instruments.[96] The sensitivity of bronchoscopy for peripheral lesions is fair, at least if multiple biopsies are taken with fluoroscopic localization using several techniques, and provided that the patients are carefully selected. Poor results are seen in patients with small lesions. Furthermore, the sensitivity for metastatic lesions is lower than for primary lung cancer (~50%).[82,96,104]

The FN rate of bronchoscopy has not been defined. It makes little sense to consider an FN rate for central visible lesions because it is unlikely that anyone would not pursue a visible endobronchial abnormality further simply because an initial bronchoscopic biopsy did not reveal a diagnosis. In the case of peripheral lesions, the FN rate can be estimated to be fairly high, particularly for smaller lesions, because of a relatively low sensitivity in these settings. Therefore, bronchoscopy is not good at *ruling out* the presence of cancer. Bronchoscopy has an important role in the diagnosis of benign conditions, but the chance of finding a benign condition in *patients who are clinically suspected to have lung cancer* is low (1%).[105] A discussion of the sensitivity of bronchoscopy in achieving a benign diagnosis in patients suspected of having a benign condition is beyond the scope of this chapter.

Transthoracic Needle Aspiration

A commonly used method of achieving a diagnosis of a pulmonary mass is to obtain a cytologic or histologic sample via a needle placed through the chest wall into the lesion. This procedure is known by a variety of terms, including *fine needle aspiration, transthoracic needle aspiration* (TTNA), and *transthoracic needle aspiration biopsy*. The needle can be placed with either fluoroscopic or CT guidance, and a variety of needles and biopsy guns is available. Usually, a needle aspiration for cytologic analy-

sis is performed, but many centers also obtain a core of tissue for histologic analysis, at least in some patients.

A variety of measures to assess the reliability of a test are used, including sensitivity, specificity, and FN and FP rates. These measures are dependent on other factors, such as the prevalence of the disease in question in the population being studied. In order for published data concerning the reliability of a test to be applicable to a particular patient prospectively, one must be sure that the patient fits into the population included in published reports. These issues are discussed in more detail in the beginning of Chapter 5. With regard to TTNA, most studies have offered little description of the patient population except to report that the study involved consecutive patients who underwent a needle aspiration for the diagnosis of a pulmonary lesion. From the prevalence of cancer, however, it can be surmised that this population is probably fairly representative of middle-aged and older patients with a pulmonary lesion in whom the appearance and presentation are at least moderately suspicious for cancer.

A TTNA of a pulmonary nodule may be performed for a number of reasons. The goal may be to rule out cancer and obviate the need for further testing, to confirm the suspicion of a benign diagnosis such as an infection, or to document a primary or metastatic cancer in a patient in whom this represents the best means of obtaining a diagnosis. The reliability of the test and the most appropriate measure of the reliability of a test depend on the question being asked. This point deserves emphasis because often there is confusion about the goal of performing a TTNA, and arguments for TTNA are sometimes made using measures of test reliability that are inappropriate for the clinical question being asked.

Various measures of the reliability of a TTNA are shown in Table 4–9. The studies included here have provided confirmation of the TTNA diagnosis according to a reasonable gold standard in ≥90% of patients. Several additional studies deserve mention because of their size (650-1390 patients), even though the criterion for confirmation of the diagnosis was more lax than that in Table 4–9.[106–109] The reliability parameters reported in these studies are slightly better than the averages in Table 4–9 (sensitivity, 86%-95%; specificity, 81%-97%; FN rate, 12%-16%). A quality review of 5274 cases of TTNA from 436 North American institutions for which histologic material was available for confirmation has also reported results similar to those in Table 4–9 (sensitivity, 89%; specificity, 96%; FP rate, 1%; FN rate, 30%).[110] In all of these studies, the results of a TTNA procedure are categorized as follows: an inadequate sample, a definite diagnosis or high suspicion of malignancy, a specific benign diagnosis, or a nonspecific or indeterminate diagnosis. In general, the cases involving an inadequate sample are excluded and the specific benign and nonspecific results are reported together.

In many patients, the presentation alone leads to a high likelihood of cancer, based on the data just given concerning the radiographic appearance and the statistics regarding SPNs. In patients in whom a TTNA represents the easiest way to confirm the suspicion of cancer, the best measure of the value of TTNA is probably the sensitivity. This measures the chance that TTNA will actually provide confirmation of the diagnosis of cancer when cancer is, in fact,

TABLE 4-9. RELIABILITY OF NEEDLE BIOPSY OF PULMONARY NODULES TO ASSESS THE PRESENCE OF CANCER

STUDY	N EVALUATED	% CONFIRMED[a]	% TECH INAD[b]	RATES FOR DIAGNOSIS OF CANCER (%)				
				Prev	Sens	Spec	FP	FN
Stanley et al[112]	440	100[c]	2	73	97	97	1	9[d]
Westcott[111]	400	100	—	73	98	94	2	5[d]
Calhoun et al[116]	397[e]	94[f]	8	76	87	(100)[g]	(0)[g]	29
Santambrogio et al[113]	220	99[h]	6	62	94	99	1	11
Charig et al[211]	196	97	—	87	85	92	1	52
Veale et al[212]	192	96	—	83	78	100	0	50
Staroselsky et al[117i]	182	100	17	77	91	95	2	25
Winning et al[213]	169	100	2	75	77	100	0	40
Thornbury et al[115]	162	100	—	55	72	98	1	47
Greene et al[214]	143	95[j]	2	83	97	96	1	12
Yankelevitz et al[215]	114	97	—	75	94	100	0	15
Average[k]					88	97	1	27

Inclusion criteria: Studies from 1980 to 2000 of ≥100 patients undergoing needle biopsy of a pulmonary lesion, reporting ≥90% confirmation of the diagnosis, with a prevalence of cancer of 10%–90%.

[a]Confirmed by gold standard, consisting of surgical biopsy, definite cancer on fine-needle aspiration, and follow-up of ≥1 year.

[b]Technically inadequate biopsy (either unable to be performed or inadequate cytological sample as assessed by cytopathologist). These patients were not considered evaluable and were excluded from calculations of results, except as indicated.

[c]A few patients followed for only 9 months.

[d]Biopsy repeated if not demonstrating cancer.

[e]Reported by number of biopsies, not patients; included technically inadequate samples in the calculated results.

[f]3-year minimum follow-up.

[g]No confirmation or follow-up of positive results.

[h]21-month minimum follow-up.

[i]Included 10% thymoma, lymphoma.

[j]5-year minimum follow-up.

[k]Not including values in parentheses.

FN, false negative rate; FP, false positive rate; Prev, prevalence; Sens, sensitivity; Spec, specificity; Tech inad, technically inadequate.

present. As shown in Table 4–9, TTNA has approximately a 90% chance (sensitivity) of providing confirmation of a suspected diagnosis of cancer in patients who have cancer. Furthermore, a positive TTNA for cancer is reliable, although larger studies consistently report a low FP rate of 1% to 2%[106,107,109,111–115] with rare exceptions.[108,116] The FP rate must be kept in mind in patients in whom a TTNA diagnosis of cancer does not fit the clinical picture or the subsequent course.

In many situations, the real value of a TTNA would be in reliably *ruling out* cancer. For example, only if a test can *reliably* rule out cancer will the approach be altered in a patient who is a good surgical candidate with an SPN that may be a resectable lung cancer. In this case, the important measure of the reliability of TTNA is the FN rate. In Table 4–9, the average FN rate is approximately 25%, although a fair amount of variability is seen. Investigators in the two studies reporting FN rates <10% frequently performed repeat TTNA (on another day) if a nonmalignant diagnosis was obtained.[111,112] In fact, in one study, TTNA was repeated 1 to 5 times in most patients (73%) in whom a benign diagnosis was obtained.[111] It is unlikely that a malignant diagnosis will be pursued as aggressively by TTNA in most institutions as it was in this study. In this particular study, the FN rate of a nonmalignant diagnosis based on the initial TTNA was 30%, which is more consistent with the majority of reports. Thus, TTNA is generally not useful in ruling out cancer because most patients and physicians would be uncomfortable with an FN rate of 20% to 30%. In all of these studies, a second aspiration was often performed immediately when the initial specimen was deemed inadequate, but this was not counted as a repeat TTNA.

A number of reports have examined methods of improving TTNA results, but in general, these have not clearly affected the FN rates (negative for a diagnosis of cancer). Repeat biopsy is an exception, as suggested by the two studies just discussed.[111,112] Having a cytopathologist present in the radiology suite during the TTNA for immediate assessment has produced mixed results. One study that assigned patients by blocks of five found that the FN rate was 10% with a cytopathologist present versus 21% without a cytopathologist present.[113] However, another study observed an FN rate of 23% with a cytopathologist present,[117] and a third study reported an FN rate of 9% but also included frequent repeat biopsy (on another day) in the face of negative results.[112] Other investigators have suggested better results with a cytopathologist present, but have not provided confirmation of the diagnosis.[118] Obtaining a tissue core as opposed to aspiration for cytology alone has also not clearly decreased the FN rate. A study specifically evaluating this found FN rates of 23% and 25% with and without core biopsies, although the ability to make a specific benign diagnosis was improved.[117] Similar findings were suggested by another study, although confirmation of benign diagnoses was frequently not sought.[119] Some studies have suggested a lower sensitivity for cancer and a higher FN rate for smaller nodules (<1.5 cm).[120,121] However, another study reported a sensitivity of 93% and an FN rate of 12% in nodules 0.5 to 1.5 cm in diameter, with no patients excluded from the study and good confirmation of results in all.[122]

A specific benign diagnosis usually implies identification of a particular infectious agent (eg, tuberculosis, fungus) or diagnosis of lesions such as hamartomas or granulomas, but some authors also include lesions such as fibrosis, pulmonary infarction, and lymph node hyperplasia.[117,119] Some authors suggest that a specific benign diagnosis is reliable,[119] but the scope of abnormalities included must engender some skepticism. Only one study that has sought confirmation of diagnoses has reported data separately for specific and nonspecific benign results.[116] In this study, the FN rate (subsequent identification of malignancy) was 6% among patients with a specific benign diagnosis on TTNA, as compared with 29% for those with a nonspecific diagnosis.[116]

A benign diagnosis on TTNA is of value primarily in patients in whom the clinical presentation strongly suggests a benign etiology. In such situations, where the chance of cancer is already thought to be low, a benign diagnosis on TTNA probably further decreases the risk of missing a malignancy, especially if a plausible specific benign diagnosis is obtained. Furthermore, a specific diagnosis will guide treatment of the condition. In these situations, it may be more important to obtain core biopsies,[117,119] but a detailed discussion of the best approach to benign pulmonary conditions is beyond the scope of this chapter. However, it must be kept in mind that the incidence of a specific benign etiology of an SPN is low, being <2% in a 1997 review of 2908 patients, most of whom were symptomatic.[105]

The risk of complications with TTNA is low. Among studies reported from 1980 to 2000 that involved >200 patients, an average of 5% of patients experienced hemoptysis, but it was usually mild and self limited.[106,107,111,112,116,118,123,124] The average rate of pneumothorax in these studies was 30%, but only 10% of patients required a chest tube.[106,107,111–113,116,118,123,124] The pneumothorax was apparent immediately in 89% and within 1 hour in 98% of 673 patients in one series.[125] The incidence of pneumothorax may be higher in patients undergoing TTNA via CT guidance (~50%), in patients with COPD (~50%), and if multiple passes of the needle must be made (40%).[126] Only two deaths (both from hemorrhage) have been reported among 4041 patients included in the reports involving >200 patients from 1980 to 2000.[106,107,111–113,116,118,123,124]

Positron-Emission Tomography Scanning

Although positron-emission tomography (PET) has been in existence since the 1960s, investigation of its clinical usefulness in the diagnosing and staging of lung cancer did not occur until approximately 1990. PET scanning provides a way to image biochemical processes in vivo through the use of an almost unlimited variety of radiotracers and radiopharmaceuticals. It provides a functional assessment of cells, as opposed to merely an anatomic assessment such as that provided by CT scan or magnetic resonance imaging (MRI).

Lung cancer has been investigated primarily with the use of fluoro[18]-2-deoxyglucose (FDG). After cell uptake and phosphorylation, this compound cannot be further metabolized by human cells, which cannot break down deoxyglucose. FDG is taken up rapidly by tumor cells, which have a higher rate of glucose uptake and glycolysis than most normal tissues. More importantly, although FDG can be dephosphorylated and excreted from normal cells, this is not readily possible in cancer cells because these cells have low levels of hexokinase, the dephosphorylating enzyme. Thus, FDG accumulates in cancer cells, whereas it is cleared from normal cells by dephosphorylation and eventual excretion in the urine.[127] Myocardium and brain tissue also contain low levels of hexokinase and thus show persistent high activity after FDG administration. Although acute hyperglycemia and high serum glucose levels can affect FDG uptake, variations of glucose within the normal range do not significantly affect the quality of PET imaging.[127,128]

PET scanning is generally done after 4 hours of fasting (in order to decrease the myocardial glucose uptake) and approximately 40 minutes after intravenous administration of FDG. Images are obtained over approximately 20 to 30 minutes.[127] The fluorine[18] isotope used has a half-life of approximately 110 minutes and requires specialized equipment (a cyclotron) for its manufacture. Because the attenuation artifacts of soft tissue structures in the body are significantly reduced in PET imaging, foci of increased activity can be seen more easily than by other nuclear medicine techniques. Another advantage of PET is the ability to perform coincidence imaging, which utilizes the unique decay property of fluorine[18] of simultaneously emitting a photon in one direction and another one 180 degrees opposite to it.[129]

Interpretation of PET images has been primarily qualitative, although several semi-quantitative and more sophisticated pharmacokinetic methods have been investigated.[130–135] However, the sensitivity, specificity, and FP and FN rates of quantitative PET scanning are not different from those of simple qualitative PET scanning,[130,132,133] and

TABLE 4–10. DETECTION OF PRIMARY LUNG CANCERS BY POSITRON-EMISSION TOMOGRAPHY SCANNING

STUDY	n	% CONFIRMED[a]	SENS (%)	SPEC (%)	FN (%)	FP (%)
Sazon et al[143]	107	93	100	52	0	13
Graeber et al[216]	96	100	97	90	7	4
Lowe et al[132]	89	98	98	69	5	13
Scott et al[144b]	62	98	94	80	20	6
Gupta et al[142]	61	95	93	88	18	5
Bury et al[147]	50	94	100	88	0	6
Average			**97**	**78**	**8**	**8**

Inclusion criteria: ≥50 patients, ≥90% with confirmation of diagnosis, prevalence of lung cancer 10%–90%.
Percentage confirmed by a surgical biopsy, follow-up of >2 years, or malignant or rigorously defined specific benign diagnosis by transthoracic needle aspiration or bronchoscopy.
[b]>20% had a "specific" benign diagnosis of granuloma.
FN, false negative rate; FP, false positive rate; Sens, sensitivity; Spec, specificity.

the quantitative evaluation does not appear at the present time to be worth the extra effort required.

Since 1990, numerous studies have investigated the role of PET in the diagnosis of pulmonary nodules and masses. Unfortunately, not all studies have employed a rigorous standard for confirmation of the PET results. We have chosen to accept as a true gold standard a surgical biopsy, a follow-up of ≥2 years, or a malignant or truly specific benign diagnosis by needle biopsy or bronchoscopy. A specific benign diagnosis by needle biopsy involves culture of an infectious agent, as in the studies that have defined a low FN rate for specific benign diagnoses,[107,116] and does not include diagnoses such as atelectasis or hemorrhage, as some authors of PET studies have done. According to this definition of a gold standard, six studies are available involving ≥50 patients in which ≥90% of the patients had adequate confirmation of the diagnosis, as shown in Table 4–10. In these studies, the average sensitivity is 97%, which means that a PET scan has a 97% chance of detecting a cancer if one is truly present. On the other hand, if a PET scan is performed and found to be negative, there is still an 8% chance that cancer is present (FN rate). Other studies involving smaller numbers of patients (30-50) or less rigorous confirmation of the diagnosis (80%-90% confirmed) have shown similar results.[135–141]

Like any test, PET scanning has some limitations. Small lesions may be missed. The technology of most current PET scanners averages the uptake over a diameter of 1.5 cm, which results in underestimation of the intensity of smaller lesions due to partial volume averaging.[133] Most of the available PET studies have primarily involved patients with lesions >2 cm in diameter, although lesions as small as 0.5 or 0.6 cm have been detected.[133,138,142,143] It is difficult to identify a size below which detection is unlikely because detection depends on both the size and the intensity of uptake of the lesion. However, many studies have reported FN scans in lesions of 1 cm or less,[133,136,138,142,144] and a number of authors have stated that, in their opinion, PET scanning is unreliable in lesions <1 cm.[135,136,138,140,142,144]

One author reported an FN rate of 18% for lesions ≤1.5 cm, as opposed to an FN rate of 13% for the entire study.[140] However, in a multicenter prospective study, the FN rate was 0 for small lesions (≤1.5 cm) and 14% for larger lesions.[132]

False negative PET results have been reported in certain tumors that may be expected to have low metabolic rates, such as carcinoid tumors[139,142] or bronchioloalveolar carcinomas.[132,136,144,145] Areas of inflammation often show higher uptake of FDG than normal lung,[134] and many of the false positive PET scans have been due to granulomas or other types of infection.[132,136,138,146,147] Some of the variability in FP rates may be related to the prevalence of granulomas in the region of the study.

Thus, PET scanning appears to be more reliable in establishing a diagnosis of an SPN than any other modality short of surgical biopsy. However, it must be remembered that most patients studied had lesions >2 cm in diameter, and the results cannot be extrapolated to smaller lesions. Furthermore, whether an FN rate of 8% is low enough to make the patient or the physician feel comfortable with observation is a matter of judgment. Because the prevalence of cancer in the patient population affects the FN and FP rates, the FN rate is likely to be lowered considerably in patients who have other characteristics that make lung cancer unlikely (eg, young age, nonsmoker). Therefore, acceptance of the results of a negative PET scan may be reasonable in patients with a low risk of cancer. Conversely, acceptance of a positive PET scan may be useful in patients with a high suspicion of cancer in whom a more definitive method of establishing a diagnosis is not feasible (eg, an older smoker with severe COPD). The costs of a PET scan and that of a TTNA are comparable.[141]

PET scanning has also been used to diagnose lung cancer recurrences. The available studies are shown in Table 4–11. The average FP rate is 10% and is better than that of any other modality. The gold standard used in all of these studies seems reasonable, with most patients having had a biopsy, clear progression, or clear lack of progression over

DATA SUMMARY: DIAGNOSIS OF PRIMARY TUMOR BY TRANSTHORACIC NEEDLE ASPIRATION OR POSITRON-EMISSION TOMOGRAPHY

	AMOUNT	QUALITY	CONSISTENCY
The sensitivity of TTNA for diagnosing cancer is 90%	High	High	Mod
The false positive rate of TTNA for diagnosing cancer is 1%	High	High	High
The false negative rate of TTNA is 25%	High	High	Mod
The incidence of a pneumothorax requiring a chest tube is 10%	High	High	High
The sensitivity of a PET scan in diagnosing cancer is 97%	High	High	High
The false positive rate of a PET scan is 8%	High	High	High
The false negative rate of PET is 8% (in solitary pulmonary nodules with an average size of 2 to 4 cm)	High	High	Mod
The specific cell type as diagnosed by sputum, TTNA, or bronchoscopy is erroneous in 20% of cases	High	High	High
The error rate of a cytologic diagnosis of non–small cell lung cancer is 1% (ie, the chance that the tumor is really small cell lung cancer)	High	High	High

Type of data rated: Plain text: descriptive statement   *Italics: controlled comparison*   **Bold: randomized comparison**

TABLE 4–11. IDENTIFICATION OF RECURRENCE OF LUNG CANCER BY POSITRON-EMISSION TESTING

STUDY	n	% CONFIRMED	PREV (%)	SENS (%)	SPEC (%)	FN (%)	FP (%)
Patz et al[148]	42	100	81	97	100	11	0
Inoue et al[217]	39	87	67	100	62	0	16
Duhaylongsod et al[141]	16	100	38	100	100	0	0
Hübner et al[134]	9[a]	100	44	75	80	20	25
Average				**93**	**86**	**8**	**10**

Inclusion criterion: All studies from 1980 to 2000.
[a]Number of lesions.
FN, false negative rate; FP, false positive rate; % Confirmed, percentage of patients confirmed by a biopsy, follow-up demonstrating clear progression of disease, or lack of change over at least 6 months; Prev (%), prevalence of recurrent cancer; Sens, sensitivity; Spec, specificity.

a period of at least 6 months. Although recent radiation and active radiation pneumonitis might well cause a false positive result, PET uptake has been observed in such instances to become normal after several weeks.[148]

More recently, a modification of standard gamma cameras to allow coincidence imaging similar to a formal PET scan has been investigated.[149–153] This technique uses FDG (made in a cyclotron) just as for a standard PET but avoids the cost of a PET camera. Preliminary studies involving 20 to 30 patients with lung cancer have indicated that the detection rate of larger primary tumors is similar to that of PET, but the signal intensity relative to the background is diminished and the ability to detect smaller foci of cancer (eg, lymph nodes) appears to be reduced by approximately 30%.[149,151–153] A multi-institutional prospective study of FDG coincidence imaging for the diagnosis of cancer in 96 patients with a pulmonary nodule found a sensitivity of 95%, a specificity of 80%, an FN rate of 33%, and an FP rate of 2% (prevalence of cancer, 90%).[150] The sensitivity in this study was slightly reduced in smaller lesions (88% in lesions of 1 to 2 cm versus 99% for lesions >2 cm).[150] In a smaller study, the sensitivity was only 20% in five cancers <2 cm in diameter.[153]

Thoracoscopy

The most definitive method of diagnosis of a pulmonary nodule is an excisional biopsy, which can often be accomplished via false negative or false positive thoracoscopy. Because the nodule is removed, there are no false negative or false positive diagnoses. In two large series (≥200 patients), the lesion was able to be excised in all patients, and only 1% required conversion to thoracotomy in order to accomplish the biopsy.[154,155] There was no mortality, a minor complication rate of 4% to 22%, and an average hospital stay of 2 to 4 days. The median hospital stay is currently 2 days, and most people are able to resume normal activities 1 week after the procedure.[156,157] In series of patients with small nodules, conversion to thoracotomy is required more frequently (primarily to locate the lesion), especially if the distance to the nearest pleural surface is ≥5 mm and the nodule is ≤1 cm in diameter.[158] Techniques such as preoperative needle localization, intraoperative ultrasound, and intraoperative needle aspiration have been recommended in such cases.[158–161]

CELL TYPE ACCURACY

In addition to establishing a diagnosis of cancer, it is useful to know the cell type of a malignant pulmonary nodule. Of greatest importance is being able to distinguish a metastatic lesion from a primary lung cancer, as well as the separation of SCLC from NSCLC, because each of these is treated in a radically different manner. Furthermore, with NSCLC, the behaviors of squamous cell cancer and adenocarcinomas are somewhat different and may influence the intrathoracic and extrathoracic staging that is to be done. Therefore, the reliability of a diagnosis of a particular cell type is an issue. The pathologist has only a cytologic sample or a small histologic biopsy to examine from most diagnostic tests, with the exception of an excisional biopsy via thoracoscopy.

Recognition that a focus of cancer in the lung is metastatic from an extrapulmonary primary site is based primarily on the clinical history and presentation, as discussed in Chapter 31. It is unrealistic to expect to be able to recognize such subtle architectural aspects of a cancer as to be able to distinguish, for example, an adenocarcinoma arising from the lung, breast, colon, ovary, or uterus. Little data addressing this has been published, but what is available indicates the error rate based on small histologic or cytologic samples approaches 50%.[124] A recent history of cancer and the presence of multiple nodules predict metastatic spread with approximately 90% reliability (see Chapter 31). In the case of an unknown primary, identification of the site of origin does not usually alter the treatment or the prognosis.

The distinction between SCLC and NSCLC is widely thought to be reliable. Data comparing the preoperative diagnosis with a final diagnosis as assessed by surgical resection or biopsy is shown in Table 4–12. Indeed, the chance that a preoperative diagnosis of NSCLC is in error (ie, the tumor is actually an SCLC) is consistently low, at approximately 1%, regardless of whether the preoperative diagnosis is based on sputum, TTNA, or bronchoscopy. On the other hand, the error rate of a diagnosis of SCLC is approximately 10%, especially in the case of TTNA. The data regarding SCLC involves a total of 160 patients for whom a surgical biopsy was available for confirmation, and it is possible that the series is biased by inclusion of patients who were taken to surgery because there was a suspicion of error in the diagnosis of SCLC. However, many of the studies involved patients seen in the 1970s, when a nonoperative approach to SCLC was not firmly established, and none of the papers indicated any known or suspected bias in this regard. Furthermore, a diagnosis of SCLC was disputed in 9% to 19% of the cases by at least a third of a panel of pathologists performing independent review of patients entered on clinical trials.[162,163] At

TABLE 4–12. RELIABILITY OF A PREOPERATIVE DIAGNOSIS OF A SPECIFIC CELL TYPE

			% ERRONEOUS CELL TYPE			
STUDY	N	TEST	4 Major Types[a]	Excluding Undifferentiated[b]	NSCLC	SCLC
Pilotti et al[63]	400	Sputum	12	12	1	12
Ng and Horak[62]	323	Sputum	8	6	0.4	0
Payne et al[75]	161	Sputum	11	7	1	8
Risse et al[70]	143	Sputum	9	5	3	3
Liang[60]	94	Sputum	7	3	—	0
Clee et al[164]	61	Sputum	8	9	2	0
Truong et al[71]	57	Sputum	22	18	—	—
Average			**11**	**9**	**1**	**4**
Zaman et al[108]	241	TTNA	—	11	1	9
Penketh et al[109]	129	TTNA	35	28	0	(75)[c]
Johnston[114]	88	TTNA	36	19	1	13
Young et al[218]	62	TTNA	23	20	1	—
Payne et al[75]	66	TTNA	38	24	0	(33)[c]
Thornbury et al[115]	62	TTNA	23	12	0	14
Average[d]			**33**	**19**	**0.5**	**12**
Ng and Horak[62]	183	Bronch-cytol	8	5	0.5	0
Payne et al[75]	126	Bronch-cytol	14	9	3	0
Matsuda et al[80]	120	Bronch-cytol	13	14	2	13
Clee et al[164]	83	Bronch-cytol	13	9	1	0
Truong et al[71]	67	Bronch-cytol	22	23	—	—
Truong et al[71]	60	Bronch-cytol	24	22	—	—
Average			**17**	**15**	**2**	**4**
Payne et al[75]	254	Bronch-biopsy	8	5	0.4	0
Cataluna et al[219]	146	Bronch-biopsy	14	12	4	22
Chuang et al[220]	107	Bronch-biopsy	38	18	2	—
Matsuda et al[80]	92	Bronch-biopsy	12	11	1	15
Average[d]			**18**	**12**	**2**	**12**
Average for all[d]			**19**	**13**	**1**	**7**

Inclusion criteria: Studies from 1980 to 2000 reporting correlation between preoperative cell type and resected histologic diagnosis in ≥ 50 patients
[a]Squamous, adenocarcinoma, large cell, and small cell carcinoma.
[b]Excluding cases of undifferentiated or large cell carcinoma by preoperative biopsy.
[c]Involves ≤5 patients.
[d]Excluding values in parentheses.
Bronch, bronchoscopy; cytol, cytology brushing, washing, or lavage; NSCLC, non–small cell lung cancer; SCLC, small cell lung cancer; TTNA, transthoracic needle aspiration.

any rate, the possibility of an erroneous diagnosis of SCLC must be kept in mind if the clinical presentation or course does not fit that of SCLC.

The error rate of a preoperative diagnosis of a specific cell type of NSCLC is approximately 20%. The error rate is particularly high in the case of TTNA (approximately 30%), whereas it is somewhat lower in the case of a diagnosis made from a sputum sample. Some authors have suggested that tumor cells that exfoliate enough to be diagnosed by sputum analysis tend to be better differentiated and more easily (and perhaps reliably) classified.[164] Nearly one-third of the misclassification of cell type results from difficulties in classifying large cell undifferentiated tumors. If these are excluded, the error rate of lung cancer cell type is 13%. Thus, if undifferentiated tumors and determinations made by TTNA are excluded, it may be reasonable to base staging decisions on the preoperatively suggested cell type.

The error rate of classifying a tumor based on a small preoperative biopsy sample compared with the gold standard of a surgical specimen must be put into context by considering the rate of disagreement between pathologists about the appropriate classification of some cases. In a study involving small biopsy samples from 691 patients (approximately evenly split between SCLC and NSCLC), at least one of three pathologists disagreed with the SCLC-NSCLC classification in 6% on central review of the same diagnostic tissue.[165] In other studies of small biopsy samples that were independently reviewed by a panel of pathologists, at least one-third of the panel members disagreed about the cell type of the lung cancer in 21% to 30% of the cases.[162,163] Such lack of agreement has also been found by others.[166] In fact, even when the resected specimen was available, at least two of five reviewing pathologists disagreed on the cell type in 6% of 100 cases of lung cancer in another study.[167]

SCREENING AND EARLY DETECTION

Sputum and Chest Radiograph

Strategies to detect early lung cancer fall into two categories: screening programs for the evaluation of asymptomatic individuals believed to be at high risk for lung cancer and early detection programs for the evaluation of patients presenting with ambiguous symptoms. Because many of the individuals who develop lung cancer have a history of chronic respiratory symptoms caused by smoking, the distinction between screening and early detection is often blurred. Traditionally, the two tests thought to be useful in the detection of early lung cancer are a CXR (particularly for peripheral cancers) and sputum cytology (particularly for central cancers). In addition, newer techniques are being studied, including chest CT, fluorescence bronchoscopy, and analysis of sputum for oncogene mutations.

Before 1980, the American Cancer Society recommended that cigarette smokers have an annual CXR. However, in a report in 1980, the American Cancer Society declared that it "does not recommend any test for the early detection of cancer of the lung."[168(p205)] This change was motivated by a desire to place more emphasis on prevention, rather than by data demonstrating a lack of benefit from screening, because the results of the major randomized screening trials had not yet become available. Following this, it became widely accepted that *no* screening tests for lung cancer were indicated because of a demonstrated lack of benefit.[169] This was clearly a misinterpretation of the data from the large screening trials. Currently, however, this data is being re-examined, and the role of screening for lung cancer has become controversial.[170]

Large studies involving CXRs in asymptomatic smokers >45 years of age have indicated that a lung cancer will be detected in 0.6%.[171] Approximately 50% of these patients are stage I, and nearly 50% can be curatively resected.[171-177] Furthermore, many studies have consistently shown that the survival is better in patients in whom lung cancer was discovered incidentally, rather than discovered because of the onset of symptoms (5-year survival, 35% versus 15%).[173-176,178-180] This data suggests that screening of high-risk individuals may result in detection of many lung cancers in an early, asymptomatic stage, thereby improving the overall survival. In addition, four large studies of screening CXRs—known as the Tokyo Metropolitan Government Study,[181] the South London Cancer Study,[182] the Veterans Administration Study,[183] and the Philadelphia Pulmonary Neoplasm Research Project[184]—were conducted during the 1950s. Although the first two of these studies suggested a benefit to screening, these were all uncontrolled, nonrandomized studies and therefore inconclusive.

The results of large randomized screening studies are listed in Table 4–13. Two of these studies (the Erfurt[175] and the North London[185] studies) did not randomize individual patients but rather assigned them randomly based on location of their residence or workplace; no differences in occupational exposures were noted. All of these studies involved men >45 years of age who were current smokers, and all except one[185] accrued patients during the 1970s. All involved an initial evaluation designed to eliminate patients with detectable lung cancers at the time of study entry (prevalence cases).

More importantly, *all* of the studies involved a CXR at regular intervals in the control group. Thus these studies were really an assessment of more intense screening versus less intense screening, which was generally an annual CXR. Two studies obtained CXRs at an interval of 3 years

in the control group,[180,185] and one study recommended, but did not require, a yearly CXR in the control group.[186] In this study,[186] approximately 50% of the control arm had yearly CXRs taken. Compliance with the screening studies ranged from 65% to 94% in the randomized studies. Two studies were designed to evaluate the addition of sputum cytology every 4 months to an annual CXR.[187,188]

The number of cases of lung cancer detected was higher in the screened patients in four out of six large randomized trials reporting this data (see Table 4–13). An example of the rate of detection is shown in Figure 4–6A. A minimally higher incidence of lung cancer was seen in the control population in the two studies involving only the addition of sputum analysis to an annual CXR.[187,188] All the studies reported that the lung cancers occurring in the screened patients were more likely to be able to be curatively resected. Furthermore, the 5-year survival of patients with lung cancer was higher among screened patients (Fig. 4–6B) in all except one study.[189] The two studies demonstrating the least difference in the proportion of resectable patients or in the 5-year survival of patients with lung cancer were the ones in which both groups received an annual CXR with the screened population also undergoing sputum analysis every 4 months.[187,188]

Thus, the data from the randomized trials is consistent in demonstrating a higher incidence, a higher rate of resectability, and better survival of patients with lung cancer in the screened patients, although the actual resection and survival rates show some variation across studies. The resection rates were fairly consistent in the U.S. studies and were higher than the studies from other countries, possibly reflecting differences in patient and physician attitudes toward resection. The survival rates parallel the resection rates.

Despite the improvement in the survival of patients with lung cancer, the mortality due to lung cancer of the entire study population was consistently the same in the screened and the control groups. A fair amount of variation is seen among studies in the actual mortality rates, although the three U.S. studies are fairly consistent. The rates in other countries may reflect differences in the incidence of lung cancer. Although each of the U.S. randomized trials had only a 50% power to detect a 20% reduction in lung cancer mortality, no consistent trend toward a reduction in mortality was seen. Because the observed trends are mixed and minimally different between arms, it is not likely that larger studies would find a difference.

Several conclusions can be made, based on the preponderance of the data from these randomized studies. Intensive screening does not lower the mortality from lung cancer in a high-risk population compared with less intensive screening. On the other hand, intensive screening leads to increased detection of lung cancers that are more likely to be resectable, leading to better survival of the patients who develop lung cancer. These conclusions are somewhat at odds with one another and are difficult to reconcile. Most commonly, the differences are ascribed to biases that are inherent in this type of study.[170] These biases include lead time bias, overdiagnosis bias, and length bias.

Lead Time Bias

Lead time bias occurs if the effectiveness of treatment is the same whether the disease is diagnosed early or late.

TABLE 4–13. RANDOMIZED LUNG CANCER SCREENING TRIALS

STUDY	N	ACCRUAL YEARS	INTERVENTION (FREQUENCY IN MO)		STUDY DURATION (y)	LUNG CANCER DETECTION RATE IN POPULATION[a]		% RESECTABLE OF PATIENTS WITH LUNG CANCER		5-y SURVIVAL OF PATIENTS WITH LUNG CANCER (%)		LUNG CANCER MORTALITY IN POPULATION[a]	
			Control	Screen		Control	Screen	Control	Screen	Control	Screen	Control	Screen
Erfurt[175 b]	143 880	1972–1977	CXR q18	CXR q6	6	.65	.95	19	28	8	14	0.8	0.6
N. London[185 b]	55 034	1960–1963	CXR q36	CXR q6	3	.38	.44	29[c]	44[c]	6	15	0.8	0.7
Hopkins[188, 189]	10 387	1973–1978	CXR q12 —	CXR q12 Sp q4	5–7	5.5	4.8	44	47	20[d]	20[d]	4.6	3.6
MSKCC[187]	10 040	1974–1978	CXR q12 —	CXR q12 Sp q4	5–8	3.8	3.7	51	53	33	37	2.7	2.7
Mayo[186]	9 211	1971–1976	CXR q12[e] Sp q12[e]	CXR q4 Sp q4	6	3.5	4.5	32	46	15	33	3.0	3.2
Czechoslovakia[180 f]	6 346	1976–1977	CXR q36[g] —	CXR q6[g] Sp[h] q6[g]	3	2.0	3.9	16	25	0	26	1.5	1.7

Inclusion criteria: Randomized trials of a screening intervention for lung cancer.
[a]Per 1000 patients/year.
[b]Groups of patients randomized rather than individual patients.
[c]$P < 0.05$.
[d]8-year survival.
[e]Yearly studies advised with ~50% compliance.
[f]Based on data from 3-year study period.
[g]Annual CXR during 3-year follow-up period.
[h]Single sputum specimen.
CXR, chest radiograph; Screen, screened arm; Sp, sputum (3 samples).

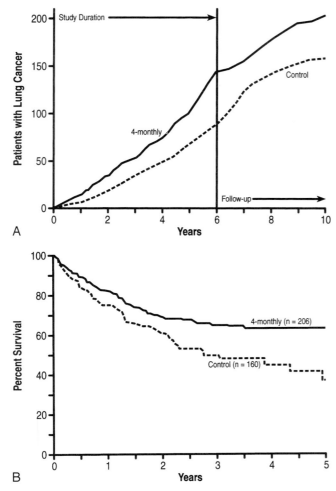

FIGURE 4–6. *A,* Cumulative incidence of lung cancer and *B,* Survival of patients diagnosed with lung cancer from the Mayo Screening Study in the group screened by chest radiograph and sputum every 4 months compared with controls, who were recommended to have an annual chest radiograph and sputum analysis. (From Cancer. 1991;67:1155–1164.[186] Copyright © 1991 American Cancer Society. Reprinted by permission of Wiley-Liss, Inc., a subsidiary of John Wiley & Sons, Inc.)

Earlier diagnosis will make the survival after diagnosis appear to be longer, but ultimately the death rate due to the disease is not altered. Lead time bias predicts that survival curves are shifted to the left by early detection but that there is no difference in the eventual plateau that is reached. Furthermore, lead time bias predicts a higher detection rate of the disease early on in the screened population, but later a compensatory increase in the control population should be seen, with the result that the final incidence at the end of an appropriate follow-up period is the same in both groups. Neither the survival curves nor the incidence curves observed in the screening studies for lung cancer are consistent with the effect of lead time bias (see Fig. 4–6A,B), making lead time bias unlikely to play a substantial role in lung cancer.

Overdiagnosis Bias

Overdiagnosis bias occurs when screening results in the diagnosis of lung cancers that are not clinically important. These are tumors that have such an indolent pattern of growth that they will never become clinically significant before the patient dies of other causes. Overdiagnosis would predict that if such tumors exist, screening will lead to a higher incidence of lung cancer and better survival of patients with a diagnosed lung cancer, but that overall mortality due to lung cancer in the population will be unaffected. In this sense, overdiagnosis fits the data observed in lung cancer screening studies. However, there is no evidence that such an indolent subgroup of lung cancers occurs except in rare circumstances (as opposed to prostate cancer, for example). The natural history of lung cancer is one of rapid death, even in early stage patients (see Table 3–4). Furthermore, among the patients detected in these screening studies, those patients who did not receive surgery had a 5-year survival of <10% (although some of these patients did receive nonsurgical treatment, including RT).[182,190,191] Finally, data from autopsy studies indicates that among patients in whom an unsuspected lung cancer is discovered at autopsy, the majority had extensive disease and lung cancer was the likely cause of death.[192] These findings suggest that the proportion of indolent tumors that remain clinically insignificant must be very small and that such tumors are not a plausible explanation for the discrepancy between increased incidence and survival and unaltered mortality as a result of intensive screening.

Length Bias

Length bias occurs when the proportion of indolent and aggressive tumors is altered by screening. It can be postulated that screening might selectively diagnose indolent tumors more frequently, whereas aggressive tumors will be discovered with equal frequency because of symptoms and rapid growth. The effect of length bias depends on the natural history of the increased proportion of indolent tumors diagnosed by screening and the effectiveness of treatment. If the natural history of the tumors is so benign that it does not affect the patient's survival with or without treatment, then the bias introduced by screening is the same as overdiagnosis bias. If the tumors discovered by screening have an impact on survival but treatment is relatively ineffective, the situation is the same as lead time bias. The third possibility is that the tumors discovered by screening have a poor prognosis if left untreated but that earlier treatment is effective. In this case, screening should result in increased survival and a reduced mortality from lung cancer in the entire population. This latter situation is actually the desired effect of screening and is not a bias. Thus, length bias results in overdiagnosis bias, lead time bias, or a true benefit, depending on the prognosis and the effectiveness of treatment of tumors that are more likely to be found by screening.

The mortality from lung cancer in the screened and control groups is similar because the increased incidence in the screened groups offsets the better survival that is seen in those patients with lung cancer. This increased incidence is the most difficult result to explain from the screening trials, if overdiagnosis is accepted as not being plausible. It is possible that the follow-up period after the study period during which screening occurred was too short to allow the control population to "catch up." The duration of follow-up was 3 years in two studies,[180,186] but it was 0 in two others.[187,188] However, the incidence curves over time (see Fig. 4–6*A*) do not suggest a trend toward a compensatory increase in the control population that did not become manifest because the follow-up was too short.

The most appropriate interpretation of the results of the randomized screening trials remains controversial and unclear. Whereas overdiagnosis may easily explain an increased incidence of cancer in screened patients without a change in the mortality, this explanation is not plausible in the case of lung cancer. A clear conclusion is also hampered by the lack of a control population that was not screened at all. Although there is data to suggest that intense screening of higher risk patients may not be better than regular screening, there is no data addressing the outcome in the absence of *any* screening tests.

In order for screening to be effective, the disease must be serious enough in the majority of patients to warrant treatment, sensitive methods of detection must be available, a sufficiently long interval must occur in which the disease is detectable and still curable, and methods of treatment must be effective. Lung cancer is certainly a serious disease, and surgery is clearly effective, although only for the minority of patients who have early stage disease. A detailed analysis of data from the screening studies has been used to construct a mathematic model of the progression kinetics of lung cancer in a screened population.[193] This model predicts that lung cancer remains in an early stage for several years. The major limitations of screening result from the limited sensitivity for the detection of early stage cancer of the screening tests used, as well as the limited effectiveness of treatment.[193] This suggests that improvements in detection may substantially alter the effectiveness of screening for lung cancer.

Screening With Chest Computed Tomography

Several groups have explored the use of CT as a screening tool to detect lung cancer.[194–197] These reports have involved low radiation dose spiral CT without intravenous contrast. CT images of the entire lung are obtained in a single breath-hold (~15-20 seconds) with a dose of radiation similar to that associated with mammography. These studies have involved volunteers, mostly heavy smokers, who are 50 to 70 years old.

Results of these studies are shown in Table 4–14. CT is clearly able to detect more nodules than CXR. Although the average size of the nodules that were malignant was 16 mm, only about one-fourth of them were seen on a CXR. This suggests that CT is approximately four times as likely to detect a nodule as CXR. The incidence of lung cancer as detected by CT was 4 in 1000 patients. This represents the prevalence of lung cancer as detected by CT because many of these patients did not have multiple scans at regular intervals.

Pulmonary nodules were detected in approximately 30% of patients.[194–196] Approximately half of these were classified as benign on the screening CT, and most of the rest were classified as benign after further investigation with a high resolution CT (HRCT). Only approximately 2% to 3% of all patients had nodules that were thought to be suspicious after further evaluation.[194,195]

The outcome of nodules not definitely diagnosed as lung cancer is not described in detail in any of the studies of screening CT. Although the nodules not biopsied were followed in all of the reported studies, the details of the follow-up were not specified. A protocol for management was defined prospectively in only one study, the Early Lung Cancer Action Project (ELCAP), conducted in the United States.[196] Patients with nodules ≤5 mm were to receive a follow-up HRCT in 3, 6, 12, and 24 months; 6- to 10-mm nodules were managed on an individual basis with biopsy, TTNA, or a follow-up HRCT; patients with nodules >10 mm were advised to have them removed by thoracoscopy.

In all of the reported studies of screening CT, few patients (average, 8%) who underwent surgical biopsy turned out not to have cancer. Furthermore, approximately 90% of all of the CT-detected lung cancers were stage I. The consistency of these findings relative to the studies of screening CXR suggests that CT is able to detect many more lung cancers than CXR, that the tumors are highly likely to be stage I, and that few patients are subjected to unnecessary surgical procedures.

In one of the studies of CT for screening, the cost per detected lung cancer was estimated to be approximately $55 000.[194] In this study, the patients (primarily smokers >50 years of age) belonged to a voluntary anti–lung cancer association that provided biannual CT scans and sputum analyses in exchange for membership dues of approximately $500. This suggests that such screening may not be out of proportion with other health maintenance interventions. However, before CT screening can be compared with other interventions in terms of incremental cost effectiveness (see Table 22–6), it must first be demonstrated that such screening can reduce lung cancer mortality. Although the data is suggestive, the experience with screening CXR is also suggestive in terms of resectability and stage distribution but has not resulted in a clear benefit in terms of mortality from lung cancer.

Fluorescence Bronchoscopy

Research in the 1980s and 1990s led to the development of a number of new tools that may lead to more effective screening, one of which is fluorescence bronchoscopy. Illumination of the endobronchial surface causes autofluorescence of the submucosa, which is less intense in areas of dysplasia or carcinoma in situ compared with normal areas.[198] During conventional white light bronchoscopy (WLB), tissue autofluorescence is not visible because its intensity is overwhelmed by the reflected and back-scattered light. The Light Induced Fluorescence Endoscope (LIFE) (Xillix Technolgies Corp, Richmond, BC, Canada) uses in vivo spectroscopy to detect autofluorescence in the green wavelength during illumination with blue light from a helium-cadmium laser (442 nm), which allows the difference in the autofluorescence of normal and dysplastic areas to be exploited.

Conventional WLB plays a limited role in the detection of premalignant lesions (dysplasia, carcinoma in situ) in the endobronchial tree. In a study of patients with carcinoma in situ detected by sputum cytology, an experienced bronchos-

TABLE 4–14. COMPUTED TOMOGRAPHY SCREENING STUDIES

STUDY	N	INCIDENCE OF CANCER (PER 1000 PATIENTS)	% CANCER OF RESECTED NODULES	AVERAGE SIZE OF CANCER (mm)	% SEEN ON CXR	% STAGE I
Ohmatsu et al[221]	9452[a]	3.7	—	15	26	82
Sone et al[195]	5483	4.8	86	17	21	84
Yasuda et al[197]	2201	3.6	—	20	38	100
Kaneko et al[194]	1369	4.3	95	16	27	93
Henschke et al[196]	1000	2.8	96	10	25	85
Average		**3.9**	**92**	**16**	**28**	**91**

Inclusion criteria: Studies of CT as a screening study for lung cancer in ≥1000 patients.
[a]Number of CT examinations.
CT, computed tomography; CXR, chest radiograph.

copist using conventional WLB could localize the source in only 29% of the patients.[199] Three studies have compared LIFE bronchoscopy to WLB in the detection of premalignant lesions, and all have found that LIFE is more sensitive in this regard. The sensitivity of LIFE bronchoscopy compared to conventional WLB for the detection of premalignant lesions was 73% versus 48% in a single-institution study of 53 patients with known or suspected lung cancer and 41 volunteers (17 current smokers, 16 ex-smokers, 8 nonsmokers).[200] In a large multicenter trial involving 173 patients known or suspected to have lung cancer, similar sensitivity for premalignant lesions was seen (67% for LIFE versus 25% for WLB).[198] The sensitivity for dysplasia was also higher for LIFE bronchoscopy compared with WLB (15% versus 6%) in a smaller study from the M.D. Anderson Cancer Center, although the rates were much lower and the difference was not statistically significant.[201] Furthermore, the two types of bronchoscopy were used in different patients in this latter study (39 patients undergoing LIFE bronchoscopy and 53 patients undergoing WLB).[201]

The prevalence of dysplasia and carcinoma in situ that was detected in these studies was surprisingly high. In the multicenter trial involving 173 patients with known or suspected lung cancer, 20% were found to have moderate or severe dysplasia or carcinoma in situ.[198] In the single institution study of 94 patients (53 with known or suspected

lung cancer and 41 volunteers), 14% had moderate or severe dysplasia and 15% had carcinoma in situ (separate from any areas of invasive cancer).[200] The rates of moderate or severe dysplasia were only slightly higher in current smokers compared with those who had quit >10 years earlier (52% versus 44%). In the third study, which involved patients with a prior smoking-related cancer, dysplasia was noted in 11% of current smokers and 7% of former smokers.[201]

The prognosis of these premalignant lesions has not been well documented because they had rarely been detected until recently. However, two studies suggest that the risk of development of invasive lung cancer is substantial. In patients with premalignant cytology noted in sputum samples, Frost et al[202] reported that 43% of 14 patients with marked dysplasia and 11% of 169 with moderate dysplasia developed lung cancer within 10 years. In a similar study, 19% of 16 uranium mine workers with severe dysplasia by sputum cytology developed lung cancer.[203]

Detection of Genetic Changes

Several new methods of sputum analysis are being investigated in an effort to detect lesions before overt invasive cancer develops. Several investigators have shown that

DATA SUMMARY: LUNG CANCER SCREENING AND EARLY DETECTION			
	AMOUNT	**QUALITY**	**CONSISTENCY**
Intense screening (every 4–6 mo) compared with regular screening (every 1–3 y) by radiograph ± sputum does not alter the mortality from lung cancer in the population	**High**	**High**	**High**
Intense screening (every 4–6 mo) compared with regular screening (every 1–3 y) by radiograph ± sputum results in better survival of those patients diagnosed with lung cancer	**High**	**High**	**High**
Approximately 50% of lung cancers diagnosed by intense screening by radiograph ± sputum are stage I	High	High	Mod
90% of lung cancers found by screening with chest CT are stage I	High	High	High
Fluorescence bronchoscopy is more sensitive than standard bronchoscopy in detecting premalignant lesions (severe dyplasia, carcinoma in situ)	*Mod*	*High*	*High*

Type of data rated: Plain text: descriptive statement   *Italics: controlled comparison*   **Bold: randomized comparison**

oncogenes can be detected in the sputum in a large proportion of patients who subsequently (1–2 years later) develop cancer.[204–206] However, these studies have been limited to retrospective analyses of patients who developed cancer and for whom previously collected sputum samples had been banked. Prospective use of detection of oncogenes in sputum is hampered by the expense and effort involved, as well as by the fact that not all lung cancers express the same oncogenes. Other studies have focused on the detection of *malignancy associated changes*.[202,207] These are morphologic changes that have been empirically associated with subsequent malignancy. The advantage of this approach is that it is amenable to automated detection by computerized analysis of sputum samples.[202,207] This would drastically decrease the cost and therefore might play a role in screening in the future. At present, however, none of these new methods of sputum analysis are even close to the kind of prospective evaluation that could lead to an established clinical role.

EDITORS' COMMENTS

The clinical presentation of patients with lung cancer is usually quite characteristic, although it is easy to dismiss many of the symptoms (eg, cough, dyspnea, weight loss) as being nonspecific or due to more common, minor ailments. However, once a CXR has been taken, the suspicion of a lung cancer is generally high. Most often, a chest CT is then obtained. Although this may not be sufficiently specific by itself, when the radiographic characteristics are combined with the history and clinical presentation, a presumptive diagnosis of either lung cancer or a benign condition can usually be made with a high degree of confidence. This does not obviate the need for further confirmation of the suspected diagnosis, but it allows the investigation to proceed in an efficient and deliberate manner. From a practical standpoint, if the chance of cancer is estimated to be >80%, it seems appropriate to proceed with a workup that is suitable for a patient with lung cancer, whereas if the chance of cancer is estimated to be <20%, a workup designed for benign etiologies is indicated. Relatively few patients fall into the in-between category, and for those, the workup is likely to proceed in a less efficient manner as various diagnoses are favored or eliminated by diagnostic interventions.

A variety of techniques are available to assist in achieving a definitive diagnosis. Selection of the most appropriate test is best done in a multidisciplinary fashion. For example, the input of a pulmonologist can be helpful in evaluating the possibility of an infectious etiology for a pulmonary mass, as well as the feasibility of achieving a diagnosis by bronchoscopy. Similarly, the input of a radiologist and a thoracic surgeon is important to assess technical factors involved in a TTNA or mediastinoscopy or thoracoscopy. Furthermore, the most appropriate test is usually determined by the presumed stage and type of lung cancer (SCLC or NSCLC). The best assessment of these factors is made by considering clinical and radiographic aspects together in a multidisciplinary discussion.

A diagnosis should be obtained by whatever means is easiest in patients who are presumed to have SCLC or who

have very clear evidence of advanced (stage IV) NSCLC. This may involve aspiration of a palpable node or nodule, sputum analysis or bronchoscopy for central lesions, or TTNA for peripheral tumors. In those patients with less clear evidence of advanced disease, the diagnosis should be attempted from the presumed site of metastasis. Patients with locally advanced or central tumors should undergo bronchoscopy and mediastinoscopy. Patients with peripheral tumors that are resectable do not need a diagnosis before thoracoscopy or lobectomy, whereas a TTNA may be useful in those who are not surgical candidates. Obviously, judgment is involved in estimating the stage, cell type, and suitability for particular treatment modalities. Each of the various diagnostic modalities has a clear role in specific situations. Unfortunately, particular diagnostic approaches are often employed in a routine fashion, without much thought having been given to the presumed stage and subsequent treatment. This is inefficient and delays appropriate care.

Sputum has a reported sensitivity of 65% overall, but the sensitivity is clearly better in central lesions (70%) compared with peripheral lesions (45%). Diagnosis by sputum cytology is not as commonly employed currently as in the past, and it is likely that the sensitivity is lower today than it was previously. This is because earlier series involved more patients with advanced tumors or central lesions. Furthermore, it must be emphasized that the reported results for sputum cytology involve multiple samples, collected fresh and processed in a laboratory with a long-term interest in optimizing the results.

Bronchoscopy is most useful for central lesions. In patients in whom the likelihood of lung cancer is uncertain, this technique can often help differentiate between an infection, an obstruction due to scarring or a foreign body, and a tumor. Often, bronchoscopy is the easiest way to confirm a diagnosis of a central cancer. Several biopsies should be taken, and brushing or transbronchial needle aspiration should be employed when direct biopsy is not feasible. However, most patients with a central lung cancer should probably undergo mediastinoscopy, provided they do not have disseminated disease. In this case, bronchoscopy can be performed more efficiently while the patient is under anesthesia, rather than as a separate procedure.

In the case of a peripheral lesion, the sensitivity of TTNA is higher than that of bronchoscopy but is limited by a high FN rate. TTNA clearly has a role in confirming the diagnosis in patients who are unresectable, either for medical reasons or because of advanced disease. TTNA may also have a role in confirming a specific benign diagnosis that is suspected by the clinical presentation. However, a thoracoscopic biopsy may be preferable because it has a much higher yield and is more definitive. TTNA has no role in patients with a lesion that is even moderately suspicious for NSCLC who appear to have limited disease and are candidates for a potential resection. Although a test that could reliably *rule out* cancer would be useful in this instance, the high FN rate of TTNA makes reliance on a negative result untenable. These patients should undergo either a thoracoscopic biopsy and subsequent lobectomy if a resectable lung cancer is confirmed, or mediastinoscopy if mediastinal node involvement is suspected.

PET scanning can be valuable in the diagnosis of a pulmonary mass, but its usefulness is limited to specific situations. PET can reliably confirm a lung cancer in patients who are too ill to tolerate thoracoscopy or a TTNA (and possible pneumothorax). However, the role of confirming a diagnosis of lung cancer in these patients is unclear because the therapeutic options are limited. The most important role of PET is probably to rule out malignancy in a patient in whom a lung cancer is felt to be relatively unlikely on clinical and radiographic grounds. The FN rate for PET is reasonably low, but it must be remembered that this applies to lesions that are >1.5 to 2 cm. The reliability of a negative PET in smaller lesions (which are much more frequent) is not well defined, but it is likely that this will change as the technology improves. In most other patients (eg, those suspected of having lung cancer who are potential surgical candidates), PET has little role in the diagnosis of the primary tumor. There may be a role for PET as a staging tool, but that is a different issue.

The appropriate management of patients with a lesion thought to have a low chance of being malignant is a major issue. A negative PET scan may be helpful, but this is only applicable for lesions >1.5 to 2 cm in size. Careful follow-up is usually done but has been limited by a poor ability to detect small changes in size over 3 to 6 months. A thoracoscopic biopsy may be a reasonable alternative to the uncertainty and expense of repeated scanning, despite being invasive. For patients with an intermediate risk of lung cancer (20%-80%), a definitive test such as thoracoscopy is generally needed, although PET scanning may also be useful.

It is unfortunate that screening for lung cancer is widely viewed as having been proven to be ineffective. In reality, the randomized studies have addressed standard screening (a CXR every 1–3 years) versus more intense screening. Furthermore, interpretation of the results is controversial, and screening for lung cancer is likely to undergo a great deal of change in the coming years. A better understanding of risk factors (eg, family history or evidence of obstructive airway disease) allows identification of individuals who are at higher risk than the population of smokers >45 years of age that was used in previous screening studies. CT can clearly detect more early stage cancers than CXR, but it remains to be seen whether screening with CT is effective in lowering lung cancer mortality and whether it is worth the price. New methods of detecting premalignant lesions not only are important in early diagnosis but also open a door to the study the development of lung cancer that could have far-reaching implications.

References

1. Bülzebruck H, Bopp R, Drings P, et al. New aspects in the staging of lung cancer: prospective validation of the International Union Against Cancer TNM classification. Cancer. 1992;70:1102–1110.
2. Fry WA, Menck HR, Winchester DP. The National Cancer Data Base report on lung cancer. Cancer. 1996;77:1947–1955.
3. Naruke T, Goya T, Tsuchiya R, et al. The importance of surgery to non–small cell carcinoma of lung with mediastinal lymph node metastasis. Ann Thorac Surg. 1988;46:603–610.
4. Janssen-Heijnen MLG, Schipper RM, Razenberg PPA, et al. Preva-lence of co-morbidity in lung cancer patients and its relationship with treatment: a population-based study. Lung Cancer. 1998;21:105–113.
5. Malmberg R, Bergman B, Branehög I, et al. Lung cancer in West Sweden 1976–1985. Acta Oncologica. 1996;35:185–192.
6. Romano PS, Mark DH. Patient and hospital characteristics related to in-hospital mortality after lung cancer resection. Chest. 1992;101:1332–1337.
7. Deslauriers J, Ginsberg RJ, Piantadosi S, et al. Prospective assessment of 30-day operative morbidity for surgical resections in lung cancer. Chest. 1994;106(suppl):329S–330S.
8. Wada H, Tanaka F, Yanagihara K, et al. Time trends and survival after operations for primary lung cancer from 1976 through 1990. J Thorac Cardiovasc Surg. 1996;112:349–355.
9. Jie C, Wever AMJ, Huysmans HA, et al. Time trends and survival in patients presented for surgery with non–small-cell lung cancer 1969–1985. Eur J Cardiothorac Surg. 1990;4:653–657.
10. Clamon G, Herndon J, Cooper R, et al. Radiosensitization with carboplatin for patients with unresectable stage III non–small-cell lung cancer: a phase III trial of the Cancer and Leukemia Group B and the Eastern Cooperative Oncology Group. J Clin Oncol. 1999;17:4–11.
11. Curran WJ Jr, Stafford PM. Lack of apparent difference in outcome between clinically staged IIIA and IIIB non–small-cell lung cancer treated with radiation therapy. J Clin Oncol. 1990;8:409–415.
12. Chute CG, Greenberg ER, Baron J, et al. Presenting conditions of 1539 population-based lung cancer patients by cell type and stage in New Hampshire and Vermont. Cancer. 1985;56:2107–2111.
13. Albain KS, Crowley JJ, LeBlanc M, et al. Survival determinants in extensive-stage non–small-cell lung cancer: the Southwest Oncology Group Experience. J Clin Oncol. 1991;9:1618–1626.
14. Simes RJ. Risk-benefit relationships in cancer clinical trials: the ECOG experience in non–small-cell lung cancer. J Clin Oncol. 1985;3:462–472.
15. Stanley KE. Prognostic factors for survival in patients with inoperable lung cancer. J Natl Cancer Inst. 1980;65:25–32.
16. O'Connell JP, Kris MG, Gralla RJ, et al. Frequency and prognostic importance of pretreatment clinical characteristics in patients with advanced non–small-cell lung cancer treated with combination chemotherapy. J Clin Oncol. 1986;4:1604–1614.
17. Ettinger DS, Cox JD, Ginsberg RJ, et al. NCCN non–small-cell lung cancer practice guidelines. Oncology. 1996;10(suppl):81–111.
18. American Society of Clinical Oncology. Clinical practice guidelines for the treatment of unresectable non–small-cell lung cancer. J Clin Oncol. 1997;15:2996–3018.
19. Brown JS, Eraut D, Trask C, et al. Age and the treatment of lung cancer. Thorax. 1996;51:564–568.
20. Janssen-Heijnen ML, Gatta G, Forman D, et al. Variation in survival of patients with lung cancer in Europe, 1985–1989. EUROCARE Working Group. Eur J Cancer. 1998;34:2191–2196.
21. Bach PB, Cramer LD, Warren JL, et al. Racial differences in the treatment of early-stage lung cancer. N Engl J Med. 1999;341:1198–1205.
22. Greenwald HP, Polissar NL, Borgatta EF, et al. Social factors, treatment, and survival in early-stage non–small cell lung cancer. Am J Public Health. 1998;88:1681–1684.
23. Guadagnoli E, Weitberg A, Mor V, et al. The influence of patient age on the diagnosis and treatment of lung and colorectal cancer. Arch Intern Med. 1990;150:1485–1490.
24. Huhti E, Sutinen S, Reinilä A, et al. Lung cancer in a defined geographical area: history and histological types. Thorax. 1980;35:660–667.
25. Ferguson MK. Diagnosing and staging of non–small cell lung cancer. Hematol Oncol Clin North Am. 1990;4:1053–1068.
26. Frost JK, Feinstein AR, Higgins GA JR, et al. Lung cancer: perspectives and prospects (NIH Conference). Ann Intern Med. 1970;73:1003–1024.
27. Feinstein AR. Symptomatic patterns, biologic behavior, and prognosis in cancer of the lung. Ann Intern Med. 1964;61:27–43.
28. Byrd RB, Carr DT, Miller WE, et al. Radiographic abnormalities in carcinoma of the lung as related to histological cell type. Thorax. 1969;24:573–575.
29. Quinn D, Gianlupi A, Broste S. The changing radiographic presentation of bronchogenic carcinoma with reference to cell types. Chest. 1996;110:1474–1479.

30. Quekel LGBA, Kessels AGH, Goei R, et al. Miss rate of lung cancer on the chest radiograph in clinical practice. Chest. 1999;115:720–724.

31. Byers TE, Vena JE, Rzepka TF. Predilection of lung cancer for the upper lobes: an epidemiologic inquiry. J Natl Cancer Inst. 1984;72:1271–1275.

32. Rubins JB, Rubins HB. Temporal trends in the prevalence of malignancy in resected solitary pulmonary lesions. Chest. 1996;109:100–103.

33. Toomes H, Delphendahl A, Manke H-G, et al. The coin lesion of the lung: a review of 955 resected coin lesions. Cancer. 1983;51:534–537.

34. Zerhouni EA, Stitik FP, Siegelman SS, et al. CT of the pulmonary nodule: a cooperative study. Radiology. 1986;160:319–327.

35. Siegelman SS, Khouri NF, Leo FP, et al. Solitary pulmonary nodules: CT assessment. Radiology. 1986;160:307–312.

36. Steele JD. The solitary pulmonary nodule: report of a cooperative study of resected asymptomatic solitary pulmonary nodules in males. J Thorac Cardiovasc Surg. 1963;46:21–39.

37. Francis DB, Zimmerman PV. Intrapulmonary coin lesions: the changing patterns. Med J Aust. 1986;144:122–123.

38. Proto AV, Thomas SR. Pulmonary nodules studied by computed tomography. Radiology. 1985;156:149–153.

39. Zwirewich CV, Vedal S, Miller RR, et al. Solitary pulmonary nodule: high-resolution CT and radiologic-pathologic correlation. Radiology. 1991;179:469–476.

40. Webb WR. Radiologic evaluation of the solitary pulmonary nodule. AJR Am J Roentgenol. 1990;154:701–708.

41. O'Keefe ME Jr, Good CA, McDonald JR. Calcification in solitary nodules of the lung. AJR Am J Roentgenol. 1957;77:1023–1033.

42. Siegelman SS, Khouri NF, Scott WW Jr, et al. Pulmonary hamartoma: CT findings. Radiology. 1986;160:313–317.

43. Swensen SJ, Brown LR, Colby TV, et al. Pulmonary nodules: CT evaluation of enhancement with iodinated contrast material. Radiology. 1995;194:393–398.

44. Yamashita K, Matsunobe S, Tsuda T, et al. Solitary pulmonary nodule: preliminary study of evaluation with incremental dynamic CT. Radiology. 1995;194:399–405.

45. Woodring JH, Fried AM, Chuang VP. Solitary cavities of the lung: diagnostic implications of cavity wall thickness. AJR Am J Roentgenol. 1980;135:1269–1271.

46. Woodring JH, Fried AM. Significance of wall thickness in solitary cavities of the lung: a follow-up study. AJR Am J Roentgenol. 1983;140:473–474.

47. Cummings SR, Lillington GA, Richard RJ. Estimating the probability of malignancy in solitary pulmonary nodules: a Bayesian approach. Am Rev Respir Dis. 1986;134:449–452.

48. Swensen SJ, Silverstein MD, Ilstrup DM, et al. The probability of malignancy in solitary pulmonary nodules: application to small radiologically indeterminate nodules. Arch Intern Med. 1997;157:849–855.

49. Gurney JW, Lyddon DM, McKay JA. Determining the likelihood of malignancy in solitary pulmonary nodules with Bayesian analysis. Part II: application. Radiology. 1993;186:415–422.

50. Edwards FH, Schaefer PS, Cohen AJ, et al. Use of artificial intelligence for the preoperative diagnosis of pulmonary lesions. Ann Thorac Surg. 1989;48:556–559.

51. Lillington GA, Cummings SR. Decision analysis approaches in solitary pulmonary nodules. Semin Respir Med. 1989;10:227–231.

52. Higgins GA, Shields TW. The solitary pulmonary nodule: ten-year follow-up of Veterans Administration–Armed Forces Cooperative Study. Arch Surg. 1975;110:570–575.

53. Geddes DM. The natural history of lung cancer: a review based on rates of tumour growth. Br J Dis Chest. 1979;73:1–17.

54. Nathan MH, Collins VP, Adams RA. Differentiation of benign and malignant pulmonary nodules by growth rate. Radiology. 1962;79:221–232.

55. Brenner MW, Holsti LR, Perttala Y. The study of graphical analysis of the growth of human tumours and metastases of the lung. Br J Cancer. 1967;21:1–13.

56. Garland LH, Coulson W, Wollin E. The rate of growth and apparent duration of untreated primary bronchial carcinoma. Cancer. 1963;16:694–707.

57. Yankelevitz DF, Gupta R, Zhao B, et al. Small pulmonary nodules: evaluation with repeat CT—preliminary experience. Radiology. 1999;212:561–566.

58. Mehta AC, Marty JJ, Lee FYW. Sputum cytology. Clin Chest Med. 1993;14:69–85.

59. Rosa UW, Prolla JC, Gastal E da S. Cytology in diagnosis of cancer affecting the lung: results in 1,000 consecutive patients. Chest. 1973;63:203–207.

60. Liang XM. Accuracy of cytologic diagnosis and cytotyping of sputum in primary lung cancer: analysis of 161 cases. J Surg Oncol. 1989;40:107–111.

61. Böcking A, Biesterfeld S, Chatelain R, et al. Diagnosis of bronchial carcinoma on sections of paraffin-embedded sputum: sensitivity and specificity of an alternative to routine cytology. Acta Cytol. 1992;36:37–47.

62. Ng ABP, Horak GC. Factors significant in the diagnostic accuracy of lung cytology in bronchial washing and sputum samples. II: sputum samples. Acta Cytol. 1983;27:397–402.

63. Pilotti S, Rilke F, Gribaudi G, et al. Sputum cytology for the diagnosis of carcinoma of the lung. Acta Cytol. 1982;26:649–654.

64. Oswald NC, Hinson KFW, Canti G, et al. The diagnosis of primary lung cancer with special reference to sputum cytology. Thorax. 1971;26:623–631.

65. Kern WH. The diagnostic accuracy of sputum and urine cytology. Acta Cytol. 1988;32:651–654.

66. Johnston WW, Frable WJ. The cytopathology of the respiratory tract: a review. Am J Pathol. 1976;84:372–424.

67. Gagneten CB, Geller CE, Saenz M. Diagnosis of bronchogenic carcinoma through the cytologic examination of sputum, with special reference to tumor typing. Acta Cytol. 1976;20:530–536.

68. Clee MD, Sinclair DJM. Assessment of factors influencing the result of sputum cytology in bronchial carcinoma. Thorax. 1981;36:143–146.

69. Laurie W, Szaloky LG. Sputum cytology in the diagnosis of bronchial carcinoma. Med J Aust. 1971;146:247–251.

70. Risse EK, van't Hof MA, Laurini RN, et al. Sputum cytology by the Saccomanno method in diagnosing lung malignancy. Diagn Cytopathol. 1985;1:286–291.

71. Truong LD, Underwood RD, Greenberg SD, et al. Diagnosis and typing of lung carcinomas by cytopathologic methods: a review of 108 cases. Acta Cytol. 1985;29:379–384.

72. Johnston WW, Bossen EH. Ten years of respiratory cytopathology at Duke University Medical Center. I: The cytopathologic diagnosis of lung cancer during the years 1970 to 1974, noting the significance of specimen number and type. Acta Cytol. 1981;25:103–107.

73. Sing A, Freudenberg N, Kortsik C, et al. Comparison of the sensitivity of sputum and brush cytology in the diagnosis of lung carcinomas. Acta Cytol. 1997;41:399–408.

74. Radke JR, Conway WA, Eyler WR, et al. Diagnostic accuracy in peripheral lung lesions: factors predicting success with flexible fiberoptic bronchoscopy. Chest. 1979;76:176–179.

75. Payne CR, Hadfield JW, Stovin PG, et al. Diagnostic accuracy of cytology and biopsy in primary bronchial carcinoma. J Clin Pathol. 1981;34:773–778.

76. Johnston WW. Ten years of respiratory cytopathology at Duke University Medical Center, III: the significance of inconclusive cytopathologic diagnoses during the years 1970 to 1974. Acta Cytol. 1982;26:759–766.

77. Risse EKJ, Vooijs GP, van't Hof MA. Diagnostic significance of "severe dysplasia" in sputum cytology. Acta Cytol. 1988;32:629–634.

78. Farber SM. Clinical appraisal of pulmonary cytology. JAMA. 1961;175:345–348.

79. Buccheri G, Barberis P, Delfino MS. Diagnostic, morphologic, and histopathologic correlates in bronchogenic carcinoma: a review of 1,045 bronchoscopic examinations. Chest. 1991;99:809–814.

80. Matsuda M, Horai T, Nakamura S, et al. Bronchial brushing and bronchial biopsy: comparison of diagnostic accuracy and cell typing reliability in lung cancer. Thorax. 1986;41:475–478.

81. Pilotti S, Rilke F, Gribaudi G, et al. Cytologic diagnosis of pulmonary carcinoma on bronchoscopic brushing material. Acta Cytol. 1982;26:655–660.

82. Zavala DC. Diagnostic fiberoptic bronchoscopy. Chest. 1975;68:12–19.

83. Popp W, Rauscher H, Ritschka L, et al. Diagnostic sensitivity of different techniques in the diagnosis of lung tumors with the flexible fiberoptic bronchoscope: comparison of brush biopsy, imprint cytology of forceps biopsy, and histology of forceps biopsy. Cancer. 1991;67:72–75.

84. Cox ID, Bagg LR, Russell NJ, et al. Relationship of radiologic position to the diagnostic yield of fiberoptic bronchoscopy in bronchial carcinoma. Chest. 1984;85:519–522.

85. Kvale PA, Bode FR, Kini S. Diagnostic accuracy in lung cancer: comparison of techniques used in association with flexible fiberoptic bronchoscopy. Chest. 1976;69:752–757.

86. Hattori S, Matsuda M, Nishihara H, et al. Early diagnosis of small peripheral lung cancer—cytologic diagnosis of very fresh cancer cells obtained by the TV-brushing technique. Acta Cytol. 1971;15:460–467.

87. Shure D, Astarita RW. Bronchogenic carcinoma presenting as an endobronchial mass. Chest. 1983;83:865–867.

88. Popovich J Jr, Kvale PA, Eichenhorn MS, et al. Diagnostic accuracy of multiple biopsies from flexible fiberoptic bronchoscopy. Am Rev Respir Dis. 1982;125:521–523.

89. Mak VHF, Johnston IDA, Hertzel MR, et al. Value of washings and brushings at fibreoptic bronchoscopy in the diagnosis of lung cancer. Thorax. 1990;45:373–376.

90. Shure D. Fiberoptic bronchoscopy—diagnostic applications. Clin Chest Med. 1987;8:1–13.

91. Bilaçeroğlu S, Günel O, Çağirici U, et al. Comparison of endobronchial needle aspiration with forceps and brush biopsies in the diagnosis of endobronchial lung cancer. Monaldi Arch Chest Dis. 1997;52:13–17.

92. Fletcher EC, Levin DC. Flexible fiberoptic bronchoscopy and fluoroscopically guided transbronchial biopsy in the management of solitary pulmonary nodules. West J Med. 1982;136:477–483.

93. Stringfield JT III, Markowitz DJ, Bentz RR, et al. The effect of tumor size and location on diagnosis by fiberoptic bronchoscopy. Chest. 1977;72:474–476.

94. Cortese DA, McDougall JC. Biopsy and brushing of peripheral lung cancer with fluoroscopic guidance. Chest. 1979;75:141–145.

95. Reichenberger F, Weber J, Tamm M, et al. The value of transbronchial needle aspiration in the diagnosis of peripheral pulmonary lesions. Chest. 1999;116:704–708.

96. McDougall JC, Cortese DA. Transbronchoscopic lung biopsy for localized pulmonary disease. Semin Respir Med. 1981;3:30–33.

97. Hanson RR, Zavala DC, Rhodes ML, et al. Transbronchial biopsy via flexible fiberoptic bronchoscope: results in 164 patients. Am Rev Respir Dis. 1976;114:67–72.

98. Naidich DP, Sussman R, Kutcher WL, et al. Solitary pulmonary nodules: CT-bronchoscopic correlation. Chest. 1988;93:595–598.

99. Gaeta M, Pandolfo I, Volta S, et al. Bronchus sign on CT in peripheral carcinoma of the lung: value in predicting results of transbronchial biopsy. AJR Am J Roentgenol. 1991;157:1181–1185.

100. de Gracia J, Bravo C, Miravitlles M, et al. Diagnostic value of bronchoalveolar lavage in peripheral lung cancer. Am Rev Respir Dis. 1993;147:649–652.

101. Pirozynski M. Bronchoalveolar lavage in the diagnosis of peripheral, primary lung cancer. Chest. 1992;102:372–374.

102. Chaudhary BA, Yoneda K, Burki NK. Fiberoptic bronchoscopy: comparison of procedures used in the diagnosis of lung cancer. J Thorac Cardiovasc Surg. 1978;76:33–37.

103. Risse EKJ, Vooijs GP, van't Hof MA. The quality and diagnostic outcome of postbronchoscopic sputum. Acta Cytol. 1987;31:166–169.

104. Poe RH, Ortiz C, Israel RH, et al. Sensitivity, specificity, and predictive values of bronchoscopy in neoplasm metastatic to lung. Chest. 1985;88:84–88.

105. Rolston KVI, Rodriguez S, Dholakia N, et al. Pulmonary infections mimicking cancer: a retrospective, three-year review. Support Care Cancer. 1997;5:90–93.

106. Khouri NF, Stitik FP, Erozan YS, et al. Transthoracic needle aspiration biopsy of benign and malignant lung lesions. AJR Am J Roentgenol. 1985;144:281–288.

107. Todd TRJ, Weisbrod G, Tao LC, et al. Aspiration needle biopsy of thoracic lesions. Ann Thorac Surg. 1981;32:154–161.

108. Zaman MB, Hajdu SI, Melamed MR, et al. Transthoracic aspiration cytology of pulmonary lesions. Semin Diag Pathol. 1986;3:176–187.

109. Penketh ARL, Robinson AA, Barker V, et al. Use of percutaneous needle biopsy in the investigation of solitary pulmonary nodules. Thorax. 1987;42:967–971.

110. Zarbo RJ, Fenoglio-Preiser CM. Interinstitutional database for comparison of performance in lung fine-needle aspiration cytology: a College of American Pathologists Q-Probe study of 5264 cases with histologic correlation. Arch Pathol Lab Med. 1992;116:463–470.

111. Westcott JL. Direct percutaneous needle aspiration of localized pulmonary lesions: results in 422 patients. Radiology. 1980;137:31–35.

112. Stanley JH, Fish GD, Andriole JG, et al. Lung lesions: cytologic diagnosis by fine-needle biopsy. Radiology. 1987;162:389–391.

113. Santambrogio L, Nosotti M, Bellaviti N, et al. CT-guided fine-needle aspiration cytology of solitary pulmonary nodules: a prospective, randomized study of immediate cytologic evaluation. Chest. 1997;112:423–425.

114. Johnston WW. Percutaneous fine needle aspiration biopsy of the lung: a study of 1,015 patients. Acta Cytol. 1984;28:218–224.

115. Thornbury JR, Burke DP, Naylor B. Transthoracic needle aspiration biopsy: accuracy of cytologic typing of malignant neoplasms. AJR Am J Roentgenol. 1981;136:719–724.

116. Calhoun P, Feldman PS, Armstrong P, et al. The clinical outcome of needle aspirations of the lung when cancer is not diagnosed. Ann Thorac Surg. 1986;41:592–596.

117. Staroselsky AN, Schwarz Y, Man A, et al. Additional information from percutaneous cutting needle biopsy following fine-needle aspiration in the diagnosis of chest lesions. Chest. 1998;113:1522–1525.

118. Conces DJ Jr, Schwenk GR Jr, Doering PR, et al. Thoracic needle biopsy: improved results utilizing a team approach. Chest. 1987;91:813–816.

119. Klein JS, Salomon G, Stewart EA. Transthoracic needle biopsy with a coaxially placed 20-gauge automated cutting needle: results in 122 patients. Radiology. 1996;198:715–720.

120. Layfield LJ, Coogan A, Johnston WW, et al. Transthoracic fine needle aspiration biopsy: sensitivity in relation to guidance technique and lesion size and location. Acta Cytol. 1996;40:687–690.

121. Li H, Boiselle PM, Shepard J-AO, et al. Diagnostic accuracy and safety of CT-guided percutaneous needle aspiration biopsy of the lung: comparison of small and large pulmonary nodules. AJR Am J Roentgenol. 1996;167:105–109.

122. Westcott JL, Rao N, Colley DP. Transthoracic needle biopsy of small pulmonary nodules. Radiology. 1997;202:97–103.

123. Berquist TH, Bailey PB, Cortese DA, et al. Transthoracic needle biopsy: accuracy and complications in relation to location and type of lesion. Mayo Clin Proc. 1980;55:475–481.

124. Simpson RW, Johnson DA, Wold LE, et al. Transthoracic needle aspiration biopsy: review of 233 cases. Acta Cytol. 1988;32:101–104.

125. Perlmutt LM, Johnston WW, Dunnick NR. Percutaneous transthoracic needle aspiration: a review. AJR Am J Roentgenol. 1989;152:451–455.

126. Sanders C. Transthoracic needle aspiration. Clin Chest Med. 1992;13:11–16.

127. Hughes JMB. 18F-fluorodeoxyglucose PET scans in lung cancer. Thorax. 1996;51(suppl 2):516–522.

128. Langen K-J, Braun U, Kops ER, et al. The influence of plasma glucose levels on fluorine-18-fluorodeoxyglucose uptake in bronchial carcinomas. J Nucl Med. 1993;34:355–359.

129. Gupta NC, Frick MP. Clinical applications of positron-emission tomography in cancer. CA Cancer J Clin. 1993;43:235–254.

130. Lowe VJ, Hoffman JM, DeLong DM, et al. Semiquantitative and visual analysis of FDG-PET images in pulmonary abnormalities. J Nucl Med. 1994;35:1771–1776.

131. Lowe VJ, Duhaylongsod FG, Patz EF, et al. Pulmonary abnormalities and PET data analysis: a retrospective study. Radiology. 1997;202:435–439.

132. Lowe VJ, Fletcher JW, Gobar L, et al. Prospective investigation of positron emission tomography in lung nodules. J Clin Oncol. 1998;16:1075–1084.

133. Valk PE, Pounds TR, Hopkins DM, et al. Staging non–small cell lung cancer by whole-body positron emission tomographic imaging. Ann Thorac Surg. 1995;60:1573–1582.

134. Hübner KF, Buonocore E, Singh SK, et al. Characterization of chest masses by FDG positron emission tomography. Clin Nucl Med. 1995;20:293–298.

135. Knight SB, Delbeke D, Stewart JR, et al. Evaluation of pulmonary lesions with FDG-PET: comparison of findings in patients with and without a history of prior malignancy. Chest. 1996;109:982–988.

136. Guhlmann A, Storck M, Kotzerke J, et al. Lymph node staging in non–small cell lung cancer: evaluation by [18F]FDG positron emission tomography (PET). Thorax. 1997;52:438–441.

137. Slosman DO, Spiliopoulos A, Couson F, et al. Satellite PET and lung cancer: a prospective study in surgical patients. Nucl Med Commun. 1993;14:955–961.

138. Dewan NA, Gupta NC, Redepenning LS, et al. Diagnostic efficacy of PET-FDG imaging in solitary pulmonary nodules: potential role in evaluation and management. Chest. 1993;104:997–1002.

139. Chin R Jr, Ward R, Keyes JW Jr, et al. Mediastinal staging of non–small-cell lung cancer with positron emission tomography. Am J Respir Crit Care Med. 1995;152:2090–2096.

140. Dewan NA, Shehan CJ, Reeb SD, et al. Likelihood of malignancy in a solitary pulmonary nodule: comparison of Bayesian analysis and results of FDG-PET scan. Chest. 1997;112:416–422.

141. Duhaylongsod FG, Lowe VJ, Patz EF Jr, et al. Detection of primary and recurrent lung cancer by means of F-18 fluorodeoxyglucose positron emission tomography (FDG PET). J Thorac Cardiovasc Surg. 1995;110:130–140.

142. Gupta NC, Maloof J, Gunel E. Probability of malignancy in solitary pulmonary nodules using fluorine-18-FDG and PET. J Nucl Med. 1996;37:943–948.

143. Sazon DA, Santiago SM, Hoo GWS, et al. Fluorodeoxyglucose–positron emission tomography in the detection and staging of lung cancer. Am J Respir Crit Care Med. 1996;153:417–421.

144. Scott WJ, Schwabe JL, Gupta NC, et al. Positron emission tomography of lung tumors and mediastinal lymph nodes using [^{18}F]fluorodeoxyglucose. Ann Thorac Surg. 1994;58:698–703.

145. Higashi K, Seki H, Taniguchi M, et al. Bronchioloalveolar carcinoma: false-negative results on FDG-PET. J Nucl Med. 1997;38(suppl):79P.

146. Dewan NA, Reeb SD, Gupta NC, et al. PET-FDG imaging and transthoracic needle lung aspiration biopsy in evaluation of pulmonary lesions: a comparative risk-benefit analysis. Chest. 1995;108:441–446.

147. Bury T, Dowlati A, Paulus P, et al. Evaluation of the solitary pulmonary nodule by positron emission tomography imaging. Eur Respir J. 1996;9:410–414.

148. Patz EF Jr, Lowe VJ, Hoffman JM, et al. Persistent or recurrent bronchogenic carcinoma: detection with PET and 2-[F-18]-2-deoxy-D-glucose. Radiology. 1994;191:379–382.

149. Weber WA, Neverve J, Sklarek J, et al. Imaging of lung cancer with fluorine-18 fluorodeoxyglucose: comparison of a dual-head gamma camera in coincidence mode with a full-ring positron emission tomography system. Eur J Nucl Med. 1999;26:388–395.

150. Weber W, Young C, Abdel-Dayem HM, et al. Assessment of pulmonary lesions with ^{18}F-fluorodeoxyglucose positron imaging using coincidence mode gamma cameras. J Nucl Med. 1999;40:574–578.

151. Lonneux M, Delval D, Bausart R, et al. Can dual-headed ^{18}F-FDG SPET imaging reliably supersede PET in clinical oncology? A comparative study in lung and gastrointestinal tract cancer. Nucl Med Commun. 1998;19:1047–1054.

152. Tatsumi M, Yutani K, Watanabe Y, et al. Feasibility of fluorodeoxyglucose dual-head gamma camera coincidence imaging in the evaluation of lung cancer: comparison with FDG PET. J Nucl Med. 1999;40:566–573.

153. Worsley DF, Celler A, Adam MJ, et al. Pulmonary nodules: differential diagnosis using ^{18}F-fluorodeoxyglucose single-photon emission computed tomography. AJR Am J Roentgenol. 1997;168:771–774.

154. Mack MJ, Hazelrigg SR, Landreneau RJ, et al. Thoracoscopy for the diagnosis of the indeterminate solitary pulmonary nodule. Ann Thorac Surg. 1993;56:825–832.

155. Mitruka S, Landreneau RJ, Mack MJ, et al. Diagnosing the indeterminate pulmonary nodule: percutaneous biopsy versus thoracoscopy. Surgery. 1995;118:676–684.

156. Hazelrigg SR, Magee MJ, Cetindag IB. Video-assisted thoracic surgery for diagnosis of the solitary lung nodule. Chest Surg Clin North Am. 1998;8:763–774.

157. Russo L, Wiechmann RJ, Magovern JA, et al. Early chest tube removal after video-assisted thoracoscopic wedge resection of the lung. Ann Thorac Surg. 1998;66:1751–1754.

158. Suzuki K, Nagai K, Yoshida J, et al. Video-assisted thoracoscopic surgery for small indeterminate pulmonary nodules: indications for preoperative marking. Chest. 1999;115:563–568.

159. Demmy TL, Wagner-Mann CC, James MA, et al. Feasibility of mathematical models to predict success in video-assisted thoracic surgery lung nodule excision. Am J Surg. 1997;174:20–23.

160. Bousamra II M, Clowry L Jr. Thoracoscopic fine-needle aspiration of solitary pulmonary nodules. Ann Thorac Surg. 1997;64:1191–1193.

161. Wicky S, Mayor B, Cuttat J-F, et al. CT-guided localizations of pulmonary nodules with methylene blue injections for thoracoscopic resections. Chest. 1994;106:1326–1328.

162. Thomas JSJ, Lamb D, Ashcroft T, et al. How reliable is the diagnosis of lung cancer using small biopsy specimens? Report of a UKCCCR Lung Cancer Working Party. Thorax. 1993;48:1135–1139.

163. Stanley KE, Matthews MJ. Analysis of a pathology review of patients with lung tumors. J Natl Cancer Inst. 1981;66:989–992.

164. Clee MD, Duguid HLD, Sinclair DJM. Accuracy of morphological diagnosis of lung cancer in a department of respiratory medicine. J Clin Pathol. 1982;35:414–419.

165. Vollmer RT, Ogden L, Crissman JD. Separation of small-cell from non–small-cell lung cancer: the Southeastern Cancer Study Group Pathologists' experience. Arch Pathol Lab Med. 1984;108:792–794.

166. Burnett RA, Howatson SR, Lang S, et al. Observer variability in histopathological reporting of non–small cell lung carcinoma on bronchial biopsy specimens. J Clin Pathol. 1996;49:130–133.

167. Roggli VL, Vollmer RT, Greenberg SD, et al. Lung cancer heterogeneity: a blinded and randomized study of 100 consecutive cases. Hum Pathol. 1985;16:569–579.

168. American Cancer Society. Report on the cancer-related health checkup: cancer of the lung. CA Cancer J Clin. 1980;30:199–207.

169. 1989 survey of physicians' attitudes and practices in early cancer detection. CA Cancer J Clin. 1990;40:77–101.

170. Strauss GM, Gleason RE, Sugarbaker DJ. Screening for lung cancer: another look; a different view. Chest. 1997;111:754–768.

171. Early lung cancer detection: summary and conclusions. Am Rev Respir Dis. 1984;130:565–570.

172. Soda H, Tomita H, Kohno S, et al. Limitation of annual screening chest radiography for the diagnosis of lung cancer: a retrospective study. Cancer. 1993;72:2341–2346.

173. Shimizu N, Ando A, Teramoto S, et al. Outcome of patients with lung cancer detected via mass screening as compared to those presenting with symptoms. J Surg Oncol. 1992;50:7–11.

174. Salomaa E-R, Liippo K, Taylor P, et al. Prognosis of patients with lung cancer found in a single chest radiograph screening. Chest. 1998;114:1514–1518.

175. Wilde J. A 10 year follow-up of semi-annual screening for early detection of lung cancer in the Erfurt County, GDR. Eur Respir J. 1989;2:656–662.

176. Satoh H, Ishikawa H, Yamashita YT, et al. Outcome of patients with lung cancer detected by mass screening versus presentation with symptoms. Anticancer Res. 1997;17:2293–2296.

177. Sobue T, Suzuki T, Matsuda M, et al. Sensitivity and specificity of lung cancer screening in Osaka, Japan. Jpn J Cancer Res. 1991;82:1069–1076.

178. Hillerdal G. Long-term survival of patients with lung cancer from a defined geographical area before and after radiological screening. Lung Cancer. 1996;15:21–30.

179. Fontana RS, Sanderson DR, Woolner LB, et al. Lung cancer screening: the Mayo program. J Occup Med. 1986;28:746–750.

180. Kubík A, Parkin DM, Khlat M, et al. Lack of benefit from semi-annual screening for cancer of the lung: follow-up report of a randomized controlled trial on a population of high-risk males in Czechoslovakia. Int J Cancer. 1990;45:26–33.

181. Hayata Y, Funatsu H, Kato H, et al. Results of lung cancer screening programs in Japan: early detection and localization of lung tumors in high risk groups. In: Band PR, ed. Recent Results of Cancer Research. Heidelberg, Germany: Springer Berlin; 1982:179–186.

182. Nash FA, Morgan JM, Tomkins JG. South London Lung Cancer Study. BMJ. 1968;2:715–721.

183. American Cancer Society–Veterans Administration Lung Cancer Screening Study Coordinating Committee. An evaluation of radiologic and cytologic screening for the early detection of lung cancer: a cooperative pilot study of the American Cancer Society and the Veterans Administration. Cancer Res. 1966;26:2083–2121.

184. Weiss W, Boucot KR. The Philadelphia Pulmonary Neoplasm Research Project: early roentgenographic appearance of bronchogenic carcinoma. Arch Intern Med. 1974;134:306–311.

185. Brett GZ. The value of lung cancer detection by six-monthly chest radiographs. Thorax. 1968;23:414–420.

186. Fontana RS, Sanderson DR, Woolner LB, et al. Screening for lung cancer: a critique for the Mayo Lung Project. Cancer. 1991;67:1155–1164.

187. Melamed MR, Flehinger BJ, Zaman MB, et al. Screening for early lung cancer: results of the Memorial Sloan-Kettering study in New York. Chest. 1984;86:44–53.

188. Tockman MS, Levin ML, Frost JK, et al. Screening and detection of lung cancer. In: Aisner J, ed. Lung Cancer: Contemporary Issues in Clinical Oncology. New York, NY: Churchill-Livingstone; 1985:25–40.

189. Tockman MS. Survival and mortality from lung cancer in a screened population: the Johns Hopkins study. Chest. 1986;89(suppl):324S–325S.

190. Flehinger BJ, Kimmel M, Melamed MR. The effect of surgical treatment on survival from early lung cancer: implications for screening. Chest. 1992;101:1013–1018.

191. Sobue T, Suzuki T, Matsuda M, et al. Survival for clinical stage I lung cancer not surgically treated: comparison between screen-detected and symptom-detected cases. Cancer. 1992;69:685–692.

192. McFarlane MJ, Feinstein AR, Wells CK. Clinical features of lung cancers discovered as a postmortem "surprise." Chest. 1996;90:520–523.

193. Flehinger BJ, Kimmel M, Polyak T, et al. Screening for lung cancer: the Mayo Lung Project revisited. Cancer. 1993;72:1573–1580.

194. Kaneko M, Eguchi K, Ohmatsu H, et al. Peripheral lung cancer: screening and detection with low-dose spiral CT versus radiography. Radiology. 1996;201:798–802.

195. Sone S, Takashima S, Li F, et al. Mass screening for lung cancer with mobile spiral computed tomography scanner. Lancet. 1998;351:1242–1245.

196. Henschke CI, McCauley DI, Yankelevitz DF, et al. Early Lung Cancer Action Project: overall design and findings from baseline screening. Lancet. 1999;354:99–105.

197. Yasuda S, Shohtsu A, Okubo K, et al. Lung cancer screening with spiral CT [abstract]. Lung Cancer. 1998;21:229–246.

198. Lam S, Kennedy T, Unger M, et al. Localization of bronchial intraepithelial neoplastic lesions by fluorescence bronchoscopy. Chest. 1998;113:696–702.

199. Woolner LB, Fontana RS, Cortese DA, et al. Roentgenographically occult lung cancer: pathologic findings and frequency of multicentricity during a 10-year period. Mayo Clin Proc. 1984;59:453–466.

200. Lam S, MacAulay C, Hung J, et al. Detection of dysplasia and carcinoma in situ with a lung imaging fluorescence endoscope device. J Thorac Cardiovasc Surg. 1993;105:1035–1040.

201. Kurie JM, Lee JS, Morice RC, et al. Autofluorescence bronchoscopy in the detection of squamous metaplasia and dysplasia in current and former smokers. J Natl Cancer Inst. 1998;90:991–995.

202. Frost JK, Ball WC Jr, Levin ML, et al. Sputum cytology: use and potential in monitoring the workplace environment by screening for biological effects of exposure. J Occup Med. 1986;28:692–703.

203. Band P, Feldstein M, Saccommano G. Reversibility of bronchial marked atypia: implication for chemoprevention. Cancer Detect Prev. 1986;9:157–160.

204. Tockman MS, Gupta PK, Myers JD, et al. Sensitive and specific monoclonal antibody recognition of human lung cancer antigen on preserved sputum cells: a new approach to early lung cancer detection. J Clin Oncol. 1988;6:1685–1693.

205. Tockman MS, Mulshine JL, Piantadosi S, et al. Prospective detection of preclinical lung cancer: results from two studies of hnRNP overexpression [abstract]. Clin Cancer Res. 1997;3:2237.

206. Mao L, Hruban RH, Boyle JO, et al. Detection of oncogene mutations in sputum precedes diagnosis of lung cancer. Cancer Res. 1994;54:1634–1637.

207. Payne PW, Sebo TJ, Doudkine A, et al. Sputum screening by quantitative microscopy: a reexamination of a portion of the National Cancer Institute Cooperative Early Lung Cancer Study [abstract]. Mayo Clin Proc. 1997;72:697.

208. Pater JL, Loeb M. Nonanatomic prognostic factors in carcinoma of the lung: a multivariate analysis. Cancer. 1982;50:326–331.

209. Lanzotti VJ, Thomas DR, Boyle LE, et al. Survival with inoperable lung cancer: an integration of prognostic variables based on simple clinical criteria. Cancer. 1977;39:303–313.

210. Lam WK, So SY, Hsu C, et al. Fiberoptic bronchoscopy in the diagnosis of bronchial cancer: comparison of washings, brushings and biopsies in central and peripheral tumours. Clin Oncol. 1983;9:35–42.

211. Charig MJ, Stutley JE, Padley SPG, et al. The value of negative needle biopsy in suspected operable lung cancer. Clin Radiol. 1991;44:147–149.

212. Veale D, Gilmartin JJ, Sumerling MD, et al. Prospective evaluation of fine needle aspiration in the diagnosis of lung cancer. Thorax. 1988;43:540–544.

213. Winning AJ, McIvor J, Seed WA, et al. Interpretation of negative results in fine needle aspiration of discrete pulmonary lesions. Thorax. 1986;41:875–879.

214. Greene R, Szyfelbein WM, Isler RJ, et al. Supplementary tissue-core histology from fine-needle transthoracic aspiration biopsy. AJR Am J Roentgenol. 1985;144:787–792.

215. Yankelevitz DF, Henschke CI, Koizumi JH, et al. CT-guided transthoracic needle biopsy of small solitary pulmonary nodules. Clin Imaging. 1997;21:107–110.

216. Graeber GM, Gupta NC, Murray GF. Positron emission tomographic imaging with flurorodeoxyglucose is efficacious in evaluating malignant pulmonary disease. J Thorac Cardiovasc Surg. 1999;117:719–727.

217. Inoue T, Kim EE, Komaki R, et al. Detecting recurrent or residual lung cancer with FDG-PET. J Nucl Med. 1995;36:788–793.

218. Young GP, Young I, Cowan DF, et al. The reliability of fine-needle aspiration biopsy in the diagnosis of deep lesions of the lung and mediastinum: experience with 250 cases using a modified technique. Diagn Cytopathol. 1987;3:1–7.

219. Cataluna JJS, Perpiná M, Greses JV, et al. Cell type accuracy of bronchial biopsy specimens in primary lung cancer. Chest. 1996;109:1199–1203.

220. Chuang MT, Marchevsky A, Teirstein AS, et al. Diagnosis of lung cancer by fibreoptic bronchoscopy: problems in the histologic classification of non–small cell carcinomas. Thorax. 1984;39:175–178.

221. Ohmatsu H, Kakinuma R, Nishiwaki Y, et al. Lung cancer screening with low-dose spiral CT [abstract]. Proc ASCO. 1999;18:463a.

CHAPTER
5

INTRATHORACIC STAGING

Frank C. Detterbeck, David R. Jones, and L. Alden Parker, Jr.

DEFINITION

Selection of the most appropriate treatment for a patient with lung cancer is determined primarily by the stage of disease. Therefore, once a diagnosis of lung cancer has been made, accurate staging is the crucial next step. Staging can be divided into extrathoracic and intrathoracic staging. *Extrathoracic staging* involves the identification of metastases to distant organs, presumably spread by hematogenous dissemination. Extrathoracic staging therefore determines the M stage of the TNM stage classification. If no distant metastases are present, then accurate *intrathoracic staging,* or determination of the clinical T and N stage, is essential.

This chapter focuses on the determination of the intrathoracic clinical stage of patients with lung cancer. The *clinical stage* is defined as the best estimation of the extent of disease using *all* staging information that is available *before the initiation of any therapy.* This includes radiographic data as well as any information available from biopsies such as that obtained during bronchoscopy, needle aspiration, or mediastinoscopy. The accuracy of the clinical stage is dependent on whether information from surgical biopsies is available, or whether it is determined by radiographic studies alone. These two clinical staging methods are often referred to as *surgical* (clinical) *staging* and *radiographic* (clinical) *staging.* The clinical stage using surgical biopsy information must not be confused with the pathologic stage, which is determined after surgical *therapy*—that is, resection—has been undertaken.

PARAMETERS FOR ASSESSING TEST RELIABILITY

A discussion of intrathoracic staging should include an assessment of when it is appropriate to perform a particular test, such as computed tomography (CT) scanning, positron-emission tomography (PET) scanning, or mediastinoscopy, as well as an analysis of the reliability of the test results. Parameters used to assess the reliability of a test and the formulas used to calculate these terms are shown in Table 5–1. However, in order to use them, it is essential to understand what each of the terms means and what the strengths and limitations of each parameter are. The *sensitivity* of a test is the chance of a positive test result in

TABLE 5–1. PARAMETERS USED TO ASSESS TEST RELIABILITY

	Disease Absent	Disease Present	Parameters Based on Test Results	
			Test Parameter	Formula
Test Negative	True Negative (N_{TN})	False Negative (N_{FN})	False Negative Rate	$\dfrac{N_{FN}}{N_{TN} + N_{FN}}$
Test Positive	False Positive (N_{FP})	True Positive (N_{TP})	False Positive Rate	$\dfrac{N_{FP}}{N_{TP} + N_{FP}}$
Disease Parameter	Specificity	Sensitivity	Accuracy	
Formula	$\dfrac{N_{TN}}{N_{TN} + N_{FP}}$	$\dfrac{N_{TP}}{N_{TP} + N_{FN}}$	$\dfrac{N_{TP} + N_{TN}}{N_{TN} + N_{FN} + N_{TP} + N_{FP}}$	
Parameters Based on Disease Status				

N_{FN}, number of false negative patients (negative by test, but positive by gold standard evaluation); N_{FP}, number of false positive patients (positive by test, but negative by gold standard evaluation); N_{TN}, number of true negative patients (negative by both test and gold standard evaluation); N_{TP}, number of true positive patients (positive by both test and gold standard evaluation).

Note: The false negative rate is equal to 100 minus the negative predictive value, and the false positive rate is equal to 100 minus the positive predictive value.

an imaginary population consisting entirely of patients who truly have the abnormality in question. *Specificity* is the proportion of negative test results in an imaginary population of patients, none of whom actually have the disease. *Accuracy* is a parameter that attempts to express sensitivity and specificity as a single number. However, so much information is lost by this process that interpretation of this number is nearly impossible.

Sensitivity and specificity have the advantage of being inherent properties of a test and are independent of the prevalence of the abnormality in a patient population.[1] In theory, they should not vary among studies, but in fact, they do because the judgment regarding when to call a test result positive or negative varies. The combination of the test itself and its interpretation covers a wide spectrum and is described in a graph known as a *receiver operating characteristic curve*.[2,3] The main shortcoming of sensitivity and specificity is that they do not measure anything that is of direct, practical use because one is never dealing with a population of patients, all of whom have (or do not have) a particular abnormality.

In actual practice, it is more important to know how to interpret a negative (or positive) test result than to know the inherent test properties in a theoretical uniform population. This is best assessed by determining the false negative (FN) or false positive (FP) rate.* The FN rate measures the percentage chance that a negative test result is falsely negative, that is, that the abnormality (eg, nodal involvement) is, in reality, present, despite a negative test result. The FP rate measures the percentage chance that a positive test result is false, that is, that the abnormality is actually not present. FN and FP rates are sometimes expressed as the percentage of their reciprocal, known as the *negative predictive value* and *positive predictive value*. This book focuses primarily on the FN and FP rates because they are simple and concrete, and because they fill the needs of the clinician who is face to face with a patient.

Assessment of the FN and FP rates requires some knowledge of the patient population because these values are influenced by the prevalence of the disease in the patient population. Application of the FN and FP rates from one study to another population is possible only if the prevalence of disease is similar. The FN and FP rates are also influenced by the sensitivity and specificity of the test. The relationship between FN and FP rates and prevalence for several levels of sensitivity and specificity is shown in Figure 5–1. The influence of prevalence on FN and FP rates is not great between 20% and 80%. The FP rate is affected dramatically as the prevalence drops below 10%, and the FN rate is affected dramatically if the prevalence is >90%.[1] Accordingly, throughout this book, we have listed FN and FP rates as well as prevalence, and we have refrained from evaluating FN and FP rates if the prevalence is ≥90% or ≤10%, respectively.

SMALL CELL LUNG CANCER

The TNM system is generally not used for staging small cell lung cancer (SCLC). An expert panel assembled to consider whether this practice should change concluded

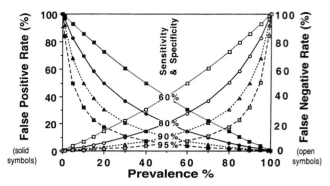

Figure 5–1. Relationship of false positive (FP) rate and false negative (FN) rate to prevalence, sensitivity, and specificity. Curves of FP and FN rates versus prevalence are depicted for different levels of sensitivity and specificity.

in 1982 that the two-stage system traditionally employed (limited and extensive stage) was more appropriate.[4] This is because SCLC is treated primarily with chemotherapy. Thoracic radiotherapy is added in those patients with *limited stage disease,* which is defined as tumor that is limited to an area of the chest that can be encompassed by a reasonable radiotherapy port. Limited disease includes patients with bilateral mediastinal node involvement, ipsilateral supraclavicular involvement, or superior vena cava obstruction. Therefore, more detailed intrathoracic staging in SCLC has little clinical importance and has not been studied extensively.

Most patients with SCLC present with radiographic evidence of mediastinal node involvement. This is shown in Table 5–2, which summarizes the chest radiograph (CXR) findings in 392 patients. Studies employing chest CT scan have also found that approximately 90% of patients have radiographic mediastinal node enlargement.[5,6] Even in patients with limited disease (N = 264), 81% were found to have positive mediastinal nodes by CT or mediastinoscopy.[7] No data is available regarding the FN or FP rate of the radiographic assessment in SCLC.

CHEST RADIOGRAPH

The accuracy of staging by CXR is commonly thought to be quite poor. However, in a multi-institutional prospective study of 170 patients with surgical confirmation of pathologic stage, prediction of T3 or T4 disease by CXR was

TABLE 5–2. RADIOGRAPHIC APPEARANCE OF SMALL CELL LUNG CANCER AT PRESENTATION

CHEST RADIOGRAPH FINDING	N	%
Central mass with hilar/mediastinal enlargement	252	64
Peripheral mass ± hilar/mediastinal enlargement	75	19
Nodal involvement only	22	6
Indirect findings (atelectasis, effusion, infiltrate)	31	8
Central mass without nodal enlargement	12	3

Inclusion criterion: Largest study reporting radiographic appearance of SCLC.
Data from Cohen MH, Matthews MJ. Small cell bronchogenic carcinoma: a distinct clinicopathologic entity. Semin Oncol. 1978;5:234–243.[161]

*This should not be confused with the *false negative fraction*, which is equal to 1 minus the sensitivity, or the *false positive fraction*, which is equal to 1 minus the specificity.

found to have an FN rate of 24% and an FP rate of 48% (prevalence, 29%).[8] Similarly, the ability to predict N2 or N3 nodal involvement by CXR had an FN rate of 21% and an FP rate of 77% (prevalence, 21%).[8] Other studies have confirmed these results.[9] These values have more similarity to the results achieved with CT scanning than one might expect (see Computed Tomography and Magnetic Resonance Imaging).

Some authors have suggested that a CXR is sufficient in patients thought to have a T1N0 lung cancer and that further evaluation (eg, with a CT scan) is not necessary before proceeding to thoracotomy.[10–12] In four studies investigating the usefulness of CT in patients who were classified as T1N0 by CXR, CT evidence of unresectability that was later pathologically confirmed was found in 15%, 16%, 19%, and 33% of 63, 31, 35, and 36 patients with T1N0 disease, respectively.[13–16] However, in two other studies of 13 and 23 patients who had a T1N0 lesion on CXR, evidence of unresectability discovered by CT was 0 and 4%.[10,12]

COMPUTED TOMOGRAPHY AND MAGNETIC RESONANCE IMAGING

A 1992 survey in England found that 44% of thoracic surgeons performed lung cancer resections having neither obtained a chest CT nor performed mediastinoscopy.[17] Furthermore, 51% of the thoracic surgeons did not routinely sample mediastinal lymph nodes at thoracotomy, thus avoiding intrathoracic staging altogether. In most Western countries, however, evaluation of lung cancer patients with a staging chest CT has become standard.[18,19] A chest CT scan provides much useful information: characteristics of the primary lesion with respect to diagnosis, extension of the tumor into adjacent structures, presence of enlarged

mediastinal lymph node metastases. In this cha obtained routinely for primarily on interpre' ing the FN and FP r

The reliability c scanning compared a number of inve ence has been fc prospective study ui nostic Oncology Group, the for assessing T3,4 disease was 56% specificity 80% versus 84%. Similarly, for un of N2,3 disease, the sensitivity of MRI versus CT was versus 52%, and the specificity 79% versus 79%.[8] Thus, there is no justification for the additional expense of an MRI scan in most instances. In the remainder of this chapter, MRI scanning is discussed only in the specific situations in which it may offer an advantage.

T STAGE

It seems likely that the radiographic assessment of T1 versus T2 disease would be accurate. Measurement of lesion size and presence of lobar atelectasis should be accurately assessed by CT, but visceral pleural involvement by tumor is difficult to detect by CT. However, only limited data about the accuracy of CT in determining the T1 or T2 status exist.[26,27] In one study of 50 cT1,2 patients, CT identification of T2 disease was found to have an FN rate of 18% and an FP rate of 47%.[26] Yet radiographic differentiation between T1 and T2 has little clinical importance because it does not significantly affect the choice of therapy.

TABLE 5–3. RELIABILITY OF COMPUTED TOMOGRAPHY PREDICTION OF T3,4 STATUS

STUDY	N	TYPE	PREV (%)	SENS (%)	SPEC (%)	FN (%)	FP (%)
Webb et al[8]	166	All	29	63	84	15	39
Fernando and Goldstraw[27]	103	All	20	52	98	11	15
Grenier et al[24]	85	All	46	43	85	36	29
Gdeedo et al[26]	74	All	14	64	79	8	65
Musset et al[22]	44	All	34	53	97	20	11
Average		**All**		**55**	**89**	**18**	**32**
Suzuki et al[32]	120	Chest wall	16	68	66	8	72
Laurent et al[23]	111	Chest wall	13	38	98	9	29
Venuta et al[34]	77	Chest wall	43	52	86	30	26
Glaze et al[30 a]	47	Chest wall	32	87	59	9	50
Pennes et al[31]	33	Chest wall	24	38	40	0	65
Nakata et al[28 b]	31	Chest wall	23	100	92	0	22
Average		**Chest wall**		**64**	**74**	**9**	**44**
Laurent et al[23]	111	Mediastinum	14	69	93	5	39
Venuta et al[34]	98	Mediastinum	46	72	75	24	29
Glazer et al[35 a, c]	80	Mediastinum	40	72	58	24	47
Baron et al[36 b]	73	Mediastinum	26	89	94	4	15
Average		**Mediastinum**		**76**	**80**	**14**	**33**

Inclusion criteria: Studies of CT evaluation of T status with ≥20 patients and ≥10%, ≤90% prevalence from 1980 to 2000.
[a]3 criteria used; positive if 2–3 present.
[b]Indeterminate scans = positive.
[c]All patients had indeterminate scans.
FN, false negative rate; FP, false positive rate; Prev, prevalence of pathologic T3,4 disease; SENS, sensitivity; SPEC, specificity; TYPE, type of T3 or T4 involvement.

e important to be able to predict T3 and
nvolvement if surgical resection is being
he results of studies addressing this issue are
ble 5–3. The reliability of CT in predicting T3
ase is not good, with an FN rate of 18% and an
of 32%. The reliability of CT in predicting involve-
in peripheral (chest wall) and central (mediastinal)
tumors is similar. In particular, the FP rate, which is
obably the most important factor in determining whether
or not to consider resection, is rather high in both subgroups (see Table 5–3).

The data regarding CT prediction of chest wall involvement shows a lot of variation, especially in the FN rate,
although it is not clear why. All studies had surgical proof
of chest wall involvement, and all included only patients
with tumors abutting the chest wall. The criteria used to
define radiographic invasion in these studies are similar,
although one study defined them vaguely.[28]

A number of radiographic findings are believed to suggest chest wall involvement by tumor. Bone destruction is
almost universally cited as a definitive sign, but few studies
have reported data regarding this.[5,29] FPs have been reported even for rib destruction.[29] The presence of pain is
the best available indicator of chest wall involvement, with
an FP rate of 17% and an FN rate of 14% in a study of 47
patients.[30] The ability of various signs to predict chest wall
involvement has been investigated most carefully by Ratto
et al[29] in 112 patients, and the results are shown in Figure
5–2. Other smaller studies (47 and 33 patients) have generally shown similar results.[30,31] The best signs of chest
wall involvement are chest pain, rib destruction, a mass
protruding through the ribs, an obtuse angle between ribs
and pleura, and length of contact of >3 cm or more than
half of the tumor diameter. Conflicting results are reported
regarding whether obliteration of the subpleural fat plane
and pleural thickening are predictive of invasion.[29–31]

One study of 120 patients found that ultrasound was
better than CT for predicting invasion of the chest wall,
with FN and FP rates of 0 and 10%, respectively.[32] MRI
has not shown any advantage in detecting involvement of
the ribs of the lateral chest wall.[8,21–24] In the case of Pancoast tumors, however, MRI scanning with sagittal and
coronal views may offer an advantage. Heelan et al[33] found
that the ability of MRI to predict brachial plexus or subcla-

vian vessel involvement in 31 patients with a Pancoast
tumor was better (FN, 6%; FP, 0%) than that of CT scanning (FN, 19%; FP, 19%).

No data has been reported regarding the ability to resect
tumor in patients with radiographic suspicion of chest wall
involvement, but it seems likely that in most cases this can
be accomplished without much difficulty. This makes it
less important to be able to predict lateral chest wall
involvement preoperatively. With Pancoast tumors, however, 30% to 50% of patients cannot be completely resected
(see Table 16–2). Unfortunately, there is no data on the
ability of scans to predict resectability of Pancoast tumors.

Mediastinal involvement by the primary tumor may be
either T3 or T4 disease and is not as likely to be resectable
as chest wall involvement. Table 5–3 lists the results of
studies investigating the value of CT in patients with tumors abutting the mediastinum. The ability of CT to rule
out mediastinal involvement in tumors abutting the mediastinum is fair (average FN rate, 14%). The more carefully
conducted studies have shown an FN rate of 24%.[34,35]
The studies in Table 5–3 with the lowest prevalence of
mediastinal involvement show the lowest FN rates, as
might be expected.[23,36]

It is probably more important to know whether CT can
accurately rule in the presence of mediastinal invasion.
Unfortunately, the ability of CT to predict mediastinal
invasion is poor in all of the studies in Table 5–3 (average
FP rate, 33%). Several other studies have also shown high
FP rates but were not included in the table because of low
prevalence of invasion (<10%) or small study size (<20
patients).[21,28,37,38] MRI has been found to have the same
reliability as CT in predicting mediastinal involvement.[8,21–25] One study suggested a slight trend to better
reliability with MRI, but the difference was not significant.[8]
A study of the value of specific radiographic signs in
predicting mediastinal tumor invasion has been carried out
by Glazer et al[35] and is shown in Figure 5–3.

More important than the prediction of mediastinal invasion per se is the ability to predict whether a tumor will be
resectable. This has been investigated in a few studies,[35,38,39]
but the data from most reports are not useful because of
either a very low prevalence of unresectable disease[38] or a
poorly defined, nonconsecutive patient population.[39] Only
one study, consisting of 80 subjects, has carefully docu-

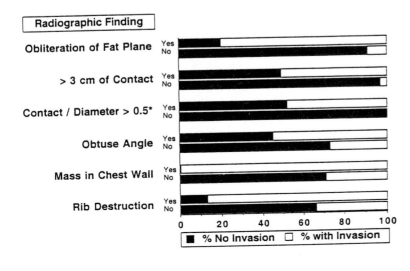

FIGURE 5–2. Computed tomography assessment of chest wall
invasion in 112 patients. *Ratio of length of contact to diameter of tumor. (Data from Ratto GB, Piacenza G, Frola C, et
al. Chest wall involvement by lung cancer: computed tomographic detection and results of operation. Ann Thorac Surg.
1991;51:182–188.[29])

found to have an FN rate of 24% and an FP rate of 48% (prevalence, 29%).[8] Similarly, the ability to predict N2 or N3 nodal involvement by CXR had an FN rate of 21% and an FP rate of 77% (prevalence, 21%).[8] Other studies have confirmed these results.[9] These values have more similarity to the results achieved with CT scanning than one might expect (see Computed Tomography and Magnetic Resonance Imaging).

Some authors have suggested that a CXR is sufficient in patients thought to have a T1N0 lung cancer and that further evaluation (eg, with a CT scan) is not necessary before proceeding to thoracotomy.[10–12] In four studies investigating the usefulness of CT in patients who were classified as T1N0 by CXR, CT evidence of unresectability that was later pathologically confirmed was found in 15%, 16%, 19%, and 33% of 63, 31, 35, and 36 patients with T1N0 disease, respectively.[13–16] However, in two other studies of 13 and 23 patients who had a T1N0 lesion on CXR, evidence of unresectability discovered by CT was 0 and 4%.[10,12]

COMPUTED TOMOGRAPHY AND MAGNETIC RESONANCE IMAGING

A 1992 survey in England found that 44% of thoracic surgeons performed lung cancer resections having neither obtained a chest CT nor performed mediastinoscopy.[17] Furthermore, 51% of the thoracic surgeons did not routinely sample mediastinal lymph nodes at thoracotomy, thus avoiding intrathoracic staging altogether. In most Western countries, however, evaluation of lung cancer patients with a staging chest CT has become standard.[18,19] A chest CT scan provides much useful information: characteristics of the primary lesion with respect to diagnosis, extension of the tumor into adjacent structures, presence of enlarged mediastinal lymph nodes, and presence of liver and adrenal metastases. In this chapter, we assume that a chest CT is obtained routinely for a variety of reasons and will focus primarily on interpretation of the CT results by investigating the FN and FP rates with respect to specific issues.

The reliability of magnetic resonance imaging (MRI) scanning compared with CT scanning has been studied by a number of investigators,[8,20–25] and, in general, no difference has been found. For example, in a multi-institutional prospective study of 170 patients by the Radiologic Diagnostic Oncology Group, the sensitivity of MRI versus CT for assessing T3,4 disease was 56% versus 63%, and the specificity 80% versus 84%. Similarly, for the assessment of N2,3 disease, the sensitivity of MRI versus CT was 48% versus 52%, and the specificity 79% versus 79%.[8] Thus, there is no justification for the additional expense of an MRI scan in most instances. In the remainder of this chapter, MRI scanning is discussed only in the specific situations in which it may offer an advantage.

T STAGE

It seems likely that the radiographic assessment of T1 versus T2 disease would be accurate. Measurement of lesion size and presence of lobar atelectasis should be accurately assessed by CT, but visceral pleural involvement by tumor is difficult to detect by CT. However, only limited data about the accuracy of CT in determining the T1 or T2 status exist.[26,27] In one study of 50 cT1,2 patients, CT identification of T2 disease was found to have an FN rate of 18% and an FP rate of 47%.[26] Yet radiographic differentiation between T1 and T2 has little clinical importance because it does not significantly affect the choice of therapy.

TABLE 5–3. RELIABILITY OF COMPUTED TOMOGRAPHY PREDICTION OF T3,4 STATUS

STUDY	N	TYPE	PREV (%)	SENS (%)	SPEC (%)	FN (%)	FP (%)
Webb et al[8]	166	All	29	63	84	15	39
Fernando and Goldstraw[27]	103	All	20	52	98	11	15
Grenier et al[24]	85	All	46	43	85	36	29
Gdeedo et al[26]	74	All	14	64	79	8	65
Musset et al[22]	44	All	34	53	97	20	11
Average		**All**		**55**	**89**	**18**	**32**
Suzuki et al[32]	120	Chest wall	16	68	66	8	72
Laurent et al[23]	111	Chest wall	13	38	98	9	29
Venuta et al[34]	77	Chest wall	43	52	86	30	26
Glaze et al[30] a	47	Chest wall	32	87	59	9	50
Pennes et al[31]	33	Chest wall	24	38	40	0	65
Nakata et al[28] b	31	Chest wall	23	100	92	0	22
Average		**Chest wall**		**64**	**74**	**9**	**44**
Laurent et al[23]	111	Mediastinum	14	69	93	5	39
Venuta et al[34]	98	Mediastinum	46	72	75	24	29
Glazer et al[35] a, c	80	Mediastinum	40	72	58	24	47
Baron et al[36] b	73	Mediastinum	26	89	94	4	15
Average		**Mediastinum**		**76**	**80**	**14**	**33**

Inclusion criteria: Studies of CT evaluation of T status with ≥20 patients and ≥10%, ≤90% prevalence from 1980 to 2000.
[a] 3 criteria used; positive if 2–3 present.
[b] Indeterminate scans = positive.
[c] All patients had indeterminate scans.
FN, false negative rate; FP, false positive rate; Prev, prevalence of pathologic T3,4 disease; SENS, sensitivity; SPEC, specificity; TYPE, type of T3 or T4 involvement.

It is much more important to be able to predict T3 and especially T4 involvement if surgical resection is being considered. The results of studies addressing this issue are shown in Table 5–3. The reliability of CT in predicting T3 or T4 disease is not good, with an FN rate of 18% and an FP rate of 32%. The reliability of CT in predicting involvement in peripheral (chest wall) and central (mediastinal) T3 tumors is similar. In particular, the FP rate, which is probably the most important factor in determining whether or not to consider resection, is rather high in both subgroups (see Table 5–3).

The data regarding CT prediction of chest wall involvement shows a lot of variation, especially in the FN rate, although it is not clear why. All studies had surgical proof of chest wall involvement, and all included only patients with tumors abutting the chest wall. The criteria used to define radiographic invasion in these studies are similar, although one study defined them vaguely.[28]

A number of radiographic findings are believed to suggest chest wall involvement by tumor. Bone destruction is almost universally cited as a definitive sign, but few studies have reported data regarding this.[5,29] FPs have been reported even for rib destruction.[29] The presence of pain is the best available indicator of chest wall involvement, with an FP rate of 17% and an FN rate of 14% in a study of 47 patients.[30] The ability of various signs to predict chest wall involvement has been investigated most carefully by Ratto et al[29] in 112 patients, and the results are shown in Figure 5–2. Other smaller studies (47 and 33 patients) have generally shown similar results.[30,31] The best signs of chest wall involvement are chest pain, rib destruction, a mass protruding through the ribs, an obtuse angle between ribs and pleura, and length of contact of >3 cm or more than half of the tumor diameter. Conflicting results are reported regarding whether obliteration of the subpleural fat plane and pleural thickening are predictive of invasion.[29–31]

One study of 120 patients found that ultrasound was better than CT for predicting invasion of the chest wall, with FN and FP rates of 0 and 10%, respectively.[32] MRI has not shown any advantage in detecting involvement of the ribs of the lateral chest wall.[8,21–24] In the case of Pancoast tumors, however, MRI scanning with sagittal and coronal views may offer an advantage. Heelan et al[33] found that the ability of MRI to predict brachial plexus or subcla-

vian vessel involvement in 31 patients with a Pancoast tumor was better (FN, 6%; FP, 0%) than that of CT scanning (FN, 19%; FP, 19%).

No data has been reported regarding the ability to resect tumor in patients with radiographic suspicion of chest wall involvement, but it seems likely that in most cases this can be accomplished without much difficulty. This makes it less important to be able to predict lateral chest wall involvement preoperatively. With Pancoast tumors, however, 30% to 50% of patients cannot be completely resected (see Table 16–2). Unfortunately, there is no data on the ability of scans to predict resectability of Pancoast tumors.

Mediastinal involvement by the primary tumor may be either T3 or T4 disease and is not as likely to be resectable as chest wall involvement. Table 5–3 lists the results of studies investigating the value of CT in patients with tumors abutting the mediastinum. The ability of CT to rule out mediastinal involvement in tumors abutting the mediastinum is fair (average FN rate, 14%). The more carefully conducted studies have shown an FN rate of 24%.[34,35] The studies in Table 5–3 with the lowest prevalence of mediastinal involvement show the lowest FN rates, as might be expected.[23,36]

It is probably more important to know whether CT can accurately rule in the presence of mediastinal invasion. Unfortunately, the ability of CT to predict mediastinal invasion is poor in all of the studies in Table 5–3 (average FP rate, 33%). Several other studies have also shown high FP rates but were not included in the table because of low prevalence of invasion (<10%) or small study size (<20 patients).[21,28,37,38] MRI has been found to have the same reliability as CT in predicting mediastinal involvement.[8,21–25] One study suggested a slight trend to better reliability with MRI, but the difference was not significant.[8] A study of the value of specific radiographic signs in predicting mediastinal tumor invasion has been carried out by Glazer et al[35] and is shown in Figure 5–3.

More important than the prediction of mediastinal invasion per se is the ability to predict whether a tumor will be resectable. This has been investigated in a few studies,[35,38,39] but the data from most reports are not useful because of either a very low prevalence of unresectable disease[38] or a poorly defined, nonconsecutive patient population.[39] Only one study, consisting of 80 subjects, has carefully docu-

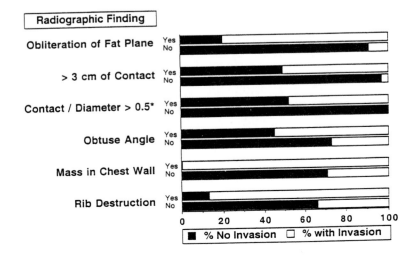

FIGURE 5–2. Computed tomography assessment of chest wall invasion in 112 patients. *Ratio of length of contact to diameter of tumor. (Data from Ratto GB, Piacenza G, Frola C, et al. Chest wall involvement by lung cancer: computed tomographic detection and results of operation. Ann Thorac Surg. 1991;51:182–188.[29])

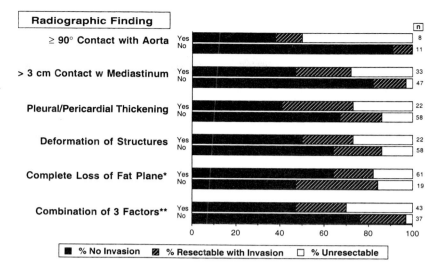

FIGURE 5–3. Computed tomography assessment of mediastinal invasion in 80 patients. *Complete loss versus focal obliteration. **Factors used were ≥90-degree contact with aorta, >3 cm contact with mediastinum, and complete loss of fat plane (2–3 positive factors, versus 0–1). (From Glazer HS, Kaiser LR, Anderson DJ, et al. Indeterminate mediastinal invasion in bronchogenic carcinoma: CT evaluation. Radiology. 1989;173:37–42.[35])

mented resectability in patients with tumors abutting the mediastinum, and the results are shown in Figure 5–3.[35] This study included only patients with *indeterminate CT scans,* defined as tumor contiguous with the mediastinum but without definite extension of tumor around the central vessels. In 94% of the patients, there was at least focal absence of a fat plane between the mass and mediastinal structures.

None of the radiographic signs investigated, either individually or in combination, is able to predict unresectability in a high proportion of the patients.[35] Therefore, patients with cT3 or cT4 disease who are otherwise surgical candidates should not be denied surgical exploration on the basis of a CT alone, although the resectability of these patients may be as low as 70%.[35] Thoracoscopy may be beneficial in correctly determining the T stage of these patients. In one study, this technique was able to correctly stage 87% of 30 cases with suspected mediastinal T4 disease.[40] Unfortunately, this study did not report data on resectability as determined by thoracoscopy. In another study employing routine thoracoscopy before thoracotomy in 286 patients, 65% of the unresectable cases could be identified.[41]

In patients with limited pulmonary reserve, it can be important to be able to predict the need for a lobectomy as opposed to a pneumonectomy. A retrospective analysis of this issue has been carried out in 26 consecutive patients with tumors that were either central or adjacent to the fissure.[42] The prediction that a pneumonectomy would not be required carried an FN rate of 20% in this population, whereas the prediction that a pneumonectomy would be necessary had an FP rate of 29%. In this study, radiographic evidence of tumor invading a central bronchus or crossing the fissure was predictive of the need for pneumonectomy (FP rates, 0 and 0), whereas radiographic invasion of the main pulmonary artery was not (FP rate, 67%).[42]

NODAL STATUS

General Concerns

The most important aspect of intrathoracic staging is accurate determination of nodal involvement. CT (and MRI) scans rely on lymph node size to predict malignant involve-

ment. Attempts have been made to improve the accuracy of radiographic nodal assessment by including morphologic features of the nodes (eg, contour and heterogeneity) in addition to size,[43] but these are complex and have not become accepted into standard practice. Thus, despite nearly 20 years of experience with CT scanning, the radiologic assessment of nodal involvement is still based solely on lymph node size. Mediastinal and intrapulmonary lymph nodes are commonly grouped into accurately defined nodal stations, as shown in Figure 5–4 (see color section at front of book). Mediastinal (N2,3) node stations are indicated by single digits, whereas intrapulmonary and hilar (N1) nodes are indicated by double digits.

The size of mediastinal lymph nodes in normal patients has been investigated in several studies.[44–46] One study analyzed actual node size from 40 normal cadavers according to the American Thoracic Society node mapping system.[45] In another study, node size assessed by CT scan was carefully documented in 56 patients who were carefully selected to have no pulmonary or systemic diseases that might affect mediastinal node size.[44] The results of these two studies are surprisingly consistent (Table 5–4) and are corroborated by other smaller studies as well.[46] The average size of a normal node in both of these studies is approximately 4 mm. Nodes in the subcarinal (station 7) and low right paratracheal (station 4R) regions are somewhat larger than those in other locations.

It is possible that patients with lung cancer, who often have chronic bronchitis, may have a "normal" node size that is different from the "normal" population investigated in the studies noted earlier. Benign nodes removed at the time of thoracotomy from patients with lung cancer had an average short axis diameter of 5 mm in one study (N = 40)[47] and 10 mm in another study (N = 364).[48] In another analysis of 44 lung cancer patients, the largest benign lymph node had an average short axis diameter of 19 mm.[49]

A transverse short axis size of 1 cm has been chosen by most radiologists as the criterion to differentiate normal from abnormal nodes. The transverse diameter is most easily assessed by the horizontal slices of a CT scan, and the transverse short axis diameter is more likely to represent the true nodal diameter as opposed to the transverse long axis, which may appear enlarged as a result of oblique

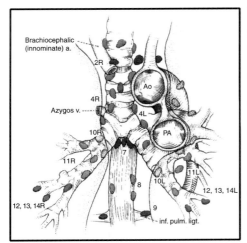

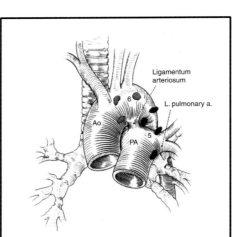

N₂ NODES
SUPERIOR MEDIASTINAL NODES

○ **1** Highest Mediastinal: Nodes lying above a horizontal line at the upper rim of the innominate vein as it crosses in front of the trachea at the midline

● **2** Upper Paratracheal: Nodes lying above a horizontal line drawn tangential to the upper margin of the aortic arch and below the inferior boundary of No. 1 nodes

● **3** Pre- and Retrotracheal: Prevascular and retrotracheal nodes may be designated 3A and 3P; midline nodes are considered to be ipsilateral

● **4** Lower Paratracheal: Nodes lying between the midline of the trachea and a horizontal line drawn tangential to the upper margin of the aortic arch and a line extending across the main bronchus at the upper margin of the upper lobe bronchus, and lying medial to the ligamentum arteriosum and contained within the mediastinal pleural envelope

AORTIC NODES

○ **5** Subaortic (A–P window): Subaortic nodes are lateral to the ligamentum arteriosum or the aorta or left pulmonary artery and proximal to the first branch of the left pulmonary artery and lie within the mediastinal pleural envelope

● **6** Para-aortic (ascending aorta or phrenic): Nodes lying anterior and lateral to the ascending aorta and the aortic arch or the innominate artery, beneath a line tangential to the upper margin of the aortic arch

INFERIOR MEDIASTINAL NODES

● **7** Subcarinal: Nodes lying caudal to the carina of the trachea, but not associated with the lower lobe bronchi or arteries within the lung

○ **8** Paraesophageal (below carina): Nodes lying adjacent to the wall of the esophagus and to the right or left of the midline, excluding subcarinal nodes

○ **9** Pulmonary Ligament: Nodes lying within the pulmonary ligament, including those in the posterior wall and the lower part of the inferior pulmonary vein

N₁ NODES

○ **10** Hilar: The proximal lobar nodes, distal to the mediastinal pleural reflection and the nodes adjacent to the bronchus intermedius on the right

◐ **11** Interlobar: Nodes lying between the lobar bronchi

● **12** Lobar: Nodes adjacent to the distal lobar bronchi

● **13** Segmental: Nodes adjacent to the segmental bronchi

● **14** Subsegmental: Nodes around the subsegmental bronchi

FIGURE 5–4. Regional lymph node stations for lung cancer staging and definitons of anatomic landmarks. (See color section following the Table of Contents.) A-P, aorto-pulmonary. (From Mountain CF, Dresler CM. Regional lymph node classification for lung cancer staging. Chest. 1997; 111:1718–1723.[162])

TABLE 5–4. MEAN NUMBER AND TRANSVERSE DIAMETER OF MEDIASTINAL NODES

NODAL STATION	NUMBER OF NODES[a]	SHORT AXIS (mm)		LONG AXIS (mm)	
		CT[b]	Autopsy[a]	CT[b]	Autopsy[a]
2R	2.5	3.5	3.7	4.5	4.8
2L	2.1	3.3	2.9	4.3	3.9
4R	4.8	5.0	4.0	6.1	6.0
4L	4.5	4.7	4.1	6.1	6.2
5	1.1	4.7	3.6	7.1	6.1
6	4.7	4.1	3.3	6.2	5.3
7	2.9	6.2	5.6	8.1	10.0
8R	1.2	4.4	3.7	5.7	5.6
8L	1.1	4.4	3.7	5.1	4.3
10R	3.5	5.9	4.5	7.7	7.9
10L	2.4	4.0	3.5	5.4	6.1
Average	**2.8**	**4.6**	**3.9**	**6.0**	**6.0**
Range	1–5	3–6	3–6	4–8	4–10

Inclusion criteria: Largest two studies reporting size of normal mediastinal nodes.
[a]Data from Kiyono et al.[45]
[b]Data from Glazer et al.[44]
CT, computed tomography.

sectioning.[44] Furthermore, in a study correlating CT findings with autopsy results, the short axis diameter was found to be the best predictor of actual nodal volume.[46] Other investigators have also found that use of the transverse short axis diameter for prediction of nodal metastases results in the highest accuracy.[50] Agreement on node size between different radiologists independently reading the same scans has been shown to be fairly good (60%-70%).[24,51-53]

Only a few studies have analyzed the effect of altering the size criteria used to classify nodes as radiographically normal or abnormal.[48,50,54-56] Not surprisingly, a threshold of 0.5 cm yields a high sensitivity (90%-95%) but at the cost of low specificity (11%-23%). A threshold of 1.5 cm decreases the sensitivity (31%-61%) but improves the specificity (83%-97%).[48,50,56] A meta-analysis of 43 studies found that the average sensitivity and specificity when a size criterion of 0.5 to 1 cm was used were 75% and 76%, respectively. Those studies using a size criterion >1 cm reported an average sensitivity of 79% and a specificity of 89%.[54] Considering these results, as well as the size of normal mediastinal lymph nodes, the 1-cm short axis size criterion adopted by most centers seems to be reasonable.

The effect of other parameters on the accuracy of CT scan interpretation of mediastinal nodes was also addressed in the meta-analysis reported by Dales et al.[54] Studies employing a fourth-generation CT scanner reported a somewhat higher sensitivity (84% versus 75%, $P < 0.05$), whereas there was little difference in the specificity (82% versus 78%, $P =$ NS). A slight (but statistically insignificant) trend toward improved sensitivity and specificity was observed with more rapid scan times (<4 seconds), thinner scan thickness (<1 cm), and more narrow scan spacing (≤1 cm). The use of contrast did not result in improved sensitivity or specificity. The most impressive result of this extensive analysis, however, is that the effect of any of these parameters was quite small. The equipment, technique, and radiographic criteria used did not seem to be the key to improving the reliability of radiologic intrathoracic staging.

The gold standard used by studies assessing the reliability of intrathoracic staging may also be an issue. The gold standard is probably a thoracotomy and complete lymph node dissection, although results appear comparable to thoracotomy and systematic node sampling, in which nodes are sampled routinely from each accessible lymph node station. A study randomizing 182 patients between these two approaches found no difference in the incidence of N2 disease, although more patients were found to have multiple station involvement in the node dissection group (59% versus 17%, $P < 0.01$).[57] Several studies, however, have found that selective sampling, in which only nodes that are visibly or palpably abnormal are biopsied, is not as accurate.[58,59] A prospective, nonrandomized study found a significant decrease in the CT sensitivity (43% versus 70%, $P = 0.05$) and specificity (61% versus 79%, $P = 0.05$) in those patients who had more node stations assessed surgically (>3 versus 1-3).[8] However, the meta-analysis of the reliability of CT scanning reported by Dales et al[54] did not find a significant difference between studies using selective sampling versus mediastinal node dissection (sensitivity of 78% versus 83% and specificity of 79% versus 75%, $P =$ NS). A comparison of the results of all larger studies with a clear description of the gold standard used does not reveal any major differences (see Involvement of Mediastinal Nodes, later).

Despite all of the caveats mentioned earlier, CT remains the most frequently used method of intrathoracic staging. The average sensitivity of CT for detection of mediastinal node involvement from a meta-analysis of 42 studies was 79%, and the specificity was 79%.[54] The interpretation of positive or negative CT findings with regard to specific issues is probably more important, and this is discussed next.

Involvement of N1 Nodes

The reliability of CT staging of N1 nodes has not been studied extensively. Table 5-5 shows results from all of the available studies involving at least 50 patients. The average FN rate was 16%, and the average FP rate was 38%. These results are similar to those reported (see later) for N2 nodes (FN, ~15%; FP, ~40%). Although the reported FN rates for N1 nodes are reasonably consistent, a fair amount of unexplained variation exists in the reported FP rates. The prevalence of disease was consistently about 30%.

TABLE 5-5. RELIABILITY OF COMPUTED TOMOGRAPHY STAGING OF N1 (HILAR) NODE INVOLVEMENT[a]

STUDY	N	PREV (%)	SENS (%)	SPEC (%)	FN (%)	FP (%)
Lewis et al[48 b]	364	28	52	92	15	32
McLoud et al[63 c]	113	39	63	58	21	62
Laurent et al[23]	111	26	69	99	10	5
Izbicki et al[37 c]	108	24	45	92	16	36
Cole et al[75 d]	96	20	32	87	16	63
Fernando and Goldstraw[27]	78	31	38	87	24	44
Ferguson et al[163 c,e]	61	28	80	67	13	47
Baron et al[36]	57	28	75	95	9	14
Average			**57**	**85**	**16**	**38**

Inclusion criterion: Studies of ≥50 consecutive patients undergoing thoracotomy, with a prevalence of N1 involvement of ≥10% and ≤90%.
[a]All studies used 1.0 cm as the size criterion, and all patients underwent thoracotomy. Intravenous contrast was routinely used except where indicated.
[b]Inconsistent use of contrast.
[c]Reported by number of nodes (not patients).
[d]Contrast not routinely used.
[e]Excluded indeterminate nodes (1-2 cm).
FN, false negative rate; FP, false positive rate; PREV, prevalence of N1 involvement; SENS, sensitivity; SPEC, specificity.

The studies reporting the lowest FN rates did not involve any pathologists as coauthors, and it may be that few N1 nodes were dissected and analyzed.[23,36] Variation is also seen in the reported sensitivity and specificity, suggesting that the judgment of the radiologists may have varied. It is likely that differentiation of abnormal hilar lymph nodes from normal hilar vessels, primary tumors, or atelectatic lung makes N1 nodal assessment by CT scan particularly susceptible to differences in judgment. The ability of thoracoscopy to assess N1 nodes also appears to be poor.[60,61]

Involvement of Mediastinal Nodes (N2,N3)

The FN and FP rates for a large number of studies of CT for assessment of mediastinal lymph nodes is shown in Table 5–6. The average FN rate is 13%, and the average FP rate 45%. The gold standard used does not appear to have a major influence. However, the variation in FN rates from 3% to 26% and in FP rates from 18% to 74% suggests that it may be possible to define certain populations of lung cancer patients in which a negative or positive CT scan *is* reliable.

The location of a mediastinal lymph node does not markedly affect the reliability of a negative or positive (>1 cm) result. Three large studies are available that report FN rates in individual node stations.[37,50,62] The pooled results, shown in Figure 5–5, suggest that there is little difference among different stations, although the FN rates may be lower for the subcarinal and lower paratracheal stations. This is surprising because these node stations have been shown to harbor the largest nodes in the normal population.[44,45] The FP rates are also relatively consistent, although nodes in the aortopulmonary window and along the left main stem bronchus seem to have lower FP rates. Similar FN and FP rates for various nodal stations were also reported in a study of 143 patients by McLoud et al.[63]

Factors influencing the FN rate of CT were carefully analyzed in the largest reported series, which prospectively analyzed 681 consecutive patients over 13 years.[64] A careful systematic mediastinal node sampling was performed in most patients. The incidence of FN CT scans for various T stages and tumor locations in this study is shown in Figure 5–6. Patients with central T3 lesions were found to have a high incidence of FN scans, whereas patients with peripheral T3,4 lesions were found to have a low FN rate.[64] The curiously low FN rate in the relatively rare patients

TABLE 5–6. RELIABILITY OF COMPUTED TOMOGRAPHY ASSESSMENT OF MEDIASTINAL NODES[a]

STUDY	N	cN0,1 (%)	PREV (%)	GOLD STANDARD	SENS (%)	SPEC (%)	FN (%)	FP (%)
Watanabe et al[145]	512	62	30	LND	69	79	14	42
Suzuki et al[69]	440	86	23	LND	33	92	18	44
Lewis et al[48]	418	56	29	LND	84	84	7	31
Ikezoe et al[164]	208	61	31	LND	74	77	13	41
Cole et al[75 b]	150	79	21	LND	26	81	19	74
Platt et al[72]	103	66	34	LND	86	92	8	23
McKenna et al[9]	102	62	25	LND	60	60	16	68
Ratto et al[105 c]	100	38	30	LND	90	50	8	56
Average					65	77	18	47
Dillemans et al[65 b]	569	—	31	Sys	69	71	26	49
Guyatt et al[51]	298	53	35	Sys	78	69	15	43
Primack et al[165]	159	70	38	Sys	63	86	21	27
Staples et al[50]	151	71	37	Sys	61	93	16[d]	43[d]
McLoud et al[63 e]	143	46	31	Sys	64	62	20	56
Izbicki et al[37]	108	~63	29	Sys	29[d]	93[d]	14[d]	72[d]
Average					61	79	19	48
Daly et al[64 b]	681	74	7	Sel	—	—	10	—
Jolly et al[166 b]	336	72	30	Sel	71	86	13	31
Whittlesey[167]	175	43	31	Sel	96	61	3	47
Matthews et al[68]	174	46	37	Sel	86	78	10	30
Rendina et al[168]	171	50	43	Sel	95	83	3	18
Brion et al[66 f]	153	65	35	Sel	89	46	12	52
Laurent et al[23]	120	61	35	Sel	79	82	12	30
Gdeedo et al[71]	100	51	32	Sel	63	57	23	59
Average					83	70	11	38
Average for all studies					69	75	13	45

Inclusion criterion: Studies of ≥100 consecutive patients reporting on reliability of CT against surgical confirmation.

[a]All patients underwent mediastinoscopy or thoracotomy or both. Results are reported per patient except where otherwise noted. CT size criterion is 1.0 cm unless noted otherwise.

[b]CT size criterion is 1.5 cm.

[c]CT size criterion is 0.8 cm.

[d]Results reported per node.

[e]Includes 10R and 10L.

[f]CT size criterion is 0.5 cm.

FN, false negative rate; FP, false positive rate; LND, lymph node dissection; Prev, prevalence; Sel, selective node sampling (suspicious nodes only); Sens, sensitivity; Spec, specificity; Sys, systematic node sampling.

False Negative Rate

False Positive Rate

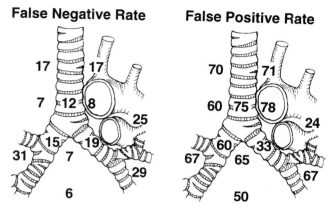

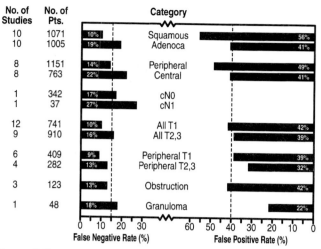

FIGURE 5–5. False negative and false positive rates (%) of chest computed tomography (CT) compared with surgical staging at each mediastinal and hilar node station. CT size criterion used was 1.0 cm. (Data taken from 363 patients [1629 nodes] from Izbicki JR, Thetter O, Karg O, et al. Accuracy of computed tomographic scan and surgical assessment for staging of bronchial carcinoma: a prospective study. J Thorac Cardiovasc Surg. 1992;104:413–420[37]; Seely JM, Mayo JR, Miller RR, et al. T1 lung cancer: prevalence of mediastinal nodal metastases and diagnostic accuracy of CT. Radiology. 1993;186:129–132[62]; and Staples CA, Müller NL, Miller RR, et al. Mediastinal nodes in bronchogenic carcinoma: comparison between CT and mediastinoscopy. Radiology. 1988;167:367–372.[50])

FIGURE 5–7. False negative and false positive rates of computed tomography (CT) assessment of mediastinal node involvement for various subgroups of patients. All patients underwent mediastinoscopy or thoracotomy or both. CT criterion was >1.0 cm. Inclusion criteria: studies reporting FN and FP rates in ≥20 patients with lung cancer in a particular category from 1980–2000. Adenoca, adenocarcinoma. (Squamous/Adenoca, data from references 37, 48, 50, 65–67, 69–71, 73; Peripheral/Central, data from references 9, 50, 65, 68–71, 73; All T1, data from references 9, 10, 14, 48, 50, 62–65, 70, 73, 165; All T2,3, data from references 9, 48, 50, 64, 65, 67, 70, 73, 165; Peripheral T1, data from references 9, 10, 50, 62, 64, 70; Peripheral T2,3, data from references 9, 50, 64, 70; cN0/cN1, data from reference 69; Obstruction, data from references 50, 63, 167; Granuloma, data from reference 50.)

with central T1 lesions (N = 25) is also remarkable. Most of these patients had early-stage disease; in fact, the prevalence of mediastinal node involvement in this study was only 7%. This low prevalence would markedly influence FP rates (not reported in this study) but would have little effect on the FN rates.

A more extensive analysis of the influence of various factors on the FN and FP rates is shown in Figure 5–7. The factors selected are all those that have been suggested or reported to influence the reliability of CT scanning. The average prevalence of mediastinal node involvement in

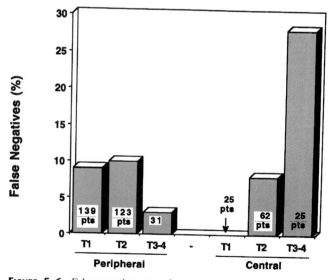

FIGURE 5–6. False negative rate of computed tomography staging of mediastinal nodes. (Modified from Daly BDT, Mueller JD, Faling LJ, et al. N2 lung cancer: outcome in patients with false-negative computed tomographic scans of the chest. J Thorac Cardiovasc Surg. 1993;105:904–911.[64])

these studies was between 23% and 41%, with the exception of the T1 and peripheral T1 groups, which had average prevalences of 17% (range, 9%-24%) and 15% (range, 9%-22%), respectively.

The FN rate is lower for squamous cell cancer than for adenocarcinoma; insufficient data is available for large cell cancer. Lower FN rates for squamous cancer were seen in 8 of the 11 series reporting on both types; in the other 3, no difference was seen.[65–67] This trend was statistically significant in only one study.[37] Unfortunately, the cell type is not always available preoperatively. Furthermore, the reliability of cell type as determined by cytology is only about 75% (see Table 4–12). These issues limit the usefulness of histology in more closely predicting the FN rate of CT.

The factor with the strongest influence on FN rates is central versus peripheral location of the tumor. This is similar to the data reported by Daly et al,[64] discussed previously. Lower FN rates for peripheral tumors were seen in five of the eight studies reporting results for both central and peripheral tumors, but the trend was in the opposite direction in the other three studies.[9,68,69] Nevertheless, the difference in FN rates in Figure 5–7 is convincing. An FN rate of 22% is probably high enough to cause uneasiness in most proponents of radiographic staging. An FN rate of 27% was found in patients who are cN1 in one study.[69]

The difference in the FN rates for T1 versus T2,3 tumors is less striking. Lower FN rates with T1 tumors were seen in seven of the nine studies reporting on both categories. When only peripheral tumors are included, the difference in FN rates is even less striking (9% for T1 versus 13% for T2,3).[9,50,64,70] There is insufficient data to analyze T3 or

TABLE 5–7. CORRELATION OF LYMPH NODE SIZE AND PRESENCE OF MALIGNANCY IN NON–SMALL CELL LUNG CANCER

STUDY	N	% MALIGNANT BY NODE SIZE		
		<1 cm	1–1.9 cm	≥2 cm
McLoud et al[63]	414	13	25	67
Cole et al[75]	404	4	33	18
Izbicki et al[67]	337	14	30	26
Whittlesey[167]	175[a]	3	32	70
Brion et al[66]	100	19	40	55
Libschitz and McKenna[74]	86[a]	14	29	71
Average		**11**	**32**	**51**

Inclusion criteria: Studies of ≥50 patients reporting mediastinal node involvement by node size.

[a]Number of patients.

N, total number of nodes (all sizes).

T4 patients further. No difference is seen in the FN rates for right-sided (12%) tumors versus left-sided (13%) tumors,[48,65,69–72] although some authors have suggested that radiographic mediastinal staging is less accurate on the left.[71]

The FP rate in a large number of series ranges from 18% to 72%, but it is generally approximately 45% (see Table 5–6). More important than the overall accuracy is whether situations can be defined in which a positive CT scan is reliable. A review of the FP rates in Figures 5–5 and 5–7 shows that no subgroup of patients with a particular nodal station, histology, T stage, or tumor location can be identified that has an acceptably low FP rate. Examination of the influence of these factors is helpful only in identifying subgroups with a somewhat higher FP rate.

Several studies have found that squamous cell cancers more often have enlarged nodes that are benign (higher FP rate) than do adenocarcinomas.[37,70,73] It is possible that atelectasis and obstruction from central tumors, which are usually squamous cancers, may cause benign lymph node enlargement.[37] A few studies have indeed suggested that the presence of obstruction or pneumonia causes benign lymph node enlargement and therefore a higher FP rate.[50,63,74] Granulomatous disease also has been suggested to cause a higher FP rate.[74] However, the average FP rates in patients with obstruction or granulomatous disease shown in Figure 5–7 do not stand out as being particularly high. More important, the FP rate in the absence of granulomatous disease or pneumonia (19%-22%) does not seem low enough to make surgical confirmation of enlarged nodes unnecessary.[50,74]

A number of studies have investigated whether there is a node size above which malignancy can be reliably predicted. The results of these studies are shown in Table 5–7. Nodes >2 cm harbor cancer an average of only 50% of the time. Even nodes >3 cm were found in two studies to have malignant involvement in 75% and 22% of all such nodes.[63,75] Although there is a surprisingly large amount of variability in the incidence of malignant involvement, it is clear from Table 5–7 that no size criteria can be established that make surgical biopsy of enlarged nodes unnecessary.

It is possible that the patients included in the studies discussed in this section and in Table 5–7 are not necessarily representative of all patients with mediastinal node involvement. The patients included in these studies have all undergone mediastinoscopy or thoracotomy and generally seem to have had discrete nodes whose size could be measured. However, some patients with locally advanced lung cancers have such extensive infiltration of the mediastinum that discrete nodes cannot be distinguished. It seems likely that these latter patients were excluded from the studies discussed earlier, perhaps because they were not subjected to mediastinoscopy or thoracotomy. Unfortunately, a discussion of such patients with extensive infiltration or even a description of which patients were excluded is not given in any of the reports on accuracy of CT assessment of the mediastinum.

DATA SUMMARY: COMPUTED TOMOGRAPHY ASSESSMENT OF T AND N STAGE	AMOUNT	QUALITY	CONSISTENCY
T Stage			
The FP rate of chest wall involvement by CT is high (45%)	High	Mod	Mod
The FP rate of mediastinal involvement by CT is high (33%)	High	Mod	Mod
N Stage			
A transverse short axis diameter of ≥1 cm is used in most studies to define an abnormal node	High	High	Mod
The FP rate of N1 involvement by CT is high (38%)	High	Mod	Poor
The FP rate of N2,3 involvement by CT is high (45%)	High	High	Mod
The FN rate of N2,3 involvement by CT is 13% overall	High	High	High
The FN rate of N2,3 involvement by CT for central tumors is high (22%)	High	High	High
The FN rate of N2,3 involvement by CT for adenocarcinoma is moderately high (19%)	High	High	High
The FN rate of N2,3 involvement by CT for T1 tumors is low (10%)	High	High	High

Type of data rated: Plain text: descriptive statement   *Italics: controlled comparison*   **Bold: randomized comparison**

POSITRON-EMISSION TOMOGRAPHY SCANNING

PET scanning allows a metabolic assessment of mediastinal lymph nodes that is inherently different from the anatomic assessment provided by CT scan or MRI. The mechanism of action is explained in Chapter 4. A number of studies have employed PET scanning before mediastinoscopy or thoracotomy. Because of the poor anatomic definition of PET scanning, these studies have generally not related accuracy to specific node stations or to T status. The gold standard used in all of these studies was lymph node biopsy via thoracotomy or mediastinoscopy. In several studies, it is clear that this has been done in a detailed fashion, with an average of 2.5 to 5 node stations per patient having been biopsied.[76–79] In others, the gold standard used is less clear. For example, in one report of mediastinal node staging by PET scanning, a total of only 22 mediastinal node stations were biopsied in the entire cohort of 42 patients.[80]

Table 5–8 shows the results of all studies involving at least 20 patients for which reasonably accurate data about mediastinal node staging via PET scan were reported. The average sensitivity is 84% and the average specificity is 93%. These results appear to be better than the sensitivity and specificity of CT scanning.[54] The average FN rate of 7% and FP rate of 16% also appear to be acceptable. Variation exists, particularly in the FP rates, and may be related to the incidence of granulomatous disease in the region in which the study was conducted. Three of the studies reporting the highest FP rates were conducted in Michigan, Iowa, and North Carolina, where granulomatous disease is common.[81–83] The prevalence of mediastinal involvement with lung cancer varied between 16% and 50% in all of these studies.

Mediastinal staging by PET scanning suffers from several limitations. There is poor anatomic localization due to the PET scan alone because most soft tissue landmarks are not well visualized on a PET scan. It is difficult to differentiate hilar nodes from mediastinal nodes. Those studies that have reported on nodal staging for hilar and mediastinal nodes together have shown an average FN rate of 19% and an FP rate of 10%.[82,84–86] Difficulties can also arise in differentiating nodal metastases from primary tumors when these are centrally located. PET scanning has been found to be less accurate in these situations.[84] Separating subcarinal node uptake from the high density uptake of the myocardium can also occasionally be difficult.[87]

Correlation of PET images with CT images is useful. Vansteenkiste et al[88] found the sensitivity of PET scan to be only 67% when used alone, but it rose to 93% when correlated with CT scan. Similarly, the FN and FP rates were 13% and 9% by PET alone versus 3% and 7% when correlated with CT scan. However, formal integration of these two modalities has not been found to be beneficial. Wahl et al[82] used fusion images of CT and PET but did not find them to add to the reliability of PET scanning.

Patients with infectious disease may exhibit FP PET scans. However, such inflammatory foci are frequently only weakly positive compared with malignant tumor involvement.[78] FN scans may arise when the lymph nodes are close to the primary tumor.[78,87] In addition, small node size may be a reason for FN scans.[78,79] Reasonable evidence was cited by one group of authors that the FN rate rose dramatically for lymph nodes <0.7 cm.[79] However, the limit of size that can be detected also depends on the intensity of the marker uptake.

In summary, PET scanning results in fairly reliable staging of the mediastinum. Its greatest limitations appear to be availability, cost, unclear reliability in small nodes, and the lack of detail compared to mediastinoscopy (N2 versus N3, single versus multiple stations positive). PET scanning does not obviate the need for CT but is best done in addition to CT scanning, thus increasing the cost.[88,89] However, the cost of PET scanning may well decrease in the future, and newer technology may make more detailed mediastinal assessment by PET scanning possible.

OTHER IMAGING TECHNIQUES

The use of scintigraphy with gallium (^{67}Ga) citrate for mediastinal staging has been controversial. A review on the use of tracer imaging in lung cancer concluded: "The discrepant nature of the results regarding the accuracy of

TABLE 5–8. ACCURACY OF POSITRON-EMISSION TOMOGRAPHY SCANNING: MEDIASTINAL NODES[a]

STUDY	N	SENS (%)	SPEC (%)	FN (%)	FP (%)	STUDY LOCATION
Saunders et al[169]	84	71	97	7	14	England
Valk et al[78]	74	83	94	8	12	California
Kernstine et al[83 b]	64	70	86	6	52	Iowa
Vansteenkiste et al[88]	50	93	97	3	7	Belgium
Steinert et al[77 b]	47	89	99	3	4	Switzerland
Sazon et al[170]	32	100	100	0	0	California
Guhlmann et al[85]	32	89	100	11	0	Germany
Chin et al[81]	30	78	81	11	36	North Carolina
Sasaki et al[79]	29	76	98	7	7	Japan
Scott et al[76]	27	100	100	0	0	Nebraska
Tatsumi et al[171]	23	78	79	15	30	Japan
Wahl et al[82]	23	82	81	13	25	Michigan
Average		**84**	**93**	**7**	**16**	

Inclusion criteria: >20 patients and histologic proof of mediastinal node status and a prevalence of mediastinal node involvement of ≥10% and ≤90%.
[a]In all studies, the gold standard used was extensive node sampling at thoracotomy or mediastinoscopy.
[b]Results reported per node (not per patient).
FN, false negative rate; FP, false positive rate; N, number of patients; SENS, sensitivity; SPEC, specificity.

TABLE 5–9. RADIONUCLEOTIDE IMAGING STUDIES IN NON–SMALL CELL LUNG CANCER: ASSESSMENT OF N2,3 NODAL INVOLVEMENT

STUDY	MARKER	FEAS	N[a]	PREV (%)	SENS (%)	SPEC (%)	FN (%)	FP (%)
Yokoi et al[172 b]	Thallium	93	105	33	80	91	10	18
Matsuno et al[173]	Thallium	100	34	18	100	86	0	25
Buccheri and Ferrigno[95]	MoAb CEA[c]	—	80	28	77	72	11	48
Vuillez et al[174]	MoAb CEA[c]	75	21	57	92	67	14	21
Rusch et al[175]	MoAb G2b[c]	96	21	43	89	58	13	38

Inclusion criteria: Data in ≥20 evaluable patients, with a prevalence of ≥10% and ≤90%.
[a]Evaluable patients.
[b]Includes 7% small cell.
[c]Monoclonal antibody to CEA or G2b.
Feas, feasibility (percentage of all patients who demonstrated sufficient marker uptake to be evaluable); FN, false negative rate; FP, false positive rate; MoAb, monoclonal antibodies; Prev, prevalence of N2,3 node involvement in evaluable patients; Sens, sensitivity; Spec, specificity.

gallium scanning for the detection of mediastinal involvement makes it difficult to translate them into a reasonable clinical approach to minimize the need for mediastinoscopy."[90(p60)] This is best illustrated by two studies involving 100 or more patients with suspected lung cancer who underwent Ga scintigraphy. One study, which found a 33% FN rate, recommended that mediastinoscopy be performed if the mediastinum was negative by Ga scan.[91] The other study, which found an FN rate of 0 but a 27% FP rate, concluded just the opposite.[92] Both studies had a similar prevalence of mediastinal node involvement (56% and 52%). As a result of the discrepant data, Ga scanning has not played a meaningful role in lung cancer staging since the advent of CT.[93,94]

More recently, other imaging techniques using radiolabeled markers have been investigated. These techniques have involved either general isotopes, such as thallium, or monoclonal antibodies (MoAbs) to specific tumor proteins. These techniques have been feasible in 70% to 90% of patients, meaning that even the primary tumor exhibited no uptake in 10% to 30% of patients. The results of those studies reporting on mediastinal staging in at least 20 evaluable patients (uptake present) are shown in Table 5–9. Although these techniques have shown reasonable effectiveness, the sensitivity, specificity, and FN and FP rates are not dramatically different from those of CT, particularly when one considers that CT is feasible in all patients. It is also notable that the group in Cuneo, Italy, which invested a lot of effort over 10 years to study MoAbs

against CEA, concluded in their most recent report that this technique offers no improvement over CT in the detection of metastases.[95]

TRANSBRONCHIAL (WANG) NEEDLE BIOPSY

Equipment and techniques have been developed to allow transbronchial aspiration of paratracheal or subcarinal lymph nodes for cytologic or histologic examination, using a flexible bronchoscope. This procedure has clearly been shown to be safe: no significant complications (ie, requiring any treatment) were encountered in 1053 patients in whom this was specifically reported.[96–102] This included 198 patients in whom larger (>20 gauge) needles were used.[97,99,101,102]

Despite this extensive experience, however, little data are available to analyze the reliability of this procedure. Not surprisingly, the FN rate is relatively high, ranging from 19% to 55% in the studies shown in Table 5–10. The studies with a higher FN rate have had a rather high prevalence, which makes estimation of FN rates less reliable. Nevertheless, considering the reported FN rates, a negative transbronchial needle aspiration probably should not obviate a need for more accurate staging, such as mediastinoscopy.

A more significant issue is whether a positive transbronchial aspiration can be relied on. FPs have been reported

TABLE 5–10. N2,3 STAGING BY TRANSBRONCHIAL NEEDLE ASPIRATION[a]

STUDY	N[b]	PREV (%)	SENS (%)	SPEC (%)	FN (%)	FP (%)
Shure and Fedullo[96]	110	—	—	100	—	0
Schenk et al[98]	73	29	38	96	19	22
Ratto et al[105]	47	30	14	100	27	0
Vansteenkiste et al[102]	72	83	—	—	45	—
Schenk et al[101]	64	86	86	—	47	—
Schenk et al[99]	29	86	80	—	55	—
Average			**55**	**99**	**39**	**7**

Inclusion criteria: Studies of ≥20 patients reporting ≥90% histologic confirmation or adequate follow-up and a prevalence of ≥10% and ≤90%.
[a]All studies incorporated precautions to minimize false positives (eg, flushing the channel, performing needle biopsy before collecting other samples). Surgical confirmation of negative results was done in all patients; positive results were confirmed in those studies for which a false positive rate and specificity are shown.
[b]Evaluable patients.
FN, false negative rate; FP, false positive rate; Prev, prevalence; Sens, sensitivity; Spec, specificity.

anecdotally[103,104] and in almost all larger series,[98,100] although the number of such cases is relatively low. The problem is that in most studies, no further confirmation was sought after a positive transbronchial aspiration result so that the number of patients in whom an assessment of the FP rate can really be made is also low. Two studies have found an FP rate of 0,[96,105] whereas one found an FP rate of 22%.[98] These three studies involved a total of 230 patients but a total of only 27 positive transbronchial needle aspirations, 2 of which (7%) were FPs. Therefore, given these results and the fact that the data are so limited, one must be somewhat cautious in accepting a positive transbronchial needle aspiration as proof of unresectability.

TRANSTHORACIC NEEDLE BIOPSY

The reported data demonstrate that a transthoracic (CT-guided) needle aspiration of mediastinal masses or nodes can be done safely.[106–108] The ability to carry out the procedure and achieve a diagnosis has been reported by several authors to be >90%.[107–110] Technical aspects that are frequently emphasized to be important in achieving a high success rate include immediate cytologic interpretation and repeat biopsy if the quality of the sample is unsatisfactory.[106–108] A wide variety of techniques and approaches can be used. Transthoracic biopsy of mediastinal nodes often involves traversing lung parenchyma, and some authors reported safely traversing such structures as the superior vena cava or pulmonary artery with fine needles.[106,107,109,110] The incidence of pneumothorax is reported to be 20% to 40%, with chest tubes being necessary in 10% to 20% of patients.[106–109] It may be possible to decrease the rate of pneumothorax markedly by careful management of the patient.[108] Hemoptysis occurs in <10% of patients and is almost always mild and self-limited.[106]

It is likely that transthoracic biopsy results are accurate, although most reports do not include any follow-up or confirmation of the diagnosis. One of the few studies to address reliability found no FPs and only 1 FN among 48 patients.[108] Transthoracic biopsy is limited by the fact that it does not allow multiple node stations to be sampled and that nodes <1.5 cm are usually not considered large enough to biopsy. The role of transthoracic needle biopsy

in mediastinal staging is usually to confirm involvement in patients with SCLC or in patients who are not surgical candidates. This technique has little role when the suspicion of mediastinal involvement is not high because of the inability to sample multiple node stations and concern about the FN rate.

MEDIASTINOSCOPY

The gold standard method of mediastinal staging is mediastinoscopy. Although this is invasive, it can be done as an outpatient procedure[111–113] with minimal morbidity (2%) and mortality (0.08%) (see Table 8–5). Paratracheal (stations 2R, 2L, 4R, 4L), pretracheal (1, 3), and anterior subcarinal nodes (7) are accessible via this approach (see Fig. 5–4 for map of node stations). Node groups that cannot be biopsied with this technique include posterior subcarinal (7), inferior mediastinal (8, 9), and aortopulmonary window and anterior mediastinal (5, 6) nodes.

The sensitivity, specificity, and FN and FP rates of mediastinoscopy from all studies including >50 patients are shown in Table 5–11. However, the specificity and FP rates cannot really be assessed because patients with a positive biopsy were not subjected to any further procedures (such as thoracotomy) to confirm the results. Nevertheless, it seems reasonable to assume that the FP rate is low. The average FN rate for the studies shown in Table 5–11 is 9%. Several authors have shown that approximately half (42%-57%) of the false-negative cases were due to nodes that were not accessible by the mediastinoscope.[50,71,114–116] The FN rate at mediastinoscopy is probably also affected by the diligence with which nodes are dissected and sampled at mediastinoscopy. Ideally, five nodal stations (stations 2R, 4R, 7, 4L, 2L) should routinely be examined, with at least one node sampled from each station unless none are present. There is no data indicating that more careful sampling at mediastinoscopy makes a difference, but extrapolation from data on occasional sampling and systematic sampling at thoracotomy suggests that this is important.[57,59]

Repeat mediastinoscopy may come to play an important role in mediastinal restaging after induction therapy. Repeat mediastinoscopy was found to be not feasible in 18% of

TABLE 5–11. RELIABILITY OF MEDIASTINOSCOPY TO ASSESS N2,3 NODE INVOLVEMENT

STUDY	N	PREV (%)	SENS (%)	SPEC[a] (%)	FN (%)	FP[a] (%)
Hammond et al[116 b]	1369	38	85	100	8	0
Coughlin et al[114]	1191	31	92	100	4	0
De Leyn et al[176]	500	39	76	100	13	0
Dillemans et al[65]	331	41	72	100	16	0
Whittlesey[167 c]	154	31	100	100	0	0
Brion et al[66 b]	153	35	67	100	15	0
Staples et al[50]	151	57	79	100	13	0
Jolly et al[166]	136	54	92	100	8	0
Gdeedo et al[71]	100	32	89	100	9	0
Ratto et al[105 b]	100	30	90	100	4	0
Average			**84**	**100**	**9**	**0**

Inclusion criteria: Studies of ≥100 consecutive patients with lung cancer undergoing mediastinoscopy ± anterior mediastinotomy and a prevalence of ≥10% and ≤90%.
[a]In all studies, patients with a positive mediastinoscopy did not undergo thoracotomy.
[b]No anterior mediastinotomy assessment of aortopulmonary window nodes) done.
[c]Unclear extent of lymph node sampling at thoracotomy when mediastinoscopy negative.
FN, false negative rate; FP, false positive rate; PREV, prevalence; SENS, sensitivity; SPEC, specificity.

140 cases because of adhesions or bleeding. The sensitivity was 74% and the FN rate 8% compared with subsequent thoracotomy.[117] No deaths and no emergency thoracotomies were encountered, but 7% of the patients suffered minor complications.[117] Similar results have been reported by others.[118] In patients with superior vena caval obstruction, mediastinoscopy has been found to be feasible in 100%, with only 6 major complications (bleeding) in 114 patients (5%).[119,120]

OTHER SURGICAL STAGING PROCEDURES

Thoracoscopy has been used to assess some node stations not accessible by mediastinoscopy (stations 5, 6, 7, 8, 9). In 40 patients with enlarged aortopulmonary window or subazygous nodes who had a negative cervical mediastinoscopy, thoracoscopy provided completely accurate staging in all, with no FNs.[121] A more traditional method of sampling nodes in the aortopulmonary window is via a parasternal mediastinotomy (Chamberlain procedure).[122–124] Particularly for left upper lobe tumors, assessment of the aortopulmonary window is important. In 34 patients with left upper lobe cancers in whom cervical mediastinoscopy was negative, 24% were found to have N2 disease in the aortopulmonary window at thoracotomy (no CT data given regarding node size).[123] However, there is no data to assess the sensitivity or FN rate of parasternal mediastinotomy.

A technique used much less commonly to assess the aortopulmonary window is *extended cervical mediastinoscopy,* in which a mediastinoscope is inserted through the suprasternal notch and directed lateral to the aortic arch.[125] In 100 consecutive patients with left upper lobe cancers, standard mediastinoscopy and extended mediastinoscopy were found to have a sensitivity of 69% and an FN rate of 11% for detection of N2,3 disease (prevalence 29%).[125] Similar results (sensitivity, 83%; FN rate, 3%) were reported in another series of 50 such patients.[126] In approximately 500 patients undergoing extended cervical mediastinoscopy, 2 major complications (1 stroke and 1 aortic injury) have been reported.[125–128]

Before the availability of CT scans, biopsy of scalene lymph nodes was commonly done and was reported to be positive in 24% of 286 patients without palpable supraclavicular adenopathy.[129] This procedure was abandoned after

the advent of radiographic (CT) and surgical (mediastinoscopy) techniques for assessing the mediastinum itself. However, a modification of this technique using the mediastinoscope has been revived as a method of detecting unsuspected supraclavicular node involvement (N3 disease) in patients with mediastinoscopically proven N2 disease who are being considered for combined-modality treatment.[130] Of 39 patients originally staged (by cervical mediastinoscopy) as N2, 15% harbored occult, nonpalpable supraclavicular disease. Of 19 patients with contralateral mediastinal node (N3) involvement, 68% also had supraclavicular involvement. This technique may become important to more accurately stage locally advanced patients being considered for aggressive multimodality treatment.

DETECTION OF OCCULT MICROMETASTASES

Several authors have investigated the detection of lymph node involvement by techniques that are more sensitive than histologic examination.[131–138] This has generally involved immunohistochemistry of paraffin-imbedded tissue using MoAbs against various tumor markers, and is commonly referred to as *detection of occult micrometastases* because these tumor cells cannot be detected by standard microscopy. The assays have a low FP rate ($\leq 3\%$) in control patients who do not have lung cancer and low FN rates in the primary tumors of patients with lung cancer.[131,136,138–140] Furthermore, these findings are corroborated by similar assays in bone marrow to detect occult distant metastases in patients with lung cancer (see Table 6–13).[139–141]

The results of studies involving detection of occult micrometastases in mediastinal lymph nodes in N0 patients are shown in Table 5–12. It can be seen that marker-positive cells are detected in a substantial number of these N0 patients. These assays have involved immunohistochemistry; however, techniques using reverse transcriptase-polymerase-chain reaction assays may be even more sensitive (but require immediate freezing at $-80°C$).[131]

The real issue, of course, is what influence the detection of occult micrometastases has on prognosis. Those studies reporting follow-up clearly show worse survival in marker-positive patients. In fact, in three studies that carried out multivariate analysis, occult marker positivity was found

TABLE 5–12. DETECTION OF OCCULT MICROMETASTASES IN MEDIASTINAL LYMPH NODES

STUDY	MARKER	N[a]	% WITH OM	MEDIAN SURVIVAL TIME (mo) OM−	OM+	P
Izbicki et al[133]	Ber-EP4	73	27	41	29	0.008
Chen et al[137]	Antikeratin	60	63	81	65	0.1
Dobashi et al[134]	p53	47[b]	45	180[c]	22	0.0001
Maruyama et al[138]	CAM 5.2	44	27	180[c]	60	0.04

Inclusion criteria: ≥ 20 evaluable N0 lung cancer patients with survival data.
[a]Evaluable patients.
[b]Data reported only for p53-positive tumors (47 of 101 patients).
[c]Estimated 5-y actuarial survival >80%.
OM, occult metastasis (per patient); OM−, micrometastasis assay–negative patients; OM+, micrometastasis assay–positive patients.

DATA SUMMARY: POSITRON-EMISSION TOMOGRAPHY, NUCLEAR IMAGING, AND INVASIVE STAGING OF N2,3 NODAL INVOLVEMENT

	AMOUNT	QUALITY	CONSISTENCY
The FN rate of PET for N2,3 nodal involvement is low (6%)	High	High	High
The FP rate of PET for N2,3 nodal involvement is low (10%)	High	High	Mod
The FN and FP rates of monoclonal antibody scanning for N2,3 involvement are similar to those of CT (FN 13%, FP 45%)	Mod	High	Mod
Transbronchial needle biopsy of N2,3 nodes can be done safely	High	High	High
The FN rate of transbronchial needle aspiration of N2,3 nodes is high (39%)	High	High	Mod
The FP rate of transbronchial needle aspiration of N2,3 nodes is 7%	Mod	Mod	Poor
The FN rate of mediastinoscopy is 9%	High	High	High

Type of data rated: Plain text: descriptive statement   *Italics: controlled comparison*   **Bold: randomized comparison.**

to carry the highest relative risk for survival with the lowest *P* value (ahead of nodal status by standard microscopy).[132,134,138] This is further strengthened by similar results in studies of occult nodal involvement in other cancers.[142,143]

The presence of occult nodal metastases in N0 patients was more strongly correlated with local recurrence (40% versus 8%, *P* = 0.001) than with distant recurrence (30% versus 16%, *P* = NS) in 59 patients in one study.[132] However, there was no correlation between the presence of occult nodal micrometastases and occult bone marrow micrometastases in this study, and these authors postulated different mechanisms for lymphatic versus hematogenous spread.[132] Other investigators have implied a correlation between occult nodal micrometastases and a higher rate of both local and distant recurrences.[134]

RADIOGRAPHIC VERSUS SURGICAL CLINICAL STAGING

It is clear that clinical staging differs markedly from pathologic staging (after resection). In a large prospective study (1984-1990, 3823 patients), clinical staging was found to agree with pathologic staging in only 56% of patients. Overstaging occurred roughly as often as understaging (24% versus 20%).[144] Almost identical findings have been reported by others,[27,48,71,145] although the incidence of overstaging and understaging depends on the population studied. In one study of cN0 patients, 19% were found to be pN1 and 24% pN2.[27] On the contrary, in another study of cN2 patients, 38% were pN0 or pN1, and 6% were found to be pN3 (Fig. 5–8A).[145]

It must be emphasized that clinical staging involves all information that is available before the initiation of therapy. The accuracy of clinical staging depends primarily on whether only information from radiographic studies is used or whether efforts have been made to obtain more precise information from surgical biopsies. Radiographic and surgical clinical staging can each be compared separately to pathologic staging. From the data reviewed earlier, radiographic staging (by CT or MRI) has an FN rate of 15% to 20% and an FP rate of 40% to 50%. Mediastinoscopy, however, has FN and FP rates of <10%. Although the morbidity of mediastinoscopy in experienced centers is low

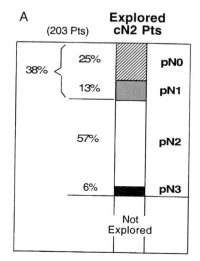

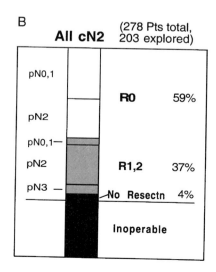

FIGURE 5–8. *A,* Comparison of clinical stage to actual pathologic stage in 203 patients with radiographic evidence of N2 disease who underwent thoracotomy. *B,* Resectability in clinical N2 patients. c, clinical stage; p, postoperative stage; R₀, complete resection (no residual disease); R₁,₂, incomplete resection (microscopic or gross residual disease). (From Watanabe Y, Shimizu J, Oda M, et al. Aggressive surgical intervention in N2 non–small cell cancer of the lung. Ann Thorac Surg. 1991;51:253–261.[145])

(see Table 8–5), the procedure is invasive and suffers from a lack of widespread availability of surgeons who are comfortable performing it.

Debate continues about whether all patients should be staged surgically with mediastinoscopy or staged radiographically without histologic confirmation of mediastinal nodal status, or whether both approaches should be combined in some manner. A randomized trial investigating the role of routine mediastinoscopy in all patients has been carried out by the Canadian Lung Oncology Group in 685 patients who by CXR had apparently operable NSCLC.[146] Patients were randomized to either routine mediastinoscopy (without a prior CT) or CT and selective mediastinoscopy (only for nodes >1 cm).

In the routine mediastinoscopy group, 81% of the patients had a negative mediastinoscopy and only 4% ever had a CT scan. In the routine CT group, 45% of the patients underwent mediastinoscopy, which was negative in 57%. The results show that both approaches have the same outcome in almost all respects: incidence of unsuspected N2 nodes found at thoracotomy (13% versus 18%), incidence of thoracotomy without complete resection (12% versus 10%), and cost of the workup and treatment in the Canadian health care system ($14 600 versus $13 900) for mediastinoscopy versus CT with selective mediastinoscopy, respectively.[146] The only significant difference was that a higher number of patients eventually found to have benign disease were subjected to thoracotomy in the routine mediastinoscopy (no routine CT scan) group (12 of 25 versus 4 of 20, $P = 0.05$).

Although these results suggest that routine mediastinoscopy in all nonmetastatic patients without a prior chest CT scan is a reasonable alternative to CT and selective mediastinoscopy, it seems doubtful that many will adopt this policy. Most centers perform mediastinoscopy only rarely or do it selectively.[17,147,148] This is in stark contrast to CT scanning, which is done routinely in most centers as an initial step to better assess the primary lesion.

Is radiographic staging alone sufficient? In patients with mediastinal node enlargement as demonstrated by CT, it is clear that reliance on radiographic staging alone will result in a major proportion of patients being subjected to inappropriate therapy. The FP rate for CT is approximately 40% in a large number of studies (see Table 5–6), and the data from one of these is illustrated graphically in Figure 5–8A. On one hand, if these patients are all rejected for surgery, a large number of pN0,1 patients will be denied resection, which remains the most effective therapy for early stage disease. On the other hand, if all patients with radiographic nodal enlargement undergo thoracotomy, approximately 40% of the entire group of cN2 patients will undergo thoracotomy without a complete resection, although those who are pN0,1 will be resected (see Fig. 5–8B and Table 17–1).[149–154] Therefore, it seems clear that radiographic staging alone will result in an error rate of approximately 40% in patients with mediastinal nodal enlargement. However, it may be reasonable to rely on radiographic staging alone in patients with lung cancer and extensive mediastinal infiltration or encasement of mediastinal structures, even though there is no actual data to confirm this.

It is more difficult to define the value of mediastinoscopy as an adjunct to CT in patients who are radiographically N0,1. There is confusion about whether the goal of intrathoracic staging is simply to identify patients with N2 disease before thoracotomy or to identify patients who cannot be completely resected because some argue that patients with N2 disease should not necessarily be denied surgical resection.[152,154–157] Unfortunately, further confusion is created in this regard by using data from one subgroup of patients as an argument to support an approach for another subgroup. For example, 5-year survival figures of 20% to 30% are often quoted in support of surgical resection of N2 patients. However, what is often forgotten is that these figures pertain only to those N2 patients in whom a complete resection is achieved and that they exclude those patients not resected or incompletely resected.

The 5-year survival of mediastinoscopy-positive patients who nevertheless are taken to thoracotomy has been reported to be 9% to 18% in studies of >20 such patients.[114,158–160] These figures include those patients who were not resected (22%-36%) or who were incompletely resected.[114,158,159] However, although it is clear that these patients were a highly select subgroup, it is not clear whether they were radiographically N0,1. Thus, the survival and resectability of radiographically N0,1 patients who might have been identified as pN2 by mediastinoscopy remain undefined.

Probably of greater significance is whether a particular policy toward mediastinoscopy in radiographically N0,1 patients has an effect on the resectability of the entire cohort of cN0,1 patients. The results of those studies reporting such data are shown in Table 5–13. There seems to be no clear difference in terms of overall resectability or the incidence of pN2 disease found at thoracotomy when different policies toward mediastinoscopy are employed. However, the data are somewhat limited, and none of these studies was undertaken to specifically address this question. One has to read between the lines to extract this data, which contributes to a sense of uneasiness in drawing firm conclusions from these results.

In the absence of a clear answer, the best approach to the dilemma of when to pursue mediastinoscopy in cN0,1 patients may be to identify a rate of pN2 disease that is unacceptably high and then to establish a policy of performing mediastinoscopy in those subgroups of patients who are likely to exceed this threshold. Where this line is drawn is influenced not only by the morbidity of mediastinoscopy and thoracotomy but also by the perceived benefits of newer multimodality treatments in patients with pN2 disease. Most thoracic surgeons would probably be willing to accept an FN rate of 10% (T1 tumors), whereas most would probably be uncomfortable with an FN rate >20% (central tumors, cN1, adenocarcinomas). These considerations should allow the establishment of a rational policy regarding surgical staging in addition to radiographic staging, even though the data falls short of providing a conclusive answer.

EDITORS' COMMENTS

Accurate intrathoracic staging is a crucial issue in lung cancer and is a prerequisite if appropriate therapy is to be selected. Some of the issues associated with intrathoracic staging are of minor importance. For example, accurate

TABLE 5–13. EFFECT OF DEFINED POLICIES REGARDING MEDIASTINOSCOPY IN PATIENTS WITH A RADIOGRAPHICALLY NEGATIVE MEDIASTINUM (cN0,1)

STUDY	N[a]	MEDIASTINOSCOPY POLICY[b]	% R_0 OF ALL PATIENTS	% pN2 AT THORACOTOMY	% R_0 OF N2
Canadian Lung Oncology Group[146]	228	Conservative	89	19	65
Daly et al[64]	500	Conservative	—	7	92
Fernando and Goldstraw[27]	103	Conservative	95	24	84[c]
Average			**92**	**17**	**80**
De Leyn et al[176]	711	Aggressive	—	15	87
Dillemans et al[65]	471	Aggressive	95	16[d]	72[e]
Gaer and Goldstraw[58]	100	Aggressive	95	24	—
Average			**95**	**18**	**80**
Coughlin et al[114]	920	All	89	—	—
Staples et al[50]	107	All	—	11	83
Average			**89**	**11**	**83**

Inclusion criteria: Studies reporting data on >100 cN0,1 patients undergoing thoracotomy in whom a consistent policy toward mediastinoscopy was used.

[a]Clinical N0,1 patients undergoing thoracotomy.

[b]Mediastinoscopy policy: conservative, no mediastinoscopy performed in cN0,1 patients (nodes <1 cm); aggressive, mediastinoscopy performed in all central, T2,3 and nonsquamous tumors; all, mediastinoscopy performed in all patients (even all cN0,1 patients).

[c]May include patients with R_1 resection.

[d]Would be 12%, except for exclusion of 23 patients who did not undergo mediastinoscopy because of contraindications.

[e]Estimated.

R_0, complete resection.

clinical staging of N1 node involvement radiographically is difficult. However, this is of little consequence in selecting appropriate therapy. Radiographic assessment of chest wall involvement is also difficult. The presence of pain seems to be both simpler and better than radiographic findings as an indicator of chest wall involvement. However, once again this is of little consequence because resection can usually be carried out when chest wall involvement is discovered at the time of thoracotomy.

Resectability in the case of mediastinal involvement is more of an issue. Because it is often difficult to ascertain this from preoperative radiographic studies, an aggressive approach is warranted. Given the high propensity for central tumors to have mediastinal node involvement despite a negative CT scan, patients with central tumors should undergo preoperative mediastinoscopy. However, if this is negative, exploration using thoracoscopy or thoracotomy is warranted because a complete resection can often be achieved despite a worrisome radiographic appearance.

The major issue in intrathoracic staging is mediastinal node involvement. Many words and much paper have been expended in discussing the usefulness of radiographic and surgical staging of the mediastinum since 1980, and the issue is still actively debated today. As in most ongoing arguments, both sides are probably right some of the time. Furthermore, the arguments put forth by each side are probably proffered with different patient populations in mind, and thus resolution is never achieved.

There is clearly a population of patients with extensive mediastinal infiltration with tumor in which the radiographic picture (together with a cytologic diagnosis of lung cancer from some site) leaves no real doubt about the presence of mediastinal involvement with cancer. What is needed is a good definition of this type of extensive disease. We propose that patients with tumor that surrounds mediastinal structures (superior vena cava, pulmonary ar-

tery, trachea, main stem bronchi) or patients in whom no discrete nodal masses can be distinguished be classified as having extensive disease. Although there are no data to document this, it seems reasonable to accept the radiographic appearance as adequate proof of malignant involvement in such cases. At any rate, it seems intuitively clear that these patients could not undergo surgical resection with a negative margin. When such patients are selected for a nonsurgical approach without histologic confirmation of mediastinal involvement, it seems highly likely that the FP rate will be low.

Patients with an abnormal mediastinum characterized by discreet areas of nodal enlargement should have surgical confirmation of this before malignant involvement is assumed. There is extensive data indicating that the FP rate of CT is high in this situation. Although transbronchial needle biopsy may allow this diagnosis to be established, it does not allow sampling of multiple nodal stations as easily as mediastinoscopy. It has been less extensively studied; furthermore, it is not clear that the morbidity of a bronchoscopy under sedation is less than that of mediastinoscopy.

In patients with left upper lobe tumors, mediastinoscopy should be combined with an assessment of the aortopulmonary window by extended mediastinoscopy, Chamberlain procedure, or thoracoscopy. Unfortunately, each of these procedures is either not easily performed or adds morbidity. Aortopulmonary window nodal involvement denotes N2 disease as much as paratracheal nodal involvement does. However, it is likely that many surgeons are more apt to look for an excuse not to sample aortopulmonary window nodes as opposed to nodes accessible by mediastinoscopy because of the increased morbidity.

Patients with a radiographically normal mediastinum are the group in which the appropriate staging (radiographic versus surgical) is least clear. With the advent of multimodality treatment for patients with N2 disease, it may be more important to accurately stage these patients preoperatively, although the optimal therapy for these cN0,1, pN2 patients is not clear. The ability of PET scans to reliably detect small foci of tumor in radiographically normal nodes is unclear, and mediastinoscopy remains the gold standard. In our own practice, we have adopted a relatively aggressive approach. Mediastinoscopy is performed in the face of a negative CT scan for central tumors as well as tumors in which a diagnosis of adenocarcinoma, large cell cancer, or small cell cancer has been made. The only patients excluded are those with peripheral lesions.

Intrathoracic staging may well change in the near future. This could be either in the direction of more detailed staging (detection of occult micrometastases) or less detailed staging (PET scanning). MoAb scans do not appear to be sensitive or specific enough to have an impact on staging, but early data for PET scanning suggest that this technique may be as sensitive and specific as mediastinoscopy. However, limitations of PET scanning include high cost, lack of wide availability, and inability to differentiate individual nodal stations or to identify millimeter-sized foci of tumor.

The detection of occult micrometastatic disease has the potential for opening up a new realm in our understanding of lung cancer. It is conceivable that in the future, occult micrometastases in bone marrow could identify patients who may benefit from chemotherapy, whereas occult micrometastases in lymph nodes would identify early-stage patients who may benefit from adjuvant mediastinal radiotherapy. However, these concepts will not be explored if mediastinoscopy is not pursued (perhaps in favor of PET scanning). Unfortunately, mediastinoscopy probably suffers from lack of availability of surgeons who are truly comfortable performing this procedure. This may be because thoracic surgery is frequently performed by surgeons who have not had extensive formal training in general thoracic surgery as opposed to general surgery or cardiac surgery. It seems unlikely that this will change in the future. Given the development of more effective chemotherapy and radiation techniques, it would be unfortunate if new methods of defining localized disease are not explored because of a preference for less invasive, yet less detailed techniques.

References

1. Vecchio TJ. Predictive value of a single diagnostic test in unselected populations. N Engl J Med. 1966;274:1171–1173.
2. Metz CE. Basic principles of ROC analysis. Semin Nuclear Med 1978;8:283–298.
3. Vining DJ, Gladish GW. Receiver operating characteristic curves: a basic understanding. Radiographics. 1992;12:1147–1154.
4. Osterlind K, Ihde DC, Ettinger DS, et al. Staging and prognostic factors in small cell carcinoma of the lung. Cancer Treat Rep. 1983;67:3–9.
5. Pearlberg JL, Sandler MA, Beute GH, et al. Limitations of CT in evaluation of neoplasms involving chest wall. J Comput Assist Tomogr. 1987;11:290–293.
6. Whitley NO, Fuks JZ, McCrea ES, et al. Computed tomography of the chest in small cell lung cancer: potential new prognostic signs. AJR Am J Roentgenol. 1984;141:885–892.
7. Shepherd FA, Ginsberg RJ, Haddad R, et al. Importance of clinical staging in limited small-cell lung cancer: a valuable system to separate prognostic subgroups. J Clin Oncol. 1993;11:1592–1597.
8. Webb WR, Gatsonis C, Zerhouni EA, et al. CT and MR imaging in staging non–small cell bronchogenic carcinoma: report of the Radiologic Diagnostic Oncology Group. Radiology. 1991;178:705–713.
9. McKenna RJ Jr, Libshitz HI, Mountain CE, et al. Roentgenographic evaluation of mediastinal nodes for preoperative assessment in lung cancer. Chest. 1985;86:206–210.
10. Pearlberg JL, Sandler MA, Beute GH, et al. T1N0M0 bronchogenic carcinoma: assessment by CT. Radiology. 1985;157:187–190.
11. Backer CL, Shields TW, Lockhart CG, et al. Selective preoperative evaluation for possible N2 disease in carcinoma of the lung. J Thorac Cardiovasc Surg. 1987;93:337–343.
12. Libshitz HI, McKenna RJ Jr, Haynie TP, et al. Mediastinal evaluation in lung cancer. Radiology. 1984;151:295–299.
13. Duncan KA, Gomersall LN, Weir J. Computed tomography of the chest in T1N0M0 non–small cell bronchial carcinoma. Br J Radiol. 1993;66:20–22.
14. Heavey LR, Glazer GM, Gross BH, et al. The role of CT in staging radiographic T1N0M0 lung cancer. Am J Radiol. 1986;146:285–290.
15. Conces DJ Jr, Klink JF, Tarver RD, et al. T1N0M0 lung cancer: evaluation with CT. Radiology. 1989;170:643–646.
16. Parker LA, Mauro MA, Delany DJ, et al. Evaluation of T1N0M0 lung cancer with CT. J Comput Assist Tomogr. 1991;15:943–947.
17. Tsang GMK, Watson DCT. The practice of cardiothoracic surgeons in the perioperative staging of non–small cell lung cancer. Thorax. 1992;47:3–5.
18. Encuentra AL, and the Bronchogenic Carcinoma Cooperative Group of the Spanish Society of Pneumology and Thoracic Surgery (GCCB-S). Criteria of functional and oncological operability in surgery for lung cancer: a multicenter study. Lung Cancer. 1998;20:161–168.
19. Feld R, Abratt R, Graziano S, et al. Pretreatment minimal staging and prognostic factors for non–small cell lung cancer (Consensus Report). Lung Cancer. 1997;17(suppl 1):S3–S10.
20. Patterson GA, Ginsberg RJ, Poon PY, et al. A prospective evaluation of magnetic resonance imaging, computed tomography, and mediastinoscopy in the preoperative assessment of mediastinal node status in bronchogenic carcinoma. J Thorac Cardiovasc Surg. 1987;94: 679–684.
21. Martini N, Heelan R, Westcott J, et al. Comparative merits of conventional, computed tomographic, and magnetic resonance imaging in assessing mediastinal involvement in surgically confirmed lung carcinoma. J Thorac Cardiovasc Surg. 1985;90:639–648.
22. Musset D, Grenier P, Carette M, et al. Primary lung cancer staging: prospective comparative study of MR imaging with CT. Radiology. 1986;160:607–611.
23. Laurent F, Drouillard J, Dorcier F, et al. Bronchogenic carcinoma staging: CT versus MR imaging-assessment with surgery. Eur J Cardiothorac Surg. 1988;2:31–36.
24. Grenier P, Dubray B, Carette MF, et al. Preoperative thoracic staging of lung cancer: CT and MR evaluation. Diagn Interv Radiol. 1989;1:23–28.
25. Poon PY, Bronskill MJ, Henkelman RM, et al. Mediastinal lymph node metastases from bronchogenic carcinoma: detection with MR imaging and CT. Radiology. 1987;162:651–656.
26. Gdeedo A, Van Schil P, Corthouts B, et al. Comparison of imaging TNM [(i)TNM] and pathological TNM [pTNM] in staging of bronchogenic carcinoma. Eur J Cardiothorac Surg. 1997;12:224–227.
27. Fernando HC, Goldstraw P. The accuracy of clinical evaluative intrathoracic staging in lung cancer as assessed by postsurgical pathologic staging. Cancer. 1990;65:2503–2506.
28. Nakata H, Ishimaru H, Nakayama C, et al. Computed tomography for preoperative evaluations of lung cancer. J Comput Tomogr. 1986;10:147–151.
29. Ratto GB, Piacenza G, Frola C, et al. Chest wall involvement by lung cancer: computed tomographic detection and results of operation. Ann Thorac Surg. 1991;51:182–188.
30. Glazer HS, Duncan-Meyer J, Aronberg DJ, et al. Pleural and chest wall invasion in bronchogenic carcinoma: CT evaluation. Radiology. 1985;157:191–194.
31. Pennes DR, Glazer GM, Wimbish KJ, et al. Chest wall invasion by lung cancer: limitations of CT evaluation. Am J Radiol. 1985;144:507–511.
32. Suzuki N, Saitoh T, Kitamura S. Tumor invasion of the chest wall in lung cancer: diagnosis with US. Radiology. 1993;187:39–42.

33. Heelan RT, Demas BE, Caravelli JF, et al. Superior sulcus tumors: CT and MR imaging. Radiology. 1989;170:637–641.
34. Venuta F, Rendina EA, Ciriaco P, et al. Computed tomography for preoperative assessment of T3 and T4 bronchogenic carcinoma. Eur J Cardiothorac Surg. 1992;6:238–241.
35. Glazer HS, Kaiser LR, Anderson DJ, et al. Indeterminate mediastinal invasion in bronchogenic carcinoma: CT evaluation. Radiology. 1989;173:37–42.
36. Baron RL, Levitt RG, Sagel SS, et al. Computed tomography in the preoperative evaluation of bronchogenic carcinoma. Radiology. 1982;145:727–732.
37. Izbicki JR, Thetter O, Karg O, et al. Accuracy of computed tomographic scan and surgical assessment for staging of bronchial carcinoma: a prospective study. J Thorac Cardiovasc Surg. 1992;104:413–420.
38. Herman SJ, Winton TL, Weisbrod GL, et al. Mediastinal invasion by bronchogenic carcinoma: CT signs. Radiology. 1994;190:841–846.
39. White PG, Adams H, Crane MD, et al. Preoperative staging of carcinoma of the bronchus: can computed tomographic scanning reliably identify stage III tumours? Thorax. 1994;49:951–957.
40. De Giacomo T, Rendina E, Venuta F, et al. Thoracoscopic staging of IIIB non–small cell lung cancer before neoadjuvant therapy. Ann Thorac Surg. 1997;64:1409–1411.
41. Roviaro GC, Varoli F, Rebuffat C, et al. Videothoracoscopic operative staging for lung cancer. Int Surg. 1996;81:252–254.
42. Quint LE, Glazer GM, Orringer MB. Central lung masses: prediction with CT of need for pneumonectomy versus lobectomy. Radiology. 1987;165:735–738.
43. Feigin DS, Friedman PJ, Liston SE, et al. Improving specificity of computed tomography in diagnosis of malignant mediastinal lymph nodes. CT: J Comput Tomogr. 1985;9:21–32.
44. Glazer GM, Gross BH, Quint LE, et al. Normal mediastinal lymph nodes: number and size according to American Thoracic Society mapping. AJR Am J Roentgenol. 1985;144:261–265.
45. Kiyono K, Sone S, Sakai F, et al. The number and size of normal mediastinal lymph nodes: a postmortem study. AJR Am J Roentgenol. 1988;150:771–776.
46. Quint LE, Glazer GM, Orringer MB, et al. Mediastinal lymph node detection and sizing at CT and autopsy. AJR Am J Roentgenol. 1986;147:469–472.
47. Arita T, Matsumoto T, Kuramitsu T, et al. Is it possible to differentiate malignant mediastinal nodes from benign nodes by size? Reevaluation by CT, transesophageal echocardiography, and nodal specimen. Chest. 1996;110:1004–1008.
48. Lewis JW Jr, Pearlberg JL, Beute GH, et al. Can computed tomography of the chest stage lung cancer?—yes and no. Ann Thorac Surg. 1990;49:591–596.
49. Kerr KM, Lamb D, Wathen CG, et al. Pathological assessment of mediastinal lymph nodes in lung cancer: implications for non-invasive mediastinal staging. Thorax. 1992;47:337–341.
50. Staples CA, Müller NL, Miller RR, et al. Mediastinal nodes in bronchogenic carcinoma: comparison between CT and mediastinoscopy. Radiology. 1988;167:367–372.
51. Guyatt GH, Lefcoe M, Walter S, et al. Interobserver variation in the computed tomographic evaluation of mediastinal lymph node size in patients with potentially resectable lung cancer. Chest. 1995;107:116–119.
52. Webb WR, Sarin M, Zerhouni EA, et al. Interobserver variability in CT and MR staging of lung cancer. J Comput Assist Tomogr. 1993;17:841–846.
53. Bollen ECM, Goei R, van't Hof-Grootenboer BE, et al. Interobserver variability and accuracy of computed tomographic assessment of nodal status in lung cancer. Ann Thorac Surg. 1994;58:158–162.
54. Dales RE, Stark RM, Raman S. Computed tomography to stage lung cancer: approaching a controversy using meta-analysis. Am Rev Respir Dis. 1990;141:1096–1101.
55. Glazer GM, Orringer MB, Gross BH, et al. The mediastinum in non–small cell lung cancer: CT-surgical correlation. AJR Am J Roentgenol. 1984;142:1101–1105.
56. Mori K, Yokoi K, Saito Y, et al. Diagnosis of mediastinal lymph node metastases in lung cancer. Jpn J Clin Oncol. 1992;22:35–40.
57. Izbicki JR, Passlick B, Karg O, et al. Impact on radical systematic mediastinal lymphadenectomy on tumor staging in lung cancer. Ann Thorac Surg. 1995;59:209–214.
58. Gaer JAR, Goldstraw P. Intraoperative assessment of nodal staging at thoracotomy for carcinoma of the bronchus. Eur J Cardiothorac Surg. 1990;4:207–210.
59. Bollen ECM, van Duin CJ, Theunissen PHMH, et al. Mediastinal lymph node dissection in resected lung cancer: morbidity and accuracy of staging. Ann Thorac Surg. 1993;55:961–966.
60. Wain JC. Video-assisted thoracoscopy and the staging of lung cancer. Ann Thorac Surg. 1993;56:776–778.
61. Roberts JR, Blum MG, Arildsen R, et al. Prospective comparison of radiologic, thoracoscopic, and pathologic staging in patients with early non–small cell lung cancer. Ann Thorac Surg. 1999;68:1154–1158.
62. Seely JM, Mayo JR, Miller RR, et al. T1 lung cancer: prevalence of mediastinal nodal metastases and diagnostic accuracy of CT. Radiology. 1993;186:129–132.
63. McLoud TC, Bourgouin PM, Greenberg RW, et al. Bronchogenic carcinoma: analysis of staging in the mediastinum with CT by correlative lymph node mapping and sampling. Radiology. 1992;182:319–323.
64. Daly BDT, Mueller JD, Faling LJ, et al. N2 lung cancer: outcome in patients with false-negative computed tomographic scans of the chest. J Thorac Cardiovasc Surg. 1993;105:904–911.
65. Dillemans B, Deneffe G, Verschakelen J, et al. Value of computed tomography and mediastinoscopy in preoperative evaluation of mediastinal nodes in non–small cell lung cancer: a study of 569 patients. Eur J Cardiothorac Surg. 1994;8:37–42.
66. Brion JP, Depauw L, Kuhn G, et al. Role of computed tomography and mediastinoscopy in preoperative staging of lung carcinoma. J Comput Assist Tomogr. 1985;9:480–484.
67. Sparup J, Friis J, Vejlsted H, et al. Computed tomography and the TNM classification of lung cancer. Scand J Thorac Cardiovasc Surg. 1990;24:207–211.
68. Matthews JI, Richey HM, Helsel RA, et al. Thoracic computed tomography in the preoperative evaluation of primary bronchogenic carcinoma. Arch Intern Med. 1987;147:449–453.
69. Suzuki K, Nagai K, Yoshida J, et al. Clinical predictors of N2 disease in the setting of a negative computed tomographic scan in patients with lung cancer. J Thorac Cardiovasc Surg. 1999;117:593–598.
70. Daly BD Jr, Faling LJ, Bite G, et al. Mediastinal lymph node evaluation by computed tomography in lung cancer: an analysis of 345 patients grouped by TNM staging, tumor size, and tumor location. J Thorac Cardiovasc Surg. 1987;94:664–672.
71. Gdeedo A, Van Schil P, Corthouts B, et al. Prospective evaluation of computed tomography and mediastinoscopy in mediastinal lymph node staging. Eur Respir J. 1997;10:1547–1551.
72. Platt JF, Glazer GM, Gross BH, et al. CT evaluation of mediastinal lymph nodes in lung cancer: influence of the lobar site of the primary neoplasm. Am J Radiol. 1987;149:683–686.
73. Rhoads AC, Thomas JH, Hermreck AS, et al. Comparative studies of computerized tomography and mediastinoscopy for the staging of bronchogenic carcinoma. Am J Surg. 1986;152:587–591.
74. Libschitz HI, McKenna RS Jr. Mediastinal lymph node size in lung cancer. AJR Am J Roentgenol. 1984;143:715–718.
75. Cole PH, Roszkowski A, Firouz-Abadi A, et al. Computerized tomography does not predict N2 disease in patients with lung cancer. Aust N Z J Med. 1993;23:688–691.
76. Scott WJ, Gobar LS, Terry JD, et al. Mediastinal lymph node staging of non–small-cell lung cancer: a prospective comparison of computed tomography and positron emission tomography. J Thorac Cardiovasc Surg. 1996;111:642–648.
77. Steinert HC, Hauser M, Allemann F, et al. Non–small cell lung cancer: nodal staging with FDG PET versus CT with correlative lymph node mapping and sampling. Radiology. 1997;202:441–446.
78. Valk PE, Pounds TR, Hopkins DM, et al. Staging non–small cell lung cancer by whole-body positron emission tomographic imaging. Ann Thorac Surg. 1995;60:1573–1582.
79. Sasaki M, Ichiya Y, Kuwabara Y, et al. The usefulness of FDG positron emission tomography for the detection of mediastinal lymph node metastases in patients with non–small cell lung cancer: a comparative study with x-ray computed tomography. Eur J Nucl Med. 1996;23:741–747.
80. Patz EF Jr, Lowe VJ, Goodman PC, et al. Thoracic nodal staging with PET imaging with ¹⁸FDG in patients with bronchogenic carcinoma. Chest. 1995;108:1617–1621.
81. Chin R Jr, Ward R, Keyes JW Jr, et al. Mediastinal staging of

non–small-cell lung cancer with positron emission tomography. Am J Respir Crit Care Med. 1995;152:2090–2096.

82. Wahl RL, Quint LE, Greenough RL, et al. Staging of mediastinal non–small cell lung cancer with FDG PET, CT, and fusion images: preliminary prospective evaluation. Radiology. 1994;191:371–377.

83. Kernstine KH, Stanford W, Mullan BF, et al. PET, CT, and MRI with Combidex for mediastinal staging in non–small cell lung carcinoma. Ann Thorac Surg 1999;68:1022–1028.

84. Bury T, Paulus P, Dowlati A, et al. Staging of the mediastinum: value of positron emission tomography imaging in non–small cell lung cancer. Eur Respir J. 1996;9:2560–2564.

85. Guhlmann A, Storck M, Kotzerke J, et al. Lymph node staging in non–small cell lung cancer: evaluation by [^{18}F]FDG positron emission tomography (PET). Thorax. 1997;52:438–441.

86. Gupta NC, Graeber GM, Rogers II JS, et al. Comparative efficacy of positron emission tomography with FDG and computed tomographic scanning in preoperative staging of non–small cell lung cancer. Ann Surg. 1999;229:286–291.

87. Scott WJ, Schwabe JL, Gupta NC, et al. Positron emission tomography of lung tumors and mediastinal lymph nodes using [^{18}F]fluorodeoxyglucose. Ann Thorac Surg. 1994;58:698–703.

88. Vansteenkiste JF, Stroobants SG, De Leyn PR, et al. Mediastinal lymph node staging with FDG-PET scan in patients with potentially operable non–small-cell lung cancer: a prospective analysis of 50 cases. Chest. 1997;112:1480–1486.

89. Graeber GM, Gupta NC, Murray GF. Positron emission tomographic imaging with flurorodeoxyglucose is efficacious in evaluating malignant pulmonary disease. J Thorac Cardiovasc Surg. 1999;117:719–727.

90. Abdel-Dayem HM, Scott A, Macapinlac H, et al. Tracer imaging in lung cancer. Eur J Nucl Med. 1994;21:57–81.

91. DeMeester TR, Golomb HM, Kirchner P, et al. The role of gallium-67 scanning in the clinical staging and preoperative evaluation of patients with carcinoma of the lung. Ann Thorac Surg. 1979;28:451–464.

92. Alazraki NP, Ramsdell JW, Taylor A, et al. Reliability of gallium scan chest radiography compared to mediastinoscopy for evaluating mediastinal spread in lung cancer. Am Rev Respir Dis. 1978;117:415–420.

93. MacMahon H, Scott W, Ryan JW, et al. Efficacy of computed tomography of the thorax and upper abdomen and whole-body gallium scintigraphy for staging of lung cancer. Cancer. 1989;64:1404–1408.

94. Ragheb AM, Elgazzar A-HH, Ibrahim AK, et al. A comparative study between planar Ga-67, T1-201 images, chest x-ray, and x-ray CT in inoperable non–small cell carcinoma of the lung. Clin Nucl Med. 1995;20:426–433.

95. Buccheri G, Ferrigno D. Therapeutic options for regionally advanced non–small cell lung cancer. Lung Cancer. 1996;14:281–300.

96. Shure D, Fedullo PF. The role of transcarinal needle aspiration in the staging of bronchogenic carcinoma. Chest. 1984;86:693–696.

97. Wang KP. Flexible transbronchial needle aspiration biopsy for histologic specimens. Chest. 1985;88:860–863.

98. Schenk DA, Bower JH, Bryan CL, et al. Transbronchial needle aspiration staging of bronchogenic carcinoma. Am Rev Respir Dis. 1986;134:146–148.

99. Schenk DA, Strollo PJ, Pickard JS, et al. Utility of the Wang 18-gauge transbronchial histology needle in the staging of bronchogenic carcinoma. Chest. 1989;96:272–274.

100. Harrow EM, Oldenburg FA Jr, Lingenfelter MS, et al. Transbronchial needle aspiration in clinical practice: a five-year experience. Chest. 1989;96:1268–1272.

101. Schenk DA, Chambers SL, Derdak S, et al. Comparison of the Wang 19-gauge and 22-gauge needles in the mediastinal staging of lung cancer. Am Rev Respir Dis. 1993;147:1251–1258.

102. Vansteenkiste J, Lacquet LM, Demedts M, et al. Transcarinal needle aspiration biopsy in the staging of lung cancer. Eur Respir J. 1994;7:265–268.

103. Cropp AJ, DiMarco AF, Lankerani M. False-positive transbronchial needle aspiration in bronchogenic carcinoma. Chest. 1984;85:696–697.

104. Carlin BW, Harrell JH II, Fedullo PF. False-positive transcarinal needle aspirate in the evaluation of bronchogenic carcinoma. Am Rev Respir Dis. 1989;140:1800–1802.

105. Ratto GB, Mereu C, Motta G. The prognostic significance of preoperative assessment of mediastinal lymph nodes in patients with lung cancer. Chest. 1988;93:807–813.

106. Westcott JL. Percutaneous transthoracic needle biopsy. Radiology. 1988;169:593–601.

107. van Sonnenberg E, Casola G, Ho M, et al. Difficult thoracic lesions: CT-guided biopsy experience in 150 cases. Radiology. 1988;167:457–461.

108. Protopapas Z, Westcott JL. Transthoracic needle biopsy of mediastinal lymph nodes for staging lung and other cancers. Radiology. 1996;199:489–496.

109. Westcott JL. Percutaneous needle aspiration of hilar and mediastinal masses. Radiology. 1981;141:323–329.

110. Moinuddin SM, Lee LH, Montgomery JH. Mediastinal needle biopsy. AJR Am J Roentgenol. 1984;143:531–532.

111. Cybulsky IJ, Bennett WF. Mediastinoscopy as a routine outpatient procedure. Ann Thorac Surg. 1994;58:176–178.

112. Vallières E, Pagé A, Verdant A. Ambulatory mediastinoscopy and anterior mediastinotomy. Ann Thorac Surg. 1991;52:1122–1126.

113. Selby JH Jr, Leach CL, Heath BJ, et al. Local anesthesia for mediastinoscopy: experience with 450 consecutive cases. Am Surg. 1978:679–682.

114. Coughlin M, Deslauriers J, Beaulieu M, et al. Role of mediastinoscopy in pretreatment staging of patients with primary lung cancer. Ann Thorac Surg. 1985;40:556–560.

115. Van Den Bosch JMM, Gelissen HJ, Wagenaar SS. Exploratory thoracotomy in bronchial carcinoma. J Thorac Cardiovasc Surg. 1983;85:733–737.

116. Hammoud ZT, Anderson RC, Meyers BF, et al. The current role of mediastinoscopy in the evaluation of thoracic disease. J Thorac Cardiovasc Surg 1999;118:894–899.

117. Meersschaut D, Vermassen F, de la Rivière AB, et al. Repeat mediastinoscopy in the assessment of new and recurrent lung neoplasm. Ann Thorac Surg. 1992;53:120–122.

118. Olsen PS, Stentoft P, Ellefsen B, et al. Re-mediastinoscopy in the assessment of resectability of lung cancer. Eur J Cardiothorac Surg. 1997;11:661–663.

119. Jahangiri M, Goldstraw P. The role of mediastinoscopy in superior vena caval obstruction. Ann Thorac Surg. 1995;59:453–455.

120. Mineo T, Ambrogi V, Nofroni I, et al. Mediastinoscopy in superior vena cava obstruction: analysis of 80 consecutive patients. Ann Thorac Surg. 1999;68:223–226.

121. Landreneau RJ, Hazelrigg SR, Mack MJ, et al. Thoracoscopic mediastinal lymph node sampling: useful for mediastinal lymph node stations inaccessible by cervical mediastinoscopy. J Thorac Cardiovasc Surg. 1993;106:554–558.

122. Jolly PC, Li W, Anderson RP. Anterior and cervical mediastinoscopy for determining operability and predicting resectability in lung cancer. J Thorac Cardiovasc Surg. 1980;79:366–371.

123. Schreinemakers HHJ, Joosten HJM, Mravunac M, et al. Parasternal mediastinoscopy: assessment of operability in left upper lobe lung cancer: a prospective analysis. J Thorac Cardiovasc Surg. 1988;95:298–302.

124. Best L-A, Munichor M, Ben-Shakkar M, et al. The contribution of anterior mediastinotomy in the diagnosis and evaluation of diseases of the mediastinum and lung. Ann Thorac Surg. 1987;43:78–81.

125. Ginsberg RJ, Rice TW, Goldberg M, et al. Extended cervical mediastinoscopy: a single staging procedure for bronchogenic carcinoma of the left upper lobe. J Thorac Cardiovasc Surg. 1987;94:673–678.

126. Lopez L, Varela A, Freixinet J, et al. Extended cervical mediastinoscopy: prospective study of fifty cases. Ann Thorac Surg. 1994;57:555–558.

127. Urschel JD, Vretenar DF, Dickout WJ, et al. Cerebrovascular accident complicating extended cervical mediastinoscopy. Ann Thorac Surg. 1994;57:740–741.

128. Ginsberg RJ, in Discussion section of Lopez L VA, Freixinet J, et al. Extended cervical mediastinoscopy: prospective study of fifty cases. Ann Thorac Surg. 1994;57:555–558.

129. Brantigan JW, Brantigan CO, Brantigan OC. Biopsy of nonpalpable scalene lymph nodes in carcinoma of the lung. Am Rev Respir Dis. 1973;107:962–974.

130. Lee JD, Ginsberg RJ. Lung cancer staging: the value of ipsilateral scalene lymph node biopsy performed at mediastinoscopy. Ann Thorac Surg. 1996;62:338–341.

131. Salerno CT, Frizelle S, Niehans GA, et al. Detection of occult micrometastases in non–small cell lung carcinoma by reverse transcriptase-polymerase chain reaction. Chest. 1998;113:1526–1532.

132. Passlick B, Izbicki JR, Kubuschok B, et al. Detection of disseminated lung cancer cells in lymph nodes: impact on staging and prognosis. Ann Thorac Surg. 1996;61:177–183.

133. Izbicki JR, Passlick B, Hosch SB, et al. Mode of spread in the early phase of lymphatic metastasis in non–small-cell lung cancer: significance of nodal micrometastasis. J Thorac Cardiovasc Surg. 1996;112:623–630.

134. Dobashi K, Sugio K, Osaki T, et al. Micrometastatic p53-positive cells in the lymph nodes of non–small-cell lung cancer: prognostic significance. J Thorac Cardiovasc Surg. 1997;114:339–346.

135. Nicholson AG, Graham ANJ, Pezzella F, et al. Does the use of immunohistochemistry to identify micrometastases provide useful information in the staging of node-negative non–small cell lung carcinomas? Lung Cancer. 1997;18:231–240.

136. Passlick B, Izbicki JR, Kubuschok B, et al. Immunohistochemical assessment of individual tumor cells in lymph nodes of patients with non–small-cell lung cancer. J Clin Oncol. 1994;12:1827–1832.

137. Chen Z-L, Perez S, Holmes EC, et al. Frequency and distribution of occult micrometastases in lymph nodes of patients with non–small-cell lung carcinoma. J Natl Cancer Inst. 1993;85:493–498.

138. Maruyama R, Sugio K, Mitsudomi T, et al. Relationship between early recurrence and micrometastases in the lymph nodes of patients with stage I non–small-cell lung cancer. J Thorac Cardiovasc Surg. 1997;114:535–543.

139. Cote RJ, Beattie EJ, Chaiwun B, et al. Detection of occult bone marrow micrometastases in patients with operable lung carcinoma. Ann Surg. 1995;222:415–425.

140. Pantel K, Izbicki J, Passlick B, et al. Frequency and prognostic significance of isolated tumour cells in bone marrow of patients with non–small-cell lung cancer without overt metastases. Lancet. 1996;347:649–653.

141. Pantel K, Izbicki JR, Angstwurm M, et al. Immunocytological detection of bone marrow micrometastasis in operable non–small cell lung cancer. Cancer Res. 1993;53:1027–1031.

142. Hayashi M, Ito I, Nakamura Y, et al. Genetic diagnosis of lymph-node metastasis in colorectal cancer. Lancet. 1995;345:1257–1259.

143. Trojani M, Mascarel I, Delsol G, et al. Micrometastases to axillary lymph nodes from carcinoma of breast: detection by immunohistochemistry and prognostic significance. Br J Cancer. 1987;55:303–306.

144. Bülzebruck H, Bopp R, Drings P, et al. New aspects in the staging of lung cancer: prospective validation of the International Union Against Cancer TNM classification. Cancer. 1992;70:1102–1110.

145. Watanabe Y, Shimizu J, Oda M, et al. Aggressive surgical intervention in N2 non–small cell cancer of the lung. Ann Thorac Surg. 1991;51:253–261.

146. The Canadian Lung Oncology Group. Investigation for mediastinal disease in patients with apparently operable lung cancer. Ann Thorac Surg. 1995;60:1382–1389.

147. Epstein DM, Stephenson LW, Gefter WB, et al. Value of CT in the preoperative assessment of lung cancer: a survey of thoracic surgeons. Radiology. 1986;161:423–427.

148. Humphrey EW, Smart CR, Winchester DP, et al. National survey of the pattern of care for carcinoma of the lung. J Thorac Cardiovasc Surg. 1990;100:837–843.

149. Martini N, Flehinger BJ, Zaman MB, et al. Results of resection in non–oat cell carcinoma of the lung with mediastinal lymph node metastases. Ann Surg. 1983;198:386–397.

150. Naruke T. Significance of lymph node metastases in lung cancer. Semin Thorac Cardiovasc Surg. 1993;5:210–218.

151. Wada H, Tanaka F, Yanagihara K, et al. Time trends and survival after operations for primary lung cancer from 1976 through 1990. J Thorac Cardiovasc Surg. 1996;112:349–355.

152. Watanabe Y, Hayashi Y, Shimizu J, et al. Mediastinal nodal involvement and the prognosis of non–small cell lung cancer. Chest. 1991;100:422–428.

153. Sawamura K, Mori T, Hashimoto S, et al. Results of surgical treatment for N2 disease [abstract]. Lung Cancer. 1986;2:96.

154. Cybulsky IJ, Lanza LA, Ryan MB, et al. Prognostic significance of computed tomography in resected N2 lung cancer. Ann Thorac Surg. 1992;54:533–537.

155. Naruke T, Goya T, Tsuchiya R, et al. The importance of surgery to non–small cell carcinoma of lung with mediastinal lymph node metastasis. Ann Thorac Surg. 1988;46:603–610.

156. Riquet M, Manac'h D, Saab M, et al. Factors determining survival in resected N2 lung cancer. Eur J Cardiothorac Surg. 1995;9:300–304.

157. Régnard JF, Magdeleinat P, Azoulay D, et al. Results of resection for bronchogenic carcinoma with mediastinal lymph node metastases in selected patients. Eur J Cardiothorac Surg. 1991;5:583–587.

158. Pearson FG, DeLarue NC, Ilves R, et al. Significance of positive superior mediastinal nodes identified at mediastinoscopy in patients with resectable cancer of the lung. J Thorac Cardiovasc Surg. 1982;83:1–11.

159. Vansteenkiste JF, DeLeyn PR, Deneffe GJ, et al. Survival and prognostic factors in resected N2 non–small cell lung cancer: a study of 140 cases. Ann Thorac Surg. 1997;63:1441–1450.

160. Kirschner PA. Lung cancer: preoperative radiation therapy and surgery. N Y State J Med. 1981:339–342.

161. Cohen MH, Matthews MJ. Small cell bronchogenic carcinoma: a distinct clinicopathologic entity. Semin Oncol. 1978;5:234–243.

162. Mountain CF, Dresler CM. Regional lymph node classification for lung cancer staging. Chest. 1997;111:1718–1723.

163. Ferguson MK, MacMahon H, Little AG, et al. Regional accuracy of computed tomography of the mediastinum in staging of lung cancer. J Thorac Cardiovasc Surg. 1986;91:498–504.

164. Ikezoe J, Kadowaki K, Morimoto S, et al. Mediastinal lymph node metastases from non–small cell bronchogenic carcinoma: reevaluation with CT. J Comput Assist Tomogr. 1990;14:340–344.

165. Primack SL, Lee KS, Logan PM, et al. Bronchogenic carcinoma: utility of CT in the evaluation of patients with suspected lesions. Radiology. 1994;193:795–800.

166. Jolly PC, Hutchinson CH, Detterbeck F, et al. Routine computed tomographic scans, selective mediastinoscopy, and other factors in evaluation of lung cancer. J Thorac Cardiovasc Surg. 1991;102:266–271.

167. Whittlesey D. Prospective computed tomographic scanning in the staging of bronchogenic cancer. J Thorac Cardiovasc Surg. 1988;95:876–882.

168. Rendina EA, Bognolo DA, Mineo TC, et al. Computed tomography for the evaluation of intrathoracic invasion by lung cancer. J Thorac Cardiovasc Surg. 1987;94:57–63.

169. Saunders CAB, Dussek JE, O'Doherty MJ, et al. Evaluation of fluorine-18-fluorodeoxyglucose whole body positron emission tomography in the staging of lung cancer. Ann Thorac Surg. 1999;67:790–797.

170. Sazon DA, Santiago SM, Hoo GWS, et al. Fluorodeoxyglucose-positron emission tomography in the detection and staging of lung cancer. Am J Respir Crit Care Med. 1996;153:417–421.

171. Tatsumi M, Yutani K, Watanabe Y, et al: Feasibility of fluorodeoxyglucose dual-head gamma camera coincidence imaging in the evaluation of lung cancer: comparison with FDG PET. J Nucl Med. 1999;40:566–573.

172. Yokoi K, Okuyama A, Mori K, et al. Mediastinal lymph node metastasis from lung cancer: evaluation with T1-201 SPECT: comparison with CT. Radiology. 1994;192:813–817.

173. Matsuno S, Tanabe M, Kawasaki Y, et al. Effectiveness of planar tomography of thallium-201 compared with gallium-67 in patients with primary lung cancer. Eur J Nucl Med. 1992;19:86–95.

174. Vuillez J-P, Brambilla E, Brichon P-Y, et al. Immunoscintigraphy using 111In-labeled F(ab')2 fragments of anti-carcinoembryonic antigen (CEA) monoclonal antibody for staging of non–small cell lung carcinoma. Eur J Cancer. 1994;30A:1089–1092.

175. Rusch V, Macapinlac H, Heelan R, et al. NR-LU-10 monoclonal antibody scanning. J Thorac Cardiovasc Surg. 1993;106:200–204.

176. De Leyn P, Schoonooghe P, Deneffe G, et al. Surgery for non–small cell lung cancer with unsuspected metastasis to ipsilateral mediastinal or subcarinal nodes (N2 disease). Eur J Cardiothorac Surg. 1996;10:649–655.

6

EXTRATHORACIC STAGING

Frank C. Detterbeck, David R. Jones, and Paul L. Molina

APPROACH TO EXTRATHORACIC STAGING

The majority of patients with small cell lung cancer (SCLC) and approximately 40% of patients with non–small cell lung cancer (NSCLC) present with distant metastases (see Fig. 4–1 and Chapter 25).[1-3] Even among those patients who are thought to have early stage (localized) disease and who undergo resection, the majority of recurrences involve extrathoracic sites (see Tables 11–5 and 12–3). This suggests that distant metastases were already present, although unrecognized, at the time of resection in those patients, emphasizing the importance of performing accurate extrathoracic staging. The fact that approximately 90% of patients with distant metastases from either SCLC or NSCLC have symptoms makes extrathoracic staging easier.[4-6]

The approach to patients with lung cancer involves many considerations and tests, which can be done in a number of different sequences. As a result, the process is not necessarily uniform and can be complex. This process has been nicely summarized by the International Association for the Study of Lung Cancer, which has divided it into three distinct steps.[7] The first step involves a clinical evaluation consisting of a history and physical examination, a chest radiograph (CXR), and blood tests. In step 2, confirmatory tests are obtained to corroborate abnormalities noted in step 1. Step 3 consists of radiographic and invasive procedures (eg, chest computed tomography [CT] and mediastinoscopy) to define the intrathoracic stage in patients who do not have distant metastases. This chapter examines issues relating to steps 1 and 2 in this process, whereas step 3 is covered in Chapter 5.

This chapter first addresses the reliability of the clinical evaluation, both as a whole and with regard to individual components of the evaluation. If metastases are suspected on the basis of the clinical evaluation or if the risk of metastases in a particular patient population remains high despite a negative clinical evaluation, the clinician is then faced with the question of which confirmatory test to obtain (eg, Should a cranial CT or magnetic resonance imaging [MRI] be done to investigate the possibility of a brain metastasis?). Once this test has been performed, the clinician must then interpret the test results (eg, What is the false positive [FP] rate of a positive cranial CT?).

In actual practice, some information is usually already available when a patient presents to be evaluated for distant metastases. A CXR and a chest CT are recommended as initial tests in all patients presenting with lung cancer by most of the current consensus statements and clinical guidelines.[7-9] In fact, these studies have usually already been obtained by the primary physician before the patient is referred for a more detailed evaluation. In addition to confirming the suspicion of lung cancer, these tests usually provide a strong suspicion of cell type (small cell versus non–small cell) and a preliminary estimation of intrathoracic stage. Therefore, although it may seem logical to first obtain a cytologic diagnosis, then to exclude extrathoracic metastases, and only thereafter to proceed with an investigation of intrathoracic stage, in actual practice a preliminary estimation of intrathoracic stage and SCLC or NSCLC categorization is usually available when the patient is first seen.

Reviews of extrathoracic staging have noted variability in the results of different studies, perhaps due to heterogeneity among the patient populations evaluated.[10,11] As mentioned earlier, a diagnosis (or at least a strong suspicion) of either SCLC or NSCLC usually exists by the time the patient undergoes a more detailed clinical evaluation. Furthermore, approximately 20% of patients have multiple, widespread metastases and an obvious clinical presentation.[5,6] Inclusion or exclusion of these groups of patients will certainly affect the outcome of an evaluation for distant metastases. The evaluation of patients with obvious metastases is less of an issue than the evaluation of patients with only a few metastases and more subtle symptoms. This chapter attempts to separate these populations in order to define homogeneous patient groups for which conclusions can be drawn.

ASSESSMENT OF THE CLINICAL EVALUATION

In order to be able to apply the results of staging studies prospectively, the patient population in a study must be defined according to clinical characteristics that can be identified preoperatively (eg, presence of symptoms or clinical stage). Furthermore, in order to be able to interpret positive or negative findings, confirmation of patients' true status with an appropriate gold standard such as follow-up, biopsy, or other tests must also be provided. Studies lacking these characteristics have limited usefulness and have been omitted. For example, data from a retrospective review of patients who underwent a brain CT is of limited use if the clinical characteristics of the patients (ie, presence of symptoms) or their true status (how many had metastases) is not provided, and such studies are not included.

Measures of reliability of a test (such as the clinical evaluation of patients with lung cancer) include sensitivity and specificity. However, the usefulness of these measures is limited because they deal with abstract patient populations that are never encountered in actual practice. For example, sensitivity addresses the question: How likely is it that the clinical evaluation will detect a metastasis *in a theoretical patient population, all of whom have metastases?* A more relevant measure is the false negative (FN) or FP rate, which directly addresses the question facing the clinician who has just completed a history and physical examination. In this patient, who has a negative (or positive) clinical examination, how likely is it that the clinical impression is falsely negative (or falsely positive)?

The FN and FP rates are influenced by a high (or low) prevalence of disease in the population. However, even in this situation, the FN and FP rates are relevant, provided the results are interpreted in a similar clinical context: In this patient *who has a presumptive diagnosis of a clinical stage I NSCLC,* how likely is it that the clinical evaluation for distant metastases is falsely negative (or falsely positive)? In other words, the definition of the patient population is crucial. Data regarding FN and FP rates must be applied prospectively to patients who are similar to those in whom the data were originally obtained. These measures of test reliability are described in more detail in Chapter 5.

SITE OF METASTASES

The most common sites of extrathoracic metastases in NSCLC are brain, bone, liver, and adrenal glands (Table 6–1). The next most common sites are lung, pleura, and subcutaneous tissue. The incidence of metastases in NSCLC and the proportion that are solitary depends on the clinical stage of the patient population. It is interesting that even in patients with relatively advanced disease, approximately two-thirds are reported to present with solitary metastases. The rate of solitary metastases is even higher in patients thought to have cI or cII disease. This may reflect a tendency not to record additional sites of metastases once one site is found.

Distant metastases are present in approximately 60% of patients with SCLC. The most common sites of metastases in SCLC are similar to those in NSCLC, with the possible exception of a lower rate of brain and adrenal metastases (see Table 6–1). SCLC also frequently involves other sites, such as the pancreas, abdominal lymph nodes, or bone marrow.[1] All of the studies of patients with SCLC in Table 6–1 have focused on patients treated on various protocols. As a result, some patients with SCLC have been excluded from these studies. However, because of the wide variety of protocols included, the data in Table 6–1 does reflect the sites and incidence of metastases in a clinically relevant population of patients, namely, patients who are candidates for treatment.

COMPONENTS OF THE CLINICAL EVALUATION

The clinical evaluation can be divided into nonspecific and organ-specific findings (Table 6–2). Attention must be paid to both categories. All of the studies regarding the reliability of the clinical evaluation have defined a positive result as *either* a nonspecific *or* an organ-specific finding. The organ-specific factors primarily involve signs and symptoms of brain and bone metastases. Symptoms or physical findings from liver metastases are rare unless the metastatic burden in the liver is overwhelming and the value of blood tests to screen for liver metastases, at least in NSCLC, is questionable (see later discussion). Adrenal metastases also rarely cause symptoms. Fortunately, the chest CT can easily be extended by a few centimeters to cover all of the liver and adrenal glands. This is commonly done and provides an assessment of these organs, as well as an assessment of the presence of pulmonary metastases. The assessment of performance status has not been formally included in the clinical evaluation but would seem to be a reasonable addition. Furthermore, additional laboratory studies (eg, electrolytes, calcium) to screen for common paraneoplastic conditions are sometimes included.

The studies that have evaluated the reliability of the clinical evaluation have used the findings noted in Table 6–2 consistently.[5,12–18] Other studies, which focused on specific findings only, have sometimes added a more detailed evaluation, such as a neurologic examination by a neurologist.[14,19,140] A large study has demonstrated variability regarding what symptoms are judged to be significant, and found that even mild symptoms were associated with a high incidence of metastases.[140] Details that were considered significant are not available in most studies.

RELIABILITY OF THE CLINICAL EVALUATION IN NON–SMALL CELL LUNG CANCER
Overall Reliability

There are not many published reports that allow assessment of the reliability of the clinical evaluation, although there

TABLE 6–1. FREQUENCY OF DISTANT METASTASES AT PRESENTATION IN PATIENTS WITH LUNG CANCER

STUDY	N	STUDY TYPE	CLINICAL STAGE	% M1 OF ALL	% Solitary Site	PERCENTAGE OF PATIENTS WITH METASTASES TO SPECIFIC SITES						
						Brain	Bone	Liver	Adrenal	Lung	Skin	Renal
Notter and Schwegler[128]	33720	Autopsy[a]	All	—	—	21	27	39	18	25	—	18
Ichinose et al[12]	309	NSCLC	cI-II	7	96	17	78	9	—	—	—	—
Salvatierra et al[14]	146	NSCLC	cI-III	30	61	43	43	41	25	0	0	5
Quint et al[22]	348	NSCLC	All	21	67	47	36	22	15	11	13	0
Sagman et al[4]	614	SCLC	All[b]	53	—	10	46	49	—	—	—	—
Richardson et al[1]	451	SCLC	All[b]	66	39	20	42	39	5	32	22[c]	—
Dearing et al[129]	411	SCLC	All[b]	66	39	16	42	38	—	—	11	—
Maurer and Pajak[31]	224	SCLC	All[b]	50	—	15	42	57	—	—	5	—
Ihde et al[2]	106	SCLC	All[b]	69	49	12	55	41	—	10	7	—

Inclusion criteria: Studies from 1980 to 2000 including ≥100 patients and providing data on incidence and site of metastases.
[a]Both SCLC and NSCLC.
[b]Patients entered on various protocols.
[c]Includes cervical lymph nodes.
NSCLC, non–small cell lung cancer; SCLC, small cell lung cancer.

TABLE 6-2. CLINICAL FINDINGS SUGGESTING METASTASIS

NONSPECIFIC FINDINGS	ORGAN-SPECIFIC FINDINGS

Weight loss ≥10%
Fatigue
Laboratory data:
  Decreased albumin
  Decreased HCT
  Increased WBC
  Increased platelets
	Brain: recent headaches, nausea, or any
	  neurologic symptom/sign
	Bone: skeletal pain/tenderness,
	  elevated ALK-P, or hypercalcemia
	Liver: right upper quadrant pain;
	  hepatomegaly; elevated ALK-P,
	  SGOT, LDH, or bilirubin
	Adrenal: none

ALK-P, alkaline phosphatase; HCT, hematocrit; LDH, lactate dehydrogenase, SGOT, serum glutamic-oxaloacetic transaminase; WBC, white blood cell (count).

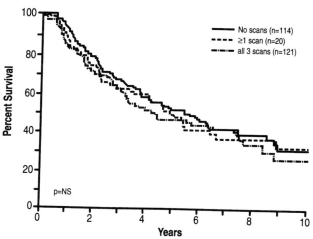

FIGURE 6-1. Survival of resected pI,II patients who had no screening scans, at least one scan, or all three scans (bone, brain, and abdominal) preoperatively. (From Hatter J, Kohman LJ, Mosca RS, et al. Preoperative evaluation of stage I and stage II non–small cell lung cancer. Ann Thorac Surg. 1994;58:1738–1741.[21])

are many reports of the detection rates of radiologic studies (in patients who may or may not have had signs and symptoms of metastases). The results of all studies of the clinical evaluation providing clear definitions and assessments of the presence of metastases are shown in Table 6–3. Most of the reports are retrospective studies; however, several are prospective.[5,14,20] These studies have been grouped according to the patient populations included. Those reports that considered only potentially operable patients excluded patients with *obvious metastases,* meaning patients who had easily palpable metastases or marked clinical symptoms. Although this definition is somewhat vague, it does seem to make sense in actual practice.

The FP rate of a positive clinical evaluation is high. More importantly, the FN rate of the clinical evaluation is about 30% when all NSCLC patients are considered and remains about 15% in potentially operable patients who are stage cI-III. Although the number of studies is limited, it appears that this is due to a high (30%) FN rate in potentially operable patients who are initially staged on the basis of the chest CT as cIII, whereas it is low (<5%) in patients initially staged as cI-II.

This is further corroborated by two reports that have focused on the survival of resected stage I-II patients.[12,21] Both studies found that the survival curves of patients who have undergone bone, brain, and abdominal scans are

superimposable on those of patients who did not (Fig. 6–1). This provides circumstantial evidence that the group of pI-II patients in whom distant scanning was omitted did not include a significant proportion who had unsuspected yet detectable distant metastases at the time of presentation. These were both retrospective, nonrandomized studies in which individual physician preference, scheduling issues, and perhaps other factors determined whether or not distant scanning was done.

It must be emphasized that it is the careful clinical evaluation that is important in these patients, not the mere presence of radiographic stage cI-II disease. The incidence of M1 disease for the entire cohort of cI-II patients (both those with and those without symptoms) has been reported to be 16% and 20% in two studies,[14,22] although it was only 4% and 7% in two other retrospective series.[12,141] Approaching this issue from a different starting point, Sider and Horejs[23] found that among 95 NSCLC patients with

TABLE 6-3. RELIABILITY OF THE CLINICAL EVALUATION[a] OF NON–SMALL CELL LUNG CANCER PATIENTS

STUDY	N	CLINICAL STAGE	PATIENT POPULATION	PREVALENCE OF METASTASES (%)[b]	SENS (%)	SPEC (%)	FP (%)	FN (%)
Michel et al[20]	110	All	All	18	95	32	76	33
Modini et al[130 c,d]	85	All	All	38	25	—	—	31
Grant et al[13 e]	37	cIII	Preop	32	—	—	—	32
Salvatierra et al[14]	146	cI-III	Preop	30	89	32	64	13
Grant et al[13 e]	114	cI-III	Preop	13	—	—	—	13
Quinn et al[5]	53	cI-III	Preop	21	75	40	72	15
Ichinose et al[12]	309	cI,II	Preop	7	96	97	—	0.4
Grant et al[13 e]	77	cI,II	Preop	4	—	—	—	4

Inclusion criteria: Studies of ≥50 patients (total) with non–small cell lung cancer providing data on the reliability of a defined clinical evaluation.
[a]Clinical evaluation includes both nonspecific and organ-specific findings as demonstrated by patient history, physical examination, and blood tests, except as otherwise indicated.
[b]Presence of metastases confirmed by biopsy, follow-up, or screening test (head, liver, adrenal computed tomography, or bone scan) in addition to confirmatory imaging studies.
[c]Includes 21% small cell.
[d]Extent of clinical evaluation unclear.
[e]Includes only patients with a negative clinical evaluation.
FN, false negative rate; FP, false positive rate; Preop, patients being considered for resection; Prev, prevalence; Sens, sensitivity; Spec, specificity.

radiographic evidence of distant metastases, 25% had stage I-II disease in the chest as seen on retrospective review of the chest CT. Most of the patients (83%) in this latter study had clinical signs and symptoms suggestive of metastases.[23]

Reliability of Individual Components

The value of assessing only one component of the clinical evaluation is somewhat questionable. It is hard to imagine conducting only part of a history and physical examination in actual practice. Moreover, the data is not detailed enough to be able to define certain components of the examination as being unhelpful. Furthermore, organ-specific factors may not be as specific as is commonly thought. Although only two authors have examined this issue, both have found that the clinical findings pointed to the site of metastasis in only 55% to 76% of cases.[5,16] In addition, some investigators have found that approximately 70% of patients with distant metastases have nonspecific symptoms.[14] These observations suggest that in a patient with any clinical finding, either nonspecific or organ-specific, consideration should be given to investigating several possible sites of metastases.

Nonetheless, many investigators have reported studies that are limited to only one component of the clinical evaluation. The results of these studies are summarized in Table 6–4. These studies have primarily addressed organ-specific symptoms, particularly with respect to the brain, bone, and liver. Little data is available to correlate these results with the intrathoracic stage of the patients, but what data is available suggests that most of the metastases occurred in cIII patients.[24,25] No data is available for clinical assessment of the adrenal glands because adrenal metastases are thought not to cause symptoms. However, the presence of adrenal metastases was found to correlate with the general clinical evaluation in 173 cI-IV patients with

lung cancer.[26] If the evaluation was negative, no adrenal metastases were found.[26]

There is little data to substantiate the value of laboratory studies in potentially operable NSCLC patients, although such studies are clearly important in the evaluation of SCLC.[27,28] Alkaline phosphatase has usually been reported as positive in only a minority of patients with bone metastases, and, conversely, only half of the patients with an elevated alkaline phosphatase have bone metastases.[16,29,30,142] An exception is the prospective study by Michel et al,[20] in which 89% of patients with bone metastases had an elevated alkaline phosphatase level. The limited data available regarding the value of liver function tests also suggests poor correlation with the presence or absence of metastases, even in patients with relatively widespread metastases.[17] No data has been reported addressing the value of a complete blood cell count in NSCLC.

It is difficult to draw clear conclusions from the data shown in Table 6–4. The FN rates for the clinical evaluation of each individual organ site are relatively low, ranging from 3% to 23%. Similar FN rates were found in a literature review.[11] Another review found that the collective rate of metastasis in asymptomatic patients (equivalent to the FN rate) was 5% for brain, 3% for bone, 2% for liver, and 8% for adrenal glands.[10] Although these rates are consistently low for individual organ sites, this data does not address the value of the clinical evaluation as a whole. It may be that these individual organ FN rates must be *added together* when the entire clinical staging evaluation is considered because most of the patients in this population have solitary metastases (see Table 6–1).

Influence of Histology on the Reliability of the Clinical Evaluation

The influence of histologic subtypes of NSCLC on the reliability of the clinical evaluation has not been studied

---

TABLE 6–4. RELIABILITY OF SPECIFIC COMPONENTS OF THE CLINICAL EVALUATION IN NON–SMALL CELL LUNG CANCER PATIENTS[a]

STUDY	N	FACTOR	CLINICAL STAGE	PATIENT POPULATION	PREV (%)	SENS (%)	SPEC (%)	FP (%)	FN (%)
Salvatierra et al[14 b]	146	Nonspec	cI-IIIa	Preop	30	71	43	65	23
Kormas et al[24 b,c]	158	Neuro	cI-III	Preop	3[d]	—	—	—	3[d]
Salvatierra et al[14 b]	146	Neuro	cI-IIIa	Preop	13	79	91	43	3
Salbeck et al[25]	151	Neuro	?	?	15[e]	41	91	55	10
Tarver et al[18]	137	Neuro	?	?	46	87	63	34	15
Jennings et al[131]	102	Neuro	?	?	23	—	—	—	23
Mintz et al[19]	66	Neuro	?	?	12	38	83	77	9
Salvatierra et al[14 b]	146	Bone	cI-IIIa	Preop	13	79	88	50	3
Michel et al[20 b]	110	Bone	cI-IV	All	8	100	54	(84)	0
Quinn et al[5]	53	Bone	cI-III	Preop	19	50	65	75	15
Salvatierra et al[14 b]	146	Liver	cI-III	Preop	12	39	84	75	9

Inclusion criteria: Studies from 1980 to 2000 reporting data on individual clinical factors in ≥50 patients with non–small cell lung cancer.
[a]Gold standard for metastases in all studies is a typical computed tomography appearance or bone scan *with* confirmatory studies, except as otherwise noted.
[b]Prospective study.
[c]Only patients with negative clinical evaluation included.
[d]6% if biopsy *and* follow-up was used as the gold standard; 77% of metastases were in IIIa patients.
[e]All in N2 patients.
[f]Questionable validity because of low prevalence.
FN, false negative rate; FP, false positive rate; Neuro, neurologic; Nonspec, nonspecific; Preop, patients being evaluated for surgery; Prev, prevalence; Sens, sensitivity; Spec, specificity; ?, unknown.

TABLE 6–5. PRESENCE OF BRAIN METASTASES IN ASYMPTOMATIC NON–SMALL CELL LUNG CANCER PATIENTS ACCORDING TO HISTOLOGIC SUBTYPE[a]

STUDY	N	CLINICAL STAGE	PATIENT POPULATION	SQUAMOUS	ADENOCARCINOMA	OTHER NON–SMALL CELL LUNG CANCER
Salbeck et al[25]	131	?	?	5	12	29
Tarver et al[18]	54	?	?	0	40	0
Kormas et al[24 b,c]	158	cI-III	Preop	2	8	27
Osada et al[49]	70	cI-III	Preop	0	0	0

Inclusion criteria: Studies reporting data by histology for asymptomatic patients in ≥50 patients.
[a]Gold standard used was a typical CT appearance for metastases, except as otherwise indicated.
[b]Gold standard: typical computed tomography *and* biopsy or follow-up.
[c]Prospective.
Preop, patients being evaluated for surgery; ?, unknown.

extensively. In one study of 146 potentially operable (cI-III) patients, the incidence of metastases was found to be 22% in squamous cancers and 40% in nonsquamous cancers, but this was not correlated to the outcome of the clinical evaluation.[14] The difference was especially apparent in patients who appeared radiographically to be stage I-II (incidence of distant metastases was 10% in squamous and 42% in nonsquamous cancers), whereas no difference was seen in cIII patients in this study (incidence of distant metastases was 33% in squamous and 37% in nonsquamous cancers).[14] In this context, approximately 25% of cI-II patients with nonsquamous cancers are actually N2,3 positive (stage III), as opposed to 10% of cI-II patients with squamous cancers (see Chapter 5).

The influence of histologic subtypes of NSCLC on the FN rate of the clinical evaluation has been reported only in regard to the presence of brain metastases. This data is shown in Table 6–5. Little detail is given about the extent of the clinical examination in most of these studies, and the results have not been correlated with intrathoracic clinical stage in most reports. The only study offering data in this regard found that 77% of brain metastases among asymptomatic patients were in patients who also had N2 nodal involvement.[24]

The data presented in Table 6–5 suggests that the incidence of brain metastases in asymptomatic patients with squamous cancers is low. The result reported for nonsquamous histologic subtypes is variable and may be related to how carefully the patient population is selected. Those studies reporting on potentially operable patients suggest that the rate of brain metastases in adenocarcinoma is <10%. The study by Kormas et al[24] was the most carefully conducted, involving prospective data and careful follow-up to discover any brain metastases that were missed by the CT done at the time of evaluation. This study found that asymptomatic metastases occurred in 14% of patients with nonsquamous tumors, but most of these patients had pN2 nodal involvement.[24]

RELIABILITY OF THE CLINICAL EVALUATION IN SMALL CELL LUNG CANCER

Most patients with SCLC are symptomatic when first seen,[4,27,31] and extensive disease (distant metastases) is consistently found at presentation in two-thirds of patients (see Table 6–1).[1,2,27] The clinical evaluation, therefore, is of little use in determining which patients do or do not need an investigation for the presence of distant metastases, and the traditional approach to SCLC has been to perform tests to detect metastatic disease in all patients.[2,28,32] The value of the clinical examination has been studied primarily to determine whether certain tests can be omitted in patients without organ-specific symptoms related to that potential metastatic site.

The traditional approach to all patients with SCLC is to perform a clinical evaluation, including a complete blood count (CBC), lactate dehydrogenase level (LDH), serum chemistry, tests of liver function, and a CXR.[28] A chest CT has usually already been performed, although a logical argument can be made to obtain this study only in patients who have been shown to have limited-stage disease in order to plan thoracic radiotherapy. Further tests to determine the presence of distant metastases consist of a bone scan, a brain CT or MRI, and a bone marrow aspirate.[28]

A compelling argument has been made to perform these tests sequentially and abort further testing once distant disease is demonstrated.[1] This would result in a significant cost savings without affecting the therapeutic management. The exact sequence of tests has little effect on the cost as long as the sequence is interrupted once extensive disease is found.[1] Beginning the investigation with a head CT in patients with neurologic symptoms and performing a biopsy of any suspicious palpable lesions seems logical and should identify approximately 60% of patients with distant disease (Fig. 6–2). The addition of a bone scan and an abdominal CT would identify >90% of extensive-stage patients.[1]

The reliability of the neurologic evaluation in a relatively unselected population of patients with SCLC has been addressed by several investigators.[33–35] The sensitivity and specificity of the clinical evaluation is approximately 75% (range, 64%-83%) and 90% (range, 81%-100%), respectively.[33–35] The absence of symptoms carries an FN rate of approximately 5% (range, 3%-9%), with a prevalence of brain metastases in these studies of approximately 20% (range, 14%-27%).[33–35] Furthermore, the majority of patients with asymptomatic brain metastases have other detectable metastases as well.[33–35] This suggests that brain CT (or MRI) has limited utility in asymptomatic patients. This should be even more true if the test is done in a select population that has been shown to have no distant metastases by other preliminary tests, as suggested by Richardson et al.[1]

A number of studies have consistently demonstrated

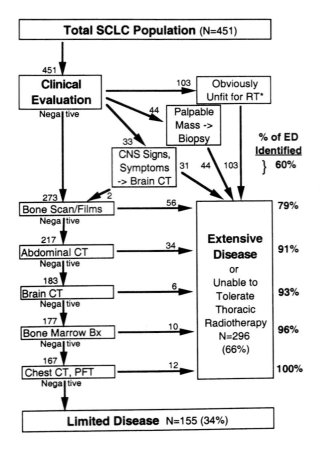

Figure 6–2. Sequential approach in patients with small cell lung cancer to determine the presence of distant metastases or inability to tolerate thoracic radiotherapy. Application of this approach retrospectively to 451 patients shows that most patients with extensive disease can be identified within the first few steps. *Pleural effusion in 92 patients, pericardial effusion in 8 patients, and bilateral chest disease in 3 patients. CNS, central nervous system; ED, extensive disease; PFT, pulmonary function tests; RT, radiotherapy. (Modified from Richardson GE, Venzon DJ, Phelps R, et al. Application of an algorithm for staging small-cell lung cancer can save one-third of the initial evaluation costs. Arch Intern Med. 1993;153:329–337.)[1]

bone marrow involvement in 20% of all patients with SCLC (range, 16%-23%).[1,2,36–38] However, these studies have also consistently found that positive bone marrow as the *only* site of extrathoracic disease occurs in <5% of patients (mean, 3%; range, 2%-4%).[1,2,36–38] Viewed slightly differently, among patients who appear to have limited disease after other staging investigations have been done, only 5% to 10% will be found to have bone marrow involvement.[1,2,36–38] Therefore, a bone marrow aspiration and biopsy is no longer a standard component of staging

SCLC[28,39] and probably should be used selectively in patients who have no other sites of metastases.

TESTS TO ASSESS THE PRESENCE OF METASTASES

If a metastasis is suspected, an imaging study must be obtained. It is important to know the reliability of the imaging study in the context of a similar group of patients

DATA SUMMARY: SITE OF METASTASES AND RELIABILITY OF THE CLINICAL EVALUATION			
	AMOUNT	**QUALITY**	**CONSISTENCY**
The most common sites of NSCLC metastases are brain, bone, liver, and adrenal glands	Mod	High	Mod
60% of SCLC patients have distant metastases	High	High	High
The most common sites of SCLC metastases are bone and liver	High	High	High
The FN rate of the clinical evaluation in cI-II NSCLC patients is <5%	Mod	Mod	High
The FN rate of the clinical evaluation for patient populations that include cIII NSCLC is approximately 15%-30%	High	Mod	High

Type of data rated: Plain text: descriptive statement   *Italics: controlled comparison*   **Bold: randomized comparison.**

in order to appropriately interpret the result. This is particularly true when only a solitary site of possible metastasis is discovered because multiple sites with an appearance that is typical for metastases leave no real doubt about the presence of stage IV disease. In order to assess the reliability of the imaging study, either a biopsy or follow-up of a positive finding must be done, and a negative imaging study must also be confirmed by follow-up. Most studies have classified a scan as FP if a lesion remains stable for ≥12 months or FN if a metastasis becomes clinically apparent within 12 months of a negative scan. The results of such studies in NSCLC patients are shown in Table 6–6. Similar data has not been reported for SCLC, probably because of the difficulty in establishing a gold standard for such a rapidly growing and widely metastatic type of cancer.

Brain

The most commonly used imaging study to detect brain metastases in lung cancer is a cranial CT scan with intravenous contrast. Radionuclide studies have been abandoned because of lower sensitivity and specificity relative to CT.[40,41] The FN and FP rates shown in Table 6–6 for cranial CT are around 5% to 10% in potentially operable, clinical stage I-III patients with NSCLC. Many of the metastases were solitary. Even in patients with more extensive disease, Patchell et al[42] found an FP rate of 11% as proven by biopsy. It must be emphasized that these figures pertain to lesions that were interpreted as being highly suspicious for metastasis and do not include findings that were indeterminate or thought unlikely to be a metastasis.

The hypothesis that MRI of the brain is superior to CT for the detection of metastases is not borne out by the literature to date. A number of studies have compared nonenhanced MRI to contrast-enhanced CT in patients at risk for cerebral metastases from a variety of cancers. These studies have consistently shown no difference between these modalities in the number of patients identified with metastases, the number of metastases found, the ability to detect small metastases, or the confidence of the radiologist in the interpretation that a metastasis is present.[43–46] However, a contrast-enhanced MRI appears to be able to detect more metastases than a nonenhanced MRI.[45,47] Despite this, none of the studies to date comparing contrast-enhanced MRI to contrast-enhanced CT have found that MRI identified more patients with brain metastases.[43,45,46,48] Two studies have reported that a greater number of metastases were detected by MRI in approximately 25% of the patients with metastases.[45,46] A third study found no difference in the number of lesions detected by contrast-enhanced MRI versus contrast-enhanced CT, although high dose contrast-enhanced MRI did detect more frequent metastases and with greater certainty than CT.[43]

Bone

The FP rate of radionuclide bone scanning is high (30%-60%; see Table 6–6). This is the case even for lesions highly suspicious for metastasis by bone scan.[20,49] This is corroborated by a study of bone scans in 276 patients with a variety of cancers, in which a suspicious lesion was found to have only an 11% chance of being a metastasis if it was solitary and a 24% chance if two suspicious lesions were apparent.[50] Therefore, a positive bone scan must be confirmed by additional studies such as plain radiographs,

TABLE 6–6. RELIABILITY OF IMAGING STUDIES TO DETECT METASTASIS IN NON–SMALL CELL LUNG CANCER[a]

STUDY	N	SITE OF METASTASIS	TYPE OF SCAN	STAGE	SOLITARY (%)[b]	PREV (%)[c]	SENS (%)	SPEC (%)	FP (%)	FN (%)
Hatter et al[21 d]	114	Brain	CT	I,II	—	8	—	—	—	8
Kormas et al[24 e]	158	Brain	CT	cI-III	100	6	50	99	(17)[f]	3
Ichinose et al[12 d]	109	Brain	CT[g]	cI-III	100	14	27	—	—	10
Ferrigno and Buccheri[132 h]	184	Brain	CT	All	48	14	92	99	4	1
Hatter et al[21 d]	117	Bone	NM[i]	pI,II	—	4	—	—	—	4
Ichinose et al[12 d]	156	Bone	NM[i]	cI-III	94	17	69	93	33	6
Salvatierra et al[14 e,j]	146	Bone	NM[i]	cI-III	61	14	—	89	42	—
Osada et al[49 j]	66	Bone	NM[k]	cI-III	—	5	—	73	(85)[f]	—
Michel et al[20 e,h]	108	Bone	NM[k]	All	89	16	80	79	60	4
Hatter et al[21 d]	124	Liver	CT	pI,II	—	0	—	—	—	0
Ichinose et al[12 d]	150	Liver	CT[g]	cI-III	50	2	67	—	—	1

Inclusion criteria: Any study of >50 lung cancer patients with an adequate gold standard in at least 90% of patients.
[a]Follow-up for 12 months was the gold standard in all studies, except as specified.
[b]Percentage of M1 patients who had a solitary metastasis.
[c]Percentage of all patients who were found to have M1 disease.
[d]Follow-up only if negative.
[e]Prospective study.
[f]Numbers in parentheses are questionable because of a low prevalence.
[g]Only nuclear medicine scans in some patients.
[h]6 months' follow-up.
[i]Criteria for positive bone scan not specified.
[j]Follow-up only if positive.
[k]Bone scan classified as positive only if highly suspicious for a metastasis (without confirmatory imaging data).
CT, computed tomography; FN, false negative rate; FP, false positive rate; NM, nuclear medicine scan; Prev, prevalence; Sens, sensitivity; Spec, specificity.

needle biopsy, or MRI scan. Although this generally results in a diagnosis that the clinician is comfortable accepting, there is little data to actually show how often the final radiographic assessment is accurate. One study addressing this issue reported no false positives on follow-up among lesions classified as metastatic by bone scan and confirmatory radiographic studies.[20]

Liver

A review of studies of lung cancer patients found that liver metastases were found in approximately 2% of asymptomatic (cI-III) patients.[10] However, benign focal liver lesions were found in approximately 2% of the "normal" population in a large series of autopsies (N = 96 625) in Los Angeles County,[51] and other smaller studies have suggested the incidence may actually be several times higher.[52–54] Approximately 90% of these lesions are hepatic cysts or hemangiomas, occurring in roughly equal proportions.[51] Hepatocellular adenomas, particularly in young women taking oral contraceptives, account for most of the remainder. Corroborating this, 17% of 1454 consecutive outpatients undergoing CT scans were found to have small (<1.5 cm) hepatic lesions.[55] In those patients with a known extrahepatic malignancy and for whom a definitive diagnosis of the hepatic lesion was achieved (confirmatory test or follow-up >6 months), 66% were found to be benign.[55] From this data it can be surmised that the chance of finding a benign hepatic lesion is at least as high as the chance of finding a liver metastasis in an asymptomatic patient with lung cancer.

Liver metastases generally appear less dense than the hepatic parenchyma on a contrast-enhanced CT, but are difficult to distinguish on an unenhanced scan. The rapid administration of intravenous contrast enhances the detection of metastases because most metastases are supplied primarily by hepatic arterial blood, whereas most of the blood flow to the liver itself is through the portal vein.[56] If scanning is delayed until equilibrium is reached (when both the aorta and inferior vena cava appear isodense), hepatic lesions become less conspicuous again. The ability to detect a liver metastasis is approximately 50% on an unenhanced scan[57–59] when lesions of all sizes are included and assessed against pathologic examination of resected hepatic specimens. The sensitivity improves to approximately 70% with appropriate use of contrast,[56,58] but after equilibrium is reached, approximately 30% of previously seen lesions are obscured.[60] Therefore, there can be little confidence that liver metastases have been excluded in lung cancer patients by a noncontrast CT or a CT scan obtained during the equilibrium phase of enhancement.

Several studies in the 1980s have compared contrast-enhanced CT to MRI for the detection of liver metastases.[58,59,61–65] Some have found CT to be superior,[58,62,63] others have found MRI to be superior,[59,64] and still others have found both techniques to be equal.[61,65]

More recently, rapid spiral CT scanning equipment has become available. This appears to have improved the quality of scans, in part due to decreased motion artifact.[56] Advances in MRI equipment and scanning techniques have improved the results using this imaging modality as

well.[56,66] Many variations of MRI parameters and pulse sequences have been investigated, but no standard technique has emerged.[56] Because the scanning techniques are continually changing, an accurate estimate of the FP and FN rates for the detection of hepatic metastases with the best current techniques is not available.[56] Furthermore, no recent studies comparing optimized MRI and spiral CT scanning techniques using surgical or pathologic correlation as a gold standard have been reported.[56] It seems likely that both techniques are significantly improved over earlier imaging methods and are probably of similar accuracy. The best imaging method for liver metastases (sensitivity, 80%-95%) is CT arterioportography,[56,65] but this is rarely used for lung cancer staging because it is invasive.

If a hepatic lesion is detected on a staging chest CT, differentiation between a benign lesion and a metastasis must be accomplished. The clinical situation and the CT appearance of the lesion usually provide some suspicion about the nature of the lesion, and it is likely this will guide the choice of further tests. The number of lesions also influences the chance that a hepatic lesion is a metastasis. In one study of 162 patients with a known malignancy in whom a definitive diagnosis of hepatic lesions was available,[55] 93% of patients with solitary lesions <1.5 cm had benign disease, compared with 76% of patients with two to four lesions and only 16% of patients with 5 or more lesions.

Hepatic cysts usually do not pose much of a problem. There is some evidence that cysts are more common in women and in the right lobe of the liver.[54] These are usually round, homogeneous lesions of water density (<10 Hounsfield units [HU]).[67] Ultrasound (US) examination appears to be able to reliably confirm the presence of a cyst in lesions >1 cm because cystic metastases are rare.[56,67]

A single photon emission computed tomography (SPECT)–tagged red blood cell scan is widely considered the procedure of choice to confirm the suspicion of a hemangioma if the lesion is >2 cm, and few false positive cases have been reported.[67–69] Hemangiomas <2 cm may be more easily detected by MRI (sensitivity, 83% versus 58%) than tagged red cell scanning, also with few false positives.[68]

Definitive confirmation of a suspected liver metastasis is best accomplished by needle biopsy.[70] A diagnosis is achieved in approximately 90% of cases using 14- to 18-gauge biopsy needles.[70–72] It is likely that there are few false positive results for metastasis, although further follow-up is usually not available. The reported FN rate is approximately 25%.[71,72] Significant complications are rare (1%-2%) and consist mainly of hemorrhage.[70,71]

The minimum size of a lesion that permits characterization by any of the imaging methods discussed is approximately 1 cm.[58,59] The sensitivity of US, contrast-enhanced CT, and MRI is poor (≤40%) for lesions that are ≤1 cm, whereas it is good (>85%) for lesions >2 cm.[58,65] Most of the published data has involved lesions that are 2 to 3 cm, and some studies have specifically excluded lesions of <1 cm.[61,68] Because the reliability of confirmatory studies is unclear for lesions <1 cm, management of patients with such lesions is probably best guided by an estimation of the chance of metastasis, given the clinical stage and presence of symptoms as outlined previously.

TABLE 6–7. INCIDENCE OF AN ABNORMAL ADRENAL GLAND IN LUNG CANCER PATIENTS[a]

STUDY	N	HISTOLOGY	CLINICAL STAGE	(%) INCIDENCE	(%)[b] METASTASES	(%)[c] SOLITARY
Silvestri et al[26]	39	SCLC, NSCLC	cI,II	0	—	—
Porte[146]	443	NSCLC	cI,III	7	56	50
Ettinghausen and Burt[82 d]	246	NSCLC	cI,III	4	40	100
Whittlesey[133]	185	NSCLC[e]	cI,III	5	60	—
Salvatierra et al[14 d]	146	NSCLC	cI,III	9	85	—
Grant et al[13]	114	NSCLC	cI,III	4	—	—
Nielsen et al[134 f]	70	NSCLC	cI,III	15	—	—
Pagani[86]	172	NSCLC	cI,IV	12	95	70
Silvestri et al[26]	173	SCLC, NSCLC	cI,IV	17	87	0
Silvestri et al[26]	134	SCLC, NSCLC	cIII,IV	19[g]	—	—
Allard et al[135 h]	91	SCLC, NSCLC	cIII,IV	22	59	—

Inclusion criteria: Studies of ≥50 patients, reporting on the status of the adrenal glands.
[a]Diagnosis proven by biopsy or follow-up in all patients.
[b]Percentage of abnormal adrenal glands shown to harbor metastases.
[c]Percentage of patients with adrenal metastasis as only site of metastasis.
[d]Prospective study.
[e]Includes 4% small cell lung cancer.
[f]Result reported per gland.
[g]Only those with metastases analyzed.
[h]Patients who had computed tomography within 3 months of death with autopsy (89% had scan within 2 months).
NSCLC, non–small cell lung cancer; SCLC, small cell lung cancer.

Adrenal Glands

Adrenal adenomas have been consistently found to occur in approximately 3.5% of autopsies of patients over the age of 30 years.[73–76] Adenomas in patients younger than 30 are rare.[73–76] More clinically applicable is the finding that 0.6% of "normal" patients undergoing upper abdominal CT scans have incidental adrenal masses.[76] This data was taken from a review of series of ≥1000 patients (total of 80 704 patients) and excluded patients suspected of having primary adrenal tumors as well as cancer patients suspected of having adrenal metastases.[76] The vast majority (70%-95%) of these adrenal masses are benign, nonfunctioning adenomas.[76,77] The average size of such adenomas is reported to be 2.4 cm, and 50% are ≤2 cm in diameter.[78]

Differentiating an adenoma from a metastasis in a patient with lung cancer is a particularly vexing problem, especially when this is the only site suspicious for metastasis. The incidence of an abnormal adrenal gland in lung cancer patients is correlated with clinical stage in Table 6–7. In stage cI-III patients, the frequency of adrenal enlargement is similar to that in the normal population, although approximately half of these lung cancer patients have an adrenal metastasis on biopsy. Other authors, who did not obtain a definite diagnosis in all patients, have reported similar results.[79–81] When the patient population includes higher-stage cancers, adrenal enlargement becomes more frequent, and the chance that an enlarged adrenal is malignant appears to increase as well. However, this data is not clear enough to define a management policy regarding abnormal adrenal glands in lung cancer patients.

Only a few studies have reported adrenal size relative to a definite diagnosis.[80–83] The normal adrenal gland is a V- or Y-shaped structure approximately 1 cm thick but may be 3 to 4 cm long.[84] It is not always clear what dimension of an abnormal gland is being reported, but it would seem logical to report the diameter of the mass in the adrenal gland. Although the number of patients is limited, the data

shown in Table 6–8 suggests that abnormal adrenal glands that are 2 cm or smaller may not require further investigation. However, even 2- to 3-cm glands appear to carry a significant rate of malignant involvement. What little data has been reported regarding the shape and density characteristics (ie, homogeneous versus heterogeneous) of abnormal adrenals suggests that these features are not useful in differentiating benign from malignant involvement.[79,80,85]

The findings cited earlier suggest that it may be reasonable to forego any further investigation of small adrenal glands (≤2 cm), particularly in clinical stage I,II patients. This is corroborated by the low rate of appearance of adrenal metastases during the early follow-up of stage pI-II patients.[12,21] Furthermore, Silvestri et al[26] found no adrenal metastases in 40 patients who had a clinical evaluation that was completely negative for any findings suggestive of metastases. However, one study has suggested an FN rate of 12% in normal adrenal glands.[84] This study involved 36 consecutive patients with NSCLC who underwent routine needle biopsy of normal adrenals. Another study by the same author involving 24 patients with SCLC found that 17% had metastatic tumor on routine fine-needle aspiration of normal-sized adrenal glands.[86] Because no data is pro-

TABLE 6–8. FREQUENCY OF ADRENAL METASTASIS RELATIVE TO SIZE IN PATIENTS WITH CLINICAL STAGE I,III NON–SMALL CELL LUNG CANCER[a]

Adrenal size (cm)	≥2	>2, ≤4	>4	<3	≥3
References[b]	81–83	81–83	81, 82	80–82, 146	80–82
N (number of adrenals)	20	20	8	41	43
Percentage malignant	10	60	75	27	74

Inclusion criteria: Studies since 1980 providing data on adrenal size and proof of diagnosis in lung cancer patients.
[a]Some small cell lung cancer patients are included in one study (Sandler et al[81]).
[b]The studies reported by Ettinghausen and Burt[82] and Burt et al[83] are from the same institution and may partially overlap.

vided in these studies regarding the radiographic stage or the outcome of the clinical evaluation in these patients, it is difficult to use these observations in defining a management policy.

Patients with an adrenal abnormality who are not in a low risk category as defined earlier (cI-II, negative clinical evaluation, adrenal ≤2 cm) should undergo further testing to establish the cause of the adrenal enlargement. A needle biopsy has been shown by multiple authors to be a safe procedure, even via transpleural or transhepatic approaches.[87–89] The overall complication rate is 8% to 9%, with a "major" complication rate, that is, requiring treatment (eg, a pneumothorax requiring a chest tube or hemorrhage requiring observation in the hospital) of 3% to 4%.[87–89] An inadequate sample is obtained in approximately 10% of cases.[87,88] The FP rate appears low, but the FN rate is 10% to 20%, even if inadequate samples are excluded (Table 6–9).

More recently, refinements of noninvasive imaging techniques have shown promising results. The pertinent issue for the lung cancer physician is how reliably these tests can diagnose an adrenal metastasis in lung cancer patients. Although these studies have generally not been done in populations of lung cancer patients, the results from populations involving mostly patients with any nonadrenal primary malignancy can probably be applied to lung cancer patients with confidence. Such results for a variety of tests are shown in Table 6–9. A technique known as *chemical shift MRI* has shown a low FN rate for metastases, although the FP rate remains substantial. Low attenuation (<10 HU) of the adrenal mass on an unenhanced CT has shown a similar low FN rate for metastases. A contrast-enhanced CT scan is also useful if delayed images (after 15–30 minutes) demonstrate low attenuation.[90–92] Perhaps most impressive is the low FN and FP rates for adrenal metastasis as defined by positron-emission tomography (PET) scanning (see Table 6–9).

The low FN rate for adrenal metastases by unenhanced CT or chemical shift MRI is further corroborated by numerous other studies, which have addressed the ability of such scans to diagnose benign adrenal adenomas (Table 6–10).[85,90,91,93–99] These latter studies have been done in less well defined populations, although generally between one-third and two-thirds of the patients have had nonadrenal malignancies. The remainder have had benign adenomas, pheochromocytomas, functioning adrenal tumors, or a variety of other adrenal lesions that prompted an imaging study. These studies have shown that the diagnosis of a benign adenoma is reliable, with a low FP rate (for adenoma) using either unenhanced or delayed-enhanced CT scanning or chemical shift MRI.[85,90,91,93–99]

Correct interpretation of the results of these tests requires attention to a number of details. If a threshold attenuation value of 18 to 20 HU is chosen for unenhanced CT in a population of cancer patients, the FN rate can rise significantly (up to 25%).[100,101] Similar changes in the FN rate have been reported when the criteria for a positive chemical shift MRI have been altered.[101] Furthermore, chemical shift MRI should not be confused with standard T1 and T2 MRI assessment of adrenal glands, which has been shown to have limited utility in lung cancer patients.[83] A full discussion of the nuances of these tests is beyond the scope of this chapter. However, it is important that physicians caring for lung cancer patients have an awareness that misinterpretations can easily occur.

It seems most appropriate to perform a needle biopsy in those adrenal lesions where the suspicion of malignancy is high. This makes best use of the low FP rate of this test. When the suspicion of an adrenal metastasis is relatively low, an unenhanced or delayed-enhanced CT or a chemical shift MRI appears to be a better choice. There is little reason to carry out both an unenhanced CT and an MRI because it has been reported that most of the lesions misclassified by one of these tests will also be misclassified

TABLE 6–9. CONFIRMATORY TESTS FOR SUSPECTED ADRENAL METASTASIS IN CANCER PATIENTS[a]

STUDY	N[b]	TEST	CRITERION	PREV (%)	SENS (%)	SPEC (%)	FP (%)	FN (%)
Welch et al[87]	277	FNA		51	81	99	1	20
Silverman et al[88 c]	83	FNA	Excl inadeq	47	89	(100)[c]	(0)[c]	9
Porte[146]	32	Unenh CT	>10 Hu	56	90	80	21	11
Schwartz et al[136 d]	42	Ch sh MRI	≤55 ASR	43	100	96	5	0
McNicholas et al[101]	37	Ch sh MRI	≤70 ASR	51	100	78	17	0
Lee et al[100]	66	Unenh CT	>10 HU	42	96	79	23	3
Boland et al[92]	44	Unenh CT	>10 HU	50	100	96	4	0
McNicholas et al[101]	37	Unenh CT	>10 HU	51	100	94	5	0
Porte[146]	32	FNA		56	100	100	0	0
Boland et al[92]	44	Del-enh CT	≥25 HU[e]	50	100	96	4	0
Boland et al[137]	24	PET	Visual	58	100	100	0	0
Erasmus et al[138 d,f]	33	PET	Visual	70	100	80	8	0

Inclusion criteria: Studies with ≥20 abnormal adrenal glands involving patient populations in which ≥80% had cancer (excluding primary adrenal cancers) and providing proof of diagnosis (biopsy or follow-up ≥6 months) on all patients.
[a]Results expressed as positive or negative for *adrenal metastasis*.
[b]Number of abnormal adrenal glands.
[c]No follow-up of malignant needle biopsies.
[d]Only patients with lung cancer.
[e]Delayed 15 minutes.
[f]Used unenhanced CT (<10 HU) as the only proof of a benign diagnosis in five patients.
ASR, adrenal-spleen ratio; Ch-sh MRI, chemical shift magnetic resonance imaging; CT, computed tomography; Del-enh CT, delayed-enhanced CT; Excl inadeq, excluding inadequate biopsies; FN, false negative rate (for absence of adrenal metastasis); FNA, percutaneous needle biopsy; FP, false positive rate (for adrenal metastasis); HU, Hounsfield units of CT attenuation; PET, positron-emission tomography; Unenh CT, unenhanced CT.

TABLE 6–10. CONFIRMATORY TESTS FOR BENIGN ADRENAL ADENOMA[a]

STUDY	N[b]	PATIENTS WITH NONADRENAL MALIGNANCY (%)	TEST	CRITERION	PREV (%)[c]	SENS (%)	SPEC (%)	FP (%)	FN (%)
Outwater et al[93]	58	~70	Ch-sh MRI	Visual	66	89	85	8	19
Reinig et al[99]	44	24	Ch-sh MRI	Visual	73	97	64	13	13
Mayo-Smith et al[94]	46	?	Ch-sh MRI	<75 ASR	65	82	100	0	22
Mitchell et al[95]	45	~30	Ch-sh MRI	Visual	60	85	100	0	29
Miyake et al[96]	36	59	Unenh CT	<15 HU	39	64	100	0	19
Singer et al[85]	24	74	Unenh CT	<10 HU	50	58	92	13	31
Outwater et al[97 d]	47	61	Unenh CT	<17 HU	64	78	100	0	17
Korobkin et al[91]	135	60	Unenh CT	<18 HU	30	85	100	0	23
Korobkin et al[98]	51	?	Del-enh CT	<30 HU[e]	80	95	100	0	17
Szolar and Kammerhuber[90]	43	56	Del-enh CT	<40 HU[f]	56	100	100	0	0

Inclusion criteria: Studies of ≥20 patients with proof of diagnosis (biopsy or follow-up ≥6 months) in all patients.
[a]Results expressed as positive or negative for adrenal adenoma.
[b]Number of abnormal adrenal glands.
[c]Prevalence of benign nonfunctioning adrenal adenoma.
[d]Used unenhanced CT (<10 HU) as proof of benign diagnosis in five patients.
[e]Delayed 60 minutes after intravenous contrast administration.
[f]Delayed 30 minutes after contrast administration.
ASR, adrenal-spleen ratio; Ch-sh MRI, chemical shift magnetic resonance imaging; CT, computed tomography; Del-enh CT, delayed rescanning after intravenous contrast administration; FN, false negative rate (for absence of adrenal adenoma); FP, false positive rate (for adrenal adenoma); HU, Hounsfield units of CT attenuation; Prev, prevalence; Sens, sensitivity; Spec, specificity; Unenh CT, unenhanced CT; ?, unknown.

by the other.[97] PET scanning appears reliable, but it may not be locally available. If doubt persists about an enlarged adrenal as an isolated site of possible metastasis, an adrenalectomy is warranted. This can be accomplished with low morbidity via a laparoscopic approach,[102] or it can be done transdiaphragmatically at the time of thoracotomy if it is on the same side as the primary tumor.[80,103,104]

Lung

Small pulmonary lesions are frequently seen in addition to the primary tumor on the chest CT. This occurred in 16% of cI-IIIa potentially operable patients with NSCLC in one large study.[105] The lesions were not calcified and ranged from 4 mm to 12 mm. A definitive diagnosis (biopsy or follow-up of >24 months) was established in only 20% of the patients, the remainder being lost to follow-up or having unavailable pathology reports. Of the lesions for which a definitive diagnosis was available, 86% were found to be benign. In another study, 10% of patients had a second lesion detected preoperatively, of which nearly 60% were found to be benign.[106] Therefore, a patient should not be denied a curative approach on the basis of a second pulmonary nodule without a definitive diagnosis. Although a fine-needle aspiration is reliable when positive, definitive diagnosis will usually require a thoracoscopic wedge biopsy (see Chapter 4).

INVESTIGATIVE ISSUES
Nuclear Medicine Scans

There has been interest in the possibility of using radiolabeled substances as a simple way to detect distant metasta-

DATA SUMMARY: INTERPRETATION OF TESTS TO ASSESS THE PRESENCE OF METASTASES

	AMOUNT	QUALITY	CONSISTENCY
The FN rate of a contrast-enhanced brain CT for metastases in NSCLC patients is <10%	High	High	High
A contrast-enhanced brain MRI does *not* detect more patients with brain metastases than a contrast-enhanced CT	High	Mod	High
The FP rate for lesions suggestive of metastases on a bone scan in NSCLC is 50%	High	Mod	Mod
Approximately 50% of enlarged adrenal glands in cI-III NSCLC patients are benign	Mod	High	Mod
Adrenal masses ≤2 cm have a 90% chance of being benign in NSCLC patients	Mod	Mod	High
An adrenal adenoma can be reliably diagnosed (<10% FP rate) by unenhanced CT, delayed enhanced CT, and chemical shift MRI	High	High	High

Type of data rated: Plain text: descriptive statement   *Italics: controlled comparison*   **Bold: randomized comparison**

TABLE 6–11. NUCLEAR MEDICINE SCANS FOR EXTRATHORACIC STAGING

STUDY	N	FEASIBILITY (%)	TEST	PREV (%)	SENS (%)	SPEC (%)	FP (%)	FN (%)
Buccheri et al[139] a	63	90	MoAb CEA	11	86	93	40	2
Leitha et al[108] b	26	84	Octreotide	50	78c	100c	0c	15c

Inclusion criteria: Studies reporting data to assess reliability of nuclear medicine tests for distant metastases in ≥20 patients with lung cancer.
aCI-IIIa non–small cell lung cancer and small cell lung cancer.
bOnly small cell lung cancer.
cMinor discrepancies in reported data between tables and text.
FN, false negative rate; FP, false positive rate; MoAb CEA, monoclonal antibody to CEA; Prev, prevalence; Sens, sensitivity; Spec, specificity.

ses.[107] These techniques have generally used either monoclonal antibodies or radiolabeled analogs of somatostatin (octreotide or pentreotide) because these latter compounds have affinity for a commonly expressed receptor in lung cancer cells.[107] Unfortunately, most of the studies to date have involved only small numbers of patients and have reported results in a preliminary, almost anecdotal fashion. Such nuclear medicine scans are able to detect 37% to 80% of known metastases.[108–110,114] An additional 10% of metastatic lesions have been found that were seen only by these scans and not by conventional imaging studies.[109,110,114] However, few studies have been reported that provide an assessment of the ability of such a scan to accurately stage lung cancer. Those studies involving at least 20 patients are shown in Table 6–11. Further investigation is needed to define the role of these techniques in staging patients with lung cancer.

Positron-Emission Tomography Scanning

Only limited data is available on the reliability of whole body PET scanning for extrathoracic staging. Several authors have reported that whole body PET scanning can detect unsuspected metastases in approximately 10% of patients with NSCLC, but these reports have not defined the patient populations (clinical stage, outcome of clinical evaluation).[111–116,144] The studies that allow some estimation of sensitivity, specificity, FN, and FP rates are shown in Table 6–12. Although these studies are hampered by short follow-up periods and vague definitions, these initial data suggests that whole body PET scanning may be a useful modality. The prospective study by Weder et al,[116] which included careful documentation of the true nature of positive PET findings in 90% of cases, found no false positives. Detection of brain metastases may be hampered by the high uptake of the radiolabeled marker used in PET scanning (FDG) by brain tissue, but some authors have reported good results for evaluation of brain metastases using PET (FP rate, 25%; FN rate, 3%).[144]

Occult Micrometastases

Monoclonal antibodies to epithelial markers expressed in cancer cells have shown that occult tumor cells are often present in distant sites, even though they cannot be seen using conventional microscopy.[117–119] These assays have been shown to have a low FP rate (<2%) in patients with benign disease, as well as a high rate of uptake in the primary tumor.[117–119] Application of these techniques to bone marrow aspirates in cI-III NSCLC patients has shown that approximately 40% of these patients harbor occult micrometastases (OMs) in the bone marrow (Table 6–13). More importantly, the presence of OMs has consistently correlated with a worse disease-free survival and a higher rate of recurrence (see Table 6–13). Furthermore, incremental worsening of disease-free survival ($P = 0.02$) was seen with an *increasing burden of OMs* (increasing numbers of OMs detected per patient) in one study.[117] The survival curves from one of these studies[125] is shown in Figure 6–3.

The presence of OMs in the bone marrow was an independent predictor of survival in the two studies that have carried out multivariate analysis.[117,119] OMs have been shown *not* to be associated with different histologic subtypes,[117,118,120] differences in differentiation,[117] T stage,[117,118] or even N stage.[117–119] One study has suggested that OMs were more common with increasing tumor grade, T stage, and N stage,[120] but these same authors subsequently refuted these findings when a larger group of patients was analyzed.[117] The lack of correlation with nodal involvement suggests that hematogenous spread of micrometastases to distant sites occurs by a different mechanism than lymphatic spread along lymph node chains.

The general consistency of the results lends credence to the argument that OMs exist and have clinical relevance. This is further corroborated by similar findings in patients with other primary tumor types.[121–123] Although it has been fairly well substantiated that the cells detected by these assays are malignant, it is not clear that they are actively growing metastases. Several authors have shown that the metastatic process in human beings and animals is inefficient and that millions of tumor cells can circulate throughout the body without the development of metastases.[124,125] It is more likely that OMs serve as a marker for metastatic potential. Indeed, newer techniques have provided evidence of tumor cells circulating in the bloodstream in lung cancer

TABLE 6–12. RELIABILITY OF POSITRON-EMISSION TOMOGRAPHY SCANNING TO IDENTIFY DISTANT METASTASES

STUDY	N	PREV (%)	SENS (%)	SPEC (%)	FN (%)	FP (%)
Bury et al[147] a	110	19	90	98	2	10
Marom et al[144] b	100	44	91	97	6	5
Weder et al[116] c	100	19	—	100	—	0
Saunders et al[111]	97	29	97	53	16	12
Bury et al[113] c	61	31	—	93	—	14
Average			93	88	8	10

Inclusion criteria: Studies of ≥50 patients with lung cancer providing data on follow-up or tissue confirmation of PET scan results for extrathoracic staging.
aData regarding bone metastases only.
bAdequacy of follow-up unclear in some cases.
FN, false negative rate; FP, false positive rate; PET, positron-emission tomography.

TABLE 6-13. EFFECT OF OCCULT MICROMETASTASES IN BONE MARROW ON SURVIVAL AND RECURRENCE RATES IN RESECTED NON–SMALL CELL LUNG CANCER[a]

STUDY	N	STAGE	PATIENTS WITH OM (%)	MEDIAN DISEASE-FREE SURVIVAL (mo)			RECURRENCE RATE (%)		
				OM+	OM−	P	OM+	OM−	P
Pantel et al[117]	66	pI	54	19	>36	0.004	75	35	0.03
Ohgami et al[118]	26	pI,II	31	13	>36	0.03	—	—	—
Pantel et al[120]	82	pI-IIIb	22	—	—	—	67	37	<0.05
Cote et al[119]	43	pI-IIIb	40	7	>36	0.0009	77	23	—
Ohgami et al[118]	39	pI-IIIb	39	9	>36	0.008	—	—	—

Inclusion criteria: Studies of ≥20 patients, investigating bone marrow occult micrometastases in non–small cell lung cancer.
[a]Studies based on immunohistochemistry of bone marrow aspirates using a monoclonal antibody against CK18 (or against AE1 and CAM5.2 in the study by Cote.[124]
OM, occult micrometastases; OM−, occult micrometastases absent; OM+, occult micrometastases present.

patients.[126] For example, one study found the presence of such circulating cells in 80% of stage IV patients (N = 10) and in 29% of stage I-III patients (N = 14) using reverse transcriptase-polymerase chain reaction (RT-PCR) to identify mRNA derived from CEA.[126] On the other hand, another study, using a similar assay (RT-PCR for CK-19 mRNA), found a high rate of detection in benign control patients.[127] Additional investigation of these techniques is clearly needed. However, the preliminary data regarding the detection of OMs suggests that these techniques may change the way staging is done in the near future.

EDITORS' COMMENTS

The most important part of staging for distant metastases is the clinical evaluation. Too often, the focus is on technologic advances. Although newer radiologic imaging techniques are clearly an improvement, they are most useful when correlated with the findings of a clinical evaluation. The evaluation must be carefully conducted, with attention given to both organ-specific and nonspecific factors.

The available data shows that a negative clinical evalua-

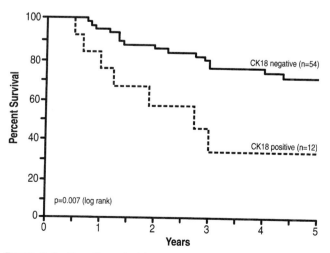

FIGURE 6-3. Overall survival in 66 node-negative patients relative to presence or absence of CK18 staining of bone marrow for occult micrometastases. Kaplan-Meier analysis, log-rank test *P* = 0.07. (From Passlick B, Kubuschok B, Izbicki JR, et al. Isolated tumor cells in bone marrow predict reduced survival in node-negative non-small cell lung cancer. Ann Thorac Surg. 1999;68:2053–2058.[145])

tion is quite reliable in patients who are clinically stage I or II on the basis of an initial CT scan. However, in the presence of radiographic evidence of mediastinal lymph node involvement, the FN rate is high enough to warrant distant organ scanning, despite a negative clinical evaluation. Controversy exists about whether a brain scan is warranted in patients with adenocarcinoma or large cell carcinoma who have a negative clinical evaluation and are radiographically stage I or II. However, such patients should undergo mediastinoscopy despite the absence of signs of mediastinal lymph node involvement. The available data suggests that a brain CT scan is probably not warranted if the mediastinoscopy is negative.

Isolated metastases are surprisingly common among clinical stage I-III "potentially operable" patients. However, incidental adrenal adenomas or benign hepatic lesions are also commonly found in this patient population. If the radiographic appearance and clinical context raise a high suspicion of metastasis, a needle biopsy is probably the best confirmatory test. Hepatic cysts and hemangiomas can be diagnosed reliably with US and tagged red blood cell scans, respectively. Adrenal lesions <2 cm have little chance of representing metastases and do not warrant further investigation unless the clinical context makes the risk of metastasis high. If the suspicion of an adrenal adenoma is high, an unenhanced or delayed-enhanced CT scan or an MRI may be the best next step. This must be interpreted with the help of a knowledgeable and astute radiologist to prevent false interpretations, however.

Bone scans carry a high FP rate and must be further investigated with other studies. It may be better to investigate patients with focal symptoms directly with plain films or MRIs of the area without obtaining a bone scan first. Imaging of the brain can be done with either contrast-enhanced MRI or contrast-enhanced CT scanning. Although it is controversial whether an MRI can pick up a greater number of lesions, MRI has not been shown to improve the chance of identifying patients with stage IV disease involving the brain. In patients who do not have multiple sites of metastatic disease, confirmation that a lesion seen on a brain scan is actually a metastasis should be obtained either by needle biopsy or, possibly, by resection. Such patients should be considered for surgical resection of the primary site and definitive treatment of the metastasis, if this is feasible.

A diagnosis of SCLC always warrants investigation for distant metastases. The clinical evaluation can identify most patients who either have extensive disease or are unsuitable for thoracic radiotherapy. Tests to identify distant metastases should be done in a sequential manner in order to curtail the number of tests that need to be performed. Although clinical contexts can be defined for each particular test where the chance of a positive finding is relatively low, the cumulative investigation shows that the majority of patients with SCLC do, in fact, have extensive disease.

References

1. Richardson GE, Venzon DJ, Phelps R, et al. Application of an algorithm for staging small-cell lung cancer can save one third of the initial evaluation costs. Arch Intern Med. 1993;153:329–337.
2. Ihde DC, Makuch RW, Carney DN, et al. Prognostic implications of stage of disease and sites of metastases in patients with small cell carcinoma of the lung treated with intensive combination chemotherapy. Am Rev Respir Dis. 1981;123:500–507.
3. Bülzebruck H, Bopp R, Drings P, et al. New aspects in the staging of lung cancer: prospective validation of the International Union Against Cancer TNM classification. Cancer. 1992;70:1102–1110.
4. Sagman U, Maki E, Evans WK, et al. Small-cell carcinoma of the lung: derivation of a prognostic staging system. J Clin Oncol. 1991;9:1639–1649.
5. Quinn DL, Ostrow LB, Porter DK, et al. Staging of non–small cell bronchogenic carcinoma: relationship of the clinical evaluation to organ scans. Chest. 1986;89:270–275.
6. Feinstein AR, Wells CK. A clinical-severity staging system for patients with lung cancer. Medicine (Baltimore). 1990;69:1–33.
7. Feld R, Abratt R, Graziano S, et al. Pretreatment minimal staging and prognostic factors for non–small cell lung cancer. Lung Cancer. 1997;17(suppl 1):S3–S10.
8. Pretreatment evaluation of non–small-cell lung cancer. The American Thoracic Society and The European Respiratory Society. Am J Respir Crit Care Med. 1997;156:320–332.
9. Ettinger DS, Cox JD, Ginsberg RJ, et al. NCCN non–small-cell lung cancer practice guidelines. Oncology. 1996;10(suppl):81–111.
10. Hillers TK, Sauve MD, Guyatt GH. Analysis of published studies on the detection of extrathoracic metastases in patients presumed to have operable non–small cell lung cancer. Thorax. 1994;49:14–19.
11. Silvestri GA, Littenberg B, Colice GL. The clinical evaluation for detecting metastatic lung cancer: a meta-analysis. Am J Respir Crit Care Med. 1995;152:225–230.
12. Ichinose Y, Hara N, Ohta M, et al. Preoperative examination to detect distant metastasis is not advocated for asymptomatic patients with stages 1 and 2 non–small cell lung cancer: preoperative examination for lung cancer. Chest. 1989;96:1104–1109.
13. Grant D, Edwards D, Goldstraw P. Computed tomography of the brain, chest, and abdomen in the postoperative assessment of non–small cell lung cancer. Thorax. 1988;43:883–886.
14. Salvatierra A, Baamonde C, Llamas JM, et al. Extrathoracic staging of bronchogenic carcinoma. Chest. 1990;97:1052–1058.
15. Hooper RG, Tenholder MF, Underwood GH, et al. Computed tomographic scanning of the brain in initial staging of bronchogenic carcinoma. Chest. 1984;85:774–776.
16. Hooper RG, Beechler CR, Johnson MC. Radioisotope scanning in the initial staging of bronchogenic carcinoma. Am Rev Respir Dis. 1978;118:279–286.
17. Gutierrez AC, Vincent RG, Bakshi S, et al. Radioisotope scans in the evaluation of metastatic bronchogenic carcinoma. J Thorac Cardiovasc Surg. 1975;69:934–941.
18. Tarver RD, Richmond BD, Klatte EC. Cerebral metastases from lung carcinoma: neurological and CT correlation: work in progress. Radiology. 1984;153:689–692.
19. Mintz BJ, Tuhrim S, Alexander S, et al. Intracranial metastases in the initial staging of bronchogenic carcinoma. Chest. 1984;86:850–853.
20. Michel F, Soler M, Imhof E, et al. Initial staging of non–small cell lung cancer: value of routine radioisotope bone scanning. Thorax. 1991;40:409–413.
21. Hatter J, Kohman LJ, Mosca RS, et al. Preoperative evaluation of stage I and stage II non–small cell lung cancer. Ann Thorac Surg. 1994;58:1738–1741.
22. Quint LE, Tummala S, Brisson LJ, et al. Distribution of distant metastases from newly diagnosed non–small cell lung cancer. Ann Thorac Surg. 1996;62:246–250.
23. Sider L, Horejs D. Frequency of extrathoracic metastases from bronchogenic carcinoma in patients with normal-sized hilar and mediastinal lymph nodes on CT. Am J Radiol. 1988;151:893–895.
24. Kormas P, Bradshaw JR, Jeyasingham K. Preoperative computed tomography of the brain in non–small cell bronchogenic carcinoma. Thorax. 1992;47:106–108.
25. Salbeck R, Grau HC, Artmann H. Cerebral tumor staging in patients with bronchial carcinoma by computed tomography. Cancer. 1990;66:2007–2011.
26. Silvestri GA, Lenz JE, Harper SN, et al. The relationship of clinical findings to CT scan evidence of adrenal gland metastases in the staging of bronchogenic carcinoma. Chest. 1992;102:1748–1751.
27. Rawson NSB, Peto J. An overview of prognostic factors in small cell lung cancer. Br J Cancer. 1990;61:597–604.
28. Feld R, Sagman U, LeBlanc M. Staging and prognostic factors: small cell lung cancer. In: Pass HI, Mitchell JB, Johnson DH, et al, eds. Lung Cancer: Principles and Practice. Philadelphia, Pa: Lippincott-Raven; 1996:495–509.
29. Merrick MV, Merrick JM. Bone scintigraphy in lung cancer: a reappraisal. Br J Radiol. 1986;59:1185–1194.
30. Kelly RJ, Cowan RJ, Ferree CB, et al. Efficacy of radionuclide scanning in patients with lung cancer. JAMA. 1979;242:2855–2857.
31. Maurer LH, Pajak TF. Prognostic factors in small cell carcinoma of the lung: a Cancer and Leukemia Group B study. Cancer Treat Rep. 1981;65:767–774.
32. Abrams J, Doyle LA, Aisner J. Staging, prognostic factors, and special considerations in small cell lung cancer. Semin Oncol. 1988;15:261–277.
33. Johnson DH, Windham WW, Allen JH, et al. Limited value of CT brain scans in the staging of small cell lung cancer. AJR Am J Roentgenol. 1983;140:37–40.
34. Levitan N, Hong WK, Byrne RE, et al. Role of computerized cranial tomography in the staging of small cell carcinoma of the lung. Cancer Treat Rep. 1984;68:1375–1377.
35. Crane JM, Nelson MJ, Ihde DC, et al. A comparison of computed tomography and radionuclide scanning for detection of brain metastases in small cell lung cancer. J Clin Oncol. 1984;2:1017–1024.
36. ten Velde GP, Kuypers-Engelen BT, Volovics A, et al. Examination of bone marrow biopsy specimens and staging of small cell lung cancer. Eur J Cancer. 1990;26:1142–1145.
37. Campling B, Quirt I, DeBoer G, et al. Is bone marrow examination in small-cell lung cancer really necessary? Ann Intern Med. 1986;105:508–512.
38. Feliu J, Barón MG, Artal A, et al. Bone marrow examination in small cell lung cancer—when is it indicated? Acta Oncol. 1991;30:587–591.
39. Shepherd FA, Ginsberg RJ, Haddad R, et al. Importance of clinical staging in limited small-cell lung cancer: a valuable system to separate prognostic subgroups. J Clin Oncol. 1993;11:1592–1597.
40. Jacobs L, Kinkel WR, Vincent RG. "Silent" brain metastasis from lung carcinoma determined by computerized tomography. Arch Neurol. 1977;34:690–693.
41. Lusins JO, Chayes Z, Nakagawa H. Computed tomography and radionuclide brain scanning: comparison in evaluating metastatic lesions to brain. N Y State J Med. 1980;80:185–189.
42. Patchell RA, Tibbs PA, Walsh JW, et al. A randomized trial of surgery in the treatment of single metastases to the brain. N Engl J Med. 1990;322:494–500.
43. Akeson P, Larsson E-M, Kristoffersen DT, et al. Brain metastases: comparison of gadodiamide injection-enhanced MR imaging at standard and high dose, contrast-enhanced CT and non–contrast-enhanced MR imaging. Acta Radiol. 1995;36:300–306.
44. Taphoorn MJB, Heimans JJ, Kaiser MC, et al. Imaging of brain metastases: comparison of computerized tomography (CT) and magnetic resonance imaging (MRI). Neuroradiology. 1989;31:391–395.
45. Sze G, Shin J, Krol G, et al. Intraparenchymal brain metastases: MR imaging versus contrast-enhanced CT. Radiology. 1988;168:187–194.
46. Davis PC, Hudgins PA, Peterman SB, et al. Diagnosis of cerebral metastases: double-dose delayed CT vs contrast-enhanced MR imaging. AJNR Am J Neuroradiol. 1991;12:293–300.
47. Healy ME, Hesselink JR, Press GA, et al. Increased detection of intracranial metastases with intravenous Gd-DTPA. Radiology. 1987;165:619–624.

48. Cole FH Jr, Thomas JE, Wilcox AB, et al. Cerebral imaging in the asymptomatic preoperative bronchogenic carcinoma patient: is it worthwhile? Ann Thorac Surg. 1994;57:838–840.

49. Osada H, Nakajima Y, Taira Y, et al. The role of mediastinal and multi-organ CT scans in staging presumable surgical candidates with non–small-cell lung cancer. Jpn J Surg. 1987;17:362–368.

50. Jacobson AF, Cronin EB, Stomper PC, et al. Bone scans with one or two new abnormalities in cancer patients with no known metastases: frequency and serial scintigraphic behavior of benign and malignant lesions. Radiology. 1990;175:229–232.

51. Craig JR, Peters RL, Edmonson HA. Tumors of the liver and intrahepatic bile ducts (second series). Washington, DC: Armed Forces Institute of Pathology; 1989.

52. Karhunen PJ. Benign hepatic tumours and tumour-like conditions in men. J Clin Pathol. 1986;39:183–188.

53. Feldman M. Hemangioma of the liver: special reference to its association with cysts of the liver and pancreas. Am J Clin Pathol. 1958;29:160–162.

54. Gaines PA, Sampson MA. The prevalence and characterization of simple hepatic cysts by ultrasound examination. Br J Radiol. 1989;62:335–337.

55. Jones EC, Chezmar JL, Nelson RC, et al. The frequency and significance of small (≤15 mm) hepatic lesions detected by CT. AJR Am J Roentgenol. 1992;158:535–539.

56. Paley MR, Ros PR. Hepatic metastases. Radiol Clin North Am. 1998;36:349–363.

57. Sugarbaker PH, Vermess M, Doppman JL, et al. Improved detection of focal lesions with computerized tomographic examination of the liver using ethiodized oil emulsion (EOE-13) liver contrast. Cancer. 1984;54:1489–1495.

58. Wernecke K, Rummeny E, Bongartz G, et al. Detection of hepatic masses in patients with carcinoma: comparative sensitivities of sonography, CT, and MR imaging. AJR Am J Roentgenol. 1991;157:731–739.

59. Reinig JW, Dwyer AJ, Miller DL, et al. Liver metastasis detection: comparative sensitivities of MR imaging and CT scanning. Radiology. 1987;162:43–47.

60. Burgener FA, Hamlin DJ. Contrast enhancement of hepatic tumors in CT: comparison between bolus and infusion techniques. AJR Am J Roentgenol. 1983;140:291–295.

61. Chezmar JL, Rumancik WM, Megibow AJ, et al. Liver and abdominal screening in patients with cancer: CT versus MR imaging. Radiology. 1988;168:43–47.

62. Glazer GM, Aisen AM, Francis IR, et al. Evaluation of focal hepatic masses: a comparative study of MRI and CT. Gastrointest Radiol. 1986;11:263–268.

63. Nelson RC, Chezmar JL, Steinberg HV, et al. Focal hepatic lesions: detection by dynamic and delayed computed tomography versus short TE/TR spin echo and fast field echo magnetic resonance imaging. Gastrointest Radiol. 1988;13:115–122.

64. Stark DD, Wittenberg J, Butch RJ, et al. Hepatic metastases: randomized, controlled comparison of detection with MR imaging and CT. Radiology. 1987;165:399–406.

65. Heiken JP, Weyman PJ, Lee JKT, et al. Detection of focal hepatic masses: prospective evaluation with CT, delayed CT, CT during arterial portography, and MR imaging. Radiology. 1989;171:47–51.

66. Soyer P, de Givry SC, Gueye C, et al. Detection of focal hepatic lesions with MR imaging: prospective comparison of T2-weighted fast spin-echo with and without fat suppression, T2-weighted breath-hold fast spin-echo, and gadolinium chelate-enhanced 3D gradient-recalled imaging. AJR Am J Roentgenol. 1996;166:1115–1121.

67. Mergo PJ, Ros PR. Benign lesions of the liver. Radiol Clin North Am. 1998;36:319–331.

68. Birnbaum BA, Weinreb JC, Megibow AJ, et al. Definitive diagnosis of hepatic hemangiomas: MR imaging versus Tc-99m-labeled red blood cell SPECT. Radiology. 1990;176:95–101.

69. Tumeh SS, Benson C, Nagel JS, et al. Cavernous hemangioma of the liver: detection with single-photon emission computed tomography. Radiology. 1987;164:353–356.

70. Molina PL, Mauro MA. Interventional computed tomography. In: Lee JKT, Sagel SS, Stanley RJ, et al, eds. Computer Body Tomography with MRI Correlation. 3rd ed. Philadelphia, Pa: Lippincott-Raven; 1998:1275–1341.

71. Martino CR, Haaga JR, Bryan PJ, et al. CT-guided liver biopsies: eight years' experience. Radiology. 1984;152:755–757.

72. Pagani JJ. Biopsy of focal hepatic lesions. Radiology. 1983;147:673–675.

73. Russi S, Blumenthal HT, Gray SH. Small adenomas of the adrenal cortex in hypertension and diabetes. Arch Intern Med. 1945;76:284–291.

74. Commons RR, Callaway CP. Adenomas of the adrenal cortex. Arch Intern Med. 1948;81:37–41.

75. Dévényi I. Possibility of normokalaemic primary aldosteronism as reflected in the frequency of adrenal cortical adenomas. J Clin Pathol. 1967;20:49–51.

76. Kloos RT, Gross MD, Francis IR, et al. Incidentally discovered adrenal masses. Endocr Rev. 1995;16:460–484.

77. Herrera MF, Grant CS, van Heerden JA, et al. Incidentally discovered adrenal tumors: an institutional perspective. Surgery. 1991;110:1014–1021.

78. Glazer HS, Weyman PJ, Sagel SS, et al. Nonfunctioning adrenal masses: incidental discovery on computed tomography. Am J Radiol. 1982;139:81–85.

79. Gilliams A, Roberts CM, Shaw P, et al. The value of CT scanning and percutaneous fine needle aspiration of adrenal masses in biopsy-proven lung cancer. Clin Radiol. 1992;46:18–22.

80. Oliver TW Jr, Bernardino ME, Miller JI, et al. Isolated adrenal masses in nonsmall-cell bronchogenic carcinoma. Radiology. 1984;153:217–218.

81. Sandler MA, Pearlberg JL, Madrazo BL, et al. Computed tomographic evaluation of the adrenal gland in the preoperative assessment of bronchogenic carcinoma. Radiology. 1982;145:733–736.

82. Ettinghausen SE, Burt ME. Prospective evaluation of unilateral adrenal masses in patients with operable non–small-cell lung cancer. J Clin Oncol. 1991;9:1462–1466.

83. Burt M, Heelan RT, Coit D, et al. Prospective evaluation of unilateral adrenal masses in patients with operable non–small-cell lung cancer: impact of magnetic resonance imaging. J Thorac Cardiovasc Surg. 1994;107:584–589.

84. Pagani JJ. Non–small cell lung carcinoma adrenal metastases: computed tomography and percutaneous needle biopsy in their diagnosis. Cancer. 1984;53:1058–1060.

85. Singer AA, Obuchowski NA, Einstein DM, et al. Metastasis or adenoma? Computed tomographic evaluation of the adrenal mass. Cleve Clin J Med. 1994;61:100–105.

86. Pagani JJ. Normal adrenal glands in small cell lung carcinoma: CT-guided biopsy. AJR Am J Roentgenol. 1983;140:949–951.

87. Welch TJ, Sheedy PF II, Stephens DH, et al. Percutaneous adrenal biopsy: review of a 10-year experience. Radiology. 1994;193:341–344.

88. Silverman SG, Mueller PR, Pinkney LP, et al. Predictive value of image-guided adrenal biopsy: analysis of results of 101 biopsies. Radiology. 1993;187:715–718.

89. Mody MK, Kazerooni EA, Korobkin M. Percutaneous CT-guided biopsy of adrenal masses: immediate and delayed complications. J Comput Assist Tomogr. 1995;19:434–439.

90. Szolar DH, Kammerhuber F. Quantitative CT evaluation of adrenal gland masses: a step forward in the differentiation between adenomas and nonadenomas? Radiology. 1997;202:517–521.

91. Korobkin M, Brodeur FJ, Yutzy GG, et al. Differentiation of adrenal adenomas from nonadenomas using CT attenuation values. AJR Am J Roentgenol. 1996;166:531–536.

92. Boland GW, Hahn PF, Peña C, et al. Adrenal masses: characterization with delayed contrast-enhanced CT. Radiology. 1997;202:693–696.

93. Outwater EK, Siegelman ES, Radecki PD, et al. Distinction between benign and malignant adrenal masses: value of T1-weighted chemical-shift MR imaging. AJR Am J Roentgenol. 1995;165:579–583.

94. Mayo-Smith WW, Lee MJ, McNicholas MMJ, et al. Characterization of adrenal masses (<5 cm) by use of chemical shift MR imaging: observer performance versus quantitative measures. AJR Am J Roentgenol. 1995;165:91–95.

95. Mitchell DG, Crovello M, Matteucci T, et al. Benign adrenocortical masses: diagnosis with chemical shift MR imaging. Radiology. 1992;185:345–351.

96. Miyake H, Takaki H, Matsumoto S, et al. Adrenal nonhyperfunctioning adenoma and nonadenoma: CT attenuation value as discriminative index. Abdom Imaging. 1995;20:559–562.

97. Outwater EK, Siegelman ES, Huang AB, et al. Adrenal masses: correlation between CT attenuation value and chemical shift ratio at MR imaging with in-phase and opposed-phase sequences. Radiology. 1996;200:749–752.

98. Korobkin M, Brodeur FJ, Francis IR, et al. Delayed enhanced CT for differentiation of benign from malignant adrenal masses. Radiology. 1996;200:737–742.

99. Reinig JW, Stutley JE, Leonhardt CM, et al. Differentiation of adrenal masses with MR imaging: comparison of techniques. Radiology. 1994;192:41–46.

100. Lee MJ, Hahn PF, Papanicolaou N, et al. Benign and malignant adrenal masses: CT distinction with attenuation coefficients, size, and observer analysis. Radiology. 1991;179:415–418.

101. McNicholas MMJ, Lee MJ, Mayo-Smith WW, et al. An imaging algorithm for the differential diagnosis of adrenal adenomas and metastases. AJR Am J Roentgenol. 1995;165:1453–1459.

102. Gagner M, Pomp A, Heniford BT, et al. Laparoscopic adrenalectomy. Ann Surg. 1997;226:238–247.

103. Mack MJ, Aronoff RJ, Acuff TE, et al. Thoracoscopic transdiaphragmatic approach for adrenal biopsy. Ann Thorac Surg. 1993;55:772–773.

104. Flores RM, Goldstein DJ, Sung RS, et al. Transthoracic, transdiaphragmatic excision of simultaneous lung and adrenal lesions. Ann Thorac Surg. 1998;65:833–835.

105. Keogan MT, Tung KT, Kaplan DK, et al. The significance of pulmonary nodules detected on CT staging for lung cancer. Clin Radiol. 1993;48:94–96.

106. Kunitoh H, Eguchi K, Yamada K, et al. Intrapulmonary sublesions detected before surgery in patients with lung cancer. Cancer. 1992;70:1876–1879.

107. Abdel-Dayem HM, Scott A, Macapinlac H, et al. Tracer imaging in lung cancer. Eur J Nucl Med. 1994;21:57–81.

108. Leitha T, Meghdadi S, Studnicka M, et al. The role of iodine-123-Tyr-3-octreotide scintigraphy in the staging of small-cell lung cancer. J Nucl Med. 1993;34:1397–1402.

109. Vansant JP, Johnson DH, O'Donnell DM, et al. Staging lung carcinoma with a Tc-99m labeled monoclonal antibody. Clin Nucl Med. 1992;17:431–438.

110. Kairemo KJA, Aronen HJ, Liewendahl K, et al. Radioimmunoimaging of non–small cell lung cancer with ¹¹¹In- and ⁹⁹ᵐTc-labeled monoclonal anti-CEA-antibodies. Acta Oncol. 1993;32:771–778.

111. Saunders CAB, Dussek JE, O'Doherty MJ, et al. Evaluation of fluorine-18-fluorodeoxyglucose whole body positron emission tomography in the staging of lung cancer. Ann Thorac Surg. 1999;67:790–797.

112. Graeber GM, Gupta NC, Murray GF. Positron emission tomographic imaging with flurorodeoxyglucose is efficacious in evaluating malignant pulmonary disease. J Thorac Cardiovasc Surg. 1999;117:719–727.

113. Bury T, Dowlati A, Paulus P, et al. Staging of non–small-cell lung cancer by whole-body fluorine-18 deoxyglucose positron emission tomography. Eur J Nucl Med. 1996;23:204–206.

114. Lewis P, Griffin S, Marsden P, et al. Whole-body ¹⁸F-fluorodeoxyglucose positron emission tomography in preoperative evaluation of lung cancer. Lancet. 1994;344:1265–1266.

115. Valk PE, Pounds TR, Hopkins DM, et al. Staging non–small cell lung cancer by whole-body positron emission tomographic imaging. Ann Thorac Surg. 1995;60:1573–1582.

116. Weder W, Schmid RA, Bruchhaus H, et al. Detection of extrathoracic metastases by positron emission tomography in lung cancer. Ann Thorac Surg. 1998;66:886–893.

117. Pantel K, Izbicki J, Passlick B, et al. Frequency and prognostic significance of isolated tumour cells in bone marrow of patients with non–small-cell lung cancer without overt metastases. Lancet. 1996;347:649–653.

118. Ohgami A, Mitsudomi T, Sugio K, et al. Micrometastatic tumor cells in the bone marrow of patients with non–small cell lung cancer. Ann Thorac Surg. 1997;64:363–367.

119. Cote RJ, Beattie EJ, Chaiwun B, et al. Detection of occult bone marrow micrometastases in patients with operable lung carcinoma. Ann Surg. 1995;222:415–425.

120. Pantel K, Izbicki JR, Angstwurm M, et al. Immunocytological detection of bone marrow micrometastasis in operable non–small cell lung cancer. Cancer Res. 1993;53:1027–1031.

121. Thorban S, Roder JD, Nekarda H, et al. Immunocytochemical detection of disseminated tumor cells in the bone marrow of patients with esophageal carcinoma. J Natl Cancer Inst. 1996;88:1222–1227.

122. Cote RJ, Rosen PR, Lesser ML, et al. Prediction of early relapse in patients with operable breast cancer by detection of occult bone marrow micrometastases. J Clin Oncol. 1991;9:1749–1756.

123. Lindemann F, Schlimok G, Dirschedl P. Prognostic significance of micrometastatic tumour cells in bone marrow of colorectal cancer cells. Lancet. 1992;340:685–689.

124. Weiss L. Metastatic inefficiency. Adv Cancer Res. 1990;54:159–211.

125. Glaves D, Huben RP, Weiss L. Haematogenous dissemination of cells from human renal adenocarcinomas. Br J Cancer. 1988;57:32–35.

126. Castaldo G, Tomaiuolo R, Sanduzzi A, et al. Lung cancer metastatic cells detected in blood by reverse transcriptase-polymerase chain reaction and dot-blot analysis. J Clin Oncol. 1997;15:3388–3393.

127. Krismann M, Todt B, Schröder J, et al. Low specificity of cytokeratin 19 reverse transcriptase-polymerase chain reaction analyses for detection of hematogenous lung cancer dissemination. J Clin Oncol. 1995;13:2769–2775.

128. Notter M, Schwegler N. Metastaseninzidenz und verteilungsmuster beim Bronchuskarzinom: autopsie-Ergebnisse über fünf Jahrzehnte (1935 bis 1984). Dtsch Med Wochenschr. 1989;114:343–349.

129. Dearing MP, Steinberg SM, Phelps R, et al. Outcome of patients with small-cell lung cancer: effect of changes in staging procedures and imaging technology on prognostic factors over 14 years. J Clin Oncol. 1990;8:1042–1049.

130. Modini C, Passariello R, Iascone C, et al. TNM staging in lung cancer: role of computed tomography. J Thorac Cardiovasc Surg. 1982;84:569–574.

131. Jennings EC, Aungst CW, Yatco R. Asymptomatic patients with primary carcinoma: computerized axial tomography study. N Y State J Med. 1980;80(7 pt 1):1096–1098.

132. Ferrigno D, Buccheri G. Cranial computed tomography as a part of the initial staging procedures for patients with non–small-cell lung cancer. Chest. 1994;106:1025–1029.

133. Whittlesey D. Prospective computed tomographic scanning in the staging of bronchogenic cancer. J Thorac Cardiovasc Surg. 1988;95:876–882.

134. Nielsen ME Jr, Heaston DK, Dunnick NR, et al. Preoperative CT evaluation of adrenal glands in non–small cell bronchogenic carcinoma. Am J Radiol. 1982;139:317–320.

135. Allard P, Yankaskas BC, Fletcher RH, et al. Sensitivity and specificity of computed tomography for the detection of adrenal metastatic lesions among 91 autopsied lung cancer patients. Cancer. 1990;66:457–462.

136. Schwartz LH, Ginsberg MS, Burt ME, et al. MRI as an alternative to CT-guided biopsy of adrenal masses in patients with lung cancer. Ann Thorac Surg. 1998;65:193–197.

137. Boland GW, Goldberg MA, Lee MJ, et al. Indeterminate adrenal mass in patients with cancer: evaluation at PET with 2-[F-18]-fluoro-2-deoxy-D-glucose. Radiology. 1995;194:131–134.

138. Erasmus JJ, Patz EF Jr, McAdams HP, et al. Evaluation of adrenal masses in patients with bronchogenic carcinoma using ¹⁸F-fluorodeoxyglucose positron emission tomography. AJR Am J Roentgenol. 1997;168:1357–1360.

139. Buccheri G, Biggi A, Ferrigno D, et al. Imaging lung cancer by scintigraphy with indium 111-labeled F(ab')2 fragments of the anticarcinoembryonic antigen monoclonal antibody FO23C5. Cancer. 1991;70:749–759.

140. Guyatt GH, Cook DJ, Griffith LE, et al. Surgeons' assessment of symptoms suggesting extrathoracic metastases in patients with lung cancer. Ann Thorac Surg. 1999;68:309–315.

141. Tanaka K, Kubota K, Kodama T, et al. Extrathoracic staging is not necessary for non–small-cell lung cancer with clinical stage T1-2 N0. Ann Thorac Surg. 1999;68:1039–1042.

142. Cowan RJ, Young KA. Evaluation of serum alkaline phosphatase determination in patients with positive bone scans. Cancer 1973;32:887–889.

143. Hochstenbag MMH, Heidendal GAK, Wouters EFM. In-111 octreotide imaging in staging of small cell lung cancer. Clin Nucl Med. 1997;22:811–816.

144. Marom EM, McAdams HP, Erasmus JJ, et al. Staging non-small cell lung cancer with whole-body PET. Radiology 1999;212:803–809.

145. Passlick B, Kubuschok B, Izbicki JR, et al. Isolated tumor cells in bone marrow predict reduced survival in node-negative non-small cell lung cancer. Ann Thorac Surg. 1999;68:2053–2058.

146. Porte HL, Ernst OJ, Delebecq T, et al. Is computed tomography–guided biopsy still necessary for the diagnosis of adrenal masses in patients with resectable non–small-cell lung cancer? Eur J Cardiothorac Surg. 1999;15:597–601.

147. Bury T, Barreto A, Daenen F, et al. Fluorine-18 deoxyglucose positron emission tomography for the detection of bone metastases in patients with non-small cell lung cancer. Eur J Nucl Med. 1998;25:1244–1247.

PART 3

GENERAL ASPECTS OF TREATMENT OF LUNG CANCER

7

PULMONARY ASSESSMENT AND TREATMENT

Kevin Martinolich and M. Patricia Rivera

The goal of this chapter is to provide an approach, based on available literature, to the pretreatment evaluation of patients scheduled to undergo surgery, radiation therapy, or chemotherapy. Both radiotherapy (RT) and chemotherapy can affect a patient's pulmonary reserve, but the loss of lung function is more sudden with surgery. Therefore, much of this chapter focuses on preoperative assessment of patients. Once it has been determined that surgery would be a good treatment approach for a patient's lung cancer, the clinician must determine whether the patient has adequate pulmonary reserve to tolerate resection and whether the patient has any preexisting medical problems that preclude surgery. This chapter presents a discussion of the tests used to evaluate this, as well as preparatory and perioperative interventions to minimize morbidity and mortality. Finally, the chapter addresses pulmonary considerations germane to treatment with RT and chemotherapy.

EFFECTS OF THORACIC SURGERY ON PULMONARY PHYSIOLOGY

The healthy person has a great deal of reserve in his or her lung function. This not only gives a person the capability to respond to periods of increased demand such as strenuous aerobic activity but also provides a person with the ability to accommodate when lung parenchyma is destroyed or must be removed. Normal tidal volume breathing makes use of only a small fraction of the vital capacity, which is the volume of a maximal exhaled breath (often referred to as the *forced vital capacity*, or FVC). The amount of air remaining in the lungs after normal exhalation is referred to as *functional residual capacity* (FRC), whereas that

remaining after maximal exhalation is known as *residual volume*. These parameters of lung function are shown in Figure 7–1A.

Spirometry is the measurement of lung volumes and is commonly also referred to as *pulmonary function testing* (PFT). These tests are inexpensive, widely available, and reproducible provided the patient is cooperative.[1,2] Spirometry is influenced by a number of factors, including gender, height, race, and age (accounting for 30%, 20%, 10% and 8% of the observed variation, respectively).[3] The most important spirometric measure in assessing lung function is the volume of air expelled during the first second of a maximal forced exhalation, known as the *forced expiratory volume in 1 second* (FEV_1). Lung function can also be evaluated by a measurement of gas exchange, either by measuring blood gas levels or by measuring the diffusing capacity of gas between the air and the blood. Finally, lung function can be assessed by determining the amount of exercise an individual is capable of, although this is also dependent on the function of other organ systems.

The long-term effects of pulmonary resection are discussed in Chapter 8. The FEV_1 is decreased by an average of 12% ≥6 months after a lobectomy, and a similar decrease is reported in the FVC. Maximal exercise capacity is also decreased by an average of 12% following lobectomy. On average, pneumonectomy results in a 31% loss of FEV_1 >6 months after resection, but maximal exercise capacity decreases only 21%. This amounts to a loss of approximately 3% per segment of lung resected.[4]

The ability to tolerate a pulmonary resection is determined primarily by whether the patient will survive the operation and the initial postoperative course, because surgery acutely alters pulmonary physiology in many ways.[5,6]

Figure 7–1. *A,* Spirometric measurements. There are four volumes, which do not overlap: inspiratory reserve volume (IRV), tidal volume (TV), expiratory reserve volume (ERV), and residual volume (RV). There are four capacities, each of which includes two or more primary volumes: total lung capacity (TLC), vital capacity (VC), inspiratory capacity (IC), and functional residual capacity (FRC).

Total lung capacity and all of its subdivisions decrease dramatically in the first few days following surgery, as summarized in Figure 7–1*B*). This data comes from a number of studies involving many patients, although some of the studies date back to the 1930s and primarily involve patients undergoing abdominal surgery.[5] However, changes following thoracic surgery are similar to those following upper abdominal surgery, suggesting that the major cause of these changes is not the loss of lung parenchyma but rather the general effects of surgery on pulmonary physiology.[6]

There are many reasons for the loss of lung volume following surgery. Thoracotomy, with or without resection, is associated with a 47% decrease in chest wall compliance when evaluated on postoperative day 3.[7] Studies have shown that the FRC is decreased by a supine posture, pain, and diaphragmatic dysfunction that occurs after surgery near the diaphragm.[6,8] The loss of FRC is particularly important when considered relative to the *closing volume,* which is the lung volume at which small airways are believed to undergo compression and closure. Once all the gas is absorbed from these alveoli, a greater effort is required to re-expand them due to the properties of surfactant. Studies have shown that the closing volume is increased with age and in patients who smoke or have chronic obstructive pulmonary disease (COPD).[5,6] The closing volume is increased further by edema in the lung parenchyma, such as that caused by intraoperative handling of the remaining lobes.[5,6] Thus many factors predispose the postoperative patient to loss of functional lung volume.

Furthermore, surgery and anesthesia affect many of the pulmonary defense mechanisms, as is shown in Table 7–1. Studies have shown that a sigh breath (defined as a breath more than three times the average tidal volume) is taken approximately 10 times per hour in normal animals and human beings. If this is prevented, compliance and FRC decrease within 30 minutes by approximately 33% and 10%, respectively.[5] This decrease is almost certainly due to airway closure because it can be reversed by hyperinfla-

tion and is corroborated by studies of dye distribution and postmortem morphologic studies.[5] Studies have shown that sighing ceases after the administration of analgesics to postoperative patients.[5] Anesthesia also decreases ciliary function, which may already be impaired due to the effects of smoking. Furthermore, thoracotomy markedly decreases the strength of coughing, as shown in Figure 7–2. In this study, administration of analgesics resulted in only a minor improvement in the strength of a cough.[9]

The combination of altered lung physiology and impaired defense mechanisms predisposes the postoperative patient to atelectasis and retained secretions, resulting in hypoxemia and an increased risk of pneumonia. Indeed, pulmonary complications are the most frequent cause of major morbidity and mortality following pulmonary resection (see Table 8–3). Accurate assessment of the risk of surgery is important in order to appropriately weigh the long-term benefits of surgical treatment relative to the short-term risks. Furthermore, accurate identification of high-risk patients allows early initiation of perioperative

TABLE 7–1. ACUTE EFFECTS OF THORACIC SURGERY ON LUNG PHYSIOLOGY

ALTERATIONS IN PHYSIOLOGY	ALTERATIONS IN DEFENSE MECHANISMS
↓ **FRC, due to** Supine posture Anesthesia Pain	↓ **Cough, due to** ↓ Lung volumes Sedation Pain
↑ **Closing volume, due to** Edema (COPD)	↓ **Sighing, due to** Analgesics Sedation
↑ **Secretions, due to** Lung manipulation Anesthesia	↓ **Ciliary clearance, due to** Anesthesia (Smoking)

Conditions in parentheses commonly cause a chronic baseline impairment in patients who undergo thoracic surgery.
COPD, chronic obstructive pulmonary disease; FRC, functional residual capacity.

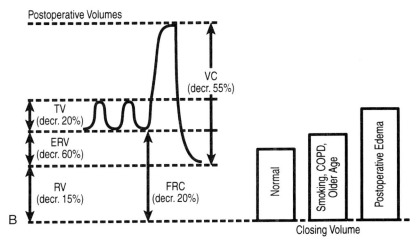

Normal Total Lung Capacity

Postoperative Volumes

VC (decr. 55%)

TV (decr. 20%)

ERV (decr. 60%)

RV (decr. 15%)

FRC (decr. 20%)

Normal

Smoking, COPD, Older Age

Postoperative Edema

B

Closing Volume

FIGURE 7–1 *Continued. B,* Effect of surgery on lung volumes and capacities, and closing volume. Data pertains to patients undergoing upper abdominal surgery. (Data from Tisi GM. Preoperative evaluation of pulmonary function. Am Rev Respir Dis. 1979;119:293–310.[5])

therapeutic interventions that may decrease the risk of complications.

PREOPERATIVE PULMONARY EVALUATION

Because of the association among smoking, COPD, and lung cancer, many patients who are diagnosed with lung cancer already have diminished pulmonary reserve. It has been suggested that >90% of lung cancer patients will have signs of COPD and at least 20% will have severe disease.[10] The list of tests that have been used to identify patients who may be safely resected is extensive (Table 7–2). Some of these tests, such as vital capacity (VC)

and maximum voluntary ventilation (MVV), have been abandoned and will not be discussed. The threshold values that have been suggested have been chosen more or less empirically. Although they are useful in identifying patients who can undergo resection with a low risk of complications, these thresholds have generally been accepted as

TABLE 7–2. COMMONLY USED TESTS AND THRESHOLD LEVELS TO DEFINE RESECTABILITY

TEST	THRESHOLD	EXTENT OF RESECTION
Spirometry		
VC	≥80%	Pneumonectomy
	≥50%	Lobectomy
MVV	>50%	—
pre-FEV$_1$	>2.0 L	Pneumonectomy
	>1.5 L	Lobectomy
	>40%	—
ppo-FEV$_1$	>800 mL	—
	>40%	—
Gas Exchange		
DLCO	>60%	Pneumonectomy
	>50%	Lobectomy
ppo-DLCO	>40%	—
PaO$_2$	>50 mmHg	—
PaCO$_2$	<45 mmHg	—
Exercise		
V̇O$_2$max	>20 mL/kg • min	Pneumonectomy
	≥15 mL/kg • min	Lobectomy
	≥50%	—
Stair climb	≥5 flights	Pneumonectomy
	≥3 flights	Lobectomy
6-min walk	>1000 ft	—

Inclusion criteria: Commonly used criteria of resectability in literature on preoperative assessment.
Adapted from a review by Bollinger CT, Perruchoud AP. Functional evaluation of the lung resection candidate. Eur Respir J. 1998;11:198–212.[108]
DLCO, diffusing capacity of lung for carbon monoxide; MVV, maximal voluntary ventilation; PaCO$_2$, partial pressure of carbon dioxide, arterial; PaO$_2$, partial pressure of oxygen, arterial; ppo, projected postoperative; pre, preresection; VC, vital capacity; V̇O$_2$max, maximum oxygen consumption.

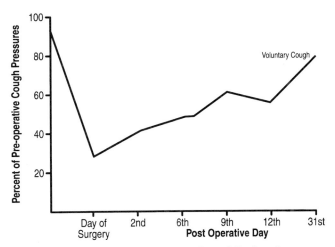

100

80

60

40

20

Percent of Pre-operative Cough Pressures

Voluntary Cough

Day of Surgery   2nd   6th   9th   12th   31st

Post Operative Day

FIGURE 7–2. Cough pressures in 24 patients following thoracotomy. Cough pressure is the pressure achieved in an intrathoracic esophageal balloon during a cough relative to ambient atmospheric pressure. (From Byrd R, Burns J. Cough dynamics in the post-thoracotomy state. Chest. 1975;67:654–657.[9])

dogma, and the risk of complications among patients who fall below these values has not been well defined.

It is difficult to predict the level of risk associated with resection in patients with limited pulmonary reserve. Most studies have grouped patients with and without complications and compared average test results between the groups. Although this may be useful to define tests that appear to be worth evaluating further, it does not provide a way to predict the risk of complications in patients with test results within a particular range. In the following section, we focus on studies that have reported the complication and mortality rates of patients with test results below commonly cited threshold values. The data is restricted to studies published between 1980 and 2000 because mortality rates have changed as a result of improvements in anesthesia, pain control, critical care, and surgery. Furthermore, the focus is on short-term morbidity and mortality because available data suggests that the long-term sequelae of resection in patients with marginal pulmonary reserve are acceptable.[11,12] The only study that has followed a larger number of patients with marginal reserve (n = 88) found identical long-term survival among operative survivors, stage for stage, compared with patients with good pulmonary function.[11]

What constitutes a prohibitive risk in a disease as lethal as lung cancer is a matter of judgment. Because the operative mortality of pulmonary resection is generally low, the pulmonary complication rate is frequently analyzed. Unfortunately, some studies have reported only the rate of all complications combined, even though complications such as wound infections or atrial fibrillation are likely to have little to do with the amount of pulmonary reserve. For the purposes of this chapter, a pulmonary complication is defined as any postoperative pulmonary condition requiring an intervention, such as antibiotics, bronchoscopy, reintubation, prolonged intensive care unit or hospital stay, or death. However, because most complications resolve eventually, the operative mortality rate may be the measure of risk that is really important in the treatment of lung cancer.

Spirometry

The most commonly used test to assess suitability for pulmonary resection is spirometry, in particular FEV_1. None of the studies have specified whether values with or without bronchodilator therapy were used, but it is probably most logical to use whatever values are higher. The *preresection FEV_1* (pre-FEV_1) is a rather crude measure because it does not take into account the amount of lung that is to be removed. Some authors have addressed this problem by suggesting different acceptable threshold levels depending on the extent of the planned resection, most commonly >2 L for a pneumonectomy and >1.5 L for a lobectomy.[13,14] More recently, the function of the amount of lung to be resected has been estimated and the estimation used to calculate the *projected postoperative FEV_1* (ppo-FEV_1), in order to provide a more accurate estimate of the postoperative pulmonary reserve.

The methods used to calculate ppo-FEV_1 are straightforward and similar to one another. In the case of a pneumo-

nectomy, the ppo-FEV_1 is calculated using the results of a quantitative radionucleotide scan that measures the relative function of the right and left lungs. Several studies have shown good correlation between the actual postoperative FEV_1 and the calculated ppo-FEV_1 using this method (r = 0.68–0.86 in studies of >20 patients).[14–17] The correlation is equally good with perfusion and ventilation scanning, reflecting intrapulmonary reflexes that maintain $\dot{V}/\dot{Q}$ (ventilation-perfusion ratio) matching.[14,16,17] Perfusion scanning is generally preferred because it is technically somewhat easier to do.[14,16,17] Older tests of differential lung function, such as the lateral position test or differential bronchospirometry through a double-lumen endotracheal tube, are no longer used because they are either poorly reproducible or invasive and cumbersome.[18]

The projected postoperative FEV_1 can also be calculated using the ratio of the number of lung segments remaining after a resection divided by the total number of pulmonary segments:

$$ppo\text{-}FEV_1 = pre\text{-}FEV_1 \cdot \frac{\text{No. of Segments Remaining}}{\text{Total No. of Segments}}$$

This method is particularly useful in the case of a lobectomy. The entire lung has 18 segments (3 in the right upper lobe [RUL], 2 in the right middle lobe [RML], 5 in the right lower lobe [RLL], 4 in the left upper lobe [LUL], and 4 in the left lower lobe [LLL]). However, some authors view it as having 19 segments, assigning an additional segment to either the LUL[14,19,20] or the LLL.[4,21] This approach has shown excellent correlation with the actual postoperative FEV_1 (r = 0.87–0.96) (Fig. 7–3).[4,14,22] The actual FEV_1 is underestimated by approximately 250 mL for a lobectomy by this method.[4] More complex formulas have been proposed, taking into account lung segments that are not ventilated or using quantitative perfusion scanning, but these do not appear to be more accurate than the simple calculation of the ratio of remaining segments to

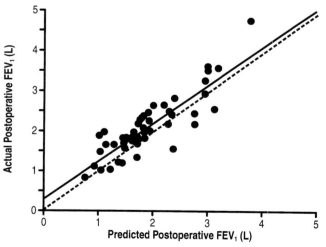

FIGURE 7–3. Correlation of actual postoperative FEV_1 (assessed an average of 8 months later) and predicted postoperative FEV_1, calculated from the preoperative FEV_1 multiplied by the proportion of segments remaining in 48 patients undergoing lobectomy. (From Zeiher B, Gross TJ, Kern JA, et al. Predicting postoperative pulmonary function in patients undergoing lung resection. Chest. 1995;108:68–72.[4])

FEV_1, forced expiratory volume in 1 second.

TABLE 7–3. INCIDENCE OF RESPIRATORY COMPLICATIONS AND MORTALITY IN HIGH RISK PATIENTS IN SERIES INVOLVING MANY LIMITED RESECTIONS

STUDY	HIGH RISK DEFINITION		% OF HIGH RISK PTS[a]	EXTENT OF RESECTION (%)			N	PULMONARY COMPLICATIONS (%)	OPERATIVE MORTALITY (%)
	Test	Threshold		Wedge[b]	Lobectomy[c]	Pneumonectomy			
Cerfolio et al[109 d]	pre-FEV$_1$	<1.2 L	100	41	52	7	85	—	4
Miller[110 d]	pre-FEV$_1$[e]	<1 L	100	100	0	0	67	—	1
Kearney et al[21]	ppo-FEV$_1$	<1 L	100	42[f]	45[f]	14[f]	47	15	4
Walsh et al[30 g]	Various[h]	—	100	52	48	0	25	44	4
Pate et al[31]	pre-FEV$_1$	<2 L	100	42	50	8	12	17	8
Morice et al[29 g]	Various[h]	—	100	50	50	0	8	25	0
Olsen et al[52]	Stair climb	<3 flights	100	46[f]	46[f]	7[f]	7	—	14

Inclusion criteria: Studies from 1980 to 2000 reporting outcomes in >5 patients classified as high risk by conventional criteria, in which > one-third underwent limited resection.
[a]Percentage of patients falling below conventional criteria of high risk, as defined in Table 7–2.
[b]Includes segmentectomy.
[c]Includes bilobectomy.
[d]Retrospective series.
[e]As well as various other criteria.
[f]Extent of resection data includes additional patients who were above threshold.
[g]May involve overlapping patients.
[h]But $\dot{V}O_2$>15 mL/kg/min in all.
FEV$_1$, forced expiratory volume in 1 second; ppo, projected postoperative; pre, preresection; Pts, patients.

the total segments.[14,16,19,23,24] A rather novel approach has been suggested by Wu et al,[25] who found excellent correlation between ppo-FEV$_1$ and actual postoperative FEV$_1$ (r = 0.93) in 38 patients using quantitative computed tomography.

The threshold value for ppo-FEV$_1$ that has been used most commonly is 800 mL, which can be traced to a suggestion made by Olsen et al in 1974.[26] This was based on personal observations of patients not undergoing surgery (no details given)[26] and on the results of a study that noted an average FEV$_1$ of 770 mL in 27 patients who had a Pco$_2$ > 40 (also patients not undergoing surgery).[27] However, subsequent studies have not substantiated 800 mL as a threshold for elevated CO$_2$.[6] Others have argued that an absolute value for ppo-FEV$_1$ does not take into account differences in the size of patients and have favored the use of a percent projected postoperative FEV$_1$ (ppo-FEV$_1$ %), which is the percentage of what is normal for a patient of a particular gender, height, race, and age.[18] Although it makes sense to use a percent predicted value, especially as the incidence of lung cancer in women is rising, the suggested values for ppo-FEV$_1$ of 30% or 40% are largely empiric and have not been well studied.[18,24,28]

It is unfortunate that the proposed thresholds for resectability have been widely accepted as defining a minimum below which the risk of resection is prohibitive. Thus, although it has been well established that a resection is safe in patients who are above the proposed thresholds, the outcome of patients who fall below these levels is not clear because few such patients have been reported who have undergone a conventional resection. Table 7–3 summarizes a number of prospective series of resection in "high-risk" patients (meaning that they fell below at least one of the traditional threshold values), in which many of the patients underwent a limited resection. Furthermore, in at least some of these studies, the "high-risk" patients were selected for operation because of good results with another evaluation, such as exercise testing.[29–31] The risk in these series appears acceptable (<10% mortality). By compari-

son, the average operative mortality in large series of patients (who are not high risk) is 3% for a lobectomy, 9% for pneumonectomy, and 4% overall (see Tables 8–1 and 8–6). The studies in Table 7–3 document that resection of high-risk patients is feasible if liberal use is made of limited resections.

Table 7–4 shows the risk of pulmonary complications and death associated with conventional resection (lobectomy, pneumonectomy) in patients who fell below traditional thresholds of resectability based on spirometry tests. It must be emphasized that this data involves only a limited number of selected patients who have undergone resection despite being below the threshold levels. Little data has been reported regarding the mortality of patients who fall below preresectional FEV$_1$ thresholds. Although the pulmonary complication and mortality rates appear to be increased in these patients, the rates do not seem to be prohibitive. On the other hand, the suggested threshold of a ppo-FEV$_1$ % of <40% of normal does correlate with a high operative mortality (30%–50%) in most studies. The mortality of conventional resection in patients with a ppo-FEV$_1$ of <35% of normal is similar.[22,28,32]

Several factors limit the ability to use the data in Table 7–4 to accurately estimate the risk of resection in prospective patients. Although few patients in these series underwent a limited resection, it remains unclear in most series how many of the "high-risk" patients underwent lobectomy or pneumonectomy because the extent of resection was reported for the entire study population. Use of threshold values based on projected postoperative values may minimize the influence of the extent of resection on mortality, however. Most of the studies in Table 7–4 involved patient populations in which relatively few patients were deemed high risk. Furthermore, it appears that the high-risk patients who underwent surgery were selected, although the selection criteria were not made clear. Although most of these series were prospective, this refers to the collection of spirometric and outcomes data and does not imply that all patients with spirometric results in particular ranges

TABLE 7–4. RISK OF RESPIRATORY COMPLICATIONS AND MORTALITY IN PATIENTS ABOVE AND BELOW SPIROMETRY TEST THRESHOLDS

STUDY	TEST	THRESHOLD	% OF HIGH RISK PTS[a]	EXTENT OF RESECTION FOR ENTIRE STUDY POPULATION (%)			PATIENTS ABOVE THRESHOLD			PATIENTS BELOW THRESHOLD		
				Wedge[b]	Lobectomy[c]	Pneumon	N	Pulmonary Complications (%)	Operative Mortality (%)	N	Pulmonary Complications (%)	Operative Mortality (%)
Olsen et al[48]	pre-FEV₁	<1.5 L[d]	All	15	70	15	11	27	—	18	22	—
Bolliger et al[54]	pre-FEV₁	<1.5 L[d]	Few	18	56	26	71	8	1	9	44	22
Duque et al[32]	pre-FEV₁	<1.3 L	Few	20	52	28	562	(33)[e]	6	30	(27)[e]	13
Dales et al[63]	pre-FEV₁	≤60%	Few	11	74	15	43[f]	21[f]	—	50	50	—
Bolliger et al[54]	pre-FEV₁	≤60%	Few	18	56	26	69	10	3	11	100	9
Duque et al[32]	ppo-FEV₁	<1 L	Few	20	52	28	542	(32)[e]	7	63	(37)[e]	6
Markos et al[24]	ppo-FEV₁	<1 L	Few	0	62	38	38	13	0	9	33	33
Wahi et al[111 g]	ppo-FEV₁	≤40%	Few	0	0	100	122	—	3	51	—	16
Nakahara et al[23]	ppo-FEV₁	≤40%	Few	0	77	23	157	16	—	15	47	—
Pierce et al[22]	ppo-FEV₁	<40%	Few	26	54	20	41	(78)[e]	10	13	(85)[e]	38
Holden et al[28]	ppo-FEV₁	<40%	All	31	44	25	6	17	0	10	60	50
Nakagawa et al[49]	ppo-FEV₁	<40%	Few	0	77	23	24	21	8	7	71	29
Markos et al[24]	ppo-FEV₁	<40%	Few	0	62	38	41	12	0	6	50	50

Inclusion criteria: Studies from 1980 to 2000 reporting outcomes in >5 high-risk patients and involving < one-third limited resections.

[a]Percentage of entire population falling below conventional criteria of resectability, as defined in Table 7–2.
[b]Includes segementectomy.
[c]Includes bilobectomy.
[d]<2 L for pneumonectomy.
[e]Any complications.
[f]For patients with pre-FEV₁ >80%.
[g]Retrospective series.

FEV₁, forced expiratory volume in 1 second; ppo, projected postoperative; pneumon, pneumonectomy; pre, preresection.

118

would necessarily undergo resection. Nevertheless, the mortality of patients with a ppo-FEV$_1$ < 40% is high, despite the fact that the patients were selected. This suggests that the resection of such patients should be undertaken only with caution, unless their risk can be estimated to be lower on the basis of other evaluations.

Gas Exchange

The requirement of a normal PaO$_2$ and PaCO$_2$ for a patient to be considered at low risk for pulmonary resection makes eminent sense. However, surprisingly little actual data exists regarding arterial blood gas measurements and the risk of pulmonary resection. Several authors have reported that resection in patients with a mildly elevated PaCO$_2$ (>45) was not associated with increased morbidity or mortality compared with patients without hypercarbia.[21,30,32,33] These patients (~80 total) were undoubtedly carefully selected and, in at least two studies, were able to complete exercise testing with a $\dot{V}O_2$ >15 mL/kg · min.[30,33] Furthermore, an elevated PCO$_2$ during exercise (>45 mm Hg) resulted in only a 9% mortality in 33 resected patients.[34] Thus hypercarbia by itself should not rule out resection if a patient is otherwise deemed suitable. Data regarding the value of PaO$_2$ has been reported in only one study, which found no difference in mortality in patients with a resting PaO$_2$ <60 or >60 mm Hg (6% versus 7%).[32]

The *diffusing capacity of lung for carbon monoxide* (DLCO; known in Europe as the transfer factor) is a measure of gas exchange. This test is readily available in most institutions, and a number of investigators have found a lower result to be associated with a higher risk of complications or mortality.[22,24,35–37] Although standards for measuring and reporting DLCO have been defined, substantial differences exist among methods that are in common use.[38] The DLCO is affected by the alveolar volume, and studies involving DLCO have used corrected values that take this into account. Furthermore, DLCO is usually reported as a percentage of the predicted normal value (DLCO %), thereby adjusting for differences in body size. DLCO is also affected by the hemoglobin level, and results that are corrected for this should be used whenever available.

A preoperative DLCO of >60% has been recommended, and morbidity and mortality are low above this number. However, this threshold should not be used to exclude patients from surgery because patients with a DLCO % below this value who undergo resection have a mortality of only about 15% (Table 7–5). It is possible to calculate a projected postoperative DLCO % using the same methods as those used to calculate a ppo-FEV$_1$. Studies have shown good correlation between the calculated ppo-DLCO and the actual measured DLCO several months later (r = 0.56–0.89 in studies of >20 patients).[17,22,24,39] The ppo-DLCO % appears to be a better indicator than pre-DLCO % of an increased risk with a standard resection, with the mortality being approximately 25% for a ppo-DLCO % of <50% and approximately 33% for a ppo-DLCO % of ≤40% (see Table 7–5). In one of the largest prospective studies evaluating the ability of tests to predict the operative mortality, the

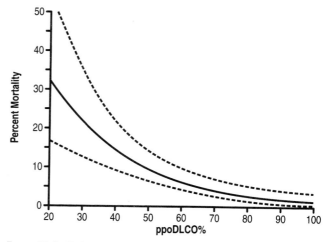

FIGURE 7–4. Estimated operative mortality of major pulmonary resection for lung cancer as a function of the projected postoperative (ppo) DLCO expressed as a percentage of predicted (normal) and corrected for alveolar volume and hemoglobin. Mortality is estimated from a logistic regression model of 334 patients, with 95% confidence limits *(dashed lines)*. (Reprinted with permission from the Society of Thoracic Surgeons [The Annals of Thoracic Surgery. 1999;67:1444–1447.].[11])

mortality increased progressively as the ppo-DLCO % decreased (Fig. 7–4).

Exercise Testing

Some patients with lung cancer report minimal limitations in normal activity despite poor spirometry results. These patients raise the suspicion that exercise testing may be a better measure than spirometry of a patient's ability to tolerate a resection. Furthermore, because exercise requires adequate functioning of both the pulmonary and the cardiac systems, exercise testing may be a better measure of a patient's ability to tolerate the physiologic stress associated with thoracic surgery. Several studies have compared the average exercise tolerance in patients with and without complications and have reported mixed results with respect to finding a significant difference. This is not entirely surprising, however, given the small size of many of these studies. Furthermore, average results in patients who retrospectively had complications do not allow prospective estimation of the risk of resection in patients who have a particular level of exercise tolerance.

During exercise, oxygen consumption, carbon dioxide production, and cardiac output all increase, and the level of work achieved reflects how well the lung, heart and vasculature interact to deliver oxygen to the tissues. With increasing workload, the amount of oxygen uptake increases, until a plateau known as $\dot{V}O_2$max, or *maximum oxygen consumption,* is reached. The $\dot{V}O_2$max is related to the type of work performed (eg, walking versus seated on a cycle ergometer), as well as the patient's age, gender, and height.[40] A predicted "normal" $\dot{V}O_2$max for an individual can be estimated, although at least two slightly different formulas have been proposed.[41,42] Furthermore, practice can significantly affect the results of exercise testing.[43] Thus, there is a need for standardization in order to allow comparison among studies. Although the measured $\dot{V}O_2$max will

TABLE 7-5. RISK OF COMPLICATIONS OR DEATH WITH SURGICAL RESECTION BY MEASUREMENTS OF GAS EXCHANGE

STUDY	TEST	THRESHOLD[a]	% OF HIGH RISK PATIENTS[b]	EXTENT OF RESECTION FOR ENTIRE STUDY POPULATION (%)			PATIENTS ABOVE THRESHOLD			PATIENTS BELOW THRESHOLD		
				Wedge[c]	Lobectomy[d]	Pneumon	N	Pulmonary Complications (%)	Operative Mortality (%)	N	Pulmonary Complications (%)	Operative Mortality (%)
Bousamra et al[37 e]	pre-DLCO	<60%[f]	Few	0	75	25	262	10	5	62	18	5
Ferguson et al[35 e]	pre-DLCO	≤60%	Few	0	69	31	145	19	5	20	45	25
Pierce et al[22]	pre-DLCO	≤60%[f]	Few	26	54	20	47	(77)[g]	17	7	(71)[g]	14
Markos et al[24]	ppo-DLCO	<50%	Few	0	62	38	32	6	0	14	43	21
Bolliger et al[39]	ppo-DLCO	<50%	All	0	46	54	14	14	0	11	27	27
Holden et al[28]	ppo-DLCO	<50%	All	31	44	25	8	50	38	8	38	25
Markos et al[24]	ppo-DLCO	<40%	Few	0	62	38	32	10	3	14	67	33
Pierce et al[22]	ppo-DLCO	≤40%	Few	26	54	20	47	(77)[g]	13	7	(71)[g]	43
Ferguson et al[36 e]	ppo-DLCO	≤40%	Few	0	75	25	?[h]	8–33	2–13	?[h]	34	22

Inclusion criteria: Studies from 1980 to 2000 reporting outcomes in >5 patients classified as high risk by conventional criteria.

[a]DLCO corrected for alveolar volume and hemoglobin, when available, and expressed as % of predicted (normal).
[b]Percentage of entire population falling below conventional criteria of resectability as defined in Table 7–2.
[c]Includes segmentectomy.
[d]Includes bilobectomy.
[e]Retrospective series.
[f]<50% for pneumonectomy.
[g]Any complication.
[h]376 patients total.

DLCO, diffusing capacity of lung for carbon monoxide; Pneumon, pneumonectomy; ppo, projected postoperative; pre, preresection.

be affected by poor motivation, in general, a symptom-limited $\dot{V}O_2$ can be assumed to be close to the true $\dot{V}O_2max$ if maximal effort criteria are achieved.[44]

As the workload increases above resting levels through exercise, the *anaerobic threshold* is reached, at which an-aerobic metabolism begins to supplement aerobic metabolism because of insufficient oxygen delivery at the cellular level. This is associated with an increase in lactic acid production and an increase in the respiratory quotient (ratio of CO_2 production to O_2 consumption). Exercise above this level can be sustained temporarily with a resultant O_2 debt, but multiorgan failure will develop if there is a persistent O_2 demand above the anaerobic threshold, such as might occur with the increased metabolic demands of the postoperative state.[45,46] The anaerobic threshold is hard to measure accurately in practice but has been estimated to occur at approximately 50% of maximum $\dot{V}O_2$.[40,42]

Because of concern that patients who are elderly or have limited pulmonary reserve might not reliably exercise to a maximal level, some authors have proposed that submaximal exercise testing be done.[47–49] In this case, $\dot{V}O_2$ must be measured at a particular level of workload (eg, 40 watts), which suffers from not being adjusted to what can be expected for an individual patient, or $\dot{V}O_2$ can be measured at the anaerobic threshold or at a particular amount of lactic acid production. These latter methods suffer from being complex and invasive and having unclear reproducibility.

A simple way of measuring exercise tolerance is to measure the distance a patient can walk or the number of flights of stairs a patient can climb before becoming exhausted. These tests are sometimes criticized for not being standardized and for measuring only low level exercise. However, stair climbing consistently results in a higher $\dot{V}O_2max$ than cycle ergometry in studies comparing these tests, and it appears that patients may be motivated to make more of a maximum effort with stair climbing than on a cycle ergometer.[28,50,51] The major limitation of these tests is that little data is available that allows mortality to be predicted on the basis of the results, although these tests have been employed for many years.

A study of 70 patients found that 97% of patients who could climb three flights had an FEV_1 >1.7 L, and 94% of those who could climb five flights had an FEV_1 >2 L.[50] This is indirect evidence that the risk of undergoing lobectomy (or pneumonectomy) is probably low if the patient can climb three (or five) flights of stairs. No mortality was reported among patients who could climb at least three flights in a study of 70 patients, but almost all of these patients were considered low risk and almost half underwent a limited resection.[52] In contrast, Holden et al[28] found an operative mortality of 27% in a study of 15 patients who could climb a minimum of three (for lobectomy) or five (for pneumonectomy) flights of stairs, but were high risk by other criteria. The ability to walk ≥2000 ft in 12 minutes was associated with a low mortality (2%) in 41 low-risk patients undergoing lobectomy or pneumonectomy,[24] but in another study, a mortality of 15% was found among 13 high-risk patients despite their being able to walk ≥1000 ft in 6 minutes.[28] Data regarding outcomes in patients who fell below these thresholds involves such limited numbers of patients that no conclusions are possible

(Table 7–6). The inability to carry out an exercise test was found by itself to correlate with a high operative mortality (21%) and complication rate (71%) in a study of low-risk patients in which 14 were unable to exercise because of musculoskeletal, neurologic, peripheral vascular, or psychiatric conditions.[53] This association of higher morbidity and mortality with an inability to exercise persisted even after correction for multiple other cardiopulmonary risk factors.[53] The value of desaturation with exercise in predicting complications or mortality appears to be limited (see Table 7–6).

The risk of respiratory complications and mortality associated with formal measurements of $\dot{V}O_2max$ is shown in Table 7–6. Most of the reported data has involved populations in which few patients were considered high risk. It is clear that the risk of resection is low in such low-risk populations when the $\dot{V}O_2max$ is >15 mL/kg/min. In groups of patients who are low risk by other criteria but have a $\dot{V}O_2max$ <15 mL/kg/min, approximately one-third can be expected to develop pulmonary complications, and the average reported mortality is 17%. Even for patients with a $\dot{V}O_2max$ <10 mL/kg/min, the risk of conventional resection does not appear to be prohibitive, but this data is limited, and these patients have undoubtedly been carefully selected.

Unfortunately, the mortality has not been defined in patients who are considered high risk by other criteria but are found to have an acceptable $\dot{V}O_2max$ (>15 mL/kg/min). Two studies have reported results for high-risk patients but have reported only the risk for those who fell below the $\dot{V}O_2max$ threshold of 15 mL/kg/min (the mortality was 18% and 27%).[28,39] Because this mortality would generally be considered increased yet still acceptable, it seems reasonable to conclude that the mortality in populations of high-risk patients who have a good $\dot{V}O_2max$ will also be acceptable. However, it is inappropriate to assume that the mortality in high-risk patients who have a good $\dot{V}O_2max$ will be the same as that of low-risk patients (by other criteria) who have a good $\dot{V}O_2max$.

It has been suggested that assessment of $\dot{V}O_2max$ as a percentage of predicted (normal) may be better than using an absolute value,[54] but at this time there is too little data regarding this to estimate the risk or even to define an appropriate threshold. Furthermore, it may be better to use the projected postoperative $\dot{V}O_2max$ than to rely on preoperative values. The one study that addressed this issue found that in high-risk patients, those with a ppo-$\dot{V}O_2max$ ≥50% had no mortality despite being high risk, whereas those with a ppo-$\dot{V}O_2max$ <50% had a mortality of 42%.[39] Two studies have shown good correlation between ppo-$\dot{V}O_2max$ and actual measured postoperative $\dot{V}O_2max$ (r = 0.65–0.9).[17,39] Finally, one study found that while a low $\dot{V}O_2max$ is associated with increased complications, both a low $\dot{V}O_2max$ and complications were predicted by various clinical factors (eg, congestive heart failure, recent myocardial infarction, arrhythmia, obesity, productive cough, wheezing, COPD).[55] The fact that these factors were a better predictor of outcome than the $\dot{V}O_2max$ suggested that the $\dot{V}O_2max$ is only a marker for the clinical factors, which are the real issue.

Using a workload of 40 watts on a cycle ergometer in 29 high-risk patients, Olsen et al[48] found that the respiratory

TABLE 7–6. RISK OF RESPIRATORY COMPLICATIONS AND DEATH FOLLOWING SURGICAL RESECTION BY MEASUREMENTS OF EXERCISE TOLERANCE

STUDY	TEST	THRESHOLD[a]	% OF HIGH RISK PATIENTS[b]	EXTENT OF RESECTION FOR ENTIRE STUDY POPULATION (%)			PATIENTS ABOVE THRESHOLD			PATIENTS BELOW THRESHOLD		
				Wedge[c]	Lobectomy[d]	Pneumon	N	Pulmonary Complications (%)	Operative Mortality	N	Pulmonary Complications (%)	Operative Mortality (%)
Bechard et al[112]	VO_2 max	<15	Many	24	56	20	28	7[e]	0	22	40[e]	13
Bolliger et al[54]	VO_2 max	<15	Few	18	56	26	64	6	1	16	38	13
Bolliger et al[39]	VO_2 max	<15	All	0	59	41	—	—	—	17	29	18
Markos et al[24]	VO_2 max	<15	Few	0	62	38	29	14	3	14	21	7
Holden et al[28]	VO_2 max	<15	All	31	44	25	—[g]	—	—	11	36	27
Pierce et al[22]	VO_2 max	<15	Few	26	54	20	44	(77)[h]	16	8	(88)[h]	25
Smith et al[113]	VO_2 max	<15	Few	27	55	18	16	19	6	6	83	17
Bechard et al[112]	VO_2 max	<10	Some	24	56	20	43	7[e]	0	7	71[e]	29
Markos et al[24]	VO_2 max	<10	Few	0	62	38	38	18	5	5	0	0
Dales et al[63]	VO_2 max	<80%	Few	11	74	15	19	37	0	27	30	—
Bolliger et al[54]	VO_2 max	<60%	Few	18	56	26	71	4	0	9	78	100
Morice et al[114]	VO_2 max	≤50%	All	—	—	—	43	12	0	—	—	—
Larsen et al[115]	VO_2 max	<50%	Few	19	54	28	92	—	2	5	—	60
Bolliger et al[39]	ppo-VO_2	<50%	All	0	59	41	18	11	0	7	43	43
Holden et al[28]	6-min walk	<1000 ft	All	31	44	25	13	31	15	—[g]	—	—
Markos et al[24]	12-min walk	<2000 ft	Few	0	62	38	41	22	2	—[g]	—	—
Holden et al[28]	Stair climb	<3L<5P[i]	All	31	44	25	15	40	27	—[g]	—	—
Markos et al[24]	Exercise desat	>4% diff	Few	0	62	38	41	24	7	—[g]	—	—
Ninan et al[116]	Exercise desat	>4% diff	Few	0	0	100	36	15	—	11	91	—
Rao et al[117]	Exercise desat	>4% diff	Few	17	69	15	184	46[j]	1	115	46[j]	2
Rao et al[117]	Exercise desat	≤90%	Few	17	69	15	234	37[j]	1	65	49[j]	3

Inclusion criteria: Studies from 1980 to 2000 reporting outcomes and involving >5 patients classified as high risk and conventional resections (lobectomy or pneumonectomy) in > two-thirds of patients.
[a]Measured in mL/kg • min, as percentage of predicted (normal) or as indicated.
[b]Percentage of entire population falling below conventional criteria of resectability, as defined in Table 7–2.
[c]Includes segmentectomy.
[d]Includes bilobectomy.
[e]Includes cardiac complications and pulmonary embolus.
[f]All but 1 able to climb >3 flights of stairs (lobectomy) or >5 flights (pneumonectomy).
[g]<5 patients.
[h]Any complication.
[i]<3 flights for lobectomy, <5 flights for pneumonectomy.
[j]Defined as prolonged need for supplemental O_2.

desat, desaturation; diff, difference between rest and exercise; Pneumon, pneumonectomy; ppo, projected postoperative; $\dot{V}O_2$ max, maximum oxygen consumption.

complication rate was increased in the patients with a *submaximal* $\dot{V}O_2$ of <10 mL/kg/min (45% versus 7%). Other investigators, who exercised 31 patients with Swan-Ganz catheters in place, have found that an O_2 delivery/ body surface area (BSA) of ≤500 mL/min/m² or a $\dot{V}O_2$/ BSA of ≤350 mL/min/m² was associated with higher surgical mortality (100% versus 0 and 45% versus 0, respectively).[49] Although these submaximal exercise tests appear to have some predictive value, they have not been validated and are complex to carry out.

Other Tests

The complexity and the variability of the results have led to the abandonment of a once-popular test involving the measurement of temporary unilateral pulmonary artery (PA) occlusion with a balloon-tipped catheter.[18] A study by Fee et al[56] suggested that an elevated pulmonary vascular resistance during exercise predicted a high mortality in 30 low-risk patients (42% versus 0), despite the fact that 40% of the patients had only a limited resection. However, other studies of pulmonary vascular resistance during exercise have not corroborated any association with increased complications or mortality.[34,48] Because these tests are complex and invasive and appear to have poor predictive value, they are of limited use. More recently, it was shown in 20 patients that clamping one PA at the time of performing pneumonectomy did not affect the PA pressure or resistance, but 25% of patients developed an abnormal right ventricular ejection fraction. This was the only measure found to correlate with late postoperative cardiopulmonary dysfunction (80% of such patients were NYHA class III or IV >6 months postoperatively).[57]

Some investigators have combined several risk factors into a composite risk index (Table 7–7). These composite indices do seem to predict a high operative mortality among groups of patients who are generally low risk. However, any such index that is discovered in one data set must be validated in another data set before it can be evaluated seriously. Only one of these indices (PPP) was validated retrospectively in another data set. Whether such composite indices will turn out to be sufficiently accurate and easy enough to use to be widely adopted remains to be seen.

Multivariate Analysis

With so many different tests having been proposed to predict the risk of complications and mortality, it is natural to ask which test is best. From the previous discussion, it appears that no single test stands out from the others. Several studies have performed a multivariate analysis of multiple tests in order to identify which ones have independent predictive value.[21,22,24,36,54,58] The three studies that have analyzed tests with regard to operative mortality have all identified ppo-D_{LCO} % as the major factor, in combination with either age[36] or ppo-FEV_1 %.[22,24] Exercise tolerance was not found to be an independent predictor, although it

must be noted that the largest study (n = 376) did not include any assessment of exercise capacity.[36]

Most of the multivariate analyses have evaluated the tests in regard to their association with complications of any type. The ppo-D_{LCO} % was commonly found to be a major factor, as well as the ppo-FEV_1 %.[21,24,36] The studies that did not find these factors to be significant generally did not examine them, although one large study found ppo-FEV_1 to be not significant (but ppo-D_{LCO} % was),[36] and one small study found neither ppo-FEV_1 % nor ppo-D_{LCO} % to be significant.[22] In this latter study (n = 54) only P_{CO_2} was found to be a significant factor for all complications and body mass index for respiratory complications.[22] Only two studies found $\dot{V}O_2$max to be a significant factor, but neither study examined ppo-FEV_1 % or ppo-D_{LCO} % (ie, only pre-FEV_1 % or pre-D_{LCO} % was assessed).[54,58]

APPROACH TO THE EVALUATION OF PATIENTS FOR PULMONARY RESECTION

Given the limited amount of data on the actual risk of resection in patients with poor pulmonary reserve and the large number of tests, it is difficult to identify one approach to evaluating patients for surgery that is optimal. Some patients are clearly not candidates for surgery because of comorbid conditions, such as poorly controlled heart failure or angina. On the other hand, some patients can be readily identified as being likely to tolerate pulmonary resection with little risk because they have adequate pulmonary reserve and are otherwise in good medical condition. For example, a patient with a pre-FEV_1 >2 L can be confidently predicted to be able to tolerate a resection based on this alone, making further testing unnecessary.

In patients who have diminished pulmonary function, more exact estimation of their reserve is necessary. It makes intuitive sense to use values that take into account the amount of lung to be removed (eg, ppo-FEV_1) as well as the effect of differences in patient gender, size, race, and age (eg, percentage of predicted normal values). Indeed, the data presented in Tables 7–4 and 7–5 suggests that the projected postoperative values expressed as a percentage of normal are better predictors of increased risk than presection values. A quantitative perfusion scan appears to be useful, at least in the case of a pneumonectomy, to predict more accurately the amount of functional lung that will be lost. The data from multivariate analysis suggests that both ppo-D_{LCO} % and ppo-FEV_1 % are major indicators of operative risk and that D_{LCO} may be the most important factor.

A suggested stepwise approach to the evaluation of patients for pulmonary resection, based on the data regarding the operative mortality, is shown in Figure 7–5. Several studies have consistently demonstrated a low mortality (<10%) in patients with a pre-FEV_1 of >60% of normal or a pre-D_{LCO} of >60% of normal. For patients falling below these presection values, several studies have consistently demonstrated a low mortality in patients with a ppo-FEV_1 of >40% of normal or a ppo-D_{LCO} of >40% of

TABLE 7-7. RISK OF RESPIRATORY COMPLICATIONS AND DEATH FOLLOWING SURGICAL RESECTION BY COMPOSITE INDICES OR PULMONARY VASCULAR RESISTANCE

STUDY	TEST	THRESHOLD	% OF HIGH RISK PATIENTS[a]	EXTENT OF RESECTION FOR ENTIRE STUDY POPULATION (%)			PATIENTS ABOVE THRESHOLD			PATIENTS BELOW THRESHOLD		
				Wedge[b]	Lobec[c]	Pneumon	N	Pulmonary Complications (%)	Operative Mortality (%)	N	Pulmonary Complications (%)	Operative Mortality (%)
Epstein et al[53]	CPRI	≥4	Few	20	73	7	46	22[d]	0	28	79[d]	14
Pierce et al[22]	PPP	<1650	Few	26	54	20	42	(76)[e]	7	12	(92)[e]	50
Markos et al[24]	PPP	<1650	Few	0	62	38	39	—	0	7	—	43
Melendez et al[118]	PRQ	<2200	Few	0	67	33	49	0	0	12	83	17
Olsen et al[48]	Exercise PVR	>190	High	15	70	15	13	23	—	13	23	—
Loddenkemper et al[34]	Exercise PAP	>35	Mod	11	58	31	175	—	12	59	—	10

Inclusion criteria: Studies from 1980 to 2000 reporting outcomes in >5 patients classified as high risk by conventional criteria.
[a]Percentage of entire study population falling below conventional criteria of resectability as defined in Table 7–2.
[b]Includes segmentectomy.
[c]Includes bilobectomy.
[d]Includes cardiac complications and pulmonary embolus.
[e]Any complication.

CPRI, combined score consisting of cardiac (congestive heart failure, recent myocardial infarction, arrhythmia, age >70 years, and so on) and pulmonary (obesity, active smoking, productive cough, wheezing, chronic obstructive pulmonary disease, P_{CO_2} >45) risk scores; FEV_1, forced expiratory volume in 1 second; Lobec, lobectomy; PAP, pulmonary artery pressure during exercise, in mm Hg; Pneumon, pneumonectomy; ppo, projected postoperative; PPP, ppo-FEV_1% · ppo-D_{LCO}%; PRQ, ppo-FEV_1% · (ppo-D_{LCO}%)/ A-a pO_2; PVR, pulmonary vascular resistance during exercise in dynes · sec · cm^{-5}.

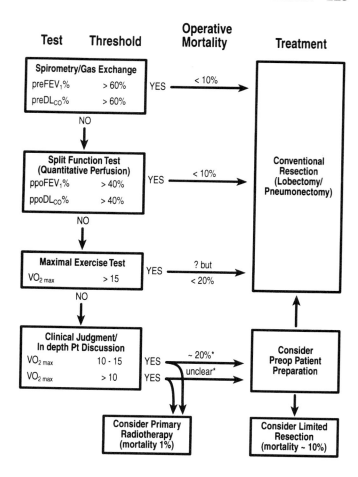

FIGURE 7–5. Suggested algorithm for evaluation of patients for pulmonary resection. *Operative mortality estimated from limited amounts of data.

DATA SUMMARY: TESTS TO PREDICT OPERATIVE RISK			
	AMOUNT	**QUALITY**	**CONSISTENCY**
Spirometry			
A ppo-FEV$_1$ <800 mL is associated with increased morbidity and mortality	Poor	Poor	—
Calculated estimates of ppo-FEV$_1$ correlate closely with actual measured FEV$_1$ postoperatively	High	High	High
A ppo-FEV$_1$ <40% of predicted (normal) is associated with an operative mortality of ~30%	High	Mod	Mod
Gas Exchange			
A preresection D$_{LCO}$ of <60% is associated with increased mortality (~15%)	Mod	Mod	High
A ppo-D$_{LCO}$<40% of normal is associated with high operative mortality (~33%)	Mod	Mod	Mod
A Pa$_{O_2}$ <60 mm Hg is associated with increased postoperative risk	Poor	Mod	—
A Pa$_{CO_2}$ <45 mm Hg is not associated with increased postoperative risk	High	Mod	High
Exercise Testing			
The inability to walk >1000 feet in a 6-minute walk test predicts a high mortality with resection	Poor	Mod	—
Patients unable to climb at least three flights of stairs have a high mortality with resection	Poor	Mod	—
The mortality in low-risk patient populations (by other tests) who have a V$_{O_2}$max of <15 mL/kg/min is approximately 15%	High	Mod	High

Type of data rated: Plain text: descriptive statement   *Italics: controlled comparison*   **Bold: randomized comparison**

normal. If either of these tests falls below this value, further investigation is needed to allow better assessment of the operative risk. A maximal exercise test demonstrating a $\dot{V}O_2max$ >15 mL/kg/min is a reasonable criterion to identify patients who should undergo resection. Although the mortality in such patients has not been clearly defined, it is likely to be acceptable (<20%).

Whether resection should be performed in patients who have a poor ppo-FEV_1 or ppo-D_{LCO} and a $\dot{V}O_2max$ of <15 mL/kg/min is a complex issue. The approach clearly requires careful clinical judgment and an in-depth discussion with the patient and family of the risks and benefits of several possible approaches. For high-risk patients with a $\dot{V}O_2max$ of 10 to 15 mL/kg/min, the mortality with conventional resection is approximately 20%, although the data documenting this is limited. It may be reasonable to accept this risk in the face of a good chance of cure. For patients with a $\dot{V}O_2max$ of <10 mL/kg/min, the risk of conventional resection is unclear. Although a few such patients have been reported who have undergone resection with a reasonable mortality, the data is too limited to allow generalization. The use of ppo-$\dot{V}O_2max$ as a percentage of normal may be a better measure to use because it is standardized to patient size and the extent of resection, just as the ppo-FEV_1 % and ppo-D_{LCO} % are, but at present too little data is available.

In patients with a poor ppo-FEV_1 or ppo-D_{LCO} and a poor $\dot{V}O_2max$, preoperative pulmonary preparation should be considered in an attempt to diminish the risk, as is discussed in the following section. More importantly, the value of alternative treatments should be weighed carefully. The mortality of limited resection is approximately 10%, but this is associated with a diminished chance of cure compared with lobectomy (see Chapter 11). Primary RT offers a low but definite chance of cure in stage I non–small cell lung cancer (NSCLC) that can be achieved with minimal mortality (see Chapter 13). The best treatment depends on the size and stage of the tumor, as well as an estimation of the risk of the treatment in an individual patient. One way to compare the outcomes may be to multiply the chance of surviving resection with the chance of cure with resection and compare it with the chance of long-term survival with an alternative therapy such as RT.

PERIOPERATIVE MANAGEMENT

Perioperative interventions are often used to diminish the risk of postoperative complications, especially in high-risk patients. Although the degree of emphysema or pulmonary fibrosis that is present cannot be altered, preoperative patient preparation can be used in an attempt to decrease sputum production, diminish airway hyperactivity, or improve aerobic conditioning. Many patients with COPD have chronic sputum production and are often colonized with bacteria.[59,60] Many individuals will also have airway hyperactivity as a result of airway inflammation.[59,61] Postoperative interventions can also be used to try to minimize the risk of retained secretions, atelectasis, and subsequent pneumonia and respiratory failure. The following section examines data regarding how effective these preoperative

and postoperative measures are in decreasing the risk of pulmonary complications.

Smoking Cessation

Smoking is frequently cited as an important risk factor for pulmonary complications[5,62] and is associated with decreased tracheobronchial clearance, increased sputum production,[6] altered pulmonary immune defenses such as depressed neutrophil chemotaxis, decreased immunoglobulin levels, and decreased macrophage adherence.[24] Several studies have found that the risk of pulmonary complications after surgery in general is approximately two to five times as high in smokers as in nonsmokers.[63–66] Warner et al[65] found an incidence of pulmonary complications of 12% in nonsmokers, 29% in those who smoked ≤1 pack per day (ppd), and 41% in those smoking >1 ppd in a retrospective analysis of 500 patients undergoing coronary artery bypass surgery. Pulmonary complications occurred in 5% of nonsmokers and 22% of smokers in another study of 410 patients undergoing a variety of surgical procedures.[66] In a prospective study of 111 patients undergoing general surgery, the incidence of pulmonary complications (broadly interpreted) correlated with the amount of smoking (8% in nonsmokers, 23% in moderate smokers, and 43% in very heavy smokers).[64] In at least two studies, the increased incidence of pulmonary complications in smokers appeared to be unrelated to the FEV_1.[64,65] Furthermore, the presence of COPD is not an independent risk factor for complications among current smokers, whereas a chronic cough appears to be an independent risk factor in another study.[66]

It stands to reason that smoking cessation might alter the risk of postoperative complications, but direct clinical evidence is limited, and the issue has not been addressed specifically in patients undergoing a thoracotomy. A large retrospective study of postoperative pulmonary complications in 500 patients undergoing coronary artery bypass surgery found that the complication rate decreased only if smoking had been stopped >8 weeks before surgery (Fig. 7–6).[65] This time frame coincides with the time it takes for functions such as tracheobronchial clearance to improve. There were no differences with respect to the amount of baseline smoking, the proportion of patients with an abnormal FEV_1, or cardiac factors among the groups in this study.[65] Unfortunately, it is impractical to postpone an operation for lung cancer for this length of time. Another study found that a mere reduction in the amount of smoking—but not stopping altogether—resulted in a 7-fold *increase* in the risk of pulmonary complications compared with patients who continued to smoke at their usual levels.[66] Nevertheless, there may be a theoretical benefit to abstention from smoking for days or even hours before surgery because the half-life of carboxyhemoglobin (COHb) is only 4 to 6 hours. In heavy smokers, as much as 15% of the circulating hemoglobin may be in the form of COHb, which decreases oxygen release by shifting the hemoglobin dissociation curve to the left. Unfortunately, there is no data to assess the clinical impact of this effect.

Pharmacology and Antibiotics

Well-defined treatment strategies have been published regarding the treatment of COPD.[59] A number of agents are

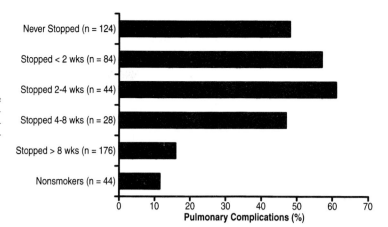

FIGURE 7–6. Effect of the duration of smoking cessation on the risk of pulmonary complications in 500 patients undergoing cardiac surgery. (From Warner MA, Divertie MB, Tinker JH. Preoperative cessation of smoking and pulmonary complications in coronary artery bypass patients. Anesthesiology. 1984;60:380–383.[65])

available, including inhaled bronchodilators, inhaled and systemic steroids, leukotriene receptor inhibitors, and theophylline. Detailed reviews regarding the general use of these agents are available.[59,67] Appropriate COPD management can result in improved lung function and improved quality of life and provides an indirect argument that such interventions may reduce the risk of complications when patients with COPD undergo surgery.

Two prospective studies have evaluated the perioperative use of inhaled bronchodilators, smoking cessation, humidified air, chest physiotherapy (PT), and antibiotics.[68,69] In one of these, 157 patients with COPD were admitted 2 to 3 days before surgery for a regimen of bronchodilators, intermittent positive-pressure breathing (IPPB), chest PT, and smoking cessation.[68] The treatment resulted in small but statistically significant improvements in FVC, MVV, and forced expiratory flow (FEF_{25-75}), and the rate of complications was decreased (19% versus 43%) relative to historic controls from the same institution with a similar mix of types of operations.[68] This corroborated an earlier retrospective analysis from the same institution of 190 patients who did and 167 who did not receive pulmonary preparation before general anesthesia, in which the pulmonary complication rate was reduced from 43% to 25%.[70] Finally, in a randomized study, half of 34 patients with abnormal PFTs were placed on a regimen of bronchodilators, antibiotics, chest PT, inhalation of humidified air, and smoking cessation.[69] A statistically significant reduction in the incidence of pulmonary complications was observed in the group that received pulmonary preparation; furthermore, the severity of the observed complications was reduced.[69]

Antibiotic use is justified when an acute infection exists, but antibiotics have been found not to be effective in preventing or treating an exacerbation of COPD in the absence of objective evidence of infection (eg, fever, leukocytosis, chest radiograph changes).[71–73] The bacteria usually involved include *Streptococcus pneumoniae, Haemophilus influenzae*, and *Moraxella catarrhalis*.[58,71] Appropriate agents include amoxicillin, erythromycin, clarithromycin, tetracycline, doxycycline, and trimethoprim-sulfamethoxazole.

In summary, a reasonable argument can be made to carry out a program of preoperative preparation in high-risk patients, although the data is limited and it is not clear which interventions are most important. Antibiotics are not indicated in the absence of infection, and it would seem that bronchodilators and steroids are of use primarily in patients who have evidence on pulmonary function tests of an improvement with such treatment.

Pulmonary Rehabilitation

It is well understood that respiratory muscle weakness often develops in patients with COPD.[74,75] There is data that supports the use of both inpatient and outpatient pulmonary rehabilitation for patients with COPD, and appropriate therapies can improve exercise tolerance and quality of life and can reduce dyspnea.[74] Whether overall survival is improved remains unclear, however, and whether the data for patients with COPD can be extrapolated to the perioperative setting is questionable.

Surprisingly little data exists regarding the use of pulmonary rehabilitation before major surgery. Pulmonary rehabilitation is considered standard care for patients awaiting lung transplantation.[76] Only one study has examined the effects of pulmonary rehabilitation (ie, exercise training) in this setting, but this study did not examine the effect on postoperative pulmonary complications.[77] Exercise resulted in a decrease in perceived dyspnea but no change in exercise tolerance as measured by 6-minute walk tests as well as tolerated work load in 28 patients awaiting transplantation.[77] Nomori et al[78] evaluated 50 patients awaiting thoracic surgery who were admitted 1 to 3 weeks before surgery and underwent deep breathing training, vigorous coughing, and training with a positive expiratory pressure device. The authors noted that both the maximum inspiratory pressure and maximum expiratory pressure improved with muscle training and that pulmonary complications were more likely to occur in patients with lower maximum inspiratory pressure and maximum expiratory pressure values. It is unclear, however, whether this intervention reduced postoperative complications because the study lacked an appropriate control group. Another small randomized study of 32 patients found that the postoperative FEV_1 was significantly improved by spirometry and inspiratory muscle training for 2 weeks preoperatively in patients undergoing lung resection[79] but did not report on complications. Thus, although pulmonary rehabilitation has been shown to be effective in patients with COPD, there is no clear-cut evidence that this intervention improves outcomes in patients undergoing pulmonary resection.

Postoperative Care

A number of maneuvers are available that focus on reversing the development of postoperative atelectasis, including incentive spirometry, IPPB, continuous positive airway pressure (CPAP), and chest PT exercises consisting of postural drainage, chest wall percussion, and assisted coughing.[80] Despite their widespread use, little data is available regarding their routine use in the post-thoracotomy setting, although an extrapolation can be made from studies of patients undergoing abdominal and cardiac surgery. Morran et al[81] noted a reduction in the incidence of pulmonary infections with the use of chest PT in 102 patients undergoing cholecystectomy (14% versus 37%, $P = 0.02$). This finding was further supported by Celli et al[82] in a randomized four-arm study of 172 patients undergoing abdominal surgery, which compared patients undergoing incentive spirometry, IPPB, and deep breathing exercises with controls. Each of the treatment groups experienced fewer respiratory complications (21%–22%) than the controls (48%), but there were no differences between any of the treatment groups. Eight randomized studies involving cardiac surgery patients were examined in a 1995 review of a variety of postoperative interventions to decrease atelectasis and retained secretions.[83] Most of these studies did not demonstrate any differences in the incidence of pulmonary complications, but five involved <50 patients and only three included a control group receiving no treatment other than routine encouragement of coughing and deep breathing.

Several small randomized studies have evaluated the usefulness of CPAP in the postoperative period.[84–86] In these studies, CPAP was delivered by face mask beginning shortly after extubation in patients undergoing upper abdominal surgery,[85] cardiac surgery,[86] or lung resection.[84] These studies generally noted early improvements in pulmonary physiologic measurements (recovery of FRC and increase in Pao_2, usually in the first 24 hours) but did not find a difference in the rate of postoperative pulmonary complications. However, these studies were extremely small, with only 9 to 13 patients per arm.

It is obvious that there is not enough data to clearly define the value of the routine use of any of the interventions commonly used to prevent or reverse atelectasis in patients following thoracotomy. Given the results of studies performed in patients undergoing abdominal surgery, it is reasonable to use these techniques in post-thoracotomy patients, particularly in those who are considered high risk. No single approach is obviously more effective than any other, and data regarding cost effectiveness is lacking. Other interventions, such as optimal pain control and early mobilization, are also important and are discussed elsewhere.[80] Furthermore, the use of interventions as a therapeutic maneuver to treat postoperative complications that have already occurred is clearly indicated by clinical experience. The efficacy of these treatments in this setting is discussed elsewhere, as well.[80]

RADIATION AND CHEMOTHERAPY

Effects of Radiotherapy

Changes in pulmonary function after radiation therapy were first described approximately 100 years ago, yet the extent of functional loss after radiation therapy has not been well defined.[87] This is particularly problematic because RT can be associated with injury to normal lung. Two forms of lung injury—acute pneumonitis and late pulmonary fibrosis—have been well described.[88–91] The incidence of symptomatic radiation pneumonitis has been reported to be between 1% and 34%, with rates of radiologic changes ranging from 13% to 100%.[89] A review of nearly 2000 patients showed rates of 8% and 43% for symptomatic pneumonitis and radiologic changes, respectively.[92] A number of studies have noted severe complication rates (grade 3 to 5) of 3% to 5%.[93,94] Issues associated with pulmonary radiation toxicity are discussed in more detail in Chapter 9.

Several authors have looked at the changes in pulmonary function after RT. In a study of 14 patients, Brady et al[87] noted a decrease in D_{LCO} that correlated with the volume and dosage delivered to the chest, but they noted little change in other measured parameters such as lung volume, lung compliance, FEV_1, and FVC. Similar results were found by Mattson et al[95] in 34 patients treated with split-course radiation. Again, the D_{LCO} was significantly decreased at 6 and 9 months after radiation treatment (21% and 27%, $P < 0.05$). Using a dose of 45 to 55 Gy for treatment of locoregional NSCLC with a 2-cm margin, Abratt and Wilcox[96] observed a mean decrease in the D_{LCO} of 14% and 12% at 6 and 12 months post-RT, respectively. Choi et al[97] noted somewhat contradictory findings. In this prospective study of 71 patients, little change was seen in spirometry measured before the initiation of postoperative RT and at yearly intervals after finishing RT. However, the baseline PFTs in this study were obtained 1 month after pulmonary resection, and D_{LCO} was not measured. Because normally a significant improvement over time is seen in PFTs compared with 1 month after surgery, the study by Choi et al[97] demonstrated that postoperative RT precluded any further improvement in pulmonary function from being realized.

Estimating pulmonary function after RT using pulmonary function tests and split-perfusion scans has been proposed. In a prospective study of 22 patients, the predicted postradiation FEV_1 was calculated using the following equation:

$$\text{Post-RT FEV}_1 = \text{Pre-RT FEV}_1 \cdot (1 - \text{Perf}_{\text{Irrad Lung}})$$

where $\text{Perf}_{\text{Irrad Lung}}$ is the fraction of total lung perfusion in the irradiated portion of the lungs.

In only two patients was the measured post-RT FEV_1 below the predicted post-RT FEV_1.[98] In a series of articles, Choi et al[99–101] noted that pretreatment lung function, extent of bronchial or pulmonary vascular obstruction by tumor, and location of treatment are important determinants of change in pulmonary function after RT. Those patients with a borderline FEV_1 of <50% of predicted, as well as those patients with an uneven distribution of perfusion to each side (suggesting atelectasis or compression by tumor), ex-

DATA SUMMARY: PERIOPERATIVE MANAGEMENT

	AMOUNT	QUALITY	CONSISTENCY
Pulmonary complications are seen in approximately 10% of non-smokers, 25% of moderate smokers, and 40% of heavy smokers after surgery (mostly general surgery)	High	Mod	High
Preoperative smoking cessation is not associated with a reduction of pulmonary complications until after 8 weeks	Poor	High	—
A regimen of preoperative preparation is associated with a reduction in the risk of pulmonary complications	*Mod*	*Mod*	*High*
Prophylactic use of postoperative interventions to diminish atelectasis and retained secretions reduces the risk of pulmonary complications	**Mod**	**Mod**	**Mod**

Type of data rated: Plain text: descriptive statement *Italics: controlled comparison* **Bold: randomized comparison**

perienced little decline in FEV_1 after radiation.[101] The authors hypothesized that loss in pulmonary function is related to the balance between injury to normal lung tissue that results from RT and the potential improvement in lung function due to relief of obstruction caused by the tumor. In general, the equation used by these authors tended to overestimate the loss of lung function.[97,98]

Effects of Chemotherapy

The lung is a common target of drug toxicity, and a variety of cancer chemotherapeutic drugs have been recognized as causative agents in the genesis of lung injury. Agents most commonly associated with pulmonary toxicity include bleomycin, BCNU, mitomycin, methotrexate, and doxorubicin when combined with RT. The pulmonary toxicity of chemotherapeutic agents has been reviewed extensively.[102–104] The incidence of clinically significant toxicity with most agents is low (<5%), with the exception of BCNU.[102,104] The pathophysiology of pulmonary toxicity is poorly understood and seems to involve different mechanisms with different agents. The diagnosis can sometimes be supported by cytologic findings but is usually made on the basis of clinical findings, which can be varied.[102,104] Pulmonary function testing in the setting of chemotherapy has centered predominantly on the effect of chemotherapy on the diffusion capacity (D_{LCO}), and this has been best studied with bleomycin. In patients with clinically significant bleomycin toxicity, both the D_{LCO} and lung volumes have decreased markedly in most cases.[105] Treatment involves discontinuation of the implicated agent and usually also the administration of steroids.[102,104]

The role of PFTs in screening for early cytotoxic drug-induced toxicity has not been studied in detail. In the case of bleomycin, several authors have sought PFT abnormalities in asymptomatic patients as a marker of subclinical damage. Although some authors have found consistent dose-related decreases in the D_{LCO} in asymptomatic patients receiving bleomycin,[106,107] others have not.[105] Because these are small studies (each with <20 patients) that have yielded conflicting results, it is difficult to make a definitive statement on the role of PFTs in screening.

EDITORS' COMMENTS

Appropriate selection of patients for surgical resection of lung cancer is crucial. On the one hand, there is no point in undertaking resection if the operative mortality is prohibitively high. On the other hand, selection of only the most ideal patients would deny many patients the option of surgery, which remains the most effective treatment for early stage lung cancer. The major issue appears to be the risk of perioperative complications and mortality, with major long-term limitations being relatively uncommon (at least with the type of patients who have been selected for surgery in the past).

There has been a gradual evolution in tests used to assess a patient's risk of perioperative complications. Assessment of preoperative measures has largely given way to projected postoperative values, which take into account the amount of functional lung to be removed. Furthermore, the use of measures expressed as a percentage of predicted (normal) allows values to be indexed to the patient's size, age, and gender. This progression has taken place most clearly with spirometric results and with measurements of diffusing capacity. A similar evolution is beginning to take place with regard to the interpretation of exercise studies. The best single test has not been defined unequivocally, but the ppo-D_{LCO} % appears to be a good candidate. Data is even more limited regarding the use of a combination of tests.

However, the real issue is that there is too little data to accurately determine threshold values for any of the tests in order to reliably identify patients who have a prohibitively high risk with a standard resection. It appears clear that a limited resection (segmentectomy or wedge resection) can be accomplished safely in most patients. It is understandable that there has been much reluctance to subject patients who fall beneath proposed thresholds to resection when the risks are unknown. However, it is time to conduct a careful prospective evaluation of the risk associated with conventional resection in patients with progressively more limited pulmonary reserve.

Preoperative preparation of patients with measures such as the use of bronchodilators appears to be useful in reducing the perioperative risk. The value of preoperative rehabilitation is unclear, and antibiotics should be used only to treat an active infection. Postoperative interventions to prevent atelectasis appear to be indicated, although the data supporting this is limited. Smoking cessation before surgery appears to be of little benefit unless smoking is stopped completely and for ≥8 weeks. It is somewhat impractical to expect patients with cancer to wait this long. Nevertheless, the diagnosis of lung cancer represents a unique opportunity to convince patients of the importance of smoking cessation.

References

1. American Thoracic Society. Standardization of spirometry. Am Rev Respir Dis. 1979;119:831.
2. American Thoracic Society. Lung function testing: selection of reference values and interpretation strategies. Am Rev Respir Dis. 1991;144:1202–1218.
3. Becklake MR. Concepts of normality applied to the measurement of lung function. Am J Med. 1986;80:1158–1164.
4. Zeiher B, Gross TJ, Kern JA, et al. Predicting postoperative pulmonary function in patients undergoing lung resection. Chest. 1995;108:68–72.
5. Tisi GM. Preoperative evaluation of pulmonary function. Am Rev Respir Dis. 1979;119:293–310.
6. Jackson C. Preoperative pulmonary evaluation. Arch Intern Med. 1988;148:2120–2127.
7. Peters RM, Wellons HA Jr, Htwe TM. Total compliance and work of breathing after thoracotomy. J Thorac Cardiovasc Surg. 1969;57:348–355.
8. Ali J, Weisel RD, Layug AB, et al. Consequences of postoperative alterations in respiratory mechanics. Am J Surg. 1974;128:376–382.
9. Byrd R, Burns J. Cough dynamics in the post-thoracotomy state. Chest. 1975;67:654–657.
10. Marshall MC, Olsen GN. The physiologic evaluation of the lung resection candidate. Clin Chest Med. 1993;14:305–320.
11. Wang J, Olak J, Ultmann RE, et al. Assessment of pulmonary complications after lung resection. Ann Thorac Surg. 1999;67:1444–1447.
12. Boysen PG, Harris JO, Block AJ. Prospective evaluation for pneumonectomy using perfusion scanning: follow-up beyond one year. Chest. 1981;80:163–166.
13. Boushy SF, Billig DM, North LB. Clinical course related to preoperative and postoperative pulmonary function in patients with bronchogenic carcinoma. Chest. 1971;59:383–391.
14. Wernly JA, DeMeester TR, Kirchner PT, et al. Clinical value of quantitative ventilation-perfusion lung scans in the surgical management of bronchogenic carcinoma. J Thorac Cardiovasc Surg. 1980;80:535–543.
15. Ladurie M, Ranson-Bitker B. Uncertainties in the expected value for forced expiratory volume in one second after surgery. Chest. 1986;90:222–228.
16. Ali MK, Mountain CF, Ewer MS, et al. Predicting loss of pulmonary function after pulmonary resection for bronchogenic carcinoma. Chest. 1980;77:337–342.
17. Corris PA, Ellis DA, Hawkins T, et al. Use of radionuclide scanning in the preoperative estimation of pulmonary function after pneumonectomy. Thorax. 1987;42:285–291.
18. Gass GD, Olsen GN. Preoperative pulmonary function testing to predict postoperative morbidity and mortality. Chest. 1986;89:127–135.
19. Giordano A, Calcagni ML, Meduri G. Perfusion lung scintigraphy for the prediction of postlobectomy residual pulmonary function. Chest. 1997;111:1542–1547.
20. Khargi K, Duurkens VAM, Verzijlbergen FF, et al. Pulmonary function after sleeve lobectomy. Ann Thorac Surg. 1994;57:1302–1304.
21. Kearney DJ, Lee TH, Reilly JJ, et al. Assessment of operative risk in patients undergoing lung resection: importance of predicted pulmonary function. Chest. 1994;105:753–759.
22. Pierce R, Copland JM, Sharpe K. Preoperative risk evaluation for lung cancer resection: predicted postoperative product as a predictor of surgical mortality. Am J Respir Crit Care Med. 1994;150:947–955.
23. Nakahara K, Monden Y, Ohno K, et al. A method for predicting postoperative lung function and its relation to postoperative complications in patients with lung cancer. Ann Thorac Surg. 1985;39:260–265.
24. Markos J, Mullan BP, Hillman DR, et al. Preoperative assessment as a predictor of mortality and morbidity after lung resection. Am Rev Respir Dis. 1989;139:902–910.
25. Wu MT, Chang JM, Chiang AA. Use of quantitative CT to predict postoperative lung function in patients with lung cancer. Radiology. 1994;191:257–262.
26. Olsen GN, Block AJ, Tobias JA. Prediction of postpneumonectomy pulmonary function using quantitative macroaggregate lung scanning. Chest. 1974;66:13–16.
27. Segall J, Butterworth B. Ventilatory capacity in chronic bronchitis in relation to carbon dioxide retention. Scand J Respir Dis. 1966;47:215–224.
28. Holden DA, Rice TW, Stelmach K. Exercise testing, 6-min walk, and stair climb in the evaluation of patients at high risk for pulmonary resection. Chest. 1992;102:1774–1779.
29. Morice RC, Peters EJ, Ryan MB. Exercise testing in the evaluation of patients at high risk for complications from lung resection. Chest. 1992;101:356–361.
30. Walsh GL, Morice RC, Putnam JB Jr, et al. Resection of lung cancer is justified in high-risk patients selected by exercise oxygen consumption. Ann Thorac Surg. 1994;58:704–711.
31. Pate P, Tenholder MF, Griffin JP. Preoperative assessment of the high-risk patient for lung resection. Ann Thorac Surg. 1996;61:1494–1500.
32. Duque JL, Ramos G, Castrodeza J, et al. Early complications in surgical treatment of lung cancer: a prospective, multicenter study. Ann Thorac Surg. 1997;63:944–950.
33. Bolliger CT, Solèr M, Stulz P. Evaluation of high-risk lung resection candidates: pulmonary haemodynamics versus exercise testing. Respiration. 1994;61:181–186.
34. Loddenkemper R, Gabler A, Gobel D. Criteria of functional operability in patients with bronchial carcinoma: preoperative assessment of risk and prediction of postoperative function. Thorac Cardiovasc Surg. 1983;31:334–337.
35. Ferguson MK, Little L, Rizzo L, et al. Diffusing capacity predicts morbidity and mortality after pulmonary resection. J Thorac Cardiovasc Surg. 1988;96:894–900.
36. Ferguson MK, Reeder LB, Mick R. Optimizing selection of patients for major lung resection. J Thorac Cardiovasc Surg. 1995;109:275–283.
37. Bousamra M, Presberg KW, Chammas JH, et al. Early and late morbidity in patients undergoing pulmonary resection with low diffusion capacity. Ann Thorac Surg. 1996;62:968–975.
38. American Thoracic Society. Single breath carbon monoxide diffusing capacity (transfer factor): recommendations for a standard technique—1995 update. Am J Respir Crit Care Med. 1995;152:2185–2198.
39. Bolliger CT, Wyser C, Roser H, et al. Lung scanning and exercise testing for the prediction of postoperative performance in lung resection candidates at increased risk for complications. Chest. 1995;108:341–348.
40. Wasserman K, Whipp B. Exercise physiology in health and disease. Am Rev Respir Dis. 1975;112:219–259.
41. Jones NL, Makrides L, Hitchcock C, et al. Normal standards for an incremental progressive cycle ergometer test. Am Rev Respir Dis. 1985;131:700–708.
42. Hansen JE, Sue DY, Wasserman K. Predicted values for clinical exercise testing. Am Rev Respir Dis. 1984;129(suppl):S49–S55.
43. Swinburn CR, Wakefield JM, Jones PW. Performance, ventilation, and oxygen consumption in three types of exercise test in patients with chronic obstructive lung disease. Thorax. 1985;40:581–586.
44. Gilbreth E, Weisman I. Role of exercise testing in preoperative evaluation of patients for lung resection. Clin Chest Med. 1994;15:389–403.
45. Shoemaker WC, Appel PL, Kram HB. Tissue oxygen debt as a determinant of lethal and non-lethal postoperative organ failure. Crit Care Med. 1988;16:1117–1120.
46. Shoemaker WC, Appel PL, Kram HB. Role of oxygen debt in the development of organ failure sepsis, and death in high-risk surgical patients. Chest. 1992;102:208–215.
47. Miyoshi S, Nakahara K, Ohno K, et al. Exercise tolerance test in

lung cancer patients: the relationship between exercise capacity and postthoracotomy hospital mortality. Ann Thorac Surg. 1987;44:487–490.

48. Olsen GN, Weiman DS, Bolton JW. Submaximal invasive exercise testing and quantitative lung scanning in the tolerance for lung resection. Chest. 1989;95:267–273.

49. Nakagawa K, Nakahara K, Miyoshi S. Oxygen transport during incremental exercise load as a predictor of operative risk in lung cancer patients. Chest. 1992;101:1369–1375.

50. Bolton JW, Weiman DS, Haynes JL. Stair climbing as an indicator of pulmonary function. Chest. 1987;92:783–788.

51. Pollock M, Roa J, Benditt J. Estimation of ventilatory reserve by stair climbing: a study in patients with chronic airflow obstruction. Chest. 1993;104:1378–1381.

52. Olsen GN, Bolton JW, Weiman DS. Stair climbing as an exercise test to predict the postoperative complications of lung resection: two years' experience. Chest. 1991;99:587–590.

53. Epstein SK, Faling LJ, Daly BDT, et al. Inability to perform bicycle ergometry predicts increased morbidity and mortality after lung resection. Chest. 1995;107:311–316.

54. Bolliger CT, Jordan P, Solèr M. Exercise capacity as a predictor of postoperative complications in lung resection candidates. Am J Respir Crit Care Med. 1995;151:1472–1480.

55. Epstein SK, Faling LJ, Daly BD. Predicting complications after pulmonary resection: preoperative exercise testing vs. a multifactorial cardiopulmonary risk index. Chest. 1993;104:694–700.

56. Fee HJ, Holmes EC, Gewirtz HS, et al. Role of pulmonary vascular resistance measurements in preoperative evaluation of candidates for pulmonary resection. J Thorac Cardiovasc Surg. 1978;195:519–524.

57. Lewis JW Jr, Bastanfar M, Gabriel F, et al. Right heart function and prediction of respiratory morbidity in patients undergoing pneumonectomy with moderately severe cardiopulmonary dysfunction. J Thorac Cardiovasc Surg. 1994;108:169–175.

58. Larsen K, Svendson UG, Milman N. Exercise testing in the preoperative evaluation of patients with bronchogenic carcinoma. Eur Respir J. 1997;10:1559–1565.

59. American Thoracic Society Statement. Standards for the diagnosis and care of patients with chronic obstructive pulmonary disease. Am J Respir Crit Care Med. 1995;152:S77–S120.

60. Reynolds HY, Swisher JW. Preoperative management of chronic bronchitis. Infect Med 1993;10:21–29.

61. Anthonisen NR, Wright EC, Hodgkin JE. Prognosis in chronic obstructive pulmonary disease. Am Rev Respir Dis. 1986;133:14–20.

62. Mohr D, Jett J. Preoperative evaluation of pulmonary risk factors. J Gen Intern Med. 1988;3:277–287.

63. Dales RE, Dionne G, Leech JA, et al. Preoperative prediction of pulmonary complications following thoracic surgery. Chest. 1993;104:155–159.

64. Chalon J, Tayyab MA, Ramanathan S. Cytology of respiratory epithelium as a predictor of respiratory complications after operation. Chest. 1975;67:32–35.

65. Warner MA, Divertie MB, Tinker JH. Preoperative cessation of smoking and pulmonary complications in coronary artery bypass patients. Anesthesiology. 1984;60:380–383.

66. Bluman LG, Mosca L, Newman N, et al. Preoperative smoking habits and postoperative pulmonary complications. Chest. 1998;113:883–889.

67. Celli B. Current thoughts regarding treatment of chronic obstructive pulmonary disease. Med Clin North Am. 1996;80:589–609.

68. Gracey DR, Divertie MB, Didier EP. Preoperative pulmonary preparation of patients with chronic obstructive disease. Chest. 1979;76:123–129.

69. Stein M, Cassara E. Preoperative pulmonary evaluation and therapy for surgery patients. JAMA. 1970;211:787–790.

70. Tarhan S, Moffitt EA, Sessler AD, et al. Risk of anesthesia and surgery in patients with chronic bronchitis and chronic obstructive pulmonary disease. Surgery. 1973;74:720–726.

71. Anthonisen NR, Manfreda J, Warren CP. Antibiotic therapy in exacerbations of chronic obstructive pulmonary disease. Ann Intern Med. 1987;106:196–204.

72. Rodnick JE, Gude JK. The use of antibiotics in acute bronchitis and acute exacerbations of chronic bronchitis. West J Med. 1988;149:347–351.

73. Schlick W. Selective indications for use of antibiotics: when and what. Eur Respir Rev. 1992;2:187–192.

74. Pulmonary rehabilitation: joint ACCP/AACVPR evidence-based guidelines. ACCP/AACVPR Pulmonary Rehabilitation Guidelines Panel. American College of Chest Physicians. American Association of Cardiovascular and Pulmonary Rehabilitation. Chest. 1997;112:1363–1396.

75. Celli B. Pulmonary rehabilitation for patients with advanced lung disease. Clin Chest Med. 1997;18:521–534.

76. Palmer S, Tapson V. Pulmonary rehabilitation in the surgical patient. Respir Care Clin N Am. 1998;4:71–83.

77. Sheldon J. Pulmonary rehabilitation prior to lung transplantation. Am J Respir Crit Care Med. 1993;147:A597.

78. Nomori H, Kobayashi R, Fuyuno G, et al. Preoperative respiratory muscle training: assessment in thoracic surgery patients with special reference to postoperative pulmonary complications. Chest. 1994;105:1782–1788.

79. Weiner P, Man A, Weiner M, et al. The effect of incentive spirometry and inspiratory muscle training on pulmonary function after lung resection. J Thorac Cardiovasc Surg. 1997;113:552–557.

80. Detterbeck FC. Postoperative management after thoracic surgery procedures. In: Moylan JA, ed. Surgical Critical Care. St. Louis, Mo: CV Mosby; 1994:409–429.

81. Morran CG, Finlay IG, Mathieson M, et al. Randomized controlled trial of physiotherapy for postoperative pulmonary complications. Br J Anaesth. 1983;55:1113–1117.

82. Celli BR, Rodriguez KS, Snider GL. A controlled trial of intermittent positive breathing, incentive spirometry, and deep breathing exercises in preventing pulmonary complications after abdominal surgery. Am Rev Respir Dis. 1984;130:12–15.

83. Thornlow DK. Is chest physiotherapy necessary after cardiac surgery? Crit Care Nurse. 1995;15:39–46.

84. Aguilo R, Togores B, Pons S, et al. Noninvasive ventilatory support after lung resection surgery. Chest. 1997;112:117–121.

85. Stock MC, Downs JB, Cooper RB, et al. Comparison of continuous positive airway pressure, incentive spirometry, and conservative therapy after cardiac operations. Crit Care Med. 1984;12:969–972.

86. Pinilla JC, Oleniuk FH, Tan L, et al. Use of a nasal continuous positive airway pressure mask in the treatment of postoperative atelectasis in aortocoronary bypass surgery. Crit Care Med. 1990;18:836–840.

87. Brady LW, German PA, Candor L. The effects of radiation therapy on pulmonary function in carcinoma of the lung. Radiology. 1965;85:130–134.

88. Rosiello R, Merrill W. Radiation-induced lung injury. Clin Chest Med. 1990;11:65–71.

89. Movsas B, Raffin TA, Epstein AH, et al. Pulmonary radiation injury. Chest. 1997;111:1061–1076.

90. Gross NJ. Pulmonary effects of radiation therapy. Ann Intern Med. 1997;86:81–92.

91. Coggle JE, Lambert BE, Moores SR. Radiation effects in the lung. Environ Health Perspect. 1986;70:261–291.

92. Roach M III, Gandara DR, Yuo H-S, et al. Radiation pneumonitis following combined modality therapy for lung cancer: analysis of prognostic factors. J Clin Oncol. 1995;13:2606–2612.

93. Perez CA, Stanley K, Rubin P, et al. A prospective randomized study of various irradiation doses and fractionation schedules in the treatment of inoperable non–oat-cell carcinoma of the lung: preliminary report by the Radiation Therapy Oncology Group. Cancer. 1980;45:2744–2753.

94. Simpson JR, Francis ME, Perez-Tamayo R, et al. Palliative radiotherapy for inoperable carcinoma of the lung: final report of a RTOG multi-institutional trial. Int J Radiat Oncol Biol Phys. 1985;11:751–758.

95. Mattson K, Holsti LR, Poppius H. Radiation pneumonitis and fibrosis following split-course radiation therapy for lung cancer. Acta Oncol. 1987;26:193–196.

96. Abratt R, Wilcox P. The effect of irradiation on lung function and perfusion in patients with lung cancer. Int J Radiat Oncol Biol Phys. 1995;31:915–919.

97. Choi N, Karanek DJ, Grillo HC. Effect of postoperative radiotherapy on changes in pulmonary function patients with stage II and IIIA lung carcinoma. Int J Radiat Oncol Biol Phys. 1990;18:95–99.

98. Rubenstein JH, Richter MP, Moldofsky PJ, et al. Prospective prediction of post-radiation therapy lung function using quantitative lung scans and pulmonary function testing. Int J Radiat Oncol Biol Phys. 1988;15:83–87.

99. Choi N. Prospective prediction of postradiotherapy pulmonary function with regional pulmonary function data: promise and pitfalls. Int J Radiat Oncol Biol Phys. 1988;15:245–247.

100. Choi N, Kanarek D, Kazemi H. Physiologic changes in pulmonary function after thoracic radiotherapy for patients with lung cancer and role of regional pulmonary function studies in predicting postradiotherapy pulmonary function before radiotherapy. Cancer Treat Symp. 1985;2:119–130.

101. Choi NC, Kanarek DJ. Toxicity of thoracic radiotherapy on pulmonary function in lung cancer. Lung Cancer. 1994;10(suppl):S219–S230.

102. Twohig K, Matthay R. Pulmonary effects of cytotoxic agents other than bleomycin. Clin Chest Med. 1990;11:31–54.

103. Rosenow EC, Myers JL, Swenson SJ. Drug-induced pulmonary disease: an update. Chest. 1992;102:239–250.

104. Kreisman H, Wolkove N. Pulmonary toxicity of antineoplastic therapy. Semin Oncol. 1992;19:508–520.

105. Van Barneveld PWC, Veenstra G, Sleijfer D. Changes in pulmonary function during and after bleomycin treatment in patients with testicular carcinoma. Cancer Chemother Pharmacol. 1985;14:168–171.

106. Comis RL, Kuppinger MS, Ginsberg SJ, et al. The role of single-breath carbon monoxide diffusing capacity in monitoring the pulmonary effects of bleomycin in germ cell tumor patients. Cancer Res. 1979;39:5076–5080.

107. White DA, Stover DE, Smith G, et al. Serial pulmonary function studies during bleomycin therapy [abstract]. Am Rev Respir Dis. 1987;135(suppl):A39.

108. Bolliger CT, Perruchoud AP. Functional evaluation of the lung resection candidate. Eur Respir J. 1998;11:198–212.

109. Cerfolio RJ, Allen MS, Trastek VF, et al. Lung resection in patients with compromised pulmonary function. Ann Thorac Surg. 1996;62:348–351.

110. Miller JI Jr. Limited resection of bronchogenic carcinoma in the patient with impaired pulmonary function. Ann Thorac Surg. 1993;56:769–771.

111. Wahi R, McMurtrey MJ, DeCaro LF, et al. Determinants of perioperative morbidity and mortality after pneumonectomy. Ann Thorac Surg. 1989;48:33–37.

112. Bechard D, Wetstein L. Assessment of exercise oxygen consumption as preoperative criterion for lung resection. Ann Thorac Surg. 1987;44:344–349.

113. Smith TP, Kinasewitz GT, Tucker WY, et al. Exercise capacity as a predictor of post-thoracotomy morbidity. Am Rev Respir Dis. 1984;129:730–734.

114. Morice RC, Walsh GL, Ali K, et al. Redefining the lowest exercise peak oxygen consumption acceptable for lung resection of high risk patients. Chest. 1996;110:161S.

115. Larsen KR, Svendsen UG, Milman N, et al. Cardiopulmonary function at rest and during exercise after resection for bronchial carcinoma. Ann Thorac Surg. 1997;64:960–964.

116. Ninan M, Sommers E, Landreneau RJ, et al. Standardized exercise oximetry predicts postpneumonectomy outcome. Ann Thorac Surg. 1997;64:328–333.

117. Rao V, Todd TRJ, Kuus A, et al. Exercise oximetry versus spirometry in the assessment of risk prior to lung resection. Ann Thorac Surg. 1995;60:603–609.

118. Melendez JA, Barrera R. Predictive respiratory complication quotient predicts pulmonary complications in thoracic surgical patients. Ann Thorac Surg. 1998;66:220–224.

GENERAL ASPECTS OF SURGICAL TREATMENT

Andy C. Kiser and Frank C. Detterbeck

Surgery plays an important role in the treatment of lung cancer. In addition, surgical procedures such as mediastinoscopy are important in the diagnosis and accurate staging of lung cancer. The decision to include surgery as part of the diagnostic or treatment plan hinges on an understanding of the anticipated benefits as well as the associated risks. The benefits of surgical staging or treatment are markedly influenced by the stage of disease and are, therefore, discussed in detail in other chapters of this book that deal with specific stages. The risk with surgical procedures, however, is largely independent of disease extent and is the focus of this chapter.

Surgical procedures involve both a risk of mortality and of complications. Complications can be classified as major or minor, but unfortunately there is no standard way they are defined. The incidence of complications or death from surgical procedures is influenced by patient selection criteria and perioperative patient management. Perioperative patient care is beyond the scope of this book and is discussed in other texts.[1] Assessment of a patient's candidacy for surgery on the basis of pulmonary reserve is addressed in detail in Chapter 7. Instead, this chapter focuses on specific nonpulmonary issues that are important in patient selection for surgical resection and addresses mortality and complications of specific thoracic surgical procedures for patients with lung cancer.

PATIENT SELECTION AND PREOPERATIVE PREPARATION

Patients who present with lung cancer have an average age of approximately 60 years and often have other medical conditions. Conditions such as diabetes, hypertension, and renal insufficiency do not affect thoracic surgical patients any differently than they affect other surgical patients and are not addressed in this chapter. Problems that affect thoracic surgical patients specifically are cardiac status and poor pulmonary reserve. These problems are addressed in the following paragraphs. Other conditions, such as malnutrition and weight loss, may occur in patients with lung cancer,[2] particularly with the use of preoperative chemotherapy, and are associated with a substantial increase in the rate of major perioperative complications.[3,4] Clinicians dealing with these patients should be aware of this, although it is not clear that any intervention can alter their outcome.

The preoperative pulmonary assessment is perhaps the most important part of the thoracic surgical patient's evaluation because respiratory failure is the most common cause of death following resection. Assessment of the patient's pulmonary reserve is discussed in depth in Chapter 7.

It is clear that measures of pulmonary reserve can be defined that predict an acceptably low operative mortality. These include a projected postoperative forced expiratory volume in 1 second (FEV1) of >1.0 L or an exercise test with an oxygen consumption ($\dot{V}O_2$) of >20 mL/min. It is more difficult to define the converse, that is, when the pulmonary reserve is so limited that the risk of surgery has become unacceptably high. This complex issue is also influenced by the postoperative management of patients.[1,5,6] The frequent use of incentive spirometry, adequate pain control, and early ambulation are important factors in reducing the incidence of atelectasis, retained secretions, and pneumonia.[1,5,6] The prediction of an unacceptably high surgical risk is further complicated by the fact that some patients may actually have better pulmonary function after resection (see Patients with Poor Pulmonary Reserve). More in-depth discussions of assessment of pulmonary reserve and perioperative management can be found in Chapter 7 and in other texts.[1]

Patients undergoing thoracic surgical procedures have been reported to have a threefold higher incidence of postoperative myocardial infarction (MI) compared with general surgical patients.[7-9] MI is the second most common cause of perioperative death after a pulmonary resection, and cardiac complications are the most common type of postoperative complications encountered (see below).[10,11] A thorough cardiovascular assessment is therefore particularly important in the preoperative evaluation of patients with thoracic malignancies. The cardiac evaluation of patients with pulmonary malignancy is the same as what should be carried out before any major surgical procedure and is discussed in detail in other texts.[12,13] In asymptomatic patients without evidence of previous cardiac disease, the risk of perioperative MI is approximately 0.1% in collected data from 46 425 patients.[9,14-16]

The cardiovascular evaluation begins with a history and physical examination, as well as an electrocardiogram (ECG) in all patients older than 45 years. Some authors believe that all thoracic surgical patients, even those without evidence of coronary artery disease, should undergo exercise treadmill testing before thoracotomy, but they do not provide data to substantiate their opinion.[12,17,18] It has been reported that 8% of asymptomatic patients over age 60 have findings suggestive of ischemia on stress thallium scanning.[17] Patients with evidence of coronary artery disease by history, ECG, or symptoms should undergo exercise thallium testing. Such patients (N = 102) have been found to have a 31% incidence of a positive stress thallium suggestive of ischemia and a 39% incidence of fixed defects suggestive of a prior MI.[17] A fixed defect is associated with only a 2% rate of cardiac complications or death with a major surgical procedure, whereas a reversible defect suggestive of ischemia carries a 30% to 50% risk of such complications.[19-21] Therefore, a reversible defect on exercise thallium testing should lead to coronary arteriography and cardiac revascularization, if indicated. Patients with a negative exercise thallium test or fixed deficits can undergo surgery with little cardiac risk.[15,17,19-22]

RISK OF THORACIC SURGICAL PROCEDURES

Mortality

Table 8–1 reviews the operative mortality for patients with lung cancer undergoing pulmonary resection for primary lung cancer. Most reports have defined *operative mortality* as any death either within 30 days of operation or occurring during the hospitalization. The reported mortality rates range between 1% and 7%, with an average of 4%. The seven largest series reviewed more than 1500 patients each and reported a mortality between 1% and 5%.[10,11,23-27] However, the mortality does not seem to be associated with the size of the study or how recently it was reported. Other studies, which are not listed in Table 8–1 because they include a substantial number of patients undergoing resection for benign disease, show similar mortality rates (1%-8%).[28-32]

Although it has been suggested that population-based data, presumed to be more representative of the general community, may show higher mortality rates than institution-based reports,[24,33] this does not seem to be true. The five population-based studies in Table 8–1 report an aver-

TABLE 8–1. OPERATIVE MORTALITY FOR PATIENTS UNDERGOING PULMONARY RESECTION FOR LUNG CANCER

STUDY	N	MORTALITY (%)[a]
Romano and Mark[24 b]	12 439	5
Wada et al[11 b]	7099	1
Harpole et al[26 c]	3516	5
van Rens et al[27]	2361	4
Ginsberg et al[10 c]	2220	4
Silvestri et al[25 b]	1583	5
Damhuis and Schutte[23 b]	1577	3
Whittle et al[33 b,d]	1290	7
Deslauriers et al[4]	1076	3
Nagasaki et al[34]	961	2
Wada et al[136]	845	2
Deslauriers et al[42]	783	4
Duque et al[36 c]	605	7
von Knorring et al[55]	598	3
Martini et al[90]	598	2
Thomas et al[37 e]	500	7
Total	38 051	
Average		**4**

Inclusion criteria: Studies reported from 1980 to 2000 including ≥500 patients resected for lung cancer.
[a]Any death either within 30 days or during hospitalization.
[b]Population-based study.
[c]Prospective study.
[d]Random 5% sample of Medicare patients (>65 years).
[e]Patients >70 years of age.

age mortality rate of 4%, which is the same as the rate in the other reports included in this table. Mortality rates as low as 1.3% have been reported even in population-based studies.[11]

An analysis of statistics from the state of South Carolina found that the mortality rate for specialists (board-certified thoracic surgeons) is lower than that for general surgeons.[25] The mortality rate for lobectomy was 3% versus 5% ($P = 0.04$) and for pneumonectomy was 12% versus 20% ($P = 0.02$) when performed by thoracic surgeons versus general surgeons, respectively. This discrepancy was not explained by differences in severity of illness or age of the patients, but the review found that only 25% of general surgeons had performed >10 pulmonary resections in a 4-year period, as opposed to 69% of thoracic surgeons.[25] An analysis of hospital statistics in California also found statistically significant ($P < 0.05$) lower mortality rates in high volume hospitals (lobectomy mortality, 4% versus 6%; pneumonectomy mortality, 11% versus 14%) for ≥9 cases per year versus <9 cases per year.[24] This difference persisted when adjusted for age, tumor characteristics, and comorbidities. Furthermore, lower mortality rates were seen in teaching hospitals, which correlated with the availability of thoracic surgeons (lobectomy and wedge mortality rate, 3% versus 4%; pneumonectomy mortality rate, 9% versus 12%; P value not reported) for high intensity teaching hospitals compared with nonteaching hospitals.[24]

The causes of death are shown in Figure 8–1. The most common cause of death by far is respiratory failure, accounting for an average of nearly 40% of deaths following pulmonary resection. A significant number of deaths were also related to the cardiac system, specifically from MI. The series by Wada et al,[11] Deslauriers et al,[4] and

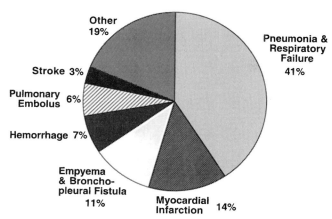

FIGURE 8–1. Cause of death in 362 patients of 14 697 who underwent resection for lung cancer. Inclusion criteria: Studies of ≥100 patients since 1980 undergoing resection for lung cancer and reporting specific causes of perioperative mortality. (Data from references 4, 10, 11, 28, 34, 37, 38, 41, 49, 55, 90, 91, 127, 139.)

Nagasaki et al,[34] critically examined primary causes of death in their reviews and most accurately reflect the primary causes of death in patients undergoing resection. The results of these series are similar to the data shown in Figure 8–1.

It is unclear whether a high risk of perioperative death can be predicted preoperatively. In a multivariate analysis, an association with any of 37 preoperative risk factors accounted for only 12% of the perioperative mortality, implying that most of the deaths were due to unpredictable, random events.[35] Among four large multivariate analyses (>250 patients),[26,35–37] three found the need for a pneumonectomy or an extended resection to be an independent risk factor for perioperative mortality.[26,36,37] In three of the four studies, a marker of vascular disease as well (premature ventricular contractions on the ECG, a history of peripheral vascular disease, or hypertension),[35–37] and two studies found age to be a significant risk factor.[26,37] A number of other factors were noted to be independent predictors of perioperative mortality in only one of the studies (male gender, low FEV_1, preoperative dyspnea, a *do-not-resuscitate* status, stage IV cancer, low serum albumin, an altered sensorium, abnormal coagulation studies, and a need for preoperative blood transfusion).[26,35–37] It must be kept in mind, though, that any such analysis of risk factors *where the patients have been carefully selected* may not demonstrate a particular factor (such as cardiac history or poor pulmonary reserve) to be significant simply because the prevalence of such patients in that series is low due to the selection process.

Acute Morbidity

The overall complication rate experienced by patients undergoing pulmonary resection is shown in Table 8–2. The average complication rate of 34% may be a consequence of the advanced age and associated medical problems often seen in these patients. The highest complication rate was seen in one study in which 75% of patients underwent an

extended resection,[38] and the next highest rates were seen in studies that included only patients undergoing pneumonectomy.[39,40]

It is unclear whether it is possible to reliably predict which patients have a high risk of complications. In a multivariate analysis of 37 preoperative factors in 423 patients undergoing resection, 72% of the postoperative complications were attributed to unpredictable, random events.[35] We examined eight large studies (>250 patients) that carefully analyzed risk factors for postoperative complications (usually with multivariate analysis).[4,26,30,31,35–37,41] All have found markers of poor pulmonary function to be associated with an increased risk of complications, although the exact criterion found to be significant was different in each case. In some studies this involved FEV1 measurements,[4,30,35,37] in others diffusing capacity of lung for carbon monoxide (DLCO) measurements,[31,41] and in another a history of respiratory disease (but measures of FEV_1 or DLCO were not significant).[26,36] Five of the eight studies found a significant association of complications with increasing age,[4,26,31,35,41] and four of the eight found that pneumonectomy was an independent risk factor for complications.[4,36,37,41] Other independent predictors of complications that were isolated findings in only one or two studies included markers of cardiac disease,[35] diabetes,[36] peripheral vascular disease,[36] weight loss >10%,[4,26] T3 tumors,[35] and incomplete resections,[35] low albumin,[26] smoking,[26] and the need for a preoperative blood transfusion.[26]

Taken together, it seems that poor pulmonary reserve, increasing age, and the need for a pneumonectomy are predictive of complications. The exact level of risk remains unclear, and it is also not clear how poor pulmonary reserve or older age should be defined. However, unpredictable,

TABLE 8–2. MORBIDITY RATES FOR PATIENTS UNDERGOING RESECTION FOR LUNG CANCER[a]

STUDY	N	MORBIDITY (%)[b]
Harpole et al[26 c]	3516	24
Deslauriers et al[4]	1076	32
Nagasaki et al[34]	961	19
Deslauriers et al[42]	783	48
Duque et al[36 c]	605	32
Thomas et al[37 d]	500	38
Ferguson et al[31]	292	48
Yano et al[41]	291	33
Harpole et al[137]	289	25
Wahi et al[40 e]	197	48
Patel et al[39 e]	197	51
Knott-Craig et al[138]	173	15
Miller et al[49]	167	21
Daly et al[139]	134	23
Izbicki et al[38 c,f]	126	60
Total	9307	
Average		**34**

Inclusion criteria: Studies published from 1980 to 2000 including ≥100 patients.
[a]Mediastinoscopy excluded.
[b]Percentage of patients who had one or more complication.
[c]Prospective study.
[d]Patients >70 years of age.
[e]Pneumonectomies only.
[f]75% extended resection.

random events also account for a sizable proportion of the postoperative complications seen.

The overall complication rates noted in Table 8–2 included both major and minor complications. Although most authors did not define or report major and minor complications separately, three of the larger series did classify complications as either major or minor.[4,34,42] Major complications, which included respiratory failure, MI, empyema, and bronchopleural fistula (BPF), were seen in 9% to 27% of patients in these series, whereas minor complications such as prolonged air leak, arrhythmias, and pleural effusion occurred in 8% to 21% of patients (Table 8–3).[4,34,42] We have defined a *major complication* as one that is life threatening, requires another operation, or significantly extends the hospital stay (by at least 3 days). Using this definition, it would seem reasonable to classify respiratory failure, pneumonia, hemorrhage, MI, empyema, and BPF as major complications. Although a prolonged air leak may extend the hospitalization, it can sometimes be managed on an outpatient basis and therefore has been included as a minor complication. Applying this classification, albeit retrospectively and somewhat arbitrarily, to the studies in Table 8–3 suggests that minor complications account for slightly more than half of the complications seen. It is difficult to define the incidence of all major or all minor complications because many of the patients experiencing complications have more than one type.

Pneumonia is reported to be the most common major complication, occurring in 6% of patients (range, 1%-22%) (see Table 8–3). Unfortunately, a clear definition of pneumonia is not provided in most of these studies. This may account for some of the variability in reported incidence rates. The incidence of pneumonia appears to be consistently elevated in pneumonectomy and extended re-

sections (see Table 8–3). Respiratory failure is also often vaguely defined but generally means a postoperative period of mechanical ventilation. The occurrence rates reported in Table 8–3 seem more consistent than those for pneumonia and are also increased with pneumonectomy or extended resections.

A respiratory complication that has received little attention in the context of pulmonary resection is adult respiratory distress syndrome (ARDS). This has not been specifically reported in most of the studies of morbidity, although it has been clearly described by many authors and carries a high mortality rate.[43-47] It is likely that many of the cases labeled *pneumonia* or *respiratory failure* (and perhaps *cardiac failure*) satisfy the criteria for acute lung injury (ALI) or ARDS. A study specifically addressing this in 1139 patients resected for lung cancer found the incidence of ALI/ARDS to be 4%.[48] The rate of occurrence paralleled the extent of resection in this study, being 1% after wedge resection, 4% after lobectomy, 6% after pneumonectomy, and 13% after extended resection.[48] Similar results have been reported by others.[43,45] Better recognition of this entity should allow a better understanding of this problem in the future.

A bronchial stump leak, often called a bronchopleural fistula (BPF), is a difficult problem to manage and is associated with a high mortality, especially after pneumonectomy. After a pneumonectomy, a bronchial stump leak is always associated with an empyema, but this is not necessarily the case after a lobectomy. Most authors have reported on the occurrence of empyema and BPF together. Where these complications are reported separately, the incidence of empyema has been reported to be 4% (range, 2%-9%),[34,36,38,39,41,42] and the incidence of BPF has been reported to be 3% (range, 1%-5%).[36,38-42,49]

TABLE 8–3. COMPLICATION RATES (%) FOR PATIENTS UNDERGOING RESECTION FOR LUNG CANCER

	STANDARD RESECTION	PNEUMONECTOMY OR EXTENDED RESECTION	ALL
N (studies)	9[a]	5[b]	**13**
N (patients)	16 953	1223	**18 176**
Major Complications (%)			
Pneumonia[c]	4	11	**6**
Respiratory failure[d]	4	9	**5**
Empyema/bronchopleural fistula	4	4	**4**
Cardiac failure[c]	1	9	**4**
Hemorrhage[e]	1	5	**2**
Myocardial infarction[c]	1	2	**1**
Pulmonary embolism	1	1	**1**
Other	2	4	**3**
Minor Complications (%)			
Arrhythmias[c]	7	20	**12**
Atelectasis/secretions[f]	5	9	**6**
Prolonged air leak[c]	5	—	**5**
Recurrent laryngeal nerve injury	2	5	**4**
Wound infection[c]	1	4	**2**
Other	3	4	**4**

Inclusion criteria: Studies reporting complications in ≥100 patients undergoing resection for lung cancer.
[a]Data from references 4, 26, 34, 36, 41, 42, 49, 139, 140.
[b]Data from references 26, 38–40, 57.
[c]As defined by author.
[d]Requiring reintubation or >24 hours of ventilation.
[e]Requiring return to the operating room.
[f]Requiring bronchoscopy.

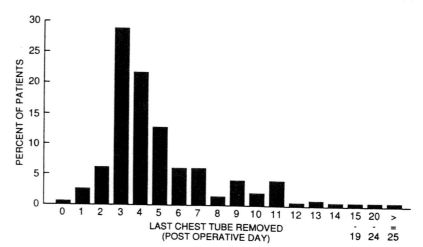

FIGURE 8–2. Duration of postoperative air leak in 197 patients undergoing pulmonary resection. (From Rice TW, Kirby TJ. Prolonged air leak. Chest Surg Clin North Am. 1992;2:803–811.[62])

The series included in Table 8–3 did not report on factors associated with the development of BPF. A review of four studies by Allen et al[50] implicated poor nutritional status, active pulmonary infections, and technical causes as risk factors for the development of this complication. A more detailed multivariate analysis of 1360 patients undergoing pulmonary resections for lung cancers associated the development of a BPF with four factors: pneumonectomy, residual carcinoma, preoperative radiation or chemotherapy, and diabetes.[51] In this study, the prevalence of BPF was 2.1%, a percentage close to the average mentioned earlier.[51] However, the mortality of patients who developed BPF in this study was 71%, which is much higher than the 11% to 13% mortality reported by others in the patients who developed BPF.[36,52,53]

Arrhythmias are the most common minor complication, occurring in 12% of patients. The vast majority (~95%) of these are minor atrial arrhythmias. In other reports that have specifically addressed arrhythmias, approximately 20% (range, 4%-40%) of patients undergoing pulmonary resection have been found to develop atrial arrhythmias, with approximately 80% occurring within 3 days of operation.[34,54-61] The lower incidence noted in Table 8–3 may represent underreporting in some studies. In two-thirds of cases, the arrhythmia is asymptomatic, and it has resolved within 3 days in three-fourths of cases.[59,60] Although many etiologies have been proposed, the true cause of atrial arrhythmias in the postoperative period is not clearly defined. The most commonly proposed mechanism of fluid overload is not supported by ECG and Swan-Ganz catheter studies.[1,58]

Older patients, patients undergoing pneumonectomy, and patients with a history of coronary artery disease are at increased risk for atrial fibrillation.[54-56,59,61] Two studies report an identical 50% incidence of arrhythmias in patients >70 years of age, compared with an incidence of 3% and 4% in patients <50 years of age.[54,59] The incidence of atrial arrhythmias in patients undergoing pneumonectomy is approximately 20% to 40% as opposed to ≤10% following wedge resection (see Table 8–3).[55-60] The mortality of patients experiencing tachyarrhythmias has been reported to be elevated (15%-25%) in some studies (but not in all)—this is probably unrelated to the arrhythmia itself.[56,58,61] von Knorring et al[55] reported a 15% to 20% incidence of cardiac arrhythmias in patients with evidence of previous MI. The role of prophylactic treatment of arrhythmias in patients undergoing thoracic surgical procedures remains controversial.[1,58,59]

The incidence of atelectasis and retained secretions has been reported to be 6% (range, 2%-13%) (see Table 8–3), but unfortunately several studies did not report how this was defined. A transient radiographic abnormality is of little interest, whereas atelectasis or secretions severe enough to warrant an intervention such as bronchoscopy is more meaningful. Those who have reported only atelectasis or retained secretions severe enough to require bronchoscopy have found that this occurred in 5% of patients (range, 2%-13%).[4,34,38,39,42,49]

A *prolonged air leak* has been defined by different authors as an air leak lasting more than 7, 10, or 14 postoperative days (see Table 8–3). A review by Rice and Kirby[62] examining the number of days of postoperative air leak in 179 patients undergoing pulmonary resection demonstrated that approximately 60% of patients had their chest tubes removed between postoperative days 3 and 5 (Fig. 8–2). However, 15% of the patients had an air leak for more than 7 days, whereas only 1.5% had a persistent air leak for more than 14 days. The authors identified male gender, higher forced vital capacity (FVC), and lower FEV_1/FVC ratio as being related to prolonged air leaks. In another study of 100 consecutive right upper lobe resections, a prolonged air leak (>7 days) was seen in 26%.[63] Only an FEV_1/FVC ratio <50% was identified as a risk factor for a prolonged air leak.[63] Prolonged air leak was reported to have occurred in an average of only 5% of patients included in Table 8–3, which seems out of proportion to the percentages reported in the two studies just mentioned (15%-25%) that specifically addressed air leaks. This low average incidence may reflect a failure to accurately report this complication in many of these retrospective studies and may reflect the lack of a consistent definition.

Injury to the left recurrent laryngeal nerve is rather rare. This injury is seen primarily after pneumonectomy or after resection of N2 tumors (see Table 8–3).

Long-Term Morbidity

Few authors have addressed the long-term morbidity of surgical therapy for lung cancer, although this clearly is an

TABLE 8–4. INCIDENCE OF CHRONIC PAIN (>3 MONTHS) FOLLOWING THORACOTOMY

STUDY	Nᵃ	TIME INTERVAL (mo)	INCIDENCE OF PAIN BY SEVERITY (% OF ALL PATIENTS)		
			Any Pain	Occasional Narcotics	Major Treatment
Conacher[141][b]	3109	>3	—	—	2
Keller et al[76][b]	238	>3	—	11	4
Kalso et al[142]	134	30	44	13	4
Kanner et al[77]	126	5	37	16	—
Landreneau et al[79]	104	>12	27	13	—
Matsunaga et al[143]	90	>6	64	—	—
Dajczman et al[75]	56	25	54	9	7
Katz et al[144]	23	18	52	—	—
Average			**46**	**12**	**4**

Inclusion criteria: Studies of ≥20 patients reporting incidence of pain >3 months following thoracotomy.
ᵃNumber of patients undergoing thoracotomy.
ᵇNo effort made to assess patients not actively complaining of pain.
Major treatment, pain requiring a treatment procedure (injections, etc.) or treatment by a chronic pain clinic; Occasional narcotics, pain severe enough to require at least occasional narcotics or other more aggressive intervention.

issue when evaluating the benefit versus cost of this therapy. The available studies generally show that the long-term cost is relatively low. The data for loss of pulmonary function, overall quality of life (QOL), and long-term postthoracotomy pain are reviewed in the following paragraphs.

The average loss of pulmonary function following surgical resection is reasonably low. The FEV_1 ≥6 months after a lobectomy has been reported to be 12% lower than preoperative values (range, 8%-17%) in eight studies of a total of 344 patients.[64–71] Similar losses after lobectomy were reported for FVC.[64,65,68,69,71] Although mean pulmonary arterial pressure with maximal exercise after lobectomy has been reported to increase from 28 to 35 mm Hg ($P < 0.05$), maximal exercise capacity decreased only 10% (range, 0%-13%).[64–66,68,71] Pneumonectomy resulted in a 31% loss of FEV_1 (range, 23%-36%) more than 6 months after resection in these studies (total of 99 patients), but maximal exercise capacity decreased only 21% (range, 16%-28%).[64–66,68,71] This amounts to a loss of 3% to 3.25% per segment of lung resected.[69] Thus, the long-term loss of lung capacity is not excessive. In fact, the losses following lobectomy are similar to those reported following radiation using conventional planning and field sizes (see Chapter 9).

QOL following surgical resection has been addressed by only a few studies.[72–74] Surgery resulted in a deterioration of various QOL parameters 1 month postoperatively compared with preoperative values (percentage of patients re-

porting "poor" score 1 month postoperatively versus preoperatively: global QOL, 17% versus 6%; activity QOL, 52% versus 26%; dyspnea 34% versus 14%).[72] Although only slight improvement in many parameters was seen at 3 months, most patients had returned to baseline or better at 6 months.[72,73]

Significant improvements have been made in the management of the acute pain associated with thoracotomy or thoracoscopy.[1] Chronic pain after thoracotomy, on the other hand, has received much less attention. A summary of available studies is shown in Table 8–4. Between one third and one-half of patients experience some chronic pain. This was reported as only mild by most patients, but occurred either daily or several times per week in half of these patients.[75] There is no suggestion that the incidence of this type of mild postoperative pain decreases over time (see Table 8–4).[75] Although 23% of patients in one study reported that pain interfered in some way with their lives,[75] only 10% to 15% require treatment with occasional narcotics, and only about 5% require more significant interventions such as nerve blocks or interventions by a chronic pain clinic (see Table 8–4). Pain occurring after a period of initial control was found to correlate with recurrent cancer in two studies.[76,77] The incidence of significant chronic pain is similar after standard thoracotomy and a muscle-sparing approach[78] or between muscle-sparing thoracotomy and video-assisted thoracic surgery (VATS) approaches.[79]

DATA SUMMARY: MORTALITY AND MORBIDITY OF SURGICAL RESECTION

	AMOUNT	QUALITY	CONSISTENCY
The average mortality of surgical resection is 4%	High	High	High
The most common cause of death is respiratory failure	Mod	High	High
The overall rate of morbidity is 33%	High	Mod	Mod
The most common morbidity is arrhythmia	High	Mod	Mod
The loss of FEV_1 after lobectomy is 13%	High	High	High
Incidence of severe chronic pain after thoracotomy is 5%	High	High	High

Type of data rated: Plain text: descriptive statement   *Italics: controlled comparison*   **Bold: randomized comparison**

SPECIFIC PROCEDURES

Mediastinoscopy

The use of mediastinoscopy to appropriately determine the extent of the disease is often a part of the diagnostic workup. Mediastinoscopy is performed under general anesthesia through a cervical incision. The pretracheal fascia is entered with a mediastinoscope, and mediastinal nodes are sampled for metastatic disease. The incidence of complications is small, with most patients currently undergoing the procedure as outpatients.[80] A report of 653 patients treated between 1961 and 1970 found a mortality rate for mediastinoscopy of 3%.[81] However, there have been only six mortalities (0.07%) in the almost 8000 cases reported since 1985 (Table 8–5). The 2% complication rate for mediastinoscopy is also low, with the most common complications being bleeding, pneumothorax, and recurrent laryngeal nerve injuries. Of the operative complications reported in the studies included in Table 8–5, only ten patients (0.12%) required emergency thoracotomy for treatment of the operative injury. No major complications have been reported following a parasternal mediastinotomy (Chamberlain procedure). In approximately 300 patients, only 1 wound infection, 1 left vocal cord paralysis, and 1 self-limited episode of venous bleeding were reported.[82–84]

Wedge Biopsy

In certain situations, removal of lung tumors by a segmentectomy or a nonanatomic wedge resection may be useful for diagnosis or as a therapeutic resection. Such resections can be performed through a thoracotomy or using video-assisted thoracoscopic surgery,[85–88] but most of the data that has been reported involves open thoracotomy. The seven series examining more than 100 patients undergoing open wedge resection report a mortality of 1% to 4%, but the authors do not report on complications

(Table 8–6).[10,11,24,27,34,89,90] The mortality rate in the 6332 patients reported in Table 8–6 ranges between 0 and 6% (average, 1.5%).

Lobectomy

Lobectomy remains the most common procedure employed for resection of lung cancer. The data reported in this section examines only patients undergoing lobectomy via open thoracotomy for cancer. The reported mortality rates are surprisingly consistent, with an average mortality rate of 2% in the 21 463 patients examined (range, 0%-8%) (see Table 8–6). Similar results have been reported by other authors who included a substantial number of patients resected for benign disease.[28,29] No data is available to suggest any differences with regard to which lobe is resected. Pulmonary and cardiac complications were the most commonly cited causes of death in these series, but the exact percentages are not clearly reported. Complications (both major and minor) were seen in 28% of lobectomy patients in one series.[42]

Pneumonectomy

An average mortality rate of 9% was seen following pneumonectomy in the series listed in Table 8–6 (range, 3%-17%). Three large population-based studies show a fair amount of variation in the mortality, ranging from the lowest to the highest reported rates (3%-17%).[11,24,25] A multi-institutional study of the Lung Cancer Study Group's experience in 1983 showed a 30-day operative mortality of 8% for 569 patients who underwent pneumonectomy for lung cancer.[10] More recently, Wada et al[11] reported on 586 patients undergoing pneumonectomy and found a mortality of only 3%. In the two studies examining side of resection, the mortality was found to be higher for right versus left pneumonectomy (13% and 14% versus 0 and 1%).[34,40] Side of resection and age (see Older Patients) may account for some of the differences in reported mortality, but it seems more likely that careful clinical judgment in patient selection is more critical for pneumonectomy than lobectomy. The causes of death following pneumonectomy have been reported to be primarily cardiac and pulmonary.[39,40] Preoperative factors associated with mortality by multivariate analysis in one study were comorbid diseases and poor pulmonary reserve (an FEV_1 <1.6 L, and an FEV_1/FVC ratio of <0.55).[39]

The study published by Wahi et al[40] examined the overall complication rates of patients who underwent a pneumonectomy for cancer and reported a 48% incidence of major and minor complications. Patel et al,[39] in a review of 197 patients who underwent pneumonectomy, reported a 49% incidence of pulmonary complications, the majority being culture-positive respiratory infections and sputum retention requiring bronchoscopy. They also reported an 8% incidence of BPF and empyema. Cardiac complications occurred in 29% of patients in this series, the majority being arrhythmias. The only preoperative factor predicting morbidity by multivariate analysis in this study was continued smoking up to the time of the operation ($P < 0.05$).[39]

TABLE 8–5. MORTALITY, MORBIDITY, AND COMMON COMPLICATIONS IN 8007 PATIENTS UNDERGOING MEDIASTINOSCOPY[a]

	NUMBER OF PATIENTS WITH COMPLICATION LISTED	%
Mortality	6	**0.07**
Morbidity	135	**1.7**
Complications		
Significant bleeding (loss of operative view requiring tamponade or thoracotomy)	47	0.6
Pneumothorax	23	0.3
Recurrent laryngeal nerve injury	12	0.3
Wound infection	10	0.2
Tracheal injury	6	0.1
Other	38	0.5

Inclusion criteria: Studies from 1980 to 2000 reporting ≥100 patients undergoing mediastinoscopy (total of 8007 patients).
[a]Data from references 80, 145–151.

TABLE 8–6. MORTALITY RATES ASSOCIATED WITH INDIVIDUAL SURGICAL PROCEDURES IN PATIENTS UNDERGOING PULMONARY RESECTION FOR LUNG CANCER[a]

STUDY	WEDGE RESECTION N	(%)	LOBECTOMY N	(%)	PNEUMONECTOMY N	(%)	EXTENDED RESECTION N	(%)
Romano and Mark[24]	4341	4	6569	4	1529	12		
Wada et al[11]	904[b]	1	5609	1	586	3		
Harpole et al[26 c]			2949	4	567	12		
van Rems[27]	158	1	1390	3	610	7		
Silvestri et al[25]			1416	4	167	17		
Ginsberg et al[10 c]	143	1	1058	3	569	8		
Damhuis and Schutte[23]			1047[d]	2[d]	530	6		
Nagasaki et al[34]	117	3	570	2	72	6		
von Knorring et al[55]			398	2	200	7		
Kohman et al[35]	31	6	298	4	94	12		
Duque et al[36]	29	0	294	4	172	13	101	10
Thomas et al[37 e]	39	0	291	8	136	8	103	13
Kadri and Dussek[152]	8	0	280	4	191	7		
Pastorino et al[153]	61	0	411	3				
Jensik et al[89]	259	1						
Martini et al[90]	122	1	125	2				
Errett et al[154]	100	3	97	2				
Wahi et al[40]					158	5	39	15
Patel et al[39]					197	9		
Busch et al[91]	20	0	47	2	13	8	25	16
Izbicki et al[38 c]			4	0	28	7	94	7
Total	6332		22 853		5819		362	
Average		**2**		**3**		**9**		**12**

Inclusion criteria: Studies published from 1980 to 2000 including ≥100 patients (total) undergoing pulmonary resection for lung cancer with procedure-specific mortality.
[a]Death either within 30 days of operation or during hospitalization.
[b]Includes patients undergoing thoracotomy without pulmonary resection.
[c]Prospective study.
[d]Includes wedge resections.
[e]Patients >70 years of age.
Extended resection, resection of lung as well as additional thoracic structures; Wedge resection, wedge resection (without video assistance).

Extended Resection

Patients with T3 disease undergoing lobectomy or pneumonectomy require resection of structures involved by the tumor (extended resection), in order to achieve complete resection (see Chapter 15). Extended resections may include portions of the chest wall, diaphragm, pericardium, or intrapericardial vessels. Patients undergoing such extended resections experience only slightly increased complication and mortality rates (see Table 8–6). Five smaller studies (total of 362 patients) reviewed the mortality associated with extended pulmonary resections and found an average mortality of 12% (both lobectomy and pneumonectomy).[36–38, 40,91] Death following extended resection was due to respiratory failure, 2; pneumonia, 2; postoperative sepsis, 2; and postoperative hemorrhage, 1 (7 deaths in 94 patients).[38] An additional study of 113 patients who underwent completion pneumonectomy showed a mortality rate of 10%.[92]

Four papers have examined the rate of complications associated with an extended lobectomy or pneumonectomy and have reported widely different rates, depending on whether minor complications were included. One large review found an overall major complication rate of 32% for patients who underwent extended resection for lung cancer.[42] In an earlier study, the major complication rate for 231 patients undergoing extended lobectomy was 20%, and for 171 patients undergoing extended pneumonectomy

it was found to be 17%.[4] A study by Wahi et al[40] examining 105 patients undergoing pneumonectomy for lung cancer demonstrated a 10% mortality and a 67% complication rate. This complication rate included both major and minor complications and was similar to the 71% overall complication rate (major plus minor) reported by Izbicki et al[38] for patients undergoing extended lung resection.

Izbicki et al[38] compared a series of 94 patients undergoing extended resection to 32 patients who had nonextended resection. Arrhythmias occurred in 23% of patients undergoing extended resection versus 13% of patients undergoing nonextended resection ($P = NS$). Pulmonary complications (pneumonia, respiratory insufficiency, atelectasis, retained secretions) also occurred more frequently in patients undergoing extended resection (36% versus 6%, $P < 0.005$).

Video-Assisted Thoracic Surgical Resections

For the patient with an undiagnosed solitary pulmonary nodule, thoracoscopic wedge resection offers a more attractive option than open thoracotomy for excision of a pulmonary nodule. A VATS wedge resection of a pulmonary nodule is usually performed under general anesthesia with the use of three to four thoracoscopic ports and an endoscopic stapling device. A review of 242 patients undergoing thoracoscopic wedge resection of indeterminate solitary pulmonary nodules reported no mortality, and complications were limited to atelectasis requiring bronchoscopy (1%), pneumonia (1%), and air leaks for >7 days (2%).[87] Allen et al[88] reported similar findings in 64 patients undergoing thoracoscopic wedge excision of indeterminate pulmonary nodules. There were no deaths and only a 6% incidence of complications (pneumothorax, 3%; atrial fibrillation, 2%; prolonged air leak, 2%). Similar results have been reported by others.[93]

Mack et al[87] reported only a 1% incidence in conversion to open thoracotomy for diagnostic resection of a pulmonary nodule by thoracoscopy. However, other studies reported a 20% to 28% incidence in conversion to open thoracotomy.[88,94] In the study by Allen et al[88] of 118 patients, the most common reasons for conversion were inability to visualize the lesion (17 patients, or 14%), nodule too large (5 patients, or 4%), pleural space obliteration or inability to collapse the lung (7 patients, or 6%), and suspicion that the mass represented a cancer (4 patients, or 3%).

In those patients who had a nodule resected by VATS, diagnosis was made in nearly 100%.[87] The average hospital stay after thoracoscopic wedge excision is 3 to 4 days versus 6 days for a resection by thoracotomy.[88,95] The total charge for thoracoscopic wedge excision in the United States is approximately $12 000, comparable to the charges for an open thoracotomy for excision of a pulmonary nodule.[88,95]

The treatment of patients with lung cancer by lobectomy with VATS has also been reported. This procedure is much more complicated, requiring thoracoscopic control of lobar arteries and veins, as well as division of the lobar bronchus.[96-98] In several studies of VATS lobectomy, the procedure could be successfully accomplished without thoracotomy in 85% of cases (range, 75%-92%).[97,99-102] Of the patients converted to thoracotomy, 9% were due to intraoperative complications (ie, bleeding), 30% because of concerns about the safety of a VATS resection, 47% for technical reasons, and 14% for oncologic reasons.[97,99-102]

Data from the larger series (≥ 100 patients) of VATS lobectomy are shown in Table 8–7. The mortality rate is acceptably low (1%). The average operative time reported in the series in Table 8–7 was 2 hours. The incidence of complications varies widely, most likely reflecting different definitions. The average hospital length of stay after a VATS lobectomy in the United States has been 5 days (range, 3-7).[85,97,99,103-105]

It is not clear that VATS resections are associated with less pain than open resections. Three nonrandomized studies comparing VATS lobectomy patients to contemporary controls found less acute pain in the VATS group,[101,102,106] but the only randomized study (only 55 patients total) found no difference in pain, length of stay, or return to work.[99]

The definition of a VATS lobectomy differs in these series, however. An access incision of varying proportions was used in most studies.[107] Some groups avoided all rib spreading,[100] whereas others spread the ribs 4 cm.[102,107] Thus, although it is fairly clear that VATS resections are feasible, it has not been shown that this approach is superior to open thoracotomy. Furthermore, there is insufficient data to date regarding 5-year survival and recurrence rates for patients after thoracoscopic lobectomy to determine the appropriateness of VATS lobectomy for cancer. Preliminary intermediate term data suggest that the 2- to 3-year survival is similar to that for open thoracotomy, stage for stage.[103,108-110]

Exploratory Thoracotomy

The mortality rate for an exploratory thoracotomy without resection is comparable to that for a pulmonary resection, although only limited data is available. The largest study of exploratory thoracotomy (150 patients) shows an operative mortality of 5%.[111] Others have reported similar mortality rates of 2% to 3%.[35,36,112] Although it is surprising how little data is available for exploratory thoracotomy, the available data suggests that the mortality rate is similar to that when a lobectomy or pneumonectomy is carried out.

SPECIFIC PATIENT POPULATIONS
Older Patients

As the elderly population increases, more physicians are caring for patients with lung cancer who are >70 years of

TABLE 8–7. SHORT-TERM OUTCOMES FOR PATIENTS UNDERGOING VIDEO-ASSISTED THORACIC SURGERY LOBECTOMY

STUDY	N	% CONVERTED	INTRAOPERATIVE BLEEDING (%)	COMPLICATIONS (%)	HOSPITAL MORTALITY (%)	LOS (d)
Yim et al[110]	214	17	1	22	0.4	(7)[a]
McKenna et al[103]	212	7	1	12	0.4	5
Lewis and Caccavale[105]	200	—	0	13	0	3
Roviaro et al[155]	171	17	3	9	1	—
Walker[108]	150	12	1	38	2	(6)[a]
Kaseda et al[109]	128	12	1	3	1	—
Brown[104]	105	8	3	7	0	3
Average[b]		**12**	**1**		**1**	**4**

Inclusion criteria: Studies of ≥100 patients undergoing video-assisted thoracic surgery lobectomy.
[a]Study done outside the United States.
[b]Excluding values in parentheses.
LOS, length of hospital stay.

age. The life expectancy of U.S. residents aged 70 is 11 years for men and 15 years for women; for those aged 80, it is 7 and 8 years, respectively.[113] The majority of these remaining years in older patients are spent in active, independent functioning.[114] On the other hand, the aging patient experiences more problems with pulmonary function due to decreased lung volumes, decreased expiratory flow rates, and loss of strength in respiratory muscles.[115,116] Furthermore, several studies have shown that older patients with lung cancer are much less likely to undergo surgical treatment,[117–120] even though the incidence of early-stage disease is higher than that for younger age groups.[117–119,121,122] Whether this reflects appropriate avoidance of surgery in older patients who are not well enough to tolerate surgery is not clear, but even among the patients with a good performance status, relatively few of the older patients were given treatment in one study.[120]

Many authors have noted an increase in perioperative morbidity and mortality after lung resection in patients >70 years (Table 8–8).[4,10,24,33–35,39,40] Four of the five largest studies have found a statistically significant increase in mortality among patients over age 70 compared with contemporary same-institution controls.[11,23,24,33] The difference in mortality with regard to age persisted when subjected to multivariate analysis or corrected for other prognostic factors in several of these studies.[23,24,33]

Whether there is an increase in mortality with age is not as important as whether the mortality in older patients is prohibitively high. A review of the reported data demonstrates that this is not the case (see Table 8–8). Even the 1133 patients over 80 years of age in the studies shown in this table were found to have an average mortality rate of 8%, and mortality for these patients was found to be as low as 2% in a population-based series from Japan.[11] Other smaller studies of 20 to 100 patients over age 80 have reported an average mortality of 14%.[123–126]

The causes of death in patients over age 70, when specifically reported, are very similar to those for younger patients undergoing pulmonary resection, with pneumonia and respiratory failure accounting for approximately half of the deaths.[11,37,127,128] The complication rate for patients ≥70 years of age was examined by six studies between 1980 and 2000, five of which found no significant difference in the overall complication rate for patients ≥70 years of age as compared with patients <70 years of age (overall complication rate, 38% versus 31% for ≥70 versus <70 years of age).[36,127–130] One study, which reported only major complications, found that these were more frequent in patients ≥70 years of age (19% versus 7%, $P < 0.01$).[131] In other studies reporting only on patients ≥80 years of age, the average complication rate was 51%.[123–126] Thus, it appears that patients over age 70 and even over age 80 experience only slightly higher mortality and complication rates than those <70 years of age, at least when they are carefully selected.

There is no doubt that the older patients are carefully selected, but it is not clear by what criteria. Preoperative pulmonary function tests have generally been reported to be worse in the older patients,[128,130,132] and these patients have more comorbid conditions.[130] However, every study reported that included information on the type of resection performed showed that fewer older patients undergo a pneumonectomy.[10,23–25,33,128] In fact, with only three exceptions,[10,23,37] the rate of pneumonectomy in patients over age 70 was ≤10% in the studies shown in Table 8–8, in contrast to 13% to 37% in patients under age 70.[10,23–25,33,128]

A closer scrutiny of the mortality in older patients demonstrates that there is little difference in the mortality rate for lobectomy. The average mortality is 3% for patients <65 to 70 years,[11,24,25,33] 5% for patients ≥65 to 70,[11,23–25,33] and 6% for patients ≥75 to 80.[11,24,33] On the other hand, the mortality for pneumonectomy has been reported to be markedly higher for patients over age 70 and especially patients over age 80 in several studies (Table 8–9). Thus,

TABLE 8–8. OVERALL MORTALITY FOR OLDER PATIENTS UNDERGOING PULMONARY RESECTION FOR LUNG CANCER

AGE CATEGORIES:	N				MORTALITY (%)			
	<60	60–69	70–79	≥80	<60	60–69	70–79	≥80
Romano and Mark[24 a]	3864	4889	3373	459	2	5	7	10
Wada et al[11]	1893	2876	2105	225	0.4	1	2	2
Ginsberg et al[10]	847	920	416	37	1	4	7	8
Damhuis and Schutte[23]	418	638	521	—	1	4	4	—
Whittle et al[33 b]	—	370	527[b]	376[b]	—	5	7[b]	10[b]
Silvestri et al[25 c]	693[c]	—	890[c]	—	3[c]	—	7[c]	—
Deneffe et al[112]	349	300	71	—	3	6	11	—
Ishida et al[128]	—	472[d]	185[e]	—	—	2	3	—
Gebitekin et al[131]	—	502[d]	145[e]	—	—	5	9	—
Duque et al[36]	—	456[d]	149[e]	—	—	9	6	—
Thomas et al[37]	—	—	464	36	—	—	7	8
Total	8064	11 423	8846	1133				
Average					**2**	**5**	**6**	**8**

Inclusion criteria: Studies from 1980 to 2000 of ≥500 patients (total) undergoing pulmonary resection for known or suspected lung cancer and reporting age-specific data.
[a]40% of patients underwent wedge or segmentectomy.
[b]Ages <75 versus ≥75.
[c]Ages <65 versus ≥65.
[d]All ages <70.
[e]All ages ≥70.

TABLE 8–9. MORTALITY FOR OLDER PATIENTS UNDERGOING PNEUMONECTOMY FOR LUNG CANCER

AGE CATEGORIES:	N			MORTALITY		
	<70	70–79	≥80	<70	70–79	≥80
Romano and Mark[24]	1197	309	24	9	19	29
Au et al[156]	625	70	—	7	21	
Gebitekin et al[131]	234	47	—	8	11	—
Patel et al[39]	165	32	—	8	13	—
Silvestri et al[25]	92	75	—	10[a]	25[a]	—
Whittle et al[33 b]	60	60[b]	34[b]	5	12[b]	26[b]
Damhuis and Schutte[23]	—	140	—	—	8[a]	—
Mizushima et al[132]	95	27	—	3	22	—
Total	2468	760	58			
Average				7	16	28

Inclusion criteria: Studies from 1980 to 2000 of ≥20 patients age ≤70 to 79 or >80 undergoing pneumonectomy for lung cancer.
[a]Age <65 versus ≥65.
[b]Age <75 versus ≥75.

it seems that one should be cautious about undertaking pneumonectomy in older patients.

Patients with Poor Pulmonary Reserve

It is difficult to determine the risk associated with surgical resection in patients with poor pulmonary reserve. Despite many studies, no universally accepted definition of what constitutes poor pulmonary reserve has emerged. Criteria that are often cited include a preoperative FEV_1 of <1.5 L, a preoperative D_{LCO} of <50%, a projected postoperative ppo FEV_1 of 800 mL, or a ppo FEV_1 of <40%.

A detailed discussion of the data regarding mortality and morbidity in patients falling above and below such proposed thresholds is provided in Chapter 7. In brief, ample data substantiates that the risk of death or complications is low in patients who fall above such thresholds. Very little data is available for patients falling below these values. A limited resection (segmentectomy or wedge by thoracotomy) can be accomplished with <10% mortality even in patients with limited pulmonary reserves. Conventional resection (lobectomy or pneumonectomy) carries a high mortality (≥25%) for patients with a ppo FEV_1 <40% or a ppo D_{LCO} <40%, even in carefully selected patients. A maximal oxygen consumption ($\dot{V}O_{2\ max}$) of <15 mL/kg/mm on an exercise tolerance test also results in a somewhat higher mortality (15%–20%).

In the coming years, firm conclusions about the amount of pulmonary reserve that precludes resection are likely to be even more confounded because of the realization that certain selected patients who are candidates for simultaneous volume reduction surgery and resection of their lung cancer may actually have *better* pulmonary function postoperatively.[133–135]

EDITORS' COMMENTS

A pulmonary resection is clearly a major intervention. The mortality rates for this procedure are quite low, however. Even with more extensive procedures, the hospital mortality rate of approximately 10%, at least when patients are carefully selected, is reasonable. Between one-third and one-half of patients are likely to develop complications. Poor pulmonary reserve, increasing age, and the need for a pneumonectomy seem to be correlated with postoperative morbidity, yet it is difficult to predict which patients will

---

DATA SUMMARY: MORTALITY OF SPECIFIC SURGICAL PROCEDURES IN SPECIFIC PATIENT POPULATIONS			
	AMOUNT	**QUALITY**	**CONSISTENCY**
Mortality for mediastinoscopy is <0.1%	High	High	High
Mortality for lobectomy is 3%	High	High	High
Mortality for pneumonectomy is 9%	High	High	High
Mortality for patients age >80 is 8%	High	High	High
Mortality for pneumonectomy in patients >70 is 16%-25%	High	High	High
Resection of selected patients with poor pulmonary reserve can be accomplished with mortality <10% if liberal use is made of limited resections	High	High	High

Type of data rated: Plain text: descriptive statement   *Italics: controlled comparison*   **Bold: randomized comparison**

develop complications. However, the data shows that this morbidity is short lived and that patients have regained their baseline status by 6 to 9 months, as measured by QOL and dyspnea assessments.

Given these results, the opinion of some physicians that pulmonary resection is a morbid procedure is unfounded. The data shows that surgery for lung cancer is a well tolerated treatment, even in elderly patients. This includes patients over age 70, those with other medical conditions, and those with limited pulmonary reserve. Advances in surgical and anesthetic techniques, as well as improvements in postoperative care, have undoubtedly contributed to these results.

Skillful patient selection is of major importance. However, the criteria that should be used remain vague. Clearer definition of the factors and criteria that influence operative morbidity and mortality should be addressed by clinical research.

References

1. Detterbeck FC. Postoperative management after thoracic surgery procedures. In: Moylan JA, ed. Surgical Critical Care. St. Louis, Mo: Mosby; 1994:409–429.
2. Bashir Y, Graham TR, Torrance A, et al. Nutritional state of patients with lung cancer undergoing thoracotomy. Thorax. 1990;45:183–186.
3. Rochester DF, Esau SA. Malnutrition and the respiratory system. Chest. 1984;85:411–415.
4. Deslauriers J, Ginsberg RJ, Dubois P, et al. Current operative morbidity associated with elective surgical resection for lung cancer. Can J Surg. 1989;32:335–339.
5. Bartlett RH, Gazzaniga AB, Geraghty TR. Respiratory maneuvers to prevent postoperative pulmonary complications: a critical review. JAMA. 1973;224:1017–1021.
6. Ali J, Weisel RD, Layug AB, et al. Consequences of postoperative alterations in respiratory mechanics. Am J Surg. 1974;128:376–382.
7. Steen PA, Tinker JH, Tarhan S. Myocardial reinfarction after anesthesia and surgery. JAMA. 1978;239:2566–2570.
8. Rao TLK, Jacobs KH, El-Etr AA. Reinfarction following anesthesia in patients with myocardial infarction. Anesthesiology. 1983;59:499–505.
9. Goldman L, Caldera DL, Nussbaum SR, et al. Multifactorial index of cardiac risk in noncardiac surgical procedures. N Engl J Med. 1977;297:847–850.
10. Ginsberg RJ, Hill LD, Eagan RT, et al. Modern thirty-day operative mortality for surgical resections in lung cancer. J Thorac Cardiovasc Surg. 1983;86:654–658.
11. Wada H, Nakamura T, Nakamoto K, et al. Thirty-day operative mortality for thoracotomy in lung cancer. J Thorac Cardiovasc Surg. 1998;115:70–73.
12. Ginsberg RJ. Preoperative assessment of the thoracic surgical patient: a surgeon's viewpoint. In: Pearson FG, Deslauriers J, Ginsberg RJ, Hiebert CA, McKneally MF, Urschel HC Jr, eds. Thoracic Surgery. New York, NY: Churchill Livingstone; 1995:29–36.
13. Anderson RW, Alexander JC Jr. Preoperative cardiac evaluation of the thoracic surgical patient and management of perioperative cardiac events. In: Shields TW, ed. General Thoracic Surgery. 4th ed. Baltimore, Md: Williams & Wilkins; 1994:288–295.
14. von Knorring J. Postoperative myocardial infarction: a prospective study in a risk group of surgical patients. Surgery. 1981;90:55–60.
15. Freeman WK, Gibbons RJ, Shub C. Preoperative assessment of cardiac patients undergoing noncardiac surgical procedures. Mayo Clin Proc. 1989;64:1105–1117.
16. Tarhan S, Moffitt EA, Taylor WF, et al. Myocardial infarction after general anesthesia. JAMA. 1972;220:1451–1454.
17. Miller JI Jr. Thallium imaging in preoperative evaluation of the pulmonary resection candidate. Ann Thorac Surg. 1992;54:249–252.
18. Miller JI Jr. Preoperative evaluation. Chest Surg Clin N Am. 1992;2:701–711.
19. Boucher CA, Brewster DC, Darling RC, et al. Determination of cardiac risk by dipyridamole-thallium imaging before peripheral vascular surgery. N Engl J Med. 1985;312:389–394.
20. Leppo J, Plaja J, Gionet M, et al. Noninvasive evaluation of cardiac risk before elective vascular surgery. J Am Coll Cardiol. 1987;9:269–276.
21. Eagle KA, Singer DE, Brewster DC, et al. Dipyridamole-thallium scanning in patients undergoing vascular surgery: optimizing preoperative evaluation of cardiac risk. JAMA. 1987;257:2185–2189.
22. Cutler BS, Leppo JA. Dipyridamole thallium 201 scintigraphy to detect coronary artery disease before abdominal aortic surgery. J Vasc Surg. 1987;5:91–100.
23. Damhuis RAM, Schutte PR. Resection rates and postoperative mortality in 7,899 patients with lung cancer. Eur Respir J. 1996;9:7–10.
24. Romano PS, Mark DH. Patient and hospital characteristics related to in-hospital mortality after lung cancer resection. Chest. 1992;101:1332–1337.
25. Silvestri GA, Handy J, Lackland D, et al. Specialists achieve better outcomes than generalists for lung cancer surgery. Chest. 1998;114:675–680.
26. Harpole Jr DH, DeCamp Jr MM, Daley J, et al. Prognostic models of thirty-day mortality and morbidity after major pulmonary resection. J Thorac Cardiovasc Surg. 1999;117:969–979.
27. van Rens MTM, de la Rivière AB, Elbers HRJ, et al. Prognostic assessment of 2,361 patients who underwent pulmonary resection for non-small cell lung cancer, stage I, II, and IIIA. Chest. 2000;117:374–379.
28. Keagy BA, Lores ME, Starek PJK, et al. Elective pulmonary lobectomy: factors associated with morbidity and operative mortality. Ann Thorac Surg. 1985;40:349–352.
29. Miller JI Jr. Physiologic evaluation of pulmonary function in the candidate for lung resection. J Thorac Cardiovasc Surg. 1993;105:347–352.
30. Kearney DJ, Lee TH, Reilly JJ, et al. Assessment of operative risk in patients undergoing lung resection: importance of predicted pulmonary function. Chest. 1994;105:753–759.
31. Ferguson MK, Reeder LB, Mick R. Optimizing selection of patients for major lung resection. J Thorac Cardiovasc Surg. 1995;109:275–283.
32. Ferguson MK, Little L, Rizzo L, et al. Diffusing capacity predicts morbidity and mortality after pulmonary resection. J Thorac Cardiovasc Surg. 1988;96:894–900.
33. Whittle J, Steinberg EP, Anderson GF, et al. Use of Medicare claims data to evaluate outcomes in elderly patients undergoing lung resection for lung cancer. Chest. 1991;100:729–734.
34. Nagasaki F, Flehinger BJ, Martini N. Complications of surgery in the treatment of carcinoma of the lung. Chest. 1982;82:25–29.
35. Kohman LJ, Meyer JA, Ikins PM, et al. Random versus predictable risks of mortality after thoracotomy for lung cancer. J Thorac Cardiovasc Surg. 1986;91:551–554.
36. Duque JL, Ramos G, Castrodeza J, et al. Early complications in surgical treatment of lung cancer: a prospective, multicenter study. Ann Thorac Surg. 1997;63:944–950.
37. Thomas P, Piraux M, Jacques LF, et al. Clinical patterns and trends of outcome of elderly patients with bronchogenic carcinoma. Eur J Cardiothorac Surg. 1998;13:266–274.
38. Izbicki JR, Knoefel T, Passlick B, et al. Risk analysis and long-term survival in patients undergoing extended resection of locally advanced lung cancer. J Thorac Cardiovasc Surg. 1995;110:386–395.
39. Patel RL, Townsend ER, Fountain SW. Elective pneumonectomy: factors associated with morbidity and operative mortality. Ann Thorac Surg. 1992;54:84–88.
40. Wahi R, McMurtrey MJ, DeCaro LF, et al. Determinants of perioperative morbidity and mortality after pneumonectomy. Ann Thorac Surg. 1989;48:33–37.
41. Yano T, Yokoyama H, Fukuyama Y, et al. The current status of postoperative complications and risk factors after a pulmonary resection for primary lung cancer: a multivariate analysis. Eur J Cardiothorac Surg. 1997;11:445–449.
42. Deslauriers J, Ginsberg RJ, Piantadosi S, et al. Prospective assessment of 30-day operative morbidity for surgical resections in lung cancer. Chest. 1994;106(suppl):329S–330S.
43. Waller DA, Gebitekin C, Saunders NR, et al. Noncardiogenic pulmonary edema complicating lung resection. Ann Thorac Surg. 1993;55:140–143.

44. Parquin F, Marchal M, Mehiri S, et al. Post-pneumonectomy pulmonary edema: analysis and risk factors. Eur J Cardiothorac Surg. 1996;10:929–933.

45. Hayes JP, Williams EA, Goldstraw P, et al. Lung injury in patients following thoracotomy. Thorax. 1995;50:990–991.

46. Verheijen-Breemhaar L, Bogaard JM, van den Berg B, et al. Postpneumonectomy pulmonary oedema. Thorax. 1988;43:323–326.

47. Zeldin RA, Normandin D, Landtwing D, et al. Postpneumonectomy pulmonary edema. J Thorac Cardiovasc Surg. 1984;87:359–365.

48. Kutlu CA, Williams E, Evans T, et al. Acute lung injury (ALI) and acute respiratory distress syndrome (ARDS) following pulmonary resection: frequency and mortality. Ann Thorac Surg. 2000;69:376–380.

49. Miller DL, McManus KG, Allen MS, et al. Results of surgical resection of patients with N2 non–small cell lung cancer. Ann Thorac Surg. 1994;57:1095–1101.

50. Allen MS, Deschamps C, Trastek VF, et al. Bronchopleural fistula. Chest Surg Clin N Am. 1992;2:823–837.

51. Asamura H, Naruke T, Tsuchiya R, et al. Bronchopleural fistulas associated with lung cancer operations: univariate and multivariate analysis of risk factors, management, and outcome. J Thorac Cardiovasc Surg. 1992;104:1456–1464.

52. Pairolero PC, Arnold PG, Trastek VF, et al. Postpneumonectomy empyema: the role of intrathoracic muscle transposition. J Thorac Cardiovasc Surg. 1990;99:958–968.

53. Mathisen DJ, Grillo HC, Vlahakes GJ. The omentum in the management of complicated cardiothoracic problems. J Thorac Cardiovasc Surg. 1988;95:677–684.

54. Kirsh MM, Sloan H. Mediastinal metastases in bronchogenic carcinoma: influence of postoperative irradiation, cell type, and location. Ann Thorac Surg. 1982;33:459–463.

55. von Knorring J, Lepäntalo M, Lindgren L, et al. Cardiac arrhythmias and myocardial ischemia after thoracotomy for lung cancer. Ann Thorac Surg. 1992;53:642–647.

56. Krowka MJ, Pairolero PC, Trastek VF, et al. Cardiac dysrhythmia following pneumonectomy: clinical correlates and prognostic significance. Chest. 1987;91:490–495.

57. Harpole DH Jr, Liptay MJ, DeCamp MM Jr, et al. Prospective analysis of pneumonectomy: risk factors for major morbidity and cardiac dysrhythmias. Ann Thorac Surg. 1996;61:977–982.

58. Amar D, Roistacher N, Burt M, et al. Clinical and echocardiographic correlates of symptomatic tachydysrhythmias after noncardiac thoracic surgery. Chest. 1995;108:349–354.

59. Asamura H, Naruke T, Tsuchiya R, et al. What are the risk factors for arrhythmias after thoracic operations? A retrospective multivariate analysis of 267 consecutive thoracic operations. J Thorac Cardiovasc Surg. 1993;106:1104–1110.

60. Curtis JJ, Parker BM, McKenney CA, et al. Incidence and predictors of supraventricular dysrhythmias after pulmonary resection. Ann Thorac Surg. 1998;66:1766–1771.

61. Cardinale D, Martinoni A, Cipolla CM, et al. Atrial fibrillation after operation for lung cancer: clinical and prognostic significance. Ann Thorac Surg. 1999;68:1827–1831.

62. Rice TW, Kirby TJ. Prolonged air leak. Chest Surg Clin N Am. 1992;2:803–811.

63. Abolhoda A, Liu D, Brooks A, et al. Prolonged air leak following radical upper lobectomy: an analysis of incidence and possible risk factors. Chest. 1998;113:1507–1510.

64. Van Mieghem W, Demedts M. Cardiopulmonary function after lobectomy or pneumonectomy for pulmonary neoplasm. Respir Med. 1989;83:199–206.

65. Nezu K, Kushibe K, Tojo T, et al. Recovery and limitation of exercise capacity after lung resection for lung cancer. Chest. 1998;113:1511–1516.

66. Larsen KR, Svendsen UG, Milman N, et al. Cardiopulmonary function at rest and during exercise after resection for bronchial carcinoma. Ann Thorac Surg. 1997;64:960–964.

67. Ginsberg RJ, Rubinstein LV, for the Lung Cancer Study Group. Randomized trial of lobectomy versus limited resection for T1 N0 non–small cell lung cancer. Ann Thorac Surg. 1995;60:615–623.

68. Markos J, Mullan BP, Hillman DR, et al. Preoperative assessment as a predictor of mortality and morbidity after lung resection. Am Rev Respir Dis. 1989;139:902–910.

69. Zeiher B, Gross TJ, Kern JA, et al. Predicting postoperative pulmonary function in patients undergoing lung resection. Chest. 1995;108:68–72.

70. Korst RJ, Ginsberg RJ, Ailawadi M, et al. Lobectomy improves ventilatory function in selected patients with severe COPD. Ann Thorac Surg. 1998;66:898–902.

71. Bolliger CT, Jordan P, Solèr M, et al. Pulmonary function and exercise capacity after lung resection. Eur Respir J. 1996;9:415–421.

72. Dales RE, Bélanger R, Shamji FM, et al. Quality-of-life following thoracotomy for lung cancer. J Clin Epidemiol. 1994;47:1443–1449.

73. Nõu E, Aberg T. Quality of survival in patients with surgically treated bronchial carcinoma. Thorax. 1980;35:255–263.

74. Hamelmann H, Thermann M, Müller-Schwefe T, et al. Surgically treated bronchial carcinoma patients—results of a systematic follow-up. Thorac Cardiovasc Surg. 1983;31:41–44.

75. Dajczman E, Gordon A, Kreisman H, et al. Long-term postthoracotomy pain. Chest. 1991;99:270–274.

76. Keller SM, Carp NZ, Levy MN, et al. Chronic post thoracotomy pain. J Cardiovasc Surg. 1994;35(suppl 1):161–164.

77. Kanner RM, Martini N, Foley KM. Nature and incidence of postthoracotomy pain [abstract]. Proc ASCO. 1982;1:152.

78. Landreneau RJ, Pigula F, Luketich JD, et al. Acute and chronic morbidity differences between muscle-sparing and standard lateral thoracotomy. J Thorac Cardiovasc Surg. 1996;112:1346–1351.

79. Landreneau RJ, Mack MJ, Hazelrigg SR, et al. Prevalence of chronic pain after pulmonary resection by thoracotomy or video-assisted thoracic surgery. J Thorac Cardiovasc Surg. 1994;107:1079–1086.

80. Cybulsky IJ, Bennett WF. Mediastinoscopy as a routine outpatient procedure. Ann Thorac Surg. 1994;58:176–178.

81. Pearson FG, Nelems JM, Henderson RD, et al. The role of mediastinoscopy in the selection of treatment for bronchial carcinoma with involvement of superior mediastinal lymph nodes. J Thorac Cardiovasc Surg. 1972;64:382–390.

82. Jolly PC, Li W, Anderson RP. Anterior and cervical mediastinoscopy for determining operability and predicting resectability in lung cancer. J Thorac Cardiovasc Surg. 1980;79:366–371.

83. Schreinemakers HHJ, Joosten HJM, Mravunac M, et al. Parasternal mediastinoscopy: assessment of operability in left upper lobe lung cancer: a prospective analysis. J Thorac Cardiovasc Surg. 1988;95:298–302.

84. Goldstraw P. Mediastinal exploration by mediastinoscopy and mediastinotomy. Br J Dis Chest. 1988;82:111–120.

85. Landreneau RJ, Sugarbaker DJ, Mack MJ, et al. Wedge resection versus lobectomy for stage I (T1 N0 M0) non–small-cell lung cancer. J Thorac Cardiovasc Surg. 1997;113:691–700.

86. Mentzer SJ, DeCamp MM, Harpole DH Jr, et al. Thoracoscopy and video-assisted thoracic surgery in the treatment of lung cancer. Chest. 1995;107:298S–301S.

87. Mack MJ, Hazelrigg SR, Landreneau RJ, et al. Thoracoscopy for the diagnosis of the indeterminate solitary pulmonary nodule. Ann Thorac Surg. 1993;56:825–832.

88. Allen MS, Deschamps C, Lee RE, et al. Video-assisted thoracoscopic stapled wedge excision for indeterminate pulmonary nodules. J Thorac Cardiovasc Surg. 1993;106:1048–1052.

89. Jensik RJ. The extent of resection for localized lung cancer: segmental resection. In: Kittle CF, ed. Current Controversies in Thoracic Surgery. Philadelphia, Pa: WB Saunders; 1986:175–182.

90. Martini N, Bains MS, Burt ME, et al. Incidence of local recurrence and second primary tumors in resected stage I lung cancer. J Thorac Cardiovasc Surg. 1995;109:120–129.

91. Busch E, Verazin G, Antkowiak JG, et al. Pulmonary complications in patients undergoing thoracotomy for lung carcinoma. Chest. 1994;105:760–766.

92. McGovern EM, Trastek VF, Pairolero PC, et al. Completion pneumonectomy: indications, complications, and results. Ann Thorac Surg. 1988;46:141–146.

93. Kaiser LR, Bavaria JE. Complications of thoracoscopy. Ann Thorac Surg. 1993;56:796–798.

94. Daniel TM, Kern JA, Tribble CG, et al. Thoracoscopic surgery for diseases of the lung and pleura: effectiveness, changing indications, and limitations. Ann Surg. 1993;217:566–575.

95. Hazelrigg SR, Nunchuck SK, Landreneau RJ, et al. Cost analysis for thoracoscopy: thoracoscopic wedge resection. Ann Thorac Surg. 1993;56:633–635.

96. Kirby TJ, Rice TW. Thoracoscopic lobectomy. Ann Thorac Surg. 1993;56:784–786.

97. Kirby TJ, Mack MJ, Landreneau RJ, et al. Initial experience with video-assisted thoracoscopic lobectomy. Ann Thorac Surg. 1993;56:1248–1253.

98. Walker WS, Carnochan FM, Tin M. Thoracoscopy assisted pulmonary lobectomy. Thorax. 1993;48:921–924.

99. Kirby TJ, Mack MJ, Landreneau RJ, et al. Lobectomy-video-assisted thoracic surgery versus muscle-sparing thoracotomy: a randomized trial. J Thorac Cardiovasc Surg. 1995;109:997–1002.

100. McKenna RJ Jr. Lobectomy by video-assisted thoracic surgery with mediastinal node sampling for lung cancer. J Thorac Cardiovasc Surg. 1994;107:879–882.

101. Yim APC, Ko K, Chau W, et al. Video-assisted thoracoscopic anatomic lung resections: the initial Hong Kong experience. Chest. 1996;109:13–17.

102. Giudicelli R, Thomas P, Lonjon T, et al. Video-assisted minithoracotomy versus muscle-sparing thoracotomy for performing lobectomy. Ann Thorac Surg. 1994;58:712–718.

103. McKenna RJ Jr, Fischel RJ, Wolf R, et al. Video-assisted thoracic surgery (VATS) lobectomy for bronchogenic carcinoma. Semin Thorac Cardiovasc Surg. 1998;10:321–325.

104. Brown WT. Video-assisted thoracic surgery: the Miami experience. Semin Thorac Cardiovasc Surg. 1998;10:305–312.

105. Lewis RJ, Caccavale RJ. Video-assisted thoracic surgical non-rib spreading simultaneously stapled lobectomy (VATS(n)SSL). Semin Thorac Cardiovasc Surg. 1998;10:332–339.

106. Landreneau RJ, Hazelrigg SR, Mack MJ, et al. Postoperative pain-related morbidity: video-assisted thoracic surgery versus thoracotomy. Ann Thorac Surg. 1993;56:1285–1289.

107. Yim APC, Landreneau RJ, Izzat MB, et al. Is video-assisted thoracoscopic lobectomy a unified approach? Ann Thorac Surg. 1998;66:1155–1158.

108. Walker WS. Video-assisted thoracic surgery (VATS) lobectomy: the Edinburgh experience. Semin Thorac Cardiovasc Surg. 1998;10:291–299.

109. Kaseda S, Aoki T, Hangai N. Video-assisted thoracic surgery (VATS) lobectomy: the Japanese experience. Semin Thorac Cardiovasc Surg. 1998;10:300–304.

110. Yim APC, Izzat MB, Liu H, et al. Thoracoscopic major lung resections: an Asian perspective. Semin Thorac Cardiovasc Surg. 1998;10:326–331.

111. Van Den Bosch JMM, Gelissen HJ, Wagenaar SS. Exploratory thoracotomy in bronchial carcinoma. J Thorac Cardiovasc Surg. 1983;85:733–737.

112. Deneffe G, Lacquet LM, Verbeken E, et al. Surgical treatment of bronchogenic carcinoma: a retrospective study of 720 thoracotomies. Ann Thorac Surg. 1988;45:380–383.

113. Yellin A, Benfield JR. Surgery for bronchogenic carcinoma in the elderly [editorial]. Am Rev Respir Dis. 1985;131:197.

114. Katz S, Branch LG, Branson MH, et al. Active life expectancy. N Engl J Med. 1983;309:1218–1223.

115. Sikes ED, Detmer DE. Aging and surgical risk in older citizens of Wisconsin. Wisc Med J. 1979;78:27–30.

116. Tisi GM. Preoperative evaluation of pulmonary function. Am Rev Respir Dis. 1979;119:293–310.

117. O'Rourke MA, Feussner JR, Feigl P, et al. Age trends of lung cancer stage at diagnosis: implications for lung cancer screening in the elderly. JAMA. 1987;258:921–926.

118. Nugent WC, Edney MT, Hammerness PG, et al. Non–small cell lung cancer at the extremes of age: impact on diagnosis and treatment. Ann Thorac Surg. 1997;63:193–197.

119. Mañé JM, Estapé J, Sánchez-Lloret J, et al. Age and clinical characteristics of 1433 patients with lung cancer. Age Ageing. 1994;23:28–31.

120. Brown JS, Eraut D, Trask C, et al. Age and the treatment of lung cancer. Thorax. 1996;51:564–568.

121. Teeter SM, Holmes FF, McFarlane MJ. Lung carcinoma in the elderly population: influence of histology on the inverse relationship of stage to age. Cancer. 1987;60:1331–1336.

122. Ershler WB, Socinski MA, Greene CJ. Bronchogenic cancer, metastases, and aging. J Am Geriatr Soc. 1983;31:673–676.

123. Naunheim KS, Kesler KA, D'Orazio SA, et al. Lung cancer surgery in the octogenarian. Eur J Cardiothorac Surg. 1994;8:453–456.

124. Pagni S, Federico JA, Ponn RB. Pulmonary resection for lung cancer in octogenarians. Ann Thorac Surg. 1997;63:785–789.

125. Osaki T, Shirakusa T, Kodate M, et al. Surgical treatment of lung cancer in the octogenarian. Ann Thorac Surg. 1994;57:188–193.

126. Shirakusa T, Tsutsui M, Iriki N, et al. Results of resection for bronchogenic carcinoma in patients over the age of 80. Thorax. 1989;44:189–191.

127. Thomas P, Sielezneff I, Ragni J, et al. Is lung cancer resection justified in patients aged over 70 years? Eur J Cardiothorac Surg. 1993;7:246–251.

128. Ishida T, Yokoyama H, Kaneko S, et al. Long-term results of operation for non–small cell lung cancer in the elderly. Ann Thorac Surg. 1990;50:919–922.

129. Morandi U, Stefani A, Golinelli M, et al. Results of surgical resection in patients over the age of 70 years with non small-cell lung cancer. Eur J Cardiothorac Surg. 1997;11:432–439.

130. Sherman S, Guidot CE. The feasibility of thoracotomy for lung cancer in the elderly. JAMA. 1987;258:927–930.

131. Gebitekin C, Gupta NK, Martin PG, et al. Long-term results in the elderly following pulmonary resection for non–small cell lung carcinoma. Eur J Cardiothorac Surg. 1993;7:653–656.

132. Mizushima Y, Noto H, Sugiyama S, et al. Survival and prognosis after pneumonectomy for lung cancer in the elderly. Ann Thorac Surg. 1997;64:193–198.

133. Ojo TC, Martinez F, Paine R III, et al. Lung volume reduction surgery alters management of pulmonary nodules in patients with severe COPD. Chest. 1997;112:1494–1500.

134. DeRose JJ Jr, Argenziano M, El-Amir N, et al. Lung reduction operation and resection of pulmonary nodules in patients with severe emphysema. Ann Thorac Surg. 1998;65:314–318.

135. DeMeester SR, Patterson GA, Sundaresan RS, et al. Lobectomy combined with volume reduction for patients with lung cancer and advanced emphysema. J Thorac Cardiovasc Surg. 1998;115:681–688.

136. Wada H, Tanaka F, Yanagihara K, et al. Time trends and survival after operations for primary lung cancer from 1976 through 1990. J Thorac Cardiovasc Surg. 1996;112:349–355.

137. Harpole DH Jr, Herndon JE II, Young WG Jr, et al. Stage I nonsmall cell lung cancer: a multivariate analysis of treatment methods and patterns of recurrence. Cancer. 1995;76:787–796.

138. Knott-Craig CJ, Howell E, Parsons BD, et al. Improved results in the management of surgical candidates with lung cancer. Ann Thorac Surg. 1997;63:1405–1410.

139. Daly RC, Trastek VF, Pairolero PC, et al. Bronchoalveolar carcinoma: factors affecting survival. Ann Thorac Surg. 1991;51:368–377.

140. Humphrey EW, Smart CR, Winchester DP, et al. National survey of the pattern of care for carcinoma of the lung. J Thorac Cardiovasc Surg. 1990;100:837–843.

141. Conacher ID. Therapists and therapies for post-thoracotomy neuralgia. Pain. 1992;48:409–412.

142. Kalso E, Perttunen K, Kaasinen S. Pain after thoracic surgery. Acta Anaesthesiol Scand. 1992;36:96–100.

143. Matsunaga M, Dan K, Manabe FY, et al. Residual pain of 90 thoracotomy patients with malignancy and non-malignancy [abstract]. Pain. 1990;(suppl 5):S148.

144. Katz J, Jackson M, Kavanagh BP, et al. Acute pain after thoracic surgery predicts long-term post-thoracotomy pain. Clin J Pain. 1996;12:50–55.

145. Puhakka HJ. Complications of mediastinoscopy. J Laryngol Otol. 1989;103:312–315.

146. Coughlin M, Deslauriers J, Beaulieu M, et al. Role of mediastinoscopy in pretreatment staging of patients with primary lung cancer. Ann Thorac Surg. 1985;40:556–560.

147. Luke WP, Pearson FG, Todd TRJ, et al. Prospective evaluation of mediastinoscopy for assessment of carcinoma of the lung. J Thorac Cardiovasc Surg. 1986;91:53–56.

148. Weissberg D. Mediastinal staging of lung cancer: the changing role of mediastinoscopy. Isr J Med Sci. 1995;31:122–124.

149. Whittlesey D. Prospective computed tomographic scanning in the staging of bronchogenic cancer. J Thorac Cardiovasc Surg. 1988;95:876–882.

150. Ginsberg RJ, Rice TW, Goldberg M, et al. Extended cervical mediastinoscopy: a single staging procedure for bronchogenic carcinoma of the left upper lobe. J Thorac Cardiovasc Surg. 1987;94:673–678.

151. Hammoud ZT, Anderson RC, Meyers BF, et al. The current role of mediastinoscopy in the evaluation of thoracic disease. J Thorac Cardiovasc Surg. 1999;118:894–899.

152. Kadri MA, Dussek JE. Survival and prognosis following resection

of primary non small cell bronchogenic carcinoma. Eur J Cardio-thorac Surg. 1991;5:132–136.

153. Pastorino U, Valente M, Bedini V, et al. Limited resection for stage I lung cancer. Eur J Surg Oncol. 1991;17:42–46.

154. Errett LE, Wilson J, Chiu RC-J, et al. Wedge resection as an alternative procedure for peripheral bronchogenic carcinoma in poor-risk patients. J Thorac Cardiovasc Surg. 1985;90:656–661.

155. Roviaro G, Varoli F, Vergani C, et al. Video-assisted thoracoscopic surgery (VATS) major pulmonary resections: the Italian experience. Semin Thorac Cardiovasc Surg. 1998;10:313–320.

156. Au J, El-Oakley R, Cameron EWJ. Pneumonectomy for bronchogenic carcinoma in the elderly. Eur J Cardiothorac Surg. 1994;8:247–250.

GENERAL ASPECTS OF RADIOTHERAPY FOR LUNG CANCER

Suzanne M. Russo and Julian G. Rosenman

This chapter provides an overview of the general concepts of radiation physics and biology that are the foundations of radiation therapy (RT), as well as those that pertain specifically to lung cancer treatment. These issues include dose, overall treatment time, fractionation, treatment volume, and toxicity. Aspects of RT that involve a specific context or group of patients are discussed in other chapters. For example, the effectiveness of RT for palliation is discussed in Chapter 29, and results and specific issues relating to the treatment of stage I, II, or III disease are discussed in Chapters 13 and 18.

GENERAL CONSIDERATIONS

RT is an important component of treatment for a large number of lung cancer patients who have a variety of clinical presentations. It is important to clearly establish the goal of therapy (curative versus palliative) for each patient. For most of the approximately 40% of patients who present with mediastinal lymph nodes (see Fig. 4–1), RT will be part of the primary treatment. RT will also be used as a palliative treatment for as many as 50% of lung cancer patients who either present with, or ultimately develop, metastatic disease. In patients with earlier-stage disease, RT is occasionally used postoperatively for close or positive surgical resection margins or if unexpected mediastinal lymphadenopathy is encountered. Finally, RT is sometimes the only tolerable treatment for patients with significant comorbid disease. Because RT is used for such

a wide range of lung cancer patients, it is important that clinicians involved in the multidisciplinary care of patients with lung cancer understand some of the methods and issues associated with RT for this disease.

How effective is RT as a treatment for non–small cell lung cancer (NSCLC)? The answer is difficult to determine from the historical data because only a few trials have compared radiation alone with best supportive care or with other nonradiation treatment modalities. Roswit et al[1] compared the use of RT with best supportive care in patients with locally advanced, nonmetastatic NSCLC and small cell lung cancer (SCLC). By today's standards, the patients were poorly staged and the treatment was mainly low-dose orthovoltage RT. Nevertheless, a small benefit was seen in the treated group as compared with the control group. Kubota et al[2] reported on 63 patients who were randomized to receive chemotherapy with or without 50 to 60 Gy of radiation and concluded that the irradiated patients had a considerably increased 2-year survival. In contrast, Johnson et al[3] compared vindesine alone with vindesine plus 60 Gy of radiation and concluded that there was no survival advantage to the RT, despite a better tumor response rate. Shepard et al[4] also reported on 31 patients with stage IIIa NSCLC who were randomized to receive RT alone or chemotherapy with cisplatin and vinblastine followed by surgery. Although the median survival times were 16 months for radiotherapy alone and 19 months for chemotherapy followed by surgery, the difference was not statistically significant in this small study. Finally, studies of RT alone have consistently shown that long-term survival is achieved in a small cohort of patients with localized NSCLC (see Chapters 13 and 18), whereas the natural history of untreated patients has consistently shown no long-term survival (see Chapter 3). We can conclude that radiation alone in locally advanced NSCLC does, indeed, cure a few patients, although the percentage is small.

In the treatment of early-stage NSCLC, most single-arm studies suggest that early-stage patients fare poorly when treated with RT as compared with surgery.[5] The few small randomized studies that have been conducted are consistent with this finding.[1,6] It may be argued that most of these patients are *medically inoperable* and are therefore not as healthy as their surgical counterparts, but demographic studies have failed to confirm that such patients have more explicit comorbidity than do their surgical counterparts.[7] Nevertheless, the poor physical condition of most of these patients may be a contributing factor to the poor results with radiation alone. In addition, patients undergoing RT for early-stage NSCLC can only be clinically staged, whereas their surgical counterparts are pathologically staged, at least in the chest, making direct comparisons of the two treatment modalities difficult.

RADIATION PHYSICS

Knowledge of radiation physics is necessary for a detailed understanding of the potential benefits and limitations of radiation treatment. Although a complete review of radiation physics is beyond the scope of this chapter, we present enough material to explain the meaning and importance of such concepts as megavoltage x-rays, fractionation schemes, radiation dosage, and three-dimensional (3-D) image-guided treatment planning.

Ionizing radiation is a form of energy that, by definition, causes ejection of an orbital electron when it is absorbed by matter. Although ionizing radiation can be particulate—involving protons, electrons, alpha particles, or neutrons—the radiation used in the treatment of lung cancer patients is primarily electromagnetic (x-rays). X-rays interact with matter in three distinct ways; the relative contribution of these three methods depends on the energy of the x-rays and has important therapeutic consequences.

Physicians are most familiar with x-rays used for diagnostic purposes, which typically have an energy in the range of 60 000 to 100 000 electron volts (60-100 keV). At this energy, x-rays interact with matter primarily by means of the photoelectric effect, whereby the energy of the photon causes the ejection of a tightly bound orbital electron. The absorption of energy by the photoelectric effect varies with the cube of the atomic number (Z), which is why high-Z tissues such as bone show up so well on a diagnostic radiograph. However Z-dependent absorption makes kilovoltage x-rays a poor choice for therapy; normal bone will inevitably receive a much higher dose than will a soft tissue tumor.

At higher energies, in the range of 1 to 20 million electron volts (1-20 MeV), ionizing radiation interacts with matter primarily by means of the Compton effect. Unlike the photoelectric effect, Compton interactions take place with loosely bound orbital electrons, and the incident x-rays do not give up all their energy to a single electron. As

a result, energy deposition by the Compton effect does not depend on Z but only on electron density. A beam of this energy is beneficial for therapy because there is no differential energy deposition between bone and soft tissue; the tumor gets at least as high a dose as any other tissue. At even higher energies, a third interactive process occurs, in which energy is absorbed by matter via the production of positron–electron pairs. During this process, the incoming photon interacts with the electromagnetic field of the atomic nucleus, but this is of only minor importance in the range of energies typically used in the medical setting.

Before 1950, therapy machines could only produce x-rays of slightly higher energy (250 keV) than those of diagnostic machines. For several reasons, use of these orthovoltage machines often resulted in substantial patient morbidity. First, orthovoltage x-rays primarily interact with matter photoelectrically and thus differentially deposit energy in high-Z tissues such as bone but not in the tumor. Second, orthovoltage x-rays have poor penetrating power compared with megavoltage x-rays. For example, a tumor at a depth of 10 cm may receive only about 40% of the entrance dose. Therefore, the surface dose will be 2.5 times the tumor dose, with the radiation dose going primarily to normal tissue rather than to the tumor. Finally, orthovoltage x-rays deposit their maximum dose within the first millimeter of tissue encountered (usually skin), as opposed to megavoltage x-rays, which partially skip or spare the first few centimeters of tissue (the exact amount of skin sparing is a function of the beam energy). High skin doses can cause skin breakdown and subsequent infection, sometimes limiting the total dose that can be given to a tumor.

This skin-sparing property of megavoltage x-rays is clinically important and deserves further explanation. The radiation dose deposited at any point within a patient is the sum of the direct effect of the primary beam and incident electrons produced elsewhere that have scattered into the area. In the megavoltage range, most of these scattered electrons are traveling in the same direction as the primary beam and are therefore scattered in the forward direction. Thus, at the skin surface there are few scattered electrons to contribute to the skin dose because only air (which produces few electrons) exists above the skin. Several centimeters deeper, the primary beam has been somewhat attenuated, but the dose from scattered electrons more than makes up for this attenuation, and the total dose increases. As the beam goes deeper still, the scattered electron dose can no longer make up for primary beam attenuation, and the dose decreases once again. The point of maximum dose (called *Dmax*) is energy dependent and varies from about 5 mm for a 1-MeV beam to >3 cm for a 20-MeV beam. For orthovoltage, Dmax is <100 μm and may be considered to be on the skin surface. Figure 9–1 illustrates two of the advantages of megavoltage compared with orthovoltage RT: the skin-sparing effect and the better dose at depth.

In the 1950s, treatment machines employing cobalt-60 (Co^{60}) for their radiation source became available. Co^{60} emits gamma rays (a name given to x-rays produced by radioactive materials) at 1.25 MeV. Because Co^{60} is in the megavoltage range, the differential absorption by bone ceased to be a problem, modest skin sparing could be achieved, and the dose at depth was improved compared with that of orthovoltage. These three improvements al-

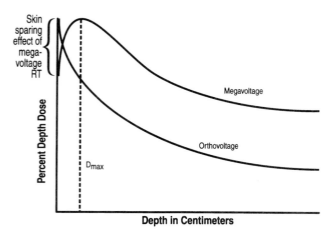

FIGURE 9–1. A comparison of the percentage depth dose for orthovoltage and megavoltage beams. Note that the skin sparing effect of megavoltage is because the maximum dose deposited by the megavoltage beams is deep to the skin. Note also the improved depth dose for megavoltage.

lowed clinicians to employ tumor doses that were considerably increased over historical values. It is fair to say that modern RT began with the introduction of this modality.

Since the early 1980s, linear accelerators with even higher energy x-rays (4–18 MeV) have become commercially available. Linear accelerators have better skin-sparing qualities than Co^{60} and a better dose at depth. In addition, a radiation beam from a linear accelerator has a sharper "edge" than a beam generated by Co^{60}, which means that tighter, more precise tumor targeting is possible. A drawback of linear accelerators is that they are among the most complicated and expensive pieces of equipment typically found in routine hospital use.

The radiation absorbed dose (formerly called a *rad*) is now measured in joules/kilogram or Grays (Gy). In the treatment of cancer, typical total radiation doses are 60 to 70 Gy, also written 6000 to 7000 cGy (100 cGy = 1 Gy). The terms *Gy* and *cGy* are preferred over the old term *rad* because the latter measure did not comply with international metric system standards. One cGy = 1 rad.

RADIATION BIOLOGY

The most important target molecule for radiation is DNA, which can be damaged directly or indirectly by intermediate radiation products such as free radicals. The inflicted injury is a combination of reversible and irreversible damage. As a result, a cell survival curve (surviving logarithm of the fraction of cells versus radiation dose) has a complex shape, which typically looks like that seen in Figure 9–2. It has an initial linear shape in the low dose range, followed by a shoulder. At higher doses, the curve becomes steeper and straight again. The experimental data are best fitted to a mathematical model using a linear quadratic equation, known as the *α,β model:*

$$\text{Surviving Fraction of Cells} = e^{-(\alpha \cdot \text{Dose} + \beta \cdot \text{Dose}^2)}$$

This model illustrates that there are two components of cell killing, one proportional to the dose ($\alpha \cdot$ Dose) and the other proportional to the dose squared ($\beta \cdot \text{Dose}^2$).

The clinical significance of the α,β model is that when radiation treatment is given so that normal tissue receives only a small dose of radiation during each treatment, most of the damage will be reversible, typically within 4 to 6 hours. However, if at the same time the tumor receives a large radiation dose (because the radiation beams are designed to overlap only on the tumor), the tumor will sustain more damage than will normal tissue (because of the higher dose) and will also have proportionally more irreversible damage because of the increased dose per fraction. This simplistic statement suggests that we should seek to break the total radiation dose into small fractions so that the damage received by normal tissue will be as reversible as possible. The problem with giving only a small dose of radiation at each treatment setting is that the total time to complete the radiation treatment will be extended. Because the tumor is presumably growing throughout the treatment course, extending the total treatment time will necessarily reduce the probability of tumor control because it increases the total amount of tumor that must be killed. Some balance is therefore needed between keeping the dose per fraction small while not increasing overall treatment time.

One approach to decreasing the dose per fraction and yet shortening overall treatment time is to use *hyperfractionation,* usually defined as more than five fractions per week. The value of twice-daily radiation has been tested in patients with SCLC with positive results[8] and in those with NSCLC with unclear results.[9–11] An extreme form of hyperfractionation, the so-called *CHART* (continuous hyperfractionated accelerated radiation therapy) regimen that used three fractions per day, has resulted in improved 2-year survival rates in patients with locally advanced NSCLC.[12]

CLINICAL RADIATION THERAPY

The use of radiation as a treatment modality involves the coordination of the radiation oncologist, radiation physicist,

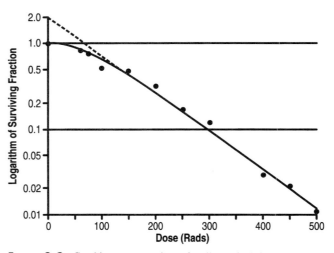

FIGURE 9–2. Graphic representation of cell survival in response to increasing doses of radiation. (From Puck and Marcus.[73] Reproduced from J Exp Med 1956;103:653–666, by copyright permission of the Rockefeller University Press.)[73]

dosimetrist, radiation therapist, and nursing staff. Because this terminology is without exact counterpart in other oncologic disciplines, the role of each of these clinicians is described briefly.

The Radiation Oncologist

The radiation oncologist is a physician who is responsible for the overall management of the patient. The first task of the radiation oncologist is to obtain a patient history and carry out a physical examination so as to be able to judge whether or not the patient should be treated with radiation. Important information that must be gathered in this process includes tumor type, stage, and patient characteristics (eg, comorbid illnesses, pulmonary reserve, and ability to tolerate treatment). Once it has been decided that the patient could benefit from radiation treatment, specific goals need to be determined. Options include an attempt at cure, palliation, or even prevention of foreseeable problems (eg, cranial prophylaxis).

If it is believed that the patient could be helped by radiation treatment, the radiation oncologist will initiate a process known as *treatment planning*. As a first step in radiation treatment planning, the radiation oncologist must define the gross tumor volume (GTV) from the appropriate radiologic studies and from the physical examination. Defining the GTV is usually straightforward, but distinguishing tumor from collapsed lung on computed tomography (CT) scans can sometimes be quite problematic. A more difficult task is that of determining the most likely areas of microscopic tumor spread, known as the *clinical tumor volume* (CTV). Tumor is usually present at least several millimeters outside the GTV because of direct microscopic spread, but it may also be present in ipsilateral hilar or mediastinal lymph nodes, distant from the primary tumor. Clinical judgment and experience are the main guides to defining the CTV. Finally, a planning target volume (PTV) is designated by adding a margin to the CTV to allow for both external and internal (cardiac and respiratory) tumor motion.

The Radiation Physicist

The radiation physicist is perhaps unique in medicine. Typically he or she holds either a master's degree or PhD in medical physics and is specifically trained to ensure that the patient receives the prescribed radiation dose. This requires constant monitoring of the treatment equipment itself and of the design of patient-specific treatment plans, which are intended to produce a high radiation dose across the PTV while limiting the dose to nearby radiation-sensitive structures. In the treatment of lung cancer, the organs of highest concern are the spinal cord, normal lung, esophagus, heart, brachial plexus, and sometimes liver. The radiation oncologist is responsible for making the final decision as to whether to implement a given treatment or to return to the computer and create alternative treatment plans.

The Radiation Dosimetrist and Radiation Therapist

The radiation dosimetrist is responsible for calculating the treatment time for each radiation beam and for maintaining the accuracy of the treatment chart. Shielding (shaping) blocks, compensators, immobilizers, and other treatment aids are constructed by the block room technician. Before a patient is actually treated, a rehearsal of the treatment known as a simulation is performed on a special piece of radiographic equipment known as an RT simulator. The simulator allows staff to accurately mimic the geometry of a linear accelerator and still obtain diagnostic-quality radiographs to verify the placement and shape of the radiation portals.

During treatment, low-quality localizing (portal) films are obtained on the linear accelerator and compared with the simulation films to ensure accurate beam placement. Portal films are usually taken once a week, but they may be taken more often in problematic cases. The radiation therapist, formerly called a *radiation therapy technologist* or technician, has the responsibility of delivering the treatment plan. Dosimetry checks and chart reviews are performed on a regular basis for quality assurance.

Nursing Staff

Close follow-up of the patient, both during and after radiation treatment, is the responsibility of the nursing staff and treating radiation oncologist. In addition to tending to general medical problems, the clinical team caring for the patient undergoing RT for lung cancer must anticipate and treat radiation-induced esophagitis, pneumonitis, and dermatitis, as well as monitor the patient's complete blood counts. Also, there must be constant review of the radiation doses delivered, especially to dose-critical organs such as the spinal cord. Typically, the patient is seen by the clinical team at least once a week during treatment for this purpose.

RADIATION TREATMENT PLANNING

Traditional or Two-Dimensional Treatment Planning

Traditionally, RT planning has been accomplished by drawing an outline of the CTV on a diagnostic chest radiograph. Defining the CTV this way is subject to many errors because it is often difficult to differentiate tumor from other structures and from collapsed lung, especially on oblique projections. Also, mediastinal lymph nodes will not be visible unless they are markedly enlarged. As a result, tumor targeting errors are not uncommon and almost certainly result in a decreased cure rate (Table 9–1).

This traditional or two-dimensional (2-D) approach to treatment planning is limiting in at least two other ways. First, even if the CTV is identified correctly on a chest radiograph acquired in the anterior-posterior direction, this information cannot be used to design a beam oriented in another direction (eg, a 30-degree oblique angle). What is

TABLE 9–1. GEOMETRIC TUMOR MISSES AND THE EFFECT ON OUTCOME IN REVIEWS OF INDIVIDUAL RADIOTHERAPY TREATMENT PLANS OF RANDOMIZED STUDIES

STUDY	N	MAJOR ERRORS (%)[a]	MINOR ERRORS (%)[b]	DID IT MATTER?[c]
RTOG 83-11[13]	832	6	22	Yes
RTOG 73-01[48]	316	12	—	Probably
EORTC 8844[71]	177	15	17	—
CALGB 8433[39]	155	23	—	Probably
SWOG 7628[72]	140	31	—	Yes

Inclusion criteria: Multi-institutional randomized trials from 1980 to 2000 reporting error rates.

[a] As defined by study (usually tumor missed in at least one radiation field).
[b] As defined by study (usually tumor <1 cm from the edge of at least one radiation field).
[c] As assessed by authors of study.

CALGB, Cancer and Leukemia Group B; EORTC, European Organization for Research and Treatment of Cancer; RTOG, Radiation Therapy Oncology Group; SWOG, Southwest Oncology Group.

needed is some way to define the CTV just once, in 3-D and then project it onto a synthesized radiograph of any desired angle. Such a system would then free the clinician to select the best beam geometry in terms of the least collateral damage to surrounding normal structures. Second, 2-D planning does not allow one to calculate the volume of normal lung (or other organs) receiving an excessive radiation dose in a given plan. Such dose-volume data is now known to correlate with radiation injury to the lung[13] and other organs.[14]

Three-Dimensional Treatment Planning

By the 1980s, a technique known as *CT-based treatment planning* made it possible to overlay CT slices with the radiation dose distribution calculated from a traditionally designed treatment plan. Using this technique, the radiation oncologist could clearly see what dose various organs would receive, including the volume of normal lung that would receive a high radiation dose. If the plan was not satisfactory, it could be modified slightly, but major changes required another patient simulation. What was needed was a way to test dozens of plans quickly and accurately without having to involve the patient each time.

Full 3-D treatment planning systems that allow one to build and manipulate 3-D patient models and to design and display entire 3-D treatment plans became available in the 1990s and are still undergoing refinement. Such systems permit one to view a treatment plan either on a succession of CT slices or on a synthetic radiograph and to make alterations to the plan interactively. Figure 9–3 (see color section at front of book) is a screen shot of one such system. The clinician can see at a glance which organs are in the radiation field, how well the tumor is covered, and how much lung is being treated. Because the system is interactive, dozens or hundreds of variations can be quickly reviewed. State-of-the-art treatment planning systems also allow data from multiple imaging studies to be used in the planning process so that positron-emission tomography

(PET) scans, for example, can be used to help define the GTV.[15] In addition, such systems allow modulation of the incident radiation beams to ensure a uniform tumor dose and the lowest possible dose to surrounding dose-critical tissue. Several centers have begun using these technologies to push radiation doses for NSCLC past the traditional levels of 60 to 70 Gy. Preliminary studies indicate that doses of 74 Gy or more are probably safe, if delivered carefully, and may be beneficial.[16,17]

ASSESSMENT OF RESPONSE TO TREATMENT

Radiographic Response

Shrinkage of lung cancer on radiographs obtained during or following treatment with RT can be readily appreciated and provides a sense of optimism to both the patient and the physician that the treatment is effective. However, several important caveats apply. First, a rapid reduction in tumor size is not prognostic for tumor control. Most mammalian cells, including lung cancers, do not express radiation damage until they enter mitosis. This means that a tumor that responds quickly to radiation may actually be growing rapidly and may recur after a short time if it is not completely destroyed. Conversely, a tumor that responds slowly to radiation may, nevertheless, be completely controlled, although it may take 6 months or more for all of the tumor to die. Second, differentiating tumor from obstructive atelectasis, radiation-induced edema, or fibrosis on radiographs or even CT can sometimes be difficult. A rapid resolution of these problems may be mistaken for tumor response. Perhaps the most encouraging radiographic sign is long-term stability at the tumor site. PET scanning, which images rapidly metabolizing cells, has shown a sensitivity of 97% to 100% and a specificity of 62% to 100% in distinguishing tumor from fibrosis[18,19] and may become an important way to follow patients after radiation therapy.

Because of these considerations, care must be taken in interpreting studies that use radiographic response as a measure of local tumor control. Using the definition of *partial response* (PR) as meaning a 50% reduction in tumor size by two perpendicular measurements and *complete response* (CR) as meaning the absence of any radiographic or clinical signs of persistent tumor, objective response rates (PR + CR) of >50% following radiation have been reported consistently.[20–23] The real issue, however, is whether radiographic response correlates with long-term survival or local control. There is little data examining this question.

Pathologic Response

A number of papers using data from either autopsy or preoperative studies have reported a *pathologic complete response rate* (pCR) of 15% to 50%,[24–28] which is defined as the absence of any microscopically visible tumor. In a series of 60 autopsies performed at different times after primary treatment with CO[60] radiation using doses from 40

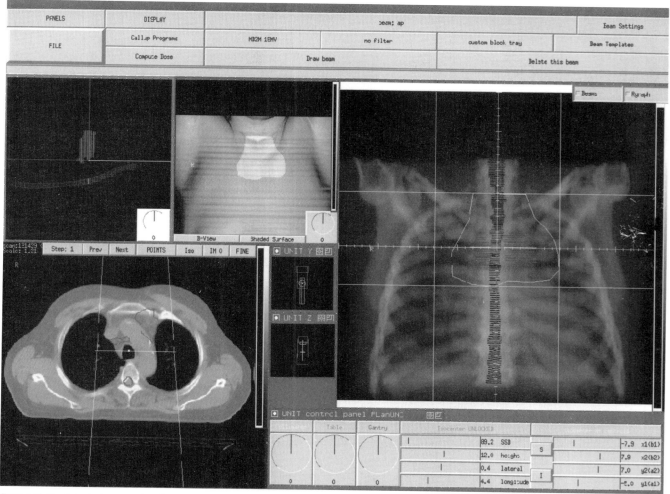

FIGURE 9–3. A typical screen shot from the three-dimensional treatment planning system used at the University of North Carolina. (See color section after the Table of Contents.)

to 70 Gy, Rissanen et al[26] found a 30% pCR at the primary tumor site. Eichhorn[25] demonstrated a 53% pCR in patients treated with 55 Gy using 2.5-Gy fractions. He also reported a 13% response rate when delivering the same dose in larger fractions (6-10 Gy). This data is supported by several series involving preoperative RT for both SCLC and NSCLC. Kirschner[28] found a 15% pCR in patients treated with 35 Gy. The Veterans Administration Lung Cancer Group[24] found a 27% pCR in 339 patients treated with 30 to 60 Gy. In an early provocative study that spurred much interest in radiation, Bloedorn et al[27] found a 54% pCR in 26 patients who received 50 to 60 Gy preoperatively. In conclusion, multiple studies have shown pCR rates of approximately 30% in patients given radiation, and the response rates appear to be slightly better with increasing doses of radiation. None of these studies correlated the pathologic response with the preoperative radiographic response.

Local Control

The value of RT, which is a local treatment modality, is best assessed by determining the rate of local tumor control.

However, as discussed earlier, the assessment of local recurrence is hampered by the difficulty of differentiating radiation-induced scarring from a recurrent tumor. More important, an analysis of recurrence patterns is hampered in most studies by a lack of clear and consistent definitions. Some studies report only first site of recurrence, whereas others report recurrence occurring at any time. After the first site of recurrence has appeared, it is likely that subsequent recurrences are underreported. With these caveats in mind, it appears that locoregional recurrence and combined recurrence (simultaneous locoregional and distant recurrence) account for approximately 75% of treatment failures. Rosenthal et al[29] found the first site of recurrence to be local in 55% of 62 patients with clinical stage II disease who were given a mean dose of 60 Gy. Reinfuss et al[30], reporting on ultimate sites of recurrence in 332 stage III patients who were given 40-Gy split-course radiation, found that 62% of patients died of locoregional recurrence, 26% died of both distant and locoregional recurrence, and only 2% died of distant disease alone. Similar results were reported by Dosoretz et al[5] in 152 patients who were clinically staged as N0. In this study, 70% of the cumulative recurrences at 4 years involved local or combined local and distant recurrences. In a study of 551 patients

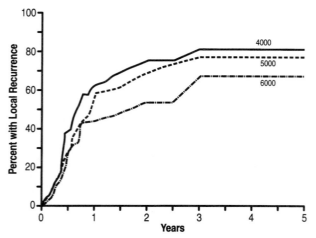

FIGURE 9–4. Chronologic appearance of recurrences within irradiated volume as first site of relapse according to treatment (dose of irradiation) in Radiation Therapy Oncology Group protocol 73-01. (From Cancer, Vol 59, No. 11, 1987, 1874–1881. Copyright © 1987 American Cancer Society. Reprinted by permission of Wiley-Liss, Inc., a subsidiary of John Wiley & Sons, Inc.[31])

(Radiation Therapy Oncology Group [RTOG] 73-01 and 73-02), Perez et al[31] found the *first* site of recurrence to be 44% local, 22% combined, and 34% distant, whereas the *ultimate* patterns of recurrence were 23% local, 54% combined, and 23% distant. It appears that local control is even worse when more careful investigations, such as bronchoscopy, are employed. Arriagada et al[32] found eventual local failure in 92% of carefully followed patients with stage IIIa and IIIb disease. In a difference that probably represents the method of assessment and reporting more than anything else, Mantravadi et al[21] found the first site of recurrence to be local in 12%, as opposed to combined recurrence in 58% and distant recurrence in only 30% of 267 patients with stage III disease.

The report by Mantravadi et al[21] suggested better locoregional control with increasing radiation doses. The authors of the Dosoretz paper[5] also made this claim strongly, but the data presented does not support it, with the exception of only four patients given a dose of at least 70 Gy. The RTOG protocols 73-01 and 73-02 demonstrated slightly better local control with increasing doses of radiotherapy (40-60 Gy) in a prospective randomized study of 551 patients, most of whom had stage IIIa and stage IIIb disease

(Figure 9–4).[31] This was statistically significant for both squamous cell and non–squamous histologic cell types.

In conclusion, the first site of recurrence in irradiated patients involves a locoregional site in at least 75% of patients. Increasing the radiation dose from 40 to 60 Gy has been shown to decrease the local failure rate. Increasing doses of radiation above 60 Gy may reduce the rate further, but this remains to be proven.

Survival

The ultimate goal of treatment for lung cancer patients is long-term survival. Although this endpoint is objective, use of this measure to identify predictors of success or failure with RT can be misleading. In many reports, few details are given regarding whether patients were adequately staged to rule out distant metastases. It should be noted that the false-negative rate of a normal history and physical examination is approximately 30% in patients with stage IIIa and IIIb disease (see Table 6–3). It would make little sense to assess the curative effect of local RT in such patients who actually have measurable distant metastases. Furthermore, given the high incidence of occult micrometastatic disease in patients with stage IIIa and IIIb disease,[33–36] it would be difficult to show an impact on overall survival by a local modality such as RT, even if there is no demonstrable M1 disease. Nevertheless, most series of patients with locally advanced lung cancer report a long-term survival rate of 5% to 10% in those treated with radiation alone.[3,9,31,37–39]

RADIOTHERAPY TREATMENT PARAMETERS

Total Dose

The dose of RT used in the curative treatment of lung cancer has generally been the in range of 60 to 66 Gy, but the optimal dose has not been defined. Four retrospective studies have demonstrated statistically significant improvement in survival following treatment with higher radiation doses. Dosoretz et al[5] found a survival benefit at 2 years for 152 cN0,1 patients treated with 60 to 69 Gy compared with 50 to 59 Gy. Unfortunately, this benefit was not

DATA SUMMARY: ASSESSMENT OF RESPONSE TO RADIOTHERAPY			
	AMOUNT	**QUALITY**	**CONSISTENCY**
Conventional RT alone results in cure in 5% to 10% of patients with locally advanced NSCLC	High	High	High
RT results in pathologic CR rates of approximately 25%	High	Poor	Mod
Local control is achieved in approximately 25% of patients with locally advanced NSCLC using conventional RT	High	Poor	Mod
Increasing RT doses from 40-60 Gy improves the local control rate	**Poor**	**High**	—
Standard RT treatment planning practices and doses result in a 15% major treatment error rate	High	Mod	High

Type of data rated: Plain text: descriptive statements   *Italics: controlled comparison*   **Bold: Randomized comparison**

sustained at 4 years. Mantravadi et al[21] analyzed 267 stage III patients and found that survival at 2 years was 21% in patients treated with 55 to 65 Gy, 11% in patients treated with 45 to 55 Gy, and only 4% in patients receiving <45 Gy. Another analysis of 427 patients, 60% of whom had stage III disease treated with split-course radiation, found a 26% 2-year survival rate in patients treated with >70 Gy compared with an 11% rate in those treated with 60 to 66 Gy.[37] An Australian retrospective study of 941 patients also found better survival (P <0.0001) with higher doses (median survival, 6 months for 20 Gy, 9 months for 30-36 Gy, and 14 months for 60 Gy).[40] However, in these retrospective nonrandomized series, the dose given may reflect that patients given lower doses had unfavorable characteristics (eg, performance status, extent of disease). This was clearly the case in at least two of these studies.[21,40]

Only two large randomized series involving different dosages are available. A slightly better survival at 2 years was seen with RT doses of 60 Gy compared with 40 and 50 Gy in 365 inoperable patients with NSCLC in RTOG study 73-01, but this was not sustained at 5 years.[31] In RTOG study 83-11, hyperfractionated RT in doses up to 79 Gy was given to 848 patients with stage III NSCLC.[9] When the entire group was analyzed, there was a slight trend toward better survival at doses >60 Gy. When only the subset of 212 favorable risk stage IIIa (N2) patients was analyzed, there was a statistically significant benefit to treatment with 69.6 Gy. However, higher radiation dosages actually resulted in poorer survival. This may be due to an imbalance of disease extent that favored the lower dose group (stage II/IIIb = 24%/24% at 60 Gy versus 8%/37% at 79 Gy).

It is rather disappointing that large randomized studies such as those conducted by the RTOG have failed to show a clear survival benefit with increasing dosages. Using the experience with other tumors in different locations suggests that oncologists may not have reached a dose at which radiation is likely to be effective in lung cancer patients, especially considering the large size of most lung cancers subjected to RT (Table 9–2). Although the randomized RTOG study 83-11[9] explored doses up to 79 Gy, there was a significant unfavorable imbalance of extent of disease at the higher doses of radiation. Therefore, this issue has really not been tested in a randomized fashion at dose levels that are likely to show a benefit. Furthermore, when one considers the high rate of distant metastases in patients with stage III NSCLC, it should not be surprising that

TABLE 9–2. RELATIONSHIP OF TYPICAL TUMOR SIZE, RADIATION DOSE, AND USUAL LOCAL CONTROL RATES FOR VARIOUS TUMORS

TUMOR EXAMPLE	DIAMETER	TYPICAL DOSE (Gy)	CONTROL RATE
Microscopic breast	<1 mm	50	Excellent
Larynx	1–2 mm	60	Excellent
Prostate	2–3 cm	≥70	Fair to good
Cervix	3–5 cm	75–85	Fair to good
Non–small cell lung cancer	5–10 cm	60–66	Poor

Inclusion criteria: Authors' assessment of efficacy of radiotherapy for different types of cancer.

the survival benefit gained by manipulation of dosage or fractionation has been of only marginal significance.

Treatment Schedule

Split-course radiation, which involves a rest period of several weeks after the delivery of the first half of the dose, may be advantageous for patients who are very ill because of their disease or a comorbid condition or who have underlying conditions that could render them intolerant of radiation. For these patients, the first half of therapy could be considered a test dose. If their condition continues to deteriorate, the radiation can be stopped at that point without subjecting them to the time necessary for an entire course of therapy. If metastatic disease develops during the break, the initial course could be considered palliative, and, again, the treatment (at least to the chest) could be aborted at that time. If the patient tolerates the treatment well and actually improves, the second course can be given without the worry that local control has been compromised by the treatment break.

Split-course radiation for curative intent is used more commonly in Europe, but is considered to be inferior in the United States because of the concern that tumor cells may repopulate during the break in radiation treatment. There is little evidence to support this theory in lung cancer patients, however. Haffty et al[41] studied split-course radiation in a 43-patient randomized trial that weakly suggested that the split-course radiation was inferior to conventional radiation. Katz and Alberts[42] found no difference in response rates, local control, or survival in 171 well-matched but nonrandomized patients treated with either continuous or split-course radiation to 55 to 65 Gy. In an earlier randomized study of 363 patients treated with 50 to 55 Gy continuous or split-course radiation, Holsti and Mattson[43] showed essentially identical survival curves. The RTOG conducted a study in the 1970s (RTOG 73-01) that randomized 365 patients with stage III lung cancer to receive either 40-Gy split-course radiation or continuous radiation.[22] Although the radiographic CR rate was lower in the split-course group, the total response rate (CR + PR) was no different in the split-course and the continuous radiation groups treated to 40 Gy. The survival rates for the two arms were also found to be essentially the same (34% versus 38% at 1 year, split-course versus continuous radiation). An analysis of the rate of recurrence within the irradiated volume suggests a minimal (nonsignificant) benefit to continuous versus split-course radiation at doses of 40 Gy (53% versus 58%, respectively).[31]

Fractionation

The term *fractionation* in RT refers to the way in which the total radiation dose is delivered. Typically, 1.8 to 2.0 Gy/day is given for 5 days each week. Hypofractionation generally means that the radiation is divided into a smaller number of fractions (larger dose per fraction) given fewer times per week. More than five fractions per week is known as *hyperfractionation,* and more than 10 Gy/week is known as *accelerated fractionation.* Frequently these two approaches are combined into hyperfractionated accelerated RT (HART). When treatment is continued unaltered over the weekend, it is known as CHART.

Various fractionation schedules have been proposed to take advantage of differences between tumor and normal tissue biology in an attempt to increase tumor control without increasing complications. However, the therapeutic ratio of radiation treatment is related to time-dose considerations in a complex fashion that is still poorly understood, and identification of the optimal regimen for a particular tumor is somewhat empirical.

Hypofractionation

Only a few studies of hypofractionation as curative treatment in lung cancer have been carried out. An early autopsy series found an inferior pCR rate with hypofractionation.[25] This was found consistently with various schedules and was more pronounced the fewer fractions that were used. More recently, the University of Maryland randomized 120 patients to 60 Gy of radiation given in 30 fractions (2.0 Gy 5 days per week × 6 weeks) versus 12 fractions (5 Gy 1 day per week for 12 weeks).[44] The CR rate was somewhat better with hypofractionation (26% versus 17%), and 2-year survival was slightly better (29% versus 23%), but these differences were not statistically significant.[44] Thus, the limited data available about hypofractionation schedules are inconclusive.

Hyperfractionation

Several studies conducted by the RTOG suggest that the survival after hyperfractionated RT is better than that after standard RT given to historical, relatively well-matched controls.[45,46] In order to investigate this issue further, a prospective randomized trial involving 452 stage IIb, IIIa, and IIIb patients has been conducted by the RTOG and the Eastern Cooperative Oncology Group (ECOG).[10,11] This study compared 60 Gy of standard fractionation RT with 69.6 Gy hyperfractionated (twice daily) RT. A third arm involved induction chemotherapy followed by standard radiation to 60 Gy (Dillman regimen). The median survival and 4-year survival were 11.4 months and 4% in the standard fractionation arm and 12.2 months and 9% in the twice-daily hyperfractionation arm, a difference that was not statistically significant.[11] However, a trial with SCLC found that 45 Gy given twice daily concurrent with chemotherapy offers improved survival compared with once-daily radiation given under the same circumstances.[8] Thus, some data suggests that hyperfractionated RT may be slightly better than standard-course treatment in SCLC, but no clear benefit has been demonstrated in NSCLC.

Accelerated hyperfractionation also employs two to three fractions of radiation per day. However, the fraction size and total dose are similar to those used in conventional treatment, and, as a consequence, the treatment time is shorter. A randomized study in 563 patients with locally advanced NSCLC reported significantly better 2-year survival with accelerated hyperfractionation compared with conventional RT (29% versus 20%, $P = 0.004$).[12] This improvement came at the price of an increase in acute esophagitis (19% versus 3%), but this resolved over the course of 1 month.[12]

Table 9–3 summarizes this data. A direct comparison of

TABLE 9–3. REPRESENTATIVE TUMOR RESPONSE RATES AND SURVIVAL IN NON–SMALL CELL LUNG CANCER WITH VARIOUS RADIATION SCHEDULES AND DOSAGES (NO CHEMOTHERAPY GIVEN)

STUDY	N	DOSE	CR + PR RATE (%)	2-YEAR SURVIVAL (%)
Perez et al[22,31]	103	40 Gy conventional RT	47	12
Perez et al[22,31]	85	60 Gy conventional RT	65	20
Komaki et al[11]	154	69.6 Gy HF RT	—	24
Saunders et al[12]	338	54 Gy CHART	—	29

Inclusion criteria: Data from major phase III trials employing different RT treatment strategies in inoperable, locally advanced non–small cell lung cancer.

CHART, continuous hyperfractionated accelerated radiotherapy; Conventional RT, five daily fractions per week; CR + PR, complete and partial response rate; HF, hyperfractionated; RT, radiotherapy.

these trials cannot be made because of issues of patient selection, disease extent, and single versus multi-institutional data. However, this table does suggest that the optimal fractionation has not been defined and that further exploration of these issues may result in an RT approach that is more beneficial than the older standard of 60 Gy in five fractions per week over 6 weeks.

Tumor Size

Several studies have suggested better response rates for patients with earlier-stage tumors[21,23,47,48] or smaller-sized tumors.[49] Survival was also found to be significantly better for an earlier T stage, as is shown in Table 9–4.[5,20,45,50–52] A number of studies have shown statistically significant better survival rates for patients with smaller tumors.[5,49,53,54] Significantly better survival was noted for those with smaller tumors (<4 cm versus ≥4 cm) by Krol et al,[49] who studied 108 patients with N0 disease treated with 60 Gy (3-year survival, 35% versus 11%; $P = 0.003$). Similar findings were noted by Dosoretz et al[5] in 152 patients who were clinically classified as N0, as well as by Coy and Kennelly.[53] Sandler et al[54] also found a significant difference in survival in tumors <3 cm in 77 cN0 patients ($P = 0.009$), but they found little difference in the rates of local recurrence. This latter finding suggests that the poorer survival with larger tumors may have less to do with the effectiveness of RT than with an increased likelihood of occult metastatic disease at the time of presentation. Other sources of data, however, indicate that the ability to suc-

TABLE 9–4. SURVIVAL AFTER PRIMARY RADIOTHERAPY RELATIVE TO T STAGE

STUDY	N	N STATUS	2-y SURVIVAL (%) T1	T2,3	T4	P
Cox et al[45]	516	cN2	21	18	12	0.06
Gauden et al[51]	347	cN0	32	21	—	0.05
Dosoretz et al[5]	152	cN0,1	55	22	—	0.006
Hazuka et al[50]	88	cN0-3	67	35	23	0.06
Noordijk et al[20]	50	cN0	69	45	—	0.06

cessfully treat patients is related to the tumor size itself, even in patients with N2,3 disease. In a study of 283 stage IIIa and IIIb patients in whom metastatic disease was excluded, a tumor size ≥ 70 cm^2 was associated with significantly worse survival (3-year survival, 0 versus 20%; $P < 0.01$), whereas no difference was found with respect to stage, age, and various other commonly cited prognostic factors.[55] In conclusion, data from several sources indicates that radiation is more effective in smaller tumors, in terms of both clinical response and survival.

Size of Radiation Fields

Although minimizing tissue damage is a complex problem, there can be little doubt that limiting radiation field sizes will reduce pulmonary toxicity. However, the desire to reduce the amount of normal lung treated must not compromise tumor coverage. No randomized controlled studies have been conducted to date to correlate the effect of field size on tumor control, but a few smaller studies report the consequences of using a limited versus an expanded radiation field in the treatment of lung cancer. In patients who are clinically N0, the results achieved without using any mediastinal radiation as reported by Krol et al[49] are not obviously different from series in which mediastinal irradiation was included.[41,56] In a retrospective analysis of 70 patients who were mostly cN1,2, those treated with limited-field irradiation to the primary tumor and ipsilateral mediastinum (median field size 90 cm^2) actually had better survival (1-year crude survival, 41% versus 19%) than patients treated with an extended field (median field size, 225 cm^2).[57,58] In a more recent analysis of 88 patients using modern beam-focusing techniques, Hazuka et al[50] found no difference in survival or local control when small fields (primary tumor and ipsilateral mediastinum) were used as opposed to larger fields (including contralateral mediastinal and hilar as well as supraclavicular areas).

In a study of 126 patients with stage IIIa,b NSCLC, the failure rate in the untreated contralateral supraclavicular area was 8%, and there were no failures in the contralateral hilum.[59] This is consistent with a study of 266 patients with IIIa,b NSCLC in whom the incidence of radiographic involvement of the supraclavicular areas was <10% (9% ipsilateral, 3% contralateral) and of the contralateral hilar lymph nodes was 4%.[60] These studies suggest that inclusion of the contralateral hilum and probably also of the supraclavicular areas adds little to the RT of IIIa,b lung cancer. These small failure rates may not warrant the use of extended-field radiation, which does not seem to improve survival and may significantly add to the morbidity of the treatment. Current practice is not to include an uninvolved contralateral hilum, but the elective inclusion of part or all of the supraclavicular fossae remains controversial.

TOXICITY OF RADIOTHERAPY

Incidence

The incidence of toxicity due to RT is generally low. The best data regarding toxicity is found in the large prospective studies conducted by the RTOG, which involved careful, systematic patient follow-up. Severe toxicity is defined as *serious* (grade 3), *life-threatening* (grade 4), or *fatal* (grade 5), according to explicit RTOG criteria. Acute toxicity usually occurs within 90 days of completing treatment and is often self-limited, whereas late toxicity is usually related to irreversible tissue damage and may develop 6 to 18 months or longer after the end of treatment.

In the RTOG 73-01 study, which involved 365 patients treated with 40 to 60 Gy of radiation, mild or moderate toxicity (grade 1 or 2) was seen in 35% of patients, grade 3 toxicity in 8%, and grade 4 toxicity in 2%.[23] No fatalities were recorded. This data includes both acute and chronic toxicities; pulmonary toxicity accounted for approximately 60% of the complications. No increase in toxicity was seen in the higher-dose groups compared with the lower-dose groups.

More detailed data is available from the RTOG 83-11 study, which used hyperfractionated (twice daily) radiation in 848 patients in doses ranging from 60 to 79.2 Gy. No significant differences in either acute or chronic toxicity were seen relative to the dose given, although a slight trend toward increased acute pulmonary toxicity was noted with increasing doses.[9] Severe acute toxicity was seen in 11% of the patients and involved grade 3 toxicity in 90% and grade 4 toxicity in 10% of patients. The acute toxicity involved pulmonary complications in 33% and esophagitis in 53%. The incidence of late toxicity increased over time, but even with adequate follow-up was seen in only 8% of all patients in the RTOG 83-11 study, despite the high doses of RT given. Seventy-five percent of the late toxicities occurred within 12 months, and almost all late toxicity had developed by 24 months. Eighty-three percent of the late complications were grade 3 and 14% were grade 4. Two fatal toxicities (0.2%) were reported in the 848 patients. Most of the late toxicities were pulmonary (82%), with cardiac toxicities accounting for another 9%.[9] Thus, even with the high doses of RT given in this study, the incidence of severe acute or late toxicity was quite low.

Pulmonary Toxicity

Radiation-induced pulmonary toxicity may occur early as acute pneumonitis or may develop many months following treatment as chronic fibrosis. Although the symptoms associated with either of these processes may range from mild to fatal and appear clinically similar, it is important to distinguish between acute and late toxicities because their pathophysiology is different. Acute radiation pneumonitis usually occurs within 90 days of treatment, is an inflammatory process that results in intra-alveolar and septal edema, and is accompanied by epithelial and endothelial desquamation. Although acute pneumonitis sometimes causes the patient to be short of breath, it usually responds quickly to corticosteroids and is self-limiting. Late effects are due to pulmonary fibrosis. As in radiation pneumonitis, the most common symptom of pulmonary fibrosis is respiratory compromise. Unlike acute toxicity, however, pulmonary fibrosis does not respond to corticosteroids and is chronic, limited to the radiated lung, and often progressive. Both acute and chronic pulmonary toxicity can be fatal. Three factors probably contribute to radiation pneumonitis: treatment volume, total radiation dose, and biologic predisposition.

Volume

A review of the data demonstrates that toxicity varies as a function of the volume of irradiated lung. Lingos et al[61] found that when small volumes of lung are irradiated in breast cancer patients, the treated lung is not associated with an increased incidence of pneumonitis. Tarbell et al[62] showed that treating entire lung volumes with low-dose radiation in patients with Hodgkin's lymphoma resulted in a 15% increase in the risk of pneumonitis. Martell et al[63] reported a retrospective analysis of 3-D dose distributions in the lungs of patients with Hodgkin's lymphoma and NSCLC. Patients who developed radiation pneumonitis had been treated with higher doses and larger volumes than patients who did not develop this disorder. Green and Weinstein[58] found that the incidence of radiation pneumonitis was 17% in patients who received extended-field radiation, as opposed to 7% in patients who received only involved-field radiation. The RTOG 83-11 study evaluated 832 patients in an attempt to relate pulmonary toxicity to lung volume treated.[13] An increase in $\geq$ grade 2 acute and late pulmonary toxicity was seen when excessive margins around the tumor or mediastinum were used (54% versus 37% for excessive margins encompassing >35 cm^2 of lung versus per protocol patients; no P value given). More accurate measures of volume toxicity will have to await evaluation of patients receiving 3-D treatment planning in whom the treated lung volume is well known. A preliminary analysis of 99 patients with NSCLC treated with RT suggests that the volume of lung that receives more than 20 Gy of radiation, the so-called V_{20}, is the best predictor of radiation pneumonitis.[64] If the V_{20} was <25% of the lung, no patients developed grade 3 radiation pneumonitis, and if the V_{20} was 25% to 37%, the risk was still only 2%. However, the risk of $\geq$ grade 3 radiation pneumonitis rose to 19% when the V_{20} exceeded 37%.[64] Similar results have been found by Marks et al.[65]

Curran et al[66] estimated the decrease in forced expiratory volume in 1 second (FEV_1) following irradiation by superimposing treatment portals and lung perfusion scans. They noted a 10% average decrease in FEV_1 after irradiation. When only the primary tumor was irradiated, the FEV_1 decreased 9%, but when the radiation field was extended to encompass the mediastinum or supraclavicular areas, the decrease in FEV_1 rose to 13%. However, Choi and Kanarek[67] found that estimates of posttreatment FEV_1 correlated well with actual values only in patients who had good baseline pulmonary function. Those patients with a borderline FEV_1 of <50% of that predicted, as well as those patients with an uneven distribution of perfusion to each side (suggesting atelectasis or compression by tumor), experienced little decline in FEV_1 after radiation.

Dose

Doses of radiation that cause either acute radiation pneumonitis or chronic fibrosis are not well known, and the tolerance limits are based mostly on consensus reports. In 1991, a consensus report published by the Collaborative Working Group for the Evaluation of Treatment Planning

TABLE 9–5. LUNG TOLERANCE TO RADIATION AS A FUNCTION OF DOSE AND VOLUME

LUNG VOLUME	TD 5/5 DOSE[a]	TD 50/5 DOSE[b]
Whole lung	17.5 Gy	24.5 Gy
2/3 lung	30 Gy	40 Gy
1/3 lung	45 Gy	65 Gy

Inclusion criteria: Taken from a recent expert-opinion consensus panel.

[a]The tolerated dose at which 5% of patients experience grade 4 pneumonitis within 5 years.

[b]The tolerated dose at which 50% of patients experience grade 4 pneumonitis within 5 years.

Data from Emami B, Lyman J, Brown A, et al. Tolerance of normal tissue to therapeutic irradiation. Int J Radiat Oncol Biol Phys. 1991;21:109–122.[14]

for External Beam Radiotherapy[14] concluded that the whole lung could tolerate approximately 17.5 Gy, with 5% of patients developing severe pneumonitis at 5 years. (This endpoint is also called the tolerance dose [TD] 5/5). TDs increased with decreasing lung volume, as shown in Table 9–5. We now know, based on 3-D planning, that the TD 5/5 dose estimate for one-third of the lung is far too low. Direct measurement of the effect of radiation dose on the lung is difficult. However, using single photon emission computed tomography (SPECT) scans, Marks et al[68] established a direct relationship between dose and degree of lung injury. Hayman et al[16] at the University of Michigan have now shown that, for selected patients, even high radiation doses do not cause clinical lung injury if the volumes are kept low.

Biologic Predisposition

Why some patients develop pulmonary toxicity and others who received the same treatment do not remains uncertain. This observation suggests that a biologic predisposition for radiation pneumonitis may exist in a subset of patients. Marks et al[65,69] showed that the extent of alteration in whole-lung function (ie, symptoms or pulmonary function changes), appeared to be related to both dose-volume and preradiation pulmonary function parameters. Anscher et al[70] showed that changes in plasma transforming growth factor-beta 1 (TGF-β_1) levels during RT appeared to be useful for identifying patients at risk for the development of symptomatic radiation pneumonitis, particularly in the subset of patients whose pretreatment TGF-β_1 levels were >7.5 ng/mL. Furthermore, most radiation oncologists recognize that patients with poor lung function will not tolerate RT well, and thus they decline to treat patients who have an FEV_1 <0.9 L.

Toxicity to Other Organs

Other toxicities that commonly occur after radiation to the thorax include acute skin reactions, acute esophagitis, pericarditis, and late esophageal strictures. Although most of the supporting data for defining tolerance limits is based on skin reactions, tolerance dose data for whole or partial radiation to multiple organ systems has been compiled. Radiation-induced injury to nonpulmonary organs is also based on treatment volume, total dose, and biologic predisposition. Thus, variability exists among patients treated

DATA SUMMARY: RADIOTHERAPY TREATMENT PARAMETERS AND TOXICITY

	AMOUNT	QUALITY	CONSISTENCY
Increasing RT doses from 40-60 Gy in patients with locally advanced NSCLC does not improve 5-year survival	Poor	High	—
Survival after split-course RT is the same as after continuous-course RT	Mod	Mod	High
Hyperfractionated RT results in a survival benefit in patients with SCLC	Poor	High	—
Hyperfractionated RT results in a nonsignificant trend toward better survival in patients with NSCLC	Poor	High	—
CHART results in better survival in patients with locally advanced NSCLC	Poor	High	—
Survival after RT is worse in patients with larger tumors	High	Poor	High
Severe (grade 3, 4) acute and late toxicity from conventional RT and HF RT occurs in 10% of patients	Mod	High	High
Fatal (grade 5) toxicity due to conventional or HF RT occurs in <1% of patients	Mod	High	High

Type of data rated: Plain text: descriptive statement *Italics: controlled comparison* **Bold: randomized comparison**

with similar radiation regimens, and there is always uncertainty in predicting the degree of toxicity in a given patient.

EDITORS' COMMENTS

RT is a major modality in the treatment of lung cancer. Since the early 1970s, RT has been the primary treatment for most patients with locally advanced NSCLC, either as an intervention with intent to cure or as a palliative measure. Furthermore, RT is used in the majority of patients with stage IV disease to palliate symptoms and improve quality of life. RT has also played a major role in the treatment of patients with SCLC, either as a potentially curative treatment together with chemotherapy in patients with limited-stage disease or as palliative treatment in patients with extensive-stage disease. It is important for clinicians to have some insight into a modality that is used for so many patients with lung cancer.

Even more important is the observation that RT is currently undergoing a profound change. The availability of the linear accelerator brought about substantial improvements in RT in the mid-1970s, and the current developments represent a similar major advance. These include technologic improvements in RT equipment such as 3-D conformal treatment planning systems, a better understanding of the physical and biologic determinants of radiation toxicity, and the advent of active chemotherapy.

Since the early 1980s, 60 Gy of RT, delivered in daily fractions 5 times per week over 6 weeks, has been accepted as the standard curative treatment for patients with locally advanced NSCLC. This regimen was adopted not so much because of demonstrated efficacy but rather because it could be delivered with the available equipment without incurring significant toxicity. For many years there was little interest in exploring higher doses or altered fractionation schemes because of fear of toxicity using conventional planning techniques. This concern was based more on anecdotal experiences than on a clear understanding of the determinants of toxicity, partly because methods to study this in a sophisticated manner were not available. Unquestioning acceptance of the status quo was also fueled by a sense of nihilism about the treatment of patients with inoperable lung cancer.

The fact that major treatment errors have been consistently reported in 15% of patients treated with conventional techniques during the 1980s and 1990s points out the limitations of conventional planning techniques, even in the hands of experienced radiation oncologists. Whether these cases really represent treatment errors may be debatable, but, at the very least, conventional planning allowed for a major disagreement among experienced radiation oncologists about the treatment plan in 15% of patients. The fact that this was found in the context of national treatment protocols, as well as the consistency of this finding, lends it credibility.

Fortunately, many radiation oncologists were not willing to accept the status quo, and, as a result, RT for lung cancer is currently on the threshold of a major advance. Much needs to be learned about how to make the best use of new techniques, and in many instances data to assess the impact of the changes is not yet available. However, it is clear from the available phase II and phase III studies that alterations in the fractionation schedule can lead to improved results with RT alone. This may be debatable in the case of hyperfractionated RT for patients with NSCLC. However, coupled with the evidence in treating patients with SCLC and the experience using CHART, there can be little doubt that manipulation of these parameters can be beneficial. Whether increasing the overall dose of RT above 70 Gy will translate into a survival benefit is not yet clear, but existing data and extrapolation from treatment of other tumor types suggest that this is a promising avenue to investigate. What is clear is that much higher doses than what had traditionally been thought safe can be given with little toxicity using 3-D planning technology.

These advances open up tremendous opportunities for further progress. 3-D planning technology provides a means to develop a more sophisticated understanding of the determinants of radiation toxicity. The ability to more accurately target complex tumors such as lung cancers, coupled with the ability to safely deliver higher doses of RT using different fractionation schemes, will lead to better local control. A better understanding of how to integrate these improved RT techniques with surgery and chemotherapy in a multidisciplinary manner will allow both local and systemic disease to be treated more effectively. The current developments in radiation oncology are exciting and have far-reaching implications for the large number of patients who will be diagnosed with lung cancer in the years to come.

References

1. Roswit B, Patno ME, Rapp R, et al. The survival of patients with inoperable lung cancer: a large-scale randomized study of radiation therapy versus placebo. Radiology. 1968;90:688–697.
2. Kubota K, Furuse K, Kawahara M, et al. Role of radiotherapy in combined modality treatment of locally advanced non–small-cell lung cancer. J Clin Oncol. 1994;12:1547–1552.
3. Johnson DH, Einhorn LH, Bartolucci A, et al. Thoracic radiotherapy does not prolong survival in patients with locally advanced, unresectable non–small cell lung cancer. Ann Intern Med. 1990;113:33–38.
4. Shepherd FA, Johnston MR, Payne D, et al. Randomised study of chemotherapy and surgery vs. radiotherapy for stage IIIa NSCLC: a National Cancer Institute of Canada clinical trials group study. Br J Cancer. 1998;78:603–605.
5. Dosoretz DE, Katin MJ, Blitzer PH, et al. Radiation therapy in the management of medically inoperable carcinoma of the lung: results and implications for future treatment strategies. Int J Radiat Oncol Biol Phys. 1992;24:3–9.
6. Morrison R, Deeley TJ, Cleland WP. The treatment of carcinoma of the bronchus: a clinical trial to compare surgery and supervoltage radiotherapy. Lancet. 1963;284:683–687.
7. Janssen-Heijnen MLG, Schipper RM, Razenberg PPA, et al. Prevalence of co-morbidity in lung cancer patients and its relationship with treatment: a population-based study. Lung Cancer. 1998;21:105–113.
8. Turrisi AT, Kim K, Sause W, et al. Observations after 5-year follow-up of Intergroup Trial 0096: four cycles of cis-platin, etoposide and concurrent 45 Gy thoracic radiotherapy given in daily or twice daily fractions followed by 25 Gy PCI. Survival differences and patterns of failure. Proc ASCO. 1998;17:457a.
9. Cox JD, Azarnia N, Byhardt RW, et al. A randomized phase I/II trial of hyperfractionated radiation therapy with total doses of 60.0 Gy to 79.2 Gy: possible survival benefit with >69.6 Gy in favorable patients with Radiation Therapy Oncology Group stage III non–small-cell lung carcinoma: report of Radiation Therapy Oncology Group 83-11. J Clin Oncol. 1990;8:1543–1555.
10. Sause WT, Scott C, Taylor S, et al. Radiation Therapy Oncology Group (RTOG) 88-08 and Eastern Cooperative Oncology Group (ECOG) 4588: preliminary results of a phase III trial in regionally advanced, unresectable non–small-cell lung cancer. J Natl Cancer Inst. 1995;87:198–205.
11. Komaki R, Scott CB, Sause WT, et al. Induction cisplatin/vinblastine and irradiation vs. irradiation in unresectable squamous cell lung cancer: failure patterns by cell type in RTOG 88-08/ECOG 4588. Int J Radiat Oncol Biol Phys. 1997;39:537–544.
12. Saunders M, Dische S, Barrett A, et al. Continuous hyperfractionated accelerated radiotherapy (CHART) versus conventional radiotherapy in non–small-cell lung cancer: a randomised multicentre trial. Lancet. 1997;350:161–165.
13. Byhardt RW, Martin L, Pajak TF, et al. The influence of field size and other treatment factors on pulmonary toxicity following hyperfractionated irradiation for inoperable non–small cell lung cancer (NSCLC)—analysis of a Radiation Therapy Oncology Group (RTOG) protocol. Int J Radiat Oncol Biol Phys. 1993;27:537–544.
14. Emami B, Lyman J, Brown A, et al. Tolerance of normal tissue to therapeutic irradiation. Int J Radiat Oncol Biol Phys. 1991;21:109–122.
15. Rosenman JG, Miller EP, Tracton G, et al. Image registration: an essential part of radiation therapy treatment planning. Int J Radiat Oncol Biol Phys. 1998;40:197–205.
16. Hayman JA, Martel MK, Ten Haken RK, et al. Dose escalation in non–small cell lung cancer (NSCLC) using conformal 3-dimensional radiation therapy (C3DRT): update of a phase I trial [abstract]. Proc ASCO. 1999;18:459a.
17. Socinski MA, Halle J, Schell MJ, et al. Induction (I) and concurrent (C) carboplatin/paclitaxel (C/P) with dose-escalated thoracic conformal radiotherapy (TCRT) in stage IIIA/B non–small cell lung cancer (NSCLC): a phase I/II trial. Proc ASCO 2000;19:496a. [Abstract.]
18. Patz EF Jr, Lowe VJ, Hoffman JM, et al. Persistent or recurrent bronchogenic carcinoma:detection with PET and 2-[F-18]-2-deoxy-D-glucose. Radiology. 1994;191:379–382.
19. Inoue T, Kim EE, Komaki R, et al. Detecting recurrent or residual lung cancer with FDG-PET. J Nucl Med. 1995;36:788–793.
20. Noordijk EM, Clement EP, Hermans J, et al. Radiotherapy as an alternative to surgery in elderly patients with resectable lung cancer. Radiother Oncol. 1988;13:83–89.
21. Mantravadi RVP, Gates JO, Crawford JN, et al. Unresectable non–oat cell carcinoma of the lung: definitive radiation therapy. Radiology. 1989;172:851–855.
22. Perez CA, Bauer M, Edelstein S, et al. Impact of tumor control on survival in carcinoma of the lung treated with irradiation. Int J Radiat Oncol Biol Phys. 1986;12:539–547.
23. Perez CA, Stanley K, Rubin P, et al. A prospective randomized study of various irradiation doses and fractionation schedules in the treatment of inoperable non–oat-cell carcinoma of the lung: preliminary report by the Radiation Therapy Oncology Group. Cancer. 1980;45:2744–2753.
24. Shields TW, Higgins GA Jr, Lawton R, et al. Preoperative x-ray therapy as an adjuvant in the treatment of bronchogenic carcinoma. J Thorac Cardiovasc Surg. 1970;59:49–61.
25. Eichhorn HJ. Different fractionation schemes tested by histological examination of autopsy specimens from lung cancer patients. Br J Radiol. 1981;54:132–135.
26. Rissanen PM, Tikka U, Holsti LR. Autopsy findings in lung cancer treated with megavoltage radiotherapy. Acta Radiol Ther Phys Biol. 1968;7:433–442.
27. Bloedorn FG, Cowley RA, Cuccia CA, et al. Combined therapy: irradiation and surgery in the treatment of bronchogenic carcinoma. AJR Am J Roentgenol. 1961;85:875–885.
28. Kirschner PA. Lung cancer: preoperative radiation therapy and surgery. N Y State J Med. 1981:339–342.
29. Rosenthal SA, Curran WJ Jr, Herbert SH, et al. Clinical stage II non–small cell lung cancer treated with radiation therapy alone: the significance of clinically staged ipsilateral hilar adenopathy (N1 disease). Cancer. 1992;70:2410–2417.
30. Reinfuss M, Skolyszewski J, Kowalska T, et al. Palliative radiotherapy in asymptomatic patients with locally advanced, unresectable, non–small cell lung cancer. Strahlenther Onkol. 1993;169:709–715.
31. Perez CA, Pajak TF, Rubin P, et al. Long-term observations of the patterns of failure in patients with unresectable non–oat cell carcinoma of the lung treated with definitive radiotherapy: report by the Radiation Therapy Oncology Group. Cancer. 1987;59:1874–1881.
32. Arriagada R, Le Chevalier T, Quoix E, et al. ASTRO plenary: effect of chemotherapy on locally advanced non–small cell lung carcinoma: a randomized study of 353 patients. Int J Radiat Oncol Biol Phys. 1991;20:1183–1190.
33. Matthews MJ, Kanhouwa S, Pickren J, et al. Frequency of residual and metastatic tumor in patients undergoing curative surgical resection for lung cancer. Cancer Chemother Rep. 1973;4:63–67.
34. Martini N, Flehinger BJ, Zaman MB, et al. Results of resection in non–oat cell carcinoma of the lung with mediastinal lymph node metastases. Ann Surg. 1983;198:386–397.
35. Mountain CF. The biological operability of stage III non–small cell lung cancer. Ann Thorac Surg. 1985;40:60–64.
36. Pantel K, Izbicki JR, Angstwurm M, et al. Immunocytological detection of bone marrow micrometastasis in operable non–small cell lung cancer. Cancer Res. 1993;53:1027–1031.
37. Würschmidt F, Bünemann H, Bünemann C, et al. Inoperable non–small cell lung cancer: a retrospective analysis of 427 patients treated with high-dose radiotherapy. Int J Radiat Oncol Biol Phys. 1994;28:583–588.
38. Le Chevalier T, Arriagada R, Quoix E, et al. Radiotherapy alone

versus combined chemotherapy and radiotherapy in nonresectable non–small-cell lung cancer: first analysis of a randomized trial in 353 patients. J Natl Cancer Inst. 1991;83:417–423.

39. Dillman RO, Seagren SL, Propert KJ, et al. A randomized trial of induction chemotherapy plus high-dose radiation versus radiation alone in stage III non–small-cell lung cancer. N Engl J Med. 1990;323:940–945.

40. Ball D, Matthews J, Worotniuk V, et al. Longer survival with higher doses of thoracic radiotherapy in patients with limited non–small cell lung cancer. Int J Radiat Oncol Biol Phys. 1993;25:599–604.

41. Haffty BG, Goldberg NB, Gerstley J, et al. Results of radical radiation therapy in clinical stage I, technically operable non–small cell lung cancer. Int J Radiat Oncol Biol Phys. 1988;15:69–73.

42. Katz HR, Alberts RW. A comparison of high-dose continuous and split-course irradiation in non–oat-cell carcinoma of the lung. Am J Clin Oncol. 1983;6:445–457.

43. Holsti LR, Mattson K. A randomized study of split-course radiotherapy of lung cancer: long-term results. Int J Radiat Oncol Biol Phys. 1980;6:977–981.

44. Slawson RG, Salazar OM, Poussin-Rosillo H, et al. Once-a-week vs conventional daily radiation treatment for lung cancer: final report. Int J Radiat Oncol Biol Phys. 1988;15:61–68.

45. Cox JD, Azarnia N, Byhardt RW, et al. N2 (clinical) non–small cell carcinoma of the lung: prospective trials of radiation therapy with total doses 60 Gy by the Radiation Therapy Oncology Group. Int J Radiat Oncol Biol Phys. 1991;20:7–12.

46. Seydel HG, Deiner-West M, Urtasun R, et al. Hyperfractionation in radiation therapy of unresectable non-oat cell carcinoma of the lung: preliminary report of a RTOG pilot study. Int J Radiat Oncol Biol Phys. 1985;11:1841–1847.

47. Graham PH, Gebski VJ, Langlands AO. Radical radiotherapy for early nonsmall cell lung cancer. Int J Radiat Oncol Biol Phys. 1994;31:261–266.

48. Perez CA, Stanley K, Grundy G, et al. Impact of irradiation technique and tumor extent in tumor control and survival of patients with unresectable non–oat cell carcinoma of the lung: report by the Radiation Therapy Oncology Group. Cancer. 1982;50:1091–1099.

49. Krol ADG, Aussems P, Noorduk EM, et al. Local irradiation alone for peripheral stage I lung cancer: could we omit the elective regional nodal irradiation? Int J Radiat Oncol Biol Phys. 1996;34:297–302.

50. Hazuka MB, Turrisi AT III, Lutz ST, et al. Results of high-dose thoracic irradiation incorporating beam's eye view display in non–small cell lung cancer: a retrospective multivariate analysis. Int J Radiat Oncol Biol Phys. 1993;27:273–284.

51. Gauden S, Ramsay J, Tripcony L. The curative treatment by radiotherapy alone of stage I non–small cell carcinoma of the lung. Chest. 1995;108:1278–1282.

52. Kaskowitz L, Graham MV, Emami B, et al. Radiation therapy alone for stage I non–small cell lung cancer. Int J Radiat Oncol Biol Phys. 1993;27:517–523.

53. Coy P, Kennelly GM. The role of curative radiotherapy in the treatment of lung cancer. Cancer. 1980;45:698–702.

54. Sandler HM, Curran WJ Jr, Turrisi AT III. The influence of tumor size and pre-treatment staging on outcome following radiation therapy alone for stage I non–small cell lung cancer. Int J Radiat Oncol Biol Phys. 1990;19:9–13.

55. Clamon G, Herndon J, Cooper R, et al. Radiosensitization with carboplatin for patients with unresectable stage III non–small-cell lung cancer: a phase III trial of the Cancer and Leukemia Group B and the Eastern Cooperative Oncology Group. J Clin Oncol. 1999;17:4–11.

56. Talton BM, Constable WC, Kersh CR. Curative radiotherapy in non–small cell carcinoma of the lung. Int J Radiat Oncol Biol Phys. 1990;19:15–21.

57. Armstrong JG, Minsky BD. Radiation therapy for medically inoperable stage I and II non–small cell lung cancer. Cancer Treat Rev. 1989;16:247–255.

58. Green N, Weinstein H. Reassessment of radiation therapy for the management of lung cancer in patients with chronic pulmonary disease. Int J Radiat Oncol Biol Phys. 1983;9:1891–1896.

59. Robinow JS, Shaw EG, Eagan RT, et al. Results of combination chemotherapy and thoracic radiation therapy for unresectable non-small cell carcinoma of the lung. Int J Radiat Oncol Biol Phys. 1989;17:1203–1210.

60. Kiricuta IC, Mueller G, Stiess J, et al. The lymphatic pathways of non–small cell lung cancer and their implication in curative irradiation treatment. Lung Cancer. 1994;11:71–82.

61. Lingos TI, Recht A, Vicini F, et al. Radiation pneumonitis in breast cancer patients treated with conservative surgery and radiation therapy. Int J Radiat Oncol Biol Phys. 1991;21:355–360.

62. Tarbell NJ, Thompson L, Mauch P. Thoracic irradiation in Hodgkin's disease: disease control and long-term complications. Int J Radiat Oncol Biol Phys. 1990;18:275–281.

63. Martell MK, Ten Haken RK, Hazuka MB, et al. Dose volume histogram and 3D treatment planning evaluation of patients with pneumonitis. Int J Radiat Oncol Biol Phys. 1994;28:575–581.

64. Graham MV, Purdy JA, Emami B, et al. Clinical dose-volume histogram analysis for pneumonitis after 3D treatment for non–small cell lung cancer. Int J Radiat Oncol Biol Phys. 1999;45:323–329.

65. Marks LB, Munley MT, Bentel GC, et al. Physical and biological predictors of changes in whole-lung function following thoracic irradiation. Int J Radiat Oncol Biol Phys. 1997;39:563–570.

66. Curran WJ, Moldofsky PJ, Solin LJ. Quantitative analysis of the impact of radiation therapy field selection on post-RT pulmonary function. Int J Radiat Oncol Biol Phys. 1988;15(suppl 1):121.

67. Choi NC, Kanarek DJ. Toxicity of thoracic radiotherapy on pulmonary function in lung cancer. Lung Cancer. 1994;10(suppl):S219–S230.

68. Marks LB, Munley MT, Spencer DP, et al. Quantification of radiation-induced regional lung injury with perfusion imaging. Int J Radiat Oncol Biol Phys. 1997;38:399–409.

69. Marks LB, Sherouse GW, Munley MT, et al. Incorporation of functional status into dose-volume analysis. Med Phys. 1999;26:196–199.

70. Anscher MS, Kong FM, Marks LB, et al. Changes in plasma transforming growth factor beta radiotherapy and the risk of symptomatic radiation-induced pneumonities. Int J Radiat Oncol Biol Phys. 1997;37:253–258.

71. Schaake-Koning C, Kirkpatrick A, Kröger R, et al. The need for immediate monitoring of treatment parameters and uniform assessment of patient data in clinical trials: a quality control study of the EORTC Radiotherapy and Lung Cancer Cooperative Groups. Eur J Cancer. 1991;27:615–619.

72. White JE, Chen T, McCracken J, et al. The influence of radiation therapy quality control on survival, response and sites of relapse in oat cell carcinoma of the lung: preliminary report of a Southwest Oncology Group study. Cancer. 1982;50:1084–1090.

73. Puck TT, Marcus PI. Action of x-rays on mammalian cells. J Exp Med. 1956;103:653–666.

GENERAL ASPECTS OF CHEMOTHERAPY

Thomas E. Stinchcombe and Mark A. Socinski

The discovery of lymphoid hypoplasia in sailors exposed to nitrogen mustard in an explosion occurring on a ship during World War II led to the use of chemotherapy to treat lymphoma. Laboratory models were developed that yielded many insights into the biology of tumors and their response to chemotherapy. The ability to successfully treat patients with lymphoma and leukemia, coupled with the National Cancer Act of 1971, led to rapid growth of the field of medical oncology. Since then, a great deal has been learned about the behavior of malignant tumors in humans, as well as the mechanism of action and limitations of chemotherapeutic agents. A brief review of many of these concepts is presented in this chapter because these principles form the framework for the current approach to the use of chemotherapy in the treatment of lung cancer.

TUMOR BIOLOGY

Animal Models

Tumor Growth

Early laboratory studies included a classic series of elegant experiments involving a murine leukemia model known as L1210.[1] Many of the characteristics demonstrated by this model have led to important concepts about the biology of cancer that still influence our thinking today. This tumor was found to grow exponentially, with a *cell growth fraction* (the proportion of actively dividing cancer cells) of nearly 100%.[1] Thus, this model exhibited a reproducible growth curve and led to adoption of the concept of exponential growth of cancers as the result of repeated cell doubling, as shown in Figure 10–1. This concept predicts a long subclinical phase and rapid host death once the

tumor has become large enough to be detected. The murine leukemia model also provided evidence that malignant tumors arose from repeated cell divisions of a single cell that had become cancerous.[1]

Sensitivity to Chemotherapy

The murine L1210 model allowed the effect of various chemotherapeutic agents to be tested. The concept of *proportional (fractional) cell kill* was established, meaning that a dose of chemotherapy will eradicate the same proportion of cancer cells each time it is administered.[1] For example, if a tumor contains 10^5 cancer cells and a dose of chemotherapy is able to eradicate 90%, the tumor burden would be reduced to 10^4 cells. A second dose of chemotherapy would eradicate another 90%, and a major clinical response to the chemotherapy would be apparent, although a cure would not have been achieved because viable cells would still remain. Six cycles of chemotherapy would

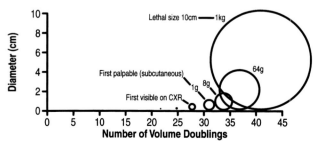

FIGURE 10–1. Exponential growth of cancers, with time expressed as number of volume doublings. (From Geddes DM. The natural history of lung cancer: a review based on rates of tumour growth. Br. J Dis Chest. 1979;73:1–17.[36])

likely result in a cure of a tumor with 10^5 cells, but the same number of doses of chemotherapy would not be successful in eradicating the tumor if the initial tumor burden had been 10^9 cells. This concept was well established by the murine leukemia model.[2]

The concept that the response rate was a crucial marker for potential cure also became firmly established in laboratory studies. The important issue is the complete response (CR) rate, because partial responses (PRs) are often followed by rapid regrowth of tumor.[3] Unless the available drugs can reliably induce a CR, cure with chemotherapy alone is extremely unlikely.[3] This concept has also fueled the eternal quest for newer, more active chemotherapeutic agents. Furthermore, analysis of laboratory tumor models led to the concept that the fastest growing tumors were the most sensitive to chemotherapy.

Dose

Laboratory models of transplanted tumors have consistently demonstrated that it is crucial to use the maximum tolerated dose (MTD) of chemotherapeutic agents.[3] Even a minor dose reduction has a dramatic impact on the cure rate, although the response rate may not be affected, as shown in Table 10–1. These laboratory studies demonstrated that a minor dose reduction markedly impairs the ability to eradicate all malignant cells, even though a large number of cells may be killed. This observation has been made almost without exception in laboratory studies.[3] An extension of this concept is the use of chemotherapy regimens involving several active agents. Ideally, these agents should be synergistic in their ability to kill cancer cells. However, the drugs should not have overlapping toxicities, so that each can be used at the MTD.

Drug Resistance

The inability to cure many cancers despite a high objective response rate led to the development of models of drug resistance. Drawing an analogy to the development of antibiotic resistance by bacteria, Goldie and Coldman[4,5] proposed that cancer cells acquire resistance to chemotherapeutic agents as a random mutational event. It was estimated that this occurred in approximately 1 in 10^3 to 10^5 cell divisions.[4] This would imply that the chance of drug resistance in small tumors would be low, whereas it would be high in larger tumors. Furthermore, this concept would predict that tumors would change from being highly

curable to being highly incurable over a short period of time. A short delay in initiating chemotherapy could have a disastrous effect on the ability to achieve a cure. Laboratory studies of cancers demonstrate many characteristics consistent with this hypothesis.[5]

Based on these considerations, mathematic modeling led to the prediction that multiple drugs would be most effective if given in as rapid a sequence as possible, such as in an alternating regimen.[6] Theoretically, and as demonstrated by some laboratory studies, eradication of all tumor cells was more likely if two different chemotherapeutic regimens were given in an alternating fashion than if several cycles of one regimen were given first, followed by several cycles of the other regimen.[5]

Human Observations

The laboratory models just discussed led to the establishment of many important principles of medical oncology. The ability of a number of different laboratory tumor models to consistently demonstrate results according to these principles provided strong evidence that a firm biologic basis for these principles existed. However, whether these insights from laboratory models can be extrapolated to the biology of cancer in human beings is unclear in most instances. As is often the case, the clinical situation appears to be much more complex.

Tumor Growth

Human tumors do not exhibit an exponential growth curve (with the possible exception of Burkitt's lymphoma).[3,7] Instead, human tumors follow a gompertzian growth curve, in which growth slows as the tumor gets larger (Figure 10–2). This has been well established by many clinical observations.[3,7] In fact, gompertzian growth is also observed in most animal models.[8–10] The maximum growth rate occurs when the tumor is approximately one third of its maximal size.[3] The gompertzian model predicts a shorter period of preclinical growth than the exponential model.[7] The mechanism causing the slowing of tumor growth is not entirely clear but appears to be more complex than simply outgrowing the available blood supply. It has become apparent that the cell cycle time of dividing cells is always the same, for normal cells as well as for tumor cells at different stages. However, the *fraction of actively dividing cells* (growth fraction) diminishes with increasing tumor size.[3,11]

The question "When do tumor cells begin to metastasize?" has given way to the question "What gives a circulating tumor cell the ability to successfully implant and grow?" Sensitive analyses have shown that circulating tumor cells are common, even in early-stage cancers. For example, circulating tumor cells were detected by reverse transcriptase–polymerase chain reaction in 40% of 71 patients with non–small cell lung cancer (NSCLC) and 30% of 15 patients with small cell lung cancer (SCLC).[12] The presence of circulating tumor cells was unrelated to tumor stage. Perhaps the expression of a factor such as angiogenesis factor is required for the establishment of distant metastases.[13] However, it appears that the situation is complex and as yet poorly understood.

TABLE 10–1. EFFECT OF ALTERATIONS IN DOSE INTENSITY ON RESPONSE AND CURE RATES IN A LABORATORY CANCER MODEL[a]

RELATIVE DOSE INTENSITY[b]	COMPLETE RESPONSE RATE (%)	CURE RATE (%)
0.60	100	60
0.47	100	44
0.44	100	10
0.31	10	0
0.27	0	0

[a]Tumors weighed 2 to 3 g.
[b]Average of dose intensity of the two drugs used.
    Data from studies involving Ridgway osteogenic sarcoma treated with a combination of cyclophosphamide and L-phenylalanine mustard. (From DeVita VT Jr, Hellman S, Rosenberg SA, eds. Cancer: Principles and Practices of Oncology. 5th ed. Philadelphia: Lippincott-Raven; 1997.[3])

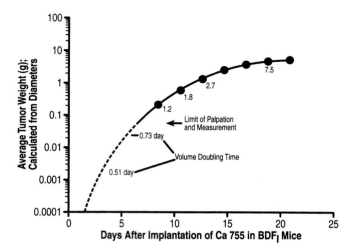

FIGURE 10–2. Gomperztian growth curve demonstrated by observed average growth rates in 100 mice following implantation of adenocarcinoma. The solid and dotted line represents a best-fit Gompertz function. (From CANCER, Vol 35, No. 1, 1975, 15–24. Copyright © 1975 American Cancer Society. Reprinted by permission of Wiley-Liss, Inc., a subsidiary of John Wiley & Sons, Inc.)[9]

Sensitivity to Chemotherapy

Approximately 10% of all human cancers account for 90% of cancers that can usually be cured with chemotherapy (leukemia, lymphoma, germ cell tumors).[3] The ability to cure human cancers with chemotherapy shows inconsistent correlation with the rapidity of tumor growth. Primarily because of the high cure rate of many leukemias and lymphomas with chemotherapy, these tumors had been assumed to be rapidly growing.[3] However, their growth rate has not been shown to be more rapid than that of many other human cancers.[3] Indeed, within a particular tumor type (eg, the diffuse aggressive lymphoma variant of non-Hodgkin's lymphoma), the tumors exhibiting a more rapid growth pattern are generally *less* responsive to chemotherapy.[3] Furthermore, many tumors (eg, SCLCs) exhibit initial dramatic sensitivity to chemotherapy, only to be followed by rapid tumor regrowth, at which time the cancer is often resistant to additional treatment and the patient dies of the disease.

The factors governing sensitivity to chemotherapy are clearly more complex than simply the rate of cancer cell growth or the percentage of actively dividing cells. It has become clear that the DNA damage caused by chemotherapeutic agents in cancer cells induces *apoptosis* (also known as programmed cell death) when these cells enter the S phase of the growth cycle. However, normal cells whose DNA has been damaged by chemotherapeutic agents are arrested in the late G_1 phase of the cell cycle, during which DNA repair is able to take place before the cell enters the S phase.[3] The factors governing the difference in fate of normal cells with damaged DNA compared with tumor cells are not entirely clear, but it appears likely that this difference plays a major role in the sensitivity of tumors to chemotherapy. A protein known as p53 facilitates both the cell cycle arrest in late G_1 and the activation of apoptosis, leading to repair of DNA when this can be accomplished (eg, normal cells) and death of the cell when this cannot be accomplished (eg, tumor cells). The loss of functional p53 is commonly found in tumors that are relatively resistant to chemotherapy, even in treatable malignancies such as lymphomas.[3] As the function of p53 is lost, the stability of the genome of the tumor cells decreases, and the tumor progresses rapidly to more unregulated growth and resistance to chemotherapy. Other proteins, such as K-Ras, tend to drive the cells into the S phase, overcoming the p53-dependent mechanisms that allow repair.[3]

Dose

Human cancers cannot be eradicated according to the principles of logarithmic cell kill as predictably as can cancers in laboratory models.[3] In responsive tumors that are difficult to cure with chemotherapy, simply adding more cycles does not seem to change the outcome. Although as a general principle the MTD of chemotherapeutic agents is recommended, in reality the dose is frequently reduced because of anticipated or perceived toxicity, particularly when chemotherapy is used in conjunction with other treatments. The impact of such dose reductions in patients is not entirely clear; however, in general, data from human studies supports at least a threshold for most chemotherapeutic agents and most tumors.[3] Furthermore, the nearly universal demonstration of the importance of dose in animal models suggests that this principle may well be transferable to the clinic setting.[3]

Most chemotherapy regimens have been designed around the kinetics of marrow recovery. In the absence of growth factors, the nadir of blood counts occurs at approximately 10 to 14 days, with recovery by day 21 to 28. Careful examination of the experience in human beings indicates that changes in the treatment schedule (interval between cycles) primarily affect the toxicity resulting from treatment and have little effect on the response or cure rates.[3]

Increasing the *dose intensity* (dose given per unit of time) over the MTD is an attractive concept, provided that toxicity can be controlled. The discovery of granulocyte and megakaryocyte colony-simulating factors provides an opportunity to increase the dose while minimizing marrow toxicity. More intense dose escalations are possible with techniques involving harvesting and reinfusion of autologous marrow stem cells. However, tumors that are relatively resistant to chemotherapy generally exhibit a relatively flat dose response curve.[3] The effect of increasing the dose intensity may be merely to increase toxicity. Whether high-dose chemotherapy has a role in the treatment of lung cancer has not been adequately studied.

Resistance

The mechanism of resistance to chemotherapy in human beings is clearly more complex than what can be explained by any of the theories proposed so far. Initially, it was thought that resistance was due to the presence of sanctuaries that rendered cancer cells impervious to the effects of chemotherapy. This included anatomic sanctuaries (eg, the blood–brain barrier) and physiologic sanctuaries (eg, a proportion of cells that were not actively dividing at the time of treatment). However, there is little data in human beings supporting this concept. Acquired resistance to specific chemotherapy drugs arising as a mutational event during the growth of the cancer is also not supported by data in human beings. Furthermore, a quite universal observation is that normal cells do not acquire resistance to chemotherapy, although this would be predicted by random mutation, which should occur at the same rate in normal cells as in tumor cells. The presence of multiple cycles of chemotherapy would exert strong pressure for selective growth of the resistant cells.

The gompertzian model of tumor growth would predict, purely on cytokinetic grounds, that the level of therapy necessary to cause a complete clinical remission may not be sufficient to eradicate all of the tumor.[14] This is because as the tumor shrinks during chemotherapy, the rate of regrowth increases. This also implies that the level of therapy necessary to cause a response in large tumors in patients with advanced disease may not be sufficient to eradicate small foci of tumor in an adjuvant setting.[14] This hypothesis, known as the *Norton–Simon hypothesis,* suggests that intensification of chemotherapy, once a remission has been induced, may be beneficial.[14]

The development of drug resistance is generally thought to be the major obstacle to curing cancer with chemotherapeutic agents.[15] It has become clear that tumor cells that demonstrate resistance to a particular drug usually also have resistance to various other drugs. This phenomenon, known as multidrug resistance (MDR), has been shown to involve upregulation of a membrane protein, which is probably involved in translocation of the drug across the cell membrane. Other such proteins have also been identified, such as multidrug resistance–associated protein (MRP) and lung cancer resistance–associated protein (LRP).[15] Assays to detect overexpression of the MDR gene have not been refined enough to be used clinically, and strategies to modulate the function of these proteins are currently only speculative.[15] Although the phenomenon of resistance is complex, it appears that a new level of understanding is beginning. This holds out some promise for novel treatment approaches in the future.

CLINICAL CONTEXT OF CHEMOTHERAPY

Chemotherapy can be used in a variety of clinical contexts. The goal of the treatment differs somewhat in these various clinical situations, as do the issues involved. Although many of the concerns are largely speculative, they are discussed briefly here because they influence the treatment strategies that are being considered.

Chemotherapy Alone

Treatment of lung cancer with chemotherapy alone is usually done in the setting of metastatic disease. It is important to define whether the goal of treatment is curative or palliative. Eradication of all tumor is certainly the ideal, but data from laboratory models, as well as clinical experience, has shown that cure is unrealistic unless a complete remission can be reliably achieved. In the case of NSCLC a CR is achieved only rarely, and treatment with curative intent is usually inappropriate. However, treatment of SCLC with chemotherapy frequently induces a CR.

Despite the frequency of CRs that has been seen in the treatment of SCLC, the tumor usually recurs, and chemotherapy alone only rarely results in a cure. In this setting, it may be useful to explore treatment approaches that address some of the hypothetical reasons for failure. New agents, particularly those with novel mechanisms of action, may be useful. Dose intensification may help overcome the cytokinetic issues predicted by the gompertzian model of tumor growth. Alternating chemotherapy regimens may overcome drug resistance. In general, however, these strategies have not shown much benefit in the treatment of human cancers, and SCLC is no exception.

When the goal of treatment is palliation, issues of toxicity and the duration and inconvenience of the treatment regimen are of major importance. The presence of measurable or evaluable disease allows chemotherapy to be discontinued in those patients in whom it is not effective (eg, those not demonstrating an objective response). In this setting, however, even PRs can be important in the palliation of symptoms or the prolongation of survival. In fact, palliation of symptoms sometimes occurs even in patients with stable disease.

Adjuvant Therapy

Chemotherapy given following definitive treatment with a local modality such as surgery is known as *adjuvant therapy.* In this case, there is no measurable disease. Chemotherapy is given to treat presumed occult microscopic systemic foci of cancer, and the residual tumor burden is extremely low. However, the gompertzian growth model predicts that tumor regrowth will be rapid, and treatment with maximal dose intensity may be of major importance. Unfortunately, particularly in the setting of adjuvant treatment following previous local therapy such as surgery, the patient's tolerance of chemotherapy may be reduced. Adjuvant therapy has generally produced at best only modest improvements in survival in the treatment of human lung cancers using current strategies and regimens.

Induction Therapy

Induction therapy in the context of the treatment of lung cancer means initial treatment with chemotherapy before the use of a local modality, such as surgery or radiotherapy (RT) for patients with localized disease. The goal of treatment is to eradicate presumed microscopic foci of systemic disease or to shrink the primary tumor before local therapy, or both. Treatment of systemic foci may be improved by the earlier administration of chemotherapy given as induction treatment rather than as adjuvant treatment. However, the same limitations and concerns apply as with adjuvant therapy regarding the use of chemotherapy to treat systemic microscopic foci of disease.

It is often argued that decreasing the size of the local tumor by induction therapy may permit less extensive local treatment, such as less extensive surgical resection or smaller radiotherapy fields. However, unless the chemotherapy is effective enough to result in the complete disappearance of tumor from parts of the local disease bed, the notion of less extensive local therapy is inappropriate. The ability to cause complete disappearance of the tumor is generally taken to mean that the therapy should be able to induce a CR with some regularity. In the setting of SCLC, this would appear to be a reasonable consideration, although how and whether the RT port should be modified is controversial. In the setting of NSCLC, CRs are unusual. However, a complete pathologic response in the mediastinum, known as *mediastinal downstaging,* can be induced by induction therapy for stage IIIa,b disease, making surgical resection a rational strategy (see Chapter 19).

Chemotherapy as a Radiation Sensitizer

Chemotherapy can be given at the same time as RT in order to exploit an interaction between the two treatments. In other words, chemotherapy can be used as a radiation sensitizer to make the tumor more sensitive to the radiation. Of course, the radiation sensitizer may make normal tissues more sensitive to the radiation as well.[16] The most common mechanism for this effect appears to be to block or slow the repair of sublethal damage caused by radiation. Many of the standard chemotherapeutic agents show some evidence of an ability to cause radiosensitization in laboratory models.[17] Some drugs, such as misonidazole, act only as radiation sensitizers, having no antitumor effect on their own. Furthermore, some drugs, such as mitomycin C and tirapazamine, are active specifically under hypoxic conditions, which make cells very resistant to radiotherapy.[16] This occurs because these agents are converted to an active form by reduction, which is inhibited in well-oxygenated tissues. Therefore, these agents enhance the effect of radiation by specifically targeting certain cells that are resistant. Some authors also consider an interaction between chemotherapy and RT to include spatial cooperation, which means that chemotherapy is treating systemic foci of cancer while radiotherapy is treating the primary tumor. However, this use of chemotherapy falls under the purview of induction or adjuvant therapy and will not be discussed further here.

When chemotherapy is used as a radiation sensitizer, the goal is to enhance the ability of RT to control the local disease. Therefore, the effectiveness of this approach should be assessed by monitoring local control. Unfortunately, assessment of local control in the setting of RT is difficult (see Chapter 9). Furthermore, although sensitization to RT can be demonstrated in laboratory models, this has been difficult to demonstrate in most human studies.[16] It is probably important to maintain adequate drug levels throughout the entire radiation treatment (by daily chemotherapy instead of a cycle of chemotherapy every 3 to 4 weeks). This has been borne out by at least one clinical study involving NSCLC, in which local control was enhanced by daily chemotherapy throughout the course of

RT.[18] There are few guidelines regarding the appropriate dose of chemotherapy as a radiation sensitizer, but the dose needed can be expected to have little relationship to the dose needed as a systemic therapeutic agent. Indeed, the issues involved in chemotherapy to enhance the effect of RT on the primary tumor and those involved in chemotherapy for the treatment of distant foci of tumor are so different that it seems unrealistic to expect to devise a treatment strategy that accomplishes both goals.

TOXICITY GRADING SYSTEM

In order to be able to compare results across studies, all of the major cooperative oncology groups have developed toxicity grading schemes. Grade 1 toxicities are mild, and grade 2 toxicities are moderate in severity. Serious treatment-related morbidity is considered a grade 3 toxicity, and life-threatening complications are classified as grade 4. In many studies, grades 3 and 4 are reported together as severe toxicities. Fatalities related to chemotherapy are rare and are designated as grade 5 toxicity. In order to promote a common system, the National Cancer Institute (NCI) published common toxicity criteria in 1998.[19] A brief list of some of the more common toxicities encountered in the treatment of lung cancer is presented in Table 10–2. There is currently a general movement toward using the NCI criteria for all protocols in order to standardize toxicity grading. However, previously published studies have used whatever grading scale was adopted by the cooperative group conducting the study.

The toxicity grading systems of the various cooperative groups have been similar in many respects. One of the few differences (as it pertains to lung cancer) is in the grading of esophagitis. In the Cancer and Leukemia Group B (CALGB) schema, grade 3 esophagitis is present if the patient is unable to eat solid foods or requires narcotics, and grade 4 esophagitis is present if parenteral or enteral support is required. On the other hand, the Radiation Therapy Oncology Group (RTOG) grading scale defines grade 3 esophagitis as "able to only swallow liquids, may have pain on swallowing; dilation required" and does not include the need for parenteral or enteral support in the toxicity grading of esophagitis. The NCI Common Toxicity Criteria define grade 3 esophagitis as requiring intravenous (IV) hydration. Thus, grade 3 toxicity under the NCI criteria would be considered grade 4 toxicity under the CALGB schema. Therefore, it is important to review the toxicity definitions in each study if comparisons are being made among and between studies.

CLASSES OF CHEMOTHERAPY AGENTS

A cursory knowledge of the commonly used chemotherapy agents is important for all physicians involved in the treatment of patients with lung cancer. A brief outline is presented here. A more complete discussion of chemotherapy agents can be found in standard medical oncology textbooks. Several characteristics of some of the more commonly used chemotherapy agents for NSCLC and SCLC are summarized in Table 10–3. Data regarding the efficacy

TABLE 10–2. NATIONAL CANCER INSTITUTE COMMON TOXICITY CRITERIA

CATEGORY	GRADE 0	GRADE 1	GRADE 2	GRADE 3	GRADE 4
Hematologic					
Hemoglobin[a]	Normal	>10	8–10	6.5–<8	<6.5
Platelets[b]	Normal	≥75	50–<75	25–<50	<25
White blood count[b]	≥4	3–<4	2–<3	1–<2	<1
Neutrophils[b]	Normal	1.5–<2	1–<1.5	0.5–<1	<0.5
Gastrointestinal					
Nausea	None	Able to eat almost normally	Able to eat, but ↓ in amount	No significant oral intake	—
Vomiting	None	1 episode/24 h	2–5 ×/24 h	6–10 ×/24 h	>10 ×/24 h
Esophagitis/ dysphagia	None	Mild dysphagia, able to eat	Dysphagia requiring soft or liquid diet	Dysphagia requiring intravenous hydration	Requires parenteral or enteral support
Diarrhea	None	↑ of 2–3 stools/d	↑ of 4–6 stools/d, moderate cramping, or nocturnal stools	↑ of 7–9 stools/d, severe cramping, or incontinence	↑ of ≥10 stools/d, bloody diarrhea, parenteral support
Neurologic					
Sensory	No change	Mild paresthesias, or loss of deep tendon reflexes	Mild to moderate objective sensory loss, moderate paresthesias	Severe objective sensory loss or paresthesias causing ↓ functioning	—
Pulmonary					
Chemotherapy-related	Normal	Asymptomatic but abnormal pulmonary function tests	Dyspnea on exertion	Dyspnea at normal level of activity	Dyspnea at rest
Late radiotherapy-related[c]	Normal	Asymptomatic, mild cough, slight CXR changes	Moderate symptoms, severe cough, patchy CXR changes	Severe symptoms, dense CXR changes	Severe respiratory insufficiency, need continuous oxygen
Renal					
Creatinine	Normal	<1.5 × normal limit	1.5–≤3 × normal limit	>3–6 × normal limit	>6 × normal limit

[a]Units g/dL.
[b]Units 10^3/mm^3.
[c]Radiation Therapy Oncology Group (RTOG) criteria.
CXR, chest radiograph.
Data from National Cancer Institute. Common Toxicity Criteria. Bethesda, Md: National Cancer Institute; 1998.[19]

of these drugs can be found in chapters dealing with specific types and stages of lung cancer.

Platinum Compounds

Cisplatin and carboplatin are two agents commonly used in the treatment of lung cancer that belong to the group known as *platins*. This group of chemotherapeutic agents acts by covalently binding to DNA by forming crosslinks between the two strands, thereby disrupting the replication of malignant cells. Cisplatin has been one of the most commonly used chemotherapeutic agents in the treatment of both SCLC and NSCLC during the 1980s and 1990s. More recently, carboplatin has been substituted for cisplatin in certain situations.

The main side effects of cisplatin are nausea and vomiting. Cisplatin has a >90% incidence of emesis if no antiemetics are given before treatment, but the incidence of emesis is reduced to <10% if premedication is used.[20] The incidence of nausea and vomiting has a bimodal distribution, with acute emesis occurring at the time of infusion and delayed emesis occurring 24 to 48 hours after infusion. One of the biggest risk factors for delayed-onset emesis is poor control of acute-onset chemotherapy emesis. Medications that are effective in preventing delayed-onset emesis are a 4- or 5-day course of dexamethasone, metoclopramide, or a serotonin receptor antagonist.

The other adverse effect associated with cisplatin exposure is nephrotoxicity. To prevent this, patients are frequently given IV fluids before administration of cisplatin. Exposure to other nephrotoxic agents, such as aminoglycosides, can potentiate this toxicity; therefore, it is important to avoid any such drugs after recent exposure to cisplatin. Cisplatin can also cause magnesium and potassium wasting, resulting in clinically significant hypomagnesemia and hypokalemia.

Carboplatin has an incidence of acute-onset emesis of approximately 30% and does not share the nephrotoxicity of cisplatin. The dose-limiting toxicity of carboplatin is myelosuppression. In NSCLC, carboplatin has frequently been used in treatment regimens in stage III and stage IV disease (see Chapters 21 and 22). Whether carboplatin has efficacy equal to that of cisplatin in SCLC is an area of ongoing research. Most authors recommend that cisplatin be used in patients with limited-stage disease who are being treated with curative intent until studies indicating equal efficacy of carboplatin are published. In extensive-stage disease, in which the intent of treatment is primarily palliation, substituting carboplatin for cisplatin in order to reduce the toxicity profile is reasonable.

Alkylating Agents

The alkylating agents act by covalently binding to the DNA in a manner similar to that for the platin compounds. These medications contain a reactive alkyl group that is

TABLE 10–3. CHARACTERISTICS OF COMMONLY USED CHEMOTHERAPEUTIC AGENTS IN THE TREATMENT OF LUNG CANCER

CLASS	MECHANISM OF ACTION	EXAMPLES	HEMATOLOGIC TOXICITY	NAUSEA/ VOMITING	OTHER MAJOR TOXICITY
Platins	Covalent binding of DNA strands	Cisplatin Carboplatin	+ + + + + +	+ + + + + + +	Renal toxicity, ototoxicity, neuropathy
Alkylating agents	Covalent binding of DNA strands	Cyclophosphamide Ifosfamide	+ + + + + + + +	+ + + + + +	Hemorrhagic cystitis, somnolence, lethargy
Vinca alkaloids	↓ Growth and ↑ destruction of microtubules	Vincristine Vinblastine Vindesine[a] Vinorelbine	+ + + + + + + +	+ + + +	Neuropathy, constipation, abdominal pain
Taxanes	↑ Tubulin polymerization	Paclitaxel Docetaxel	+ + + + +	+ + + +	Neuropathy, myalgias, arthralgias, fluid retention
Topoisomerase inhibitors	Inhibit enzyme that initiates DNA replication	Etoposide Teniposide[a] Topotecan Irinotecan	+ + + + + + + + + + + + + +	+ + + + + + + +	Alopecia, mucositis, diarrhea (especially with irinotecan)
Antimetabolites	Inhibit purine synthesis Base substitution in DNA	Methotrexate Edatrexate Gemcitabine	+ + + + + +	+ + +	Mucositis, nephrotoxicity Hepatotoxicity, rash, fever
Antibiotics	Intercalation in DNA strands	Doxorubicin Mitomycin C	+ + + +	+ + + + + +	Cardiomyopathy Pulmonary toxicity

[a]Not available in the United States.

+, number of + signs refers to an increasing propensity for toxicity relative to other agents.

capable of forming bonds with DNA and preventing DNA replication. Cyclophosphamide and ifosfamide are members of this class of drugs that are commonly used in the treatment of lung cancer. The main toxicity associated with these two medications is myelosuppression. Although the incidence of nausea and vomiting with these agents is generally moderately high (30%-90% incidence of emesis without any premedication), this can be readily controlled with a single antiemetic medication. A less common side effect occasionally seen with cyclophosphamide is syndrome of inappropriate antidiuretic hormone (SIADH). Both cyclophosphamide and ifosfamide may damage the uro-epithellium, causing hemorrhagic cystitis. In general, the doses of cyclophosphamide necessary to cause damage to the uro-epithelium are higher than those used in the treatment of lung cancer. Ifosfamide is often given with mesna, a chemoprotectant, and hydration, which protects the ureters and bladder from the damage caused by ifosfamide. In general, cyclophosphamide is infrequently used in treating lung cancer because of the development of newer agents, whereas the role of ifosfamide is an area of active investigation.

Vinca Alkaloids

Microtubules form the mitotic spindle on the chromosome that is responsible for the separation of the replicated chromosomes during cell division. Microtubules consist of two different types of tubulin proteins, the α-subunit and the β-subunit. The production and destruction of microtubules is a continuously occurring process, and interference with either the production or the destruction of microtubules disrupts the mitotic process and leads to the death of dividing cells. *Vinca alkaloids* and the taxanes are two groups of drugs that act by this mechanism.

Vinca alkaloids are believed to have two sites of action on the tubulin molecule. At one site, they bind to the tubulin and prevent its further growth; at the other site, their binding causes disruption of the physical structure of the microtubule and its subsequent disintegration.[21] Drugs that are part of this class of medications include vincristine, vinblastine, vindesine, and vinorelbine. Vindesine is currently approved for treatment of NSCLC in Europe but not in the United States. All of these medications can cause mild and reversible alopecia and Raynaud's phenomenon. A neuropathy consisting of loss of sensation and deep tendon reflexes in the extremities is a common toxicity after multiple treatments. Extravasation during the infusion of these drugs may cause tissue necrosis and cellulitis.

Taxanes

Paclitaxel and docetaxel belong to a class of chemotherapeutic agents known as *taxanes*. These drugs bind to the β-tubulin subunit of microtubules, inducing uncontrolled polymerization of tubulin. This upsets the delicate balance of tubulin growth and disassembly that is necessary for the cell to successfully complete the mitotic cycle. Both medications were originally approved for the treatment of metastatic breast cancer but have been found to be useful in a number of other cancers, including lung cancer. Both of them have also been found to enhance the cytotoxic effects of RT, which may be of clinical benefit in combined-modality treatment.

A hypersensitivity reaction during infusion is one of

the more common side effects associated with paclitaxel. Premedication with dexamethasone, diphenhydramine, and a histamine receptor type 2 (H₂) antagonist is recommended before infusion. If a hypersensitivity reaction does occur, the patient can be rechallenged with the paclitaxel infusion running at a slower rate after a second course of premedication, provided there has been no respiratory distress or hemodynamic instability. The other major side effect of paclitaxel use is a sensory neuropathy. This complication usually occurs after multiple treatments and can be severe enough to necessitate discontinuing the medication. Other side effects include transient myalgias, alopecia, and inflammation of the skin over previous sites of irradiation (radiation recall). Docetaxel also can cause a hypersensitivity reaction during infusion and can cause a peripheral neuropathy as well. Docetaxel is more myelosuppressive than paclitaxel. A side effect unique to docetaxel is a capillary leak syndrome, resulting in fluid retention with edema, pleural effusions, weight gain, and ascites. This is generally a cumulative toxicity, and dexamethasone is often given for several days surrounding the docetaxel infusion to prevent the fluid retention syndrome. Docetaxel also can cause a feeling of general malaise and fatigue.

Topoisomerase Inhibitors

The topoisomerase enzymes I and II make either single- or double-stranded cuts in the DNA double helix that allow replication of the opposite strand of the DNA. These enzymes are critical to the modification and maintenance of the DNA structure. Drugs capable of inhibiting these enzymes have shown significant antitumor activity. Irinotecan (CPT-11) was originally developed for the treatment of colon cancer, but there has been interest in exploring the activity of this agent in treating NSCLC. The major toxicity associated with this medication is severe diarrhea, which can require hospitalization and can be fatal in a debilitated patient. This side effect can be avoided by early and aggressive treatment of abdominal cramping and diarrhea with loperamide. Patients may require up to 32 mg of loperamide in a 24-hour period. The other major side effect associated with this medication is myelosuppression. At present, irinotecan is not approved for treatment of NSCLC, but many clinical protocols are exploring its activity in this disease. Another topoisomerase I inhibitor available in the United States is topotecan. This medication has shown significant activity in the treatment of SCLC and is currently often used for salvage chemotherapy. The main side effects associated with topotecan are myelosuppression and alopecia.

Etoposide is a topoisomerase II inhibitor that is part of the standard chemotherapy for SCLC. It may be given orally or IV. The use of the oral agent avoids a clinic visit for a patient, but requires that the patient be reliable. The oral formulation of this drug has been used as a single agent in the palliative treatment of SCLC in patients with a poor performance status, but it has been shown to have a lower response rate and median survival than combination chemotherapy.[22] The main side effect associated with etoposide is myelosuppression. Teniposide is a topoisomerase II inhibitor used in Europe that has activity and toxicity

profiles similar to those of etoposide but is not approved for use in the United States.

Antimetabolites

This class of medications works by inhibiting one of several enzymes necessary for DNA synthesis or by substituting for a nucleotide base in DNA or RNA, thereby blocking transcription. Gemcitabine is the drug in this class that is used most often in the treatment of NSCLC. This medication is a pyrimidine antagonist that is incorporated into DNA and slows the elongation of the DNA, which is ultimately fatal to the affected cell. Gemcitabine is often used in the treatment of metastatic NSCLC. The major toxicity associated with this medication is myelosuppression. Edatrexate is another drug in this class that is currently entering clinical trials involving NSCLC. This medication is an analog of methotrexate that inhibits dihydrofolate reductase, which is important in purine synthesis.

Antibiotics

Doxorubicin and mitomycin C are two chemotherapy agents used in treating lung cancer that are classified as antibiotics, reflecting their original use. Doxorubicin intercalates between DNA strands and is a topoisomerase II inhibitor. Mitomycin C is activated in vivo to an alkylating agent that crosslinks DNA strands, thereby halting DNA synthesis. Both agents are currently used less frequently than in the 1980s. Doxorubicin is part of a standard combination regimen (cyclophosphamide, doxorubicin, vincristine) used in treating SCLC, but this combination has largely been replaced by the etoposide/cisplatin regimen. Likewise, although mitomycin C has substantial activity in NSCLC, it has largely been supplanted by more active agents with superior toxicity profiles. The major toxicities of doxorubicin are myelosuppression, mucositis, and extravasation injury. Cardiomyopathy may also occur, but this is rare (<5%) if the cumulative dose is <450 mg/m². Mitomycin C can cause a cumulative myelosuppression, pneumonitis, and a microangiopathic hemolytic–uremic syndrome.

Evolution of Chemotherapy Agents for Lung Cancer

The chemotherapy agents used in the treatment of NSCLC can be broadly divided into three groups, often called *three generations* of chemotherapy drugs (Table 10–4). These correspond roughly to agents used in the 1970s, 1980s, and 1990s. The first generation drugs consisted primarily of alkylating agents and antimetabolites. These agents exhibited poor activity, were not associated with a survival benefit, and are no longer used in NSCLC. The use of cisplatin-based regimens marked the era of second generation chemotherapy. Cisplatin-based regimens exhibited better anticancer activity and were associated with a survival

TABLE 10–4. CHEMOTHERAPY AGENTS USED IN THE TREATMENT OF NON–SMALL CELL LUNG CANCER

FIRST GENERATION	SECOND GENERATION	THIRD GENERATION
Cyclophosphamide	Cisplatin	Paclitaxel
Doxorubicin	Carboplatin	Docetaxel
Methotrexate	Etoposide	Vinorelbine
Procarbazine	Vindesine	Gemcitabine
CCNU/BCNU	Vinblastine	Irinotecan
5-Fluorouracil	Mitomycin C	Topotecan
	Ifosfamide	Edatrexate

benefit for patients with stage III and IV NSCLC in a large number of randomized trials conducted in the 1980s. During the 1990s, a number of newer agents became available that appeared to produce better response rates than the second generation agents. Studies involving these newer agents (often in combination with second generation agents) suggested better survival than with second generation agents alone (see Chapters 21 and 22). Furthermore, the toxicity of third generation agents is generally lower than that of second generation drugs. Currently, both second and third generation agents are in common use.

A wide variety of chemotherapeutic agents produce high response rates in SCLC. Because even the regimens that were available in the 1970s are still in use, the treatment of SCLC cannot be easily grouped into eras or generations of drugs. The newer agents are also active in SCLC, but regimens involving some of the earlier agents are still in use today as well (see Chapters 24 and 25). The focus of research has been on alterations in the schedule of administration of chemotherapy regimens (eg, dose intensity) and the optimal way to combine chemotherapy with RT, as much as on the identification of regimens with superior activity.

SUPPORTIVE THERAPY

Antiemetics

The development of effective antiemetic therapy has alleviated one of the most common and dreaded adverse effects of chemotherapy. The emesis related to chemotherapy is divided into two categories: acute emesis occurring within 24 hours of receiving chemotherapy and delayed emesis occurring more than 24 hours later. New medications have greatly improved the ability to control acute emesis (Table 10–5). Progress in controlling delayed-onset chemotherapy emesis has been slower, however, and this remains a problem with some patients.

The development of serotonin receptor antagonists was a major breakthrough in the treatment of acute nausea, and use of these medications has become routine with moderately or highly emetogenic treatment regimens. The addition of corticosteroids further improves the effectiveness of the serotonin receptor antagonists, and such a combination of medications has consistently yielded the greatest antiemetic protection in multiple randomized controlled trials.[23] Premedication with corticosteroids alone can be used with chemotherapeutic agents with intermediate risk for acute emesis, and low-risk chemotherapeutic agents frequently do not require any antiemetic premedication.[23] Other agents used as antiemetics for low-risk chemotherapeutic agents include dopamine receptor antagonists and benzodiazepines, especially when a component of anxiety or anticipatory emesis contributes to the patient's symptoms.

Preventive medication for delayed-onset chemotherapy emesis caused by cisplatin and other highly emetogenic chemotherapy treatments is recommended in the American Society for Clinical Oncology (ASCO) guidelines, but it is not recommended for the intermediate-risk regimens.[23] The preventive treatment is usually a corticosteroid taper over 4 to 5 days, either alone or in combination with metoclopramide.[23] Scheduled doses of prochlorperazine as a single agent are often used to prevent delayed-onset nausea and vomiting, but randomized clinical trials supporting this common practice are lacking. Although serotonin receptor antagonists have been used in the prevention of delayed emesis, they have not been shown to be clearly superior to the combination of metoclopramide and corticosteroids.[23] Another medication that can be useful in this setting is dronabinol, which is the principal psychoactive substance in marijuana. However, this medication may have central nervous system effects such as euphoria, anxiety, or paranoia. Dronabinol should be used primarily if the patient has failed to benefit from standard therapy.[23]

Growth Factors

Neutropenia is defined as an absolute neutrophil count $<500/\mu L$. The current standard of care involves hospitalization and treatment with intravenous antibiotics if an absolute neutrophil count below this level is accompanied by a fever. Despite these interventions, the mortality rate from febrile neutropenia ranges from 0% to 6% for patients with all types of solid tumors and from 3% to 6% for patients with SCLC.[24] Furthermore, neutropenia can cause significant treatment delays and the need for chemotherapy dose reductions. Dose reductions to prevent neutropenia may substantially diminish the chances of eradicating the

TABLE 10–5. COMMONLY USED ANTIEMETICS

SEROTONIN RECEPTOR ANTAGONISTS	CORTICOSTEROIDS	DOPAMINE ANTAGONISTS	BENZODIAZEPINES
Dolasetron	Dexamethasone	Metoclopramide	Lorazepam
Granisetron	Methylprednisolone	Prochlorperazine	Alprazolam
Ondansetron			
Tropisetron			

disease. Because of these concerns, granulocyte colony–stimulating factor (G-CSF) and granulocyte-macrophage colony-stimulating factor (GM-CSF) were developed. These medications have been proved to shorten the duration of neutropenia,[25,26] but their exact role and their cost-benefit ratio are still being defined.

The current ASCO guidelines recommend that G-CSF or GM-CSF be given prophylactically to reduce the likelihood of febrile neutropenia when the incidence of this complication is expected to be >40%.[24] A randomized study found that the use of G-CSF reduced the incidence of febrile neutropenia from 77% to 40% in patients with SCLC when six cycles of chemotherapy were given.[26] There was also a reduction in the number of confirmed infections, days of treatment with intravenous antibiotics, and days of hospitalization. The ASCO guidelines also recommended the use of growth factors after one episode of febrile neutropenia.[24] This recommendation is based on studies that indicate that patients who have had one episode of febrile neutropenia are at risk for experiencing a second episode.[24] Furthermore, growth factors are generally indicated if a patient with febrile neutropenia has a tissue infection such as cellulitis or sinusitis, an abscess, or pneumonia.[24] The use of growth factors is not recommended for patients with febrile neutropenia who do not have a confirmed infection.[24]

The use of platelet growth factors, such as interleukin-11 (IL-11), has been an area of interest because thrombocytopenia is often a dose-limiting toxicity of chemotherapeutic agents that can lead to dose reductions or delays in treatment. IL-11 is currently approved by the Food and Drug Administration (FDA) in the United States to reduce the incidence of life-threatening thrombocytopenia. IL-11 (50 μg/kg/day after two cycles of chemotherapy) reduced the need for platelet transfusion from 68% to 41% ($P = 0.04$) in a study in patients with metastatic breast cancer.[27] The main toxicities of this medication are fluid retention, a decrease in the hematocrit related to hemodilution, and atrial arrhythmias. Another medication that is being developed is thrombopoietin, which is a recombinant pegylated form of human megakaryocyte growth and development factor. This medication is currently being evaluated in phase I trials. The role and exact benefit of both of these medications have yet to be defined, but this is an area of ongoing research and drug development.

Erythropoietin, a growth factor that increases the production of red blood cells, is used to reduce the need for blood transfusions. This medication is already widely used for patients with renal insufficiency, and it is beginning to establish a role in the prevention of chemotherapy-induced anemia. A study involving 2370 patients treated at 621 community cancer centers suggested that erythropoietin can improve the anemia associated with cancer chemotherapy.[28] Furthermore, patients responding to erythropoietin therapy experienced a statistically significant improvement in quality of life, independent of tumor response to chemotherapy. Although this study generated considerable interest in erythropoietin, the role of this drug remains unclear because of its expense and the fact that the benefit has not been proved in a randomized controlled trial. It is possible that the same improvement in quality of life may be realized with less expense by the more frequent use of blood transfusions.

Chemotherapy Protectants

Several drugs have been investigated that are intended to prevent a specific toxicity. The goal of these therapies is to protect normal tissues from the effects of chemotherapeutic agents without diminishing the effectiveness of the agents in eradicating tumor cells. Because they may affect both the risk and the efficacy of the chemotherapy, these medications should be evaluated in carefully designed clinical trials before they gain widespread use.

Mesna is a thiol compound that binds to metabolites of cyclophosphamide and ifosfamide to form stable nontoxic compounds. Mesna is rapidly cleared from the plasma by the kidneys, resulting in a high concentration of mesna in the urine. As a result, some of the genitourinary toxicities are diminished. Because mesna has a short intravascular half-life, it does not interfere with the cytotoxic activity on the malignant cells, and it does not protect against other adverse effects of cyclophosphamide and ifosfamide. Mesna is recommended with the use of ifosfamide and high-dose cyclophosphamide.[29]

Amifostine is another thiol compound that is believed to protect cells from damage by oxygen-derived free radicals when it is converted to its active form by the endothelial cell enzyme alkaline phosphatase. Less activation of amifostine occurs in cancers because of a low pH and poor tumor vascularity.[29] Patients who received amifostine had a significantly lower incidence of grade 4 neutropenia and grade 3 peripheral neuropathy and a lower incidence of moderate renal toxicity in a randomized controlled trial of 242 patients with ovarian cancer who received cyclophosphamide and cisplatin.[30] This study also found that only 9% of patients had to discontinue therapy in the amifostine treatment arm versus 24% in the placebo arm, with no difference in median survival between the two arms. As a result of this and other studies, current clinical guidelines recommend consideration of the use of amifostine with cisplatin chemotherapy to prevent nephrotoxicity and with alkylating agent chemotherapy to prevent neutropenia.[29]

There is some evidence that amifostine may reduce the incidence of peripheral neuropathy, which is a major toxicity of some newer agents used in treating lung cancer, such as paclitaxel. Amifostine was associated with a reduction in peripheral neuropathy due to cisplatin therapy in a randomized study, but the incidence of grade 3 peripheral neuropathy was low in both study arms, and the benefit was relatively modest (7% versus 13%).[30] However, amifostine did not provide protection from paclitaxel-related neurotoxicity in a small randomized study involving 40 women with metastatic breast cancer.[31] Current ASCO guidelines state that the data is insufficient to recommend the routine use of amifostine to prevent cisplatin or paclitaxel-related neuropathy.

Amifostine was approved by the FDA for use as a radioprotectant in the treatment of head and neck cancers. The average duration of ≥grade 3 mucositis was decreased with amifostine (23 days versus 45 days; $P < 0.02$) in a randomized study involving accelerated RT.[32] There is also accumulating evidence that amifostine can decrease the incidence of mucositis and xerostomia associated with RT to the head and neck region.[33] This data and that of other trials have led to speculation that amifostine may act as an esophageal protectant in patients receiving combined chemoradiotherapy.[34] An ongoing phase III trial (RTOG 9801) is studying the effects of amifostine with concurrent chemotherapy (carboplatin, paclitaxel) and twice-daily RT.

Treatment of Anorexia

It was previously thought that cancer patients lost weight because of the caloric demands of a rapidly growing tumor. However, as our understanding of tumor biology has improved, it has become clear that much of the weight loss is related to an alteration in the metabolism of normal cells as well as to decreased appetite. Alterations in the levels of cytokines (eg, tumor necrosis factor, IL-1, IL-2) have been implicated as a cause of cancer-related cachexia. In many cases, the patient is not bothered by the poor appetite and weight loss, but these symptoms frequently result in a significant amount of distress to family members and other caregivers.

The two medications used most commonly to stimulate the appetite are megestrol acetate and corticosteroids. A randomized control trial compared a corticosteroid (dexamethasone), an anabolic corticosteroid (fluoxymesterone), and megestrol acetate.[35] An average weight gain of approximately 2 kg was seen, and only 4% to 10% of patients gained more than 10% of weight over baseline levels with each of these medications, with no significant differences among the three drugs. By subjective assessment, appetite was improved by both dexamethasone and megestrol acetate. The patients treated with dexamethasone had a significantly higher incidence of myopathy, cushingoid changes, and peptic ulcers, whereas the patients treated with megestrol acetate had a nonsignificantly higher rate of deep vein thrombosis (5% versus 1%; $P = 0.06$). The patients treated with dexamethasone also had a higher rate of drug discontinuation than the patients treated with megestrol acetate (36% versus 25%; $P = 0.03$). At present, both megestrol acetate and a corticosteroid can be used for appetite stimulation, but the absolute weight gain with both medications is relatively modest.

Often family members will raise the question about the role of a gastric feeding tube. Placement of a gastric feeding tube should be reserved for special situations because there has been no demonstrated benefit to aggressive nutritional support with regard to life expectancy or symptomatic improvement. A feeding tube may be useful in patients who have a mechanical obstruction that prevents them from eating and a relatively slow-growing tumor. A feeding tube may also be useful in order to maintain hydration and nutritional intake during periods of temporary mucositis occurring while the patient is receiving aggressive chemotherapy, or RT, or both. In general, however, a feeding tube does not affect quality or quantity of life unless the problem causing the poor nutritional intake is temporary or due to local problems in a patient who has a significant life expectancy.

EDITORS' COMMENTS

Extensive research has led to an understanding of many details of the cause of cancer and what governs the growth and spread of malignant tumors. Unfortunately, the sum result at present is that of a complex puzzle in which the overall picture is still unclear even though a number of individual pieces have been fitted together. Thus, many of the insights that have been gained do not yet have a clear impact in clinical practice. Nevertheless, a general knowledge of the currently favored paradigms is useful in providing a backdrop for the treatment of lung cancer.

Many questions about the behavior of cancers still remain unanswered. For example, what governs the ability of cancer cells to form systemic metastatic foci is unknown, although it seems clear that the process is much more complex than simply the release of a cancer cell into the bloodstream. Reliance on the paradigm of progression of a cancer from a localized stage to one involving regional lymph nodes, and finally to hematogenous dissemination, is waning. Instead, it appears that the ability of cancer cells to grow and metastasize is governed by complex biologic mechanisms that are not necessarily static throughout the growth of a malignant tumor and may be an expression of acquisition of progressively more genetic defects. The interplay of various oncogenes also appears to have an effect on the way a cell responds to damage by chemotherapeutic agents—by undergoing either apoptosis or cell cycle arrest, during which repair can take place. The mechanism for resistance to chemotherapy is poorly understood but appears to be much more complex than simply an intrinsic or acquired genetic mutation. Why the cure rates of some tumors, such as SCLC, are low, despite high complete response rates, also remains unclear.

However, on a more concrete level, it is clear that active chemotherapeutic agents are available for both SCLC and NSCLC. The ability to cure disseminated disease with chemotherapy alone is still poor, and better agents are needed—perhaps with novel mechanisms of action, as suggested by new insights into tumor biology. However, in limited-stage disease, there is good evidence that currently available chemotherapeutic agents can destroy cancer cells in the primary tumor and, more important, can decrease the development of distant recurrences. Furthermore, it is clear that many patients with apparently localized lung cancers actually have occult foci of systemic disease. This makes it important to know how best to integrate chemotherapy with a local treatment such as RT or surgery. Progress is being made in these areas, as discussed elsewhere in this book.

In a majority of patients with lung cancer, the goals of therapy are palliative. Although prolongation of survival can be achieved, the major hope is that chemotherapy can palliate disease-related symptoms and improve overall quality of life. A number of new chemotherapeutic agents are available that have increased antitumor activity and often have better toxicity profiles as well. Supportive care measures that decrease the morbidity of chemotherapy are also important in increasing the therapeutic gain from chemotherapy. The development of effective antiemetics and growth factors has been a major achievement.

References

1. Skipper HE, Schabel FM Jr, Wilcox WS. On the criteria and kinetics associated with "curability" of experimental leukemia. Cancer Chemother Rep. 1964;35:1–111.

2. DeVita VT. Cell kinetics and the chemotherapy of cancer. Cancer Chemother Rep. 1971;2:23–33.

3. DeVita VT Jr. Principles of cancer management: chemotherapy. In: DeVita VT Jr, Hellman S, Rosenberg SA, ed. Cancer: Principles and Practice of Oncology. 5th ed. Philadelphia: Lippincott-Raven; 1997:333–347.

4. Goldie JH, Coldman AJ. A mathematical model for relating the drug sensitivity of tumors to their spontaneous mutation rate. Cancer Treat Rep. 1979;63:1727–1733.

5. Goldie JH, Coldman AJ. The genetic origin of drug resistance in neoplasms: implications for systemic therapy. Cancer Res. 1984;44:3643–3653.

6. Goldie JH, Coldman AJ, Gudauskas GA. Rationale for the use of alternating non–cross-resistant chemotherapy. Cancer Treat Rep. 1982;66:439–449.

7. Norton L. A Gompertzian model of human breast cancer growth. Cancer Res. 1988;48:7067–7071.

8. Gunduz N, Fisher B, Saffer EA. Effect of surgical removal on the growth and kinetics of residual tumor. Cancer Res. 1979;39:3861–3865.

9. Schabel FM Jr. Concepts for systemic treatment of micrometastases. Cancer. 1975;35:15–24.

10. Simpson-Herrin L, Sanford AH, Holmquist JP. Effects of surgery in the cell kinetics of residual tumor. Cancer Treat Rep. 1976;60:1744–1760.

11. Young RC, DeVita VT. Cell cycle characteristics of human solid tumors in vivo. Cell Tissue Kinet. 1970;8:285–290.

12. Peck K, Sher Y-P, Shih J-Y, et al. Detection and quantitation of circulating cancer cells in the peripheral blood of lung cancer patients. Cancer Res. 1998;58:2761–2765.

13. Folkman J. Clinical applications of research on angiogenesis. N Engl J Med. 1995;333:1757–1763.

14. Norton L, Simon R. The Norton-Simon hypothesis revisited. Cancer Treat Rep. 1986;70:163–169.

15. Beck WT, Dalton WS. Mechanisms of drug resistance. In: DeVita VT Jr, Hellman S, Rosenberg S, eds. Cancer: Principles and Practice of Oncology. 5th ed. Philadelphia: Lippincott-Raven; 1997:498–512.

16. Tannock I. Treatment of cancer with radiation and drugs. J Clin Oncol. 1996;14:3156–3174.

17. Vokes EE, Weichselbaum RR. Concomitant chemoradiotherapy: rationale and clinical experience in patients with solid tumors. J Clin Oncol. 1990;8:911–934.

18. Schaake-Koning C, van den Bogaert W, Dalesio O, et al. Effects of concomitant cisplatin and radiotherapy on inoperable non–small-cell lung cancer. N Engl J Med. 1992;326:524–530.

19. National Cancer Institute. Common Toxicity Criteria. Bethesda, Md: National Cancer Institute; 1998.

20. Roila F, Tonato M, Cognetti F, et al. Prevention of cisplatin-induced emesis: a double-blind multicenter randomized crossover study comparing ondansetron and ondansetron plus dexamethasone. J Clin Oncol. 1991;9:674–678.

21. Perry MC, ed. The Chemotherapy Source Book. 2nd ed. Philadelphia: Williams & Wilkins; 1997.

22. Girling DJ. Comparison of oral etoposide and standard intravenous multidrug chemotherapy for small-cell lung cancer: a stopped multicentre randomised trial (Medical Research Council Lung Cancer Working Party). Lancet. 1996;348:563–566.

23. Gralla RJ, Osoba D, Kris MG, et al. Recommendations for the use of antiemetics: evidence-based clinical practice guidelines. J Clin Oncol. 1999;17:2971–2994.

24. American Society of Clinical Oncology. Recommendations for the use of hematopoietic colony-stimulating factors: evidence-based, clinical practice guidelines. J Clin Oncol. 1994;12:2471–2508.

25. Antman KS, Griffin JD, Elias A, et al. Effect of recombinant human granulocyte-macrophage colony-stimulating factor on chemotherapy-induced myelosuppression. N Engl J Med. 1988;319:593–598.

26. Crawford J, Ozer H, Stoller R, et al. Reduction by granulocyte colony-stimulating factor of fever and neutropenia induced by chemotherapy in patients with small-cell lung cancer. N Engl J Med. 1991;325:164–170.

27. Issacs C, Robert NJ, Bailey FA, et al. Randomized placebo control trial of recombinant interleukin-11 to prevent chemotherapy-induced thrombocytopenia in patients with breast cancer receiving dose-intensive cyclophosphamide and doxorubicin. J Clin Oncol. 1997;15:3368–3377.

28. Demetri GD, Fletcher CD, Mueller E, et al. Quality of life benefit in chemotherapy patients treated with epoetin alfa is independent of disease response or tumor type: results from a prospective community oncology study. J Clin Oncol. 1998;16:3412–3425.

29. American Society of Clinical Oncology. American Society of Clinical Oncology clinical practice guidelines for the use of chemotherapy and radiotherapy protectants. J Clin Oncol. 1999;17:3333–3355.

30. Kemp G, Rose P, Lurain J, et al. Amifostine pretreatment for protection against cyclophosphamide-induced and cisplatin-induced toxicities: results of a randomized control trial in patients with advanced ovarian cancer. J Clin Oncol. 1996;14:2101–2112.

31. Gelmon K, Eisenhauer E, Bryce C, et al. Randomized phase II study of high dose paclitaxel with or without amifostine in patients with metastatic breast cancer. J Clin Oncol. 1999;17:3038–3047.

32. Bourhis J, Wibault P, Luboinski B, et al. A randomized phase II study of very accelerated radiotherapy with and without amifostine in advanced head and neck carcinoma [abstract]. Proc ASCO. 1999;18:393a.

33. Buntzel J. Selective cytoprotection with amifostine in concurrent radiochemotherapy for head and neck cancer. Ann Oncol. 1998;9:505–509.

34. Roychowdhury DF, Redmond K, Desai P, et al. A phase II trial of amifostine with paclitaxel, carboplatin and concurrent radiation therapy for unresectable non–small cell lung cancer [abstract]. Proc ASCO. 1999;18:522a.

35. Loprinzi CL, Kugler JW, Sloan JA, et al. Randomized comparison of megestrol acetate versus dexamethasone versus fluoxymesterone for treatment of cancer anorexia/cachexia. J Clin Oncol. 1999;17:3299–3306.

36. Geddes DM. The natural history of lung cancer: a review based on rates of tumour growth. Br J Dis Chest. 1979;73:1–17.

PART 4

EARLY STAGE NON–SMALL CELL LUNG CANCER

SURGERY FOR STAGE I NON-SMALL CELL LUNG CANCER

David R. Jones and Frank C. Detterbeck

DEFINITION AND STAGING ISSUES

Stage I non–small cell lung cancer (NSCLC) is defined as a T1 or T2 tumor without nodal involvement. Although this definition is clear, the nuances of how this is determined are often overlooked. The most important distinction is whether patients are classified as stage I using clinical staging or pathologic staging. Clinical staging involves all information available *before any treatment is carried out.* Most often, this involves radiographic staging: a clinical stage I (cI) patient has no evidence of N1, N2, or N3 nodal enlargement on computed tomography (CT) scan as well as no evidence of distant metastases by history and physical examination. However, because CT carries a false negative (FN) rate for mediastinal nodes of 10% to 25% (see Table 5–7), more accurate clinical staging includes mediastinoscopy. Unfortunately, most studies of cI patients have not reported in detail how staging was performed.

Pathologic staging is based on information available after surgical resection. Although this is clearly more accurate than clinical staging, it has the drawback of being an after-the-fact assessment. At the point that decisions about the course of treatment for patients are made, only clinical staging is available. It is important not to extrapolate the results of pathologically staged patients to clinically staged patients.

Even though pathologic staging seems straightforward, the care with which it is done affects the accuracy. First, it is important that lymph nodes are actually pathologically assessed. Although this may seem to be obvious, a 1990 survey of thoracic surgeons reported that 45% did not routinely sample mediastinal lymph nodes at thoracotomy unless they were grossly abnormal.[1] Such an intraoperative gross assessment was found to be unreliable, however, in a study of 575 cI patients, which found that the surgeon

did not detect 68% of involved N2 nodes by intraoperative inspection or palpation.[2] In two additional studies of 100 and 379 patients in whom the nodes were carefully assessed intraoperatively, the surgeon's visual inspection and palpation resulted in a 41% false positive and a 10% to 11% FN rate.[3,113] These results make it clear that mediastinal nodes should be biopsied in order to obtain accurate pathologic staging. It is embarrassing how often examination of operative and pathology reports will disclose so-called *pathologic stage I* patients where mediastinal nodes were not sampled by the surgeon and N1 nodes were not assessed by the pathologist.

Assessment of N1 nodes alone is not sufficient to classify a patient as pathologically N0. Multiple studies have consistently shown that approximately one-third (average, 29%; range, 24%-36%) of resected pN2 patients have no involvement of their N1 nodes (so-called *skip metastases*).[2, 4–13] This is strikingly similar to the 24% incidence of segmental lymph channels that drain directly into mediastinal nodes that was reported in a study of 260 cadavers.[14] Adenocarcinomas and other nonsquamous tumor histologies may be more likely to have skip metastases than squamous cell tumors.[8]

The surgical technique used to biopsy the mediastinal lymph nodes is probably not of major importance. On one hand, *systematic mediastinal node sampling* involves opening the mediastinal pleura and performing routine biopsy of nodes in regions 2, 4, and 7 on the right and 4, 5, 6, and 7 on the left.[15–17] Nodes from the other stations are explored and removed only if suspicious for cancer. *Radical lymphadenectomy,* on the other hand, consists of removing all tissue en bloc from the superior and inferior mediastinal compartments and completely exposing the trachea, superior vena cava, innominate vein, aorta, recurrent laryngeal nerve, and esophagus.[2,8,18–20] Whether such a radical lymphadenectomy is associated with any increased morbidity or longer operative times is controversial.[21,22] A prospective, randomized study comparing these two techniques in 182 patients with operable NSCLC found no difference in the percentage of patients with N1 or N2 disease.[6] However, radical lymphadenectomy identified significantly more patients with multilevel nodal involvement compared with lymph node sampling (57% versus 17%; $P = 0.007$).[6] This suggests that radical lymphadenectomy is not necessary to accurately determine the pathologic N stage of a patient, although additional detail among N2 patients may be gained.

Although it is important to biopsy mediastinal lymph nodes to adequately stage the tumor, there is little evidence that a radical lymphadenectomy is of therapeutic benefit. Two randomized studies have found no differences in recurrence rates or survival in patients undergoing lymphadenectomy versus lymph node sampling (in 115 patients with $\leq$2 cm stage pI NSCLC, and 182 cI-IIIa patients.)[21,22] However, two retrospective studies have found conflicting results.[16,114] In 125 patients with pT1N0M0 NSCLC, approximately half of whom underwent lymph node dissection based on the personal policies of the surgeons at their respective institutions, 5-year survival was worse in patients undergoing lymphadenectomy (70% vs. 90%, $P < 0.05$).[16] In contrast, better median survival was found after lymphadenectomy compared with node sampling in a retrospective review of 355 patients enrolled in a study of adjuvant therapy for resected patients with pII,IIIa NSCLC (53 months versus 29 months, $P = 0.003$).[114] The American College of Surgeons Oncology Group initiated a randomized study in 1999 to re-evaluate the therapeutic benefit of lymphadenectomy in patients with N0,1 NSCLC (ACoSOG Z0030).

NATURAL HISTORY

Little information is available regarding the natural history of patients who are clinically stage I and who do not receive any treatment. The only clear description of such a group was by Vrdoljak et al,[23] who found a median survival of 17 months in 19 patients with cT2N0 NSCLC. The 2-year survival was 20%, and all patients had died by 3 years. Thus the natural history of even stage I lung cancer, when untreated, appears to be rapid progression to death in essentially all patients.

OUTCOME OF CLINICAL STAGE I PATIENTS

Few authors have reported on the final pathologic stage of patients initially classified as clinical stage I patients. Of seven studies addressing this issue, an average of 73% (range, 61%-81%) of cI patients are found to be pathologically N0, 11% (range, 6%-23%) are found to be pathologically N1, and another 14% (range, 12%-21%) are pathologically N2.[2,8,21,24–27] The incidence of pN2 disease is similar to the FN rates for mediastinal node involvement on CT scan (see Table 5–7). This is not surprising because almost all of these patients were clinically staged by CT without undergoing mediastinoscopy.[2,8,21,24,25] Furthermore, <1% of

the cI patients in these studies were found to be M1.[2,8,24,25]

There is no information on how often cI patients were found to be unresectable, but presumably this rate is low. In a population-based study of 676 cI,II patients <70 years of age, 19% did not undergo surgery because of co-morbidity, and 47% of 437 patients >70 years did not undergo resection because of either age or co-morbidity.[28] The extent of pulmonary parenchyma excision necessary to achieve a complete resection (R_0) in resected pT1,2N0 NSCLC is a lobectomy in 73% (range, 55%-83% in studies of >100 cI patients).[29–34] Approximately 6% (range, 4%-8%) of patients require a bilobectomy, 11% (range, 4%-19%) require a pneumonectomy, and 11% (range, 4%-26%) undergo a segmentectomy or wedge resection for various reasons.[29–34] A pneumonectomy may be required more frequently (27%) for a T2N0 tumor compared with a T1N0 lesion (2%).[31]

The survival of clinical stage I patients is shown in Table 11–1. Survival for cT1N0 patients is good, but the outcome decreases markedly for cT2N0 patients. Particularly for the latter group, the survival of clinically staged patients is much worse than that of pathologically staged patients. A comparison of the numbers of clinical and pathologic stage T1,2N0 patients indicates a possible explanation. Two large series suggest that more of the cT2N0 patients are reassigned to different TNM categories after pathologic assessment than is true for cT1N0 patients.[18,35]

OUTCOME OF PATHOLOGIC STAGE I PATIENTS

Surgical resection is widely accepted as the treatment of choice for stage I lung cancer. Resection is intuitively appealing because a complete resection with an adequate

TABLE 11–1. SURVIVAL OF RESECTED CLINICAL STAGE I PATIENTS

STUDY	N	T STAGE	5-YEAR SURVIVAL
Naruke et al[18]	821	T1,T2	50
Bülzebruck et al[103]	506	T1,T2	37
Suzuki et al[104]	365	T1,T2	67
Average			**51**
Mountain[39] a	687	T1	61
Naruke et al[18]	349	T1	65
Asamura et al[8]	337	T1	77
Suzuki et al[104]	198	T1	77
Sugi et al[21]	115	T1 b	(83) b
Average c			**70**
Mountain[39] a	1189	T2	38
Naruke et al[18]	479	T2	42
Suzuki et al[104]	167	T2	54
Average			**47**

Inclusion criteria: Studies of ≥100 clinical stage I patients.
a Includes 4% SCLC.
b All tumors <2 cm.
c Excluding values in parentheses.

margin in stage I lung cancers can be accomplished with low morbidity and mortality rates (see Table 8–1). A large number of studies have reported on the survival of resected, pathologic stage I patients. The results are shown in Table 11–2, with an overall 5-year survival of approximately 65%. The reported survival has been found consistently to be between 55% and 75%, with few exceptions.[36,37,106] Survival curves from one of the largest series (Memorial Sloan-Kettering) are shown in Figure 11–1. A variety of prognostic factors have been investigated, and these are discussed in the following sections.

T Status

The T status of stage I tumors has prognostic significance. Every series comparing T stage in Table 11–2 found better survival of T1 compared with T2 patients, and this difference was significant in each of those reports in which the significance was calculated. Figure 11–1 is typical of many published reports of survival of T1 and T2N0 patients. The survival difference of approximately 15% for T1 versus T2 was found to be statistically significant for both squamous cell carcinoma ($P = 0.001$) and adenocarcinoma ($P = 0.009$) in an analysis from the Mayo Clinic.[38] Recognizing this survival difference, the most recent revision of the International System for Staging Lung Cancer has classified T1N0 lesions separately (stage Ia) from T2N0 tumors (stage Ib).[39]

The relative significance of the T classification based on tumor size versus visceral pleural involvement is unclear. The four studies that have examined this have shown conflicting results.[33,34,40,41] Martini et al[40] found a significant difference in survival between tumors ≤3 cm and those >3 cm ($P < 0.04$), but visceral pleural involvement did not affect survival. Padilla et al[34] also found no significant effect of visceral pleural involvement. In contrast, Harpole et al,[33] using multivariate analysis, found visceral pleural involvement to be a predictor of early recurrence and cancer death. In a fourth study of 243 stage I patients, Ichinose et al[41] found the difference in survival by tumor

size (<3 cm or >3 cm, 84% versus 66%) not to be significant by multivariate analysis (despite significance by univariate analysis), whereas visceral pleural involvement was significant (5-year survival, 89% versus 66%, $P = 0.004$). Thus, the prognostic value of visceral involvement is unclear. It may be that the significance of pleural involvement is an association with larger tumors, as suggested by the largest study.[40] When size was controlled, pleural invasion no longer had prognostic value.[40] The only study addressing stage I tumors that are T2 by virtue of lobar bronchial obstruction found no significant difference in survival (5-year survival, 87% in 26 patients with proximal involvement versus 71% in 128 patients without; $P = $ NS).[34]

Thus, the T stage significantly influences survival, with approximately 15% to 20% worse 5-year survival with T2 cancers. The prognostic value of visceral pleural involvement remains to be determined. Other factors such as molecular markers may be of greater importance in the future. For example, one study found the T factor to be of only marginal significance by multivariate analysis ($P = 0.08$) when the degree of differentiation and the DNA ploidy were included.[29]

Size

Several authors, particularly in Japan, have questioned the choice of 3 cm as the breakpoint for a difference in survival.[8,24,42] Indeed, several studies have shown a difference in survival (statistically significant in some reports)[24,34] for N0 tumors using 2 cm as the breakpoint,[24,33,34,42] although others have found no difference.[8] Using multivariate analysis, Harpole et al[33] found the 3 cm breakpoint to be slightly better than 2 cm, although several other factors (symptoms, vascular invasion, visceral pleural invasion) were of much greater prognostic benefit. Results from the largest study are shown in Figure 11–2. They strongly suggest that the effect of tumor size is a continuum, and the breakpoint chosen is arbitrary. Thus, there seems to be no compelling reason to abandon 3 cm as the breakpoint between T1 and T2 tumors.

Histology

Some authors have suggested that stage I squamous cell cancers have an improved survival compared with adenocarcinomas.[30-32,43,44] In fact, only one study in Table 11–2 reported a trend toward worse survival with squamous cell cancer.[18] However, statistically significant better survival for squamous cancers was only seen in one of eight studies.[43] The preponderance of contemporary reports have found no difference in survival based on tumor histology for stage I tumors.[8,18,29,33,34,38,40] This provides strong evidence that tumor histology is not a significant prognostic factor in stage I NSCLC. The small difference in average survival in the data shown in Table 11–2 supports this conclusion.

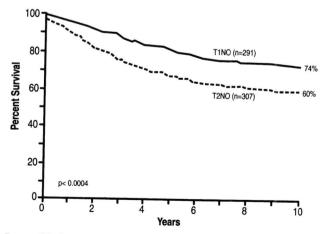

FIGURE 11–1. Survival by T factor in resected stage I non–small cell lung cancer in 598 patients. (From Martini N, Bains MS, Burt ME, et al. Incidence of local recurrence and second primary tumors in resected stage I lung cancer. J Thorac Cardiovasc Surg. 1995;109:120–129.)[40]

TABLE 11-2. SURVIVAL AFTER RESECTION OF PATHOLOGIC STAGE I NON–SMALL CELL LUNG CANCER

STUDY	N	5-YEAR SURVIVAL (%)				5-YEAR SURVIVAL (%)		
		ALL	T1	T2	P (T1:T2)	Squamous Cell Cancer	Adenocarcinoma ± Large Cell	P (ADENOCARCINOMA: SQUAMOUS)
van Rens[117]	1249	—	63	46	0.0001	—	—	—
Mountain and Dresler[35]	1060	—	67	57	0.05	—	—	—
Thomas et al[44 a]	907	68	65	—	—	69	62	NS
Naruke[7]	798	—	—	—	—	—	—	—
Inoue et al[105]	751	—	80	65	0.001	—	—	—
Mountain et al[43]	725	68	75	60	0.0004	83[a]	69[a]	0.02
Martini et al[40]	598	75	82	68	—	74	74	—
Jie et al[106]	568	47	—	—	—	—	—	—
Naruke et al[18]	536	65	76	57	—	64	69	—
Pastorino et al[36 b]	515	48	62	44	0.0008	52	45	NS
Williams et al[30]	461	71	80	62	—	70	65[c]	—
Bülzebruck et al[103]	439	58	—	—	—	—	—	—
Kotlyarov and Rukosuyer[37 d]	403	43	54	38	—	—	—	—
Maggi et al[13]	373	65	—	—	—	—	—	—
Read et al[31 c]	372	63	73	49	—	62	42	—
Fujisawa[118]	369	70	—	—	—	—	—	—
Adebonojo[119]	342	—	77	62	0.006	—	—	—
Pairolero et al[38 f]	328	69	70	58	0.01	—	—	NS
Harpole et al[33]	289	63	70[g]	50[g]	0.001	68	61	NS
Average		63	71	55		68	61	

Inclusion criteria: All reported series from 1980 to 2000 involving ≥250 patients undergoing resection of pathologic stage I non–small cell lung cancer.

[a] T1N0 patients only.
[b] 10% limited resection.
[c] Excludes bronchoalveolar cell cancer.
[d] Includes 9% small cell.
[e] Disease-free survival, excluding operative mortality; 21% had limited resection.
[f] Unclear extent of operative staging.
[g] T stage based on size only.

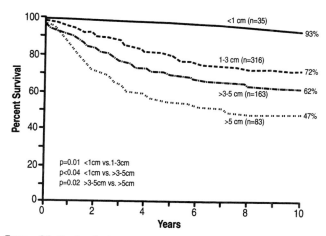

FIGURE 11–2. Survival by tumor size in centimeters. (From Martini N, Bains MS, Burt ME, et al. Incidence of local recurrence and second primary tumors in resected stage I lung cancer. J Thorac Cardiovasc Surg. 1995;109:120–129.[40])

Tumor Differentiation, Vascular Invasion

Several studies suggest that survival may be better in patients with well differentiated tumors.[33,41,45,46] In a detailed study of 243 resected stage I patients, Ichinose et al[41] found that the degree of tumor differentiation was a statistically significant factor by multivariate analysis (5-year survival, 87% versus 71%; $P = 0.02$ for well differentiated versus moderately or poorly differentiated pI tumors). This study did not find the histologic grade to be of significance in stage II (63 patients) or IIIa (108 patients).[41] A similar study limited to small (≤2 cm) peripheral adenocarcinomas also found that the degree of differentiation was a significant prognostic factor by multivariate analysis.[46] Chung et al[45] also found better survival among 66 stage I patients with well differentiated tumors (2-year survival, 89%, 71%, and 50% for well, moderately, and poorly differentiated cancers, respectively; no significance reported). Harpole et al[33] found tumor differentiation to be a significant predictor ($P < 0.05$, univariate analysis) of 5-year survival after resection of stage I NSCLC in 289

patients. This was not significant, however, in a multivariate analysis. The degree of differentiation has also been found to correlate with the incidence of distant metastases after complete resection for stage I or II adenocarcinoma of the lung.[47]

The presence of vascular invasion by the tumor is associated with decreased survival.[33,41,45,48,49] This was statistically significant by multivariate analysis in three large studies (106, 243, and 249 patients) of patients with stage I NSCLC,[33,41,49] but not in a fourth study (N = 277).[50] Five-year survival in stage I patients was 79% in the absence of vascular invasion and 48% in its presence in one of these studies,[41] 79% and 47% in another,[49] and 68% and 35% in a third.[33] Macchiarini et al[48,51] also found vascular invasion to be of major prognostic significance in multivariate analysis in a smaller study of pathologic stage I tumors, but a later, larger study found this to be not significant.[50] An earlier study involving 551 N0 patients with NSCLC or small cell lung cancer found blood vessel invasion to have no prognostic relevance.[52]

Other Factors

A large number of other prognostic factors have been examined mostly in small studies that have evaluated only one factor and which have generally yielded conflicting results.[36,53] The largest multivariate study, involving 10 molecular markers in 408 stage I patients, found that five different factors had independent prognostic significance (angiogenesis factor VIII, apoptosis factor p53, metastatic adhesion factor CD-44, growth factor erb-b2, and cell cycle factor rb).[54] A multivariate analysis of different markers in 151 patients with stage I NSCLC identified tumor DNA ploidy as a predominant prognostic factor.[29] Patients with aneuploid tumors had significantly decreased 2-, 3-, and 5-year survivals compared with patients with diploid tumors ($P < 0.04$). In another study of 106 patients with pathologic stage I NSCLC, angiogenesis and blood vessel invasion were significant prognostic factors by multivariate analysis.[49] In a third multivariate analysis of 101 consecutive patients, the presence of tumor angiogenesis had dramatic prognostic importance ($P = 0.00001$), completely overshadowing the value of other variables (T,N stage,

DATA SUMMARY: SURVIVAL AND PROGNOSTIC FACTORS IN STAGE I NSCLC			
	AMOUNT	**QUALITY**	**CONSISTENCY**
The 5-year survival of cT1N0 patients is 70%	High	High	High
The 5-year survival of cT2N0 patients is 45%	Mod	High	High
The 5-year survival of pI patients is 65%	High	High	Mod
The 5-year survival of pT1N0 patients is 70%	High	High	High
The 5-year survival of pT2N0 patients is 55%	High	High	Mod
There is no significant difference in survival of pI patients between squamous and adenocarcinoma	High	High	High
Tumor differentiation may be a significant prognostic factor	High	Mod	Mod
Vascular invasion may be a significant prognostic factor	High	Mod	Mod

Type of data rated: Plain text: descriptive statement   *Italics: controlled comparison*   **Bold: randomized comparison**

grade).[55] The presence of angiogenesis correlated dramatically with the development of distant (but not nodal) metastases. A number of studies in other tumor types have shown similar results.[55] However, none of the biologic markers has been studied extensively enough to permit any firm conclusions to be drawn.[36,53]

Some authors have found statistically significant better survival for women with stage I NSCLC as compared with men,[30,33,115] whereas others have noted the opposite trend.[34] It is probably most revealing that gender did not retain any significant prognostic value in multivariate analysis in two large studies (>250 patients).[33,115] Conflicting results have also been noted regarding survival after lobectomy versus pneumonectomy in stage I tumors.[30,33,56,116] There is some suggestion that pneumonectomy is associated with higher stage tumors.[31,57] The only study to report stage and procedure-specific survival found no difference between lobectomy and pneumonectomy for each stage.[57]

OCCULT CANCER

The majority of NSCLCs are visible radiographically at the time of diagnosis. Occasionally, however, sputum cytology diagnoses a lung cancer that is radiographically occult. These cases have been identified primarily as a result of two large screening studies in the United States[58,59] and an ongoing screening project in Japan.[60,61] Fiberoptic bronchoscopy with systematic inspection and brushing of each segmental bronchus is the recommended method to localize the tumor.[58–62] Approximately 25% (range, 22%-28%) of these tumors are not visible by bronchoscopy, and an additional 30% (range, 26%-38%) have only minute abnormalities that are easily overlooked.[59,61,62] It is often necessary to repeat the bronchoscopy two or three times to achieve an accurate diagnosis.[63] Most (58%) of the cancers are located in segmental or larger bronchi, 30% in subsegmental bronchi, and only 13% in even more distal areas.[61]

Squamous cell cancer has consistently been found to be involved almost exclusively in cases of occult lung cancers.[58,61,64] The majority (52%-94%) of these tumors are pT1N0M0 lesions, including 14% to 35% involving carcinoma in situ.[58–60] Only a few patients (5%-17%) have had N1 involvement, and even fewer are found to be higher stage.[58–60] Approximately 10% (range, 7%-10%) of patients are found to have synchronous primary tumors,[61,64] which emphasizes the importance of a systematic and meticulous bronchoscopic examination in these patients. Furthermore, the risk of subsequent development of a metachronous second primary lung cancer has been found to be 2% to 5% per patient per year.[59,60] As a result, at 5 years 11% to 32% of patients with occult lung cancer have been found to develop a second lung cancer, 50% of which are also occult.[58–60] These patients should undergo LIFE (light-induced fluorescence endoscopy) bronchoscopy, which has been shown by a multi-institutional trial to have significantly improved sensitivity in detecting areas of moderate or severe dysplasia and carcinoma in situ (9% versus 56%, $P < 0.05$).[65] The 5-year survival for resected patients with occult lung cancer has been found to be 80% to 90%.[59,60]

SPECIFIC SURGICAL ISSUES

Extent of Surgical Resection

In 1940, Ochsner and DeBakey stated that "any procedure short of total removal of the involved lung [for the treatment of lung cancer] is irrational."[66(p993)] This approach generally prevailed, but in 1958 Churchill et al reported on a series of resections where "lobectomy was considered reasonable when there was evidence of diminished pulmonary or cardiac reserve . . . and the lesion could be totally excised."[67(p301)] As the techniques of hilar dissection were understood and established, lobectomy became the procedure of choice. Thus it was only natural that the efficacy of more limited resections would be explored, either as a compromise procedure in poor risk patients or as the procedure of choice.

It is important to distinguish between different types of limited resection. A *segmental resection* involves isolation of the bronchus, artery, and vein of an anatomic segment of the lung and complete removal of the segment. This is usually done in experienced centers and carries a risk of prolonged air leak from the dissected lung.[68] A *segmentectomy* is a different operation from a *wedge resection*, where staples are placed, not necessarily respecting the segmental anatomic planes of the involved lung, to excise a lesion. Particularly with the advent of video-assisted thoracic surgery (VATS), the temptation to "wedge out" peripheral tumors is great. Only a nonanatomic wedge resection is generally possible via thoracoscopy, and this is not necessarily comparable to a formal segmentectomy.

Several nonrandomized studies have been reported in an attempt to compare limited resection to lobectomy.[33,40,42,69–73] Two of these studies[42,70] involved only segmentectomy in 68 and 46 patients (most of whom would have also tolerated a lobectomy) and compared them with patients undergoing lobectomy at the same institutions during the same period. One study found a significant 5-year survival difference (46% versus 66%, $P = 0.03$),[42] whereas the other did not (93% versus 88%).[70] The study showing a survival difference noted that this was most marked in tumors >3 cm.[42] The other study was limited to highly selected patients with peripheral T1 lesions that were not spiculated.[70] Both studies reported that local recurrences were significantly more frequent after segmentectomy (23% versus 5% and 9% versus 1%, $P < 0.05$).[42,70]

Six additional studies have compared lobectomy to wedge resection as a compromise operation in poor risk patients.[33,40,69,71–73] In one study of 598 patients, 5-year survival was 77% after lobectomy versus 59% after limited resection (N = 62, $P = 0.02$),[40] In another study of 244 consecutive stage I patients, 5-year survival was found to be 73% after lobectomy and pneumonectomy versus 48% after limited resection (N = 58, $P = 0.003$).[72] A third study (219 patients) reported 5-year survival to be 70% after lobectomy, compared with 58% (N = 42, $P = 0.005$) after open wedge and 65% after a VATS wedge (N = 60, $P = $ NS).[71] The fourth study, involving 197 consecutive stage I patients, reported a 5-year survival of 75% after lobectomy and 69% after wedge resection (N = 100, $P = $ NS).[69] The reported survival in this latter study is quite astounding, because only 14% of the patients were T1N0,

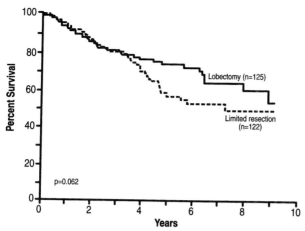

FIGURE 11–3. Survival of 247 T1N0 patients randomized to lobectomy or limited resection. $P = 0.062$, one-tailed log rank test. (From Rubinstein LV, Ginsberg RJ. Reply to "Randomized trial of lobectomy versus limited resection for T1 N0 non-small cell lung cancer," 1995 article by the Lung Cancer Study Group. Ann Thorac Surg. 1996;62:1249–1250.[75])

and 25% were T1N1. There was no difference in the stage distribution between the two groups.[69] In the remaining two studies (involving 61 and 75 patients with limited resections), the difference was minimal.[33,73]

The only prospective, randomized trial of lobectomy versus limited resection for pT1N0 NSCLC was carried out by the Lung Cancer Study Group (LCSG).[74,75] The study involved a highly select group of 247 patients with T1 tumors who underwent careful segmental, lobar, hilar, and mediastinal lymph node staging and who were all fit enough to tolerate a lobectomy. The limited resection (N = 122) involved a formal segmentectomy in approximately two-thirds of the patients and a wedge with at least a 2-cm margin in the remainder. The survival curves were similar for the first 3 years, but at 5 years there was a significant survival benefit to the lobectomy group (5-year survival, 73% versus 56%; $P = 0.06$) (Fig. 11–3). The recurrence-free survival was also significantly better in the lobectomy group ($P = 0.04$). The rate of distant recurrences was the same in both groups, but the limited resection patients experienced a 3-fold higher rate of locoregional recurrence (5.4% versus 1.9% per person per year, $P = 0.009$).[75]

The LCSG trial was designed to prove that a lesser resection would afford a chance of survival and a local recurrence rate similar to that for a lobectomy. The authors were greatly concerned about avoiding a false negative conclusion, that is, failing to detect a potential benefit for lobectomy. Therefore, the trial was designed from the outset with a one-sided statistical significance level of 0.10. Because the overall survival was better with lobectomy at a P value of 0.06, this was interpreted as a statistically significant benefit for lobectomy. Although one might question this design, these statistical considerations were clearly defined at the outset, and the design was approved by the LCSG and the National Institutes of Health. Furthermore, the other differences noted were all statistically significant at the usual $P = 0.05$ level.[74,75]

In summary, the data from seven of eight nonrandomized comparisons shows better survival after lobectomy than after limited resection.[33,40,42,69,71–73] The magnitude of the differences is relatively small, and only three studies found a statistically significant difference.[40,42,72] Furthermore, a carefully conducted, prospective, randomized trial found better survival after lobectomy.[74,75]

A 2- to 4-fold higher local recurrence rate was seen in all five nonrandomized trials that evaluated recurrence patterns.[33,40,42,70,71] More importantly, the only prospective, randomized trial also found a 3-fold increase in local recurrence.[74,75] Therefore, a lobectomy must be considered the operation of choice in the treatment of stage I lung cancer.

Outcome After Limited Resection

Although lobectomy remains the procedure of choice for patients with stage I NSCLC, definition of the outcome after limited resection is important for those patients who are thought not to be suitable candidates for lobectomy. In analyzing the survival after limited resection, it is important to distinguish between a limited resection carried out as an optional alternative in patients who would be able to tolerate a lobectomy and a limited resection carried out as a compromise in poor risk patients. Unfortunately, the reason that patients are selected for limited resection is often alluded to only vaguely. Furthermore, it is not clear what degree of comorbid pulmonary, cardiac, or other disease is necessary to make a patient a poor risk for lobectomy, yet still a candidate for a limited resection (usually accomplished via open thoracotomy). For example, in only one of the studies of limited resection as a compromise procedure were the pulmonary parameters cited at a level that is commonly accepted as prohibitively low for a lobectomy (preoperative forced expiratory volume in 1 second [FEV_1] <1.0 L).[76] In other studies, parameters that characterized poor risk patients could be questioned (average age, 70[69,71] and average preoperative FEV_1 of 1.56 L,[69] or an average preoperative FEV_1 of 65% predicted).[71] Nevertheless, it must be accepted that these patients were thought to be a poor risk by the authors of the studies, who were experienced and respected thoracic surgeons.

The results of all series of ≥ 20 patients undergoing limited resection are shown in Table 11–3. The average 5-year survival of 47% for patients undergoing a compromise operation is fairly good, although there is a fair amount of variation between studies. Several additional, smaller (<20 patients) studies have reported similar results.[42,70,77,78] The highest survival, reported by Errett et al,[69] is astounding, given the stage of disease of many of the patients. The relatively low survival reported by Miller and Hatcher[76] involved only patients with severely impaired pulmonary function. The differences do not seem to be related to the type of limited resection performed or to the extent of nodal staging performed. The reported rate of non-cancer-related late deaths has varied from 0% to 50%, but at an average of 22% it is not higher than for resected stage I patients in general (see below).[69–71,74,77,78]

Local recurrence is reported to occur in 15% (range, 6%-24%) of all patients[40,68,70,71,74,76–78] and accounts for at least half of all recurrences in most studies,[40,70,71,74] with only two exceptions.[76,78] Of the patients who experience a local recurrence, consistently fewer than one-third are able

TABLE 11–3. SURVIVAL AFTER LIMITED RESECTION IN CLINICAL STAGE I NON–SMALL CELL LUNG CANCER

STUDY	N	RESECTION TYPE	LN STAGING	SELECTION	% pT1	% pN0	5-YEAR SURVIVAL
Jensik[68]	259	Segment	?	Optional	74	92	55
Ginsberg et al[74,75]	122	Segment[a]	Yes	Optional	100	100	56
Kulka and Forrai[107]	107	?	?	Optional	?	?	60
Tsubota et al[108]	55[b]	Segment	Yes	Optional	100	95	91[c]
Kodama et al[70]	46	Segment	Yes	Optional	100	100	93
Warren and Faber[42]	38[b]	Segment	Yes	Optional[d]	100	100	65
Kutschera[109]	27	Segment	No	Optional	?	?	32
Average							**65**
Harpole et al[33]	75	Wedge	?	Both	98[c]	100	61[c]
Warren and Faber[42]	66	Segment	Yes	Both	77	100	46
Martini et al[40]	62	Wedge	Yes	Both	89	100	59
Average							**55**
Landreneau et al[71]	102	Wedge[f]	Yes	Compromise	100	100	61
Errett et al[69]	100	Wedge	Yes[d]	Compromise	12	45	69
Strauss et al[72]	58	?	?	Compromise	90	100	48
Miller and Hatcher[76]	32	Wedge[a]	?	Compromise	87	97	31
Kutschera[109]	30	Segment	No	Compromise	?	?	20
Pastorino et al[73]	28	?	Yes	Compromise	56	100	53
Average							**47**

Inclusion criteria: Studies of limited resection in >20 patients.
[a]In 67%.
[b]≤2 cm.
[c]Disease-free survival.
[d]Implied.
[e]Estimated.
[f]60% video-assisted thoracic surgery.
Both, both resections as optional alternative and as a compromise procedure; Compromise, limited resection as compromise procedure in poor risk patients; LN staging, Was lymph node (N1, N2) staging done in most patients?; Optional, limited resection as an optional alternative in patients able to tolerate lobectomy; Segment, segmentectomy; Selection, criteria for selection of type of resection in most (>75%) of the patients; ?, unknown.

to undergo a second resection.[33,42,68,70] In one small study of 17 patients, the local recurrence rate was reduced from 35% to 11% in the patients who were given postoperative radiation.[77] The role of postoperative radiation after wedge resection is currently being investigated in a phase II trial by the Cancer and Leukemia Group B (CALGB Protocol No. 9335).

In summary, although the local recurrence rates may be somewhat higher, the 5-year survival after a limited resection as a compromise operation is fairly good. It appears that the survival of clinical stage I patients after limited resection as a compromise is approximately twice what is seen after treatment with radiation alone (see Table 13–3). Thus the data favors limited resection over conventional radiation as the second choice treatment after lobectomy.

Video-Assisted Thoracic Surgery Lobectomy

The introduction of VATS has resulted in application of this technology to perform major pulmonary resections, including lobectomy and pneumonectomy. Proponents of VATS lobectomy have reasoned that this minimally invasive approach will result in shorter hospital stays, decreased perioperative morbidity, decreased pain, and lower hospital costs.[79–82] The results of how well a VATS approach to lobectomy achieves these proposed benefits are conflicting, however. Although some authors[79,82] found less postoperative pain with VATS, others[83] found no significant difference when compared with a muscle-sparing thoracotomy. Length of hospitalization and costs are also not clearly reduced by VATS (see Table 8–7).

The only prospective, randomized study comparing VATS lobectomy with muscle-sparing thoracotomy and lobectomy for clinical stage I NSCLC was reported by Kirby et al in 1995.[83] This small, three-center trial randomized only 55 patients over 2 years. VATS lobectomy was not associated with a significant decrease in chest tube drainage, length of hospital stay, postthoracotomy pain, or faster recovery and return to work when compared with a muscle-sparing thoracotomy and lobectomy.[83]

The majority of the VATS lobectomy literature has centered on the technique and feasibility of the operation.[79–82,84–86] A VATS lobectomy for cancer has prompted concern about violating surgical oncologic principles.[81] As discussed previously, mediastinal and hilar node sampling is crucial to adequately stage the tumor. With advances in technology, however, it does appear that surgeons can perform adequate nodal sampling using a VATS technique.[79–81,84]

Long-term studies that allow comparison of the survival after VATS versus open lobectomy are not yet available. Intermediate-term results have been published and suggest that survival after VATS lobectomy is the same as that after conventional lobectomy.[87–89] These studies have each included >100 patients with NSCLC and have reported 3-year survival in pathologic stage I patients of >90%.[87–89]

CAUSES OF DEATH

Examination of the causes of death after resection of stage I NSCLC reveals that approximately half of the patients die from recurrence of their original lung cancer (Table 11–4). Approximately 10% die of a new malignancy, most often a new lung cancer, and approximately 30% die of unrelated, nonmalignant causes. Thus, only about 60% of deaths are related to recurrence of the original lung cancer. Extrapolation of this finding to the overall survival results shown in Table 11–2 suggests that the disease-free survival after resection of stage I NSCLC is approximately 80%.

RECURRENCE PATTERNS

Approximately one-third of all resected pathologic stage I patients will develop a recurrence (Table 11–5). Several risk factors for recurrence in stage I NSCLC have been identified. These include the T status (T2 more likely to recur than T1), histology (adenocarcinoma more likely to recur than squamous), visceral pleural invasion, vascular invasion, symptoms at the time of initial presentation, and an elevated CEA level.[32,33,38,44,48,56,90] The location of the tumor (central versus peripheral), extent of formal pulmonary resection (lobectomy versus pneumonectomy), or side of operation (left versus right) is not associated with an increased risk of recurrence.[32] Martini et al[40] suggested that mediastinal lymph node dissection decreased the risk of locoregional recurrence.

The majority of recurrences in stage I NSCLC are distant and occur in 12% to 27% of all patients (see Table 11–5). The risk of locoregional recurrence is 5% to 12% of all patients undergoing resection.[33,38,40,56,90,91] No difference is apparent in the recurrence patterns for stage Ia and Ib

tumors[33,38,92] or histology[40,92] in most studies. The most commonly involved distant sites for recurrence are brain, bone, and liver.[47,48,90] Adenocarcinoma is more likely to recur in the brain than squamous cell histology.[40,91,92]

Most recurrences (60%) are detected within the first 24 months after resection.[33,38,40] The likelihood of recurrent disease decreases thereafter but is still 7% to 9%[40,44,93] in patients who are clinically disease-free after 5 years. The risks of developing a nonpulmonary cancer after resection of a stage I NSCLC is between 5% and 23%.[33,40,44] In addition, the incidence of developing a new primary lung cancer after resection of a stage I NSCLC is approximately 5% to 10%.[38,40,56,93] Although the rate of recurrence decreases with time, the risk of developing a new lung primary or a nonpulmonary malignancy does not diminish.

Most of the patients who experience a recurrence will die of it, and <10% will have successful control of their disease.[38,40] However, a new primary lung cancer can often be successfully treated; in one study, 52% of patients with a second primary lung cancer were alive 2 years after detection of the new primary lung cancer (see Chapter 30).[38] These observations have prompted many investigators to suggest continued patient surveillance even beyond 5 years in patients with resected stage I NSCLC.[38,40,44]

VALUE OF FOLLOW-UP

Routine follow-up after a resection for lung cancer is commonly done, but there is little data to evaluate the efficacy. A survey of 1294 thoracic surgeons who perform lung cancer resections found that 60% carry out routine follow-up of their patients.[94] This generally consists of a clinic visit and a chest radiograph (CXR) three or four times a year during the first year, two or three times during the second year, and once or twice each year thereafter. Blood tests were obtained only about one-third of the time, and other tests or scans were rarely done.[94] Potential benefits of careful follow-up include psychological support for the patient, knowledge of the eventual outcome after resection, early detection of a new primary lung cancer,

TABLE 11–4. CAUSE OF DEATH IN PATHOLOGIC STAGE I NON–SMALL CELL LUNG CANCER

				% OF ALL DEATHS[a]			
STUDY	N	FOLLOW-UP (mo)	% DEAD[a]	Recurrence	New Primary[b]	Other Cancer[c]	Noncancer
Thomas et al[44 d]	907	96	—	—	—	—	30
Martini et al[40]	598	91	48	49	12	9	30
Read et al[31]	384	—	55	42	11	——47——	
Pairolero et al[38 e]	346	84	50[f]	66	10[g]	——24[g]——	
Harpole et al[33]	289	61	64	——57——		——43——	
Little et al[56]	96	78	22	57	14	0	29
Macchiarini et al[48 d]	95	100	32	73	7	3	17
Average				**57**	**11**	——**33**——	

Inclusion criteria: Studies of >50 stage 1 patients reporting late cause of death.
[a]Excluding operative deaths.
[b]New primary lung cancer.
[c]Other primary nonpulmonary cancer.
[d]Only T1N0.
[e]Includes 5% T1N1.
[f]Includes operative deaths.
[g]Estimated.

TABLE 11–5. FIRST SITE OF RECURRENCE AFTER RESECTION OF PATHOLOGIC STAGE I NON–SMALL CELL LUNG CANCER

STUDY	N	MEDIAN FOLLOW-UP (mo)	% OF ALL PATIENTS		% OF ALL RECURRENCES		
			New Primary[a]	Recurrence	LR	LR/D	D
Thomas et al[44] [b]	907	96	3[c]	23[c]	39	—	61
Martini et al[40]	598	91	10	27	28	3	69
Feld et al[92] [d]	390	41	5	34	30	—70—	
Pairolero et al[38] [d]	346	84	10	29	25	14	61
Harpole et al[33]	289	61	2	37	31	18	51
Ramacciato et al[110]	202	—	—	48	45	—	55
Walsh et al[95]	190	76	—	24	22	15	63
Al-Kattan et al[90]	123	54	1	41	39	—	61
Little et al[56]	96	78	3	16	27	—	73
Immerman et al[111]	77	—	—	39	31	—	70
Lafitte et al[112] [e]	70	>60	—	41	38	3	57
Average			**5**	**33**	**32**	—68—	

Inclusion criteria: Studies of >50 pathologic stage I patients reporting recurrence patterns.
[a]New primary lung cancer.
[b]Only T1N0.
[c]Estimated.
[d]Includes 5%–8% T1N1.
[e]Only T2N0.
D, distant; LR, local or regional; LR/D, both local-regional and distant.

and early detection of a recurrence permitting a potentially curative treatment or more effective palliation to be initiated. There is no data to assess the value of the first two points. The value of early detection of a recurrence or a new lung cancer depends on the ability of follow-up to succeed in identifying these situations early, as well as the ability of treatment to alter the prognosis.

The detection of recurrences of lung cancer during follow-up after resection has been analyzed in two studies involving 346 and 358 patients, the majority of whom were pI.[38,95] Recurrences were found in approximately one-third of the patients during follow-up, which consisted of a clinic visit and a CXR every 3 to 4 months for 2 years and every 6 to 12 months thereafter. Despite the frequent visits, 36% to 45% of recurrences were found outside of a planned follow-up visit because of symptoms, 21% to 40% were found during a planned follow-up visit because of symptoms, and only 24% to 31% of recurrences were found while patients were still asymptomatic.[38,95] The clinical history was the most important component of the visit in symptomatic patients because the diagnosis was discovered by physical examination in only 7%, by CXR in 36%, and by other tests (eg, CT or bone scan) in the remainder.[95] Among asymptomatic patients, the CXR was the most important, detecting 76% of recurrences, whereas physical examination found only 3% to 6% of recurrences.[38,95] Patients with local recurrences are more likely to be asymptomatic (60%) than those with distant metastases (21%).[38]

A possible benefit to detection of a recurrence before the onset of symptoms is suggested by the observation in one study that the median survival after diagnosis of recurrence is 16 months in asymptomatic patients as compared with 8 months in symptomatic patients ($P = 0.008$).[95] Lead time bias does not account for this difference because the survival is also significantly different for these two groups if measured from the time of the original resection. A slight trend toward better survival in patients with local versus distant recurrences has been noted in two studies,

but the differences were not statistically significant.[38,95] In both asymptomatic and symptomatic patients, the same proportion (30%) could be treated with a potentially curative approach.[95] A curative treatment of a recurrence resulted in better 5-year survival (25% versus 15% from the time of the *original* resection, $P = 0.03$).[95]

Multivariate analysis reveals, however, that the most important prognostic factor for survival in patients with a recurrence was a disease-free interval of >12 months (relative risk of death, 4.5; $P = 0.0001$).[95] Potentially curative versus palliative treatment was less significant (relative risk, 1.6; $P = 0.04$), and other factors including the site of recurrence, the presence of symptoms, or initial tumor stage were not significant.[95] These results suggest that the tumor biology is most important and that our ability to alter the prognosis of recurrences by early detection and treatment is limited. This is corroborated by a retrospective analysis that found no difference in survival between patients receiving intensive versus nonintensive follow-up after lung cancer resection.[96]

None of these studies addressed the value of a regular CXR for the detection of a new primary lung cancer in patients with a prior lung cancer. The large screening trials that have been reported also do not address this issue because they have investigated the role of sputum cytology and not CXR to detect lung cancer.[97–99] More importantly, the incidence of new primary lung cancer of 2% per patient per year (see Chapter 30) is much higher than that of the populations in the screening studies. In fact, there are few patient populations with such a high risk of the development of a cancer. An analogy can be made to patients with Barrett's esophagus, who have a similar risk for the development of esophageal cancer and who have been found to benefit from screening esophagoscopy.[100,101]

Although further investigation of the role of follow-up of resected lung cancer patients is clearly needed, a rational approach must be formulated based on data currently available. The benefit of follow-up is primarily to provide sup-

DATA SUMMARY: LIMITED RESECTION, RECURRENCE PATTERNS IN STAGE I NSCLC			
	AMOUNT	**QUALITY**	**CONSISTENCY**
The 5-year survival after limited resection is slightly worse than after lobectomy	*High*	*Mod*	*Mod*
Local recurrence is 2 to 4 times higher after limited resection than after lobectomy	*High*	*High*	*High*
Limited resection as a compromise procedure in patients with poor pulmonary reserve has a 5-year survival of 50%	High	Poor	Mod
Intermediate-term survival after VATS lobectomy is similar to that after open lobectomy	*Mod*	*Mod*	*High*
Recurrence accounts for 57% of deaths in resected stage I NSCLC	High	High	Mod
70% of recurrences involve distant metastases	High	High	High
The risk of a new primary lung cancer is 2% per year	High	High	High
Despite frequent follow-up, 70% of patients with recurrence have symptoms at presentation	Mod	High	High

Type of data rated: Plain text: descriptive statement   *Italics: controlled comparison*   **Bold: randomized comparison**

port to the patient, evaluate the outcome of treatment, and detect new primary cancers because the data discussed earlier suggests that the benefit of early detection of a recurrence is limited. Obviously, patients should be seen whenever symptoms arise or reassurance and support are needed. How frequently patients should be seen for detection of a new primary lung cancer is unclear. An analysis of a screening study has suggested that the average period between the time that a lung cancer has become detectable by CXR and the development of symptoms is about 7 to 8 months.[102] Therefore, a CXR at least once a year is probably a minimum.

EDITORS' COMMENTS

Surgery is clearly well established as an effective treatment for patients with localized stage I lung cancer. The 5-year survival for patients with pI NSCLC is 65%, and the disease-free survival is approximately 80%. Although this leaves some room for improvement, this is more an issue of better staging than of the ability of surgery to cure localized disease. Analysis of recurrence patterns and data on the incidence of occult micrometastases clearly suggests that we need to improve our ability to define localized disease. At the very least, careless pathologic staging on the part of surgeons (by not sampling mediastinal nodes) and pathologists (by not commenting on intrapulmonary nodes) should be avoided in order to better understand the biology of NSCLC and to select patients for possible adjuvant treatment.

It is important that clinicians be accurate in their use of data. The results of pathologically staged patients are frequently quoted in making a treatment plan for a patient, even though only clinical staging data is applicable to that patient. More accurate use of the available data will greatly reduce some of the confusion and defuse some of the arguments surrounding the treatment of early stage lung cancer.

A number of prognostic factors in stage I NSCLC have been identified. The most important factor in stage I patients is the T status. The size of a tumor clearly affects prognosis; the effect of pleural invasion is mild and less well defined. The histologic subtype of NSCLC plays a very minor role, at best. The role of tumor differentiation and vascular invasion appears to be more important, although the data for these factors is somewhat limited. There continues to be much hope that molecular biologic characterization of lung cancers will provide keys to predicting which tumors are more likely to metastasize, but this has not been achieved so far.

A lobectomy is clearly the type of resection that should be done whenever possible for stage I NSCLC. Although the data supporting lobectomy over a limited resection involves only one randomized study, the fact that an increased local recurrence rate has been found consistently among all studies makes it quite clear that lobectomy is superior. The optimal treatment for patients who are not able to tolerate a lobectomy because of poor pulmonary reserve is less clear. The operative mortality of resection in these patients is much lower than what is commonly thought, as outlined in Table 7–3. Although the long-term survival after limited resection as a compromise operation is lower than that after a lobectomy, a limited resection is probably the treatment of choice, provided the patient is deemed able to tolerate a surgical approach.

VATS lobectomy has received a great deal of attention, and its role in the treatment of lung cancer is gradually being defined. Operative mortality is acceptably low, and preliminary survival data suggests that the outcomes are similar to those for open resection. However, it is technically demanding and associated with a low but not insignificant rate of intraoperative bleeding. Furthermore, as discussed in Chapter 8, the benefits in terms of patient comfort are much less than what most physicians and patients think. Whether a slight benefit in terms of morbidity versus the difficulty in performing VATS lobectomy will allow this procedure to become widely used in the future (in selected patients with small peripheral tumors) is not clear.

Follow-up of resected patients with stage I NSCLC is important. A diagnosis of cancer is a difficult fact to live with, even if it is stage I, and reassurance by the treating physician is tremendously helpful. Furthermore, the delivery of appropriate care requires assessment of our results. Reviewing hard data is important in this regard, but seeing individual patients in follow-up allows a different type of assessment to be made that is invaluable, although hard to measure. In addition, few patient populations have as high a risk of development of a new cancer as resected patients with lung cancer. Although pessimism exists regarding the value of screening for lung cancer in general, this outlook is inappropriate in resected patients. The general screening data is often misinterpreted (screening CXRs have never been evaluated) and, furthermore, cannot be extrapolated to a group of patients whose risk of lung cancer is several orders of magnitude greater. As a result of these considerations, resected patients at our institution are seen four times in the first year, twice in the second year, and annually thereafter.

References

1. Tsang GMK, Watson DCT. The practice of cardiothoracic surgeons in the perioperative staging of non–small cell lung cancer. Thorax. 1992;47:3–5.
2. Takizawa T, Terashima M, Koike T, et al. Mediastinal lymph node metastasis in patients with clinical stage I peripheral non–small-cell lung cancer. J Thorac Cardiovasc Surg. 1997;113:248–252.
3. Gaer JAR, Goldstraw P. Intraoperative assessment of nodal staging at thoracotomy for carcinoma of the bronchus. Eur J Cardiothorac Surg. 1990;4:207–210.
4. Naruke T, Goya T, Tsuchiya R, et al. The importance of surgery to non–small cell carcinoma of lung with mediastinal lymph node metastasis. Ann Thorac Surg. 1988;46:603–610.
5. Ishida T, Tateishi M, Kaneko S, et al. Surgical treatment of patients with nonsmall-cell lung cancer and mediastinal lymph node involvement. J Surg Oncol. 1990;43:161–166.
6. Izbicki JR, Passlick B, Karg O, et al. Impact on radical systematic mediastinal lymphadenectomy on tumor staging in lung cancer. Ann Thorac Surg. 1995;59:209–214.
7. Naruke T. Significance of lymph node metastases in lung cancer. Semin Thorac Cardiovasc Surg. 1993;5:210–218.
8. Asamura H, Nakayama H, Kondo H, et al. Lymph node involvement, recurrence, and prognosis in resected small, peripheral, non–small-cell lung carcinomas: are these carcinomas candidates for video-assisted lobectomy? J Thorac Cardiovasc Surg. 1996;111:1125–1134.
9. Martini N, Flehinger BJ, Zaman MB, et al. Results of resection in non–oat cell carcinoma of the lung with mediastinal lymph node metastases. Ann Surg. 1983;198:386–397.
10. Yoshino I, Yokoyama H, Yano T, et al. Skip metastasis to the mediastinal lymph nodes in non–small cell lung cancer. Ann Thorac Surg. 1996;62:1021–1025.
11. Riquet M, Manac'h D, Saab M, et al. Factors determining survival in resected N2 lung cancer. Eur J Cardiothorac Surg. 1995;9:300–304.
12. Tateishi M, Fukuyama Y, Hamatake M, et al. Skip mediastinal lymph node metastasis in non–small cell lung cancer. J Surg Oncol. 1994;57:139–142.
13. Maggi G, Casadio C, Mancuso M, et al. Resection and radical lymphadenectomy for lung cancer: prognostic significance of lymphatic metastases. Int Surg. 1990;75:17–21.
14. Riquet M, Hidden G, Debesse B. Direct lymphatic drainage of lung segments to the mediastinal nodes. J Thorac Cardiovasc Surg. 1989;97:623–632.
15. Thomas PA, Piantadosi S, Mountain CF. Should subcarinal lymph nodes be routinely examined in patients with non–small cell lung cancer? J Thorac Cardiovasc Surg. 1988;95:883–887.
16. Funatsu T, Matsubara Y, Ikeda S, et al. Preoperative mediastinoscopic assessment of N factors and the need for mediastinal lymph node dissection in T1 lung cancer. J Thorac Cardiovasc Surg. 1994;108:321–328.
17. Sorensen JB, Badsberg JH. Prognostic factors in resected stages I and II adenocarcinoma of the lung: a multivariate regression analysis of 137 consecutive patients. J Thorac Cardiovasc Surg. 1990;99:218–226.
18. Naruke T, Tomoyuki G, Tsuchiya R, et al. Prognosis and survival in resected lung carcinoma based on the new international staging system. J Thorac Cardiovasc Surg. 1988;96:440–447.
19. Watanabe Y, Shimizu J, Tsubota M, et al. Mediastinal spread of metastatic lymph nodes in bronchogenic carcinoma: mediastinal nodal metastases in lung cancer. Chest. 1990;97:1059–1065.
20. Martini N, McCormack P. Therapy of stage III (nonmetastatic disease). Semin Oncol. 1983;10:95–110.
21. Sugi K, Nawata K, Fujita N, et al. Systematic lymph node dissection for clinically diagnosed peripheral non–small-cell lung cancer less than 2 cm in diameter. World J Surg. 1998;22:290–294.
22. Izbicki JR, Thetter O, Habekost M, et al. Radical systematic mediastinal lymphadenectomy in non–small cell lung cancer: a randomized controlled trial. Br J Surg. 1994;81:229–235.
23. Vrdoljak E, Mise K, Sapunar D, et al. Survival analysis of untreated patients with non–small-cell lung cancer. Chest. 1994;106:1797–1800.
24. Koike T, Terashima M, Takizawa T, et al. Clinical analysis of small-sized peripheral lung cancer. J Thorac Cardiovasc Surg. 1998;115:1015–1020.
25. Gdeedo A, Van Schil P, Corthouts B, et al. Comparison of imaging TNM [(i)TNM] and pathological TNM [pTNM] in staging of bronchogenic carcinoma. Eur J Cardiothorac Surg. 1997;12:224–227.
26. Fernando HC, Goldstraw P. The accuracy of clinical evaluative intrathoracic staging in lung cancer as assessed by postsurgical pathologic staging. Cancer. 1990;65:2503–2506.
27. Oda M, Watanabe Y, Shimizu J, et al. Extent of mediastinal node metastasis in clinical stage I non–small-cell lung cancer: the role of systematic nodal dissection. Lung Cancer. 1998;22:23–30.
28. Janssen-Heijnen MLG, Schipper RM, Razenberg PPA, et al. Prevalence of co-morbidity in lung cancer patients and its relationship with treatment: a population-based study. Lung Cancer. 1998;21:105–113.
29. Ichinose Y, Hara N, Ohta M, et al. Is T factor of the TNM staging system a predominant prognostic factor in pathologic stage I non–small-call lung cancer? A multivariate prognostic factor analysis of 151 patients. J Thorac Cardiovasc Surg. 1993;106:90–94.
30. Williams DE, Pairolero PC, Davis CS, et al. Survival of patients surgically treated for stage I lung cancer. J Thorac Cardiovasc Surg. 1981;82:70–76.
31. Read RC, Schaefer R, North N, et al. Diameter, cell type, and survival in stage I primary non–small-cell lung cancer. Arch Surg. 1988;123:446–449.
32. Gail MH, Eagan RT, Feld R, et al. Prognostic factors in patients with resected stage I non–small cell lung cancer: a report from the Lung Cancer Study Group. Cancer. 1984;54:1802–1813.
33. Harpole DH Jr, Herndon JE II, Young WG Jr, et al. Stage I nonsmall cell lung cancer: a multivariate analysis of treatment methods and patterns of recurrence. Cancer. 1995;76:787–796.
34. Padilla J, Calvo V, Peñalver JC, et al. Surgical results and prognostic factors in early non–small cell lung cancer. Ann Thorac Surg. 1997;63:324–326.
35. Mountain CF, Dresler CM. Regional lymph node classification for lung cancer staging. Chest. 1997;111:1718–1723.
36. Pastorino U, Andreola S, Tagliabue E, et al. Immunocytochemical markers in stage I lung cancer: relevance to prognosis. J Clin Oncol. 1997;15:2858–2865.
37. Kotlyarov EV, Rukosuyev AA. Long-term results and patterns of disease recurrence after radical operations for lung cancer. J Thorac Cardiovasc Surg. 1991;102:24–28.
38. Pairolero PC, Williams DE, Bergstralh EJ, et al. Postsurgical stage I bronchogenic carcinoma: morbid implications of recurrent disease. Ann Thorac Surg. 1984;38:331–338.
39. Mountain CF. Revisions in the International System for Staging Lung Cancer. Chest. 1997;111:1710–1717.

40. Martini N, Bains MS, Burt ME, et al. Incidence of local recurrence and second primary tumors in resected stage I lung cancer. J Thorac Cardiovasc Surg. 1995;109:120–129.

41. Ichinose Y, Yano T, Asoh H, et al. Prognostic factors obtained by a pathologic examination in completely resected non–small-cell lung cancer: an analysis in each pathologic stage. J Thorac Cardiovasc Surg. 1995;110:601–605.

42. Warren WH, Faber LP. Segmentectomy versus lobectomy in patients with stage I pulmonary carcinoma. J Thorac Cardiovasc Surg. 1994;107:1087–1094.

43. Mountain CF, Lukeman JM, Hammar SP, et al. Lung cancer classification: the relationship of disease extent and cell type to survival in a clinical trials population. J Surg Oncol. 1987;35:147–156.

44. Thomas P, Rubinstein L, and the Lung Cancer Study Group. Cancer recurrence after resection: T1 N0 non–small cell lung cancer. Ann Thorac Surg. 1990;49:242–247.

45. Chung CK, Zaino R, Stryker JA, et al. Carcinoma of the lung: evaluation of histological grade and factors influencing prognosis. Ann Thorac Surg. 1982;33:599–604.

46. Takizawa T, Terashima M, Koike T, et al. Lymph node metastasis in small peripheral adenocarcinoma of the lung. J Thorac Cardiovasc Surg. 1998;116:276–280.

47. Stenbygaard LE, Sorensen JB, Olsen JE. Metastatic pattern in adenocarcinoma of the lung: an autopsy study from a cohort of 137 consecutive patients with complete resection. J Thorac Cardiovasc Surg. 1995;110:1130–1135.

48. Macchiarini P, Fontanini G, Hardin MJ, et al. Blood vessel invasion by tumor cells predicts recurrence in completely resected T1 N0 M0 non–small-cell lung cancer. J Thorac Cardiovasc Surg. 1993;106:80–89.

49. Duarte IG, Bufkin BL, Pennington MF, et al. Angiogenesis as a predictor of survival after surgical resection for stage I non–small-cell lung cancer. J Thorac Cardiovasc Surg. 1998;115:652–659.

50. Lucchi M, Fontanini G, Mussi A, et al. Tumor angiogenesis and biologic markers in resected stage I NSCLC. Eur J Cardiothorac Surg. 1997;12:535–541.

51. Macchiarini P, Fontanini G, Hardin JM, et al. Most peripheral, node-negative, non–small-cell lung cancers have low proliferative rates and no intratumoral and peritumoral blood and lymphatic vessel invasion: rationale for treatment with wedge resection alone. J Thorac Cardiovasc Surg. 1992;104:892–899.

52. Shields TW. Prognostic significance of parenchymal lymphatic vessel and blood vessel invasion in carcinoma of the lung. Surg Gynecol Obstet. 1983;157:185–190.

53. Apolinario RM, van der Valk P, de Jong JS, et al. Prognostic value of the expression of p53, bcl-2, and bax oncoproteins, and neovascularization in patients with radically resected non–small-cell lung cancer. J Clin Oncol. 1997;15:2456–2466.

54. D'Amico TA, Massey M, Herndon JE III, et al. A biologic risk model for stage I lung cancer: immunohistochemical analysis of 408 patients with the use of ten molecular markers. J Thorac Cardiovasc Surg. 1999;117:736–743.

55. Matsuyama K, Chiba Y, Sasaki M, et al. Tumor angiogenesis as a prognostic marker in operable non–small cell lung cancer. Ann Thorac Surg. 1998;65:1405–1409.

56. Little AG, DeMeester TR, Ferguson MK, et al. Modified stage I (T1N0M0, T2N0M0), nonsmall cell lung cancer: treatment results, recurrence patterns, and adjuvant immunotherapy. Surgery. 1986;100:621–628.

57. Shah R, Sabanathan S, Richardson J, et al. Results of surgical treatment of stage I and II lung cancer. J Cardiovasc Surg. 1996;37:169–172.

58. Martini N, Melamed MR. Occult carcinomas of the lung. Ann Thorac Surg. 1980;30:215–223.

59. Cortese DA, Pairolero PC, Bergstralh EJ, et al. Roentgenographically occult lung cancer. J Thorac Cardiovasc Surg. 1983;86:373–380.

60. Saito Y, Sato M, Sagawa M, et al. Multicentricity in resected occult bronchogenic squamous cell carcinomas. Ann Thorac Surg. 1994;57:1200–1205.

61. Sato M, Saito Y, Usada K, et al. Occult lung cancer beyond bronchoscopic visibility in sputum-cytology positive patients. Lung Cancer. 1998;20:17–24.

62. Usuda K, Saito Y, Nagamoto N, et al. Relation between bronchoscopic findings and tumor size of roentgenographically occult bronchogenic squamous cell carcinoma. J Thorac Cardiovasc Surg. 1993;106:1098–1103.

63. Saito Y, Nagamoto N, Ota S, et al. Results of surgical treatment for roentgenographically occult bronchogenic squamous cell carcinoma. J Thorac Cardiovasc Surg. 1992;104:401–407.

64. Woolner LB, Fontana RS, Cortese DA, et al. Roentgenographically occult lung cancer: pathologic findings and frequency of multicentricity during a 10-year period. Mayo Clin Proc. 1984;59:453–466.

65. Lam S, Kennedy T, Unger M, et al. Localization of bronchial intraepithelial neoplastic lesions by fluorescence bronchoscopy. Chest. 1998;113:696–702.

66. Ochsner A, DeBakey M. Surgical considerations of primary carcinoma of the lung: review of the literature and report of 19 cases. Surgery. 1940;8:992–1023.

67. Churchill ED, Sweet RH, Scannell JG, et al. Further studies in the surgical management of carcinoma of the lung. J Thorac Surg. 1958;36:301–308.

68. Jensik RJ. The extent of resection for localized lung cancer: segmental resection. In: Kittle CF, ed. Current Controversies in Thoracic Surgery. Philadelphia, Pa: WB Saunders; 1986:175–182.

69. Errett LE, Wilson J, Chiu RC-J, et al. Wedge resection as an alternative procedure for peripheral bronchogenic carcinoma in poor-risk patients. J Thorac Cardiovasc Surg. 1985;90:656–661.

70. Kodama K, Doi O, Higashiyama M, et al. Intentional limited resection for selected patients with T1 N0 M0 non–small-cell lung cancer: a single-institution study. J Thorac Cardiovasc Surg. 1997;114:347–353.

71. Landreneau RJ, Sugarbaker DJ, Mack MJ, et al. Wedge resection versus lobectomy for stage I (T1 N0 M0) non–small-cell lung cancer. J Thorac Cardiovasc Surg. 1997;113:691–700.

72. Strauss G, Kwiatkowski D, De-Camp M, et al. Extent of surgical resection influences survival in stage IA non–small cell lung cancer (NSCLC). Proc ASCO. 1998;17:462a.

73. Pastorino U, Valente M, Bedini V, et al. Limited resection for stage I lung cancer. Eur J Surg Oncol. 1991;17:42–46.

74. Ginsberg RJ, Rubinstein LV, for the Lung Cancer Study Group. Randomized trial of lobectomy versus limited resection for T1 N0 non–small cell lung cancer. Ann Thorac Surg. 1995;60:615–623.

75. Rubinstein LV, Ginsberg RJ. Reply to "Randomized trial of lobectomy versus limited resection for T1 N0 non–small cell lung cancer," 1995 article by the Lung Cancer Study Group. Ann Thorac Surg. 1996;62:1249–1250.

76. Miller JI, Hatcher CR Jr. Limited resection of bronchogenic carcinoma in the patient with marked impairment of pulmonary function. Ann Thorac Surg. 1987;44:340–343.

77. Yano T, Yokoyama H, Yoshino I, et al. Results of a limited resection for compromised or poor-risk patients with clinical stage I non–small cell carcinoma of the lung. J Am Coll Surg. 1995;181:33–37.

78. Crabbe MM, Patrissi GA, Fontenelle LJ. Minimal resection for bronchogenic carcinoma: should this be standard therapy? Chest. 1989;95:968–971.

79. Walker WS, Carnochan FM, Pugh GC. Thoracoscopic pulmonary lobectomy: early operative experience and preliminary clinical results. J Thorac Cardiovasc Surg. 1993;106:1111–1117.

80. McKenna RJ Jr. Lobectomy by video-assisted thoracic surgery with mediastinal node sampling for lung cancer. J Thorac Cardiovasc Surg. 1994;107:879–882.

81. Landreneau RJ, Mack MJ, Dowling RD, et al. The role of thoracoscopy in lung cancer management. Chest. 1998;113:6S–12S.

82. Giudicelli R, Thomas P, Lonjon T, et al. Video-assisted minithoracotomy versus muscle-sparing thoracotomy for performing lobectomy. Ann Thorac Surg. 1994;58:712–718.

83. Kirby TJ, Mack MJ, Landreneau RJ, et al. Lobectomy-video-assisted thoracic surgery versus muscle-sparing thoracotomy: a randomized trial. J Thorac Cardiovasc Surg. 1995;109:997–1002.

84. Kaseda S, Hangai N, Yamamoto S, et al. Lobectomy with extended lymph node dissection by video-assisted thoracic surgery for lung cancer. Surg Endosc. 1997;11:703–706.

85. Lewis RJ. Simultaneously stapled lobectomy: a safe technique for video-assisted thoracic surgery. J Thorac Cardiovasc Surg. 1995;109:619–625.

86. Yim APC, Liu H-P. Thoracoscopic major lung resection—indications, technique, and early results: experience from two centers in Asia. Surg Laparosc Endosc. 1997;7:241–244.

87. Walker WS. Video-assisted thoracic surgery (VATS) lobectomy: the

Edinburgh experience. Semin Thorac Cardiovasc Surg. 1998;10:291–299.

88. McKenna RJ Jr, Fischel RJ, Wolf R, et al. Video-assisted thoracic surgery (VATS) lobectomy for bronchogenic carcinoma. Semin Thorac Cardiovasc Surg. 1998;10:321–325.

89. Kaseda S, Aoki T, Hangai N. Video-assisted thoracic surgery (VATS) lobectomy: the Japanese experience. Semin Thorac Cardiovasc Surg. 1998;10:300–304.

90. Al-Kattan K, Sepsas E, Fountain SW, et al. Disease recurrence after resection for stage I lung cancer. Eur J Cardiothorac Surg. 1997;12:380–384.

91. Thomas PA, Piantadosi S, for The Lung Cancer Study Group. Postoperative T1 N0 non–small cell lung cancer. J Thorac Cardiovasc Surg. 1987;94:349–354.

92. Feld R, Rubinstein LV, Weisenberger TH, et al. Sites of recurrence in resected stage I non–small-cell lung cancer: a guide for future studies. J Clin Oncol. 1984;2:1352–1358.

93. Thomas PA Jr, Rubinstein L. Malignant disease appearing late after operation for T1N0 non–small-cell lung cancer. J Thorac Cardiovasc Surg. 1993;106:1053–1058.

94. Naunheim KS, Virgo KS, Coplin MA, et al. Clinical surveillance testing after lung cancer operations. Ann Thorac Surg. 1995;60:1612–1616.

95. Walsh GL, O'Connor M, Willis KM, et al. Is follow-up of lung cancer patients after resection medically indicated and cost-effective? Ann Thorac Surg. 1995;60:1563–1572.

96. Virgo KS, McKirgan LW, Caputo MCA, et al. Post-treatment management options for patients with lung cancer. Ann Surg. 1995;222:700–710.

97. Strauss GM, Gleason RE, Sugarbaker DJ. Screening for lung cancer: another look; a different view. Chest. 1997;111:754–768.

98. Melamed MR, Flehinger BJ, Zaman MB, et al. Screening for early lung cancer: results of the Memorial Sloan-Kettering study in New York. Chest. 1984;86:44–53.

99. Fontana RS, Sanderson DR, Woolner LB, et al. Lung cancer screening: the Mayo program. J Occup Med. 1986;28:746–750.

100. Peters JH, Clark GWB, Ireland AP, et al. Outcome of adenocarcinoma arising in Barrett's esophagus in endoscopically surveyed and nonsurveyed patients. J Thorac Cardiovasc Surg. 1994;108:813–822.

101. Streitz JM Jr, Andrews CW Jr, Ellis FH Jr. Endoscopic surveillance of Barrett's esophagus: does it help? J Thorac Cardiovasc Surg. 1993;105:383–388.

102. Walter SD, Kubik A, Parkin DM, et al. The natural history of lung cancer estimated from the results of a randomized trial of screening. Cancer Causes Control. 1992;3:115–123.

103. Bülzebruck H, Bopp R, Drings P, et al. New aspects in the staging of lung cancer: prospective validation of the International Union Against Cancer TNM classification. Cancer. 1992;70:1102–1110.

104. Suzuki K, Nagai K, Yoshida J, et al. Prognostic factors in clinical stage I non–small cell lung cancer. Ann Thorac Surg. 1999;67:927–932.

105. Inoue K, Sato M, Fujimura S, et al. Prognostic assessment of 1310 patients with non–small-cell lung cancer who underwent complete resection from 1980 to 1993. J Thorac Cardiovasc Surg. 1998;116:407–411.

106. Jie C, Wever AMJ, Huysmans HA, et al. Time trends and survival in patients presented for surgery with non–small-cell lung cancer 1969–1985. Eur J Cardiothorac Surg. 1990;4:653–657.

107. Kulka F, Forrai I. The segmental and atypical resection of primary lung cancer [abstract]. Lung Cancer. 1986;2:81.

108. Tsubota N, Ayabe K, Doi O, et al. Ongoing prospective study of segmentectomy for small lung tumors. Ann Thorac Surg. 1998;66:1787–1790.

109. Kutschera W. Segment resection for lung cancer. Thorac Cardiovasc Surg. 1984;32:102–104.

110. Ramacciato G, Paolini A, Volpino P, et al. Modality of failure following resection of stage I and stage II non–small cell lung cancer. Int Surg. 1995;80:156–161.

111. Immerman SC, Vanecko RM, Fry WA, et al. Site of recurrence in patients with stages I and II carcinoma of the lung resected for cure. Ann Thorac Surg. 1981;32:23–27.

112. Lafitte JJ, Ribet ME, Prévost BM, et al. Postresection irradiation for T2 N0 M0 non–small cell carcinoma: a prospective, randomized study. Ann Thorac Surg. 1996;62:830–834.

113. Suzuki K, Nagai K, Yoshida J, et al. Clinical predictors of N2 disease in the setting of a negative computed tomographic scan in patients with lung cancer. J Thorac Cardiovasc Surg. 1999;117:593–598.

114. Keller SM, et al, and the ECOG membership, Adak S, Wagner H, Johnson DH. Complete mediastinal lymph node dissection improves survival in patients with resected stages II and IIIa non-small cell lung cancer. Ann Thorac Surg. 2000; in press.

115. Ferguson MK, Wang J, Hoffman PC, et al. Sex-associated differences in survival of patients undergoing resection for lung cancer. Ann Thorac Surg. 2000;69:245–250.

116. Ferguson MK, Karrison T. Does pneumonectomy for lung cancer adversely influence long-term survival? J Thorac Cardiovasc Surg. 2000;119:440–448.

117. van Rens MTM, de la Rivière AB, Elbers HRJ, et al. Prognostic assessment of 2,361 patients who underwent pulmonary resection for non-small cell lung cancer, stage I, II, and IIIA. Chest. 2000;117:374–379.

118. Fujisawa T, Iizasa T, Saitoh Y, et al. Smoking before surgery predicts poor long-term survival in patients with stage I non-small-cell lung carcinoma. J Clin Oncol. 1999;17:2086–2091.

119. Adebonojo SA, Bowser AN, Moritz DM, Corcoran PC. Impact of revised stage classification of lung cancer on survival: a military experience. Chest. 1999;115:1507–1513.

SURGERY FOR STAGE II NON-SMALL CELL LUNG CANCER

Frank C. Detterbeck and Thomas M. Egan

DEFINITION

NATURAL HISTORY

OUTCOME OF CLINICAL STAGE II PATIENTS

OUTCOME OF PATHOLOGIC STAGE II PATIENTS
  T Factors
  N Factors
  Histology
  Other Factors

RECURRENCE PATTERNS

SLEEVE RESECTION

EDITORS' COMMENTS

DEFINITION

Stage II non–small cell lung cancer (NSCLC) includes primarily T1 or T2 tumors with N1 (intrapulmonary) lymph node involvement. According to the most recent revision of the staging classification, T3N0 tumors are also included in the IIb group.[1] However, the biologic implications of direct invasion of chest wall or mediastinum without nodal involvement (T3N0) may not be the same as that of primary tumors that have spread to intrapulmonary lymph nodes (T1,2N1), even though the survival with current treatment approaches may be similar. Furthermore, T3N0 tumors account for a relatively small proportion of stage II tumors, comprising only approximately 20% of resected pII patients in three large series.[1–3] Therefore, this chapter focuses on the data regarding T1,2 patients with N1 nodal involvement. T3N0 tumors are discussed in Chapter 15.

Patients with T1,2N1 lung cancers comprise a relatively small proportion of patients with lung cancer. Patients staged clinically (c) as cT1,2N1 comprise only 7% (range, 5%-10%) of large series of clinically staged patients.[1–3] Patients with pathologically (p) staged pT1,2N1 tumors account for an average of 15% (range, 9%-19%) of all resected patients among surgical series of >1000 patients.[1–5] In a population-based series of 1534 patients, the incidence of clinical stage II NSCLC was found to be 31%, but some of the patients in this series were probably understaged because many were staged by chest radiograph alone.[6]

Because the number of stage II patients is small, results for this group have often been lumped together with either stage I or stage IIIa patients. Analysis of the data pertaining to stage II lung cancer is also hampered by the fact that stage II has been significantly affected by revisions of the staging system. The 1979 American Joint Committee on Cancer staging system included only T2N1 patients in stage II,[7] whereas the revision in 1986 included T1N1 and T2N1 patients,[8] and the most recent revision added T3N0 patients to stage II as well.[1] Other staging issues are also important, such as the difference between clinical staging and pathologic staging and the extent of intraoperative mediastinal and intrapulmonary node assessment. Although these issues are discussed in Chapter 11, they apply to stage II patients as well.

NATURAL HISTORY

Little data has been reported specifically addressing the outcome of stage II patients who did not receive any curative treatment. Among 31 untreated patients with histologically proven NSCLC who were staged as cT2N1, the median survival was found to be 11 months.[9] The 2-year survival was only 6%, and all patients were dead by 30 months. This small group of patients received supportive care but no chemotherapy, surgery, or radiation except for palliation.[9] Thus the chance of survival beyond 1 to 2 years with stage II lung cancer appears to be negligible without treatment.

OUTCOME OF CLINICAL STAGE II PATIENTS

No data has been reported on how often patients who are clinically staged as T1,2N1 also are found to be pathologic stage T1,2N1. Data from the reliability of computed tomography to predict N1 nodal involvement shows that radiographic assessment of N1 nodes carries a 40% false positive rate and a 15% false negative rate (see Table 5–6). In addition, there is at least a 15% to 25% chance of finding pN2 involvement at operation if mediastinal node sampling is thorough (see Table 5–7). Furthermore, no data addresses the likelihood that a complete resection will be accomplished in patients who are cII. Thus, although there is no direct data, indirect data suggests that clinical assessment of stage II disease is inaccurate in 30% to 40% of cases.

The long-term outcome of resected patients who were

TABLE 12–1. SURVIVAL OF CLINICAL STAGE II PATIENTS UNDERGOING RESECTION

STUDY	N	T STAGE	5-y SURVIVAL (%)
Bülzebruck et al[2]	373	T1, T2	24
Naruke et al[3]	248	T1, T2	31
Naruke et al[3]	32	T1	34
Mountain[1]	29	T1	34
Mountain[1]	250	T2	24
Naruke et al[3]	212	T2	32
Average			**30**

Inclusion criteria: Studies of >20 patients with clinical stage II non–small cell lung cancer.

clinically staged as T1,2N1 (irrespective of the final pathologic stage) is shown in Table 12–1. The 5-year survival is consistently reported to be approximately 30%. All of these studies included a small number of patients (~5%) who were found on resection to have small cell cancer.

OUTCOME OF PATHOLOGIC STAGE II PATIENTS

Surgery is widely accepted as the standard treatment for patients with stage II NSCLC. Table 12–2 lists the 5-year survival of resected patients from studies involving at least 100 stage II patients. The reported 5-year survival of approximately 40% is quite consistent among studies. Other reports, involving smaller numbers of patients, have shown similar results.[10–13]

T Factors

The T stage appears to be a significant prognostic factor among stage II NSCLC patients (Fig. 12–1 and Table 12–2). Every report in Table 12–2 comparing T1N1 with T2N1 patients has shown a trend to better survival for T1N1 patients, and the difference was statistically significant in three of the four studies that analyzed this factor.[1,3,4,14] An analysis of the Lung Cancer Study Group

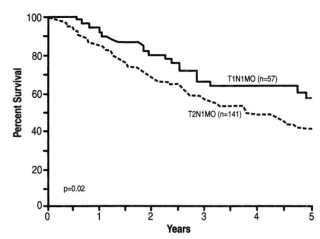

FIGURE 12–1. Survival of resected patients with T1N1M0 and T2N1M0 non–small cell lung cancer ($P = 0.02$). (From Inoue K, Sato M, Fujimura S, et al. Prognostic assessment of 1310 patients with non–small-cell lung cancer who underwent complete resection from 1980 to 1993. J Thorac Cardiovasc Surg. 1998;116:407–411.)[4]

experience found that the survival difference between T1N1 and T2N1 patients was observed both for squamous and nonsquamous cancers.[15] The survival difference of approximately 15% is similar to the difference seen between T1 and T2 tumors among stage I patients (see Table 11–2).

The prognostic significance of T2 status on the basis of tumor size versus T2 status because of pleural involvement is unclear. Only two studies have specifically addressed these factors. One study found a trend toward worse survival for larger tumors, and a statistically significant difference for tumors ≥5 cm versus <5 cm.[14] Pleural involvement was also associated with worse survival (33% versus 41%),[14] but this was not statistically significant, despite an earlier report from the same institution that did find statistically poorer survival in patients with pleural involvement.[16] However, a report from another institution found no survival difference with respect to size (>3 cm or <3 cm)

TABLE 12–2. SURVIVAL AFTER RESECTION OF PATHOLOGIC STAGE II (N1) NON–SMALL CELL LUNG CANCER

STUDY	N	5-y SURVIVAL (%) All	T1	T2	P (T1:T2)	5-y SURVIVAL (%) Sq	Ad	P (Sq:Ad)
van Rens[49]	625	—	52	33	<0.02	—	—	—
van Velzen[43]	369	—	—	38	—	41[a]	18[a]	0.0006[a]
Mountain[1 b]	364	42[c]	55	39	<0.05	—	—	—
Naruke[35 b]	304	47	52	45	—	—	—	—
Bülzebruck et al[2]	256	35	—	—	—	—	—	—
Naruke et al[3 b]	221	43	53	38	<0.05	48	40	—
Martini et al[14]	214	39	40	38	NS	44	34	NS
Inoue et al[4]	197	—	57	42	0.02	—	—	—
Mountain et al[15 a, b]	185	—	—	—	—	53[a]	25[a]	0.01[a]
Jie et al[36]	144	32	—	—	—	—	—	—
Maggi et al[19]	132	46	—	—	—	—	—	NS
Average		**41**	**52**	**39**		**47**	**29**	

Inclusion criteria: Reported series from 1980 to 2000 of ≥100 resected pII non–small cell lung cancer patients. In the case of two studies from the same institution in 2000 which the patients from one study were included among those of the other study, only the most inclusive (latest) study is shown, except as indicated.
[a]T2 only.
[b]Some patients reported a second time in another study by the same author.
[c]Estimated.
Ad, adenocarcinoma; NS, not significant; Sq, squamous.

in 63 stage II patients,[11] whereas visceral pleural involvement was a statistically significant predictor of worse survival by multivariate analysis (5-year survival, 35% versus 56%; $P < 0.05$).[11]

N Factors

Significantly poorer survival has been observed when multiple N1 nodes are involved than when only a single node is involved (5-year survival, 31% versus 45%; $P = 0.016$) (Fig. 12–2).[14] Patients with multiple positive nodes are more likely to have adenocarcinoma, and the positive nodes in patients with adenocarcinoma are more often grossly normal despite microscopic tumor involvement.[16,17] Multivariate analysis demonstrated that the number of N1 nodes involved was a significant independent prognostic factor (as was tumor size, but *not* histologic type) in a study of 214 N1 patients.[14] However, another study of 117 patients with T1-4N1 NSCLC did not find the number of N1 nodes to be of prognostic value.[42]

Patients with lobar node involvement (stations 12 and 13) have better survival than those with hilar involvement (stations 10 and 11), as shown in Figure 12–3.[10] In fact, this was the only significant prognostic factor by multivariate analysis in this study, although T status was almost significant at $P = 0.052$ (the number of nodes involved was not analyzed).[10] Three additional studies have found better survival for patients with lobar compared with hilar nodal involvement (5-year survival, 67% vs. 30%; $P = 0.016$ in 58 T1N1 patients[18]; 57% versus 30%, $P = 0.003$ in 391 T2N1 patients[43]; and 54% versus 39%, $P = 0.02$ in 256 T1-4N1 patients[44]). Only one study of 117 T1-4N1 patients found no prognostic significance associated with the level of N1 involvement.[42]

Involvement of N1 nodes by direct extension from the primary tumor was found to carry the same prognosis as involvement of nodes that were physically separated from the primary tumor in two studies (involving 256 T1-4N1 patients[44] and 391 T2N1 patients[43]). However, N1 involvement by direct extension from the primary tumor had significantly better survival in 58 T1N1 patients (5-year survival, 69% versus 31%; $P = 0.004$).[18] One small study

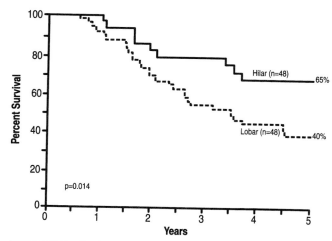

FIGURE 12–3. Survival after resection of patients with N1 disease according to the level of involved N1 nodes: lobar node metastasis (stations 12, 13) versus hilar node metastasis (stations 10, 11) ($P = 0.014$). (From Yano T, Yokoyama H, Inoue T, et al. Surgical results and prognostic factors of pathologic N1 disease in non–small-cell carcinoma of the lung—significance of N1 level: lobar or hilar nodes. J Thorac Cardiovasc Surg. 1994;107:1398–1402.)[10]

(43 patients) found a marked difference in survival between patients with macroscopically detectable N1 involvement and those with only microscopic involvement (5-year survival, 28% versus 76%; $P = 0.001$ by multivariate analysis).[45]

Histology

All studies analyzing the influence of histology in stage II NSCLC have shown a trend toward better survival for squamous cell cancers (Fig. 12–4 and Table 12–2). However, approximately half of these studies found that the difference was not statistically significant.[10,14,19] Significantly better survival was found in patients with squamous cancers among both T1N1 and T2N1 tumors.[15] Two smaller studies also found significantly better survival in patients with squamous cancers.[11,12] The histologic type was a significant prognostic factor by multivariate analysis in two[11,43] of the four studies that have examined this.[10,11,14,43]

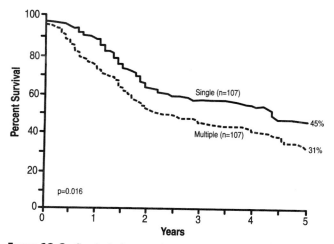

FIGURE 12–2. Survival after resection of T1,2N1 lung cancer by number of involved N1 nodes. (From Martini N, Burt ME, Bains MS, et al. Survival after resection of stage II non–small cell lung cancer. Ann Thorac Surg. 1992;54:460–466.)[14]

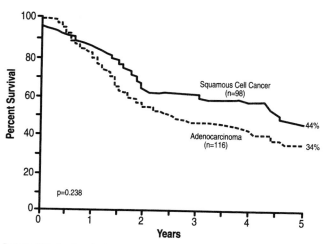

FIGURE 12–4. Survival after resection of T1,2N1 lung cancer by histology. (From Martini N, Burt ME, Bains MS, et al. Survival after resection of stage II non–small cell lung cancer. Ann Thorac Surg. 1992;54:460–466.)[14]

TABLE 12–3. FIRST SITE OF RECURRENCE IN RESECTED pII NON–SMALL CELL LUNG CANCER

STUDY	N	% OF ALL PATIENTS		% OF ALL RECURRENCES		
		New 1°	Recurrence	Local	Local and Distant	Distant
Martini et al[14]	214	3	55	21	—	79
Yano et al[10]	78	—	46	23	5	72
Ramacciato et al[37 a]	68	—	63	40	—	60
van Velzen et al[18 b]	58	—	51	24	38	38
Walsh et al[38]	47	—	50	35	13	52
Baldini et al[47]	46	—	57	19	15	65
Ferguson et al[39]	34	—	44	13	7	80
Iascone et al[40]	32	—	66	29	—	71
Immerman et al[20 c]	22	—	(64)	(64)	—	(36)
Average[d]			**54**	**26**	**74**	

Inclusion criteria: Studies of ≥20 pII non–small cell lung cancer patients from 1980 to 2000 reporting sites of recurrence.
[a]Cumulative sites of recurrence.
[b]T1N1 only.
[c]Extent of mediastinal node staging was limited.
[d]Excluding values in parentheses.
New 1°, new primary lung cancer.

Other Factors

Other factors have not been found to be of prognostic significance in stage II NSCLC, although this has received only limited attention. Histologic differentiation, vascular invasion, and lymphatic invasion had no discernible effect on survival in one study of 63 patients.[11]

RECURRENCE PATTERNS

Approximately 75% of recurrences of stage II NSCLC involve distant recurrences (Table 12–3). Only one study reported a high rate of local recurrences, but this was likely due to positive N2 nodes that were poorly assessed in this study.[20] The proportion of distant recurrences was slightly higher in stage II adenocarcinomas than in squamous cancers in one study (87% versus 66%, no *P* value reported).[14] The incidence of new primary lung cancer in stage II patients has been analyzed infrequently, but appears to be less common in stage II than in stage I patients, probably due to the poorer survival of stage II patients. The cause of death among stage II patients has been reported to be due to recurrence in 72% and 77% of patients in two studies.[14,18]

SLEEVE RESECTION

Occasionally, a central tumor is amenable to a sleeve resection as an alternative to a pneumonectomy. The usual indication for this type of procedure is a tumor that is so proximal in a lobar orifice that a standard lobectomy is not feasible. A portion of the bronchus from which the lobar bronchus arises (eg, a portion of the right main stem and bronchus intermedius in the case of a right upper lobe tumor) is resected in order to achieve a complete resection. This usually involves a bronchial sleeve resection or occasionally only a V (wedge) resection of the bronchus, but sometimes a wedge or sleeve resection of the pulmonary artery (PA) is also necessary. The function of the remaining lobes is preserved by creating an anastomosis between the proximal and distal bronchial (or PA) ends after the tumor has been resected. The necessity of performing a more extensive resection is usually dictated by the proximity of the primary tumor itself at the lobar bronchial orifice, but occasionally, nodal involvement around the bronchus or PA branches precludes standard lobectomy.

Staging of tumors resected by a sleeve resection using the TNM classification is difficult. Because of their proximal location in a lobar orifice, most of these cancers can

DATA SUMMARY: SURGERY FOR STAGE II (N1) NON–SMALL CELL LUNG CANCER			
	AMOUNT	**QUALITY**	**CONSISTENCY**
The 5-year survival of cII patients is 30%	Mod	High	High
The 5-year survival of pII patients is 40%	High	High	High
The 5-year survival of T1N1 patients is 15% higher than for T2N1 patients	High	High	Mod
Patients with hilar N1 involvement have worse survival than those with lobar involvement	High	Mod	High
The 5-year survival of patients with squamous cancer is 15% better than with adenocarcinoma	Mod	Mod	Mod
75% of recurrences in resected pII (N1) patients involve distant metastases	High	High	High

Type of data rated: Plain text: descriptive statement   *Italics: controlled comparison*   **Bold: randomized comparison**

be presumed to be T2 but may occasionally be classified as T3 tumors if they are located within 2 cm of the carina. Most often, there is either no nodal involvement or only N1 disease. Staging is difficult because most studies have not reported details of T and N staging (especially in relation to outcomes) and because the stage grouping for these types of tumors has changed with each revision of the staging system. Because the available studies span nearly 3 decades, significant differences exist among patients included in a particular stage classification in these studies. Retrospective rearrangement of the data to a consistent definition is not possible.

Tumors that are amenable to a sleeve resection do not lend themselves to discussion in the context of a particular stage. Interpretation of outcomes in the absence of a stage designation is difficult. However, classification of patients according to stage is problematic because of the changing stage grouping. In any case, most such tumors are likely to be classified *clinically* as stage II. For these reasons, these tumors are discussed in this chapter, even though the final pathologic staging may range from pT1N0 to pT4N2.

Tumors amenable to sleeve resection most commonly involve the upper lobes. In a number of studies reporting this data (830 patients total), on average, the tumors were located in the right upper lobe in 53%, the right upper and middle lobes in 7%, the right lower lobe in 9%, the left upper lobe in 19%, and the left lower lobe in 8%. Sleeve bronchial resections without loss of pulmonary parenchyma were involved in 3% of cases.[21–28,46] Because of the proximal bronchial location, it is not surprising that the vast majority of these tumors are squamous cell cancers. Studies involving sleeve resection have often included a few patients (<5%) with carcinoid and adenoid cystic tumors.

The average operative mortality for sleeve resections of 4% (Table 12–4) is essentially the same as that for standard lobectomy (see Chapter 8). A review involving 91 deaths among 1915 bronchoplastic procedures found that early mortality was due to respiratory failure in 21%, cardiac event in 20%, pneumonia in 15%, pulmonary embolus in 14%, bronchopleural or bronchovascular fistula in 13%, and empyema in 2%.[29] The incidence of complications was also relatively low in this review. Pneumonia occurred in 10%, atelectasis in 5%, benign stricture in 5%, bronchopleural fistula in 3%, bronchovascular fistula in 2%, and pulmonary embolus and empyema in 2% each.[29] Thus, the morbidity and mortality of sleeve resection are not different from those of a standard lobectomy.

Because of the different stages of tumors involved, it makes little sense to examine the 5-year survival of patients undergoing sleeve resection as a group. However, analysis of these results with respect to stage is also difficult for reasons outlined earlier. Reported data by stage is shown in Table 12–4. The average survival is 58% for stage I tumors, 45% for stage II, and 33% for stage IIIa. Although the reported results for stage I are reasonably consistent, there is a wide range of reported outcomes for stages II and III. This may be due to inclusion of varying numbers of patients who are T3N0 as opposed to those with N1 or N2 disease. Furthermore, the number of patients who had an incomplete resection is not reported in many studies. When the data relative to nodal status (as opposed to stage group) is examined, there continues to be a wide range of reported survivals for patients with N1 and N2 disease.

Again, it is not clear how many patients have had incomplete resections, and the mix of patients with T1 or T2 versus T3 or even T4 disease cannot be ascertained.

In the opinion of some authors, peribronchial nodal disease (N1) that precludes a standard lobectomy is a contraindication to sleeve resection.[30] However, there is no reported data that justifies this stance. The reported outcomes in Table 12–4 would justifies proceeding with a sleeve resection. Furthermore, one study of sleeve resections found no difference in survival among patients with proximal N1 disease versus those with more distal N1 disease.[23] In fact, the data in Table 12–4 indicates that even when N2 involvement is discovered at thoracotomy, a sleeve resection is worthwhile because a reasonable number of these patients are found to be long-term survivors.

There is little data examining the outcomes of patients undergoing a bronchial sleeve resection compared with a PA or a double (bronchial and PA) sleeve resection. Naruke[31] found the overall survival (all stages) to be 24% after a double sleeve resection versus 41% after a bronchial sleeve resection. However, this figure is difficult to interpret because no data is available regarding the T and N status of these patients. Other studies have suggested no difference in survival between these groups when stratified by stage, although the specific survival of patients undergoing double sleeve or PA sleeve resections is not reported.[32,46] Intuitively, it is likely that the extent of the tumor (T and N stage) is the determining factor for survival, rather than the operative techniques required to achieve a complete resection.

Little data is available regarding the distance from the gross tumor to the resection margin that is necessary. None of the studies involving sleeve resection has reported data regarding this. The only study that carefully analyzed this issue found that 50% of patients had a microscopically positive margin when the distance to the gross tumor was <0.5 cm, whereas it was 15% with a distance of 0.5 to 1 cm and 5% with a distance of 1 to 2 cm.[33] Furthermore, positive peribronchial nodal margin carries a worse prognosis than a positive bronchial margin.[22,34]

Sleeve resection has the advantage of preserving the pulmonary function of lobes that are uninvolved with cancer. On one hand, it may be the only option in patients with limited pulmonary reserve, who can undergo sleeve resection as a compromise procedure despite not being able to tolerate a pneumonectomy. On the other hand, because of the low operative morbidity and mortality and good long-term results, sleeve resection is often performed as an alternative to pneumonectomy. Two authors have suggested that the outcome of patients who undergo sleeve resection as a compromise operation (5-year survival, 20% and 31%) is worse than that of patients who undergo sleeve resection as an elective alternative to pneumonectomy (5-year survival, 55% and 60%).[22,24] No details are available to assess whether these patients are comparable with respect to stage, nodal status, or completeness of resection.

Overall, the 5-year survivals for patients undergoing a sleeve resection are essentially the same as for those undergoing a standard resection, stage for stage. This is especially true because series of sleeve resections include few patients with T1 tumors. Given the acceptable operative morbidity and mortality and long-term outcomes, sleeve

TABLE 12–4. OUTCOMES OF PATIENTS UNDERGOING SLEEVE RESECTIONS FOR CANCER

STUDY	N	% Ro	% COMPROMISE[a]	% OPERATIVE MORTALITY[b]	% LOCAL RECURRENCE[c]	5-y SURVIVAL (%) I[d]	II[d]	IIIa	5-y SURVIVAL (%) N0	N1	N2
Vogt-Moykopf et al[32]	248[e]	—	—	12	16	—35—		13	—	—	—
Van Schil et al[48f]	145	100	13	5	—	59[g]	22[g]	42[g]	59[g]	21[g]	44[g]
Mehran et al[21]	142	87	8	2	23	63	48	14	57	47	0
Naruke[31]	111	70	—	1	—	54	62	39	50	46	33
Faber et al[26h]	101	—	—	2	(9)[i]	36	18	15	36	—23—	
Firmin et al[27]	90	—	—	1	(4)[i]	—	—	—	71	—17—	
Gaissert et al[22]	72	—	49	4	14	42	52	45	57	38	43
Deslauriers et al[41]	72	93	—	0	16	66	58	71	67	63	—
Rendina et al[46j]	52	94	—	—	—	83	56	22	56	37	19
Van den Bosch et al[30]	50	—	—	—	—	—	—	—	64	0	—
Average[k]				**3**	**17**	**58**	**45**	**33**	**57**	**36**	**28**

Inclusion criteria: Studies of ≥50 patients undergoing a sleeve resection (excluding sleeve pneumonectomy) for non–small cell lung cancer (in ≥95% of patients, except as indicated).

[a]Percentage of patients undergoing sleeve resection as a compromise, because not able to tolerate pneumonectomy.
[b]As defined by authors.
[c]Percentage of all patients experiencing a recurrence in the chest.
[d]Most studies have reported data using the 1976 staging system (T1N1 included in stage I; only T2N1 in stage II).
[e]Patients undergoing sleeve bronchoplasty *or* pulmonary arterioplasty resections or both.
[f]Includes 9% carcinoid tumors.
[g]Squamous only.
[h]Includes 8% small cell lung cancer.
[i]Suture line recurrence only.
[j]All had PA sleeve resection.
[k]Excluding values in parentheses.
Ro, complete resection with no residual; local recurrence, intrathoracic recurrence in *all* patients.

resection can certainly be justified as an alternative to pneumonectomy.

EDITORS' COMMENTS

It is important to keep in mind that patients who appear radiographically to have stage II NSCLC do not necessarily have the same pathologic stage of lung cancer after resection. Approximately one-third of patients classified as cII-(N1) will be classified as pI, whereas a similar number of patients not thought to have N1 involvement will be classified as pII (N1) after resection. The more important issue, however, is that the false negative rate for mediastinal node involvement in patients who are clinical stage II is probably on the order of 20% to 30%. Therefore, such patients should undergo mediastinoscopy before thoracotomy.

Surgical resection should be the primary treatment when-ever feasible for cancers localized to the lung parenchyma, such as T1,2N1 tumors. The operative mortality rate is quite low, and lobectomy is usually sufficient to remove the primary tumor and all involved nodes. Even in patients with hilar lymph node involvement, a sleeve lobectomy will usually suffice to resect the tumor with an adequate margin, thus preserving lung tissue without compromising the chance for cure. The operative mortality and long-term survival of sleeve lobectomy is similar to that of standard lobectomy, and the long-term survival is also similar to that of a standard lobectomy or pneumonectomy. This makes sleeve resection a viable alternative in order to preserve lung function.

Local control of stage II NSCLC with surgery is quite good. However, 50% of patients have a recurrence, mostly involving distant sites. This raises the question of the addition of chemotherapy, either before or following surgi-

DATA SUMMARY: RESULTS OF SLEEVE RESECTION

	AMOUNT	QUALITY	CONSISTENCY
The operative mortality for a sleeve lobectomy is 4%	High	High	High
The 5-year survival after sleeve resection in patients who are N0 is 60%	High	High	High
The 5-year survival after sleeve resection in patients who are N1 is 40%	High	High	Mod
The 5-year survival after sleeve resection in selected patients who are N2 is 30%	High	High	Mod
The long-term survival of patients undergoing sleeve resection as a compromise procedure is lower than that of patients who could tolerate a pneumonectomy	Mod	High	High

Type of data rated:　　Plain text: descriptive statement　　*Italics: controlled comparison*　　**Bold: randomized comparison**

cal resection. Intuitively, such a combined modality approach makes sense, but the current data is insufficient to either support or refute a survival benefit to this strategy. Further investigation is needed in order to improve the survival of stage II NSCLC patients.

References

1. Mountain CF. Revisions in the International System for Staging Lung Cancer. Chest. 1997;111:1710–1717.
2. Bülzebruck H, Bopp R, Drings P, et al. New aspects in the staging of lung cancer: prospective validation of the International Union Against Cancer TNM classification. Cancer. 1992;70:1102–1110.
3. Naruke T, Tomoyuki G, Tsuchiya R, et al. Prognosis and survival in resected lung carcinoma based on the new international staging system. J Thorac Cardiovasc Surg. 1988;96:440–447.
4. Inoue K, Sato M, Fujimura S, et al. Prognostic assessment of 1310 patients with non–small-cell lung cancer who underwent complete resection from 1980 to 1993. J Thorac Cardiovasc Surg. 1998;116:407–411.
5. Humphrey EW, Smart CR, Winchester DP, et al. National survey of the pattern of care for carcinoma of the lung. J Thorac Cardiovasc Surg. 1990;100:837–843.
6. Chute CG, Greenberg ER, Baron J, et al. Presenting conditions of 1539 population-based lung cancer patients by cell type and stage in New Hampshire and Vermont. Cancer. 1985;56:2107–2111.
7. American Joint Committee on Cancer, Task Force on Lung. Staging of lung cancer 1979. Chicago, Ill: American Joint Committee on Cancer; 1979.
8. Mountain CF. A new international staging system for lung cancer. Chest. 1986;89(suppl):225S–233S.
9. Vrdoljak E, Mise K, Sapunar D, et al. Survival analysis of untreated patients with non–small-cell lung cancer. Chest. 1994;106:1797–1800.
10. Yano T, Yokoyama H, Inoue T, et al. Surgical results and prognostic factors of pathologic N1 disease in non–small-cell carcinoma of the lung-significance of N1 level: lobar or hilar nodes. J Thorac Cardiovasc Surg. 1994;107:1398–1402.
11. Ichinose Y, Yano T, Asoh H, et al. Prognostic factors obtained by a pathologic examination in completely resected non–small-cell lung cancer: an analysis in each pathologic stage. J Thorac Cardiovasc Surg. 1995;110:601–605.
12. Shah R, Sabanathan S, Richardson J, et al. Results of surgical treatment of stage I and II lung cancer. J Cardiovasc Surg. 1996;37:169–172.
13. Riquet M, Manac'h D, Le Pimpec Barthes F, et al. Prognostic value of T and N in non–small cell lung cancer three centimeters or less in diameter. Eur J Cardiothorac Surg. 1997;11:440–444.
14. Martini N, Burt ME, Bains MS, et al. Survival after resection of stage II non–small cell lung cancer. Ann Thorac Surg. 1992;54:460–466.
15. Mountain CF, Lukeman JM, Hammar SP, et al. Lung cancer classification: the relationship of disease extent and cell type to survival in a clinical trials population. J Surg Oncol. 1987;35:147–156.
16. Martini N, Flehinger BJ, Nagasaki F, et al. Prognostic significance of N1 disease in carcinoma of the lung. J Thorac Cardiovasc Surg. 1983;86:646–653.
17. Izbicki JR, Thetter O, Karg O, et al. Accuracy of computed tomographic scan and surgical assessment for staging of bronchial carcinoma: a prospective study. J Thorac Cardiovasc Surg. 1992;104:413–420.
18. van Velzen E, Snijder RJ, de la Riviere AB, et al. Type of lymph node involvement influences survival rates in T1N1M0 non–small cell lung carcinoma. Chest. 1996;110:1469–1473.
19. Maggi G, Casadio C, Mancuso M, et al. Resection and radical lymphadenectomy for lung cancer: prognostic significance of lymphatic metastases. Int Surg. 1990;75:17–21.
20. Immerman SC, Vanecko RM, Fry WA, et al. Site of recurrence in patients with stages I and II carcinoma of the lung resected for cure. Ann Thorac Surg. 1981;32:23–27.
21. Mehran RJ, Deslauriers J, Piraux M, et al. Survival related to nodal status after sleeve resection for lung cancer. J Thorac Cardiovasc Surg. 1994;107:576–583.
22. Gaissert HA, Mathisen DJ, Moncure AC, et al. Survival and function after sleeve lobectomy for lung cancer. J Thorac Cardiovasc Surg. 1996;111:948–953.
23. Van Schil PE, de la Rivière AB, Knaepen PJ, et al. TNM staging and long-term follow-up after sleeve resection for bronchogenic tumors. Ann Thorac Surg. 1991;52:1096–1101.
24. Frist WH, Mathisen DJ, Hilgenberg AD, et al. Bronchial sleeve resection with and without pulmonary resection. J Thorac Cardiovasc Surg. 1987;93:350–357.
25. Keszler P. Sleeve resection and other bronchoplasties in the surgery of bronchogenic tumors. Int Surg. 1986;71:229–232.
26. Faber LP, Jensik RJ, Kittle CF. Results of sleeve lobectomy for bronchogenic carcinoma in 101 patients. Ann Thorac Surg. 1984;37:279–285.
27. Firmin RK, Azariades M, Lennox SC, et al. Sleeve lobectomy (lobectomy and bronchoplasty) for bronchial carcinoma. Ann Thorac Surg. 1983;35:442–449.
28. Fugimura S, Kondo T, Imai T, et al. Prognostic evaluation of tracheo-bronchial reconstruction for bronchogenic carcinoma. J Thorac Cardiovasc Surg. 1985;90:161–166.
29. Tedder M, Anstadt MP, Tedder SD, et al. Current morbidity, mortality, and survival after bronchoplastic procedures for malignancy. Ann Thorac Surg. 1992;54:387–391.
30. Van den Bosch JMM, Bergstein PGM, Laros CD, et al. Lobectomy with sleeve resection in the treatment of tumors of the bronchus. Chest. 1981;80:154–157.
31. Naruke T. Bronchoplastic and bronchovascular procedures of the tracheobronchial tree in the management of primary lung cancer. Chest. 1989;96:53S–56S.
32. Vogt-Moykopf I, Fritz T, Meyer G, et al. Bronchoplastic and angio-plastic operation in bronchial carcinoma: long-term results of a retrospective analysis from 1973 to 1983. Intern Surg. 1986;71:211–220.
33. Kayser K, Anyanwu E, Bauer H-G, et al. Tumor presence at resection boundaries and lymph-node metastasis in bronchial carcinoma patients. Thorac Cardiovasc Surg. 1993;41:308–311.
34. Kaiser LR, Fleshner P, Keller S, et al. Significance of extramucosal residual tumor at the bronchial resection margin. Ann Thorac Surg. 1989;47:265–269.
35. Naruke T, Tschiya R, Kondo H, et al. Implications of staging in lung cancer. Chest. 1997;112(suppl):242S–248S.
36. Jie C, Wever AMJ, Huysmans HA, et al. Time trends and survival in patients presented for surgery with non–small-cell lung cancer 1969–1985. Eur J Cardiothorac Surg. 1990;4:653–657.
37. Ramacciato G, Paolini A, Volpino P, et al. Modality of failure following resection of stage I and stage II non–small cell lung cancer. Int Surg. 1995;80:156–161.
38. Walsh GL, O'Connor M, Willis KM, et al. Is follow-up of lung cancer patients after resection medically indicated and cost-effective? Ann Thorac Surg. 1995;60:1563–1572.
39. Ferguson MK, Little AG, Golomb HM, et al. The role of adjuvant therapy after resection of T1 N1 M0 and T2 N1 M0 non–small cell lung cancer. J Thorac Cardiovasc Surg. 1986;91:344–349.
40. Iascone C, DeMeester TR, Albertucci M, et al. Local recurrence of resectable non–oat cell carcinoma of the lung: a warning against conservation treatment for N0 and N1 disease. Cancer. 1986;57:471–476.
41. Deslauriers J, Gaulin P, Beaulieu M, et al. Long-term clinical and functional results of sleeve lobectomy for primary lung cancer. J Thorac Cardiovasc Surg. 1986;92:871–879.
42. Sawyer TE, Bonner JA, Gould PM, et al. Factors predicting patterns of recurrence after resection of N1 non–small cell lung carcinoma. Ann Thorac Surg. 1999;68:1171–1176.
43. van Velzen E, Snijder RJ, de la Rivière AB, et al. Lymph node type as a prognostic factor for survival in T2 N1 M0 non–small cell lung carcinoma. Ann Thorac Surg. 1997;63:1436–1440.
44. Riquet M, Manac'h D, Le Pimpec-Barthes F, et al. Pronostic significance of surgical-pathologic N1 disease in non–small cell carcinoma of the lung. Ann Thorac Surg. 1999;67:1572–1576.
45. Yoshino I, Nakanishi R, Osaki T, et al. Unfavorable prognosis of patients with stage II non–small cell lung cancer associated with macroscopic nodal metastases. Chest. 1999;116:144–149.
46. Rendina EA, Venuta F, De Giacomo T. Sleeve resection and prosthetic reconstruction of the pulmonary artery for lung cancer. Ann Thorac Surg. 1999;68:995–1002.
47. Baldini EH, DeCamp MM Jr, Katz MS, et al. Patterns of recurrence and outcome for patients with stage II non–small cell lung cancer. Am J Clin Oncol. 1999;22:8–14.
48. Van Schil PE, de la Rivière AB, Knaepen PJ, et al. TNM staging and long-term follow-up after sleeve resection for bronchogenic tumors. Ann Thorac Surg. 1991;52:1096–1101.
49. van Rens MTM, de la Rivière AB, Elbers HRJ, et al. Prognostic assessment of 2,361 patients who underwent pulmonary resection for non–small cell lung cancer, stage I, II, and IIIA. Chest. 2000;117:374–379.

RADIOTHERAPY FOR STAGE I,II NON–SMALL CELL LUNG CANCER

Harold Johnson and Jan S. Halle

PATIENT SELECTION	RECURRENCE PATTERNS	RADIOTHERAPY DOSE
TREATMENT PARAMETERS	PROGNOSTIC FACTORS	EDITORS' COMMENTS
SURVIVAL		

Surgery is the mainstay of treatment for patients with early-stage (I and II) non–small cell lung cancer (NSCLC). Nevertheless, radiotherapy (RT) plays an important role in the management of patients who would otherwise be treated surgically but who either are medically unable to or choose not to undergo surgery. This chapter reviews the data regarding RT alone given as a curative treatment for stage I,II NSCLC. Not all studies have clearly identified whether RT was given with curative or palliative intent. For the purposes of this chapter, RT involving <45 Gy is assumed to be palliative. One might argue that 45 to 50 Gy is also too low to be curative, but at the time that many of these studies were conducted, this was considered to be a reasonable curative dose. It is interesting to note that all of the studies cited in the tables in this chapter were published within the 1990s, with the exception of one published in 1989. Most treatment has been done with external-beam radiation therapy, which is the focus of this chapter. However, other approaches such as radioactive seed implantation using iodine-125, percutaneous high-dose-rate brachytherapy, and endobronchial high-dose-rate brachytherapy have been used occasionally.[1,2]

Since the 1960s, a number of retrospective studies of primary RT for stage I,II NSCLC have been published. It is intuitively obvious that these results cannot be readily compared with those of surgical series because of differences in the patient population. Although patients who have elected RT by choice may be similar, those excluded from surgery because of significant comorbid illnesses have additional factors that may influence their survival. In addition, patients treated with RT for clinical stage I,II NSCLC cannot be compared with patients who are pathologically staged as stage I,II after a resection. Furthermore, almost all patients treated with RT have undergone only radiographic mediastinal staging. Approximately 15% of patients with a radiographically negative mediastinum are actually stage III if clinical staging includes mediastinoscopy or other invasive techniques (see Table 5–7). The incidence of distant metastases should be relatively low in the presence of a negative clinical examination (see Table 6–3). Unfortu-

nately, details about the patients with respect to these issues have not been reported in most studies of primary RT. These caveats must be kept in mind when comparing treatment results for stage I,II NSCLC.

PATIENT SELECTION

It is important to define the population of patients treated with RT alone. Various characteristics of patients in the reported studies are summarized in Table 13–1. In most studies, the majority of patients are stage I, although a few studies[3,4] included primarily stage II patients. The average median age of patients treated with RT is 70 years (range, 60-74 years). This is somewhat older than the average age of patients treated surgically, which is approximately 64 years in several large series (23,295 patients total).[5–8] In fact, the average age of patients treated with RT is slightly older than the average age of 66 years for all patients who are diagnosed with lung cancer (see Fig. 4–2). Despite these differences, the average age differs from that in surgical series by only a few years.

Most patients treated with RT alone had a good performance status (defined as a Karnofsky score of 80-100 or a Zubrod score of 0-1). Only an average of 17% of patients (range, 0-43%) had a poor performance status (PS). The presence of comorbidity is more difficult to evaluate because of unclear definitions and because comorbidity is often not reported. However, only 15% of patients were treated with RT because they refused surgery. The vast majority of patients were thought to be unsuitable for surgery, most often because of poor pulmonary reserve. This is somewhat in conflict with the data that the vast majority of patients had a good PS. It also raises the question of whether some of the patients who underwent RT alone for stage I,II NSCLC because of poor pulmonary reserve or advanced age might be considered surgical candidates based on current criteria for surgical suitability (see Chapter 7) and the development of minimally invasive surgical techniques (see Chapter 8). At any rate, it is clear that the great majority of patients treated with RT alone

TABLE 13–1. CHARACTERISTICS OF PATIENTS TREATED WITH RADIOTHERAPY ALONE FOR STAGE I,II NON–SMALL CELL LUNG CANCER

STUDY	N	STAGE I (%)	MEDIAN AGE (y)	POOR PS[a] (%)	REASON SURGERY NOT PERFORMED (%)[b]					
					Refused	Age	Pulmonary	Cardiac	Comorbidity	Other
Gauden et al[9]	347	100	70	13	—	—	—	—	—	—
Dosoretz et al[18, 20]	245	70[d]	74[d]	17[d]	11	0	60	8	64[c] ———— 6	15
Burt et al[10]	175	76[e]	65	—	—	—	—	—	—	—
Morita et al[21]	149	100	75	—	17	28	39	—	16	—
Sibley et al[15]	141	100	70	—	1	—	69	—	—	30
Hayakawa et al[3]	116	36[e]	—	28	4	30	42	10	7	7
Krol et al[11]	108	100	74	0[f]	6	—	66	34	6	7
Graham et al[14]	103	90	67	13	—	—	—	—	—	—
Sandler et al[22]	77	100	72	16	17	5	78[c] ————			
Talton et al[23]	77	78[g]	65	0[f]	—	—	—	—	—	—
Kupelian et al[19]	71	63[g]	—	43	—	—	—	—	—	—
Jeremic et al[26]	67	0[h]	60	13	36	—	16	37	—	10
Rosenthal et al[4]	62	0[h]	68	34	—	—	—	—	—	—
Kaskowitz et al[16]	53	100	73	9	19	—	—	—	—	—
Average			**70**	**17**	**14**	**16**	**49**	**22**	**9**	**15**

Inclusion criteria: Studies of ≥50 patients with stage I,II non–small cell lung cancer treated with radiotherapy alone with curative intent.
[a]Performance status ≥2 or ≤70.
[b]Percentages may exceed 100% because some patients had more than one reason.
[c]"Medical reasons."
[d]Data based on first 152 patients.
[e]Chest computed tomography done in <50% of patients.
[f]PS ≤60.
[g]All N0 (study includes T3,4N0 patients).
[h]All stage II.
PS, performance status.

had comorbid conditions or were thought by the treating physicians to be too old for surgery. Despite the comorbid factors, the planned RT could be delivered in almost all of the patients (Table 13–2).

TREATMENT PARAMETERS

Table 13–2 summarizes the RT treatment parameters used in the studies of curative RT. Consistent with the exclusion of studies involving noncurative (low-dose) RT, the vast majority of studies involved a median dose of ≥60 Gy. Only three studies used doses <60 Gy in a majority of patients,[9,10,26] but two studies used a somewhat larger fraction size (2.5-3.5 Gy/day) and the other used twice-daily RT. Because of a greater radiobiologic effect of larger fraction sizes (see Chapter 9), the effect of the smaller total doses is offset to some degree. All of the studies used a megavoltage radiation source.

TABLE 13–2. TREATMENT PARAMETERS IN STUDIES OF CURATIVE RADIOTHERAPY FOR STAGE I,II NON–SMALL CELL LUNG CANCER

STUDY	N	RT DOSE (Gy)		RT TO MEDIASTINUM (%)	PATIENTS COMPLETING PLANNED RT (%)
		Total	Fraction		
Gauden et al[9]	347	50	2.5	100	100
Burt et al[10]	175	50–55[a]	~2.5–3.5	0	—
Dosoretz et al[18]	152	50–69[a]	—	>50[b]	—
Morita et al[21]	149	55–75[c]	2	44	—
Sibley et al[15]	141	50–80[c]	1.2[d]–3	73	100
Würschmidt et al[24]	132	60–70	2–2.5	—	—
Hayakawa et al[3]	116	60–74	2	100	100
Krol et al[11]	108	60–65	2.5–3	0	98
Graham et al[14]	103	60[e]	2–2.5	80	—
Sandler et al[22]	77	60[e]	—	90	—
Talton et al[23]	77	60	2	100	100
Kupelian et al[19]	71	63[e]	—	72	100
Jeremic et al[26]	67	69.6[d]	1.2[d]	100	—
Rosenthal et al[4]	62	60[e]	—	—	—
Kaskowitz et al[16]	53	50–79[a]	—	89	—

Inclusion criteria: Studies of ≥50 patients with stage I,II non–small cell lung cancer treated with radiotherapy alone with curative intent.
[a]In >95% of patients.
[b]Listed as "the majority."
[c]Median dose 64 Gy.
[d]Hyperfractionated RT.
[e]Median dose.
RT, radiotherapy.

TABLE 13–3. SURVIVAL OF PATIENTS WITH STAGE I,II NON–SMALL CELL LUNG CANCER TREATED WITH CURATIVE RADIOTHERAPY

STUDY	N	STAGE I (%)	OVERALL SURVIVAL			CANCER-SPECIFIC SURVIVAL			FREEDOM FROM LOCAL RECURRENCE	
			MST	2-y (%)	5-y (%)	MST	2-y (%)	5-y (%)	2-y (%)	5-y (%)
Gauden et al[9]	347	100	28	54	27	20[a]	41[a]	23[a]	—	—
Morita et al[21]	149	100	27	55	22	—	—	—	—	—
Sibley et al[15]	141	100	18	39	13	30	60	32	—	—
Krol et al[11]	108	100	23	49	15	31	58	31	(71)[b, c]	66[c]
Graham et al[14]	103	90	16	35	14	—	—	—	—	—
Sandler et al[22]	77	100	20	35	12	15	33	18	53	42
Kaskowitz et al[16]	53	100	21	43	6	20	54	13	65	0
Average[d] (cI)			**22**	**44**	**16**	**23**	**49**	**23**		
Dosoretz et al[18,20]	245	70	16	34	7	11[a]	27[a]	9[a]	—	—
Burt et al[10]	175	76	17	37	15	18	40	20	—	—
Würschmidt et al[24]	132	66	17	30	13	—	—	—	—	—
Hayakawa et al[3]	116	36	19	43	20	—	—	—	70[e]	60[e]
Talton et al[23]	77	78[f]	(15)[g]	(36)[g]	(17)[g]	—	—	—	—	—
Kupelian et al[19]	71	63	16	33	12	17	47	32	66	56
Jeremic et al[26]	67	0	27	53	25	26[a]	52[a]	31[a]	69	61
Rosenthal[4]	62	0	18	33	12	—	—	—	—	—
Average[d] (cI-II)			**17**	**36**	**15**	**18**	**42**	**23**		
Average[d] (all studies)			**20**	**41**	**15**	**20**	**45**	**23**	**65**	**48**

Inclusion criteria: Studies of ≥50 patients with stage I,II non–small cell lung cancer treated with radiotherapy alone with curative intent.
[a] Disease-free survival.
[b] 3-year rate.
[c] Only patients with an initial complete response reported.
[d] Excluding values in parentheses.
[e] Estimated.
[f] All N0 (study includes T3,4N0 patients).
[g] Absolute (crude) survival.
MST, median survival time (in months).

The majority of studies included the mediastinum in the treatment field in most patients, and only two studies clearly omitted radiation of the mediastinum.[10, 11] This is because, until recently, standard practice in radiation oncology was to include the mediastinum provided that treatment could be accomplished without significant morbidity. However, the false-negative rate of normal mediastinal lymph nodes on a computed tomography (CT) scan in patients with cI,II tumors is consistently reported to be approximately 15% (see Table 5–7). Several authors have questioned whether the rate of failure in the mediastinum is high enough in cI,II lung cancer to warrant routine mediastinal irradiation.[11–13]

SURVIVAL

The survival of patients with stage I,II NSCLC treated with RT is summarized in Table 13–3. Overall survival rate at 5 years is approximately 15%, with a median survival period of approximately 18 months. As can be seen from the table, the results among studies are consistent. Representative survival curves from two of the larger studies are shown in Figures 13–1 and 13–2. There is no obvious relationship between survival data and the minor differences in patient selection criteria noted in the studies in Table 13–1. Likewise, checking these survival figures against the dose information and mediastinal treatment data from Table 13–2 does not reveal any clear trends. The

survival rates of stage cI and stage cII patients are also similar, although there is a slight trend to better median and 2-year survival in studies that involve only patients with stage cI cancer compared with those involving patients with stage cI and cII tumors. In those studies that have reported specifically on patients with stage cII NSCLC, the average 5-year survival is 19%.[3,4,26]

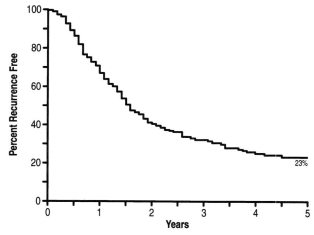

FIGURE 13–1. Overall survival of 347 patients with clinical stage I non–small cell lung cancer treated with radiotherapy with curative intent. (From Gauden S, Ramsay J, Tripcony L. The curative treatment by radiotherapy alone of stage I non–small cell carcinoma of the lung. Chest. 1995; 108:1278–1282.[9])

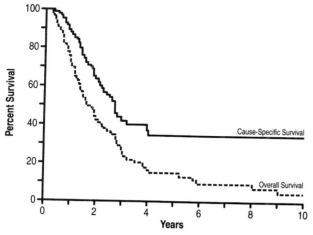

FIGURE 13–2. Overall and cancer-specific survival of 141 patients with clinical stage I NSCLC treated with radiotherapy with curative intent. (Reprinted from *International Journal of Radiation Oncology, Biology, Physics,* Vol 38, Sibley GS, Jamieson TA, Marks LB, et al, Radiotherapy alone for medically inoperable stage I non–small-cell lung cancer: the Duke experience, 521–525, Copyright 1997, with permission from Elsevier Science.[15])

The lack of an identifiable impact of patient and treatment characteristics on survival may be due to the fact that, on average, the studies spanned a 10-year period (range, 3-17 years), with most patients being treated between 1980 and 1990. During the long accrual times, it is likely that the policies regarding selection, staging, and treatment (eg, three-dimensional [3-D] conformal RT planning techniques) gradually changed. The lack of identifiable trends does not necessarily mean that no such trends exist but only that they are not identifiable with the currently available data.

In patients with comorbid conditions, the issue of whether survival is limited by the lung cancer or by the patient's general condition must be examined. Many studies have reported cancer-specific survival, in which patients dying of noncancer causes are censored. Some studies have reported disease-free survival, which is similar except that patients who are alive with a recurrence of cancer or who have died of a noncancer cause despite a recurrence are censored in the cancer-specific analysis but not in the disease-free analysis. However, the number of patients who

develop a recurrence but remain alive or die of other causes appears to be low, and the survival data reported by these two methods is similar. Considering these methods together, the average 5-year cancer-specific or disease-free survival is approximately 25%, or about 10% better than the overall survival.

Several studies have reported cause of death, as shown in Table 13–4. This data confirms that lung cancer is the predominant cause of death, as is suggested by the relatively small difference between the overall and cancer-specific survival data. There is some variability in the data reported, with cancer being the cause of death for an average of 73% of patients but ranging from 46% to 88% of patients. It is possible that the cause of death is not always reliably reported, with death being ascribed to a likely cause, such as lung cancer, without consideration of whether recurrent cancer was really even present. However, these patients also had other medical conditions that might be viewed as likely causes of death. At any rate, we have to accept the results as they are reported. Furthermore, the proportion of noncancer deaths may be related to the length of follow-up. Noncancer causes of death have been specifically reported in only one study, with 9% of deaths due to pulmonary disease and 15% due to a cardiac condition.[14] Mortality related to RT was reported in one study[15] and accounted for <2% of deaths.

Although a comparison of treatment by surgery and treatment by RT is inappropriate because of differences in the patient population, it is interesting to compare the outcomes of the two different patient groups treated with these therapies. The 5-year survival of *clinical* stage I patients treated with surgery is 50% (see Table 11–1) and that of *clinical* stage II patients undergoing resection is 30% (see Table 12–1). Although disease-free survival for patients with clinical stage I NSCLC treated with surgery has not been specifically reported, it can be estimated to be approximately 70% from the fact that about 60% of deaths after resection of pathologic stage I lung cancers are due to a recurrence (see Table 11–4). The causes of death following surgery or RT for stage cI,II NSCLC are surprisingly similar.

RECURRENCE PATTERNS

Assessment of local control after RT is not entirely straightforward. RT can cause fibrosis that can be difficult to

TABLE 13–4. CAUSE OF DEATH IN PATIENTS WITH STAGE I,II NON–SMALL CELL LUNG CANCER TREATED WITH CURATIVE RADIOTHERAPY

STUDY	N	N DEATHS	MEDIAN FOLLOW-UP (mo)	DIED OF Cancer (%)	Other Cause (%)
Gauden et al[9]	347	—	>29	88	12
Dosoretz et al[20]	245	—	—	88	12
Morita et al[21]	149	116	91	81	19
Sibley et al[15]	141	108	24	46	54
Krol et al[11]	108	93	—	66	34
Graham et al[14]	103	93	≥60[a]	72	28
Sandler et al[22]	77	61	—	84	16
Kupelian et al[19]	71	57	36	60	40
Kaskowitz et al[16]	53	49	—	71	29
Average				**73**	**27**

Inclusion criteria: Studies of ≥50 patients with stage I,II non–small cell lung cancer treated with radiotherapy alone with curative intent.
[a]With the exception of two patients.

differentiate from tumor (see Chapter 9). Another issue is whether to classify a persistent abnormality as stable local disease or as no evidence of cancer. Because objective data such as a biopsy result is lacking, the assessment of local control is subjective and open to bias. Whether this results in an overestimation or an underestimation of the rate of local recurrence is open to speculation. In addition to difficulties in determining when a local recurrence has happened, there are difficulties regarding the best way to present the data. A simple recording of the rate of local failure is dependent on the length of follow-up. Plotting an actuarial freedom from local progression is problematic in a situation in which there are competing events such as distant recurrences or noncancer deaths. Because patients with these latter events are censored and may not be observed long enough for local recurrence to occur, actuarial freedom from progression tends to underestimate the chance of local recurrence. Finally, recording the recurrence rate along with the proportion of local recurrences is hampered by the fact that some studies report only first recurrences, whereas others report cumulative recurrence patterns.

Studies reporting actuarial freedom from local recurrence have found a 5-year rate of approximately 50% (see Table 13–3). Moderate consistency exists among studies, with the exception of one study,[16] which reported a puzzling 5-year freedom from local recurrence rate of 0, despite a 2-year rate of 65%. Studies that have reported recurrence patterns are shown in Table 13–5. Approximately 60% of patients have been found to develop a recurrence, and about 70% of these involve a local recurrence, either as an isolated event or simultaneous with distant recurrences. One study reported a conspicuously high proportion of mixed recurrences (both local and distant), leading to the suspicion that it was really cumulative recurrences that were reported.[11] Exclusion of this study leads to an average proportion of mixed recurrences of 16% and of distant recurrences of 32%.

The proportion of regional (mediastinal) recurrence after RT for stage cI,II NSCLC, either as an isolated event or in conjunction with other sites, is low (see Table 13–5). Most of the studies of clinical stage I,II patients delivered radiation to the mediastinal lymph nodes as well as to the primary tumor. However, there is no difference in the mediastinal recurrence rate in the study in which patients received radiation only to the primary tumor.[11] Three studies, reporting on smaller numbers of stage I patients who did not receive mediastinal irradiation (26, 36, and 49 patients), also reported 10% regional recurrences, which is the same rate as that for patients at the same institution who received mediastinal irradiation.[12,15,17]

PROGNOSTIC FACTORS

A number of studies have evaluated the survival of patients with T1 versus T2 tumors (Table 13–6). Although a general trend toward poorer survival with a T2 tumor is seen, the difference is statistically significant by univariable analysis in only about half of the studies. Cancer-specific survival at 5 years is fairly well correlated with the T status, with the average survival in three studies being 47% for T1, 24% for T2, and 11% for T3 tumors.[10,18,19] A nonsignificant trend toward better local control of T1 tumors was reported in one study.[19]

In contrast, tumor size correlated significantly with survival in all studies that have examined this relationship (Table 13–7). A possible explanation is that patients with larger primary tumors may be more likely to have more advanced cancers (stage cII instead of cI), but this does not appear to be the case. Three of the four studies included only stage I patients, and in the fourth, the association of survival with tumor size was highly significant, whereas the association with nodal status was not (N0 versus N1).[3] A more likely explanation appears to be that it is more difficult to control larger tumors with RT, at least at the doses that have been employed. Local control is worse with larger tumors in each of the studies that have analyzed this factor. However, the differences are modest, statistical significance is found inconsistently, and evaluation of local control is fraught with potential biases.

A number of larger studies have performed multivariable analysis in order to identify prognostic factors in patients with early-stage NSCLC treated with RT.[3,4,10,14–16,19,20] Unfortunately, different studies have examined different factors; a clear consensus is not possible. However, it seems

TABLE 13–5. RECURRENCE PATTERNS AFTER RADIOTHERAPY GIVEN WITH CURATIVE INTENT FOR STAGE I,II NON–SMALL CELL LUNG CANCER

STUDY	N	RT TO MEDIASTINUM (%)	MEDIAN FOLLOW-UP (mo)	% WITH RECURRENCE	% OF FIRST RECURRENCES			
					Local	Reg/Med	Mixed	Distant
Dosoretz et al[18]	152	>50	—	66	——55——		15	30
Morita et al[21a]	149	44	91	61	——79——			21
Sibley et al[15]	141	73	24	39	42	7	12	38
Krol et al[11]	108	0	—	73	40	3	54	4
Kupelian et al[19]	71	72	36	44	—	—	—	—
Rosenthal et al[4b]	62	—	>24	85	——64——		—	36
Kaskowitz et al[16]	53	>89	—	67	46	6	22	25
Average				**62**	**43**	**5**	**26**	**26**

Inclusion criteria: Studies of ≥50 patients with stage I,II non–small cell lung cancer treated with RT alone with curative intent.
[a]Recurrence pattern as the cause of death.
[b]Stage II patients only.
Reg/Med, regional/mediastinal; RT, radiotherapy.

TABLE 13–6. EFFECT OF T STATUS ON OVERALL SURVIVAL AND LOCAL CONTROL

STUDY	N	STAGE I (%)	MST (mo)		SURVIVAL 2-y (%)		5-y (%)		P
			T1	T2	T1	T2	T1	T2	
Freedom From Local Recurrence									
Kupelian et al[19]	71	63	—	—	89	60	68	60	NS
Overall Survival									
Gauden et al[9]	347	100	29	21	59	48	32	21	.05
Morita et al[21]	149	100	—	—	—	—	—	—	NS
Hayakawa et al[3]	116	36	12	21	43	52	0	25	(.04)a
Graham et al[14]	103	90	—	—	—	—	29	4	.01
Jeremic et al[26]	67	0	32	19	68	42	40	13	.003
Rosenthal et al[4]	62	0	27	18	—	—	—	—	NS
Noordijk et al[25]	50	100	37	17	67	43	27b	15b	.06
Average (overall survival)			**27**	**19**	**59**	**46**	**26**	**16**	

Inclusion criteria: Studies of ≥50 patients with stage I,II non–small cell lung cancer treated with radiotherapy alone with curative intent.
aStatistically significant better survival for T2 versus T3; study included only eight patients with T1 tumors.
b4-year survival.
MST, median survival time (in months); NS, not significant.

clear that PS is a major determinant of survival, with a PS ≥2 having been found to be significantly correlated with poorer survival in all studies that have examined this.[3,4,19,20] Tumor size >5 cm has also consistently been found to be an important factor.[3,14,19,20] T status (T1 versus T2) was significant in one multivariate analysis,[16] but not in three others.[3,4,15] Two of four studies[14,20] found weight loss to be significant,[4,10] and one of six[15] found age >70 years to be significant as a prognostic factor.[3,4,10,16,20] The histologic subtype was significant in one of five studies[15] (poorer survival with non–squamous cell carcinoma),[3,4,10,20] whereas gender has consistently been found *not* to correlate with survival.[3,4,10] Nodal status was not significant in the one study that examined this factor.[3] Thus, PS and tumor size are the only two clearly demonstrated prognostic factors, and T status, weight loss, age, and histologic type are of questionable prognostic value.

RADIOTHERAPY DOSE

The optimal dose of RT for definitive treatment of early-stage stage lung cancer has not been determined. As shown in Table 13–1, the dose of RT used in the majority of cases was ≥60 Gy, which has traditionally been considered an acceptable dose. However, there is currently much interest in exploring the benefits and limitations of higher doses[13] (see Chapter 9). Initial data indicates that higher doses are well tolerated, provided the field size is not excessive (see Chapter 9). However, the limited data currently available for stage I,II NSCLC does not clearly suggest a dose response within the ranges examined (50–80 Gy). A trend toward better local control with higher doses of RT was suggested in two studies, but the differences were not statistically significant.[11,15] A nonsignificant trend toward better survival was seen in one study,[10] but either no differ-

TABLE 13–7. EFFECT OF PRIMARY TUMOR SIZE ON SURVIVAL

STUDY	N	SIZE (cm)	MST (mo)		SURVIVAL 2-y (%)		5-y (%)		P
			≤	>	≤	>	≤	>	
Freedom From Local Recurrence									
Hayakawa et al[3]	116	5	—	—	80	61	65	61	.06
Krol et al[11]	108	4	—	—	(72)a	(50)a	—	—	NS
Sandler et al[22]	77	3	—	—	62	45	46	36	NS
Kupelian et al[19]	71	4	—	—	77	49	62	49	.003
Averageb (freedom from local recurrence)					**73**	**52**	**58**	**49**	
Overall Survival									
Morita et al[21]	149	4	—	—	—	—	25	17	.05
Hayakawa et al[3]	116	5	31	14	55	27	22	13	.005
Sandler et al[22]	77	3	20	16	44	31	20	4	.009
Noordijk et al[25]	50	4	25	12	64	20	20	(<8)	.0007
Averageb (overall survival)			**25**	**14**	**54**	**26**	**22**	**11**	

Inclusion criteria: Studies of ≥50 patients with stage I,II non–small cell lung cancer treated with radiotherapy alone with curative intent.
a3-year survival.
bExcluding values in parentheses.
≤, less than or equal to size threshold; >, greater than size threshold; MST, median survival time (in months); NS, not significant.

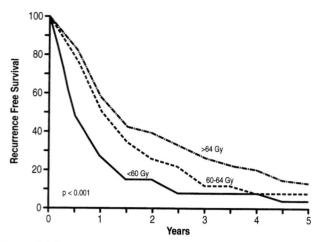

FIGURE 13–3. Percentage of patients without recurrence by dose of radiotherapy given. (From Dosoretz DE, Katin MJ, Blitzer PH, et al. Medically inoperable lung carcinoma: the role of radiation therapy. Semin Radiat Oncol. 1996;6:98–104.[20])

ence[3,21] or a trend toward worse survival[11] was seen in other reports. One frequently quoted study[18] reported progressively better disease-free survival with increasing doses of RT (from <50 to ≥70 Gy; $P = 0.014$). However, this is based on a short-term difference (at 1–2 years), with no difference in 5-year disease-free survival being observed[20] (Fig. 13–3). Hyperfractionated RT (69.6 Gy) in 49 cI and 67 cII patients has been reported in two studies[17,26] to result in an overall survival of 30% and 25% and an actuarial rate of local control of 55% and 61%. It is difficult to assess the impact of the RT schedule in comparison with other studies because these patients were somewhat younger (median age, 63 years) and had a better PS.[17,26] Thus, the existing data does not offer much guidance regarding the optimal dose of RT.

Radiation treatment parameters (ie, dose, volume) have also been examined by multivariate analysis, although these are not pretreatment patient characteristics that can be used to guide patient selection. The results of these studies are not helpful in suggesting an optimal treatment approach. One study found RT treatment factors to be significant,[14] whereas another did not.[10] However, neither study specified these treatment factors. The total dose of RT was not significantly associated with survival by multivariate analysis in three studies,[15,16,19] although it was associated with significantly better outcomes in one study[20] and marginally associated with better local control in another ($P = 0.07$).[15]

EDITORS' COMMENTS

Surgery is the treatment of choice for patients with early-stage NSCLC. Randomized studies comparing surgery with RT are so old that the data is no longer relevant, given the changes in staging and surgical and radiation treatment that have occurred. However, the overall survival of patients with clinical stage I tumors treated with surgery is 50%, whereas that of patients with such tumors treated with RT is 15%. Local recurrence is seen in 5% to 10% of all patients with pI tumors undergoing lobectomy and in 45% of all patients with cI tumors undergoing RT. The differences that certainly exist between patients selected for surgery and those referred for RT hamper this comparison. Nevertheless, the 5-year survival after surgery is 40%, even among those patients who undergo a wedge resection as a compromise operation because of comorbid factors precluding a lobectomy.

Although surgery is the treatment of choice, RT clearly has a role as a curative treatment in early-stage lung cancer. The data regarding the natural history of untreated NSCLC indicates a 2-year survival of <10%, even in patients with cI cancers. The fact that only approximately 50% of the patients treated with RT are found to develop a local

DATA SUMMARY: RADIOTHERAPY FOR STAGE cI,II NON–SMALL CELL LUNG CANCER			
	AMOUNT	**QUALITY**	**CONSISTENCY**
Of patients with cI,II NSCLC treated with RT for cure, 15% voluntarily declined surgery	High	High	High
Of patients with cI,II NSCLC treated with RT for cure, 80% have a good PS (0,1 or 80–100)	High	High	High
Overall 5-year survival of cI,II patients after curative RT is 15%	High	High	High
The 5-year cancer-specific survival of cI,II patients after curative RT is 25%	High	High	High
Approximately 70% of deaths are due to lung cancer	High	High	Mod
A local recurrence is involved in approximately 70% of recurrences	High	High	High
The rate of mediastinal recurrence is low (<10%) if RT is given to the primary tumor only	Mod	Mod	High
There is no significant association between better survival and higher doses of RT in the range of 50 to 80 Gy that has been used for curative RT of stage cI,II NSCLC	Mod	High	Mod

Type of data rated:　　Plain text: descriptive statement　　*Italics: controlled comparison*　　**Bold: randomized comparison**
PS, performance status.

recurrence supports the use of RT as a curative modality, although there are potential biases in reporting this data in patients with competing risks of death. Indeed, there is some discrepancy in reporting local recurrence rates. On the one hand, the rate of *freedom* from local recurrence at 5 years is reported to be 45%, whereas only 45% of all patients experience a local recurrence based on an analysis of recurrence patterns.

Ninety percent of the patients receiving RT for cI,II NSCLC have comorbid conditions. However, the nature and severity of these illnesses have not been defined. Given the overall nihilism about the treatment of lung cancer, there is potential variability in what constitutes a condition that precludes surgery. The fact that 80% of patients treated with RT had a good PS, as well as the fact that intercurrent deaths account for only 30% of deaths, suggests that these patients were not as ill as might be assumed. Prospective selection of patients for RT versus supportive care should be based only on the PS and the size of the primary tumor because these are the only clearly identified prognostic factors.

Clinical and radiographic staging of patients appears to be reasonable. Extrathoracic staging of patients with cI,II NSCLC is probably not necessary if the clinical evaluation is negative. Treatment of a radiographically negative mediastinum is not necessary in cI,II patients. If there is doubt about the status of the mediastinal lymph nodes, it may be reasonable to perform mediastinoscopy or positron emission tomography (PET), although the reliability of PET in detecting small (<1 cm) nodes has not been clearly defined.

Alterations in RT treatment parameters should be explored. Dose escalation is attractive, and it is clear that much higher doses can be given safely with modern techniques. The available data is not strongly suggestive of a dose response for RT in this setting, but this data involves only a limited number of studies, and only a limited range of doses has been employed. The data regarding hyperfractionated RT and continuous hyperfractionated accelerated radiation therapy (CHART) suggests that alterations in treatment parameters can alter outcome in patients with lung cancer. These issues are not currently being addressed adequately in early-stage patients who are not surgical candidates.

References

1. Pisch J, Harvey JC, Panigrahi N, et al. Iodine-125 volume implant in patients with medically unresectable stage I lung cancer. Endocurie-therapie/Hyperthermia Oncology. 1996;12:165–170.
2. Imamura F, Chatani M, Nakayama T, et al. Percutaneous brachytherapy for small-sized non–small cell lung cancer. Lung Cancer. 1999;24:169–174.
3. Hayakawa K, Mitsuhashi N, Furuta M, et al. High-dose radiation therapy for inoperable non–small cell lung cancer without mediastinal involvement (clinical stage N0, N1). Strahlenther Onkol. 1996;172:489–495.
4. Rosenthal SA, Curran WJ Jr, Herbert SH, et al. Clinical stage II non–small cell lung cancer treated with radiation therapy alone: the significance of clinically staged ipsilateral hilar adenopathy (N1 disease). Cancer. 1992;70:2410–2417.
5. Romano PS, Mark DH. Patient and hospital characteristics related to in-hospital mortality after lung cancer resection. Chest. 1992;101:1332–1337.
6. Damhuis RAM, Schutte PR. Resection rates and postoperative mortality in 7,899 patients with lung cancer. Eur Respir J. 1996;9:7–10.
7. Wada H, Nakamura T, Nakamoto K, et al. Thirty-day operative mortality for thoracotomy in lung cancer. J Thorac Cardiovasc Surg. 1998;115:70–73.
8. Ginsberg RJ, Hill LD, Eagan RT, et al. Modern thirty-day operative mortality for surgical resections in lung cancer. J Thorac Cardiovasc Surg. 1983;86:654–658.
9. Gauden S, Ramsay J, Tripcony L. The curative treatment by radiotherapy alone of stage I non–small cell carcinoma of the lung. Chest. 1995;108:1278–1282.
10. Burt PA, Hancock BM, Stout R. Radical radiotherapy for carcinoma of the bronchus: an equal alternative to radical surgery? Clin Oncol. 1989;1:86–90.
11. Krol ADG, Aussems P, Noorduk EM, et al. Local irradiation alone for peripheral stage I lung cancer: could we omit the elective regional nodal irradiation? Int J Radiat Oncol Biol Phys. 1996;34:297–302.
12. Hayakawa K, Mitsuhashi N, Saito Y, et al. Limited field irradiation for medically inoperable patients with peripheral stage I non–small cell lung cancer. Lung Cancer. 1999;26:137–142.
13. Sibley GS. Radiotherapy for patients with medically inoperable stage I non–small cell lung carcinoma: smaller volumes and higher doses—a review. Cancer. 1998;82:433–438.
14. Graham PH, Gebski VJ, Langlands AO. Radical radiotherapy for early non–small cell lung cancer. Int J Radiat Oncol Biol Phys. 1994;31:261–266.
15. Sibley GS, Jamieson TA, Marks LB, et al. Radiotherapy alone for medically inoperable stage I non-small-cell lung cancer: the Duke experience. Int J Radiat Oncol Biol Phys. 1998;40:149–154.
16. Kaskowitz L, Graham MV, Emami B, et al. Radiation therapy alone for stage I non–small cell lung cancer. Int J Radiat Oncol Biol Phys. 1993;27:517–523.
17. Jeremic B, Shibamoto Y, Acimovic L, et al. Hyperfractionated radiotherapy alone for clinical stage I non–small cell lung cancer. Int J Radiat Oncol Biol Phys. 1997;38:521–525.
18. Dosoretz DE, Katin MJ, Blitzer PH, et al. Radiation therapy in the management of medically inoperable carcinoma of the lung: results and implications for future treatment strategies. Int J Radiat Oncol Biol Phys. 1992;24:3–9.
19. Kupelian PA, Komaki R, Allen P. Prognostic factors in the treatment of node-negative nonsmall cell lung carcinoma with radiotherapy alone. Int J Radiat Oncol Biol Phys. 1996;36:607–613.
20. Dosoretz DE, Katin MJ, Blitzer PH, et al. Medically inoperable lung carcinoma: the role of radiation therapy. Semin Radiat Oncol. 1996;6:98–104.
21. Morita K, Fuwa N, Suzuki Y, et al. Radical radiotherapy for medically inoperable non–small cell lung cancer in clinical stage I: a retrospective analysis of 149 patients. Radiother Oncol. 1997;42:31–36.
22. Sandler HM, Curran WJ Jr, Turrisi AT III. The influence of tumor size and pre-treatment staging on outcome following radiation therapy alone for stage I non–small cell lung cancer. Int J Radiat Oncol Biol Phys. 1990;19:9–13.
23. Talton BM, Constable WC, Kersh CR. Curative radiotherapy in non–small cell carcinoma of the lung. Int J Radiat Oncol Biol Phys. 1990;19:15–21.
24. Würschmidt F, Bünemann H, Bünemann C, et al. Inoperable non–small cell lung cancer: a retrospective analysis of 427 patients treated with high-dose radiotherapy. Int J Radiat Oncol Biol Phys. 1994;28:583–588.
25. Noordijk EM, Clement EP, Hermans J, et al. Radiotherapy as an alternative to surgery in elderly patients with resectable lung cancer. Radiother Oncol. 1988;13:83–89.
26. Jeremic B, Shibamoto Y, Acimovic L, et al. Hyperfractionated radiotherapy for clinical stage II non–small cell lung cancer. Radiother Oncol. 1999;51:141–145.

ADJUVANT THERAPY OF RESECTED NON–SMALL CELL LUNG CANCER

Mark A. Socinski, Frank C. Detterbeck, and Julian G. Rosenman

The term *adjuvant therapy* refers to the addition of treatments delivered after surgery (postoperatively) in order to improve cure rates over surgery alone. It is logical that such therapy would be directed at those patients who are at high risk for a recurrence following surgery, which may involve either a local or a systemic recurrence. The purpose of this chapter is to review the role of adjuvant radiotherapy (RT) and chemotherapy in curatively resected non–small cell lung cancer (NSCLC). A brief section on adjuvant immunotherapy and non–cisplatin-based chemotherapy is also included, but the main emphasis is on cisplatin-based trials. Preoperative treatment, otherwise known as induction or neoadjuvant therapy, is covered in Chapter 19.

Two general strategies have been employed with regard to adjuvant therapy of NSCLC. Adjuvant RT employs the use of a second local modality, and it would seem obvious that this approach addresses only the risk of local recurrence. The second adjuvant approach has been the use of systemic therapy, which is designed to eradicate systemic micrometastatic disease. Studies examining patterns of relapse in this population have convincingly shown that the majority of patients experience relapse at distant sites (see Tables 11–5 and 12–3).[1,2] Studies employing sensitive immunohistochemical or polymerization chain reaction (PCR) techniques have also shown that distant micrometastatic disease is often present in early stage patients, although it is radiographically and histologically occult (see Table 6–13).[3–5] This suggests that NSCLC is a good model to test the concept of adjuvant systemic therapy. Both immunotherapy and chemotherapy have been studied in this setting.

Several points deserve comment as one considers the issue of adjuvant treatment of NSCLC and the interpretation of available data. The first point is the accuracy of staging. In reports involving adjuvant therapy, it is not always clear what preoperative staging investigations have been performed. In addition, it is often unclear to what extent intraoperative mediastinal node staging was performed. Both of these points raise the concern that the population of patients entered into clinical trials of adjuvant therapy may be more heterogeneous than was previously thought. Furthermore, randomized trials have not consistently stratified for variables known to have prognostic importance, raising the possibility of an imbalance in the distribution of these variables.

A second issue that hampers the interpretation of data regarding adjuvant therapy is that the chemotherapy that was used is suboptimal, in terms of both the choice of agents and the doses received. The cisplatin-based trials available for analysis were carried out mainly in the 1980s. As will be discussed later, the drug regimens that were used are no longer considered active regimens for this disease. Furthermore, the drug delivery and dose intensity were compromised in this population of patients. This is due to the side effects of the agents used, the poorer quality of supportive care available at that time compared to modern-day standards, and the fact that the chemotherapy was given to patients who were still recovering from major thoracic operations.

ADJUVANT RADIOTHERAPY

Thirteen randomized trials have been published comparing surgery alone with surgery plus adjuvant RT in early stage resected NSCLC.[6–20] Two trials carried out in the 1960s used low-voltage RT equipment and are not pertinent in the modern era,[6,13] and several other trials have been reported only in a preliminary fashion without detailed data.[11,12,14–16] For these reasons, they will not be considered in this chapter. Data from the remaining seven studies is shown in Table 14–1.

It is striking that there was no significant survival benefit in any of the seven modern randomized trials of adjuvant RT listed in Table 14–1.[7–10,17–20] Even among subgroups of different N stages, adjuvant RT did not result in a significant survival benifit in any of the studies or subgroups analyzed. All of these studies were of a reasonable size

TABLE 14–1. RANDOMIZED CLINICAL TRIALS OF SURGERY ALONE VERSUS SURGERY PLUS ADJUVANT RADIOTHERAPY

STUDY	N EVALUABLE	STAGE	RT DOSE (GY)	5-y SURVIVAL (%)			LOCAL RECURRENCE (%)		
				S	S/RT	P	S	S/RT	P
Dautzenberg et al[20]	728	I–III	60	**42**	30	0.002	**34**	28	NS
Stephens et al[8]	308	II, III	40	19	**22**	NS	**44**	34	NS
LCSG[9]a	210	II, III	50	37	**38**	NS	19b	1b	0.001
Mayer et al[19]	155	I–III	50–56	20	**30**	NS	24	6	0.01
Dautzenberg et al[20]	221	I	60	**56**	43	0.07	—	—	—
Van Houtte[7]c	175	N0	60	**43**	24	NS	21	5	0.002
Lafitte et al[10]d	132	N0	45–60	**52**	35	NS	17	15	NS
Mayer et al[9]	39	N0	50–56	32	**60**	NS	13	4	NS
Stephens et al[8]	183	N1	40	**25**	18	NS	49	40	NS
Dautzenberg et al[20]	180	II	60	**50**	24	0.003	—	—	—
Mayer et al[19]	67	N1	50–56	22	**42**	NS	26	8	NS
Dautzenberg et al[20]	337	III	60	**30**	24	NS	—	—	—
Stephens et al[8]	106	N2	40	14	**35**	NS	41	29	NS
Debevec et al[17]	74	N2	30	18	**33**	NS	16	28	NS
Mayer et al[19]	49	N2	50–56	6	**29**	NS	26	4	0.05

Inclusion criteria: Studies of adjuvant RT from 1980 to 2000 involving ≥50 patients (total). The higher of the two arms is indicated in bold type.
aOnly squamous cell.
bIncludes only isolated local recurrences (simultaneous local plus distant recurrences are excluded).
cIncludes 8% small cell lung cancer and <5% T3N0.
dOnly T2N0.
LCSG, Lung Cancer Study Group; NS, not significant; S, surgery; S/RT, surgery plus radiotherapy.

(≥50 patients) and involved modern RT (megavoltage) delivered to the mediastinum after a complete resection. Two of the trials involved rather low doses of RT (30–40 Gy),[8,17] and one study used only a cobalt radiation source and large treatment fields.[7] However, most of these studies treated at least some of the patients using cobalt RT, which is not optimal by current standards, although it does involve megavoltage radiation.[8–10,20,21]

In fact, a trend toward *poorer* survival with adjuvant RT was seen in the subgroup of N0 patients in three of four studies that analyzed this, although the differences were not statistically significant.[7,10,20] In one of these studies, this might be attributed to large treatment fields and inferior equipment, which may have caused an increased number of early deaths.[7] Among patients with N1 node involvement, survival trends were mixed,[8,19,20] but a trend toward better survival with adjuvant RT was found among patients with N2 disease in three of four studies.[8,17–19]

Taking a different approach, Sawyer et al[22] performed a retrospective (nonrandomized) analysis of adjuvant RT in 224 completely resected IIIa (N2) patients who were stratified into low-, medium-, or high-risk categories by pathologic prognostic factors (T stage, number and location of N1 and N2 nodes involved, and so on). Adjuvant RT was found to improve survival and decrease local recurrence to a progressively greater degree as the risk of recurrence increased. The benefits were statistically significant for the medium- and high-risk groups. Although such retrospective data must be validated by other studies, it does suggest that selection of patients at higher risk of recurrence may allow definition of a group for which RT is useful.

All of the trials and subgroups examined in Table 14–1 have shown a trend toward better local control after adjuvant RT, with one exception.[17] The difference was found to be statistically significant in approximately half of the studies.[7,9,19] Analysis of smaller subgroups based on nodal status also demonstrated a consistent trend to better local control with adjuvant RT, although statistical significance was often not achieved. The reason for the one exception, which involved a relatively small study of N2 patients, is not clear.[17] However, it is interesting to note that the studies that found the smallest differences in the local recurrence rate involved the lowest doses (30–40 Gy) of adjuvant RT.[8,17]

Further analysis of the effect of adjuvant RT on local recurrence is hampered by vague reporting of data. The effect of adjuvant RT is best assessed by examining the cumulative rate of local recurrence, regardless of the appearance of additional systemic metastases. Although it is plausible that a local recurrence may lead to subsequent distant metastases, the chance of locoregional disease arising *as a result of* a distant metastasis is exceedingly slim. Unfortunately, it is often not clear whether only the first site of recurrence is reported or *any* local recurrence, regardless of the sequence of presentation. Furthermore, in the often-quoted Lung Cancer Study Group (LCSG) trial,[9] the local recurrence rate reported involved only isolated local recurrences and excluded simultaneous local and distant recurrences. This raises the question of whether a local recurrence in an irradiated patient may have prompted a more thorough search for additional systemic disease, making the reported local-only recurrence rate in the RT group particularly low. The fact that a large amount of variability in reported recurrence rates is seen between studies, even within a particular stage group, underscores the lack of a consistent definition of this endpoint.

Nevertheless, the data in Table 14–1 indicates that adjuvant RT decreases the chance of local recurrence. Despite this, none of the trials found a statistically significant effect on survival, although a trend was seen toward worse survival with adjuvant RT in N0 patients and toward better survival in N2 patients. Considering that most recurrences after resection of NSCLC are distant, regardless of the

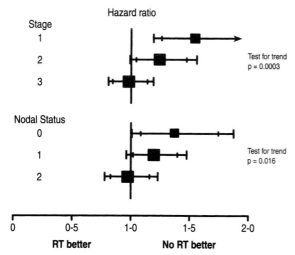

FIGURE 14–1. Hazard ratio for survival with or without postoperative radiotherapy (RT) by stage and nodal subgroup. (From PORT Meta-Analysis Trialists Group. Postoperative radiotherapy in non–small-cell cancer: systemic review and meta-analysis of individual patient data from nine randomised controlled trials. Lancet. 1998;352:257–263, © by The Lancet Ltd., 1998.)[21]

stage (see Tables 11–5, 12–3, and 17–5), the lack of a dramatic impact on survival with the use of a second local modality is not surprising. Given the lower overall incidence of recurrences in early stage patients, it may be that the toxicity of RT outweighs any benefit, whereas the higher incidence of recurrence in patients with N2 disease may allow better local control and result in a slight survival advantage.

A 1998 study[21] reported a meta-analysis of adjuvant RT involving 2128 patients in nine published and unpublished randomized trials. This study found a 21% increased risk of death with postoperative RT ($P = 0.001$). The detriment to survival was most marked in N0 patients, whereas there was no difference in patients with N2 disease (Fig. 14–1).[21] The difference was due to an increase in noncancer deaths with RT (19% versus 11%), although data on cause of death was incomplete. RT resulted in a 24% decrease in the risk of local recurrence. However, this is probably an overestimation because the higher death rate with adjuvant RT decreases the number of patients who live long enough to develop a local recurrence.

The meta-analysis has been criticized because it included older studies, which used larger treatment fields and inferior RT equipment.[23] Indeed, in eight of the nine studies analyzed, at least some of the patients were treated using a cobalt RT source.[21] However, eight of the nine studies involved patients treated in the 1980s and 1990s, and 65% of the patients were from studies that began during or after 1985. Thus, although the RT used in these trials may not represent the best techniques currently available, it may be fairly representative of what has been done even more recently in a majority of centers.

There is reason to think that modern RT techniques using three-dimensional (3-D) planning and different treatment schedules and fields will result in lower toxicity (see Chapter 9). Such modern RT may lead to better survival because even the conventional RT used in the trials listed in Table 14–1 resulted in better local control. However, a survival benefit has yet to be demonstrated. Better definition of

patients who are most likely to benefit (eg, N2 patients, patients with multiple positive node stations, or patients with close surgical margins) may also improve results. Finally, integration of adjuvant RT in a treatment strategy that addresses the risk of systemic recurrence as well may prove to be useful. To address this latter question, the Cancer and Leukemia Group B (CALGB) is conducting a trial (CALGB 9734) that randomizes resected IIIa (N2) patients to adjuvant chemotherapy followed by RT versus adjuvant chemotherapy alone.

ADJUVANT IMMUNOTHERAPY

In 1972, Ruckdeschel et al[24] reported that patients who developed postoperative empyemas outlived patients who did not develop this complication, and they attributed this effect to a nonspecific regional immune response. Following this observation, four randomized trials involving ≥50 patients were performed using nonspecific immune stimulants including intrapleural bacillus Calmette-Guérin (BCG),[25,26] *Corynebacterium parvum*,[27] or intradermal BCG.[28] None of these trials suggested a benefit to this approach.

Preliminary reports using more modern immunotherapeutic agents such as interferon,[29] interleukins,[30] and tumor necrosis factor[31] have not shown significant activity in NSCLC. Therefore, these agents are not optimal candidates for adjuvant therapy, and it is unlikely that they will be tested in this setting. Specific immunotherapy using vaccines has been studied by Takita et al.[32] These investigators randomized patients with stage I and II squamous cell carcinoma to either intradermal injections of squamous cell carcinoma-associated antigen and complete Freund adjuvant versus surgery alone. Five-year survival was improved in the immunotherapy group compared with the surgery alone group (75% versus 34%). This trial included only 85 patients and, therefore, must be confirmed in a larger study.

Two randomized trials involving interleukin-2 (IL-2) and adoptive immunotherapy in conjunction with surgery, chemotherapy, and radiation have shown promising results.[33,34] Both studies involved primarily stage IIIa patients, although some stage II and some T4 (stage IIIb) patients were included as well. The adoptive immunotherapy involved either lymphocyte-activated killer cells (LAKs)[34] or tumor-infiltrating lymphocytes[33] grown in tissue culture in the presence of IL-2 and then reinfused. The groups were well matched with respect to prognostic factors. In both studies, survival was significantly better in patients given immunotherapy (5-year survival, 58% versus 32%, $P = 0.01$[34]; 3-year survival, 38% versus 20%, $P = 0.05$).[33] Thus, these newer methods of enhancing the immune response to tumor cells may be more effective than the general immune stimulation attempted in the past, but further research is necessary.

ADJUVANT CHEMOTHERAPY

The predominant pattern of recurrence following curative resection of early stage NSCLC is systemic[1, 2] (see Tables 11–5 and 12–3). This observation led to the use of systemic chemotherapy as an adjuvant treatment following surgical resection. These early trials employed alkylating agents that are now considered, at best, marginally effective in this disease. The advent of cisplatin-based combination regimens thought to be of greater effectiveness in metastatic disease led to a number of trials employing these combinations in earlier stage disease. These two classes of agents are considered separately. The strongest evidence of an effect of chemotherapy in NSCLC has come from the meta-analysis performed by the Non–Small Cell Lung Cancer Collaborative Group.[35] This study suggested that there may be a survival benefit for patients receiving adjuvant cisplatin-based chemotherapy, and this will be discussed following discussion of the individual trials.

Non–Cisplatin-Based Adjuvant Chemotherapy

The early era of adjuvant chemotherapy trials employed alkylating agents that were marginally effective or ineffective in the treatment of NSCLC. Many of these early trials suffered from the inclusion of patients with small cell lung cancer, lack of proper nodal staging, and inadequate stratification for prognostic factors. Six major randomized trials were published before 1975, none of which found a survival benefit.[36–41] These trials involved between 189 and 1192 patients, who had undergone either a curative or a palliative resection. The chemotherapy regimens involved either cyclophosphamide (oral, intravenous, or intrapleural) or nitrogen mustard (intrapleural or intravenous).

The major trials published since 1975 using alkylating agents, shown in Table 14–2, did not find a survival benefit.[42–46] These trials ranged in size from 518 to 865 evaluable patients (involving either two or three arms). The cumulative experience showed no survival benefit from adjuvant chemotherapy. A meta-analysis of these six trials found a hazard ratio (HR) that favored surgery alone (HR = 1.15, P = 0.005).[35] This 15% increase in the risk of death translates to an absolute detriment of chemotherapy of 4% at 2 years and 5% at 5 years. This cumulative experience strongly suggests that alkylating agents have no role in the adjuvant therapy of surgically resected NSCLC.

Cisplatin-Based Adjuvant Chemotherapy

Since 1980, 14 randomized trials have been reported using so-called second generation chemotherapy for NSCLC that is based on cisplatin.[34,47–59] The patient population included in these trials ranged from stage I to IIIa. Two predominant strategies have been employed in the design of these trials. The first design involves trials that compared surgery alone to surgery plus chemotherapy and included mainly patients with predominantly node-negative disease. The second design involves trials that compared surgery plus RT with the same treatment with adjuvant chemotherapy and included mainly patients with predominantly node-positive disease. These two groups of studies will be considered separately, as they were in the Non–Small Cell Lung Cancer Collaborative Study Group meta-analysis[35] and the review by George et al.[60]

Predominantly Node-Negative Trials

In this category of trials, 1407 evaluable patients were included in six randomized clinical trials.[47–52] These trials, none of which included additional adjuvant RT, are summarized in Table 14–3. The composite 5-year survival rate was 64% for the chemotherapy arm and 57% for the surgery-alone arm. An analysis[60] of the first five of these trials[47–51] found that the results of surgery alone and surgery plus chemotherapy were consistent between studies, with no evidence of heterogeneity between the studies. Overall, this analysis[60] found a 5.6% 5-year survival advantage for chemotherapy, which was marginally significant (standard error, 3.0%; P = 0.06).

When the trials are examined individually, the treatment effects at 5 years range from a 13% benefit for chemotherapy[47] to a 1% benefit for surgery alone.[51] Two studies found a statistically significant benefit to adjuvant chemotherapy,[47,50] two found a favorable but nonsignificant trend,[48,52] and two found no difference at all between the treatment arms.[49,51] Survival figures from the largest study, which involved two different adjuvant treatment arms, are shown in Figure 14–2A.[47] Survival curves from another large study, conducted by LCSG from 1980 to 1986, are shown in Figure 14–2B.[49] This latter study represents the most thoughtfully planned and carefully conducted trial and involved 269 evaluable patients with T2N0 or T1N1 NSCLC.[49]

All of the trials included in Table 14–3 have flaws that hamper analysis. Only one of the trials stratified patients according to known prognostic factors, and this study failed

TABLE 14–2. RANDOMIZED CLINICAL TRIALS EMPLOYING NON-CISPLATIN ADJUVANT CHEMOTHERAPY IN RESECTED NON–SMALL CELL LUNG CANCER

| | N | | | 5-y SURVIVAL (%) | | |
STUDY	EVALUABLE	STAGE	CHEMOTHERAPY	S	S + Chemo	P
Shields et al[44]	865	I-III	CcHu	46	35	NS
Trakhtenberg et al[43]	720	I-III	MxFC	34	34	NS
Karrer et al[46]	518	I-IV	CMxVb	26[a]	27[a]	NS
Girling et al[42 b]	492	I-III	Bs	34	28	NS
Girling et al[42 b]	483	I-III	C	34	27	NS
Shields et al[45 b]	285	I-III	CMx	24	26	NS
Shields et al[45 b]	275	I-III	C	24	25	NS
Average				**32**	**29**	

Inclusion criteria: Randomized trials of non-cisplatin adjuvant chemotherapy in ≥250 patients.
[a]5-year survival for stage III subgroup.
[b]Three-arm trial
Chemo, chemotherapy; NS, not significant; S, surgery.
Chemotherapy abbreviations: Bs, busulphan; C, cyclophosphamide; F, 5-fluorouracil; Hu, hydroxyurea; Mx, methotrexate; U, CCNU; Vb, vinblastine.

TABLE 14–3. PREDOMINANTLY NODE-NEGATIVE ADJUVANT CHEMOTHERAPY TRIALS IN NON–SMALL CELL LUNG CANCER

STUDY	N EVALUABLE	% N0	CHEMOTHERAPY	5-y SURVIVAL (%)		
				S	S + Chemo	P
Imaizumi et al[48]	309	71	CAUft	58	**62**	NS[a]
Feld et al[49]	269	84	CAP	55	**55**	NS
Wada et al[52]	225	83	MVdP/Uft	71	**77**	NS
Wada et al[47]	207	73	CVdUft	49	**61**	0.08
Wada et al[47]	201	75	Uft	49	**64**	0.02
Niiranen et al[50]	110	100	CAP	56	**67**	0.05
Ichinose et al[51]	86	60	*PAP*/CAP-M/PVd	62	61	NS
Average				**57**	**64**	

Inclusion criteria: Randomized trials from 1980 to 2000, of ≥50 patients and involving cisplatin-based adjuvant chemotherapy. The higher of the two arms is indicated in bold type. Italics are used for regimens that are conventionally known by an abbreviation in which the letters used to denote chemotherapeutic agents in the regimen are *different* from the letters commonly used for those agents in other regimens or as single agents.

[a]$P = 0.04$ when stratification imbalances are corrected in Cox proportional hazards model (randomization failed to stratify pN status, and the chemotherapy arm had significantly more advanced tumors).

NS, not significant; Chemo, chemotherapy; S, surgery.
Chemotherapy abbreviations: CAUft: cisplatin 66 mg/m² × 1, doxorubicin 26 mg/m² × 1, Uft 8 mg/kg/d × 6 mo.
CAP (Feld et al): cyclophosphamide 400 mg/m², doxorubicin 40 mg/m², cisplatin 60 mg/m² q 3 wk × 4.
MVdP/Uft: mitomycin C 8 mg, vindesine 2–3 mg/m², cisplatin 80 mg/m² q wk × 2, then Uft 400 mg/d × 1 y.
CVdUft: cisplatin 50 mg/m² × 1, vindesine 2–3 mg/m² q 1–2 weeks × 2, Uft 400 mg/d × 1 y.
Uft: uracil/tegafur 400 mg/d × 1 y.
CAP (Niiranen et al): cyclophosphamide 400 mg/m², doxorubicin 40 mg/m², cisplatin 40 mg/m² q 4 wk × 6.
PAP/CAP-M/PVd: Three chemotherapy treatment arms—cisplatin 60 mg/m², doxorubicin 30 mg/m², pepleomycin 5 mg/m²; cyclophosphamide 400 mg/m², doxorubicin 30 mg/m², cisplatin 60 mg/m², mitomycin C 3 mg/m²; cisplatin 80–100 mg/m², vindesine 3 mg/m².

to stratify for T or N status.[49] As a result, imbalances were found between the treatment arms in three of the five studies. In the two largest studies, the surgery-alone arms were favored by inclusion of fewer N2,3 patients (14% versus 23%, $P = 0.02$, in the study by Imaizumi et al[48]; 9% versus 15% and 16%, $P =$ NS, in the study by Wada et al[47]). In the third study, the surgery-alone arm included more resections involving a pneumonectomy (39% versus 20%, P not given), although the patients were well matched with regard to stage, performance status (PS), and histology.[50]

Attempts to correct for these imbalances have been made but must be viewed with caution because the results are not protected by the randomization process. In the study by

Imaizumi et al,[48] the survival difference became statistically significant in favor of adjuvant chemotherapy when adjusted for the imbalances. In the study by Wada et al,[47] adjuvant chemotherapy remained a statistically significant prognostic factor even when other factors are taken into account by multivariate analysis. The significance of the imbalance in the third study[50] is questionable because other studies[61] have found no difference in outcomes relative to the extent of the resection (see Chapters 11, 12, and 17). Furthermore, pneumonectomy was not associated with a higher rate of noncancer deaths in this study, and subset analysis by type of resection demonstrated a consistent trend in favor of adjuvant chemotherapy.

The studies in Table 14–3 are relatively small, with only

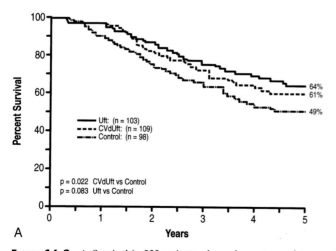
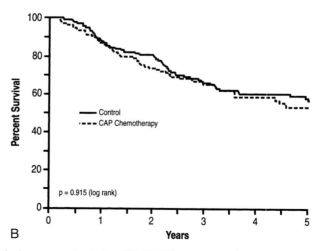

FIGURE 14–2. *A,* Survival in 323 patients who underwent complete resection and who were randomized to Uft, CVdUft, or surgery alone. *B,* Survival in 269 resected patients randomized to postoperative CAP versus surgery alone. CAP, cyclophosphamide/doxorubicin/cisplatin; CVdUft, cisplatin, vindesine, uracil/tegafur; Uft, uracil/tegafur. (*A,* From Wada H, Hitomi S, Teramatsu T, et al. Adjuvant chemotherapy after complete resection in non-small-cell lung cancer. West Japan Study Group for Lung Cancer Surgery. J Clin Oncol. 1996;14[4]1048–1054.[47] *B,* From Feld R, Rubinstein L, Thomas PA, et al. Adjuvant chemotherapy with cyclophosphamide, doxorubicin, and cisplatin in patients with completely resected stage I non-small-cell lung cancer. [LCSG 801]. J Natl Cancer Inst. 1993;85:299–306, by permission of the Oxford University Press, Oxford, England.[49])

two having more than 300 evaluable patients.[47,48] A planned study size was defined in only two of the reports.[47,49] In one of them, this was not based on a statistical power to detect a significant difference,[47] whereas in the other, the size chosen was sufficient to detect only a 2-fold difference in median survival (with a power of 90%).[49]

The dose of cisplatin used in the studies in Table 14–3 is relatively low, ranging from 40 to 80 mg/m². The number of cycles of cisplatin chemotherapy given ranges from one to six. In those studies involving only one cycle, daily oral uracil/tegafur (UFT) was given for 1 year.[47,48] The suggestion of a survival benefit using this drug in these two studies is intriguing. However, these results are also surprising, given the fact that 5-fluorouracil, the more commonly used analog of this drug, has not demonstrated significant activity in NSCLC (see Chapter 10).

Predominantly Node-Positive Trials

Eight randomized trials of adjuvant cisplatin-based chemotherapy have been reported that have involved primarily node-positive (N1,2) patients.[34,53–59] These trials, involving a total of 1298 evaluable patients, are summarized in Table 14–4. The composite 2-year survival rates for the control and adjuvant chemotherapy arms were 46% and 55%, respectively. An analysis of six of these trials[60] has been carried out, but one large trial,[59] which was reported only in abstract form, could not be included in the analysis. Two trials reported notably higher survival rates in the chemotherapy arms,[34,57] whereas one trial had an unusually high survival rate in the control arm.[57] Because of this, there was evidence of statistical heterogeneity among the

trials in each of the two treatment arms.[60] If the two trials with unusually high survival are excluded, the 2-year survival rates drop to 33% and 39% and the remaining trials appear statistically homogeneous.[60] The 5-year survival averages 26% and 31% in the surgery-alone and adjuvant chemotherapy arms, respectively, although the results are variable.

When examined individually, the effect of adjuvant chemotherapy in the six predominately node-positive trials included in the review[60] described earlier ranges from a 26% advantage for chemotherapy[34] to a 13% benefit for surgery alone.[55] Besides the two extreme treatment effects (which also had the smallest sample sizes), the effects of the four other trials are clustered between a 4% and 11% benefit for adjuvant chemotherapy at 2 years. Overall, an 8% 2-year survival advantage is seen with chemotherapy, which is marginally significant ($P = 0.06$).[60] Five of the six trials demonstrated at least a trend to better survival with adjuvant chemotherapy at 2 years, and three of six trials found significantly better survival at 5 years. Representative recurrence-free survival curves from two of these studies are shown in Figure 14–3A and B.

A large trial conducted by the Eastern Cooperative Oncology Group was reported in preliminary form,[59] but the data currently available does not permit inclusion in the detailed composite analysis just presented. This study involved 351 evaluable patients (54% stage IIIa, 46% stage II) who were randomized to either postoperative RT (50 Gy) or concurrent RT with etoposide and cisplatin (4 cycles). No differences were seen in the median survival (38 versus 38 months) or the 5-year survival (39% versus

TABLE 14–4. PREDOMINANTLY NODE-POSITIVE ADJUVANT CHEMOTHERAPY TRIALS IN NON–SMALL CELL LUNG CANCER

STUDY	N EVALUABLE	% NODE POSITIVE	RT (BOTH ARMS)	CHEMOTHERAPY TREATMENT	2-y SURVIVAL (%)			5-y SURVIVAL (%)		
					S	S + Chemotherapy	P	S	S + Chemotherapy	P
Keller et al[59]	358	100	50	EP	60	60	NS	**41**	39	NS
Dautzenberg et al[54]	267	97	60	*COPAC*	33	**41**	NS	**19**	18	NS
Ohta et al[57]	181	75	—	PVd	59	**63**	NS	**42**	35	NS
Lad et al[56]	164	92	40	CAP	32	**40**	NS	13[a]	**26**[a]	0.002
Holmes et al[53,93 b,c]	130	87	—	CAP	30	**41**	0.08	18[a]	**29**[a]	0.03
Pisters et al[55]	72	100	40	PVd	**44**	31	NS	**30**	17	NS
Kimura et al[34]	69	84	—	MVdP, 1L-2, LAK	51	**82**	0.004	32	**58**	0.01
Park et al[58]	57	100	50–56	MVbP	60	**83**	0.09	57	**70**	0.09
Average					**46**	**55**		**32**	**37**	

Inclusion criteria: Randomized trial of ≥50 patients involving adjuvant cisplatin-based chemotherapy in resected patients, the majority of whom were node positive (N1 and/or N2). The higher of two arms is indicated in bold type.
[a]Disease-free survival (overall survival data not available).
[b]The control arm involved surgery plus treatment with BCG, which has been shown in other trials to have no effect.[22]
[c]Only adenocarcinoma and large cell carcinoma.
NS, not significant. S, surgery.
Chemotherapy abbreviations:
EP: Etoposide 120 mg/m² and cisplatin 60 mg/m² q mo × 4.
COPAC: Two alternating regimens q 4 weeks—course 1, 3: doxorubicin 40 mg/m², vincristine 1.2 mg/m², cisplatin 75 mg/m² and lomustine; course 2, 4: vincristine 1.2 mg/m², cisplatin 75 mg/m², and cyclophosphamide 600 mg/m².
PVd (Ohta et al): Cisplatin 80 mg/m² and vindesine 3 mg/m² q mo × 3.
CAP (Lad et al): Cytoxan 400 mg/m², doxorubicin 40 mg/m², cisplatin 40 mg/m² q mo × 6.
CAP (Holmes et al): Cytoxan 400 mg/m², doxorubicin 40 mg/m², cisplatin 40 mg/m² q mo × 6.
PVd (Pisters et al): Cisplatin 120 mg/m² q 1 mo × 4, vindesine 3 mg/m² q wk × 5.
MVdP, IL-2, LAK : Mitomycin C 8 mg/m² on d1, vindesine 3 mg/m² on d1, d8, and two cycles of cisplatin 80 mg/m² on d1, followed by interleukin 2 (IL-2) and lymphokine-activated killer (LAK) cells q 2–3 mo × 2 y.
MVbP: Mitomycin C 10 mg/m², vinblastine 6 mg/m², cisplatin 100 mg/m² q 3 wk × 3.

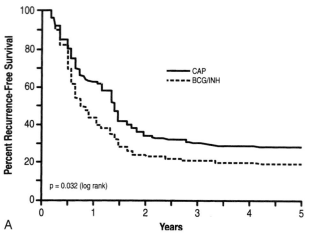
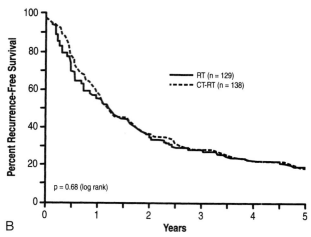

Figure 14–3. *A,* Recurrence-free survival of 130 stage II, III patients with completely resected adenocarcinoma or large cell undifferentiated lung cancer randomized to chemotherapy (CAP) or immunotherapy (BCG/INH). BCG/INH, bacillus Calmette-Guérin/isoniazid; CAP, cyclophosphamide/doxorubicin/cisplatin. *B,* Survival of resected patients (71% stage III) randomized to postoperative radiotherapy (RT) or chemoradiotherapy (CT-RT). (*A* from Holmes EC. Postoperative chemotherapy for non–small-cell lung cancer. *CHEST.* 1993;103[1 suppl]:30S–34S.[93] *B* From Dautzenberg B, Chastang C, Arriagada R, et al. Adjuvant radiotherapy versus combined sequential chemotherapy followed by radiotherapy in the treatment of resected nonsmall cell lung carcinoma: a randomized trial of 267 patients. Cancer. 1995;76:779–786.)[54]

33%). In the combined modality arm, 64% of the patients received the planned treatment, compared with 84% in the RT-only arm.

Major differences exist between the trials, but these differences do not explain the different results. Half of the trials involved adjuvant RT (40–60 Gy) given to all patients.[54–56,58,59] Two of these trials involved a major cohort of patients (39% and 100%) who had undergone an incomplete resection.[55,56] However, in these trials, an incomplete resection included patients with negative margins in whom the highest mediastinal lymph node was found to be positive—a definition that is not considered appropriate currently.[55,56] The trials have included varying numbers of N1, N2, and T3N0 patients. However, none of these factors consistently explain the reported survival differences.

Several issues relative to the trial design hamper interpretation of the results. Only three of eight trials reached their accrual goal,[56,57,59] with the remainder being stopped early due to accrual issues. Two trials were designed to have sufficient power to detect a 20% survival difference[57] and a 2-fold difference in median survival time,[56] but they were not large enough to detect smaller differences. The third trial[59] did not have enough power to detect a 15% difference in survival because of the mix of patients and the results of the control group. However, the observed results in this trial suggested no benefit at all to adjuvant therapy.[59] Most of the studies stratified patients according to prognostic factors,[34,53,55,56,59] but three of these studies did not include a stratification for PS or N stage.[34,53,56] As a result, imbalances favoring surgery alone (40% versus 29% T3N0-1, *P* = NS)[57] or favoring adjuvant chemotherapy (23% versus 12% with a PS ≤70, no *P* value given)[54] existed in some of the studies. The planned dose of cisplatin ranged from 40 to 120 mg/m^2 in these eight trials, and between one and six cycles were to be given. However, compliance with the planned regimen was poor.

Taken together, the trials of adjuvant chemotherapy in predominantly node-positive patients do not demonstrate a clear benefit. However, the trials are underpowered to de-

tect a 5% or 10% benefit (which would be clinically important), and in fact, an 8% benefit at 2 years is suggested by the data. Furthermore, the trials involve heterogeneous patient populations and are open to criticism regarding issues of stratification and adequate drug delivery to the patients randomized to adjuvant chemotherapy.

Meta-Analysis of Adjuvant Chemotherapy

The Non–Small Cell Lung Cancer Collaborative Group analyzed the trials of adjuvant cisplatin-based chemotherapy in a slightly different manner.[35] Trials were divided based on whether surgery alone or surgery plus RT was used as the local treatment strategy, regardless of nodal involvement. Eight randomized trials of surgery versus surgery plus chemotherapy were included, involving 1394 patients. The hazard ratio estimates for most trials favored chemotherapy, and an overall hazard ratio for death of 0.87 was found (*P* = 0.08). This 13% reduction in the risk of death implies a survival benefit of 3% at 2 years and 5% at 5 years with adjuvant chemotherapy (Fig. 14–4). The 95% confidence intervals for absolute survival were consistent with a 0.5% detriment to a 7% benefit of chemotherapy at 2 years and a 1% detriment to a 10% benefit at 5 years. Although suggestive, this information is insufficient to draw definitive conclusions.

Six trials employing surgery and RT versus surgery and RT plus chemotherapy, involving only 668 patients, were available for analysis.[35] The hazard ratio for survival was 0.94 (*P* = 0.46), suggesting a 6% reduction in the risk of death favoring chemotherapy. This translates into a 2% survival benefit at both 2 and 5 years with adjuvant chemotherapy in addition to surgery and RT, with confidence intervals ranging from a 3% to 4% detriment to an 8% benefit at those time points. The small number of patients included in trials of this design precludes the identification of small but clinically meaningful differences in survival.

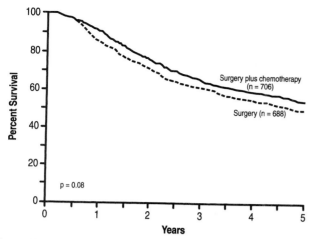

FIGURE 14–4. Survival by meta-analysis of surgery alone versus surgery plus cisplatin-based chemotherapy in eight trials involving 1394 patients. The difference at 5 years is 5% (*P* = 0.08). (This figure was first published in the BMJ [Stewart LA, for the Non–Small Cell Lung Cancer Collaborative Group. Chemotherapy in non–small cell lung cancer: a meta-analysis using updated data on individual patients from 52 randomised clinical trials. BMJ. 1995;311:899–909] and is reproduced by permission of the BMJ.)[35]

Pitfalls in the Trials of Adjuvant Cisplatin-Based Chemotherapy

Three major shortcomings of the trials of adjuvant chemotherapy for NSCLC warrant further discussion: the type and dose of chemotherapy used, the poor compliance with the planned chemotherapy, and the number of patients studied. Many other issues exist with specific trials, such as lack of appropriate stratification, inclusion of heterogeneous patient populations, and closure of trials before the planned accrual goal. These latter issues have already been addressed in the preceding pages.

The majority of adjuvant chemotherapy trials reported since 1980 have involved cisplatin-based chemotherapy regimens that are not considered optimal in the modern era. The dose of cisplatin used was ≤60 mg/m² in 10 of 14 trials, whereas doses of 75 to 120 mg/m² are typically used currently. The regimen most frequently studied (CAP) contains (in addition to cisplatin) the agents cyclophosphamide and doxorubicin, which have inferior single-agent activity compared with a number of agents now available. Furthermore, cisplatin is now used much less frequently in the treatment of NSCLC because of the incidence of nausea and renal toxicity. Newer agents, such as vinorelbine,[62] paclitaxel,[63] and gemcitabine[64] have been shown to be well tolerated and to improve survival in advanced NSCLC.

The ability to deliver adjuvant chemotherapy in the postoperative setting has also been an issue. Table 14–5 summarizes data regarding compliance in the randomized studies involving cisplatin-based chemotherapy. Approximately 10% of patients randomized to receive adjuvant therapy never received a single dose, and nearly 25% received fewer than two cycles. Slightly >50% of the patients received the planned adjuvant treatment. Given such compliance figures, the existing trials hardly seem to be a fair test of adjuvant chemotherapy in resected NSCLC. The poor compliance is probably due to a combination of the toxicity of cisplatin-based regimens, the antiemetic and supportive care measures available in the 1980s, and the compromised postoperative state of the patients. Advances in the outpatient delivery and supportive care of patients with agents such as more effective antiemetics (5HT3 [serotonin] inhibitors), growth factors (filgrastim), cytoprotective agents (amifostine), and appropriate hydration schedules may allow more effective delivery of more active agents in the postoperative setting. Trials evaluating these new agents in this setting are ongoing.

A great deal of caution must be used in interpreting the results of randomized trials that do not show a statistically significant benefit, as providing proof that there is no treatment effect (see Chapter 2). A negative trial can show only

TABLE 14–5. CHEMOTHERAPY COMPLIANCE IN THE CISPLATIN-BASED TRIALS IN NON–SMALL CELL LUNG CANCER

STUDY	NO. OF CYCLES PLANNED	% OF PATIENTS RECEIVING		
		No Chemotherapy	**<2 Cycles**	**All Cycles**
Feld et al[49]	4	20	34	53
Niiranen et al[50]	6	13	—	57
Ichinose et al[51]	≥2[a]	—	—	70[b]
Keller et al[59]	4	—	13	69
Dautzenberg et al[54]	4	12	20	76
Ohta et al[57]	3	0	16	41
Lad et al[56]	6	7	19	51
Holmes et al[53]	6	24	—	58[c]
Kimura and Yamaguchi[34]	2[d]	(0)[e]	(0)[e]	(100)[e]
Pisters et al[55]	4	0	25	36
Park et al[58]	3	—	—	86
Average[f]		**11**	**21**	**60**

Inclusion criteria: Randomized studies of adjuvant chemotherapy reporting compliance data.
[a]Two cycles of chemotherapy were planned, but more cycles were allowed.
[b]Received more than two cycles.
[c]Percentage of total planned dosage.
[d]Two cycles of chemotherapy and 2 years of immunotherapy.
[e]Unclear whether patients receiving less than two cycles were excluded from analysis.
[f]Excluding values in parentheses.

that there is no treatment effect greater than a certain minimum threshold, which is determined by the number of patients included, the baseline survival (or other outcome measure) of the control group, the desired power of detection (usually 80%), and the desired level of statistical significance (usually 95%, or $P \leq 0.05$). When the number of patients included in a trial is small, the threshold survival difference that can be excluded by a negative trial is often high (ie, an increase in the survival rate of 20%-40%). It is important to determine what survival difference is clinically worthwhile, that is, sufficient to warrant acceptance as appropriate therapy. Most clinicians would consider an increase in the survival rate of 10% to be clinically important, and most patients would probably consider an increase in the survival rate of 5% to be worth pursuing, provided the toxicity was reasonable.[65,66] If the minimum threshold detectable by a trial is well above what is clinically important, an open mind toward a possible treatment benefit should be maintained despite the negative result. Of course, it is equally important not to ascribe too much importance to trends that are not statistically significant.

When several smaller trials suggest a consistent trend that is not statistically significant in the individual trials, the technique of meta-analysis can be useful. However, there are many pitfalls in conducting a meta-analysis,[67] and the magnitude of the survival difference that can be detected (or excluded) is still determined by the number of patients included. Table 14–6 summarizes the number of patients studied and the number needed to detect a 5% or 10% survival benefit and compares these with other cancer types. So few patients have been included in published adjuvant chemotherapy to date that, even with meta-analysis, it is difficult to draw a conclusion. A survival benefit is strongly suggested by the available data, but a firm conclusion is not possible because of insufficient numbers of patients. The British meta-analysis, which attempted to minimize publication bias by including unpublished trials, also found a strong suggestion of a survival benefit.[35]

The small number of patients with NSCLC enrolled in adjuvant chemotherapy trials is in marked contrast to the situation in breast and colon cancer. In these two types of cancer, adjuvant therapy after resection is well accepted.

The increase in survival seen in these cancer types is approximately 5% to 10%. However, adjuvant therapy in these situations has become well accepted because the statistical significance of the benefit is strong simply because many more patients have been studied. A number of adjuvant chemotherapy trials in NSCLC have finished accrual or are ongoing, particularly in Europe.[60] When these results become available, a better assessment of the benefit of adjuvant chemotherapy should be possible.

INCOMPLETE RESECTION

The goal of surgery is to "get it all" and to perform a complete resection. In the past, the incidence of a positive surgical margin was 20% to 40%,[68–70] and the incidence of a *palliative resection,* in which gross tumor was knowingly left behind, was also high (44%).[68] Because of a better ability to plan a resection (computed tomography scanning, mediastinoscopy), as well as the availability of intraoperative frozen section assessment, the incidence of a positive margin or a palliative resection in most more recent studies is <5%,[56,71–77] although a few authors have reported an incidence of 10% to 15%.[78–80]

In discussing the subject of incomplete resection, it is worth distinguishing several different types of incomplete resection. At one extreme is the *exploratory thoracotomy,* in which practically no tumor is removed other than perhaps for a biopsy. This cannot be considered a resection and is excluded from further discussion in this section. In a *palliative resection,* a small amount of gross tumor (either of the primary or of nodal disease) is knowingly left behind. This is classified as a resection with gross residual disease (R_2) in the American Joint Committee on Cancer (AJCC) staging system.[81] A resection with microscopic residual disease, that is, a positive resection margin that is discovered on the final pathologic analysis, is classified as R_1. Such a positive margin may involve the bronchial resection line, peribronchial (lymphatic) tissue, or the edge of resected mediastinal nodes. In addition, a resection in which the highest mediastinal node removed was found to have cancer was formerly also considered an incomplete resection because of the assumption that higher, unresected nodes were likely to harbor cancer as well. This latter

TABLE 14–6. SIZE OF TRIALS OF ADJUVANT CHEMOTHERAPY VERSUS SURGERY ALONE

PARAMETER	NON–SMALL CELL LUNG CANCER[a]		OTHER TYPES OF CANCER	
	Node Negative	Node Positive	Colon[b]	Breast[c]
Largest randomized trial	309	351	1526	—
N (total of patients in randomized trials)	1407	1298	21 000	75 000
Increase in survival rates[d]	6%	8%[e]	5%[f]	6%[g]
P value from meta-analysis	0.06[h]	0.06[h]	(0.02)[f]	0.00001
N needed to detect a 10% benefit[i]	290	360	—	—
N needed to detect a 5% benefit[i]	1560	1380	—	—

[a]Cisplatin-based chemotherapy.
[b]Based on review by Macdonald.[94]
[c]Based on meta-analysis by the Early Breast Cancer Trialists' Collective Group.[95]
[d]Absolute difference in percentage of 5-year survival of patients treated with adjuvant therapy versus surgery alone.
[e]2-year survival difference.
[f]3-year survival, based on largest single study.[96]
[g]10-year survival difference in meta-analysis.
[h]Based on meta-analysis by George et al.[60]
[i]Assuming 80% power, $\alpha = 0.05$, assuming baseline survival of 50% for node-negative and 30% for node-positive patients.

DATA SUMMARY: ADJUVANT THERAPY

	AMOUNT	QUALITY	CONSISTENCY
Adjuvant radiotherapy improves local control	High	High	Mod
Adjuvant radiotherapy does not improve survival	High	High	High
Adjuvant alkylating agent chemotherapy has no impact on survival	High	Mod	High
Adjuvant cisplatin-based chemotherapy in predominantly node-negative patients results in a trend toward better 5-year survival	High	Mod	Mod
Adjuvant cisplatin-based chemotherapy in predominantly node-positive patients results in mixed survival trends	**High**	**Mod**	**(High)**[a]
The planned adjuvant chemotherapy was able to be given in only 60% of patients	High	High	Mod
The size of adjuvant chemotherapy trials has been insufficient to rule out a 10% improvement in survival	High	High	High

Type of data rated: Plain: descriptive statement   *Italics: controlled comparison*   **Bold: randomized comparison**
[a]By definition, the term *mixed trends* suggests high consistency.

concept has fallen out of favor[78] and is not recognized by the AJCC system.

The long-term outcome of patients undergoing resection with gross tumor remaining (R_2) has been consistently reported to be 0, despite additional adjuvant therapies (199 patients total).[36,82–84] Furthermore, there is no difference in survival among patients undergoing a palliative resection, an exploratory thoracotomy, or no operation at all in a series reported by Hara et al (Fig. 14–5).[82] All of these patients were clinically stage III, and most (>90%) received additional therapy (radiation and chemotherapy).

The fate of patients with a microscopically positive final margin appears to be much better. Two older studies have found an absolute 5-year survival rate of 23% and 26% in patients with a microscopically positive bronchial (submucosal) margin,[36,70] and several more recent studies reported 5-year survival rates of 22% to 36% (183 patients total).[75–77,84] The outlook appears to be much worse if a positive bron-

chial margin involves peribronchial (nodal) tissues.[74] An older report indicates a 5-year survival of only 4% in this instance.[36] Other papers have also suggested that a positive peribronchial margin correlates with mediastinal node involvement and a poor prognosis.[73,74,85]

The incidence of a positive bronchial margin was found to correlate with the distance from the resection line to the gross tumor in a prospective study of 120 patients operated on in 1992.[80] A histologically positive margin was found in 72% of patients with a gross margin of 0 to 2 mm, 30% with 2 to 5 mm, 15% with 5 to 10 mm, 5% with 10 to 20 mm, and 0 in 56 patients with a gross distance of >20 mm from the resection line to the gross tumor.[80] A positive margin was also correlated with increasing nodal status in this study (0 in N0, 18% in N1, 32% in N2,3 tumors).

A microscopically positive resection margin involving the chest wall, diaphragm, or mediastinal tissues (excluding peribronchial nodal tissues) was associated with a relatively good 5-year survival of 30% in 31 patients in one study.[84] This is similar to the reported 5-year survival for completely resected patients with T3 disease (see Table 15–3), although it must be noted that these incompletely resected patients were all treated with adjuvant RT (40–60 Gy).[84] In patients who were incompletely resected because the highest mediastinal lymph node was found to harbor cancer (although the surgical resection margins were negative) the 5-year survival was found to be 12%.[84] This is similar to that of resected patients with multiple positive N2 stations (see Table 17–3).

There is little data regarding the efficacy of adjuvant therapy in incompletely resected patients. Postoperative RT is commonly employed for patients with a positive resection margin. It makes sense to use RT in such patients because it has been shown to decrease local recurrence in completely resected patients. Furthermore, in a retrospective analysis, Sawyer et al[86] found progressively greater benefit to adjuvant RT as the risk of recurrence increased, although this study did not include incompletely resected patients. Several reports cite an intrathoracic recurrence rate of approximately 15% to 30% following adjuvant radiation as evidence of benefit from postoperative radiation.[87–89] However, this argument is rather weak in light of the fact that the vast majority of recurrences are distant

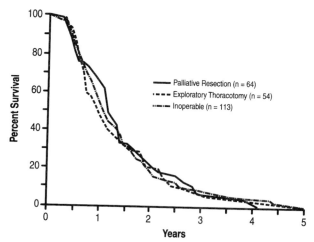

FIGURE 14–5. Comparison of survival among patients with stage III non–small cell lung cancer undergoing palliative resection or exploratory thoracotomy, or with inoperable carcinoma. (From Hara N, Ohta M, Tanaka K, et al. Assessment of the role of surgery for stage III bronchogenic carcinoma. J Surg Oncol, Copyright © 1984 John Wiley & Sons. Reprinted by permission of Wiley-Liss, Inc., a subsidiary of John Wiley & Sons, Inc.)[82]

even in apparently localized lung cancer.[1,2] Slater et al[89] reported on 28 patients with a positive resection margin who received at least 50 Gy postoperatively. Nine patients had gross residual disease and 19 had microscopic residual disease, with an overall 5-year survival rate of 46%. The 5-year survival of 12 N0 patients was 78%. It is difficult to imagine that the survival, especially that of the N0 patients who were incompletely resected, would have been as good without postoperative RT. Another report of 31 N0 patients with a microscopically positive margin who were given adjuvant RT found a 23% 5-year survival rate.[88] By comparison, earlier reports of patients with a positive resection margin who received no postoperative therapy have found an absolute 5-year survival of 13% to 23%.[36,70] Thus, the evidence supporting postoperative radiation in incompletely resected patients is meager, although this therapy makes sense intuitively.

Surprisingly, there is better data regarding adjuvant chemotherapy than for adjuvant RT in incompletely resected patients.[56,90,91] One of the randomized trials (LCSG 791) included earlier (in the context of adjuvant chemotherapy in node positive patients) specifically targeted only incompletely resected patients (with gross residual in 16%, microscopic residual in 84%, and highest node positive in 32%).[90] Patients were randomized to receive either radiation (split course 20 Gy plus 20 Gy) or concurrent radiation (20 Gy plus 20 Gy) and chemotherapy (CAP every month for 6 months). Seventy-four percent of these patients had N2 disease, and 92% had stage IIIa disease. Recurrences were significantly reduced by adjuvant chemotherapy ($P = 0.002$), as shown in Figure 14–6. This difference was true for all histologic types and nodal status and was most pronounced in patients with macroscopic residual or T3 disease.[90] Both the local and distant recurrence rates were decreased by approximately half with the combination therapy.[56]

Adjuvant immunotherapy has been shown to be of benefit in one randomized trial of 105 incompletely resected patients.[92] The patients were well matched with regard to stage, histologic type, and type of incomplete resection. The patients were randomized to receive standard postoperative treatment alone or the same treatment in addition to immunotherapy with interleukin 2 (IL-2) and lymphokine-activated killer cells (LAKs) given every 2 months for 2 years. Standard therapy consisted of 40 to 60 Gy of RT in most patients, chemotherapy (cisplatin, vindesine, mitomy-

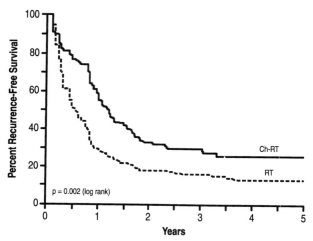

FIGURE 14–6. Recurrence-free survival (including second primaries) for 164 incompletely resected patients treated with radiotherapy alone (RT) or chemotherapy plus radiotherapy (Ch-RT). $P = 0.002$, log rank test. CAP, cyclophosphamide/doxorubicin/cisplatin. (From Holmes EC. Postoperative chemotherapy for non–small-cell lung cancer. *CHEST*. 1993; 103[1 suppl]:30S–34S.)[93]

cin C for 2 cycles) in some patients, and intrapleural chemotherapy in those patients with pleural dissemination. The 5-year survival was better in the group given immunotherapy (39% versus 13%, $P < 0.01$).[34]

EDITORS' COMMENTS

It is clear that adjuvant RT in resected patients improves local control but does not provide a survival benefit. In fact, a survival detriment is suggested when adjuvant RT is used in patients who are N0. Given the low local recurrence rates in such patients, it may well be that the toxicity of RT outweighs any benefit. However, it is crucial to realize that the techniques of RT used in these studies (large fields, cobalt radiation) are inferior to current optimal treatment (precise targeting through 3-D planning). There is good reason to expect that modern RT results both in less toxicity and greater efficacy. It is likely that the results of the studies throughout the 1980s and 1990s cannot be generalized to modern RT, given the technologic transformation that is occurring in radiation oncology.

The available data on adjuvant RT does permit the con-

DATA SUMMARY: INCOMPLETE RESECTION

	AMOUNT	QUALITY	CONSISTENCY
Incomplete resection in gross residual disease (R₂) yields no 5-year survivors	High	Mod	High
Incomplete resection with microscopic residual disease (R₁) yields a 5-year survival of 30%	Mod	Mod	High
Adjuvant radiotherapy for incompletely resected patients results in better survival	Poor	Poor	—
Adjuvant chemotherapy for incompletely resected patients results in better survival	**Poor**	**High**	—

Type of data rated: Plain: descriptive statement   *Italics: controlled comparison*   **Bold: randomized comparison**

clusion that this treatment should be used in patients in whom the risk of local recurrence is high, and that it should be omitted in others. Patients who are at high risk are probably most clearly defined by a close or microscopically positive margin. A perceived high risk may be due merely to the fact that N2 disease has been encountered, and in fact the data suggests a small survival benefit in this group. Furthermore, as more effective therapy for systemic disease is developed, the issue of local control will become more important.

The role of adjuvant chemotherapy in the day-to-day care of patients with resected early stage NSCLC remains controversial. The data discussed in this chapter does not lend itself to a definitive conclusion either way. It is known that surgical resection alone does not result in a cure in many patients with stage I-IIIa NSCLC, and most of the recurrences are at distant sites. Adjuvant chemotherapy makes intuitive sense, and a benefit was suggested by both of the composite analyses done so far.[35,60] However, proof of a benefit is not available at this time, and each physician must come to a conclusion about whether or not to recommend adjuvant chemotherapy based on his or her own interpretation of the data.

Many developments suggest that adjuvant chemotherapy will play a much larger role in the near future. A major problem with adjuvant chemotherapy has been the difficulty of administering it in the postoperative period, but it is likely that compliance in the coming years will be better than what has been reported in the past. Newer chemotherapy agents have less toxicity, and, equally as important, better supportive care allows side effects to be managed more effectively. Newer chemotherapy drugs have been shown to be more effective in stage IV disease, and some are now being investigated in an adjuvant setting. Because the response rate to a chemotherapeutic agent has consistently always been higher the earlier the stage of disease in which it is used, it is likely that a greater effect on survival may be seen. However, until the role of adjuvant chemotherapy is defined more clearly, all patients should be entered in clinical trials designed to answer these questions.

References

1. Martini N, Burt ME, Bains MS, et al. Survival after resection of stage II non–small cell lung cancer. Ann Thorac Surg. 1992;54:460–466.
2. Martini N, Bains MS, Burt ME, et al. Incidence of local recurrence and second primary tumors in resected stage I lung cancer. J Thorac Cardiovasc Surg. 1995;109:120–129.
3. Pantel K, Izbicki J, Passlick B, et al. Frequency and prognostic significance of isolated tumour cells in bone marrow of patients with non–small-cell lung cancer without overt metastases. Lancet. 1996;347:649–653.
4. Ohgami A, Mitsudomi T, Sugio K, et al. Micrometastatic tumor cells in the bone marrow of patients with non–small cell lung cancer. Ann Thorac Surg. 1997;64:363–367.
5. Cote RJ, Beattie EJ, Chaiwun B, et al. Detection of occult bone marrow micrometastases in patients with operable lung carcinoma. Ann Surg. 1995;222:415–425.
6. Paterson R, Russell MH. Clinical trials in malignant disease, IV: lung cancer. Value of post-operative radiotherapy. Clin Radiol. 1962;13:141–144.
7. Van Houtte P, Rocmans P, Smets P, et al. Postoperative radiation therapy in lung cancer: a controlled trial after resection of curative design. Int J Radiat Oncol Biol Phys. 1980;6:983–986.
8. Stephens RJ, Girling DJ, Bleehen NM, et al. The role of postoperative radiotherapy in non–small-cell lung cancer: a multicentre randomised trial in patients with pathologically staged T1-2, N1-2, M0 disease. Br J Cancer. 1996;74:632–639.
9. Weisenburger TH, Gail M, for The Lung Cancer Study Group. Effects of postoperative mediastinal radiation on completely resected stage II and stage III epidermoid cancer of the lung. N Engl J Med. 1986;315:1377–1381.
10. Lafitte JJ, Ribet ME, Prévost BM, et al. Postresection irradiation for T2 N0 M0 non–small cell carcinoma: a prospective, randomized study. Ann Thorac Surg. 1996;62:830–834.
11. Israel L, Bonadonna G, Sylvester R, et al. Controlled study with adjuvant radiotherapy, chemotherapy, immunotherapy, and chemoimmunotherapy in operable squamous carcinoma of the lung. In: Muggia F, Rozencweig M, eds. Lung Cancer: Progress in Therapeutic Research. New York, NY: Raven Press; 1979:443–452.
12. Israel L, Depierre A, Sylvester R. Influence of postoperative radiotherapy on epidermoid carcinoma with regard to nodal status: preliminary results of the EORTC protocol 08741. Recent Results Cancer Res. 1979;68:242–243.
13. Bangma PJ. Postoperative radiotherapy. In: Deeley TJ, ed. Carcinoma of the Bronchus: Modern Radiotherapy. London, England: Butterworth; 1971:163–170.
14. Mei W, Xianzhi G, Weibo Y, et al. Randomized clinical trial of postoperative irradiation after surgery for non–small cell lung carcinoma (NSCLC) (abstract). 1st ALCW Abstracts/Lung Cancer 1994;10:388–389.
15. Jiang G-L, Qian H, Fu X-L, Xia S-J. The indications for postoperative radiotherapy in non–small cell lung cancer (abstract). 1st ALCW Abstracts/Lung Cancer 1994;10:388.
16. Ricci SB, Milani F, Gramaglia A, et al. Surgery (S) vs surgery + radiotherapy (S + RT) in T_2-N_{1-2} non–small cell lung carcinoma (NSCLC): an analysis of mean term data (abstract). Lung Cancer. 1991;7:99.
17. Debevec M, Bitenc M, Vidmar S, et al. Postoperative radiotherapy for radically resected N2 non–small-cell cancer (NSCLC): randomised clinical study 1988–1992. Lung Cancer. 1996;14:99–107.
18. Smolle-Juettner FM, Mayer R, Pinter H, et al. "Adjuvant" external radiation of the mediastinum in radically resected non–small cell lung cancer. Eur J Cardiothorac Surg. 1996;10:947–951.
19. Mayer R, Smolle-Juettner F-M, Szolar D, et al. Postoperative radiotherapy in radically resected non–small cell lung cancer. Chest. 1997;112:954–959.
20. Dautzenberg B, et al, for the Groupe d'Etude et de Traitement des Cancers Bronchiques. A controlled study of postoperative radiotherapy for patients with complete resected non–small cell lung carcinoma. Cancer. 1999;86:265–273.
21. PORT Meta-Analysis Trialists Group. Postoperative radiotherapy in non–small-cell lung cancer: systemic review and meta-analysis of individual patient data from nine randomised controlled trials. Lancet. 1998;352:257–263.
22. Sawyer TE, Bonner JA, Gould PM, et al. Effectiveness of postoperative irradiation in stage IIIA non–small cell lung cancer according to regression tree analyses of recurrence risks. Ann Thorac Surg. 1997;64:1402–1408.
23. Munro AJ. What now for postoperative radiotherapy for lung cancer? Lancet. 1998;352:250–251.
24. Ruckdeschel JC, Codish SD, Stranahan A, et al. Postoperative empyema improves survival in lung cancer: documentation and analysis of a natural experiment. N Engl J Med. 1972;287:1013–1017.
25. Gail MH. A placebo-controlled randomized double-blind study of adjuvant intrapleural BCG in patients with resected T1N0, T1N1, or T2N0 squamous cell carcinoma, adenocarcinoma, or large cell carcinoma of the lung (LCSG Protocol 771). Chest. 1994;106(suppl):287S–292S.
26. McKneally MF, Mauer C, Liniger L, et al. Four year follow-up of the Albany experiment with intrapleural BCG in lung cancer. J Thorac Cardiovasc Surg. 1981;81:485–492.
27. Ludwig Lung Cancer Study Group. Adverse effect of intrapleural Corynebacterium parvum as adjuvant therapy in resected stage I and II non–small cell carcinoma of the lung. J Thorac Cardiovasc Surg. 1985;89:842–847.
28. Souter RG, Gill PG, Gunning AJ, et al. Failure of specific active immunotherapy in lung cancer. Br J Cancer. 1981;44:496–501.
29. Yang SC, Grimm EA, Roth JA. Immunotherapy of lung cancer. Chest Surg Clin N Am. 1991;1:191–204.

30. Owen-Schaub LB, Gutterman JU, Grimm EA. Synergy of tumor necrosis factor and interleukin-2 in the activation of human cytotoxic lymphocytes: effect of tumor necrosis factor alpha and interleukin-2 in the generation of human lymphokine-activated killer cell cytotoxicity. Cancer Res. 1988;48:788–792.

31. Jakubowski AA, Casper ES, Gabrilove JL, et al. Phase I trial of intramuscularly administered tumor necrosis factor in patients with advanced cancer. J Clin Oncol. 1989;7:298–303.

32. Takita H, Hollinshead AC, Adler RH, et al. Characterization of cellular infiltrates in the rat urinary bladder following BCG and thiotepa intravesical therapy. J Surg Oncol. 1991;46:9–14.

33. Ratto GB, Zino P, Mirabelli S, et al. A randomized trial of adoptive immunotherapy with tumor-infiltrating lymphocytes and interleukin-2 versus standard therapy in the postoperative treatment of resected nonsmall cell lung carcinoma. Cancer. 1996;78:244–251.

34. Kimura H, Yamaguchi Y. Adjuvant chemo-immunotherapy after curative resection of Stage II and IIIA primary lung cancer. Lung Cancer. 1996;14:301–314.

35. Stewart LA, for the Non–Small Cell Lung Cancer Collaborative Group. Chemotherapy in non–small cell lung cancer: a meta-analysis using updated data on individual patients from 52 randomised clinical trials. BMJ. 1995;311:899–909.

36. Shields TW, Robinette CD, Keehn RJ. Bronchial carcinoma treated by adjuvant cancer chemotherapy. Arch Surg. 1974;109:329–333.

37. Higgins GA, Humphrey EW, Hughes FA, et al. Cytoxan as an adjuvant to surgery for lung cancer. J Surg Oncol. 1969;3:221–228.

38. Slack HH. Bronchogenic carcinoma: nitrogen mustard as a surgical adjuvant and factors influencing survival. Cancer. 1970;25:987–1002.

39. Miller AB. Study of cytotoxic chemotherapy as an adjuvant to surgery in carcinoma of the bronchus. BMJ. 1971;2:421–428.

40. Brunner KW, Marthaler T, Muller W. Effects of long term adjuvant chemotherapy with cyclophosphamide (NSC-26271) for radically resected bronchogenic carcinoma. Cancer Chemother Rep. 1973;4:125–132.

41. Hughes FA, Higgins G. Veterans Administration Surgical Adjuvant Lung Cancer Chemotherapy Study: present status. J Thorac Cardiovasc Surg. 1962;44:295–308.

42. Girling DJ, Stott H, Stephens RJ, et al. Fifteen-year follow-up of all patients in a study of postoperative chemotherapy for bronchial carcinoma. Br J Cancer. 1985;52:867–873.

43. Trakhtenberg AK, Zakharchenkov AV, Zhiglov MA, et al. Combined treatment including postoperative chemotherapy in lung cancer patients. Neoplasma. 1988;35:351–358.

44. Shields TW, Higgins GA Jr, Humphrey EW, et al. Prolonged intermittent adjuvant chemotherapy with CCNU and hydroxyurea after resection of carcinoma of the lung. Cancer. 1982;50:1713–1721.

45. Shields TW, Humphrey EW, Eastridge CE, et al. Adjuvant cancer chemotherapy after resection of carcinoma of the lung. Cancer. 1977;40:2057–2062.

46. Karrer K, Pridun N, Denck H. Chemotherapy as an adjuvant to surgery in lung cancer. Cancer Chemother Pharmacol. 1978;1:145–159.

47. Wada H, Hitomi S, Teramatsu T, et al. Adjuvant chemotherapy after complete resection in non–small-cell lung cancer. J Clin Oncol. 1996;14:1048–1054.

48. Imaizumi M, et al, for The Study Group of Adjuvant Chemotherapy for Lung Cancer (Chubu, Japan). A randomized trial of postoperative adjuvant chemotherapy in non–small cell lung cancer (the second cooperative study). Eur J Surg Oncol. 1995;21:69–77.

49. Feld R, Rubinstein L, Thomas PA, et al. Adjuvant chemotherapy with cyclophosphamide, doxorubicin, and cisplatin in patients with completely resected stage I non–small-cell lung cancer. (LCSG 801). J Natl Cancer Inst. 1993;85:299–306.

50. Niiranen A, Niitamo-Korhonen S, Kouri M, et al. Adjuvant chemotherapy after radical surgery for non–small cell lung cancer: a randomized study. J Clin Oncol. 1992;10:1927–1932.

51. Ichinose Y, Hara N, Ohta M, et al. Postoperative adjuvant chemotherapy in non–small cell lung cancer: prognostic value of DNA ploidy and postrecurrent survival. J Surg Oncol. 1991;46:15–20.

52. Wada H, et al, and the West Japan Study Group for lung cancer surgery (WJSG). Postoperative adjuvant chemotherapy with PVM (cisplatin + mitomycin C) and UFT (Uracil + Tegafur) in resected stage I–II NSCLC (non–small cell lung cancer): a randomized clinical trial. Eur J Cardiothorac Surg. 1999;15:438–443.

53. Holmes EC, Gail M, for the Lung Cancer Study Group. Surgical adjuvant therapy for stage II and stage III adenocarcinoma and large-cell undifferentiated carcinoma. J Clin Oncol. 1986;4:710–715.

54. Dautzenberg B, Chastang C, Arriagada R, et al. Adjuvant radiotherapy versus combined sequential chemotherapy followed by radiotherapy in the treatment of resected nonsmall cell lung carcinoma: a randomized trial of 267 patients. Cancer. 1995;76:779–786.

55. Pisters KMW, Kris MG, Gralla RJ, et al. Randomized trial comparing postoperative chemotherapy with vindesine and cisplatin plus thoracic irradiation with irradiation alone in stage III (N2) non–small cell lung cancer. J Surg Oncol. 1994;56:236–241.

56. Lad T, Rubinstein L, Sadeghi A, et al. The benefit of adjuvant treatment for resected locally advanced non–small-cell lung cancer. J Clin Oncol. 1988;6:9–17.

57. Ohta M, Tsuchiya R, Shimoyama M, et al. Adjuvant chemotherapy for completely resected stage III non–small-cell lung cancer: results of a randomized prospective study. J Thorac Cardiovasc Surg. 1993;106:703–708.

58. Park JH, Shim YM, Baek HJ, Kim M-S, Choe DH, Cho K-J, Lee C-T, Zo JI. Postoperative adjuvant therapy for stage II non–small cell lung cancer. Ann Thorac Surg. 1999;68:1821–1826.

59. Keller SM, Adak S, Wagner H, et al. Prospective randomized trial of postoperative adjuvant therapy in patients with completely resected stages II and IIIa non–small cell lung cancer: an intergroup trial (E3590) [abstract]. Proc ASCO. 1999;18:465a.

60. George S, Schell MJ, Detterbeck FC, et al. Adjuvant chemotherapy for resected non–small cell carcinoma of the lung: why we still don't know. Oncologist. 1998;3:35–44.

61. Ferguson MK, Karrison T. Does pneumonectomy for lung cancer adversely influence long-term survival? J Thorac Cardiovasc Surg. 2000;119:440–448.

62. Wozniak AJ, Crowley JJ, Balcerzak SP, et al. Randomized trial comparing cisplatin with cisplatin plus vinorelbine in the treatment of advanced non–small-cell lung cancer: a Southwest Oncology Group study. J Clin Oncol. 1998;16:2459–2465.

63. Bonomi P, Kim KM, Fairclough D, et al. Comparsion of survival and quality of life in advanced non–small-cell lung cancer patients treated with two dose levels of paclitaxel combined with cisplatin versus etoposide with cisplatin: results of an Eastern Cooperative Oncology Group trial. J Clin Oncol 2000; 18:623–631.

64. Sandler A, Nemunaitis J, Dehnam C, et al. Phase III trial of gemcitabine plus cisplatin versus cisplatin alone in patients with locally advanced nonsmall cell lung cancer. J Clin Oncol. 2000; 18:122–130.

65. Slevin ML, Stubbs L, Plant HJ, et al. Attitudes to chemotherapy: comparing views of patients with cancer with those of doctors, nurses, and general public. BMJ. 1990;300:1458–1460.

66. Brundage MD, Davidson JR, Mackillop WJ. Trading treatment toxicity for survival in locally advanced non–small cell lung cancer. J Clin Oncol. 1997;15:330–340.

67. L'Abbé KA, Detsky AS, O'Rourke K. Meta-analysis in clinical research. Ann Intern Med. 1987;107:224–233.

68. Overholt RH, Neptune WB, Ashraf MM. Primary cancer of the lung: a 42-year experience. Ann Thorac Surg. 1975;20:511–519.

69. Matthews MJ, Kanhouwa S, Pickren J, et al. Frequency of residual and metastatic tumor in patients undergoing curative surgical resection for lung cancer. Cancer Chemother Rep. 1973;4:63–67.

70. Soorae AS, Stevenson HM. Survival with residual tumor on the bronchial margin after resection for bronchogenic carcinoma. J Thorac Cardiovasc Surg. 1979;78:175–180.

71. Jolly PC, Hutchinson CH, Detterbeck F, et al. Routine computed tomographic scans, selective mediastinoscopy, and other factors in evaluation of lung cancer. J Thorac Cardiovasc Surg. 1991;102:266–271.

72. Mountain CF. Prognostic implications of the international staging system for lung cancer. Semin Oncol. 1988;15:236–245.

73. Kaiser LR, Fleshner P, Keller S, et al. Significance of extramucosal residual tumor at the bronchial resection margin. Ann Thorac Surg. 1989;47:265–269.

74. Liewald F, Hatz RA, Dienemann H, et al. Importance of microscopic residual disease at the bronchial margin after resection for non–small cell lung carcinoma of the lung. J Thorac Cardiovasc Surg. 1992;104:408–412.

75. Gebitekin C, Gupta NK, Satur CM, et al. Fate of patients with residual tumour at the bronchial resection margin. Eur J Cardiothorac Surg. 1994;8:339–342.

76. Heikkilä L, Harjula A, Suomalainen RJ, et al. Residual carcinoma in bronchial resection line. Ann Chir Gynaecol. 1986;75:151–154.

77. Law MR, Hodson ME, Lennox SC. Implications of histologically reported residual tumour on the bronchial margin after resection for bronchial carcinoma. Thorax. 1982;37:492–495.

78. Lacasse Y, Bucher HC, Wong E, et al. "Incomplete resection" in non–small cell lung cancer: need for a new definition. Ann Thorac Surg. 1998;65:220–226.

79. Maggi G, Casadio C, Giobbe R, et al. The value of selective mediastinoscopy in predicting resectability of patients with bronchogenic carcinoma. Int Surg. 1992;77:280–283.

80. Kayser K, Anyanwu E, Bauer H-G, et al. Tumor presence at resection boundaries and lymph-node metastasis in bronchial carcinoma patients. Thorac Cardiovasc Surg. 1993;41:308–311.

81. American Joint Committee on Cancer. AJCC Cancer Staging Handbook, 5th ed. Philadelphia: Lippincott-Raven; 1998.

82. Hara N, Ohta M, Tanaka K, et al. Assessment of the role of surgery for stage III bronchogenic carcinoma. J Surg Oncol. 1984;25:153–158.

83. Maggi G, Casadio C, Cianci R, et al. Results of surgical resection of Stage IIIA (N2) non small cell lung cancer, according to the site of the mediastinal metastases. Intern Surg. 1993;78:213–217.

84. Kimura H, Yamaguchi Y. Survival of noncuratively resected lung cancer. Lung Cancer. 1994;11:229–242.

85. Gaissert HA, Mathisen DJ, Moncure AC, et al. Survival and function after sleeve lobectomy for lung cancer. J Thorac Cardiovasc Surg. 1996;111:948–953.

86. Sawyer TE, Bonner JA, Gould PM, et al. The impact of surgical adjuvant thoracic radiation therapy for patients with nonsmall cell lung carcinoma with ipsilateral mediastinal lymph node involvement. Cancer. 1997;80:1399–1408.

87. Emami B, Kim T, Roper C, et al. Postoperative radiation therapy in the management of lung cancer. Radiology. 1987;164:251–253.

88. Emami B, Kaiser L, Simpson J, et al. Postoperative radiation therapy in non–small cell lung cancer. Am J Clin Oncol. 1997;20:441–448.

89. Slater JD, Ellerbroek NA, Barkley HT Jr, et al. Radiation therapy following resection of non–small cell bronchogenic carcinoma. Int J Radiat Oncol Biol Phys. 1991;20:945–951.

90. Sadeghi A, Payne D, Rubinstein L, et al. Combined modality treatment for resected advanced non–small cell lung cancer: local control and local recurrence. Int J Radiat Oncol Biol Phys. 1988;15:89–97.

91. Lad T. The comparison of CAP chemotherapy and radiotherapy to radiotherapy alone for resected lung cancer with positive margin or involved highest sampled paratracheal node (stage IIIA). Lung Cancer Study Group 791. Chest. 1994;106:302S–306S.

92. Kimura H, Yamaguchi Y. Adjuvant immunotherapy with interleukin 2 and lymphokine-activated killer cells after noncurative resection of primary lung cancer. Lung Cancer. 1995;13:31–44.

93. Holmes EC. Postoperative chemotherapy for non–small-cell lung cancer. Chest. 1993; 103:30S–34S.

94. Macdonald JS. Adjuvant therapy for colon cancer. CA Cancer J Clin. 1997;47:243–256.

95. Early Breast Cancer Trialists' Collaborative Group. Systemic treatment of early breast cancer by hormonal, cytotoxic, or immune therapy. Lancet. 1992;339:71–85.

96. International Multicentre Pooled Analysis of Colon Cancer Trials (IMPACT). Efficacy of adjuvant fluorouracil and folinic acid in colon cancer. Lancet. 1995;356:939–944.

PART 5

Locally Advanced Non–Small Cell Lung Cancer

T3 NON–SMALL CELL LUNG CANCER (STAGE IIB-IIIA)

Frank C. Detterbeck and Andy C. Kiser

DEFINITION

In the 1986 international staging system for lung cancer, any T3N0,1 tumor was classified as stage IIIa.[1] Because of better survival exhibited by T3N0 tumors, especially those involving the chest wall, the 1997 modification of the staging system classifies T3N0 tumors as stage IIb.[2] It does appear that currently the overall survival of T3N0 patients is similar to that of T2N1 (stage IIb) patients, and the survival of T3N1 patients is similar to that of T1,2N2 (stage IIIa) patients.[2] However, it is not intuitive that the biologic behavior of T3N0 and T2N1 tumors is the same. Issues related to recurrence patterns and appropriate selection of treatment modalities may be different. The biologic behavior of T3N1 tumors may also be different from that of T3N0 cancers. However, data for T3N1 tumors is usually reported together with data for T3N0 tumors. Therefore, T3N0,1 tumors are reviewed as a separate group in this chapter, even though the survival of some of these patients may be similar to that of T2N1 or T1,2N2 patients. T3N2 tumors are probably more similar to other N2 lesions, which are discussed in Chapter 17.

The behavior and survival of different categories of T3N0,1 tumors may also be different.[3] Tumors are classified as T3 because of any one of the following factors:

1. Peripheral extension into the chest wall or diaphragm
2. Extension centrally into mediastinal structures (mediastinal pleura, pericardium, phrenic nerve, azygous vein, or right or left pulmonary artery)
3. Tumor involvement of a main stem bronchus within 2 cm of the carina
4. Involvement of the lower brachial plexus at the apex of the chest (Pancoast tumors)

These structures are generally resectable without requiring major reconstruction. This is in contrast to T4 tumors, which invade more vital structures such as the aorta, heart, great vessels, trachea, esophagus, or vertebral bodies. This chapter reviews the published data regarding the treatment of T3 tumors divided into the following categories of disease:

1. Extension into the chest wall
2. Extension into the mediastinum
3. Proximity to the carina and involving the main stem bronchus

Pancoast tumors are discussed in detail in Chapter 16 and are mentioned only briefly here.

INCIDENCE

A number of large series have reported that T3N0,1 patients comprise about 5% of all non–small cell lung cancer (NSCLC) patients and about 10% of resected NSCLC patients.[1,4–8] In surgical series involving patients with T3 disease who are found to be pathologically N0,1, approximately 60% of the patients have N0 disease and 40% N1 disease (Table 15–1). Such surgical series have found that an additional 30% of the cT3N0,1 primary tumors actually had N2 involvement histologically.[6,7,9–11] However, because patients with clinical N2 disease are excluded from these series, this provides only a partial estimate of the incidence of T3N2 disease. Thus, it appears that pT3N0,1 patients comprise a relatively small group, with most of these patients having N0 disease.

The distribution of the type of T3 tumors is shown in Table 15–1. The two largest groups are tumors invading the chest wall and those invading mediastinal structures. Although patients with chest wall involvement are a large group, they make up only half of all patients with T3 disease. Furthermore, both the biologic behavior of peripheral T3 versus central T3 tumors and the surgical implications of resecting adjacent peripheral versus central structures may be quite different. Therefore, survival and prognostic factors for each category of T3 disease are reviewed separately in this chapter.

TABLE 15–1. DISTRIBUTION OF T3 TUMORS (SURGICAL SERIES)

STUDY	N	pNO[a]	pN1[a]	CHEST WALL	PANCOAST	MEDIASTINUM	MAIN STEM BRONCHUS
Pitz et al[6]	233	55%	45%	50%	—	20%	30%
Watanabe et al[28]	102	69%	31%	68%		20%[b]	12%
Mountain[52]	80	80%	20%	39%	15%	46%	
Izbicki et al[10]	77	44%	56%	46%	0%	48%	6%
Average		**62%**	**38%**	**45%**	**8%**	**29%**	**16%**

Inclusion criteria: Surgical series involving at least 75 unselected patients with T3 disease.
[a]Excluding N2 patients.
[b]Pericardium only.

CLINICAL STAGING

No data is available that specifically addresses the incidence of distant metastases in patients with T3 disease. Given the higher incidence of a false negative clinical history and physical examination in patients with locally advanced tumors (see Table 6–3), it would seem reasonable to perform distant organ scans in these patients, at least in those with central tumors and possible lymph node involvement. The reliability of radiographic intrathoracic staging is discussed in detail in Figs. 5–6 and 5–7. Briefly, the false negative rate of a radiographically normal mediastinum is particularly high in central T3 lesions. Thus, it seems reasonable for such patients to undergo mediastinoscopy, regardless of the computed tomography (CT) findings with respect to mediastinal lymph nodes. Furthermore, the ability to predict true T3 disease (invasion into adjacent structures) on the basis of CT scans is poor. A thoracotomy may be required to determine whether there is no invasion (T2 disease), resectable invasion (T3 disease), or unresectable extension (T4 disease).

RESECTABILITY

Only a few studies assessing the resectability rate are available concerning patients clinically thought to have T3N0,1 disease. About 70% of such clinically staged patients undergo complete resection (R_0), and about 15% undergo exploratory thoracotomy alone without resection (Table 15–2). It can also be seen that about 20% of patients actually have lower-stage (T2N0,1) disease, whereas about 20% have higher-stage disease (including N2 disease). Mediastinoscopy was not routinely used as part of the clinical staging in any of these studies.

More information is available on the resectability of pathologically staged patients who have undergone resection (Table 15–3). Again, approximately 80% of patients achieve a complete resection. The rate of complete resection appears to be somewhat higher (84%) for patients with T3 disease involving the chest wall as opposed to those with mediastinal or bronchial involvement (66%). Approximately 25% of resected patients have been found to be pathologically T3N2. The only studies that used routine mediastinoscopy found this to be accurate in excluding patients with N2 disease as well as in optimizing the complete resection rate.[12, 13]

RESULTS FOR ALL T3 PATIENTS

Few studies have reported survival of T3 patients based on clinical (pretherapy) staging. Mountain[14] reported only a 6% 5-year survival for 95 patients clinically staged as T3 (including all N categories). More recently, Mountain[2] reported a 5-year survival of 22% for 107 cT3N0 patients and 9% for 40 cT3N1 patients. In another series of 171 patients, the 5-year survival was 22% for cT3N0 patients and 36% for cT3N1 patients.[4] It is also surprising how few studies have reported on the survival of pathologically staged T3 patients as a general group. The data from such studies from 1980 to 2000 involving at least 20 patients is shown in Table 15–4. The reported 5-year survival of resected T3 patients in general is approximately 40%. More information is available, however, on specific categories of resected T3 disease, especially on patients with chest wall involvement.

TABLE 15–2. RESECTABILITY OF CLINICAL T3 NON–SMALL CELL LUNG CANCER TUMORS

STUDY	TYPE OF T3	N	RESECTABILITY		Exploratory Thoracotomy (%)	FINAL p STAGE	
			R_0 (%)	$R_{1,2}$ (%)		Lower (<T3) (%)	Higher (>T3N0,1) (%)
Ratto et al[16 a]	Chest wall	112	77	12	11	25	26
Albertucci et al[22 b,c]	Chest wall	37	70	30	—	19[c]	19[d]
Burt et al[35 d]	Mediastinum	196	78		22	8	?

Inclusion criterion: Studies of ≥20 cT3 patients.
[a]Clinically adjacent to chest wall.
[b]Report includes only patients undergoing resection.
[c]Vague reporting.
[d]Includes both T3 and T4.

p, pathologic; R_0, complete resection; $R_{1,2}$, microscopic or grossly incomplete resection; <T3, patients with pT1 or pT2 disease; >T3N0,1, patients with pT4 or pN2,3 disease; ?, unknown.

TABLE 15–3. RESECTABILITY OF PATHOLOGICALLY STAGED T3 NON–SMALL CELL LUNG CANCER[a]

STUDY	T3 TYPE	N	RESECTABILITY (%)		% >T3N0,1
			R₀	R₁,₂	
Watanabe et al[28]	All	137	64	36	43
Nakahashi et al[11]	All	78	77	23	27
Downey[17]	Ch w	334	65	35	29
Pitz et al[7]	Ch w	125	69	31	23
Ratto et al[16]	Ch w	99	87	13	26[b]
Casillas et al[30]	Ch w	97	81	19	24
Ricci et al[53]	Ch w	55	91	9	41
Allen et al[12 c]	Ch w	52	98	2	(0)[c]
Albertucci et al[22]	Ch w	37	70	30	19[d]
Patterson et al[31]	Ch w	35	86	14	14
López et al[51]	Ch w	35	83	17	17
Paone et al[19]	Ch w	32	87	13[d]	16
Harpole et al[13 c]	Ch w	22	100	0	(9)[e]
Martini et al[36 f,g]	Med	102	(45)[f]	(55)[f]	—[g]
Burt et al[35 f]	Med	100	(49)[f]	(51)[f]	(30)[f]
Pitz et al[6]	Med	33	64	36	18
Pitz et al[6]	MSB	68	68	32	25
Average[h]			**79**	**21**	**25**

Inclusion criterion: Studies of ≥20 patients.
[a]All studies based on patients undergoing resection, except where indicated.
[b]Based on all patients undergoing thoracotomy.
[c]Negative mediastinoscopy required.
[d]Vague reporting.
[e]Selected mediastinoscopy-positive patients resected after induction therapy.
[f]Includes both T3 and T4.
[g]N2 excluded.
[h]Excluding values in parentheses.
Ch w, chest wall; Med, mediastinum; MSB, main stem bronchus; R₀, complete resection; R₁,₂, microscopic or grossly incomplete resection; >T3N0,1, patients with pT4 or pN2,3 disease.

CHEST WALL INVOLVEMENT

A number of series of patients with chest wall involvement have been reported. All series from 1980 to 2000 reporting actuarial survival of at least 20 resected patients with NSCLC invading the chest wall only are listed in Table 15–5. The studies are arranged according to the rate of

TABLE 15–4. 5-YEAR SURVIVAL OF RESECTED pT3 PATIENTS

STUDY	N	ALL T3	T3N0	T3N1
Naruke et al[4]	327	38	—	—
van Rens[57]	226	—	33	25
Mountain[2]	142	—	38	25
Okada[37]	132	—	48	32
Wada et al[44 a]	116	46	—	—
Maggi[27]	93	35	—	—
Inoue et al[33 b]	85	—	34	38
Mountain[52]	80	39	—	—
van Velzen et al[54]	80	—	—	28
Watanabe et al[28 a,b]	56	50	—	—
Sabanathan et al[55]	51	—	42	6
Nakahashi et al[15]	47	—	33	0
Average		**42**	**38**	**22**

Inclusion criterion: Studies of ≥20 resected patients.
[a]Only pT3N0,1 patients.
[b]Only patients who were completely resected.

complete resection. The average survival for all patients (including some T3N2 patients) is 34%. It is difficult to compare series because the inclusion criteria, as well as the method of reporting, are not consistent. However, there appears to be a trend to higher survival in those studies reporting on only completely resected patients (40%) compared with those including incompletely resected patients (24%).

The importance of a complete resection has been emphasized by a number of studies (see Fig 15–1A).[7,10,15-19] Most authors have reported no survivors beyond 2 years with microscopically or grossly positive margins,[16,18,19] but a few studies have reported 5-year survival of 4% to 10% despite incomplete resection of T3 (chest wall) tumors.[7,10,15,17] Another major factor influencing survival appears to be the nodal status,[17,20–23] as seen in Figure 15–1B. The average survival of T3N0 patients is 41%, whereas that of T3N1 patients drops dramatically to 17%. The survival of T3N0 (chest wall) patients undergoing complete resection has been consistently reported to be 50% to 60%,[13,16,17,20,22–24] with few exceptions.[7]

The depth of invasion, as determined histologically, also appears to be a significant factor influencing survival in

DATA SUMMARY: T3 TUMORS

	AMOUNT	QUALITY	CONSISTENCY
T3 tumors comprise about 5% of non–small cell lung cancer	Mod	High	High
Approximately 40% of T3 tumors involve the chest wall	Mod	High	High
Patients with central T3 tumors should undergo mediastinoscopy even if the mediastinum appears radiographically normal	Poor	Mod	—
Patients with peripheral T3 tumors do not need mediastinoscopy if the mediastinum appears radiographically normal	Poor	Mod	—
Approximately 80% of clinical T3 patients are able to be completely resected	Mod	Mod	High
Approximately 20% of clinical T3 patients are found to be only pT2	Mod	Mod	High
Approximately 20% of clinical T3 patients are found to be pT4 or pN2	Mod	Mod	High
The resectability of chest wall tumors is somewhat higher than that of central T3 tumors	Mod	High	High

Type of data rated: Plain text: descriptive statement   *Italics: controlled comparison*   **Bold: randomized comparison**

TABLE 15–5. SURVIVAL OF RESECTED T3 PATIENTS WITH CHEST WALL INVOLVEMENT

STUDY	R₁,₂ (%)	N (ALL T3)	All T3	T3N0	T3N1
Downey[17]	0	175	36	49	27
Okada[37]	0	94	39	—	—
Pitz et al[7 a]	0	86	29	36	23
Trastek et al[21 a,b]	0	73	40	38	29[c]
Piehler et al[23 a,d]	0	66	33	54	7[c]
Mountain[52]	0	31	39	—	—
Watanabe et al[28 a,e]	0	24	43	—	—
Harpole et al[13]	0	22	54	60	—
Allen et al[12]	2	52	26	29	11
Ricci et al[53]	9	55	15	22	12
Paone et al[19]	13	32	35	?	0
Patterson et al[31]	14	35	38	—	—
López et al[51 f]	17	28	28	36	—
Ratto et al[16]	18	—	—	47	(22)[g]
Casillas et al[30 a]	19	97	23	34	8
van Velzen et al[54]	21	24	—	—	23
Albertucci et al[22]	30	37[h]	30	41	29
Shah et al[20 d,i]	?	51	(37)[j]	(45)[j]	(38)[j]
Inoue et al[33]	?	24	26	—	—
Average[k]			**34**	**41**	**17**

Inclusion criterion: Studies of ≥20 resected T3 patients.
[a]Excludes operative mortality.
[b]Only patients with parietal pleura (not rib) involvement, but 47% also had invasion of mediastinal structures.
[c]N1 + N2.
[d]Includes 3% small cell.
[e]All N0,1.
[f]Includes 29% Pancoast.
[g]4-year survival.
[h]Includes seven patients who were cT3 but pT2.
[i]Includes 10% Pancoast.
[j]Absolute survival.
[k]Excluding values in parentheses.
R₁,₂, incompletely resected; ?, unknown.

most studies (Fig. 15–2A,B),[13,16,25–27] although the largest series found no difference among patients who were completely resected.[17] However, an earlier study from the same institution involving a subset of these patients found a difference (5-year survival of completely resected patients with involvement of parietal pleura versus chest wall of 48% versus 16%, $P = 0.02$).[18]

The technique of resection of lesions that are not obviously deeply invasive into the ribs is a matter of some debate. For such lesions, Downey et al[17] advocate an attempt at an extrapleural resection without rib resection, as long as this does not appear to violate tumor. Indeed, with this technique they have reported good survival of 80 patients who had invasion of only the parietal pleura in whom a complete resection was achieved (see Fig. 15–2A). No information is available about how often extrapleural resection was attempted but found to result in an incomplete resection. Others have had better results using a more aggressive approach.[21,22,28,29] In a series from the Mayo Clinic, 5-year survival was 75% when chest wall was resected versus 30% when the resection was performed by extrapleural dissection ($P = 0.057$)[21] (Fig. 15–3A). Albertucci et al[22] also found better survival after en bloc rib resection, even in those patients who were subsequently found to have had only parietal pleural involvement with tumor (see Fig. 15–3B). This was statistically significant for the entire group of patients (34 patients, all N status)

as well as for only those who were N0 (21 patients). Cangemi et al[29] reported 5-year survival of 14% in 23 patients treated by extrapleural resection versus 43% in 8 patients undergoing chest wall resection ($P = NS$).

The ability to determine the adequacy of an extrapleural resection at the time of operation appears to be poor. The incidence of finding a positive final margin in patients who have undergone an extrapleural resection has been variously reported, ranging from 12% to 62%.[18,22] Moreover, when the involved chest wall is resected discontinuously rather than en bloc (because a positive margin is discovered intraoperatively), the survival is significantly worse[7,16] (Fig. 15–4A,B). Because there is little additional morbidity or mortality to chest wall resection,[13,17,21,23,24,29,30] it seems to be prudent to err on the side of rib resection, although extrapleural resection of lesions that are only loosely attached to the parietal pleura (perhaps only by adhesions) may be reasonable in selected instances.

No controlled studies have investigated the use of adjuvant radiotherapy (RT) after chest wall resection. Intuitively, it seems that the addition of another local modality would be of little benefit when a complete resection with

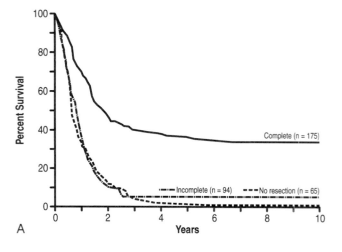

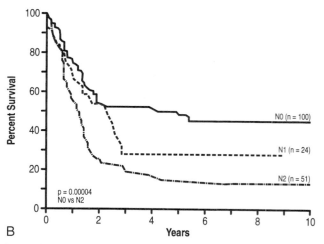

FIGURE 15–1. A, Survival of patients with non–small cell lung cancer (NSCLC) invading the chest wall. B, Survival following complete resection in patients with NSCLC invading parietal pleura or chest wall by nodal status. Reprinted with permission from the Society of Thoracic Surgeons [The Annals of Thoracic Surgery. 1999;68:188–193].[17]

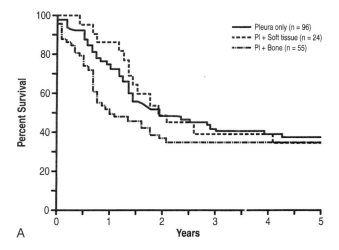

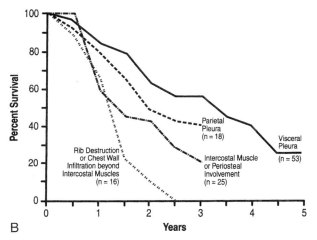

FIGURE 15–2. *A,* Survival following complete resection in patients with non–small cell lung cancer invading parietal pleura or chest wall (*P* = NS). Pl, pleura. *B,* Survival according to the depth of chest wall infiltration (*P* < 0.01 for visceral pleura involvement versus rib destruction). *A,* Reprinted with permission from The Society of Thoracic Surgeons [The Annals of Thoracic Surgery. 1999;68:188–193].[17] *B,* Reprinted with permission from the Society of Thoracic Surgeons [The Annals of Thoracic Surgery. 1991;51:182–188].)[16]

an adequate margin has been achieved. In the largest series, there was no difference in 5-year survival for completely resected patients with or without additional RT (52% versus 48%, *P* = NS).[17] However, in a retrospective review of 35 patients (30 with complete resection, 5 with incomplete resection), the survival was better in the 22 patients who were radiated postoperatively (5-year survival 56% versus 30%, *P* value not calculated), and the local recurrence rate was lower (0% versus 27%).[31] Adjuvant radiation in patients who were incompletely resected has not resulted in long-term survival,[16,18,22] and local recurrence rates of 30% to 40% at the site of a positive margin have been seen, despite the use of radiation (dose not reported).[18,22]

One can speculate that a complete resection for T3N0 patients with diaphragmatic involvement might result in survival similar to that for T3N0 patients with chest wall involvement. Such patients are exceedingly rare, and little data is available. Only three studies of a total of 27 patients

with diaphragmatic involvement have been published.[32–34] Seven patients with N2 disease had a median survival of 23 months, and all had died of cancer by 3½ years. Of the 21 patients with N0,1 disease, three died of unrelated causes within 1 year, and 12 died of cancer within 2½ years.[32–34] The actuarial 5-year survival for T3N0 patients was reported to be 27% in the largest series.[34] The liver was the most common site of recurrence.[34]

TUMORS INVADING THE MEDIASTINUM

The results of studies reporting survival of patients with tumors invading the mediastinum are shown in Table 15–6. It is immediately apparent that the number of studies and patients is limited. The average 5-year survival in these series is 25%. The largest series involves only patients who

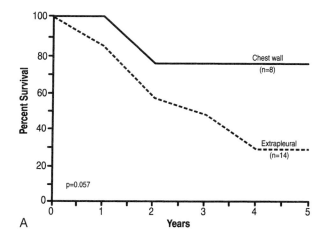

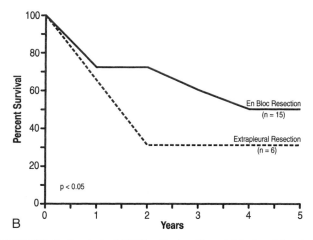

FIGURE 15–3. Survival of T3N0 patients with parietal pleural involvement with tumor, according to the type of resection. *A,* Survival of 22 patients from the Mayo Clinic (*P* = 0.057). *B,* Survival of 21 patients from Italy (*P* < 0.05). (*A,* From Trastek VF, Pairolero PC, Piehler JM, et al. En bloc (non–chest wall) resection for bronchogenic carcinoma with parietal fixation. J Thorac Cardiovasc Surg. 1984;87:352-358.[21] *B,* From Albertucci M, DeMeester TR, Rothberg M, et al. Surgery and the management of peripheral lung tumors adherent to the parietal pleura. J Thorac Cardiovasc Surg. 1992;103:8–13.)[22]

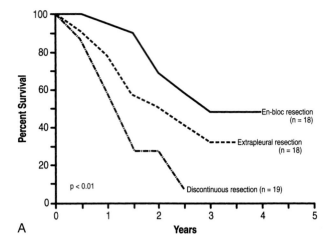

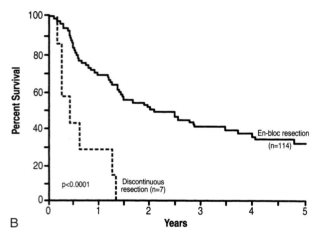

FIGURE 15–4. *A,* Survival of patients with tumors extending to the chest wall, according to the type of resection (*P* < 0.01 for en bloc versus discontinuous resection). *B,* Survival of patients with tumors extending to the chest wall who underwent en bloc resection versus patients in which the tumor was opened (*P* < 0.0001). (*A,* Reprinted with permission from the Society of Thoracic Surgeons [The Annals of Thoracic Surgery. 1991;51:182–188].[16] *B,* From Pitz CC, Brutel de la Riviere A, Elbers HR, et al. Surgical treatment of 125 patients with non–small cell lung cancer and chest wall involvement. Thorax. 1996;51:846–850, with permission from the BMJ Publishing Group.[7])

TABLE 15–6. SURVIVAL OF RESECTED T3 PATIENTS WITH INVOLVEMENT OF THE MEDIASTINUM

STUDY	ALL T3	
	N	5 y (%)
Burt et al[35 a]	49	9
Martini et al[36 a,b,c]	46	30
Pitz et al[6 d,e]	40	25
Inoue et al[33 b]	39	37[f]
Total	174	
Average		**25**

Inclusion criterion: Studies of ≥20 resected patients.
[a]Only completely resected.
[b]All N0 or N1.
[c]17% T4.
[d]Excludes operative mortality.
[e]28% incompletely resected.
[f]Estimated.

with mediastinal invasion as well as main stem bronchial involvement found a small difference between N0 and N1 disease (45% versus 37%, *P* = 0.03) and a trend to better survival for patients with squamous cell cancer.[6] The most important factor appears to be the completeness of the resection[6,36] (see Fig. 15–5*B*).

No controlled studies concerning the use of adjuvant radiation for T3 mediastinal tumors have been performed. In a retrospective review using interstitial brachytherapy, Martini et al[36] found a 5-year survival of 20% with incomplete resection and adjuvant radiation (N = 10), compared with 7% with incomplete resection and no radiation (N = 15) and 0% with radiation alone (N = 30). This suggests that radiation may be of benefit with a positive margin. However, there is no data to support its use as a routine adjuvant treatment when a complete resection has been achieved.

MAIN STEM BRONCHUS INVOLVEMENT

The data on 5-year survival in patients with involvement of the main stem bronchus within 2 cm of the carina is shown in Table 15–8. This includes all series from 1980 to

TABLE 15–7. 5-YEAR SURVIVAL FOLLOWING RESECTION OF T3,4N0,2 PATIENTS WITH MEDIASTINAL INVOLVEMENT

SITE	N	5-y SURVIVAL (%)
Pericardium	25	11
Pulmonary artery	37	4
Pulmonary veins	23	7
Phrenic nerve	13	7
Esophagus	7	14
Left atrium	3	0
Superior vena cava or aorta	37	0
Recurrent nerve	6	0

Inclusion criteria: Largest study reporting survival separately based on type of mediastinal T3 involvement.
Data from Burt ME, Pomerantz AH, Bains MS, et al. Results of surgical treatment of stage III lung cancer invading the mediastinum. Surg Clin North Am. 1987;67:987–1000.[35]

were completely resected and shows an average survival of only 9% but includes patients with T3 and T4 disease.[35] The most common mediastinal tissues involved in patients with T3 disease are the main pulmonary vessels, the pericardium, and the mediastinal pleura or fat.[35,36] As shown in Table 15–7, there does not appear to be a marked difference in survival based on the structures involved.

Only a few studies provide data about the influence of nodal involvement.[6,35,36] Two are from Memorial Sloan-Kettering and involve both completely resected and incompletely resected patients. Nodal status appears to influence early survival, but this does not seem to hold up at 5 years (Fig. 15–5*A*). No difference was noted between patients who were N0 or N1.[35,36] Surprisingly, patients with adenocarcinoma had more favorable results than those with squamous cell cancers in this study (5-year survival 30% versus 14%, *P* = 0.002).[36] Another study that involved patients

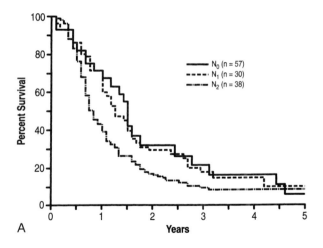

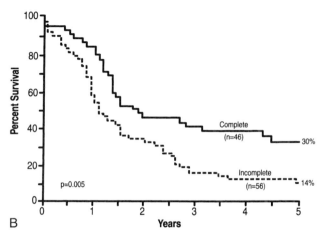

FIGURE 15–5. *A,* Survival of operated patients with T3 mediastinal disease, according to pathologic nodal status. *B,* Survival of operated patients with T3,T4 mediastinal disease by extent of resection (complete resection group with 17% T4; incomplete resection group with 67% T4). (*A,* From Burt ME, Pomerantz AH, Bains MS, et al. Results of surgical treatment of stage III lung cancer invading the mediastinum. Surg Clin North Am. 1987;67:987–1000.[35] *B,* Reprinted with permission from the Society of Thoracic Surgeons [The Annals of Thoracic Surgery. 1994;58:1447–1451].[36])

2000 involving at least 20 patients, but the number of patients on whom data is reported is limited. Although tumors involving the main stem bronchus are frequently resected, patients with these tumors are usually reported in the context of sleeve resections. These reports contain a variety of stages of patients and have generally not defined the T, N, and M status; therefore, these studies are of limited value here. The average 5-year survival in those series reporting stage and survival data is 22%, although two small studies reported long-term survival of $\geq 80\%$ with T3 main stem bronchial involvement.[15,37] This is similar to that seen in patients with mediastinal involvement. The largest series shows a 5-year survival of only 12%.[38] No data is available to analyze the influence of nodal status, resection margin, or other factors that may be related to survival in patients with main stem bronchus involvement. In the overall series of 101 central T3 patients reported by Pitz et al,[6] 68% of whom had main stem

bronchus involvement, complete resection (R_0) was important (5-year survival 35% versus 18%, $P = 0.05$), as well as nodal status (5-year survival for R_0 resections: 45% for N0; 37% for N1, $P = 0.03$; and 0% for N2, $P = 0.02$).

PANCOAST TUMORS

Tumors arising in the apex of the chest and involving the brachial plexus are also classified as T3 tumors. These tumors can also involve T4 structures such as the subclavian vessels or the vertebral bodies. In most surgical series of Pancoast tumors, approximately 30% of patients have T4 lesions. The average 5-year survival for a large number of resected patients, including some T4 and some N2 patients, is approximately 30%[39] (see Table 16–2). In T3N0,1 patients in whom a complete resection with negative margins is achieved, the 5-year survival has been reported to be 41%.[40] Thus, the survival of patients with Pancoast tumors is intermediate between central T3 tumors (with mediastinal or main stem bronchial involvement) and chest wall tumors.

COMPARISON OF DIFFERENT T3 CATEGORIES

The apparent differences in survival of patients with central versus peripheral T3 tumors may be a reflection of differences in the biologic behavior. The usual pattern of spread of lung cancers appears to be via the lymphatic channels through the lung, then to the mediastinum, and finally by distant hematogenous dissemination. By this hypothesis, peripheral T3 tumors (chest wall, Pancoast) may be less likely to involve mediastinal nodes or to have undergone hematogenous dissemination at the time of diagnosis. This might be particularly true for those patients who are resected and pathologically staged as T3N0,1.

Alternatively, the apparent differences in survival may be due to inaccurate staging. Central T3 tumors appear to have a higher rate of radiographically occult mediastinal node involvement, and therefore the staging of central T3 tumors may be particularly unreliable when surgical staging is not done. Because details of the adequacy of surgical staging are not given in most reports, it is possible that the apparent differences in survival between patients with

TABLE 15–8. SURVIVAL OF RESECTED T3 PATIENTS WITH INVOLVEMENT OF THE MAIN STEM BRONCHUS

	ALL T3	
STUDY	**N**	**5-y (%)**
Vogt-Moykopf et al[38] [a]	97	12
Pitz et al[6] [b]	75	40
Deslauriers et al[56]	31	14
Total	203	
Average		**22**

Inclusion criterion: Studies of ≥ 20 patients.
[a]Small cell in 15%.
[b]Excludes operative mortality.

TABLE 15–9. RECURRENCES AFTER RESECTION OF T3 TUMORS

STUDY	% R_0	TYPE OF T3	N	RECURRENCE % OF ALL PATIENTS	% OF ALL RECURRENCES		
					L	L+D	D
Pitz et al[6]	100	MSB/med	64	53	24	3	74
Harpole et al[13]	100	Chest wall	22	41	11	44	45
López et al[51]	83	Chest wall	35	36	17	—	83
Martini et al[36]	45	Med	96	81	49	10	41
Trastek et al[21 a]	100	Chest wall[b]	73	61	43	3	53

Inclusion criterion: Studies reporting recurrence data on ≥20 patients.
[a]Extrapleural dissection only; no patients had rib resection.
[b]47% also had invasion of mediastinal structures.
D, distant; L, local; L + D, simultaneous local and distant; med, mediastinum; MSB, main stem bronchus; R_0, complete resection.

peripheral T3 and those with central T3 tumors could be due to inaccurate staging.

One might also speculate that the differences in survival are due to differences in the ability to achieve a complete surgical resection. One can easily obtain a wide margin around peripheral tumors involving the chest wall. However, the presence of many vital structures within the mediastinum limits the ability to get a wide margin around central T3 tumors. Similarly, it is difficult to achieve a wide margin when resecting Pancoast tumors. Unfortunately, there is little data either to substantiate or to refute this hypothesis. Certainly, those patients with chest wall tumors or Pancoast tumors who achieve a complete resection exhibit relatively good survival. Unfortunately, no data is available on the incidence of complete resections or their impact on survival in central T3 tumors.

One can speculate that lung cancers involving the chest wall have a better biologic behavior (less nodal spread) and can be more easily completely resected. Pancoast tumors may also have less propensity to nodal spread but pose difficulties in obtaining an R_0 (complete) resection and thus exhibit worse survival. The further reduction in survival of central T3 tumors might be due to both nodal metastases and lack of achievement of a complete resection.

T3N2 TUMORS

N2 nodal status appears to have a profound effect on survival of lung cancers, regardless of the T stage, and this is discussed in detail in Chapter 17. There is evidence that T3N2 tumors have a particularly poor prognosis. This seems to be the case even when the N2 status is discovered only at thoracotomy.[19,22] Although 5-year postoperative survival of >20% in T3N2 patients has been reported,[41–43] many other studies of T3 disease have reported no survivors at all after resection of T3N2 lesions.[6,16,19,20,22,29] The 5-year survival in 23 studies reporting on resected T3N2 patients (with all types of T3 involvement) ranges from 0 to 29%, with an average of 10%.[6,7,9,11,16,19,20,22,27,29,33,35,41–50] Given such poor survival, it seems that surgical resection as the primary treatment for T3N2 disease should be undertaken only in select circumstances.

RECURRENCE PATTERNS

Little information is available on recurrence patterns after resection of T3N0,1 lesions. The available data is shown in Table 15–9. Two studies in which most patients had a complete resection found distant recurrence to be most common.[6,51] Three other studies found a much more even distribution between local and distant recurrences.[13,21,36] In one of these studies, the majority of patients had an incomplete resection.[36] In another study, which involved tumors invading the chest wall, only extrapleural dissection was done.[21] Although the authors reported pathologically clear margins, the high local recurrence rate suggests that this type of excision may have been inadequate.

EDITORS' COMMENTS

In our opinion, T3 tumors should be considered as a separate group because the biologic behavior is probably different from that of T2N1 (stage IIb) or T1,2N2 (stage IIIa) tumors, even though the current 5-year survival rate may be similar to the rate for these groups. The major decision point is whether or not a complete resection can be accomplished. Certainly, patients with T3 lesions involving the chest wall in whom a complete resection can be done should undergo surgery. However, patients with tumors involving the mediastinal structures or main stem bronchus should be approached with caution. These patients must be carefully selected by appropriate staging studies before treatment planning.

Peripheral T3 tumors are approached the same way as most lung cancers in terms of staging. The history and physical examination is used to determine whether distant organ scanning is necessary. Enlarged mediastinal nodes should be biopsied, but a normal mediastinum with a peripheral T3 lesion probably does not warrant mediastinoscopy. On the other hand, all central T3 lesions should undergo mediastinoscopy, even if the mediastinum appears radiographically normal. This is true for tumors involving the main stem bronchus as well as tumors involving mediastinal structures. This pretreatment surgical staging should be conducted carefully to ensure that patients are not inappropriately subjected to surgical resection.

Patients with tumors involving the chest wall should undergo resection, in most cases. Every effort must be made to ensure that the resection is complete. In our opinion, an adequate margin of chest wall is approximately 2 cm above or below the most closely involved ribs. A greater margin (~5 cm) should be obtained along the length of the ribs. Occult extension of tumor within the marrow is frequently a cause for positive margins. Particu-

DATA SUMMARY: T3 TUMORS

	AMOUNT	QUALITY	CONSISTENCY
T3 (Chest Wall) Tumors			
The 5-year survival of all T3 (chest wall) patients is 40%	High	High	High
The 5-year survival of completely resected T3N0 (chest wall) patients is 50% to 60%	High	High	High
The 5-year survival of T3N1 (chest wall) patients is 20%	High	Mod	Mod
The depth of chest wall invasion affects survival	Mod	High	Mod
En bloc resection of chest wall results in better survival in patients with parietal pleural invasion	*Mod*	*High*	*High*
T3 (Mediastinum) Tumors			
The 5-year survival of T3 (mediastinum) patients is 27%	Mod	Mod	Mod
N0 versus N1 status has little prognostic effect	Mod	Poor	High
T3 (Main Stem Bronchus) Tumors			
The 5-year survival of T3 (bronchus) patients is 28%	Mod	Mod	Mod
T3 (Pancoast) Tumors			
The 5-year survival of T3 (Pancoast) patients is 30%	High	High	High
T3N2 Tumors			
Patients with T3N2 tumors have poor survival (~10%) after resection	High	Mod	High

Type of data rated: Plain text: descriptive statement   *Italics: controlled comparison*   **Bold: randomized comparison**

larly when there is clear rib invasion, a large lengthwise margin (5-10 cm) is probably warranted. If a lesion appears to be attached to the chest wall by adhesions, an extrapleural resection is reasonable. However, if there is suspicion of tumor extension into the parietal pleura, then an excision of the involved ribs should be undertaken. No adjuvant or neoadjuvant therapy is used with chest wall T3N0 tumors in our practice.

Central T3 tumors (main stem bronchus or mediastinal invasion) represent a more difficult group. For patients who have minimal mediastinal involvement, such as involvement of a small portion of mediastinal pleura or pericardium, surgery alone is a reasonable option. In actual practice, such patients are most likely to have the presence of T3 disease discovered at the time of thoracotomy. Every effort should be made to achieve a complete resection, which should not be difficult in such instances. More extensive central T3 disease, which is generally suspected preoperatively, should be approached with caution. In such patients, we would perform a head CT or magnetic resonance imaging and bone scan even in the face of a normal history and physical examination, and then proceed to mediastinoscopy if no distant metastases were found. If mediastinoscopy is negative and it appears likely that a complete resection can be achieved, then surgery for such patients appears to be indicated. Although primary resection is a reasonable option, it is also reasonable to consider preoperative therapy in such patients, with the understanding that this approach has not yet been studied adequately. However, such neoadjuvant therapy—particularly radiation above 45 Gy—may increase the morbidity following resection. If resection is to be undertaken, every effort must be made to ensure that a complete resection is achieved.

In cases in which there is significant doubt that a complete resection can be achieved, combination chemotherapy and radiation without resection should be strongly considered. Unfortunately, an exploratory thoracotomy is often necessary to establish, with confidence, resectability of central T3 lesions. If patients have been otherwise carefully scrutinized (negative distant organ scanning and negative mediastinoscopy), an exploration is reasonable despite the chance that the patient's cancer may turn out to be unresectable.

Patients with documented T3N2 disease have a poor prognosis. Such patients should be approached with combined modality treatment. It is unlikely that surgical resection is of benefit in such patients, and it should be undertaken only in very selected cases. The best treatment for these patients is probably chemotherapy and radiation.

References

1. Mountain CF. A new international staging system for lung cancer. Chest. 1986;89(suppl):225S–233S.
2. Mountain CF. Revisions in the International System for Staging Lung Cancer. Chest. 1997;111:1710–1717.
3. Detterbeck FC, Socinski MA. IIB or not IIB: the current question in staging non–small cell lung cancer. Chest. 1997;112:229–234.
4. Naruke T, Tomoyuki G, Tsuchiya R, et al. Prognosis and survival in resected lung carcinoma based on the new international staging system. J Thorac Cardiovasc Surg. 1988;96:440–447.
5. Bülzebruck H, Bopp R, Drings P, et al. New aspects in the staging of lung cancer: prospective validation of the International Union Against Cancer TNM classification. Cancer. 1992;70:1102–1110.
6. Pitz CCM, de la Riviere AB, Elbers HRJ, et al. Results of resection of T3 non–small cell lung cancer invading the mediastinum or main bronchus. Ann Thorac Surg. 1996;62:1016–1020.
7. Pitz CCM, de la Riviere AB, Elbers HRJ, et al. Surgical treatment of 125 patients with non–small cell lung cancer and chest wall involvement. Thorax. 1996;51:846–850.
8. Kotlyarov EV, Rukosuyev AA. Long-term results and patterns of disease recurrence after radical operations for lung cancer. J Thorac Cardiovasc Surg. 1991;102:24–28.
9. Watanabe Y, Shimizu J, Oda M, et al. Aggressive surgical intervention in N2 non–small cell cancer of the lung. Ann Thorac Surg. 1991;51:253–261.
10. Izbicki JR, Knoefel T, Passlick B, et al. Risk analysis and long-term survival in patients undergoing extended resection of locally advanced lung cancer. J Thorac Cardiovasc Surg. 1995;110:386–395.
11. Nakahashi H, Yasumoto K, Sugimachi K. Results of surgical treat-

ment of patients with T3 non–small cell lung cancer. Ann Thorac Surg. 1996;61:273–274.

12. Allen MS, Mathisen DJ, Grillo HC, et al. Bronchogenic carcinoma with chest wall invasion. Ann Thorac Surg. 1991;51:948–951.

13. Harpole DH Jr, Healey EA, DeCamp M Jr, et al. Chest wall invasive non–small cell lung cancer: patterns of failure and implications for a revised staging system. Ann Surg Oncol. 1996;3:261–269.

14. Mountain CF. Value of the new TNM staging system for lung cancer. Chest. 1989;96(suppl):47S–49S.

15. Nakahashi H, Yasumoto K, Ishida T, et al. Results of surgical treatment of patients with T3 non–small cell lung cancer. Ann Thorac Surg. 1988;46:178–181.

16. Ratto GB, Piacenza G, Frola C, et al. Chest wall involvement by lung cancer: computed tomographic detection and results of operation. Ann Thorac Surg. 1991;51:182–188.

17. Downey RJ, Martini N, Rusch VW, et al. Extent of chest wall invasion and survival in patients with lung cancer. Ann Thorac Surg. 1999;68:188–193.

18. McCaughan BC, Martini N, Bains MS, et al. Chest wall invasion in carcinoma of the lung: therapeutic and prognostic implications. J Thorac Cardiovasc Surg. 1985;89:836–841.

19. Paone JF, Spees EK, Newton CG, et al. An appraisal of en bloc resection of peripheral bronchogenic carcinoma involving the thoracic wall. Chest. 1982;81:203–207.

20. Shah SS, Goldstraw P. Combined pulmonary and thoracic wall resection for stage III lung cancer. Thorax. 1995;50:782–784.

21. Trastek VF, Pairolero PC, Piehler JM, et al. En bloc (non–chest wall) resection for bronchogenic carcinoma with parietal fixation. J Thorac Cardiovasc Surg. 1984;87:352–358.

22. Albertucci M, DeMeester TR, Rothberg M, et al. Surgery and the management of peripheral lung tumors adherent to the parietal pleura. J Thorac Cardiovasc Surg. 1992;103:8–13.

23. Piehler JM, Pairolero PC, Weiland LH, et al. Bronchogenic carcinoma with chest wall invasion: factors affecting survival following en bloc resection. Ann Thorac Surg. 1982;34:684–691.

24. Pairolero PC, Trastek VF, Payne WS. Treatment of bronchogenic carcinoma with chest wall invasion. Surg Clin North Am. 1987;67:959–964.

25. Mishina H, Suemasu K, Yoneyama T, et al. Surgical pathology and prognosis of the combined resection of chest wall and lung in lung cancer. Jpn J Clin Oncol. 1978;8:161–168.

26. Albain KS, Hoffman PC, Little AG, et al. Pleural involvement in stage IIIM0 non–small-cell bronchogenic carcinoma: a need to differentiate subtypes. Am J Clin Oncol. 1986;9:255–261.

27. Maggi G. Results of radical treatment of stage IIIa non–small-cell carcinoma of the lung. Eur J Cardiothorac Surg. 1988;2:329–335.

28. Watanabe Y, Shimizu J, Oda M, et al. Results of surgical treatment in patients with stage IIIA non–small-cell lung cancer. Thorac Cardiovasc Surg. 1991;39:44–49.

29. Cangemi V, Volpino P, D'Andrea N, et al. Results of surgical treatment of stage IIIA non–small cell lung cancer. Eur J Cardiothorac Surg. 1995;9:352–359.

30. Casillas M, Paris F, Tarrazona V, et al. Surgical treatment of lung carcinoma involving the chest wall. Eur J Cardiothorac Surg. 1989;3:425–429.

31. Patterson GA, Ilves R, Ginsberg RJ, et al. The value of adjuvant radiotherapy in pulmonary and chest wall resection for bronchogenic carcinoma. Ann Thorac Surg. 1982;34:692–697.

32. Weksler B, Bains M, Burt M, et al. Resection of lung cancer invading the diaphragm. J Thorac Cardiovasc Surg. 1997;114:500–501.

33. Inoue K, Sato M, Fujimura S, et al. Prognostic assessment of 1310 patients with non–small-cell lung cancer who underwent complete resection from 1980 to 1993. J Thorac Cardiovasc Surg. 1998;116:407–411.

34. Rocco G, Rendina EA, Meroni A, et al. Prognostic factors after surgical treatment of lung cancer invading the diaphragm. Ann Thorac Surg. 1999;68:2065–2068.

35. Burt ME, Pomerantz AH, Bains MS, et al. Results of surgical treatment of stage III lung cancer invading the mediastinum. Surg Clin North Am. 1987;67:987–1000.

36. Martini N, Yellin A, Ginsberg RJ, et al. Management of non–small cell lung cancer with direct mediastinal involvement. Ann Thorac Surg. 1994;58:1447–1451.

37. Okada M, Tsubota N, Yoshimura M, et al. How should interlobar pleural invasion be classified? Prognosis of resected T3 non–small cell lung cancer. Ann Thorac Surg. 1999;68:2049–2052.

38. Vogt-Moykopf I, Fritz T, Meyer G, et al. Bronchoplastic and angioplastic operation in bronchial carcinoma: long-term results of a retrospective analysis from 1973 to 1983. Intern Surg. 1986;71:211–220.

39. Detterbeck FC. Pancoast (superior sulcus) tumors. Ann Thorac Surg. 1997;63:1810–1818.

40. Ginsberg RJ, Martini N, Zaman M, et al. Influence of surgical resection and brachytherapy in the management of superior sulcus tumor. Ann Thorac Surg. 1994;57:1440–1445.

41. Martini N, Flehinger BJ, Zaman MB, et al. Results of resection in non–oat cell carcinoma of the lung with mediastinal lymph node metastases. Ann Surg. 1983;198:386–397.

42. Mountain CF. Surgery for stage IIIa-N2 non–small cell lung cancer. Cancer. 1994;73:2589–2598.

43. Neptune WB. Primary lung cancer surgery in stage II and stage III. Arch Surg. 1988;123:583–585.

44. Wada H, Tanaka F, Yanagihara K, et al. Time trends and survival after operations for primary lung cancer from 1976 through 1990. J Thorac Cardiovasc Surg. 1996;112:349–355.

45. Régnard JF, Magdeleinat P, Azoulay D, et al. Results of resection for bronchogenic carcinoma with mediastinal lymph node metastases in selected patients. Eur J Cardiothorac Surg. 1991;5:583–587.

46. Ishida T, Tateishi M, Kaneko S, et al. Surgical treatment of patients with nonsmall-cell lung cancer and mediastinal lymph node involvement. J Surg Oncol. 1990;43:161–166.

47. Maggi G, Casadio C, Cianci R, et al. Results of surgical resection of stage IIIA (N2) non–small cell lung cancer, according to the site of the mediastinal metastases. Intern Surg. 1993;78:213–217.

48. Nakanishi R, Osaki T, Nakanishi K, et al. Treatment strategy for patients with surgically discovered N2 stage IIIA non–small cell lung cancer. Ann Thorac Surg. 1997;64:342–348.

49. Vansteenkiste JF, DeLeyn PR, Deneffe GJ, et al. Survival and prognostic factors in resected N2 non–small cell lung cancer: a study of 140 cases. Ann Thorac Surg. 1997;63:1441–1450.

50. Naruke T. Significance of lymph node metastases in lung cancer. Semin Thorac Cardiovasc Surg. 1993;5:210–218.

51. López L, Pujol JL, Varela A, et al. Surgical treatment of stage III non–small cell bronchogenic carcinoma involving the chest wall. Scand J Thorac Cardiovasc Surg. 1992;26:129–133.

52. Mountain CF. Expanded possibilities for surgical treatment of lung cancer: survival in stage IIIa disease. Chest. 1990;97:1045–1051.

53. Ricci C, Rendina EA, Venuta F. En bloc resection for T3 bronchogenic carcinoma with chest wall invasion. Eur J Cardiothorac Surg. 1987;1:23–28.

54. van Velzen E, de la Riviere AB, Elbers HJJ, et al. Type of lymph node involvement and survival in pathologic N1 stage III non–small cell lung carcinoma. Ann Thorac Surg. 1999;67:903–907.

55. Sabanathan S, Richardson J, Mearns AJ, et al. Results of surgical treatment of stage III lung cancer. Eur J Cardiothorac Surg. 1994;8:183–187.

56. Deslauriers J, Mehran RJ, Guimont C, et al. Staging and management of lung cancer: sleeve resection. World J Surg. 1993;17:712–718.

57. van Rens MTM, de la Rivière AB, Elbers HRJ, et al. Prognostic assessment of 2,361 patients who underwent pulmonary resection for non–small cell lung cancer, stage I, II, and IIIA. Chest. 2000;117:374–379.

PANCOAST TUMORS

Frank C. Detterbeck, David R. Jones, and Julian G. Rosenman

DIAGNOSIS

CLINICAL STAGING

PALLIATION

TREATMENT WITH RADIATION
ALONE

TREATMENT WITH
COMBINATION RADIATION
AND SURGERY
Prognostic Factors
Sequencing and Dosing of
Combined Modality Therapy
Postoperative Radiation
Extent of Pulmonary Resection

RECURRENCE PATTERNS

CHEMOTHERAPY

EDITORS' COMMENTS

Patients with lung cancers arising in the apex of the chest generally exhibit a characteristic syndrome that is named after Henry Pancoast, a radiologist who reported on seven such cases in 1932.[1] These tumors often invade the lower portion of the brachial plexus, the upper thoracic ribs and vertebral bodies, the stellate ganglion, and the subclavian vessels. They characteristically produce arm pain and eventually numbness and weakness, particularly in the T1 and C8 nerve root distribution, as well as Horner's syndrome (Fig. 16–1). These tumors appear to invade the apical chest wall and surrounding structures early and metastasize to lymph nodes much later.

Before 1950, Pancoast tumors were found to be uniformly fatal, despite attempts at treatment with radiation or surgery.[2] What little information is available on the natural history of this disease indicates that the average survival is between 10 and 14 months after diagnosis, with most patients experiencing severe, unrelenting arm pain.[3] Thus, it is not surprising that palliative radiation of Pancoast tumors has frequently been used, and it has become clear

that in some instances radiation alone can be curative. The treatment of Pancoast tumors has been greatly affected by a report from Shaw et al[4] in 1961, in which a combination of preoperative radiation and surgical resection was used in 18 patients. At the time of the report, 12 of these patients were alive without disease up to 51 months following resection. However, follow-up was <1 year in half of the patients and <2 years in 89%.

DIAGNOSIS

In current reports, adenocarcinoma accounts for approximately two-thirds of cases of Pancoast tumors, and squamous cell cancers make up most of the remainder, with <10% being due to large cell cancers.[5,6] The incidence of small cell cancer is <5%.[7] Other lesions producing a Pancoast syndrome have been described, and these include lymphoma and plasmacytoma, as well as infections such as Staphylococcus, Cryptococcus, Echinococcus, and Acti-

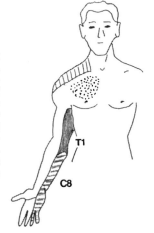
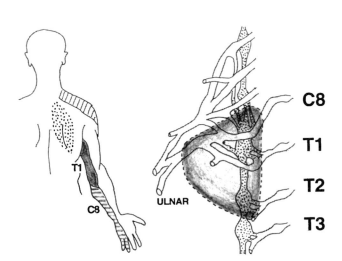

FIGURE 16–1. Nerve involvement in a typical Pancoast tumor (C8,T1,T2 lower trunk of brachial plexus, sympathetic chain). The dermatomes of C8 and T1 are illustrated, as well as areas of referred pain in the scapular and pectoral regions (mediated through different fibers of the sympathetic chain). (Reprinted with permission from the Society of Thoracic Surgeons [The Annals of Thoracic Surgery. 1997;63:1810–1818].)[59]

nomycosis.[7-10] It is standard practice in most institutions to obtain a histologic diagnosis before beginning treatment, although the incidence of lesions other than non–small cell lung cancer (NSCLC) causing Pancoast syndrome is probably small.[11] Fiberoptic bronchoscopy has achieved a diagnosis in only 30% to 40% of patients.[12-14] This is not surprising, considering the peripheral nature of these tumors. Many reports have indicated a >90% success rate using fine needle aspiration,[11,13,15] and this is generally considered to be the diagnostic procedure of choice.

CLINICAL STAGING

Little data is available to define the appropriate intrathoracic or extrathoracic staging of Pancoast tumors. Magnetic resonance imaging (MRI) scanning can provide better detail of tumor involvement around the brachial plexus and vertebral bodies than computed tomography (CT) scan.[16] The false negative rate of CT in staging mediastinal lymph nodes in peripheral T3 and T4 tumors was reported to be low by Daly et al.[17] This is the only study addressing this issue, but interpretation is difficult because the study was not limited to Pancoast tumors.

Almost no data is available about mediastinal node staging in Pancoast tumors because mediastinoscopy has not been used routinely in any of the series reported; in only one study was it done in many of the patients.[18] The incidence of N2 node involvement at the time of resection (usually after preoperative radiation) is approximately 20% in most series.[5,19,20] Because N2 patients exhibit poor survival, a pretreatment, or at least a preoperative mediastinoscopy, seems reasonable. No data is available about the false negative rate of a normal history and physical examination in excluding distant metastases in Pancoast patients.

PALLIATION

Palliation is important in a disease in which most patients present with severe arm pain. In general, good palliation is achieved in approximately 80% of patients with either radiation alone or radiation and surgery. Van Houtte et al[21] reported good palliation in 75% of patients with radiation alone. Others, using a combination of radiation and surgery, have reported excellent palliation in approximately 80% and good palliation in approximately 90% of patients.[19,22-26] The duration of palliation, when indicated, was usually either at least 1 year or the length of patient survival. There is some evidence that palliation with radiation alone may be more readily achieved when higher doses (>50 Gy) are used.[21,27] Administering higher doses increases the concern about causing a brachial plexopathy, but no data on the incidence of this complication is available.

TREATMENT WITH RADIATION ALONE

A number of series of patients with Pancoast tumors treated with radiation alone have been published, and the results of all series from 1980 to 1999 involving at least 20 patients are summarized in Table 16–1. It is unclear in most of these studies whether the radiation was given in a curative attempt or simply to palliate symptoms. Certainly in many studies, the disease appears to have been advanced, and the long-term survival is low.[6,12,13,18] However, the doses of radiation given were generally at least 50 to 60 Gray (Gy), which is higher than the doses generally used for palliation alone. Those studies that appear to have selected patients who had a reasonable chance of cure report 5-year survival rates of approximately 20%.[21,22,26,28]

Little information is available on prognostic factors in patients with Pancoast tumors as they pertain to treatment with radiation alone. The survival has not been correlated with T, N, and M stage. In fact, most reports have not even commented on the T stage, nor have they provided detailed information on the N stage. Van Houtte et al[21] reported that scalene lymph node involvement and radiographic evidence of rib destruction were poor prognostic factors, but no statistical significance was calculated. Ahmad et al[26] also suggested poorer survival when rib destruction was present, but analysis of the results is difficult because 25% of the patients underwent surgery in addition to radiation. Among patients treated with curative intent, Millar et al[28] found no survival difference with regard to vertebral body or rib involvement, but they did find a significantly poorer survival if any nodal involvement was present (3-year survival, 24% versus 10%, $P = 0.003$). Herbert et al[29] found no difference in survival among 30 patients with regard to stage (cIIIa versus cIIIb) or nodal status.

Komaki et al[6] reported on a variety of prognostic factors in a group of 85 patients with Pancoast tumors who were treated with a variety of therapies, although approximately two thirds of these patients were treated with radiation alone. Patients with a Karnofsky performance status of ≥80 clearly exhibited longer survival than patients with a poor performance status ($P < 0.0001$). Patients with <5% weight loss also had a better prognosis (2-year survival,

DATA SUMMARY: DIAGNOSIS OF PANCOAST TUMORS			
	AMOUNT	**QUALITY**	**CONSISTENCY**
Over 95% of patients with Pancoast syndrome have non–small cell lung cancer	Mod	High	High
Fine-needle aspiration has a >90% success rate in achieving a diagnosis	High	High	High

Type of data rated: Plain text: Descriptive statement   *Italics: controlled comparison*   **Bold: randomized comparison**

TABLE 16–1. SURVIVAL AFTER RADIOTHERAPY ALONE FOR PANCOAST TUMORS

STUDY	NO. OF PATIENTS TREATED	% OF ALL PATIENTS SEEN	RT (DOSE IN GRAY)	STAGE	SELECTION CRITERIA	OVERALL SURVIVAL FOR TREATED PATIENTS		
						MST (mo)	2 y (%)	5 y (%)
Millar et al[28]	78	60	~20	?	Palliative	4	6	**4**
Komaki et al[6]	56	66	70–72	52% IIIb	Inoperable, unfit	12	22	**8**
Hagan et al[39]	39	53	Palliative	38% M1	Inoperable, unfit	—	—	**7**
Attar et al[53]	37	35	60	32% IIIb, 59% IV	Inoperable, mets	6	17	**0**
Neal et al[31]	32	44	65	50% IIIb	Inoperable, unfit	14	29	**14**
Herbert et al[29]	30	Most	30–71	47% N2,3	None	10	10	—
Anderson et al[13]	27	49	45–60	?	Unfit, mets	8	—	**0**
Stanford et al[18]	25	47	Palliative	56% N2, 20% M1	Inoperable	8	12	**(5)**[a]
Schraube and Late[32]	22	46	30–61	68% IIIb	Inoperable, unfit	17	23	**0**
Strojan et al[54]	21	48	45–54	?	?	10	8	—
Average[b]						**10**	**16**	**5**
Millar et al[28c]	53	40	~60	M0	Good risk	18	35	**15**
Ahmad et al[26]	48	76	30–60	5% M1, 30% N2	—	—	28[d]	**17**[d]
Komaki et al[22]	36	100	40–64	33% N2	—	14	—	**23**
Van Houtte et al[21]	31	—	20–70	?	M0	17	25	**18**
Average						**16**	**29**	**18**

Inclusion criteria: Studies from 1980 to 2000 of ≥20 patients with Pancoast tumors treated with radiation alone.
[a]4-year survival.
[b]Excluding values in parentheses.
[c]Includes 19% who had surgical resection.
[d]Data for 63 patients, 48 of whom received RT alone, 15 of whom had RT plus surgery.

mets, distant metastases present; MST, median survival time; % of all patients seen, percentage of patients treated out of the total number of patients with Pancoast tumors seen at that institution during the study period; RT, radiotherapy; unfit, deemed unfit for surgical resection; ?, unknown.

47% versus 17%, $P < 0.0003$). Patients with vertebral involvement had a worse survival (2-year disease-free survival, 15% versus 40%, $P < 0.0006$). Similarly, patients who were stage cIIIa did better than those who were cIIIb (2-year disease-free survival, 47% versus 21%, $P = 0.004$).[6] However, these patients received a variety of treatments, and each of these prognostic factors clearly affected their selection for the type of treatment. Treatment involving surgery was clearly associated with longer survival (2-year survival, 52% versus 22%; 5-year survival, 40% versus 8%; $P < 0.004$). However, it is difficult to draw any conclusions about how to select patients for treatment or to compare treatment with radiation alone to that with surgery and radiation because information about prognostic factors within each group is not available.

In general, local control with radiation alone has been achieved in approximately one-half of patients.[7] There is some evidence that local control is higher with higher doses of radiation. Van Houtte et al[21] found that local control was better with doses above 50 Gy. Similar results were reported by Komaki et al[6] for those patients treated with radiation alone (local control for patients receiving >65 Gy or <65 Gy: 69% versus 38%; $P < 0.05$). However, Herbert et al[29] found no evidence of a dose response among <50 Gy, 50 to 60 Gy, and >60 Gy.

In an earlier study, Komaki et al[22] found that local control was improved with larger (>12 cm²) field sizes (52% versus 36%, no P value calculated). Better control was also found in patients who received continuous radiation as opposed to split course radiation (50% versus 18%, $P = 0.05$).[6] However, it is not clear that this is an independent predictor because split course radiation was more commonly used during earlier years.

DATA SUMMARY: PANCOAST TUMORS—TREATMENT WITH RADIOTHERAPY ALONE

	AMOUNT	QUALITY	CONSISTENCY
Curative radiotherapy in "good-risk" patients has a 5-year survival of 15%–20%	High	High	High
Negative Prognostic Factors			
Rib destruction is a poor prognostic factor	Mod	Mod	Mod
Vertebral body invasion *may be* a poor prognostic factor	Poor	Poor	—
N2,3 node involvement *may be* a poor prognostic factor	Poor	Poor	—
Better local control *may be* achieved with higher doses of radiotherapy	*Mod*	*Poor*	*High*

Type of data rated: Plain text: descriptive statement   *Italics: controlled comparison*   **Bold: randomized comparison**

TABLE 16–2. SURVIVAL AFTER COMBINATION RADIOTHERAPY AND SURGERY IN PANCOAST TUMORS[a]

STUDY	NO. OF PATIENTS TREATED	% OF ALL PATIENTS SEEN	TREATMENTS[b]	STAGE	% COMPLETELY RESECTED	% LIMITED RESECTION	OVERALL SURVIVAL FOR TREATED PATIENTS		
							MST (MO)	2 y (%)	5 y (%)
Hilaris et al[36]	129	—	20–40/S/RT	15% N2, 18% N3	—	—	20	38	25
Ginsberg et al[5]	124	—	~40/S	16% N2, 19% T4	56	68	17	40	26
Paulson[11]	78	—	—	—	—	—	14	38	31
Maggi et al[19]	60	83	30/S ± RT	8% N2, 28% T4	60	68	17	30	17
Sartori et al[33]	42	75	30–40/S	12% N2, 31% T4	—	83	14	33	25
Neal et al[31]	41	56	30–50/S	24% T4	<70	—	13	17	15
Ricci et al[55]	41	73	30/S ± RT	12% T4, 7% MI	54	44	—	—	22
Hagan et al[39]	34	47	40/S	12% N2,3, 18% T4	79	—	21	42	33
Dartevelle et al[35]	29	—	S/56	3% N2, 45% T4	—	48	24	50	30
Anderson et al[13]	28	51	30–45/S	18% N2	71	—	25	—	34
Attar et al[53]	28	27	30–60/S	38% IIIb	—	4	22	43	27
Komaki et al[6]	25	29	±30/S/50–60	36% IIIb	—	—	43	54	40
Harpole et al[56]	25	—	30–56/S[c]	20% N2	88	—	36	53	(38)[d]
Fuller and Chambers[30]	21	88	55–65/S	—	43	33	—	48	38
Wright et al[24]	21	—	30–45/S/± 20	All N0, 43% T4	76	18	24	52	27
Schraube and Latz[32]	20	42	18–40/S	35% IIIb, 5% M1	—	—	15	43	18
Average[e]							**22**	**42**	**27**

Inclusion criteria: All studies from 1980 to 2000 of ≥20 patients.
[a]Staging was radiographic for all except Anderson and Wright.
[b]Numbers represent dose of RT in Gray.
[c]Six had preoperative chemotherapy alone; 12 had preoperative chemotherapy and radiotherapy.
[d]4-year survival.
[e]Excluding values in parentheses.
MST, median survival time; RT, radiotherapy; S, surgery; % completely resected, percentage of patients completely resected (negative margins) out of all patients treated; % limited resection, percentage of patients who underwent surgery who had a wedge or segmentotomy.

TREATMENT WITH COMBINATION RADIATION AND SURGERY

The results of all studies from 1980 to 2000 reporting data on at least 20 patients with Pancoast tumors treated with radiation and surgery are shown in Table 16–2. The treatment has generally involved approximately 30 Gy of radiation preoperatively, although in some studies, as many as half of the patients received only postoperative radiation. The table lists data for all patients selected for treatment with preoperative radiation and surgery. In general, the number of patients who did not undergo thoracotomy because of progressive disease was small. The rate of complete resection was approximately 70%. The tumors of the remaining 30% of patients were either not resected at all, or, more commonly, they were resected but were found to have a microscopically positive margin at the time of final histological examination. Staging was generally done radiographically, and approximately 18% to 40% of patients were found to have N2 disease at the time of thoracotomy.

Five-year survival ranged from 8% to 50% for all patients who began the treatment regimen. It is not clear from examining the stage of disease why there should be such variation. A consistent definition of Pancoast tumors was used in all of the studies. Some of those studies reporting poor results (5-year survival, ≤25%) appeared to have been relatively nonselective; that is, most of the patients seen at the institution were selected for this treatment approach. In addition, in a large number of the resected patients, only a limited pulmonary resection (wedge or segmentectomy) was performed. On the other hand, some of those reporting good results (5-year survival, ≥40%)

appeared to have been fairly selective, and resections generally involved a lobectomy. However, there are several exceptions to this trend.[30-32]

Those patients who were completely resected with negative margins (R₀) showed a somewhat better 5-year survival of approximately 40% (Table 16–3). However, there is still a great deal of variation in the 5-year survival. No information is available for these patients regarding nodal status or the type of resection performed (lobectomy versus limited resection).

Prognostic Factors

By definition, Pancoast tumors are T3 lesions because they invade the parietal pleura and brachial plexus. Invasion of

TABLE 16–3. PANCOAST TUMORS TREATED WITH RADIATION AND SURGERY: SURVIVAL OF PATIENTS WHO WERE RESECTED WITH A NEGATIVE MARGIN

STUDY	N	SURVIVAL		
		MST (mo)	2 y (%)	5 y (%)
Rusch[38]	126	41	58	44
Maggi et al[19]	36	19	43	25
Muscolino et al[20]	11	23	49	35
Average[b]		**28**	**50**	**34**

Inclusion criteria: All studies from 1980 to 2000 reporting survival of completely resected patients.
[a]Absolute survival.
[b]Excluding values in parentheses.
MST, median survival time; N, number of patients completely resected.

the subclavian vessels or invasion of the vertebral bodies is defined as T4 disease and has been considered to be a poor prognostic factor in patients undergoing surgical resection. Of 22 patients with vertebral body involvement, Ginsberg et al[5] found only two 5-year survivors (9%) following resection. Others have reported no 5-year survivors,[24,33] although follow-up was incomplete in one study.[24] Komaki et al[6] reported two 4-year survivors out of 18 patients (11%), although it appears that most of these patients were treated with radiation alone. Anderson et al[13] reported significantly worse survival ($P = 0.001$) with vertebral body invasion in seven patients, but no actual survival data was given. A more aggressive approach is being explored by some groups, involving complete vertebrectomy and spinal reconstruction.[24] A 2-year actuarial survival of 54% has been reported in 17 such patients.[34] Thus, although vertebral body invasion may not preclude successful resection entirely, it is certainly a major negative prognostic factor.

Subclavian artery involvement is also a major negative prognostic factor. One study reported one of four patients alive at 2 years or longer,[24] and another reported one of five patients alive at 2 years.[33] Only Dartevelle et al,[35] whose anterior approach makes resection of Pancoast tumors with vascular involvement easier, reported 5-year survival after subclavian vessel resection (30% actuarial 5-year survival for 12 patients).

Some controversy exists about the importance of actual rib destruction by tumor. Shahian et al[23] reported no difference in survival with or without rib involvement (5-year survival, 53% versus 56%). Sartori et al[33] found 2-year survival with rib involvement to be slightly inferior to survival without rib involvement (45% versus 55%, no P value calculated). Komaki et al[6] found 2-year survival with rib involvement to be significantly inferior to survival without rib involvement (25% versus 37%, $P = 0.014$), although many of their patients were treated with radiation only. Muscolino et al[20] found no 2-year survivors among five patients with first rib involvement, but four of five had either N2 disease or incomplete resection. An example of the negative prognostic implications of vertebral body,

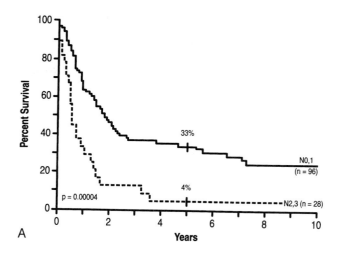

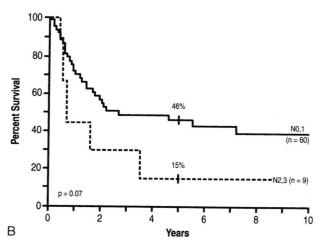

FIGURE 16–3. *A,* Survival by nodal status for entire patient cohort. *B,* Survival by nodal status for completely resected patients. (Reprinted with permission from the Society of Thoracic Surgeons [The Annals of Thoracic Surgery. 1994;57:1440–1445].)[5]

subclavian vessel, or rib involvement is shown in Figure 16–2.

Mediastinal lymph node involvement has been found to be a strong negative prognostic factor in a large number of studies involving resection of Pancoast tumors.[5,11,13,20,23,33,36,37] One study suggested that there was no difference in survival of N2 versus N0 patients, but this study involved only five N2 patients.[19] An example of the difference in survival, taken from one of the largest studies, is shown in Figure 16–3. Similar survival curves were found by other large series.[33,36,38] Although the 15% 5-year survival for N2,3 patients shown in Figure 16–3*B* may seem reasonable, *this is a select group* because only approximately one-third of the N2 patients actually underwent a complete resection. In fact, in six studies totaling 75 resected N2,3 patients, only six (8%) were found to be 4-year survivors.[5,11,23,33,36,37] Pretreatment mediastinoscopy was not performed routinely in any of these studies. Therefore, the N2 involvement was found at the time of thoracotomy, often after preoperative radiation. Although such N2,3 involvement does not absolutely preclude long-term survival, it certainly represents a

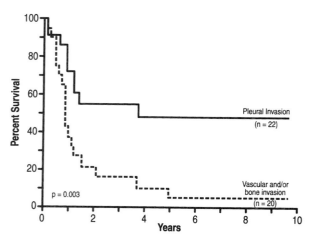

FIGURE 16–2. Survival of patients with Pancoast's tumor who had only pleural invasion compared with those with vascular invasion, bone invasion, or both ($P = 0.003$). (From Sartori F, Rea F, Calabró F, et al. Carcinoma of the superior pulmonary sulcus: results of irradiation and radical resection. J Thorac Cardiovasc Surg. 1992;104:679–683.)[33]

major negative prognostic factor similar to that for other T3N2 tumors.

There is some evidence that patients with ipsilateral supraclavicular node (N3) involvement have a better prognosis than patients with ipsilateral mediastinal node (N2) involvement.[5,36] Ginsberg et al[5] found a 5-year survival of 14% of patients with N3 node involvement as opposed to 0% in patients with N2 node involvement. Similarly, Hilaris et al[36] found a median survival of 13 months for 23 N3 patients, as compared with 9 months for 19 N2 patients. Both of these studies are from the same institution, and there is some overlap between the patient cohorts. Other studies have not differentiated between patients with N2 and N3 node involvement. It may be that for Pancoast tumors, ipsilateral supraclavicular node involvement represents local limited nodal extension, whereas in other lung cancers, supraclavicular node involvement represents extensive nodal metastases.

The presence of Horner's syndrome appears to be a negative prognostic factor in resected patients.[5,13,33,39] Sartori et al[33] found a 5-year survival of 8% in 15 patients with Horner's syndrome, as opposed to 35% in 27 patients without the syndrome ($P = 0.05$). Ginsberg et al[5] found a 5-year survival of 13% in 30 patients with Horner's syndrome, in contrast to 26% for the overall population of 124 Pancoast patients (no P value calculated). It is not clear that histology plays a role. Hilaris et al[36] found better survival among 129 patients with adenocarcinomas than patients with squamous cell cancers (median survival time, 25 months versus 14 months, $P = 0.005$). However, Shahian et al[23] found the opposite trend in a much smaller group of 18 patients, with a 5-year survival of 75% for patients with squamous cell cancers versus 53% for those with adenocarcinomas ($P = NS$).

Sequencing and Dosing of Combined Modality Therapy

Ever since the report by Shaw et al[4] in 1961, 30 to 40 Gy of preoperative radiation has commonly been used. However, the sequencing and dosage of combined modality therapy have never been examined in a randomized fashion. Ginsberg et al[5] stated that in their experience with 124 patients, preoperative radiation was no more effective than postoperative radiation. However, no actual data was provided that demonstrated this. A review suggested that preoperative radiation produces results similar to postoperative radiation, but it did not include corroborating data.[7]

The most controlled data available examining the value of preoperative radiation is shown in Figure 16–4. The patients for whom data is shown in this figure are stratified by nodal involvement, which appears to be the most important prognostic factor. The data in this figure show that preoperative radiation, when controlled for nodal involvement, appears to be of benefit for each nodal stage. The use of preoperative radiation was a significant prognostic factor in univariate analysis (median survival with versus without preoperative radiation, 23 months versus 14 months; $P = 0.05$) and in multivariate analysis.[36] The only other significant factor in the multivariate analysis was the mediastinal node status. The use of brachytherapy and postoperative radiation did not make a significant differ-

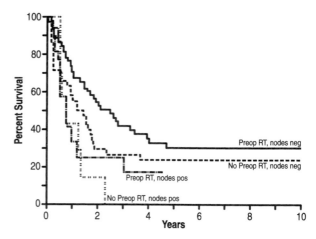

FIGURE 16–4. Survival according to mediastinal node status in 128 patients with superior sulcus tumor who did or did not receive preoperative radiation. Preop, preoperative; nodes neg/pos, mediastinal nodes negative or positive for cancerous involvement; RT, radiotherapy. (From Hilaris BS, Martini N, Wong GY, et al. Treatment of superior sulcus tumor [Pancoast tumor]. Surg Clin North Am. 1987;67:965–977.)[36]

ence. This was a retrospective study, however. No information can be gleaned from this report about other factors that may have affected the results and may have led to erroneous conclusions concerning preoperative radiation.

Higher doses of radiation have been used only sporadically. Attar et al[12] found an increased morbidity with the use of 55 Gy preoperatively in 13 patients (23% bronchopleural fistula; 15% mortality). However, Fuller et al[30] used the same dose of radiation preoperatively on 21 patients and found no major complications and only 1 death (8%), which was due to a stroke. Higher doses of radiation do not appear to enhance resectability or survival in these reports.[12,30]

Given the location of Pancoast tumors, it is not surprising that in a significant number of attempted resections, achieving a complete resection with an adequate margin is difficult. The most common sites of residual gross or microscopic tumor are along the cords of the brachial plexus, the neural foramina, the vertebral bodies, and the subclavian vessels.[19,20] Not surprisingly, this has a significant effect on 5-year survival[5,19,20,23,38,40] (Fig. 16–5). The largest series reported a 5-year survival of 44% in completely resected versus 14% in incompletely resected patients.[38]

Niwa et al[40] reported a 2-year survival of 60% in 11 completely resected (R_0) patients, as opposed to 0 of 10 patients with a positive margin ($P < 0.01$). Muscolino et al[20] found no 2-year survivors among four incompletely resected (R_1) patients. Maggi et al[19] reported a 2-year survival of 43% in 36 completely resected patients, as opposed to 11% in 24 patients with a positive surgical margin ($P < 0.025$). Shahian et al[23] found a slight difference in survival for R_0 versus R_1 resection (5-year survival, 62% versus 50%), but there was no statistical significance in this small study (N = 18). From Ginsberg's analysis, it appears that there is little difference between an incomplete resection and no resection at all, which is similar to the findings for resection of NSCLCs in general.[5,41] The results reported by Maggi et al,[19] Niwa et al,[40] and Muscolino et al[20] appear to corroborate this, although the good 5-year

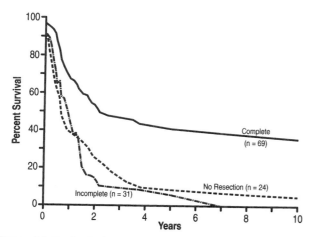

FIGURE 16–5. Survival of 124 patients with superior sulcus tumors. (Incomplete resection curve estimated from reported data of overall group and those with complete resection or no resection.) (Adapted with permission from the Society of Thoracic Surgeons [The Annals of Thoracic Surgery. 1994;57:1440–1445].)[5]

survival reported by Shahian et al[23] with a microscopically positive margin is somewhat at odds with this. At any rate, it appears that every attempt should be made intraoperatively to achieve a complete resection.

Postoperative Radiation

Although postoperative radiation has been used in a number of institutions, its use has generally been inconsistent, and this hampers interpretation of the results. In a large series of completely resected patients from the Memorial Sloan-Kettering Cancer Center who received postoperative brachytherapy, a trend toward worse survival with brachytherapy was seen, but the difference was not statistically significant (Fig. 16–6).[5] This implies a selection bias in this retrospective series, as well as little benefit to the brachytherapy.

In the patients who had incomplete resections in this

same center, postoperative brachytherapy was used in practically all patients, but it appears to have been of little benefit (see Fig. 16–5). In the series by Maggi et al,[19] the patients with incomplete resections also had a poor survival rate. Although not stated explicitly, it appears that only about half of these patients received postoperative external beam radiotherapy (RT). Similarly, the use of brachytherapy in the series reported by Hilaris et al[36] made no difference in survival (median survival, 19 months versus 16 months, P = NS). This series included 129 patients, all of whom had thoracotomy but only 63% of whom had a resection. On the other hand, Shahian et al[23] reported a 5-year survival of 50% in nine patients who had a positive margin, all of whom were treated with postoperative radiation (usually 30-35 Gy, after a preoperative dose of 30-40 Gy). A 5-year survival of 50% was also reported by Hagan et al[39] among 14 patients with either a close or positive margin, all of whom received postoperative RT. Thus, the available data does not clearly show a benefit to postoperative radiation in either completely resected or incompletely resected patients.

Extent of Pulmonary Resection

Pancoast tumors have often been viewed as exhibiting early local invasion with a late propensity to spread along lymph node chains,[11] and controversy exists about whether a wedge resection or formal lobectomy should be performed. Shahian et al[23] reported a better 5-year survival in nine patients undergoing limited resection (63% versus 49%), but the difference was not statistically significant. The only larger study addressing this question was reported by Ginsberg et al[5] (Fig. 16–7). In 69 patients who underwent a complete en bloc resection, a survival benefit was seen in patients who underwent a formal lobectomy (60% versus 33%, P = 0.039). Furthermore, the local recurrence rate was reduced after complete resection involving a lobectomy (23% versus 38%, no P value calculated).[5] Thus, it appears that every attempt should be made to perform a

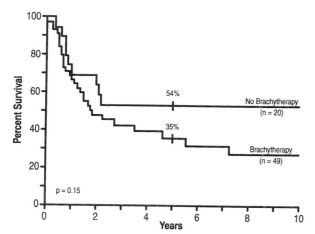

FIGURE 16–6. Survival according to the use of brachytherapy in completely resected patients. (Reprinted with permission from the Society of Thoracic Surgeons [The Annals of Thoracic Surgery. 1994;57:1440–1445].)[5]

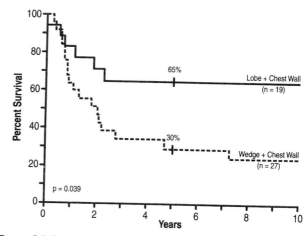

FIGURE 16–7. Survival for completely resected patients according to the extent of pulmonary resection. (Reprinted with permission from the Society of Thoracic Surgeons [The Annals of Thoracic Surgery. 1994;57:1440–1445].)[5]

DATA SUMMARY: PANCOAST TUMORS TREATED WITH RADIOTHERAPY AND SURGERY

	AMOUNT	QUALITY	CONSISTENCY
RT and surgery results in a 5-year survival of 30% (20%–40%)	High	High	Mod
The 5-year survival for completely resected (R_0) patients is 40%	High	High	Mod
About one-third of patients in RT and surgery series are T4	High	High	Mod
About 10%–20% of patients in RT and surgery series are N2,3	High	High	Mod
The rate of complete (R_0) resection is 66%	High	High	Mod
Prognostic Factors for RT and Surgery			
Vertebral body invasion is a poor prognostic factor	High	Mod	High
Subclavian artery invasion is a poor prognostic factor	Mod	Mod	Mod
Rib involvement is a poor prognostic factor	Mod	Mod	Poor
N2,3 node involvement is a poor prognostic factor	High	High	High
Ipsilateral N3 involvement may be a better prognostic factor than N2 involvement	Poor	High	High
Horner's syndrome is a poor prognostic factor	Mod	High	High
Technical Aspects of RT and Surgery			
Preoperative RT is better than initial surgery ± RT	*Poor*	*Mod*	—
An incomplete (R_{1-2}) resection is of little benefit	High	High	Mod
Postoperative RT is not beneficial in patients with an R_0 resection	*Poor*	*Poor*	—
Postoperative RT is not beneficial in patients with an R_{1-2} resection	*High*	*Poor*	*Mod*
Lobectomy may result in better survival than limited resection	*Mod*	*Mod*	*Poor*

Type of data rated: Plain text: descriptive statement   *Italics: controlled comparison*   **Bold: randomized comparison**

complete resection of the tumor, including a lobectomy, rather than a wedge resection.

RECURRENCE PATTERNS

A summary of recurrence patterns is shown in Table 16–4. However, this data must be viewed with caution because in most studies, recurrence data is inconsistently and loosely reported. For example, recurrences have generally been reported with little regard to length of follow-up or number of patients at risk. In addition, these studies rarely state clearly whether *recurrence* means the first site of recurrence, any recurrence at any time, or recurrence as a cause of death. The data shown in Table 16–4 represents an effort to glean whatever information can be obtained from all of the papers on Pancoast tumors reporting any recurrence data, but some inaccuracies may be present because of the inconsistent and ambiguous way the data has been reported in individual papers.

From the data in Table 16–4, it is apparent that approximately two-thirds of patients experience a recurrence.

TABLE 16–4. RECURRENCE PATTERNS IN PANCOAST TUMORS

STUDY	N	TREATMENT	DEF OF RECUR	% OF ALL PATIENTS RECUR	LR	LR + D	D	(%) OF ALL RECUR LR	LR + D	D
Hilaris et al[36]	129	RT/S[b]	First	81	36	—	45	**44**	—	**56**
Ginsberg et al[5]	124	RT/S	First	76	51	4	21	**67**	5	**28**
Rusch[38]	101	RT/S	First	67	32	4	25	**52**	7	**41**
Komaki et al[6]	85	RT[a]	First	58	39	—	19	**67**	—	**33**
Komaki et al[22]	36	RT	Any	70	28	25	17	**40**	36	**24**
Van Houtte et al[21]	31	RT	Any	71	32	13	26	**45**	18	**37**
Beyer et al[57]	28	RT/±S[c]	Any	77	52	20	8	**65**	25	**10**
Harpole et al[56]	25	Ch/RT/S	Any	52	4	4	44	**8**	8	**84**
Maggi et al[19]	60	RT/S	Death	65	15	—	50	**23**	—	**77**
Devine et al[58]	50	RT/S[d]	Death	70	40	8	22	**57**	11	**31**
Sartori et al[33]	42	RT/S	Death	54	21	—	33	**39**	—	**61**

Inclusion criteria: Studies from 1980 to 2000 of ≥20 Pancoast patients, reporting recurrence data.
[a]36% had thoracotomy but no resection.
[b]30% had RT/S.
[c]46% had only RT.
[d]20% had only RT.
Ch, chemotherapy; D, distant only; Def, definition; LR, locoregional only; LR + D, combination of locoregional and distant; Recur, recurrence; RT, radiotherapy; S, surgery.

When first site of recurrence is analyzed, it appears that the recurrence is locoregional in approximately two-thirds of patients, as well. Not surprisingly, when any recurrence at any time is reported, recurrences are distributed much more evenly among the categories, with many more patients having both local and distant recurrences. However, locoregional recurrence still remains the most common single category. Distant recurrences appear to be much more important as a cause of death, although approximately one-third of patients die of local disease.

It is difficult to draw any further conclusions. The two studies that have shown surprisingly low overall recurrence rates have employed both preoperative and postoperative RT as well as resection.[23,30] In one of these studies, the local recurrence rate appeared to be low,[23] but this was not the case in the other study.[30] Furthermore, postoperative brachytherapy was employed in most patients at Memorial Sloan-Kettering but without an apparent benefit in either the overall recurrence rate or the percentage of local recurrences.[5]

There is no obvious difference in the local recurrence rate between studies that have employed radiation alone as the primary modality and studies that have used both RT and surgery. Maggi et al[19] reported local recurrence as the cause of death in only 3% of 36 patients who had undergone complete tumor resection. However, Ginsberg et al,[5] who reported first site of recurrence, found that even in 69 completely resected patients with negative margins, two-thirds of the recurrences were locoregional. Thus, it is not clear that good locoregional control can be achieved even with preoperative radiation and a complete resection.

The most common site of distant metastases appears to be the brain, accounting for 40% to 80% of distant recurrences.[5,6,19,22,36,37] In one carefully analyzed study of 68 patients treated with radiation alone, 53% of the patients developed brain metastases by 3 years.[25] Bone metastases appear to be the second most common site of distant disease.[6,36,37] New primary lung tumors have been described sporadically.[19,21,30,33]

CHEMOTHERAPY

An extensive body of literature exists relating to chemotherapy with radiation and/or surgery in IIIa,b disease (non-Pancoast) involving mediastinal nodes (N2,3), including randomized studies that show improved survival.[42–45] In particular, the use of concurrent chemotherapy and radiation has resulted in better local control, presumably due to the radiation-sensitizing effects of the chemotherapy.[46–49]

Such an approach followed by resection has yielded exciting results (2-year survival, 40%) in non-Pancoast patients with pathologically proven mediastinal node involvement.[50]

Concurrent chemotherapy (cisplatin, etoposide) and radiation (45 Gy) followed by surgery has been used in 111 patients with Pancoast tumors in a more recently completed multi-institutional protocol.[51] Three deaths occurred during the induction chemotherapy, and the operative mortality was 2%, which is similar to series not involving chemotherapy. Resection was carried out in 75% of all patients entered in the trial, and the 2-year survival was 55% for all patients. Of the patients undergoing surgery, 34% had no pathologically identifiable tumor remaining, and 31% had only minimal microscopic foci. The rate of complete resection was 92% of those undergoing surgery, which is much higher than the rate in other series. Local recurrence accounted for only 23% of all recurrences, while combined recurrences accounted for 10% and distant recurrences 66%. Almost two-thirds of the distant recurrences involved the brain only.[51] The high rate of complete resection, a high pathologic complete response, a low local recurrence rate, and good intermediate-term survival were corroborated by another, smaller study involving 17 patients.[52]

EDITORS' COMMENTS

The defining characteristic of a Pancoast tumor, in our opinion, is the invasion of the apical chest wall, making it difficult to achieve an R_0 resection. Therefore, we consider all patients with a mass arising in the apex of the chest with no intervening lung to have Pancoast tumors. This is true whether or not the patient is having pain typical of Pancoast syndrome. Because actual rib involvement can be difficult to see radiographically, we do not require evidence of rib destruction but rather proximity close enough to the apical structures (ribs, subclavian vessels, brachial plexus) to make resection difficult. We generally obtain a tissue diagnosis by fine-needle biopsy because it is easy to do, but we would be willing to forego this in a patient with a typical appearance and presentation because the incidence of lesions other than NSCLC in this setting is <5%.

We biopsy any palpable supraclavicular nodes and perform mediastinoscopy, even in the face of a negative mediastinum by CT scan. Patients who are being considered for resection undergo an MRI for better planning of the operative approach. We obtain brain and bone scans only if there is suspicion of distant metastasis by history and physical examination. Patients with distant metastases or who are

DATA SUMMARY: PANCOAST TUMORS—RECURRENCE PATTERNS			
	AMOUNT	QUALITY	CONSISTENCY
About two-thirds of patients experience a recurrence	High	High	Mod
About two-thirds of recurrences are local	High	High	Mod
There is little difference in the recurrence pattern between RT alone and RT and surgery	*Mod*	*Poor*	*High*
About two-thirds of deaths are due to systemic disease	High	Mod	Mod

Type of data rated: Plain text: descriptive statement   *Italics: controlled comparison*   **Bold: randomized comparison**

otherwise not candidates for a curative approach receive 30 Gy of radiation to the primary tumor in 300 cGy fractions. Patients who have mediastinal node involvement but are otherwise good candidates are treated with a curative approach involving combination RT and chemotherapy such as would be done for patients with other unresectable locally advanced lung cancers. Patients with Pancoast tumors have traditionally been excluded from trials involving locally advanced NSCLC, but there is no basis for excluding such N2-positive Pancoast patients from what has become standard therapy for locally advanced lung cancer.

The data for chemoradiotherapy followed by surgery shows that the rate of complete resection and the local control rate are improved compared with surgery alone. Although randomized studies are not available, the data is suggestive that chemoradiotherapy is also associated with better survival. This is corroborated by studies involving non-Pancoast stage III NSCLC. Because randomized studies are not likely ever to be able to be conducted in Pancoast tumors, we believe that the available data establishes chemoradiotherapy followed by surgery as the new standard of care.

In patients who are not candidates for chemotherapy, we recommend treatment with a classic combination therapy approach of 46 Gy of radiation (200 cGy fractions) followed by resection. The mediastinum is not radiated. Resection should involve a lobectomy, and every attempt must be made intraoperatively to achieve an R_0 resection. We prefer the classic posterior approach for tumors involving the posterior ribs and the anterior (Dartevelle) approach in patients with tumors involving the anterior half of the first rib or if there is a suspicion of subclavian vessel involvement. Postoperative radiation is not routinely given, except for palliative reasons or if the patient did not receive preoperative radiation. Patients who have a positive resection margin may be given postoperative radiation but with the realization that there is little evidence to suggest that this is beneficial.

We consider a combined modality approach to be reasonable in patients with minimal subclavian vessel or vertebral body involvement. Surgery should not be considered in patients for whom there are significant doubts about the ability to achieve a complete (R_0) resection. This assessment should be based on the original MRI scan; shrinkage of the tumor after radiation does not change which tissues should be resected. However, with preoperative chemoradiotherapy, the ability to achieve a complete resection is improved. It is reasonable, in our opinion, to consider surgery for patients with supraclavicular node involvement if the mediastinal nodes and distant organ scans are negative. However, the benefit of an operative approach in this situation is not clear, and this fact must be presented to the patient.

References

1. Pancoast HK. Superior pulmonary sulcus tumor: tumor characterized by pain, Horner's syndrome, destruction of bone and atrophy of hand muscles. JAMA. 1932;99:1391–1396.
2. Walker JE. Superior sulcus pulmonary tumor (Pancoast syndrome). J Med Assoc Ga. 1946;35:364–365.
3. Paulson DL. Carcinoma of the lung. Curr Probl Surg. 1967;4:1–64.
4. Shaw RR, Paulson DL, Kee JL Jr. Treatment of the superior sulcus tumor by irradiation followed by resection. Ann Surg. 1961;154:29–40.
5. Ginsberg RJ, Martini N, Zaman M, et al. Influence of surgical resection and brachytherapy in the management of superior sulcus tumor. Ann Thorac Surg. 1994;57:1440–1445.
6. Komaki R, Mountain CF, Holbert JM, et al. Superior sulcus tumors: treatment selection and results for 85 patients without metastasis (M0) at presentation. Int J Radiat Oncol Biol Phys. 1990;19:31–36.
7. Komaki R. Preoperative radiation therapy for superior sulcus lesions. Chest Surg Clin N Am. 1991;1:13–33.
8. Mills PR, Han LY, Dick R, et al. Pancoast syndrome caused by a high grade B cell lymphoma. Thorax. 1994;49:92–93.
9. Mitchell DH, Sorrell TC. Pancoast's syndrome due to pulmonary infection with Cryptococcus neoformans variety gattii. Clin Infect Dis. 1992;14:1142–1144.
10. Gallagher KJ, Jeffrey RR, Kerr KM, et al. Pancoast syndrome: an unusual complication of pulmonary infection by Staphylococcus aureus. Ann Thorac Surg. 1992;53:903–904.
11. Paulson DL. The "superior sulcus" lesion. In: Delarue N, Eschapasse H, eds. International Trends in General Thoracic Surgery. Philadelphia, Pa: WB Saunders; 1985:121–131.
12. Attar S, Miller JE, Satterfield J, et al. Pancoast's tumor: irradiation or surgery? Ann Thorac Surg. 1979;28:578–586.
13. Anderson TM, Moy PM, Holmes EC. Factors affecting survival in superior sulcus tumors. J Clin Oncol. 1986;4:1598–1603.
14. Maxfield RA, Aranda CP. The role of fiberoptic bronchoscopy and transbronchial biopsy in the diagnosis of Pancoast's tumor. N Y State J Med. 1987;87:326–329.
15. Walls WJ, Thornbury JI, Naylor B. Pulmonary needle aspiration biopsy in the diagnosis of Pancoast tumors. Radiology. 1974;111:99–102.
16. Heelan RT, Demas BE, Caravelli JF, et al. Superior sulcus tumors: CT and MR imaging. Radiology. 1989;170:637–641.
17. Daly BDT, Mueller JD, Faling LJ, et al. N2 lung cancer: outcome in patients with false-negative computed tomographic scans of the chest. J Thorac Cardiovasc Surg. 1993;105:904–911.
18. Stanford W, Barnes RP, Tucker AR. Influence of staging in superior sulcus (Pancoast) tumors of the lung. Ann Thorac Surg. 1980;29:406–409.
19. Maggi G, Casadio C, Pischedda F, et al. Combined radiosurgical treatment of Pancoast tumor. Ann Thorac Surg. 1994;57:198–202.
20. Muscolino G, Valente M, Andreani S. Pancoast tumours: clinical assessment and long term results of combined radiosurgical treatment. Thorax. 1997;52:284–286.
21. Van Houtte P, MacLennan I, Poulter C, et al. External radiation in the management of superior sulcus tumor. Cancer. 1984;54:223–227.
22. Komaki R, Roh J, Cox JD, et al. Superior sulcus tumors: results of irradiation of 36 patients. Cancer. 1981;48:1563–1568.
23. Shahian DM, Neptune WB, Ellis FH Jr. Pancoast tumors: improved survival with preoperative and postoperative radiotherapy. Ann Thorac Surg. 1987;43:32–38.
24. Wright CD, Moncure AC, Shepard JO, et al. Superior sulcus lung tumors: results of combined treatment (irradiation and radical resection). J Thorac Cardiovasc Surg. 1987;94:69–74.
25. Komaki R, Derus SB, Perez-Tamayo C, et al. Brain metastasis in patients with superior sulcus tumors. Cancer. 1987;59:1649–1653.
26. Ahmad K, Fayos JV, Kirsh MM. Apical lung carcinoma. Cancer. 1984;54:913–917.
27. Morris RW, Abadir R. Pancoast tumor: the value of high dose radiation therapy. Radiology. 1979;132:717–719.
28. Millar J, Ball D, Worotniuk V, et al. Radiation treatment of superior sulcus lung carcinoma. Australas Radiol. 1996;40:55–60.
29. Herbert SH, Curran WJ Jr, Stafford PM, et al. Comparison of outcome between clinically staged, unresected superior sulcus tumors and other stage III non–small cell lung carcinomas treated with radiation therapy alone. Cancer. 1992;69:363–369.
30. Fuller DB, Chambers JS. Superior sulcus tumors: combined modality. Ann Thorac Surg. 1994;57:1133–1139.
31. Neal CR, Amdur RJ, Mendenhall WM, et al. Pancoast tumor: radiation therapy alone versus preoperative radiation therapy and surgery. Int J Radiat Oncol Biol Phys. 1991;21:651–660.
32. Schraube P, Latz D. Wertigkeit Strahlentherapie bei der Behandlung des Pancoast-Tumors der Lunge. Strahlenther Onkol. 1993;169:265–269.

33. Sartori F, Rea F, Calabrï F, et al. Carcinoma of the superior pulmonary sulcus: results of irradiation and radical resection. J Thorac Cardiovasc Surg. 1992;104:679–683.

34. Gandhi S, Walsh GL, Komaki R, et al. A multidisciplinary surgical approach to superior sulcus tumors with vertebral invasion. Ann Thorac Surg. 1999;68:1778–1785.

35. Dartevelle PG, Chapelier AR, Macchiarini P, et al. Anterior transcervical-thoracic approach for radical resection of lung tumors invading the thoracic inlet. J Thorac Cardiovasc Surg. 1993;105:1025–1034.

36. Hilaris BS, Martini N, Wong GY, et al. Treatment of superior sulcus tumor (Pancoast tumor). Surg Clin North Am. 1987;67:965–977.

37. Miller JI, Mansour KA, Hatcher CR Jr. Carcinoma of the superior pulmonary sulcus. Ann Thorac Surg. 1979;28:44–47.

38. Rusch VW, Parekh KR, Leon L, et al. Factors determining outcomes after surgical resection of T3 and T4 lung cancers of the superior sulcus. J Thorac Cardiovasc Surg. 2000; 119:1147–1153.

39. Hagan MP, Choi NC, Mathisen DJ, et al. Superior sulcus lung tumors: impact of local control on survival. J Thorac Cardiovasc Surg. 1999;117:1086–1094.

40. Niwa H, Masaoka A, Yamakawa Y, et al. Surgical therapy for apical invasive lung cancer: different approaches according to tumor location. Lung Cancer. 1993;10:63–71.

41. Hara N, Ohta M, Tanaka K, et al. Assessment of the role of surgery for stage III bronchogenic carcinoma. J Surg Oncol. 1984;25:153–158.

42. Roth JA, Fossella F, Komaki R, et al. A randomized trial comparing perioperative chemotherapy and surgery with surgery alone in resectable stage IIIA non–small-cell lung cancer. J Natl Cancer Inst. 1994;86:673–680.

43. Rosell R, Gómez-Codina J, Camps C, et al. A randomized trial comparing preoperative chemotherapy plus surgery with surgery alone in patients with non–small-cell lung cancer. N Engl J Med. 1994;330:153–158.

44. Dillman RO, Seagren SL, Propert KJ, et al. A randomized trial of induction chemotherapy plus high-dose radiation versus radiation alone in stage III non–small-cell lung cancer. N Engl J Med. 1990;323:940–945.

45. Le Chevalier T, Arriagada R, Quoix E, et al. Radiotherapy alone versus combined chemotherapy and radiotherapy in nonresectable non–small-cell lung cancer: first analysis of a randomized trial in 353 patients. J Natl Cancer Inst. 1991;83:417–423.

46. Schaake-Koning C, van den Bogaert W, Dalesio O, et al. Effects of concomitant cisplatin and radiotherapy on inoperable non–small-cell lung cancer. N Engl J Med. 1992;326:524–530.

47. Soresi E, Clerici M, Grilli R, et al. A randomized clinical trial comparing radiation therapy v radiation therapy plus cis-Dichlorodiammine platinum (II) in the treatment of locally advanced non–small cell lung cancer. Semin Oncol. 1988;15:20–25.

48. Jeremic B, Shibamoto Y, Acimovic L, et al. Randomized trial of hyperfractionated radiation therapy with or without concurrent chemotherapy for stage III non–small-cell lung cancer. J Clin Oncol. 1995;13:452–458.

49. Jeremic B, Shibamoto Y, Acimovic L, et al. Hyperfractionated radiation therapy with or without concurrent low-dose daily carboplatin/ etoposide for stage III non–small-cell lung cancer: a randomized study. J Clin Oncol. 1996;14:1065–1070.

50. Rusch VW, Albain KS, Crowley JJ, et al. Surgical resection of stage IIIA and stage IIIB non–small-cell lung cancer after concurrent induction chemoradiotherapy: a Southwest Oncology Group trial. J Thorac Cardiovasc Surg. 1993;105:97–106.

51. Rusch V. Induction chemoradiation and surgical resection for NSCLC of the superior sulcus. J Thorac Cardiovasc Surg. In press.

52. Martínez-Monge R, Herreros J, Aristu JJ, et al. Combined treatment in superior sulcus tumors. Am J Clin Oncol. 1994;17:317–322.

53. Attar S, Krasna MJ, Sonett JR, et al. Superior sulcus (Pancoast) tumor: experience with 105 patients. Ann Thorac Surg. 1998;66:193–198.

54. Strojan P, Debevec M, Kovac V. Superior sulcus tumor (SST): management at the Institute of Oncology in Ljubljana, Slovenia, 1981–1994. Lung Cancer. 1997;17:249–259.

55. Ricci C, Rendina EA, Venuta F, et al. Superior pulmonary sulcus tumors: radical resection and palliative treatment. Int Surg. 1989;74:175–179.

56. Harpole DH Jr, Healey EA, DeCamp M Jr, et al. Chest wall invasive non–small cell lung cancer: patterns of failure and implications for a revised staging system. Ann Surg Oncol. 1996;3:261–269.

57. Beyer DC, Weisenburger T. Superior sulcus tumors. Am J Clin Oncol. 1986;9:156–161.

58. Devine JW, Mendenhall WM, Million RR, et al. Carcinoma of the superior pulmonary sulcus treated with surgery and/or radiation therapy. Cancer. 1986;57:941–943.

59. Detterbeck FC. Pancoast (superior sulcus) tumors. Ann Thorac Surg. 1997;63:1810–1818.

SURGICAL TREATMENT OF STAGE IIIA(N2) NON–SMALL CELL LUNG CANCER

Frank C. Detterbeck and David R. Jones

DEFINITION OF PATIENT GROUPS

NATURAL HISTORY

PREOPERATIVE PATIENT SELECTION

Resectability
Benefit of Resection

OPERATIVE FACTORS
Prognostic Factors
Surgical Issues

RECURRENCE PATTERNS

EDITORS' COMMENTS

Stage IIIa non–small cell lung cancer (NSCLC) is a heterogeneous group. Until 1997, this stage included T3N0 lesions, and most published reports of resected stage IIIa patients include such patients. Largely because of extensive evidence that patients with T3N0,1 lesions exhibit different survival from the patients who are stage IIIa by virtue of N2 disease,[1–5] this subset was removed from stage IIIa in the most recent revision of the staging system.[6] T3N1 patients are still included, but the biologic behavior of this group may also be different from that of patients with mediastinal node involvement. Because of this, the treatment of patients with T3N0,1 disease is reviewed separately in Chapter 15, and this discussion deals only with patients with T1-3N2 disease.

The published data about surgically treated stage IIIa(N2) patients primarily involves retrospective analyses of long-term survival of such patients. This data must be examined carefully before using it to make generalizations because it suffers from several shortcomings. Most importantly, attention must be given to the effect of a *diminishing denominator,* meaning that as an increasingly select subgroup is culled from a population, the survival of the subgroup (but not the population as a whole) becomes more and more favorable. The criteria that define the subgroup are also important. Often, in retrospective series, the characteristic that is used to define the subgroup is the fact that the survival was better. In other series, only vague descriptions are provided. Such data is of limited use to prospectively guide the management of patients. The patients included in a study must be clearly defined by criteria that can be readily identified preoperatively.

The main purpose of examining data about patient outcomes is to be able to prospectively select patients more appropriately. The first part of this chapter reviews issues regarding how patient groups are defined preoperatively. The second part of this chapter focuses on data that pertains to patient selection. The third part of this chapter deals with the influence of prognostic factors on patient survival.

These latter factors generally cannot be identified preoperatively, and therefore are not useful in determining patient selection.

DEFINITION OF PATIENT GROUPS

Many differences exist among the patients classified as stage IIIa(N2) in different reports. The greatest difference is probably between stage IIIa(N2) patients in surgical series and those in nonsurgical series. Surgical series have generally involved only a small subgroup of all N2 patients, whereas patients treated with radiation alone have excluded only a small proportion of patients. Most surgical reports have classified patients on the basis of postoperative pathologic staging data, whereas nonsurgical series have relied almost exclusively on radiographic criteria alone. Furthermore, performance status (PS) is a major independent prognostic factor in stage IIIa(N2) patients, both in surgical series[7] and in nonsurgical reports.[8–10] It is likely that the N2 patients selected for resection have a better PS and less weight loss than those in nonsurgical reports, but most studies have not included this data.

The use of data from pathologically staged patients is problematic when applied prospectively to preoperative patients. Such data is, by necessity, retrospective and involves a mixture of only some of the patients initially thought to be cN2 and some patients thought to be cN0,1. Therefore, the outcome data of a cohort of postoperatively defined pN2 patients cannot easily be applied to a preoperative group of patients. Prediction of outcome for a preoperatively defined group of patients requires survival data specific for that group, rather than for a collection of some patients from several preoperative groups, all of whom eventually were found to be pN2.

Only one author reported on an entire cohort of patients with clinical N2 disease (Fig. 17–1).[4] Of 278 patients with cN2 disease in this study, 27% were found to be pN0,1.

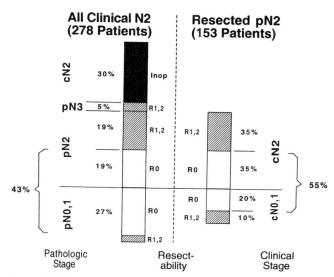

All Clinical N2 (278 Patients)

Resected pN2 (153 Patients)

FIGURE 17–1. Distribution of all patients seen from 1980 to 1990 with cN2 node involvement with respect to pathologic stage and resectability, and clinical stage and resectability of all resected patients with pathologic disease. Inop, inoperable patients; R_0, complete resection; $R_{1,2}$, incomplete resection with either microscopic (R_1) or gross (R_2) residual tumor. (Data from Watanabe Y, Shimizu J, Oda M, et al. Aggressive surgical intervention in N2 non–small cell cancer of the lung. Ann Thorac Surg. 1991;51:253–261.[4])

Of the entire cohort of cN2 patients, 73% underwent an operation and 43% underwent a curative (complete) resection, if one includes the patients who turned out to be pN0,1. However, only 19% of the entire group of 278 patients were found to be pN2 and to have undergone a complete resection (R_0). The survival results reported in this study, on the other hand, were based on a larger number of pN2 patients because of the inclusion of an additional group of patients (37% of the pN2, R_0 group) who were preoperatively staged as cN0,1.[4] In other words, the survival data was based on a mixture of a minority of the initial cohort of cN2 patients as well as other patients who were not part of this initial cohort but who were found to be pN2. This illustrates some of the problems in trying to apply data about resected pN2 patients prospectively to preoperative patients.

The reliability of preoperative staging is a major issue in patient selection. Reliance on radiographic evidence of N2 node enlargement is only a gross estimate of actual N2 status.[11] Node enlargement carries a 40% false positive rate, and normal sized nodes by computed tomography (CT) have a 10% to 25% false negative rate when compared with pathologic stage (see Table 5–7, Fig. 5–7). The use of preoperative staging by mediastinoscopy decreases the variability markedly. The uncertainty associated with groups of patients staged by CT alone is eliminated. Furthermore, the number of patients whose preoperative (clinical) stage changes (from cN2 to pN0,1) with surgical resection diminishes greatly because the false negative rate for mediastinoscopy is approximately 10% (see Table 5–12). Unfortunately, in many studies, mediastinoscopy is used selectively, and clear criteria defining when it is done are not provided.

Even when mediastinoscopy is carried out, there may be nuances in how it is performed that affect its accuracy. Whether a careful systematic sampling of all accessible nodal stations or merely a biopsy of one or two nodes is done may be important. No study has been reported comparing the extent of node sampling at mediastinoscopy. However, extrapolation from data on node assessment techniques at thoracotomy suggests that the chance of finding N2 node involvement is two to three times as high with systematic sampling as opposed to only selective biopsy.[12] Unfortunately, details of the extent of surgical staging are rarely available in reports of stage IIIa(N2) patients.

The reported data for resected stage IIIa(N2) patients involves only particular subgroups of N2 patients. Because of the unreliability of radiographic staging and the variation in the use of mediastinoscopy, the definition of a preoperative group of stage IIIa(N2) patients is difficult. The complexity of this situation is illustrated in Figure 17–2. Many points of potential crossover exist where patients initially classified with one group can be reassigned to the opposite group by the addition of further parameters.

At least six different groups of patients can be identified on the basis of preoperative staging parameters. For the sake of simplicity, these staging parameters include CT evidence of normal or enlarged N2 nodes and whether mediastinoscopy was positive, negative, or not done. These groups are labeled 1 through 6 in Figure 17–2. This figure

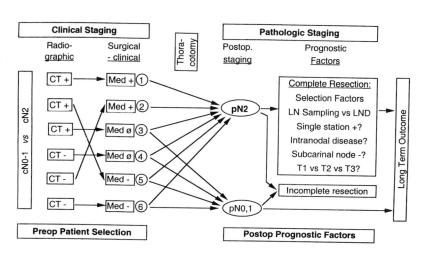

FIGURE 17–2. Relationship of preoperative selection factors and prognostic factors to long-term outcome in resected IIIa(N2) patients with non–small cell lung cancer. Preoperative selection groups: 1 and 2, N2 involvement proved histologically by mediastinoscopy; 3, N2 disease suspected radiographically; 4, unsuspected N2 disease (computed tomography negative), but N2 disease possible because mediastinoscopy not performed; 5 and 6, obscure, no N2 disease identifiable preoperatively by mediastinoscopy. LN Sampling vs LND, lymph node sampling versus lymph node dissection; Med −, mediastinoscopy negative; Med Ø, mediastinoscopy not performed; Med +, mediastinoscopy positive for N2 involvement; Postop, postoperative; Preop, preoperative.

is meant to provide a general overview in order to decrease some of the confusion caused by attempting to compare studies that have included different patient cohorts. Most studies of resected stage IIIa(N2) patients have included patients from several of these preoperative groups. Clear outcomes for a particular category by itself are not available, but general trends can be identified.

Comparison of the data regarding stage IIIa(N2) patients from different reports is impossible unless some common denominators are identified. The overall survival data from published reports varies considerably, largely because of differences in the denominator used. Some authors report on the survival of all N2 patients who present to an institution, others on all those seen by a surgical service, others on all patients who have undergone thoracotomy, others on patients undergoing resection, and still others on only those patients undergoing a complete resection. Certainly those patients who are not resected or in whom gross disease is left behind (classified as R_2) cannot be considered surgically treated the same way as patients resected with a negative margin (R_0).

What is reported as a complete resection without residual disease (R_0) by the surgeons and pathologists in different institutions is probably reasonably similar. This is also a figure that is available in most studies of surgical treatment of stage IIIa(N2) patients. Definition of margins may be difficult if lymph nodes are not resected en bloc, and some earlier reports classified patients as having a positive margin if the highest mediastinal node removed was positive, even if the margins themselves were negative. However, such instances appear to be uncommon. Nevertheless, it seems likely that there is less variation in what constitutes a complete resection than in what constitutes an incomplete resection or in which patients are excluded from surgery.

Reviewing the data for completely resected patients seems to be the best way to compare surgically treated N2 patients. The reported survival of unresected or incompletely resected stage IIIa(N2) patients is extremely poor,[11,13–15] and inclusion of varying numbers of such patients in overall results makes comparisons impossible. Because most reports do not separate resections resulting in microscopic (R_1) or gross residual (R_2) disease, and because there is evidence that patients with R_1 disease fare poorly,[7,16] R_1 and R_2 patients are grouped together here. This chapter focuses primarily on the data for stage IIIa(N2) patients who have undergone complete resection with no residual disease (R_0).

Comparison to nonsurgical reports and assessment of the impact of surgery on the entire group of N2 patients is not possible, however, by looking only at the completely resected (R_0) subgroup. The proportion of the entire population of N2 patients presenting to an institution who eventually undergo complete resection with no residual tumor (R_0) is an important parameter in making such a comparison. Unfortunately, this information is available in only a few reports. The impact of whether a liberal or restrictive policy is used to select N2 patients for surgery can be assessed by examining the resectability rate (proportion of operated patients who undergo complete resection) of different reports. Therefore, these parameters are also examined in this chapter.

NATURAL HISTORY

To assess the benefit of treatment, it is important to compare it with the natural history of untreated patients. As demonstrated by several studies, the natural history of stage IIIa(N2) NSCLC is a median survival of approximately 7 months and a 1-year survival of approximately 10% (see Table 3–4).[17–20] In 100 clinical stage IIIa patients, Reinfuss et al[17] found that the median survival was 7 months, the 1-year survival was 9%, and all patients had died by 2 years. Similarly, in another study of 17 patients clinically determined to be stage IIIa, the median survival was 8 months, 1-year survival was 24%, and all patients were dead within 18 months.[18] In 112 patients who were surgically staged as IIIa(N2) but not resected, median survival was 7 months and 1-year survival 10%.[19] Approximately half of these patients were treated with radiotherapy (RT) but with no apparent survival benefit. Thus, the natural history of stage IIIa(N2) patients is marked by consistently short survival, and no 5-year survivors without treatment have been reported.

PREOPERATIVE PATIENT SELECTION

There is a wide disparity of opinions about which stage IIIa(N2) patients should be selected for surgical treatment. In some countries, such as Japan, most patients with non-metastatic disease undergo thoracotomy, regardless of CT scan staging and often without mediastinoscopy.[11,13] At the other extreme, many physicians, particularly in the United States, believe that there is no role for surgery in stage IIIa(N2) patients and employ extensive preoperative work-ups, including CT and mediastinoscopy, to exclude these patients from surgery whenever possible.[21] This results in a lot of variation in which patients are subjected to thoracotomy.

One can define at least four different approaches to the selection of stage IIIa(N2) patients for surgical treatment. At one extreme are those who have undergone minimal selection. This group includes patients with proven N2 disease (by mediastinoscopy) who have undergone attempted resection nevertheless (groups 1 and 2 in Fig. 17–2). Another group of minimally selected patients is patients with suspected N2 disease by CT scan who have not undergone mediastinoscopy (group 3 in Fig. 17–2). A more select group is patients with unsuspected disease who have a clinically negative mediastinum by CT scan (cN0,1) but who have not undergone mediastinoscopy (group 4 in Fig. 17–2). The most select group is patients with obscure N2 disease in whom preoperative mediastinoscopy was negative (groups 5 and 6 in Fig. 17–2). In this latter group, N2 involvement is not discovered until thoracotomy.

A hybrid, less well defined approach has been taken by a number of institutions where mediastinoscopy is performed selectively on some patients. The patients undergoing thoracotomy at these institutions were thought not to have N2 disease, but it is often not clear whether this was thought because of a negative CT scan (cN0,1), a negative mediastinoscopy, both, or neither (based on other, not explicitly stated, reasons). This approach includes groups 4, 5, and 6 in Figure 17–2 but may also include some patients in group 3.

Of course, when patients are selected preoperatively, the final pathologic status is not known. In practically all of the approaches discussed, some of the patients will be found to be pN0,1. Surgical resection in these pN0,1 patients is clearly indicated. Furthermore, reported survival data for stage IIIa(N2) patients involves only pN2 patients and does not include patients who may have been suspected to have N2 disease but are pN0,1. Therefore, these cN2 but pN0,1 patients are not considered further.

Resectability

The first concern with patients selected for surgical resection is whether they are actually able to be completely resected. Studies that address this issue relative to patient selection are shown in Table 17–1. The reports listed in this table fall into two broad categories: those that are relatively selective and those that are not. The difference is defined primarily by radiographic criteria for inclusion (cN2 versus cN0,1). Those patients undergoing mediastinoscopy are not reported in enough detail to allow their consideration separately here. Those reports in which many patients with a positive mediastinoscopy are nevertheless subjected to thoracotomy are included in the nonselective group, whereas the selective group includes both series that staged patients as cN0,1 solely on the basis of CT findings, and those that also obtained pathologic confirmation of cN0,1 status by a negative mediastinoscopy. The selective studies involve mostly patients from group 4 (and possibly

5 and 6) in Figure 17–2, whereas the nonselective studies involve mostly groups 3 and 4 (and sometimes 1 and 2).

The percentage of all N2 patients seen who underwent curative resection in the two groups is similar in those series that provide this data. The most striking difference is the number of patients who were subjected to thoracotomy but in whom a complete resection was not achieved. Those institutions that operated on patients who were radiographically N2 found that a complete resection could not be accomplished in an average of 37% of the pN2 patients. In contrast, those institutions that selected patients for operation by a negative CT scan and sometimes also a negative mediastinoscopy found that an average of only 15% of patients subjected to thoracotomy were not completely resected. Thus a less rigorous approach to stage IIIa(N2) patients in terms of selection for surgical treatment does not seem to increase the number of complete resections (R_0) as much as it increases the number of patients who merely have an exploratory thoracotomy.

Benefit of Resection

Data on the influence of patient selection on the long-term survival of completely resected stage IIIa(N2) patients is presented in Table 17–2. The studies are grouped according to the approaches defined earlier for patient selection using radiographic and mediastinoscopy criteria. This table allows comparisons between studies to be made. In addition, several reports, which are also included in the table, have compared two groups of patients in the same study. These have the advantage of contemporary patient popula-

TABLE 17–1. RATE OF COMPLETE RESECTION AMONG REPORTS OF STAGE IIIa(N2) PATIENTS

STUDY	N (pN2, R_0)	RADIOGRAPHIC STAGE	MEDIASTINOSCOPY PERFORMED?	% THORACOTOMY WITHOUT R_0 RESECTION	% R_0 RESECTION OF ALL cN2 PATIENTS	5-y SURVIVAL (R_0 PATIENTS) (%)
Naruke[13]	339	All	No	38	—	23
Martini et al[29, 66]	151	All	No	33	21	29
Wada et al[28]	119	All	No	30	—	31
Watanabe et al[27]	84	All	No	48	28	24
Sawamura[74]	71	All	No	36	—	(35)[a]
Suzuki[11]	167	All	Rarely	25	—	36
Cybulsky et al[26]	73	All	Rarely	41	—	—
Riquet et al[16]	207	All	Selected patients[b]	36	—	20
Pearson et al[25]	76	All	All patients[b]	46	19	24[c]
Average[d]				**37**	**23**	**27**
Maggi et al[33]	236	cN0-2[e]	Selected patients[f]	15	—	19
Goldstraw et al[32]	127	cN0,1	Selected patients[f]	15	28	20
Nakanishi et al[40]	45	cN0,1	Selected patients	15	—	21
Daly et al[23]	33	cN0,1	Selected patients[f]	11	15	31
Vansteenkiste et al[7]	113	cN0,1	Many patients[g]	19	—	25
Average				**15**	**22**	**23**

Inclusion criteria: Studies reporting data on ≥20 pN2, completely resected patients from 1980 to 2000.
[a]4-year survival.
[b]Some mediastinoscopy positive patients went on to thoracotomy.
[c]Estimated.
[d]Excluding the values in parentheses.
[e]Most patients were cN0,1 or mediastinoscopy negative.
[f]Mediastinoscopy was negative in those patients included in which it was performed.
[g]Included 14% very select cases in which mediastinoscopy was positive; the remainder were mostly negative by mediastinoscopy, some negative by computed tomography only.
R_0, complete resection (negative margin).

TABLE 17–2. SURVIVAL OF COMPLETELY RESECTED pN2 PATIENTS ACCORDING TO SELECTION CRITERIA USED

STUDY	N (pN2, R₀)	ADJUVANT THERAPY	RADIOGRAPHIC STAGE	MEDIASTINOSCOPY PERFORMED?	MEDIASTINOSCOPY RESULTS	5-y SURVIVAL (R₀ PATIENTS) (%)	AVERAGE (%)
Pearson et al[25]	51	RT	—	All patients	Positive	15	17
Coughlin et al[22]	28	?	—	All patients	Positive	18	
Régnard et al[53]	191	RT	cN2	Rarely[a]	—	23	
Naruke[13]	339	?	cN2	No	—	23	
Watanabe et al[27]	53	None	cN2	No	—	20	21
Wada et al[28]	119	±RT ± Chemo	cN2	No	—	31	
Martini et al[29]	33	RT	cN2	No	—	8	
Martini et al[29]	118	RT	cN0,1	No	—	33	
Watanabe et al[27]	31	None	cN0,1	No	—	33	32
Daly et al[23]	33	RT	cN0,1	Rarely[a, b]	—	31	
Mountain[31]	307	± Chemo	cN0-2[c]	Selected patients	Negative[c]	31	
Maggi et al[33]	236	RT	cN0-2	Selected patients	Negative	19	
Miller et al[24]	147	± RT ± Chemo	cN0-2	Selected patients	Negative[a]	24	23
Goldstraw et al[32]	127	None	cN0-2	Selected patients	Negative[c]	20	
Nakanishi et al[40]	45	± Chemo ± RT	cN0-2[d]	Selected patients	Negative[c]	21	
Vansteenkiste et al[7]	58	±RT	—	All patients	Negative	32[e]	37
Pearson et al[25]	25	±RT	—	All patients	Negative	41	

Inclusion criteria: Studies reporting on ≥20 pN2, completely resected patients.
[a]<3% mediastinoscopy positive patients included.
[b]Mediastinoscopy done in <15%.
[c]Vaguely reported.
[d]All patients were either radiographically N0,1 or had negative mediastinoscopy.
[e]15% had an incomplete resection.
Chemo, chemotherapy; R₀, complete resection (negative margin); RT, radiotherapy; Selected patients, mediastinoscopy performed in at least all patients with radiographic N2 disease; in most series also in patients with T3 tumors and central tumors; ?, unknown.

tions at the same institution and thus are less prone to bias. In practically all of the reports in Table 17–2, resection explicitly included a radical lymph node dissection.[7,22–24] The exceptions are evenly distributed among the different approaches to patient selection, and no differences in survival among these studies and those employing radical node dissection are apparent.

Limited data is available regarding the survival of patients who were positive by mediastinoscopy but were nevertheless resected. This is probably because a positive mediastinoscopy result is not likely to be ignored by those institutions that take the trouble to do preoperative mediastinoscopy. In 1982, Pearson convincingly demonstrated that survival of NSCLC patients with N2 disease discovered at mediastinoscopy was inferior to that of patients with N2 disease discovered at thoracotomy, although no calculation of statistical significance was made[25] (Fig. 17–3). The 5-year survival for completely resected patients was 15% versus 41%, and for all patients evaluated, it was 9% versus 24%. Although the survival rates are inferior to those for patients with a negative mediastinoscopy, it is notable that 15% of those patients with a positive mediastinoscopy who were completely resected were, in fact, 5-year survivors. Coughlin et al[22] reported a similar 5-year survival of 18% in a select group of mediastinoscopy-positive patients. Vansteenkiste et al[7] also reported a 15% 5-year survival, despite the inclusion of patients who were not completely resected (36% of total). They noted that resection of N2 positive patients was undertaken only in very select cases. If one assumes that none of the incompletely resected patients survived 5 years, then the esti-

mated survival of the completely resected patients would be approximately 24%.[7] It should be noted that in the series by Pearson et al[25] and Coughlin et al,[22] mediastinoscopy-positive patients who underwent complete resection represented 13% and 10% of all cN2 patients seen.

The results for patients with radiographic N2 disease are varied, ranging from 8% to 31% in Table 17–2. It is not clear why this is the case. Perhaps some of these studies

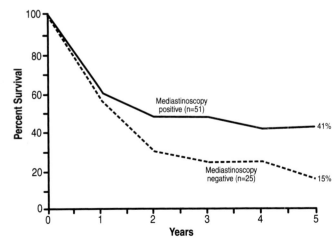

FIGURE 17–3. Survival of patients undergoing complete resections for N2 lesions of the lung, according to outcome of mediastinoscopy. (From Pearson FG, DeLarue NC, Ilves R, et al. Significance of positive superior mediastinal nodes identified at mediastinoscopy in patients with resectable cancer of the lung. J Thorac Cardiovasc Surg. 1982;83:1–11.[25])

included a mix of cN0,1 patients and cN2 patients, although this is not reported. Two other studies of cN2 patients found a 5-year survival of 7%.[11,26] These are not included in Table 17–2 because the survival figures include the nearly 40% of patients who were incompletely resected. Three of the studies with relatively good survival are from Japan,[13,27,28] whereas the two United States studies show a 5-year survival of <10%.[26,29]

Although it is not clear what value should be accepted as the 5-year survival for pN2 patients who have "bulky" radiographically positive nodes, it is fairly clear that these patients have a worse prognosis than those with radiographically negative nodes. All three studies[4,26,29] that performed internal comparisons (comparisons between cN0,1 and cN2 patients at the same institution and during the same time period) showed better survival in those patients who were radiographically N0,1, although it was statistically significant in only one of the two studies in which this was calculated.[26] It should be noted that all the patients reported in these retrospective series did have pathologically confirmed N2 disease at thoracotomy. However, applying such radiographic selection in a prospective fashion remains problematic because approximately 40% of those who appear by CT to be cN2 are actually pN0,1[4,30] and therefore should not be denied surgery based on CT appearance alone. Conversely, if many radiographic N2 patients are subjected to thoracotomy, approximately 40% will have an incomplete or no resection and will derive no benefit from surgery, as shown in Table 17–1.

The 5-year survival of pN2 patients who by pretreatment staging (CT or mediastinoscopy) are cN0,1 is approximately 25% to 35% (see Table 17–2). Those patients who are cN0,1 by radiographic staging alone have an average 5-year survival of 32%. The studies that required a negative mediastinoscopy in all patients show a slightly better survival of 37%. It is interesting that the additional requirement of a negative mediastinoscopy seems to have improved the survival slightly but not dramatically compared with patients who are cN0,1 by radiographic staging alone.

In light of this finding, it is puzzling that the hybrid group, in which patients were presumably either cN0,1 or mediastinoscopy negative, is consistently lower than that of patients who are explicitly cN0,1 or mediastinoscopy negative. The average survival of this more mixed group in which most patients are presumed to be cN0,1 (by either CT or mediastinoscopy) is 23%. Closer scrutiny of these reports using either radiographic staging or mediastinoscopy reveals that the staging criteria used were rather vague in almost all of them. Often, the criteria for a positive CT were not defined[24,31] or were applied only to certain nodal stations.[32] In others, the policy used clearly evolved over the course of the study.[33] Thus the poorer survival results could be due to less well defined staging criteria that resulted in a less select group of patients undergoing resection.

Table 17–2 suggests that more highly selected patients exhibit better survival. Less highly selected patients, such as those who are mediastinoscopy positive or have radiographic N2 disease, do not seem to fare as well after resection. Those who are radiographically N0,1 by strict criteria do better, and those who have a negative mediastinoscopy have a rather acceptable 5-year survival rate of nearly 40%.

However, if one considers the entire population of stage IIIa(N2) patients, then surgery as the primary treatment modality is disappointing. If only 25% of all patients undergo complete resection and only approximately 25% of these patients are 5-year survivors, then surgery as the primary treatment for all N2 patients results in a 5-year survival of only 6%. This is similar to the 5-year survival in reported series of stage IIIa patients treated with RT alone, in which most of the N2 patients seen have generally been accepted for treatment (see Chapter 18).

However, it is well documented that the select group of N2 patients who undergo a complete resection has a reasonable survival (20%–40%). This is clearly better than the uniformly dismal survival from natural history studies. The natural history data, although limited, shows such

DATA SUMMARY: NATURAL HISTORY AND PATIENT SELECTION FOR RESECTION

	AMOUNT	QUALITY	CONSISTENCY
The natural history of stage IIIa(N2) patients is a median survival of 7 months	Mod	High	High
When many clinical N2 patients are taken to surgery, a complete resection is achieved in 60%	High	High	High
When only clinical N0,1 patients are taken to surgery, a complete resection is achieved in 85%	High	High	High
The proportion of *all* clinical N2 patients who are able to be completely resected is 25%, regardless of the criteria used to select patients for surgery	High	Mod	High
The 5-year survival of completely resected pN2 patients is approximately 25%	High	High	High
Patients who are radiographically N0,1 or negative by mediastinoscopy have a 5-year survival of 30% to 40%	High	High	High
Patients who have radiographic or mediastinoscopic evidence of N2 disease have a 5-year survival after complete resection of 20%	High	High	Mod

Type of data rated: Plain text: descriptive statement   *Italics: controlled comparison*   **Bold: randomized comparison**

consistently short survival that it appears convincing that surgery does, in fact, benefit this select group, rather than simply being a marker for a more favorable subgroup who would have done well regardless of the treatment provided.

In summary, widely disparate policies are used by different institutions to select stage IIIa(N2) patients for surgical treatment. The differences are primarily in the extent of the preoperative workup used to rule out N2 disease, and surgical resection is reserved for N2 disease discovered at thoracotomy, with few exceptions. The less rigorous policies do not seem to result in greater numbers of patients who are completely resected, but they result in higher rates of thoracotomy without R_0 resection. The 5-year survival after complete resection in more carefully selected patients (cN0,1, mediastinoscopy negative) appears to be somewhat better.

OPERATIVE FACTORS
Prognostic Factors

A number of prognostic factors have been identified that influence the survival of patients who have undergone

resection for N2 disease. These are listed in Table 17–3. In general, these factors are not known until after the resection has taken place; thus, these factors are not particularly useful in selecting which patients should undergo thoracotomy. This data about the relative influence of each prognostic factor involves comparisons within studies; in other words, in each study, patients with the factor are compared with others without it (contemporary controls from the same institution).

The most consistent findings, as well as the finding with the largest survival difference, is whether or not a complete resection was achieved. All 11 studies that have addressed this have shown a clear trend, and statistical significance was found whenever this was analyzed. The average 5-year survival of incompletely resected patients is 5%. Authors of only one study stated that no difference was found, but they did not provide any actual data.[26] Thus it is clear that incompletely resected patients do not fare well and that patients should be carefully selected to avoid a high incidence of thoracotomy without a complete resection.

Another fairly consistent finding is that patients with only a single N2 station involved have a better prognosis

TABLE 17–3. PROGNOSTIC FACTORS IN RESECTED IIIa(N2) NSCLC PATIENTS[a]

FACTOR (REFERENCES)	5-YEAR SURVIVAL (%)				TREND	P < 0.05	n+/n−
	Positive		Negative				
	Mean	(Range)	Mean	(Range)			
Incomplete resection (7, 11[b], 13, 16, 24, 27, 32, 33, 40, 46, 53)	5	(0–13)	24	(18–36)	→11/11	9/9	577/1782
Multiple positive node stations (7, 11[b], 16, 24, 27, 29, 31, 32[c], 33, 40, 53[d], 75[e])	15	(3–27)	27	(16–37)	→12/12	7/11	802/1119
Extracapsular extension (7, 33, 35, 46[d])	16	(11–18)	27	(20–38)	→4/4	2/3	207/317
Contiguous to primary tumor (53[d])	12		22		→1/1	0/1	92/162
Subcarinal node, ie, Stations 7–9 vs. 1–4 (7, 11[b], 24[f], 27, 29[f], 32[f], 33, 38[b], 39, 40, 53[d], 75)	15	(0–27)	29	(19–45)	→11/12 ←1/12	4/11	602/778
Aortopulmonary node, ie, Stations 5,6 vs 1–4 (7, 11[b], 24[f], 39[f], 40, 75)	30	(0–80)	25	(19–36)	→2/6 ←4/6	0/5	179/368
High paratracheal nodes, ie, Stations 1–2 vs. all other (24, 38[b], 39[d])	18	(8–25)	24	(18–36)	→2/3 ←1/3	0/2	97/203
N1 node positive (45, 50[d])	19	(13–22)	31	(24–35)	→2/2	0/2	173/92
Nonsquamous histology (4, 7, 11[b], 13, 29, 31, 32, 40, 46[d], 74)	24	(4–34)	26	(0–45)	→6/10 ←4/10	1/8	912/613
T status (4, 7, 13, 28[d], 29, 31, 33, 40, 46[d], 53[d], 77, 78)	T1 38 (20–48)	T2 25 (14–34)	T3 13 (0–29)		←12/12	6/8 (T1 vs. T3)	(T1) 344 (T2) 1344 (T3) 509

Inclusion criteria: Studies reporting actuarial data on prognostic factors on ≥20 patients for a particular category.
[a] All data is from studies of complete resections or mostly complete resections (≥80%), except where indicated.
[b] <80% completely resected, using definition that includes highest negative lymph node.
[c] Vague reporting.
[d] Versus all other.
[e] Compared five different regions, rather than stations.
[f] Compared only patients with single station positive.
n+, number of patients with the respective prognostic factor; n−, number of patients without the respective prognostic factor; P < 0.05, number of studies showing statistical significance/number of studies for which this was given; Trend, number of studies with trend in the direction of the arrow/total number of studies; →, better survival with factor absent (negative); ←, better survival with factor present (positive).

than those with multiple station involvement. All 12 of the studies that have analyzed this supported this finding, although statistical significance was shown in only 7. One other study found no difference, although no details were given.[26] A meta-analysis of pN2 patients that included studies involving both completely resected and incompletely resected patients also concluded that single node station involvement was favorable (5-year survival estimate, 30% versus 21%, $P = 0.0008$).[34]

Patients with intranodal microscopic disease have been found by several investigators to have a more favorable prognosis compared with those with extracapsular extension.[26,32,33,35,36] However, some authors have not noted this,[2,26] and the meta-analysis found only a nonsignificant trend to better survival with intranodal disease.[34]

Both intranodal disease and involvement of only a single node station have been called *signs of minimal N2 disease* and have been suggested as selection criteria for resection after a positive mediastinoscopy. Although multiple node station positivity can be determined by a careful mediastinoscopy, the ability of pathologists to determine extracapsular extension consistently from mediastinoscopy biopsies is poor.[37] Thus the usefulness of these factors as selection criteria in actual practice is questionable.

Controversy has existed about whether subcarinal or aortopulmonary (AP) window nodal involvement carries a particularly poor or good prognosis.[38] In reference to subcarinal involvement, 11 out of 12 studies show a trend toward poorer survival in this patient group. However, Goldstraw et al[32] found the opposite to be true. The influence of single station versus multiple station N2 involvement may be a confounding factor in many of these studies. Three studies compared only patients with single level involvement, and all found a trend toward worse survival if subcarinal disease was present.[27,38,40] One of these authors found a 5-year survival of 23% versus 45% ($P =$ NS),[27] another 0 versus 36% ($P =$ NS),[40] and another 14% versus 19% ($P =$ NS; estimated from hazard function)[38] for patients with versus patients without subcarinal node involvement. The meta-analysis estimated 5-year survival to be 18% and 29% in patients with and without subcarinal node involvement ($P = 0.0007$).[34] Maggi et al[33] suggested that the inferior survival may not be due to a difference in the biologic behavior of tumors involving subcarinal nodes but may exist because it is more difficult to consistently biopsy subcarinal nodes by mediastinoscopy as opposed to other mediastinal nodes.

Patterson et al[41] suggested that N2 patients with only AP window (station 5) nodal involvement have a better prognosis. This is based on a 5-year survival rate of 42% in 23 patients of 34 undergoing a curative resection, but no data for a control group was presented. These patients were all negative at mediastinoscopy. Survival rate is not clearly better than that for other completely resected patients with single station positive, mediastinoscopy negative N2 disease. Indeed, those studies that have included a control group have all shown conflicting trends and a lack of statistical significance. The average reported survival is essentially the same with AP window node involvement versus paratracheal involvement. Other reports that have analyzed this, but reported the data in a manner that did 25not allow inclusion in Table 17–3, have also found no difference in the survival of N2 positive patients who had or did not have AP window node involvement.[42,43]

Involvement of high paratracheal nodes (stations 1,2) has been thought to signify involvement of the last nodal station before hematogenous spread. A worse survival for patients with involvement of these nodes has been seen in a few studies but not consistently and without statistical significance.[24,38,39]

Many authors have shown that approximately 30% of resected patients with N2 node involvement do not have N1 node involvement (so-called *skip metastases*).[2,16,29,44–51] Yoshino et al[45] found no difference in 33 such patients in terms of T status or the incidence of radiographic N2 disease. Patients with skip metastases were more likely to have fewer N2 nodes involved. However, even among only those patients with a single N2 station involved, patients without N1 involvement showed better survival than those with positive N1 nodes (38% versus 15%, $P = 0.09$), suggesting that perhaps the number of nodes involved (all categories of nodes) has prognostic significance. Tateishi et al[50] found a similar trend. Martini et al[29] found "no difference" in survival of the 27% of patients with skip metastases but provided no details.

It is not clear that histology is a prognostic factor in surgically treated N2 disease. Although a trend to slightly better survival for squamous cell cancer patients was seen in six studies,[2,4,7,31,32,52] the opposite was found in four other reports.[11,29,40,46] In only one of these studies was any statistical significance found.[32] Other authors have also reported finding no difference.[26,28,33] A meta-analysis of pN2 patients suggested that patients with squamous cancer exhibited better survival than patients with nonsquamous NSCLC (28% versus 20%, $P = 0.0015$).[34]

A consistent trend has been seen favoring patients with an earlier T stage in all 12 studies that have analyzed this (Table 17–3). This appears to hold true for T1 versus T2 as well as T2 versus T3. Although 5-year survival rates over 20% (as high as 29%) after resection of T3N2 disease have been reported,[29,31] several authors have shown survival figures of <10%.[7,40,46] The average 5-year survival for T3N2 patients noted in the 10 studies in Table 17–3 is 13%. A meta-analysis estimated 5-year survival to be 41% for T1, 22% for T2, and 12% for T3N2 patients ($P = 0.0001$).[34] Other series, which did not contain control groups, have reported similar survivals for T3N2 patients ranging from 0% to 29%, with an average of 7%.[28,54–64] Although it is not clear why such variation in the survival of T3N2 patients has been seen, it does appear clear that one should be selective before undertaking resection in patients suspected to have T3N2 disease.

In summary, the factors that most clearly convey a poorer prognosis are incomplete resection, multiple node station involvement, and higher T stage. Extracapsular node involvement, subcarinal node involvement, and nonsquamous histology appear to be somewhat weaker negative prognostic factors. The effect of other putative prognostic factors among resected pN2 patients appears to be limited.

Three studies have analyzed prognostic factors using multivariate analysis.[7,11,36] One of these studies found clinical N2 disease, larger tumor size, multiple N2 node involvement, and incomplete resection to be independent predictors of poor survival in 222 patients.[11] Another study (140 patients) found clinical N2 disease, T3,4 disease, multiple node station involvement, performance status 1 or

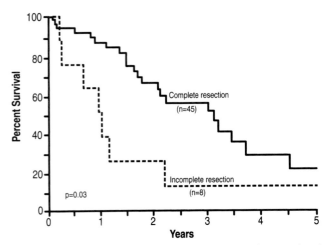

FIGURE 17–4. Survival of resected N2 patients undergoing complete (n = 45) or incomplete (n = 8) resection (P = 0.03). (Reprinted with permission from the Society of Thoracic Surgeons [The Annals of Thoracic Surgery. 1997;64:342–348].[40])

2, and nonsquamous histology to be associated with poor survival.[7] Interestingly, the completeness of the resection, the factor with the lowest P value in univariate analysis (25% vs 4%, P = 0.002), did not emerge as an independent factor in multivariate analysis.[7] The third study, which involved only 48 cN0,1 completely resected patients, found that peripheral tumors and the need for a pneumonectomy were independent prognostic factors of poorer survival.[36] The results of this third study are somewhat counterintuitive and may not hold up in a larger group of patients.

Surgical Issues

Most patients with stage IIIa(N2) disease who undergo thoracotomy were not suspected preoperatively to have N2 disease. This raises the question of what the surgeon should do when so-called *surgically discovered* N2 disease is found. A frozen section can be readily obtained in most cases to confirm the presence of N2 disease intraoperatively. Because the natural history is poor and a 5-year survival with resection of up to 40% can be achieved in such surgically discovered N2 patients, it seems reasonable to proceed with resection when N2 disease is discovered at thoracotomy. Although radiation and chemotherapy might have been an alternative, the patient has already been subjected to the morbidity of a thoracotomy. Reported data does not indicate an appreciable increase in the morbidity or mortality of exploratory thoracotomy versus resection[27,65]; therefore, there is no reason to abandon the resection provided the tumor can be completely resected.

Every effort should be made to obtain a complete resection. There is no reason to perform a microscopically or grossly incomplete (R_1 or R_2) resection. In a large series of patients with stage III disease, Hara et al[14] showed identical poor survival among patients undergoing incomplete resection, exploratory thoracotomy alone, or no thoracotomy (see Fig. 14–5). Other authors have also confirmed poor survival after incomplete resection.[66] More recent studies comparing incomplete with complete resection have all consistently shown poor survival for incomplete resection

(see Table 17–3). The best survival reported is 13% (Fig. 17–4).[40]

Controversy exists about whether a lobectomy or pneumonectomy should be performed if N2 disease is encountered. Some surgeons believe that a pneumonectomy should always be performed if N2 disease is encountered, to more completely remove tumor-bearing lymphatics. On the other hand, others believe the survival after a pneumonectomy in the presence of N2 disease is so poor that only a lobectomy is justified. Unfortunately, this issue has not clearly been addressed by any study. Some studies have shown slightly better survival after pneumonectomy,[7,32] whereas others have shown slightly worse survival.[24,26,36,40,60] However, the tumors of patients requiring pneumonectomy were more extensive.[36,60] A meta-analysis of resected N2 patients also concluded that there is no difference in survival between lobectomy and pneumonectomy in N2 patients.[34] Therefore, although a complete resection with negative margins should be done, a recommendation to either perform or avoid a pneumonectomy simply because of the presence of N2 disease cannot be made.

There continues to be controversy about the therapeutic benefit of mediastinal node dissection but with little data. A formal mediastinal node dissection involves removal of all of the node-bearing tissues, leaving only the skeletonized trachea, phrenic nerves, aorta, and superior vena cava behind.[4] It does appear that a careful mediastinal node dissection can be carried out safely and that it approximately doubles the rate of discovery of N2 node involvement relative to a limited mediastinal node sampling.[12,67] However, a systematic node sampling achieves the same rate of positive node involvement as a formal node dissection.[12,68] Izbicki et al[47,68] studied 182 randomized patients without bulky adenopathy, of whom approximately half underwent systematic node sampling and the others an extensive node dissection. Although the final staging was the same in both groups, multiple levels of N2 node involvement were found significantly more often in the

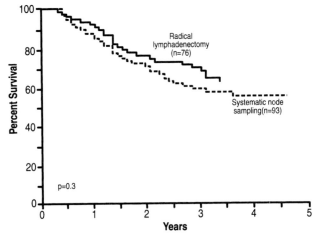

FIGURE 17–5. Survival (including 30-day mortality) of patients undergoing radical systematic lymphadenectomy (n = 76, *solid line*) and systemic node sampling (n = 93, *dashed line*) (P = 0.3). (From Izbicki JR, Passlick B, Pantel K, et al. Effectiveness of radical systematic mediastinal lymphadenectomy in patients with resectable non–small cell lung cancer. Ann Surg. 1998;227[1]:138–144.[70])

TABLE 17–4. STAGE IIIa NON–SMALL CELL LUNG CANCER RECURRRENCE PATTERNS

STUDY	THERAPY (RT DOSE IN GY)	HOW STAGED	NO. OF PATIENTS	% OF ALL RECURRENCES			% WITHOUT RECURRENCE
				L	L + D	D	
Reinfuss et al[17]	None	Radiographic	118	**73**	27	**0**	0
Reinfuss et al[17]	RT(40s)	Radiographic	170	**62**	26	**2**	2
Perez et al[71a]	RT(40)	Radiographic	97	**39**	34	**27**	21
Mantravadi et al[72]	RT(45–55)	Radiographic	161	**15**	52	**33**	15
Perez et al[71a]	RT(60)	Radiographic	84	**17**	40	**43**	23
Martini et al[29]	S/RT	Pathologic	151	**13**	4	**77**	32
Mountain[73]	S/RT	Pathologic	92	**3**	14	**83**	25

No inclusion critera; selected reports judged by the authors to be representative of a particular treatment approach.
[a]Excluding patients who died in <1 year.
D, distant; L, local; R, radiotherapy; s, split course RT; S, surgical resection.

node dissection group (59% versus 17%, $P = 0.007$).[68] This staging data suggests that less extensive node removal at thoracotomy might leave tumor behind in some instances.

Naruke[13] showed better 5-year survival in each stage of lung cancer when a careful mediastinal node dissection was performed. However, those patients who did not undergo node dissection had either "advanced disease that precluded a complete resection" or were "elderly or high-risk" patients. Furthermore, the 5-year survival of 24% in stage IIIa(N2) NSCLC patients reported by Watanabe et al,[4] who are strong proponents of extensive mediastinal node dissection, did not appear to be different from that reported by other authors who did not do a node dissection,[25,29,31] although comparisons between studies are difficult at best. In a nonrandomized study of a somewhat different population of 125 T1N0 patients, Funatsu et al[69] found inferior survival in those patients who had a radical node dissection compared with a careful sampling alone (5-year survival, 70% versus 90%; $P < 0.05$). The only controlled, randomized study that addressed node dissection in N2 patients is the study by Izbicki et al[47,68,70] mentioned earlier. In 169 randomized stage I-IIIa patients, the survival curves with careful lymphadenectomy were identical to those with node sampling (Fig. 17–5), although a lower total recurrence rate after lymphadenectomy was seen in the subgroup of 46 patients with stage II,IIIa disease (41% versus 79%, $P = 0.04$).[70]

RECURRENCE PATTERNS

A summary of recurrence patterns after various treatments for patients with N2 disease is shown in Table 17–4. It can be seen that both local and distant disease is a significant problem, but this varies somewhat with the treatment received. Without treatment, most patients die of local disease.[17] Radiation, particularly higher doses, seems to decrease the proportion of patients with local recurrence alone.[17,71,72] Patients treated with surgery and postoperative radiation have the lowest proportion of local failures.[29,73] It must be emphasized, however, that the stage IIIa(N2) patients in the group selected for surgery are not necessarily comparable to radiographically staged patients selected for RT alone.

A more extensive summary of recurrence patterns after surgery as the primary treatment for N2 disease is shown in Table 17–5. Many of the patients received adjuvant treatment, but it is not clear that this had a major impact. Further data about adjuvant treatment is available in Chapter 14. When the studies are ordered with respect to the percentage of patients with a complete resection, it appears

TABLE 17–5. RECURRENCE PATTERNS IN RESECTED pN2 PATIENTS

STUDY	N	% R₁,₂ RESECTION	DEFINITION OF RECUR	% RECUR OF ALL PATIENTS	% OF ALL RECURRENCES			ADJUVANT THERAPY
					L	L + D	D	
Mountain[73]	92	0[a]	First	75	**3**	14	**83**	RT
Martini et al[29]	151	0	First[a]	68	**14**	4	**82**	RT
Yoshino et al[45]	110	11	First	50[a]	**24**	5	**71**	None[a]
Riquet et al[a16]	237	13	Any	53	**16**	6	**78**	±RT
Nakanishi et al[40]	88	18	First	52	**33**	—	**67**	±Chemo ± RT
Miller et al[24]	167	20	First[a]	69	**20**	22	**58**	±RT ± Chemo
Cybulsky et al[26]	124	41	Any[a]	63	**35**	–	**56**	±RT ± Chemo
Average					**20**	**10**	**70**	

Inclusion criteria: Studies reporting recurrence data on ≥50 resected pN2 patients.
[a]Vague reporting.
Any, recurrence at any time; Chemo, chemotherapy; D, distant; First, first site of recurrence; L, local; Recur, recurrence; RT, radiotherapy; % R₁,₂, percentage of incompletely resected patients with microscopic (R₁) or gross (R₂) residual disease.

DATA SUMMARY: PROGNOSTIC FACTORS AND SURGICAL ISSUES			
	AMOUNT	**QUALITY**	**CONSISTENCY**
Incompletely resected patients have a 5-year survival rate of <10%	High	High	High
Patients with multiple node stations involved have poorer survival than patients with single station involvement	High	High	High
Extracapsular nodal extension of tumor is an unfavorable prognostic indicator	High	High	High
Involvement of a subcarinal node is a negative prognostic indicator	High	Mod	High
Aortopulmonary window node involvement has no particular prognostic significance	High	Mod	Mod
Involvement of high paratracheal nodes may be a poor prognostic indicator	Mod	Mod	Mod
Histology carries no particular prognostic significance among patients with pIIIa(N2) non–small cell lung cancer	High	High	Mod
Higher T stage is a negative prognostic factor	High	High	High
Mediastinal node dissection has not been shown to produce a survival advantage	Poor	High	—
The majority of recurrences after resection of N2 disease are distant	High	Mod	High

Type of data rated: Plain text: descriptive statement   *Italics: controlled comparison*   **Bold: randomized comparison**

that more incomplete ($R_{1,2}$) resections correlate with a higher incidence of local recurrences, although the overall incidence of recurrences is less clearly affected.

EDITORS' COMMENTS

A local therapy such as surgery clearly has a role for some patients with stage IIIa(N2) disease. The two dominant issues are how to select patients who will benefit and what to recommend to patients in the current era, given the results of multimodality treatment for lung cancer.

Patient selection on the basis of radiographic appearance leaves much to be desired. Although patients with "bulky" N2 disease clearly do poorly as a group, a large number of these patients do not actually have N2 disease. It would be inappropriate to exclude these patients simply on the basis of radiographic appearance. On the other hand, if all patients with bulky N2 disease undergo thoracotomy, the nearly 40% incidence of thoracotomy without effective resection (R_0) is too high, in our opinion. Therefore, it seems most appropriate to evaluate patients further by performing mediastinoscopy. Patients who have a positive mediastinoscopy are not accepted for surgery as primary therapy in our practice. Although long-term survival of mediastinoscopy-positive patients can occasionally be achieved, the chance of this is low. Especially with the results of multimodality treatment, surgery alone for these patients is not justified, in our opinion.

Published results of multimodality therapy for stage III NSCLC are as good as those for primary surgery. However, the patients undergoing multimodality treatment appear to be less well selected, in that they often have unfavorable characteristics (bulky N2 disease, mediastinoscopy positive). It seems reasonable that better selected patients may derive even more benefit from multimodality treatment.

Therefore, in our practice, patients who have been shown to have N2 disease preoperatively do not undergo primary surgery but are offered multimodality protocol treatment.

Surgery for stage IIIa(N2) patients, therefore, is reserved for those patients in whom N2 disease is discovered at the time of thoracotomy. When this is encountered, it appears justified to carry out the resection, provided a complete resection can be accomplished safely. This involves removal of all known or suspected disease. By extrapolation, this would involve removal of all accessible mediastinal lymph nodes. In other words, mediastinal lymph node dissection is done for N2 disease, realizing that there is no data showing that this is of therapeutic benefit.

After resection of stage IIIa(N2) disease, adjuvant therapy should be considered. Although conclusive proof of its efficacy is lacking, there are several indications that this may be beneficial. Further discussion of this can be found in Chapter 14. Because the role and exact nature of this therapy are not entirely clear, patients should be enrolled in a protocol for postoperative treatment, rather than treated off protocol.

References

1. Green MR, Lilenbaum RC. Stage IIIA category of non–small-cell lung cancer: a new proposal. J Natl Cancer Inst. 1994;86:586–588.
2. Naruke T, Goya T, Tsuchiya R, et al. The importance of surgery to non–small cell carcinoma of lung with mediastinal lymph node metastasis. Ann Thorac Surg. 1988;46:603–610.
3. Mountain CF. Expanded possibilities for surgical treatment of lung cancer: survival in stage IIIa disease. Chest. 1990;97:1045–1051.
4. Watanabe Y, Shimizu J, Oda M, et al. Aggressive surgical intervention in N2 non–small cell cancer of the lung. Ann Thorac Surg. 1991;51:253–261.
5. Ichinose Y, Yano T, Asoh H, et al. Prognostic factors obtained by a pathologic examination in completely resected non–small-cell lung cancer: an analysis in each pathologic stage. J Thorac Cardiovasc Surg. 1995;110:601–605.

6. Mountain CF. Revisions in the International System for Staging Lung Cancer. Chest. 1997;111:1710–1717.
7. Vansteenkiste JF, DeLeyn PR, Deneffe GJ, et al. Survival and prognostic factors in resected N2 non–small cell lung cancer: a study of 140 cases. Ann Thorac Surg. 1997;63:1441–1450.
8. Stanley KE. Prognostic factors for survival in patients with inoperable lung cancer. J Natl Cancer Inst. 1980;65:25–32.
9. Cox JD, Azarnia N, Byhardt RW, et al. N2 (clinical) non–small cell carcinoma of the lung: prospective trials of radiation therapy with total doses 60 Gy by the Radiation Therapy Oncology Group. Int J Radiat Oncol Biol Phys. 1991;20:7–12.
10. Rosenthal SA, Curran WJ Jr, Herbert SH, et al. Clinical stage II non–small cell lung cancer treated with radiation therapy alone: the significance of clinically staged ipsilateral hilar adenopathy (N1 disease). Cancer. 1992;70:2410–2417.
11. Suzuki K, Nagai K, Yoshida J, et al. The prognosis of surgically resected N2 non–small cell lung cancer: the importance of clinical N status. J Thorac Cardiovasc Surg. 1999;118:145–153.
12. Bollen EC, van Duin CJ, Theunissen PH, et al. Mediastinal lymph node dissection in resected lung cancer: morbidity and accuracy of staging. Ann Thorac Surg. 1993;55:961–966.
13. Naruke T. Significance of lymph node metastases in lung cancer. Semin Thorac Cardiovasc Surg. 1993;5:210–218.
14. Hara N, Ohta M, Tanaka K, et al. Assessment of the role of surgery for stage III bronchogenic carcinoma. J Surg Oncol. 1984;25:153–158.
15. Watanabe Y, Shimizu J, Oda M, et al. Results of surgical treatment in patients with stage IIIA non–small-cell lung cancer. Thorac Cardiovasc Surg. 1991;39:44–49.
16. Riquet M, Manac'h D, Saab M, et al. Factors determining survival in resected N2 lung cancer. Eur J Cardiothorac Surg. 1995;9:300–304.
17. Reinfuss M, Skolyszewski J, Kowalska T, et al. Palliative radiotherapy in asymptomatic patients with locally advanced, unresectable, non–small cell lung cancer. Strahlenther Onkol. 1993;169:709–715.
18. Vrdoljak E, Mise K, Sapunar D, et al. Survival analysis of untreated patients with non–small-cell lung cancer. Chest. 1994;106:1797–1800.
19. Paul A, Marelli D, Wilson JAS, et al. Does the surgical trauma of "exploratory thoracotomy" affect survival of patients with bronchogenic carcinoma? Can J Surg. 1989;32:322–327.
20. Roswit B, Patno ME, Rapp R, et al. The survival of patients with inoperable lung cancer: a large-scale randomized study of radiation therapy versus placebo. Radiology. 1968;90:688–697.
21. Shields TW. The significance of ipsilateral mediastinal lymph node metastasis (N2 disease) in non–small cell carcinoma of the lung: a commentary. J Thorac Cardiovasc Surg. 1990;99:48–53.
22. Coughlin M, Deslauriers J, Beaulieu M, et al. Role of mediastinoscopy in pretreatment staging of patients with primary lung cancer. Ann Thorac Surg. 1985;40:556–560.
23. Daly BDT, Mueller JD, Faling LJ, et al. N2 lung cancer: outcome in patients with false-negative computed tomographic scans of the chest. J Thorac Cardiovasc Surg. 1993;105:904–911.
24. Miller DL, McManus KG, Allen MS, et al. Results of surgical resection of patients with N2 non–small cell lung cancer. Ann Thorac Surg. 1994;57:1095–1101.
25. Pearson FG, DeLarue NC, Ilves R, et al. Significance of positive superior mediastinal nodes identified at mediastinoscopy in patients with resectable cancer of the lung. J Thorac Cardiovasc Surg. 1982;83:1–11.
26. Cybulsky IJ, Lanza LA, Ryan MB, et al. Prognostic significance of computed tomography in resected N2 lung cancer. Ann Thorac Surg. 1992;54:533–537.
27. Watanabe Y, Hayashi Y, Shimizu J, et al. Mediastinal nodal involvement and the prognosis of non–small cell lung cancer. Chest. 1991;100:422–428.
28. Wada H, Tanaka F, Yanagihara K, et al. Time trends and survival after operations for primary lung cancer from 1976 through 1990. J Thorac Cardiovasc Surg. 1996;112:349–355.
29. Martini N, Flehinger BJ, Zaman MB, et al. Results of resection in non–oat cell carcinoma of the lung with mediastinal lymph node metastases. Ann Surg. 1983;198:386–397.
30. Daly BD Jr, Faling LJ, Bite G, et al. Mediastinal lymph node evaluation by computed tomography in lung cancer: an analysis of 345 patients grouped by TNM staging, tumor size, and tumor location. J Thorac Cardiovasc Surg. 1987;94:664–672.
31. Mountain CF. Surgery for stage IIIa-N2 non–small cell lung cancer. Cancer. 1994;73:2589–2598.
32. Goldstraw P, Mannam GC, Kaplan DK, et al. Surgical management of non–small-cell lung cancer with ipsilateral mediastinal node metastasis (N2 disease). J Thorac Cardiovasc Surg. 1994;107:19–28.
33. Maggi G, Casadio C, Cianci R, et al. Results of surgical resection of stage IIIA (N2) non–small cell lung cancer, according to the site of the mediastinal metastases. Int Surg. 1993;78:213–217.
34. Vansteenkiste JF, De Leyn PR, Deneffe GJ, et al. Clinical prognostic factors in surgically treated stage IIIA-N2 non–small cell lung cancer: analysis of the literature. Lung Cancer. 1998;19:3–13.
35. Suemasu K, Naruke T. Prognostic significance of extranodal cancer invasion of mediastinal lymph nodes in lung cancer. Jpn J Clin Oncol. 1982;12:207–212.
36. van Klaveren RJ, Festen J, Otten HJ, et al. Prognosis of unsuspected but completely resectable N2 non–small cell lung cancer. Ann Thorac Surg. 1993;56:300–304.
37. Theunissen PHMH, Bollen ECM, Koudstaal J, et al. Intranodal and extranodal tumour growth in early metastasised non–small cell lung cancer: problems in histological diagnosis. J Clin Pathol. 1994;47: 920–923.
38. Thomas PA, Piantadosi S, Mountain CF. Should subcarinal lymph nodes be routinely examined in patients with non–small cell lung cancer? J Thorac Cardiovasc Surg. 1988;95:883–887.
39. Naruke T, Suemasu K, Ishikawa S. Lymph node mapping and curability at various levels of metastasis in resected lung cancer. J Thorac Cardiovasc Surg. 1978;76:832–839.
40. Nakanishi R, Osaki T, Nakanishi K, et al. Treatment strategy for patients with surgically discovered N2 stage IIIA non–small cell lung cancer. Ann Thorac Surg. 1997;64:342–348.
41. Patterson GA, Piazza D, Pearson FG, et al. Significance of metastatic disease in subaortic lymph nodes. Ann Thorac Surg. 1987;43:155–159.
42. Gozzetti G, Mastrorilli G, Bragaglia RB, et al. Surgical management of N2 lung cancer [abstract]. Lung Cancer. 1986;2:96.
43. Bülzebruck H, Bopp R, Drings P, et al. New aspects in the staging of lung cancer: prospective validation of the International Union Against Cancer TNM classification. Cancer. 1992;70:1102–1110.
44. Takizawa T, Terashima M, Koike T, et al. Mediastinal lymph node metastasis in patients with clinical stage I peripheral non–small-cell lung cancer. J Thorac Cardiovasc Surg. 1997;113:248–252.
45. Yoshino I, Yokoyama H, Yano T, et al. Skip metastasis to the mediastinal lymph nodes in non–small cell lung cancer. Ann Thorac Surg. 1996;62:1021–1025.
46. Ishida T, Tateishi M, Kaneko S, et al. Surgical treatment of patients with nonsmall-cell lung cancer and mediastinal lymph node involvement. J Surg Oncol. 1990;43:161–166.
47. Izbicki JR, Thetter O, Habekost M, et al. Radical systematic mediastinal lymphadenectomy in non–small cell lung cancer: a randomized controlled trial. Br J Surg. 1994;81:229–235.
48. Watanabe Y, Shimizu J, Tsubota M, et al. Mediastinal spread of metastatic lymph nodes in bronchogenic carcinoma: mediastinal nodal metastases in lung cancer. Chest. 1990;97:1059–1065.
49. Asamura H, Nakayama H, Kondo H, et al. Lymph node involvement, recurrence, and prognosis in resected small, peripheral, non–small-cell lung carcinomas: are these carcinomas candidates for video-assisted lobectomy? J Thorac Cardiovasc Surg. 1996;111:1125–1134.
50. Tateishi M, Fukuyama Y, Hamatake M, et al. Skip mediastinal lymph node metastasis in non–small cell lung cancer. J Surg Oncol. 1994;57:139–142.
51. Maggi G, Casadio C, Mancuso M, et al. Resection and radical lymphadenectomy for lung cancer: prognostic significance of lymphatic metastases. Int Surg. 1990;75:17–21.
52. Sawamura K, Mori T, Hashimoto S, et al. Results of surgical treatment for N2 disease [abstract]. Lung Cancer. 1986;2:96.
53. Régnard JF, Magdeleinat P, Azoulay D, et al. Results of resection for bronchogenic carcinoma with mediastinal lymph node metastases in selected patients. Eur J Cardiothorac Surg. 1991;5:583–587.
54. Paone JF, Spees EK, Newton CG, et al. An appraisal of en bloc resection of peripheral bronchogenic carcinoma involving the thoracic wall. Chest. 1982;81:203–207.
55. Ratto GB, Piacenza G, Frola C, et al. Chest wall involvement by lung cancer: computed tomographic detection and results of operation. Ann Thorac Surg. 1991;51:182–188.
56. Shah SS, Goldstraw P. Combined pulmonary and thoracic wall resection for stage III lung cancer. Thorax. 1995;50:782–784.
57. Burt ME, Pomerantz AH, Bains MS, et al. Results of surgical treat-

ment of stage III lung cancer invading the mediastinum. Surg Clin North Am. 1987;67:987–1000.

58. Nakahashi H, Yasumoto K, Sugimachi K. Results of surgical treatment of patients with T3 non–small cell lung cancer. Ann Thorac Surg. 1996;61:273–274.

59. Pitz CCM, de la Riviere AB, Elbers HRJ, et al. Surgical treatment of 125 patients with non–small cell lung cancer and chest wall involvement. Thorax. 1996;51:846–850.

60. Maggi G. Results of radical treatment of stage IIIa non–small-cell carcinoma of the lung. Eur J Cardiothorac Surg. 1988;2:329–335.

61. Albertucci M, DeMeester TR, Rothberg M, et al. Surgery and the management of peripheral lung tumors adherent to the parietal pleura. J Thorac Cardiovasc Surg. 1992;103:8–13.

62. Pitz CC, de la Riviere AB, Elbers HR, et al. Results of resection of T3 non–small cell lung cancer invading the mediastinum or main bronchus. Ann Thorac Surg. 1996;62:1016–1020.

63. Cangemi V, Volpino P, Giuliani A, et al. The role of surgery in stage IIIa non–small cell lung cancer. Panminerva Med. 1994;36:62–65.

64. Neptune WB. Primary lung cancer surgery in stage II and stage III. Arch Surg. 1988;123:583–585.

65. Sabanathan S, Richardson J, Mearns AJ, et al. Results of surgical treatment of stage III lung cancer. Eur J Cardiothorac Surg. 1994;8:183–187.

66. Martini N, Flehinger BJ, Zaman MB, et al. Prospective study of 445 lung carcinomas with mediastinal lymph node metastases. J Thorac Cardiovasc Surg. 1980;80:390–399.

67. Gaer JAR, Goldstraw P. Intraoperative assessment of nodal staging at thoracotomy for carcinoma of the bronchus. Eur J Cardiothorac Surg. 1990;4:207–210.

68. Izbicki JR, Passlick B, Karg O, et al. Impact on radical systematic mediastinal lymphadenectomy on tumor staging in lung cancer. Ann Thorac Surg. 1995;59:209–214.

69. Funatsu T, Matsubara Y, Ikeda S, et al. Preoperative mediastinoscopic assessment of N factors and the need for mediastinal lymph node dissection in T1 lung cancer. J Thorac Cardiovasc Surg. 1994;108:321–328.

70. Izbicki JR, Passlick B, Pantel K, et al. Effectiveness of radical systematic mediastinal lymphadenectomy in patients with resectable non–small cell lung cancer. Ann Surg. 1998;227:138–144.

71. Perez CA, Stanley K, Rubin P, et al. A prospective randomized study of various irradiation doses and fractionation schedules in the treatment of inoperable non–oat-cell carcinoma of the lung: preliminary report by the Radiation Therapy Oncology Group. Cancer. 1980;45:2744–2753.

72. Mantravadi RVP, Gates JO, Crawford JN, et al. Unresectable non–oat cell carcinoma of the lung: definitive radiation therapy. Radiology. 1989;172:851–855.

73. Mountain CF. The biological operability of stage III non–small cell lung cancer. Ann Thorac Surg. 1985;40:60–64.

74. Sawamura K. Cited by Frytak S, Eagan RT, Sawamura K, et al. Treatment of "limited" stage III non–small cell carcinoma of the lung. Cancer Invest. 1988;6:193–207.

75. Conill C, Astudillo J, Verger E. Prognostic significance of metastases to mediastinal lymph node levels in resected non–small cell lung carcinoma. Cancer. 1993;72:1199–1202.

76. Frytak S, Eagan RT, Sawamura K, et al. Treatment of "limited" stage III non–small cell carcinoma of the lung. Cancer Invest. 1988;6:193–207.

77. Adebonojo SA, Bowser AN, Moritz DM, Corcoran PC. Impact of revised stage classification of lung cancer on survival: a military experience. Chest. 1999;115:1507–1513.

78. van Rens MTM, de la Rivière AB, Elbers HRJ, et al. Prognostic assessment of 2,361 patients who underwent pulmonary resection for non–small cell lung cancer, stage I, II, and IIIA. Chest. 2000;117:374–379.

18

RADIOTHERAPY ALONE FOR STAGE IIIA,B NON–SMALL CELL LUNG CANCER

Jay A. Clark, Julian G. Rosenman, and Frank C. Detterbeck

RESULTS WITH CONVENTIONAL RADIOTHERAPY

PATIENT SELECTION ISSUES
Extent of Staging
Performance Status and Weight Loss
IIIa Versus IIIb Disease
Multivariate Analysis
Conclusions Regarding Patient Selection

RADIOTHERAPY TREATMENT ISSUES
Dose
Volume
Split Course Radiotherapy
Hypofractionation
Hyperfractionation
Continuous Hyperfractionated Accelerated Radiotherapy

Hyperfractionated Accelerated Radiotherapy
Three-Dimensional Conformal Radiotherapy
Local Control

EDITORS' COMMENTS

For many decades, radiotherapy (RT) alone was the standard treatment for stage IIIa,b non–small cell lung cancer (NSCLC). This chapter examines the data regarding the use of RT alone when given with curative intent for locally advanced NSCLC. RT that is given explicitly for palliation is discussed in Chapter 29. Unfortunately, the intent of treatment in many studies is not clear, especially in many older reports. Studies involving RT doses of <40 Gy are arbitrarily assumed to have been done with a palliative intent and are excluded. Furthermore, studies involving both RT and chemotherapy for IIIa and IIIb disease are discussed in Chapters 19 and 21 and are not included here.

RT alone clearly results in the cure of some patients with stage IIIa,b NSCLC, although the 5-year survival is low. On the other hand, the natural history of untreated patients with this disease demonstrates no survivors beyond 2 years (see Table 3–4).[1] Although RT does cure some patients, there is clearly much room for improvement in terms of survival as well as local control. This chapter examines issues related to patient selection and the delivery of radiation in order to define factors that influence the ability of RT to cure locally advanced lung cancer.

The data reported in this chapter is taken primarily from prospective, multi-institutional, randomized trials. Such results are used not only to examine the differences between the randomized arms within a phase III trial but also to establish a solid baseline for particular RT approaches that are used in a similar fashion among several different trials. Multi-institutional trials involve clearly defined patient populations and data that has been carefully scrutinized in

terms of quality and completeness. Furthermore, these trials are probably more able to be generalized to the general medical community. Single institution and phase II trials are included where the data points out a new direction that may lead to a survival benefit.

RESULTS WITH CONVENTIONAL RADIOTHERAPY

RT given at 1.8 to 2.0 Gy per day, five fractions per week, to a total dose of approximately 60 Gy using traditional two-dimensional treatment planning was considered to be standard treatment by most radiation oncologists during the 1980s and 1990s. Data from prospective, multi-institutional studies involving conventional radiation in well defined patient groups is shown in Table 18–1. These results are consistent with one another, and the average 1-, 2-, 3-, and 5-year overall survival rates are 44%, 18%, 9%, and 6%, respectively. Average median survival is approximately 11 months. The data from other nonrandomized trials of ≥100 patients has shown identical results.[2–4]

It is clear that there is room for significant improvement in the treatment of stage IIIa,b patients with NSCLC using RT alone. Better results using RT alone may come through patient selection by defining which patients are most likely to achieve a benefit. In addition, alterations in the way RT is given may result in improved survival. These issues are examined in the following sections.

TABLE 18-1. OVERALL SURVIVAL WITH CONVENTIONAL RADIOTHERAPY[a] ALONE FOR IIIa,b NON–SMALL CELL LUNG CANCER

STUDY	N	TOTAL DOSE (Gy)	DOSE PER FRACTION (Gy)	SURVIVAL		
				MST (mo)	2-y (%)	5-y (%)
Saunders et al[37]	225	60	2	13	20	7[b]
Le Chevalier et al[29]	167	65	2.5	10	14	4
Holsti and Mattson[40]	158	50	1.7	—	(12)[c, d]	(6)[c, d]
Sause et al[38]	149	60	2	11	21	5
Perez et al[41]	129	60	2	12	24	—
Simpson et al[28]	123	60	2	—	15	—
Miller[39]	117	58	2	9	18	4
Blanke et al[31]	111	60–65	1.8–2	11	13	2
Johnson et al[32]	104	60	1.8	9	13	3
Average[e]				11	17	4

Inclusion criteria: Conventional radiotherapy arms of prospective randomized trials involving ≥100 patients with IIIa,b non–small cell lung cancer from 1980 to 2000.
[a]Defined as 50–65 Gy of radiotherapy given once a day, Monday through Friday.
[b]4-year survival.
[c]Absolute (not actuarial) survival.
[d]Disease-free survival.
[e]Excluding numbers in parentheses.
MST, median survival time (months).

PATIENT SELECTION ISSUES

Extent of Staging

One of the issues that can potentially affect survival of patients treated with RT alone is the extent of distant staging. Advancements in diagnostic imaging may more accurately identify those patients who have localized disease. Certainly, patients who have unsuspected distant metastases cannot be expected to be cured with thoracic RT alone, and there is evidence that approximately 30% of patients with stage cIIIa,b disease harbor radiographically detectable distant metastases even when asymptomatic (see Table 6–3). Reliance on an absence of symptoms of distant metastases alone, without radiographic studies to look for silent metastases, may therefore adversely affect outcome data.

Table 18–2 lists the survival results of multi-institutional trials according to whether a negative clinical examination was considered sufficient for patient inclusion or whether distant organ scanning was required. There was no difference in median or long-term survival. The reason for this is unclear. It may be that a radiologic evaluation for distant metastases was performed in most of the patients undergoing limited staging, even though it was not required. Alter-

TABLE 18-2. OVERALL SURVIVAL IN TRIALS EMPLOYING EXTENSIVE INVESTIGATION OF DISTANT METASTASES VERSUS LIMITED STAGING

STUDY	N	STAGING	MST (mo)	2-y (%)	5-y (%)
LeChevalier et al[29]	167	Extensive	10	14	4
Blanke et al[31]	111	Extensive[a]	11	13	2
Johnson et al[32]	104	Extensive[b]	9	13	3
Dillman et al[10]	77	Extensive[b]	10	13	7
Slawson et al[21]	63	Extensive	10	23	—
Average			10	15	4
Holsti and Mattson[40]	158	Limited	—	(12)[c]	(6)[c]
Sause et al[38]	149	Limited[d]	11	21	5
Perez et al[41]	129	Limited	12	24	—
Simpson et al[28]	123	Limited	8	15	—
Morton et al[33]	58	Limited[a, f]	10	16	7
Soresi et al[11]	50	Limited[d]	11	25	—
Average			11	20	5

Inclusion criteria: Data from prospective, randomized trials from 1980 to 2000, providing information about whether extensive staging or limited staging was performed, in ≥50 patients with IIIa,b non–small cell lung cancer treated with conventional radiotherapy given with curative intent (50–65 Gy, once daily).
[a]Bone scan excluded.
[b]Brain imaging excluded.
[c]Absolute disease-free survival.
[d]Chest computed tomography included.
[e]4-year survival.
[f]Included bone scan.
Extensive staging, clinical workup including chest/upper abdominal computed tomography, bone scan, and brain imaging; Limited staging, clinical workup with chest radiography only; MST, median survival time.

natively, the clinical evaluation may, in fact, be accurate in determining the absence of distant metastases for these patients. However, it is most likely that the results with conventional RT alone are so poor that a difference relative to the extent of staging cannot be detected.

Performance Status and Weight Loss

It is generally believed that patients with a poor performance status (PS) or with weight loss have a worse prognosis when they are treated with RT for cure than patients who are relatively asymptomatic. PS has been found to be the best predictor of survival in advanced stage patients (see Table 22–1), and the same is probably true of stage IIIa,b patients as well. As a result, almost all studies of curative RT have included only a small number of patients with a poor PS ($\leq$70) or weight loss ($\geq$5%), and the actual outcome of such patients treated with conventional RT is undefined. In addition, patients with extensive comorbidity or poor pulmonary reserve are believed to have poor outcomes, although specific data is not available because such patients are excluded from reported studies.

Three phase III studies of RT have included a majority (50%-58%) of patients with a PS $\leq$70, weight loss $\geq$5%, or both.[5–7] These studies have employed either low dose RT (36 or 45 Gy) or 65 Gy hyperfractionated RT.[6] The average median and 2-year survival in these studies was 10 months and 18%, respectively, which is not appreciably different from that of conventional RT arms (55-65 Gy, daily fractions) in phase III trials that have excluded patients with poor PS or weight loss altogether (median survival time, 11 months; 2-year survival, 19%).[8–11] The validity of such a comparison is questionable, however, because of the markedly different RT regimens used.

Several studies employing retrospective multivariate analysis have consistently demonstrated that PS is a major independent prognostic factor among locally advanced patients treated with RT.[12,13] Weight loss has been inconsistently found to be an independent prognostic factor.[12–14] The results of multivariate analysis are discussed further in the next section. In conclusion, it is clear that PS is a major independent prognostic factor in stage IIIa,b patients

treated with RT, although the actual outcome of patients with a poor PS has not been defined.

IIIa Versus IIIb Disease

One of the primary purposes of a staging system is to distinguish patient groups that have a different prognosis. However, most patients with locally advanced NSCLC have been treated with the same RT approach regardless of whether they are classified as cIIIa or cIIIb, and the TNM staging system is criticized for not providing useful prognostic information for patients treated with RT.[14] A summary of studies examining this issue is shown in Table 18–3. The majority of these studies have demonstrated that stage IIIa patients have better survival, and in fact, the difference was statistically significant in all of these. Only one study found that there was no difference.[14]

These studies involved both retrospective series and prospective randomized trials in which the survival of IIIa and IIIb patients was examined separately. Whether there was an association between the stage of the disease and other potential prognostic factors (eg, performance status) or treatment factors (eg, RT dose) was generally not analyzed. The study by Curran and Stafford[14] did analyze other factors and found that patients were well matched with respect to age, gender, PS, weight loss, histologic type, and grade. However, significantly more patients with stage IIIa than with IIIb disease received an RT dose $\geq$55 Gy (79% versus 58%, $P = 0.01$). Despite this, the stage IIIa patients in this retrospective analysis did not survive longer than the IIIb patients. The reason that this study found no difference, while all other comparisons of IIIa and IIIb patients demonstrated a difference, is not clear.

Multivariate Analysis

A multivariate analysis of 77 prognostic factors was reported in 1980, involving >5000 patients from several Veterans Administration (VA) Lung Group Protocols from 1968 to 1978.[12] The three factors that had statistically significant prognostic value were PS, extent of disease, and weight loss. However, it is not clear that this data is

TABLE 18–3. SURVIVAL OF PATIENTS WITH LOCALLY ADVANCED NON–SMALL CELL LUNG CANCER TREATED WITH RADIOTHERAPY ALONE, ACCORDING TO STAGE (IIIa VERSUS IIIb)

STUDY	N	TYPE	MST (mo)		2-y SURVIVAL %		P
			IIIa	IIIb	IIIa	IIIb	
Cox et al[34a]	516	Randomized	9	7	18	11	<0.03
Jeremic et al[6a,b]	131	Randomized	25	13	54	17	<0.0001
Kreisman et al[35b]	112	Randomized	17	11	32	13	<0.005
Rosenthal[3]	656	Retrospective	11	10	22	18	<0.05
Würschmidt[2]	233	Retrospective	14	11	28	6	<0.02
Reinfuss[4]	170	Retrospective	11	5	16	3	<0.05
Curran[14]	306	Retrospective	9	10	17	18	NS
Average			**14**	**10**	**27**	**12**	

Inclusion criteria: Studies of $\geq$100 patients from 1980 to 2000 treated with >40 Gy RT and reporting stage IIIa,b-specific results
[a]Includes patients receiving hyperfractionated RT.
[b]Includes patients receiving chemotherapy and RT; however, the difference between IIIa and IIIb is reported to be similar in patients treated with RT alone.
MST = mean survival time; NS, not significant; RT, radiotherapy.

TABLE 18–4. RECURSIVE PARTITIONING ANALYSIS OF PROGNOSTIC FACTORS

PROGNOSTIC CLASS	KARNOFSKY PS	N STAGE	AGE	RT DOSE	WEIGHT LOSS	PLEURAL EFFUSION	MST (mo)	2-y (%)
Group I	80–100 80–100	N0 N1–3	— <70	— >66 Gy	— <5%	— —	13	25
Group II	80–100 80–100	N1–3 N1–3	<70 <70	>66 Gy ≤66 Gy	≥5% —	— —	8	13
Group III	80–100 ≤70	N1–3 —	≥70 —	— —	— —	— None	6	8
Group IV	≤70	—	—	—	—	Present	3	5

Inclusion criteria: Largest multivariate analysis of prognostic factors in patients treated with RT alone with curative intent.
MST, median survival time; PS, performance status; RT, radiotherapy.
Data from Scott C, et al.[13]

applicable to current patients with locally advanced NSCLC treated with RT given with curative intent. Not all of the patients in the VA series had stage IIIa,b disease, and the treatment primarily involved RT that would be considered palliative by today's standards.

A multivariate analysis of nine pretreatment variables in a cohort of 1592 NSCLC patients treated on various Radiation Therapy Oncology Group (RTOG) protocols has been carried out.[13] The factors examined included age, gender, PS, weight loss, T stage, N stage, race, histology, and presence of pleural effusion. Independent prognostic factors by Cox multivariate analysis were found to be PS, N stage, age, weight loss, and whether a pleural effusion was present.[13] The T-stage and gender were of marginal significance ($P = 0.05$-0.1).

The same cohort of 1592 patients was also analyzed using recursive partitioning analysis.[13] This analysis identified the PS as the most important factor, followed by age and weight loss (among those with a PS of 80-100). The RT dose received (>64 Gy or ≤64 Gy) also had prognostic value, but this does not represent a patient characteristic that can be used to prospectively guide selection of patients

for treatment. Four distinct prognostic classes were identified, as shown in Table 18–4 and Figure 18–1. The 2-year survival varied from 25% for the most favorable class to 5% for the least favorable (PS ≤ 70 with a pleural effusion). The four prognostic groups identified by recursive partitioning analysis were validated in an independent data set involving 282 patients.[13]

Conclusions Regarding Patient Selection

By what criteria, then, should patients with stage IIIa,b NSCLC be selected for RT with an intent to cure? Review of the data cited earlier leaves this issue somewhat unclear, in part because the survival of these patients is generally poor when treated with conventional RT alone. PS is a major prognostic factor, as is clearly demonstrated by the multivariate analyses discussed earlier. The clinical stage (IIIa versus IIIb) is also of importance, although this has received less attention. The prognostic value of weight loss is controversial. The recursive partitioning analysis discussed earlier provides the best guidance because it is by far the largest study, has been validated in another data set, and quantifies the outcomes of specific patient groups.[13]

Aggressive RT in patients with locally advanced, nonmetastatic NSCLC who have a good PS (Karnofsky PS ≥80) and who are <70 years old can be easily justified. Whether patients with a good PS who are >70 years should be treated aggressively is not clear. Patients with a PS of ≤70 have a median survival of only 6 months at best,[13] and it seems that the goal of treatment for these patients should be palliation rather than cure. Although those studies that included a majority of patients with poor prognostic factors reported median survivals of approximately 10 months, almost half of the patients in these studies did not have poor prognostic factors.[5–7] Furthermore, the definition of unfavorable prognostic factors in these studies is not entirely clear. The multivariate analysis provides good data indicating that the median survival of patients with a PS of ≤70 is ≤6 months.

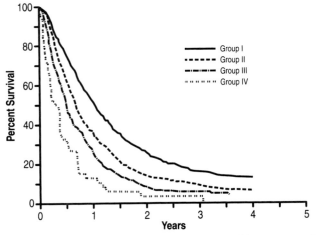

FIGURE 18–1. Survival of 1592 patients with inoperable, nonmetastatic non–small cell lung cancer, separated by recursive partitioning analysis into four prognostic groups. (From Scott C, Sause WT, Byhardt R, et al. Recursive partitioning analysis of 1592 patients on four radiation therapy oncology group studies in inoperable non–small cell lung cancer. Lung Cancer. 1997;17(suppl 1):S59–S74.)[13]

RADIOTHERAPY TREATMENT ISSUES

Dose

Based on concepts proposed by Fletcher[15] in 1973, in which doses of up to 100 Gy were hypothesized to be

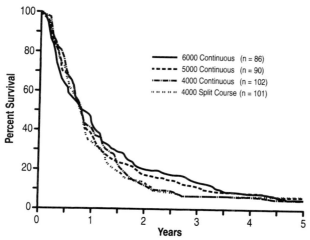

FIGURE 18–2. Survival of 551 patients with inoperable nonmetastatic non–small cell lung cancer, randomized to four different radiotherapy regimens. (From CANCER, Vol 59, No. 11, 1987, 1874–1881. Copyright © 1987 American Cancer Society. Reprinted by permission of Wiley-Liss, Inc., a subsidiary of John Wiley & Sons, Inc.)[16]

required to control large carcinomas, the doses currently accepted as standard for the treatment of locally advanced NSCLC may be inadequate. Corroborating this hypothesis is indirect data that suggests that doses of 40 to 50 Gy are tumoricidal only for microscopic disease (see Chapter 9). In light of these considerations, it is actually remarkable that 5% to 10% of patients with locally advanced lung cancer treated with 50 to 60 Gy of conventional RT are cured of their disease.

A number of arguments have been presented suggesting that increasing the total dose of RT for NSCLC might be beneficial (see Chapter 9). However, data showing a survival benefit in locally advanced NSCLC is limited, at best. RTOG conducted a randomized trial of 365 patients given 40 Gy split course and 40, 50, or 60 Gy of continuous RT (Fig. 18–2). Although there were slight differences in the median survival (37, 41, 41, and 47 weeks), there was no difference in the 5-year survival (5%-6% in all arms).[16] Another randomized study of hyperfractionated RT explored doses varying from 60 to 79 Gy in 884 patients.[17] No statistically significant difference was seen between the trial arms, although this trial was designed as a randomized phase II study to investigate toxicity rather than survival. There was a suggestion that survival was better at 69 Gy, but the argument that this was due to the dose is weakened by the fact that higher doses exhibited worse survival. Furthermore, there were differences in the stage of patients in the various arms even though the trial was randomized, because patients for the various arms were not all accrued at the same time (stage II:IIIb, 24%:24% at 60 Gy versus 8%:37% at 79 Gy).[17] It may be that the effect of increasing the dose of RT in NSCLC has not been adequately tested in randomized studies at dose ranges that are high enough to make a difference in terms of survival.

In summary, although there is no clear data showing that a higher dose of RT results in improved survival, there is reason to maintain an open mind and explore this issue further. The advent of 3-dimensional (3-D) RT planning systems appears to allow higher doses to be delivered with

less normal tissue toxicity, and there are suggestions that altering the dose and the way that RT is delivered (eg, hyperfractionation, continuous hyperfractionated accelerated radiation therapy [CHART]) may result in a survival benefit. Thus the standard of 60 to 65 Gy using standard fractionation still stands, but further investigation of higher doses in the context of a study protocol is warranted.

Volume

There is no evidence that larger radiation fields that include radiographically uninvolved contralateral hilar or supraclavicular lymph nodes are beneficial. Conventional RT treatment plans cover the primary tumor, ipsilateral hilum, and mediastinum plus a 2-cm margin. Beam arrangements have typically been anterior-posterior/posterior-anterior to spinal cord tolerance (~45 Gy) followed by opposed oblique portals blocking the spinal cord out of the radiation beam to higher doses. Controversy has long existed regarding the necessity of including *uninvolved* nodes (negative by either mediastinoscopy or by imaging studies) within the radiation portals. The rationale for omitting coverage of uninvolved lymph nodes is based on the argument that the majority of local failures are located within areas of gross disease and that escalation of the RT dose to the gross tumor can be achieved more safely if the volume of normal tissue receiving radiation is reduced.

The data on this subject is sparse. The University of Michigan omitted uninvolved nodes from their radiation portals in a study in which 3-D conformal RT (CRT) treatment planning was used to escalate dose to the gross tumor volume. Robertson et al[18] found that none of the 48 patients (18 patients stage I, II, 28 patients stage III, and 2 patients with mediastinal recurrence after surgery) failed in the radiographically uninvolved, high risk, untreated mediastinum as the sole site of failure. Another study involving 126 patients treated with chemotherapy and RT (40 Gy concurrent) found that only 8% failed in untreated contralateral supraclavicular nodes, and none failed in the untreated contralateral hilum.[19] Because there is no data suggesting a high rate of failure if radiographically uninvolved nodal regions are not radiated, it is reasonable to cover uninvolved nodes only if the inclusion of these areas does not involve a significant volume of additional normal lung.

Split Course Radiotherapy

Split course radiation typically involves a 2- to 4-week break after 25 to 30 Gy of RT before an additional 25 to 30 Gy of RT is given over a total treatment period of 6 to 11 weeks. Many investigators believe that split course treatment is inferior because the break gives the tumor time to undergo accelerated repopulation. Despite the potential radiobiologic advantages to continuous course irradiation, there is no clinical data to suggest that split course RT results in decreased long-term survival. Three prospective, randomized trials have compared split course to continuous course RT (Table 18–5). None of these three trials found

TABLE 18–5. OVERALL SURVIVAL OF RANDOMIZED TRIALS OF SPLIT VERSUS CONTINUOUS COURSE RADIOTHERAPY

STUDY	N	TOTAL DOSE (Gy)	DOSE PER FRACTION (Gy)	RT SCHEDULE	SURVIVAL		
					MST (mo)	2-y (%)	5-y (%)
Holsti and Mattson[40a]	205	55	2.5–3	Split	10	12	2
Perez et al[16]	101	40	4	Split	9	10	5
Lee et al[36b]	102	50	1.75–2	Split	—	11	2
Holsti and Mattson[40a]	158	50	2	Continuous	10	12	6
Perez et al[16]	102	40	2	Continuous	9	15	4
Lee et al[36b]	86	50	1.75–2	Continuous	—	10	4

Inclusion criteria: Results of trials from 1980 to 2000 that randomized ≥100 patients with IIIa,b non–small cell lung cancer to either split or continuous RT.
[a]Includes 13% small-cell lung cancer.
[b]Includes 31% small-cell lung cancer.
MST = median survival time; RT, radiotherapy.

any survival differences between these two approaches. However, results of these trials and other trials involving split course RT give the impression that patients have generally tolerated the split course treatment better than the continuous course of RT.

Split course RT is attractive to many radiation oncologists when the intent of treatment is unclear. Patients who present with severe symptoms or poor PS can be given a palliative dose of RT as a first course of treatment. When the patient returns for follow-up approximately 2 weeks after completion of the first course, an assessment of suitability for a second course of radiation can be made. If the patient has become symptomatically worse or if metastatic disease is detected, the patient can forego any further radiation to the chest. If there has been symptomatic improvement after the first course of radiation, it is reasonable to add a second course of RT in an attempt to cure.

No data is available regarding whether an early response (to the first course of RT) predicts an improved outcome among patients receiving both courses of RT. Data from continuous course regimens indicates that patients who achieve a response to RT have a better prognosis than nonresponders.[20] Extrapolation of this data suggests that basing a decision for a second course of RT on clinical or radiographic response to the first course of RT has some validity. However, it is not clear that a lack of response to the first course justifies withholding further RT, at least when there has not been evidence of disease progression.

In summary, a split course schedule is a reasonable approach for patients with poor PS or a shorter life expectancy as a test to determine how the patient will respond clinically to the treatment. The first course can be given over a 2- to 3-week period and, in itself, may be an adequate palliative dose of RT. This first course would then be followed by a 2- to 4-week break, followed by reassessment for a second 2- to 3-week course of treatment.

Hypofractionation

Hypofractionated radiation, in which large doses per fraction are delivered once or twice a week, has long been frowned on by the radiation oncology community because large dose fractions are thought to be associated with severe long-term radiation morbidity. Only one randomized trial has been conducted involving hypofractionated RT given with curative intent in locally advanced NSCLC. The University of Maryland randomized 120 patients treated with a total of 60 Gy of RT, given either once weekly (5 Gy per weekly fraction for 12 weeks) or as conventional radiation (2 Gy per daily fraction 5 days a week for 6 weeks).[21] No significant difference in overall survival was found between once-a-week and conventional RT (1-year survival, 59% versus 49%; 2-year survival, 29% versus 23%). Not surprisingly, patients on the once-a-week arm had less acute morbidity from the radiation. Somewhat surprising, however, was the finding that there was no increase in late morbidity (average follow-up, 3 years) in the hypofractionated arm.[21]

In contrast to the Maryland study, RTOG randomized 108 patients to 6 Gy given twice weekly to a total dose of 36 Gy with or without the hypoxic cell sensitizer misonidazole.[7] Median survival times in both arms were poor at 7 months, which may have been largely a reflection of the patient population (60% of the patients had a Karnofsky PS of 60-80). The most striking finding was the late radiation morbidity. Three patients developed esophageal stricture, which led to perforation and death in one case. Pneumonitis was reported in three patients and led to death in one of them. There were two cases of severe pulmonary fibrosis and two cases of radiation myelopathy. The large fractions led to severe morbidity in 10% of patients and would probably have been higher with more long-term survivors.[7]

Hyperfractionation

The definition of *hyperfractionation* is delivery of more than one radiation treatment per day (see Chapter 9). Typically, the total daily dose of radiation is 10% to 15% higher than conventional fractionation and the total treatment dose is usually slightly higher than conventional RT, while the overall treatment time remains unchanged. With the use of smaller doses per fraction, yet overall higher doses, the late effects of radiation on normal tissues may be reduced while the tumor control probability may be increased compared with standard continuous fractionation (see Chapter 9).

TABLE 18–6. OVERALL SURVIVAL AFTER CONVENTIONAL AND HYPERFRACTIONATED RADIOTHERAPY FOR IIIa,b NON–SMALL CELL LUNG CANCER

STUDY	N	TOTAL DOSE (Gy)	DOSE PER FRACTION (Gy)	RT SCHEDULE	SURVIVAL		
					MST (mo)	2-y (%)	5-y (%)
Saunders et al[37]	225	60	2	Every day	13	20	7[a]
Le Chevalier et al[29]	167	65	2.5	Every day	10	14	4
Sause et al[38]	149	60	2	Every day	12	21	5
Perez et al[41]	129	60	2	Every day	12	24	—
Simpson et al[28]	123	60	2	Every day	8	15	—
Miller et al[39]	117	58	2	Every day	9	18	4
Blanke et al[31]	111	60–65	2	Every day	10	13	2
Johnson et al[32]	104	60	2	Every day	9	13	3
Average (Conventional)					11	17	4
Saunders et al[37]	338	54	1.5	Three times a day	16	29	14[a]
Cox et al[17]	220	69.6	1.2	Twice a day	10	20	8[a]
Cox et al[17]	211	74.4	1.2	Twice a day	9	15	—
Cox et al[17]	207	79.2	1.2	Twice a day	11	20	—
Sause et al[38]	152	69.6	1.2	Twice a day	12	24	6
Cox et al[17]	127	64.8	1.2	Twice a day	6	14	8[a]
Average (Hyperfractionated)					11	20	9[a]

Inclusion criteria: Conventional fractionation (once daily) or hyperfractionation (twice or three times a day) RT arms in prospective, randomized trials from 1980 to 2000 involving ≥100 patients.
[a]4-year survival.
MST, median survival time; RT, radiotherapy.

The data from hyperfractionated RT arms in various phase III prospective trials is summarized in Table 18–6 and compared with conventional fractionation. These results suggest that hyperfractionated RT may lead to a modest improvement in survival when compared with standard fractionation to 60 Gy. However, these trials have not generally randomized patients between hyperfractionated RT and conventional RT, and thus differences in patient population and prognostic factors may confound the results.

One randomized, prospective trial comparing hyperfractionated irradiation with standard fractionation on a head-to-head basis has been carried out.[22] Patients in this trial, performed by the RTOG and the Eastern Cooperative Oncology Group (ECOG), were required to have a Karnofsky PS of ≥70 and minimal weight loss. A trend to better survival was seen at 1 year in the hyperfractionation arm versus the standard RT arm (51% versus 46%, P = NS). Median survival was 12.3 months in the hyperfractionated arm versus 11.4 months in the standard arm (P = NS). Toxicity was acceptable in both arms.[22] In an update of this trial,[9] the overall survival was approximately 5% better with hyperfractionated RT compared with standard RT (2-year survival, 24% versus 20%; 4-year survival, 9% versus 4%), but the difference was not statistically significant (Fig. 18–3).

Continuous Hyperfractionated Accelerated Radiation Therapy

Because many tumors will rapidly proliferate in response to treatment,[23] it has been hypothesized that decreasing the overall treatment time may counter the effects of accelerated repopulation of a tumor and improve control rates. Combining this concept of decreasing the overall treatment

time with giving smaller doses per fraction to minimize long-term morbidity led to the introduction of CHART. A randomized trial of conventional RT (60 Gy at 2 Gy per day over 6 weeks) versus CHART (54 Gy at 1.5 Gy twice a day over 12 days) has been carried out in 563 good PS patients with locally advanced NSCLC (Fig. 18–4).[8] A statistically significant survival benefit was found in the

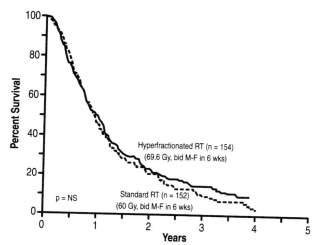

FIGURE 18–3. Survival of 300 patients with inoperable locally advanced non–small cell lung cancer, randomized to conventional RT (60 Gy in 2-Gy fractions over 6 weeks) versus hyperfractionated RT (69.6 Gy in 1.2-Gy fractions given twice daily over 6 weeks) in RTOG 88-08/ECOG 4588 study. Data from a third arm, involving chemotherapy and RT, is not included. RT, radiotherapy. (Adapted from *International Journal of Radiation Oncology, Biology, Physics,* Vol 39, Komaki R, Scott CB, Sause WT, et al, Induction cisplatin/vinblastine and irradiation vs. irradiation in unresectable squamous cell lung cancer: failure patterns by cell type in RTOG 88-08/ECOG 4588, 537–544, Copyright 1997, with permission from Elsevier Science.)[9]

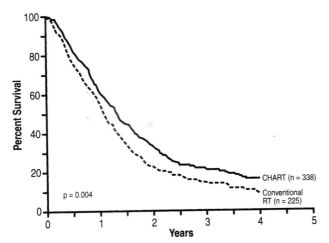

FIGURE 18–4. Survival of 563 patients with locally advanced non–small cell lung cancer, randomized to conventional radiotherapy (60 Gy in 2-Gy fractions over 6 weeks) versus continuous hyperfractionated accelerated radiotherapy (54 Gy in 1.5-Gy fractions given three times per day over 12 consecutive days). (From Saunders M, Dische S, Barrett A, et al. Continuous hyperfractionated accelerated radiotherapy [CHART] versus conventional radiotherapy in non–small-cell lung cancer: a randomised multicentre trial. Lancet. 1997;350[9072]:161–165, © by The Lancet Ltd, 1997.)[8]

CHART arm (2-year overall survival, 29% versus 20%; $P = 0.004$) Although severe acute esophagitis was more prevalent in the CHART group (19% versus 3%), the long-term morbidity was not affected.

Hyperfractionated Accelerated Radiation Therapy

Hyperfractionated accelerated radiation therapy (HART) is also being studied.[24,25] HART is similar to CHART with the exception that no radiation is given on the weekends. No phase III trials comparing HART with conventional RT or chemoradiation have been reported. ECOG is currently conducting a phase III trial investigating HART.

Three-Dimensional Conformal Radiotherapy

The arguments indicating that 3-D CRT treatment planning will play an important role in improving the results of RT are compelling. 3-D CRT allows more precise tumor targeting while minimizing the amount of radiation delivered to the surrounding normal tissues (see Chapter 9). This is a prerequisite for safe escalation of the total dose of RT, especially in lung cancer. Investigators at the University of Michigan have reported the use of 3-D CRT treatment planning to escalate RT doses to as high as 100 Gy in patients with NSCLC.[18] The preliminary data that has been reported indicates that this can be done without significant toxicity.[18,26,27] There were no instances of severe radiation pneumonitis among 48 patients treated with 63 to 92.4 Gy (to radiographically abnormal areas only). It is important to note that the volume of normal tissue irradi-

ated was kept to a minimum in this study. 3-D treatment planning holds promise for improved local control rates and potentially improved survival rates, but no long-term survival data is available regarding the use of 3-D CRT in lung cancer.

Local Control

The issue of local control is difficult to analyze from the literature because of the low doses of RT used and the various ways local control is defined. The assessment of local control has traditionally been evaluated by radiographic follow-up. This is hampered by the difficulty of differentiating radiation-induced scarring from recurrent tumor. More importantly, however, analysis of recurrence patterns between studies is difficult because of a lack of clear and consistent definitions. Lack of radiographic tumor progression, radiographic complete response, and endoscopic pathologic complete response have all been used as definitions of local control in the literature. Some studies report only *first* site of recurrence, whereas others report recurrences occurring *at any time*. After the first site of recurrence has appeared, it is likely that subsequent recurrences are underreported.

Nevertheless, with these caveats in mind, it appears that locoregional recurrence is involved in approximately 75% of recurrences.[4,16,28–30] Reinfuss et al,[4] considering ultimate sites of recurrence in 332 patients with stage III disease who were given 40 Gy split course irradiation, found that 62% died of locoregional recurrence, 26% died of both distant and locoregional recurrence, and only 2% died of distant disease alone. In a study of 551 patients from RTOG 73-01 and 73-02, Perez et al[16] found the *first* site of recurrence to be 44% local, 22% combined, and 34% distant, whereas the *ultimate* patterns of recurrence were 23% local, 54% combined, and 23% distant. It appears that local control is worse when more careful investigations, such as bronchoscopy, are employed. Le Chevalier et al[29] found bronchoscopic local failure in 83% of patients with IIIa and IIIb disease who received 65 Gy. Therefore, local control with the use of RT has significant room for improvement.

Several studies have indicated that increased doses result in better local control. The randomized trial of stage IIIa,b patients given 40, 50, or 60 Gy of RT (RTOG 73-01) found lower cumulative local recurrence rates at higher doses (33%, 39%, and 49% for 60, 50, and 40 Gy, respectively)[16] (see Fig. 9–4). Better local control (58%) relative to historic controls is suggested by RTOG 83-12, which delivered 75 Gy in 25 fractions to 59 patients with Karnofsky PS ≥ 60.[30]

EDITORS' COMMENTS

Even if one accepts the general belief that chemoradiation is superior to radiation alone for the treatment of locally advanced NSCLC, one still needs to treat a significant cohort of patients who either cannot or will not consent to chemotherapy with RT alone. Such patients are not necessarily incurable. These patients represent a spectrum, rang-

DATA SUMMARY: RADIOTHERAPY FOR IIIA,B NON–SMALL CELL LUNG CANCER

	AMOUNT	QUALITY	CONSISTENCY
Conventional RT (60 Gy, 5 daily fractions per week) results in a 5% 5-year survival in stage IIIa,b non–small cell lung cancer	High	High	High
Survival of cIIIa patients treated with RT alone is better than that of cIIIb patients	High	Mod	High
Performance status ≤70 and age ≥70 are markers of limited survival (median ≤6 months) in patients treated with RT alone	Poor	High	—
Survival results with split course RT are equivalent to continuous course RT	**Mod**	**High**	**High**
CHART results in an increased survival by approximately 10% compared to conventional RT	**Poor**	**High**	—
Increasing the RT dose (daily fractions) between 40-60 Gy results in no improvement in long-term survival	**Poor**	**High**	—

Type of data rated: Plain: descriptive statement   *Italics: controlled comparison*   **Bold: randomized comparison**

ing from those who are healthy but elect not to receive chemotherapy to those who cannot tolerate chemotherapy because of comorbid conditions. The first group of patients may do best with continuous RT, perhaps delivered twice a day. The second cohort may benefit most from a split course approach that reduces acute morbidity, shortens treatment time, and allows patients who experience a decline in general well being to drop out of therapy after the first course.

It seems incontestable that proper tumor targeting is essential for cure. A growing body of experience suggests that 3-D treatment planning improves the ability to achieve this goal compared with two-dimensional planning. In addition, the traditional dose of 60 Gy for the treatment of NSCLC seems entirely too low when compared with doses given to other types of primary tumors of similar volume or smaller (uterine, cervix, prostate, and head and neck cancers). It is clear that the use of 3-D treatment planning will permit much higher radiation doses to be given safely. It is likely that 3-D treatment planning, higher doses, and altered fractionation schedules will lead to better local control, and hopefully also better survival.

Despite many years of collective experience in treating NSCLC with radiation, there remain a significant number of things we have yet to learn. We do not have reliable predictors for radiation pneumonitis. We do not know to what extent coverage of radiographically uninvolved nodes is important. The significant problem of discriminating between tumor and collapsed or edematous lung still remains. Finally, the optimal radiation dose and the dose fractionation for the treatment of NSCLC have yet to be determined.

References

1. Vrdoljak E, Mise K, Sapunar D, et al. Survival analysis of untreated patients with non–small-cell lung cancer. Chest. 1994;106:1797–1800.
2. Würschmidt F, Bünemann H, Bünemann C, et al. Inoperable non–small cell lung cancer: a retrospective analysis of 427 patients treated with high-dose radiotherapy. Int J Radiat Oncol Biol Phys. 1994;28:583–588.
3. Rosenthal SA, Curran WJ Jr, Herbert SH, et al. Clinical stage II non–small cell lung cancer treated with radiation therapy alone: the significance of clinically staged ipsilateral hilar adenopathy (N1 disease). Cancer. 1992;70:2410–2417.
4. Reinfuss M, Skolyszewski J, Kowalska T, et al. Palliative radiotherapy in asymptomatic patients with locally advanced, unresectable, non–small cell lung cancer. Strahlenther Onkol. 1993;169:709–715.
5. Trovo MG, Minatel E, Franchin G, et al. Radiotherapy versus radiotherapy enhanced by cisplatin in stage III non–small cell lung cancer. Int J Radiat Oncol Biol Phys. 1992;24:11–15.
6. Jeremic B, Shibamoto Y, Acimovic L, et al. Hyperfractionated radiation therapy with or without concurrent low-dose daily carboplatin/etoposide for stage III non–small-cell lung cancer: a randomized study. J Clin Oncol. 1996;14:1065–1070.
7. Simpson JR, Bauer M, Wasserman TH, et al. Large fraction irradiation with or without misonidazole in advanced non–oat cell carcinoma of the lung: a phase III randomized trial of the RTOG. Int J Radiat Oncol Biol Phys. 1987;13:861–867.
8. Saunders M, Dische S, Barrett A, et al. Continuous hyperfractionated accelerated radiotherapy (CHART) versus conventional radiotherapy in non–small-cell lung cancer: a randomised multicentre trial. Lancet. 1997;350:161–165.
9. Komaki R, Scott CB, Sause WT, et al. Induction cisplatin/vinblastine and irradiation vs. irradiation in unresectable squamous cell lung cancer: failure patterns by cell type in RTOG 88-08/ECOG 4588. Int J Radiat Oncol Biol Phys. 1997;39:537–544.
10. Dillman RO, Seagren SL, Propert KJ, et al. A randomized trial of induction chemotherapy plus high-dose radiation versus radiation alone in stage III non–small-cell lung cancer. N Engl J Med. 1990;323:940–945.
11. Soresi E, Clerici M, Grilli R, et al. A randomized clinical trial comparing radiation therapy v radiation therapy plus cis-dichlorodiammine platinum (II) in the treatment of locally advanced non–small cell lung cancer. Semin Oncol. 1988;15:20–25.
12. Stanley KE. Prognostic factors for survival in patients with inoperable lung cancer. J Natl Cancer Inst. 1980;65:25–32.
13. Scott C, Sause WT, Byhardt R, et al. Recursive partitioning analysis of 1592 patients on four Radiation Therapy Oncology Group studies in inoperable non–small-cell lung cancer. Lung Cancer. 1997;17(suppl 1):S59–S74.
14. Curran WJ Jr, Stafford PM. Lack of apparent difference in outcome between clinically staged IIIA and IIIB non–small cell lung cancer treated with radiation therapy. J Clin Oncol. 1990;8:409–415.
15. Fletcher GH. Clinical dose-response curves of human malignant epithelial tumours. Br J Radiol. 1973;46:1–12.
16. Perez CA, Pajak TF, Rubin P, et al. Long-term observations of the patterns of failure in patients with unresectable non–oat cell carcinoma of the lung treated with definitive radiotherapy: report by the Radiation Therapy Oncology Group. Cancer. 1987;59:1874–1881.
17. Cox JD, Azarnia N, Byhardt RW, et al. A randomized phase I/II trial of hyperfractionated radiation therapy with total doses of 60.0 Gy to 79.2 Gy: possible survival benefit with >69.6 Gy in favorable patients with Radiation Therapy Oncology Group stage III non–small-cell lung carcinoma: report of Radiation Therapy Oncology Group 83-11. J Clin Oncol. 1990;8:1543–1555.

18. Robertson JM, Ten Haken RK, Hazuka MB, et al. Dose escalation for non–small cell lung cancer using conformal radiation therapy [abstract]. Int J Radiat Oncol Biol Phys. 1997;37:1079–1085.

19. Robinow JS, Shaw EG, Eagan RT, et al. Results of combination chemotherapy and thoracic radiation therapy for unresectable non–small cell carcinoma of the lung. Int J Radiat Oncol Biol Phys. 1989;17:1203–1210.

20. Perez CA, Stanley K, Rubin P, et al. A prospective randomized study of various irradiation doses and fractionation schedules in the treatment of inoperable non–oat-cell carcinoma of the lung: preliminary report by the Radiation Therapy Oncology Group. Cancer. 1980;45:2744–2753.

21. Slawson RG, Salazar OM, Poussin-Rosillo H, et al. Once-a-week vs conventional daily radiation treatment for lung cancer: final report. Int J Radiat Oncol Biol Phys. 1988;15:61–68.

22. Sause WT, Scott C, Taylor S, et al. Radiation Therapy Oncology Group (RTOG) 88-08 and Eastern Cooperative Oncology Group (ECOG) 4588: preliminary results of a phase III trial in regionally advanced, unresectable non–small-cell lung cancer. J Natl Cancer Inst. 1995;87:198–205.

23. Wilson GD, McNally NJ, Dische S, et al. Measurement of cell kinetics in human tumours in vivo using bromodeoxyuridine incorporation and flow cytometry. Br J Cancer. 1988;58:423–431.

24. Mehta MP, Tannehill SP, Adak S, et al. Phase II trial of hyperfractionated accelerated radiation therapy for nonresectable non–small-cell lung cancer: results of Eastern Cooperative Oncology Group 4593. J Clin Oncol. 1998;16:3518–3523.

25. Fu XL, Jiang GL, Wang LJ, et al. Hyperfractionated accelerated radiation therapy for non–small cell lung cancer: clinical phase I/II trial. Int J Radiat Oncol Biol Phys. 1997;39:545–552.

26. Graham MV, Purdy JA, Emami B, et al. Clinical dose-volume histogram analysis for pneumonitis after 3D treatment for non–small cell lung cancer (NSCLC). Int J Radiation Oncology Biol Phys. 1999;45:323–329.

27. Hayman JA, Martel MK, Ten Haken RK, et al. Dose escalation in non–small cell lung cancer (NSCLC) using conformal 3-dimensional radiation therapy (C3DRT): update of a phase I trial (Abstract). Proc ASCO. 1999;18:459a. [Abstract.]

28. Simpson JR, Bauer M, Perez CA, et al. Radiation therapy alone or combined with misonidazole in the treatment of locally advanced non–oat cell lung cancer: report of an RTOG prospective randomized trial. Int J Radiat Oncol Biol Phys. 1989;16:1483–1491.

29. Le Chevalier T, Arriagada R, Quoix E, et al. Radiotherapy alone versus combined chemotherapy and radiotherapy in nonresectable non–small-cell lung cancer: first analysis of a randomized trial in 353 patients. J Natl Cancer Inst. 1991;83:417–423.

30. Graham MV, Purdy JA, Emami B, et al. Preliminary results of a prospective trial using three dimensional radiotherapy for lung cancer. Int J Radiat Oncol Biol Phys. 1995;33:993–1000.

31. Blanke C, Ansari CB, Mantravadi R, et al. Phase III trial of thoracic irradiation with or without cisplatin for locally advanced unresectable non–small-cell lung cancer: a Hoosier Oncology Group protocol. J Clin Oncol. 1995;13:1425–1429.

32. Johnson DH, Einhorn LH, Bartolucci A, et al. Thoracic radiotherapy does not prolong survival in patients with locally advanced, unresectable non–small cell lung cancer. Ann Intern Med. 1990;113:33–38.

33. Morton RF, Jett JR, McGinnis WL, et al. Thoracic radiation therapy alone compared with combined chemoradiotherapy for locally unresectable non–small cell lung cancer: a randomized, phase III trial. Ann Intern Med. 1991;115:681–686.

34. Cox JD, Azarnia N, Byhardt RW, et al. N2 (clinical) non–small cell carcinoma of the lung: prospective trials of radiation therapy with total doses 60 Gy by the Radiation Therapy Oncology Group. Int J Radiat Oncol Biol Phys. 1991;20:7–12.

35. Kreisman H, Lisbona A, Olson L, et al. Effect of radiologic stage III substage on nonsurgical therapy of non–small cell lung cancer. Cancer. 1993;72:1588–1596.

36. Lee RE, Carr DT, Childs DS Jr. Comparison of split-course radiation therapy and continuous radiation therapy for unresectable bronchogenic carcinoma: 5 year results. AJR Am J Roentgenol. 1976;126:116–122.

37. Saunders M, Dische S, Barrett A, et al. Continuous, hyperfractionated, accelerated radiotherapy (CHART) versus conventional radiotherapy in non–small cell lung cancer: mature data from the randomised multicentre trial. Radiother Oncol. 1999;52:137–148.

38. Sause W, Kolesar P, Taylor IV S, et al. Final results of phase III trial in regionally advanced unresectable non–small cell lung cancer (Radiation Therapy Oncology Group, Eastern Cooperative Oncology Group, and Southwest Oncology Group). Chest. 2000;117:358–364.

39. Miller TP, Crowley JJ, Mira J, et al. A randomized trial of chemotherapy and radiotherapy for stage III non–small cell lung cancer. Cancer Therapeutics. 1998;1:229–236.

40. Holsti LR, Mattson K. A randomized study of split-course radiotherapy of lung cancer: long term results. Int J Radiat Oncol Biol Phys. 1980;6:977–981.

41. Perez CA, Bauer M, Emami BN, et al. Thoracic irradiation with or without levamisole (NSC #177023) in unresectable non–small cell carcinoma of the lung: a phase III randomized trial of the RTOG. Int J Radiat Oncol Biol Phys. 1988;15:1337–1346.

INDUCTION THERAPY AND SURGERY FOR I-IIIA,B NON–SMALL CELL LUNG CANCER

Frank C. Detterbeck and Mark A. Socinski

TOXICITY OF INDUCTION
THERAPY

RESPONSE TO INDUCTION
THERAPY

PATIENT SELECTION

RESULTS WITH INDUCTION
CHEMOTHERAPY AND
SURGERY
  *Results in Stage I,II Non–Small
    Cell Lung Cancer*
  *Results in Stage IIIa,b Non–Small
    Cell Lung Cancer*

PROGNOSTIC FACTORS

MEDIASTINAL RESTAGING

RECURRENCE PATTERNS AFTER
INDUCTION CHEMOTHERAPY

ROLE OF RADIATION IN
ADDITION TO CHEMOTHERAPY
AND SURGERY

RADIOTHERAPY ALONE AS
INDUCTION THERAPY BEFORE
SURGERY

ROLE OF SURGERY IN
ADDITION TO CHEMOTHERAPY
AND RADIATION

EDITORS' COMMENTS

There is little doubt that microscopic systemic foci of occult metastatic tumor are present in many patients with localized (stage I-IIIa,b) non–small cell lung cancer (NSCLC), given the frequent appearance of distant recurrences after resection of an early stage primary tumor (see Tables 11–5 and 12–3) and the data demonstrating occult micrometastases in nodes and bone marrow using immunohistochemical markers (see Tables 5–12 and 6–13). This makes combination treatment involving chemotherapy in addition to surgery and radiation an attractive concept. In theory, there are many reasons to give chemotherapy first, as an induction treatment prior to a definitive local therapy such as surgery or radiation. These include the presence of a smaller number of tumor cells, a lower chance that any of these cells have developed drug resistance, and better blood supply of the primary tumor preoperatively than postoperatively (see Chapter 10).

This chapter examines data from phase II and phase III studies of induction (or *neoadjuvant*) chemotherapy in addition to surgery and radiation for patients with stage I-IIIa,b NSCLC. Many induction treatment regimens have also involved postoperative (*adjuvant*) treatment. Treatment approaches that involve *only* adjuvant therapy are discussed in Chapter 14. Combination treatment involving chemotherapy and radiation *without surgery* is covered in Chapter 21. This chapter includes a discussion of induction therapy for early stage (Ib, IIa,b) NSCLC, but the vast majority of these studies have been comprised of patients with stage IIIa and IIIb disease.

It is difficult to compare one study of patients with stage IIIa,b disease with another because of issues of patient selection. The possibility that different patient populations were selected is an issue in comparing any clinical studies, but it is a particularly difficult problem in stage IIIa,b NSCLC because the terminology used to describe these patients is crude, at best. The TNM staging system is the obvious place to start, and it does indeed provide a way to differentiate patients with N2 and N3 disease. However, stage IIIa also includes patients with T3N1 disease and, until the staging system revision in 1997, included T3N0 disease as well. The proportion and outcome of such subclasses is often not reported in detail and may be an issue because the effect of combination therapy on tumors involving mediastinal nodes may be different from the effect on peripheral tumors involving parietal pleura and no lymph nodes.

A more difficult issue is the fact that no simple way has emerged to describe the amount of tumor in mediastinal nodes. There is data to suggest that the prognosis is different for patients with involvement of a single nodal station compared with those with multiple mediastinal nodal stations and for patients with large, easily visible mediastinal nodes as opposed to patients with normal-sized nodes that harbor microscopic foci of malignant cells (see Chapter 17). Furthermore, whether radiographic or surgical staging of the mediastinum was used to categorize the patients as stage III is also in question. The false positive rate of

TABLE 19-1. TOXICITY OF INDUCTION THERAPY BEFORE SURGICAL RESECTION IN STAGE IIIa,b NON-SMALL CELL LUNG CANCER

STUDY	N	INDUCTION CHEMO	INDUCTION RT (Gy)	ADJUVANT THERAPY	ALL TREATMENT MORTALITY[a] (%)	GRADE 3,4 INDUCTION TOXICITY[a] (%)						ALL INDUCTION MORTALITY[a] (%)	SURGICAL COMPLICATIONS[b] (%)			SURGICAL MORTALITY[b] (%)
						WBC	Plat	Infect	N&V	Eso	Pulm		BPF	ARDS	Pneum	
Martini et al[14]	136	MVP × 2-3	—	Chemo ± RT[c]	5	39	66	6	5	—	1	1	5	3	—	4
Sugarbaker et al[21]	74	PVb × 2	—	Chemo + 54-60	5	—	—	10	11	—	—	1	—	—	9	3
Aristu et al[22]	55	MVP × 1-6	—	IORT + 45	8	11	—	—	—	0	—	2	—	—	—	10
Darwish et al[17]	46	EP × 2-3	—	±56	2	—	—	—	0	0	—	2	—	—	—	0
Takita et al[23]	41	PACCO × 2	—	RT[c]	2	—	—	—	—	—	—	—	—	—	—	—
Average					**4**							**2**				**4**
Bonomi et al[25]	128	PF/EPF × 4	c40	—	7	~60		—	—	—	—	2	4	2	—	5
Albain et al[1]	126	EP × 2	c45	—	10	5		6	6	12	—	4	2	—	2	9
Weiden et al[20]	85	PF × 2	c30	—	5	12	2	—	4	5	0	6	2	—	6	7
Weitberg et al[16]	53	EP × 2	c54	Chemo	4	—	—	—	—	—	—	0	—	—	—	6
Palazzi et al[24]	43	EP × 2	c40[d]	—	9	68	29	24	39	—	—	—	—	—	—	10
Strauss et al[18]	41	PFVb × 2	c30	Chemo/c30	15							7				
Average					**8**							**4**				**7**
Eberhardt et al[4]	94	EP × 3	cHF45[e]	—	6	60	31	5	9	40	3	2	5	3	3	7
Thomas et al[6]	54	CbIE × 2	cHF45	—	9	14	5	6	—	8	9	2	10	3	8	8
Pisch et al[19]	47	EPF × 2	cHF40[d]	—	6	—	—	—	2	19	—	6	—	—	—	0
Rice et al[5]	45	PT qd	cHF30	Chemo/cHF30	4	—	—	—	5	20	—	0	3	3	3	5
Rice et al[3]	42	EPF qd	cHF27	Chemo/cHF27	12	—	—	—	—	19	—	2	0	11		11
Choi et al[2]	42	PFVb × 2	cHF42[e]	Chemo/cHF18	7	23	2	—	—	(14)[f]	3	2	0	—	3	5
Average					**7**					21		**4**				**6**
Average[g]					**7**	**32**	**23**	**10**	**9**	**21**	**3**	**2**	**3**	**3**	**3**	**6**
Average for all[g]					**7**	**32**	**23**	**10**	**9**	**14**	**3**	**3**	**3**	**3**	**5**	**6**

Inclusion criteria: Prospective phase II trials of induction therapy and surgery in ≥40 patients from 1980 to 2000.

[a]% of all patients treated.
[b]% of all operated patients.
[c]Dose not given.
[d]Split course RT.
[e]Includes prophylactic cranial irradiation.
[f]Grade 4.
[g]Excluding value in parentheses.

All induction mortality, all mortality (from any cause) during the induction treatment until surgery; All surgery mortality, all mortality occurring within 30 days of or during hospitalization for surgery; All treatment mortality, all mortality occurring during the induction treatment; ARDS, adult respiratory distress syndrome; BPF, bronchopleural fistula (stump breakdown); All induction mortality, all mortality, including induction therapy–related and surgical mortality as well as unrelated death occurring during the period of treatment; occurring during treatment, including induction therapy–related and surgical mortality as well as unrelated death occurring during the period of treatment; Pulm, pulmonary toxicity; RT, radiotherapy; WBC, c, concurrent; Chemo, chemotherapy; Eso, esophagitis; HF, hyperfractionated; IORT, intraoperative RT; N&V, nausea and vomiting; Plat, platelet count; Pneum, pneumonia; white blood count.

Chemotherapy regimens: CbIE, carboplatin, ifosfamide, etoposide; EP, etoposide, cisplatin; EPF, etoposide, cisplatin, 5-fluorouracil; MVP, mitomycin C, vincristine, cisplatin; PACCO, cisplatin, doxorubicin, cyclophosphamide, CCNU, and vincristine; PF, cisplatin, 5-fluorouracil; PFVb, cisplatin, 5-fluorouracil, vinblastine; PT, cisplatin, teniposide; PVb, cisplatin, vinblastine.

enlarged mediastinal nodes has been shown consistently to be approximately 40% (see Table 5–7), yet some studies involving induction therapy and surgery for stage IIIa,b disease have accepted radiographic staging for varying proportions of the patients.

Another issue that is important specifically in the discussion of induction therapy and surgery is the use of the terms *resectable* and *unresectable*. These terms are often used to describe the patients included in a study, yet they are not defined. Much variation exists regarding what is considered resectable at different institutions and in different countries. Furthermore, it is often unclear whether the term *unresectable* means that a tumor is technically unresectable—that is, unable to be removed with either no residual (R_0) or microscopic residual (R_1) disease—or whether it is biologically unresectable, meaning that removal of the tumor does not affect the course of the patient's disease. The latter definition is, of course, subject to change as improvements in the effectiveness of nonsurgical treatment modalities occur. Finally, it is often unclear whether categorization of patients as resectable or unresectable applies to the situation at the time of presentation or after induction therapy has caused the tumor to shrink. Because of these ambiguities, this chapter avoids use of the terms *resectable* and *unresectable* to prospectively describe patient populations. Instead, the terms are restricted to describing how often a complete resection (R_0) could be technically achieved when surgery was performed (after induction therapy).

TOXICITY OF INDUCTION THERAPY

Since the advent of active chemotherapy for NSCLC around 1980, a large number of phase II trials have been carried out investigating the feasibility of induction chemotherapy with or without radiation before surgical resection. Although these studies have involved a wide variety of induction therapy regimens, they have uniformly shown that the treatment is well tolerated. The average treatment-related mortality occurring at any time during the induction, operative, or postoperative recovery phase is 7%, as shown in Table 19–1. This finding is consistent among studies, regardless of the induction regimen. The mortality rate during the induction treatment alone is only 3%. The mortality of surgical resection after induction therapy is similar to that after surgery alone (see Chapter 8).

In one large study of induction chemoradiotherapy, 49% of patients experienced a grade 3 (serious) and 13% a grade 4 (life-threatening) toxicity by the World Health Organization standard definitions.[1] Table 19–1 presents a variety of specific toxicity rates. By far the most common grade 3,4 toxicities are hematologic, but these are defined primarily by laboratory values and do not necessarily affect how patients feel. The rates of hematologic toxicity vary widely, most likely due to differences in the chemotherapeutic agents used, the dosages given, and the supportive agents available. Nausea and vomiting have generally been fairly mild. Esophagitis has been rare in patients treated with chemotherapy alone and low in patients treated with concurrent conventionally fractionated RT as well. The rate of grade 3,4 esophagitis in patients receiving concurrent

hyperfractionated RT is approximately 20%, but it is usually brief and self-limited (lasting approximately 1 week).[2–5]

Concern about higher surgical morbidity and mortality after induction therapy appears unfounded, according to the data in Table 19–1. The overall operative mortality does not appear to be increased. The rates of bronchial stump breakdown, pneumonia, and adult respiratory distress syndrome are also similar to those seen in primary resections. However, the reported series generally involved a single-institution experience, and it is likely that careful selection and technical precautions to avoid an increased rate of complications play a role. Many authors with experience express concern about an increased risk of complications following induction therapy[6–11] and recommend that extra precautions be taken, such as coverage of bronchial stumps with muscle flaps.[6,7,12]

RESPONSE TO INDUCTION THERAPY

The tumor response to treatment can be measured in a variety of ways. An objective radiographic response is defined as either the complete radiographic disappearance of all tumor (*complete response* [CR]) or a $\geq 50\%$ reduction in the tumor size (*partial response* [PR]). Using these definitions, the objective response rate to induction treatment is reported to be approximately 50% to 70%, with an average of 65% (Table 19–2). The addition of radiotherapy (RT) to induction chemotherapy does not appreciably improve the radiographic response rates. However, some of the more aggressive regimens, such as those using hyperfractionated RT, have shortened the overall induction treatment time. This means that the response to treatment is assessed earlier, perhaps before the maximal response is realized. Disease progression during induction treatment has been found to be relatively infrequent in most series, being seen in an average of only 7% of patients.

An average of 16% of patients are found not to have viable cancer cells remaining, that is, a pathologic CR (pCR), on histologic examination of the resected tumor at the time of thoracotomy. The pCR rate may be influenced by how meticulously the tissue is sectioned by the pathologist. The pCR rate at the primary tumor site was reported as 39% in one study.[4] The CR rate in mediastinal nodal tissue was found to be approximately 50% in several studies in which initial surgical staging was employed. This is often called *downstaging*. However, the rate of clearance of tumor from the mediastinal nodes varies greatly (from 16%–77%). The reasons for this are not clear. It does not appear to be related to the type of induction therapy or to the stage of patients included (N2 versus N3).

The radiographic response does not reliably predict the pathologic response rate. In studies of >20 patients that have reported such data, a pCR was noted in approximately two-thirds of patients (range, 33%–100%) who had a radiographic CR,[4,13–17] in 17% of patients (range, 0%–35%) with a radiographic PR,[4,13–18] and in 0% to 10% of patients with radiographic stable disease.[4,13–15,17,18]

Although surgery was planned following induction therapy in all of the prospective studies shown in Table 19–2, the criteria for proceeding with this plan were variable. In some studies, only patients showing a response to induction

TABLE 19–2. RESPONSE TO INDUCTION THERAPY IN PROSPECTIVE PHASE II TRIALS IN STAGE IIIa,b NON–SMALL CELL LUNG CANCER

STUDY	N	INDUCTION CHEMO	INDUCTION RT (Gy)	ADJUVANT THERAPY	% SURGICALLY STAGED	DISEASE PROGRESSION (%)	RADIOGRAPHIC RESPONSE RATE (%)	% pCR/ THORACOTOMY N2,3 Nodes	% pCR/ THORACOTOMY All Sites	% R0	SURVIVAL MST (mo)	SURVIVAL 5-y (%)
Martini et al[14]	136	MVP × 2-3	—	Chemo ± RT[a]	0	9	77	—	17	65	19	17
Sugarbaker et al[21]	74	PVb × 2	—	Chemo + 54-60	100	9	—	16	0	45	15	—
Aristu et al[22]	55	MVP × 1-6	—	IORT + 45	Few	4	64	—	10	33	—	—
Darwish et al[17]	46	EP × 2-3	—	± 56	Few	7	82	—	11	16	21	—
Takita et al[23]	41	PACCO × 2	—	RT[a]	Few	18	60	—	—	41	18	—
Average						**9**	**71**		**10**	**49**	**18**	
Bonomi et al[25]	128	PF/EPF × 4	c40	—	Some	5	67	—	17	77	22	—
Albain et al[1]	126	EP × 2	c45	—	100	8	59	53	21	69	15	21[b]
Weiden et al[20]	85	PF × 2	c30	—	60	4	56	—	15	34	13	—
Weitberg et al[16]	53	EP × 2	c54	Chemo	94	0	87	—	45	51	24	—
Palazzi et al[24]	43	EP × 2	c40[c]	—	—	—	70	—	23	28	14	—
Strauss et al[18]	41	PFVb × 2	c30	Chemo/c30	93	4	46	—	23	59	16	18
Average						**4**	**64**		**24**	**53**	**17**	
Eberhardt et al[4]	94	EP × 3	Chemo/cHF45[d]	—	100	4	54	77	26	53	19	28
Thomas et al[6]	54	CbIE × 2	Chemo/cHF45	—	100	7	69	—	18	63	20	30
Pisch et al[19]	47	EPF × 2	cHF40[c]	—	Few	—	—	—	0	34	18	—
Rice et al[5]	45	PT qd	cHF30	Chemo/cHF30	100	13	53	35	13	71	22	—
Rice et al[3]	42	EPF qd	cHF27	Chemo/cHF27	100	2	57	33	6	79	21	—
Choi et al[2]	42	PFVb × 2	cHF42[d]	Chemo/cHF18	100	7	74	67	10	81	25	37
Average						**4**	**61**	**47**	**12**	**64**	**21**	
Average for all						**7**	**65**	**47**	**16**	**56**	**19**	**25**

Inclusion criteria: Prospective phase II trials of induction therapy and surgery in ≥40 patients from 1980 to 2000.

[a] Dose not given.
[b] 6-year survival.
[c] Split course RT.
[d] Includes prophylactic cranial irradiation.

c, concurrent; Chemo, chemotherapy (usually same as induction regimen); disease progression, local cancer growth or appearance of distant metastases during induction treatment; HF = hyperfractionated; IORT, intraoperative RT; MST, median survival time (months); % pCR/thoracotomy, percentage of patients undergoing thoracotomy who had a pathologic complete response (no tumor found); radiographic response rate, radiographic response rate to induction treatment, that is, percentage with a complete response (CR) or a partial response (PR, ≥50% reduction); R_o, completely resected patients; RT = radiotherapy (dose in Grays).

Chemotherapy regimens: CbIE, carboplatin, ifosfamide, etoposide; EP, etoposide, cisplatin; EPF, etoposide, cisplatin, 5-fluorouracil; MVP, mitomycin C, vincristine, cisplatin; PACCO, cisplatin, doxorubicin, cyclophosphamide, CCNU, and vincristine; PF, cisplatin, 5-fluorouracil; PFE, cisplatin, 5-fluorouracil, etoposide; PFVb, cisplatin, 5-fluorouracil, vinblastine; PT, cisplatin, teniposide; PVb, cisplatin, vinblastine.

therapy underwent surgery,[19,20] in others, patients with radiographic stable disease also underwent thoracotomy,[1–3,5,6,14, 16,17,21] and in still others, it seems that no specific criteria were used.[18,22–25] Only one study employed surgical restaging (repeat mediastinoscopy).[4] Furthermore, not all patients who underwent thoracotomy were able to be completely resected (R_0 resection). Of the patients begun on induction therapy, an average of 64% were completely resected (see Table 19–2); however, this rate varies from 28% to 81%. The variability is not explained by differences in the induction regimen or stage of patients included in the study. Rather, it appears to be related to how aggressively surgical resection was pursued after induction therapy in these patients who had fairly extensive tumors. In those series in which no explicit criteria for proceeding with a resection were defined[18,22–25] or only responding patients were resected,[19,26] an average of 49% of all patients were completely resected, whereas in those studies in which resection was planned for all patients except those with progressive disease,[1–3,5,14,16,17,21] an average of 65% were completely resected.

PATIENT SELECTION

A variety of inclusion criteria and staging methods have been used in the prospective phase II studies of induction therapy before surgical resection. Table 19–3 provides a summary of these factors. Most of these prospective studies have involved surgical staging (mediastinoscopy) in the vast majority of patients. Although a few studies have included some patients with T3N0 disease, the majority of patients have had N2,3 node involvement. It is clear that these studies included patients with fairly extensive stage IIIa,b disease whose prognosis with surgery alone was poor.

The patients included in induction therapy studies have consistently been relatively young, with a median age of 57 years. Other characteristics have not been reported in many studies. In those studies reporting weight loss, an average of 14% (range, 0%–31%) have had >5% weight loss.[16,21,22,24,25] The majority of patients included had a performance status (PS) of 0 or 1. In those studies reporting PS in detail, the proportion of patients with a PS of 0 ranged from 2% to 81%.[4,6,16,18,24]

RESULTS WITH INDUCTION CHEMOTHERAPY AND SURGERY

Results in Stage I,II Non–Small Cell Lung Cancer

Few of the studies of induction chemotherapy have included many patients who were stage I or II, although some studies have included a minority of patients who had

TABLE 19–3. STAGE OF PATIENTS INCLUDED IN PROSPECTIVE PHASE II INDUCTION THERAPY TRIALS

| | | | | PATIENT CHARACTERISTICS | | | | OUTCOMES | | | | |
| | | | | | Proportion (%) | | | | | | Survival | |
STUDY	n	Median Age	% Surgically Staged	T3N0	N2,3	T4/ N3	Radiographic Response Rate (%)	pCR (%)	% R_0 Resection	MST (mo)	5 y (%)
Bonomi et al[25]	128	57	Some	42[a]	41[a,b]	16[a,c]	67	17	77	22	—
Strauss et al[18]	41	57	93	12	80[b]	0	46	23	59	16	18
Martini et al[14]	136	55	0	0	100[a,b]	0	77	17	65	19	17
Sugarbaker et al[21]	74	52	100	0	100[b]	0	—	0	45	15	—
Weitberg et al[16]	53	62	44	4	94	0	87	45	51	24	—
Darwish et al[17]	46	58	0	0	100[a,b]	0	82	11	61	21	—
Choi et al[2]	42	57	100	0	100[b]	0	74	10	81	25	37
Weiden et al[20]	85	58	60	—	57[b]	13[c]	56	15	34	13	—
Rice et al[5]	45	59	100	0	98	21	53	13	71	22	—
Average							**68**	**17**	**58**	**19**	**24**
Albain et al[1]	126	58	100	0	87	40	59	21	69	15	21[d]
Eberhardt et al[4]	94	55	100	6	85	42	54	26	53	19	28
Rice et al[3]	42	55	100	0	93	45	57	6	79	21	—
Thomas et al[6]	54	57	100	0	96	50	69	18	63	20	30
Aristu et al[22]	55	62	Few	20[a]	—	55[a]	64	10	33	—	—
Pisch et al[19]	47	59	Few	2[a]	89[a]	49[a]	—	0	34	18	—
Palazzi et al[24]	43	58	—	7	74	58	70	23	28	14	—
Takita et al[23]	41	56	Few	7[a]	83[a]	66[a]	60	—	41	18	—
Average							**62**	**15**	**50**	**19**	**26**
Average for all		57					**65**	**16**	**56**	**18**	**25**

Inclusion criteria: Prospective phase II trials of induction therapy and surgery in ≥40 patients from 1980 to 2000.
[a] By radiographic staging only.
[b] Only N2.
[c] Only T4; no N3 patients.
[d] 6-year survival.

MST, median survival time; pCR, pathologic complete response; R_0, completely resected patients; Radiographic response rate, radiographic response rate to induction treatment, such as percentage with a complete (CR) or partial response (PR, ≥50% reduction in size).

DATA SUMMARY: TOXICITY AND RESPONSE TO INDUCTION THERAPY

	AMOUNT	QUALITY	CONSISTENCY
Mortality (from any cause) during induction therapy and surgical resection occurs in 7% of patients	High	High	High
Disease progression during induction therapy is seen in 7% of patients	High	High	High
With appropriate precautions, resection after induction therapy can be accomplished without increased operative mortality (average, 6%)	High	High	High
A radiographic objective response to induction therapy is seen in 65% of patients	High	High	High
A pathologic complete response (pCR) to induction therapy is seen in 15% of all patients resected	High	High	High
A pCR is seen in two-thirds of resected patients who demonstrated a radiographic CR	High	High	Poor
A pCR in the mediastinal nodes (*downstaging*) is seen in 50% of all resected patients	High	High	Mod
A complete resection (R_0) can be accomplished in 60% of all patients for whom induction therapy and surgery is planned	High	Mod	Mod

Type of data rated: Plain text: descriptive statement   *Italics: controlled comparison*   **Bold: randomized comparison**

T3N0 tumors, which were classified as stage IIIa until the staging system revision in 1997. A prospective phase II study of 94 patients with stage Ib, IIa,b and T3N1 disease, known as the Bimodality Lung Oncology Team (BLOT) trial, has finished accrual.[27] This study involved preoperative and postoperative treatment with carboplatin and paclitaxel. The radiographic response rate was 56%, disease progression was seen in 3%, and 86% of all patients underwent a complete resection. The planned induction therapy could be given in 96% of the patients, whereas only 64% of those eligible for postoperative chemotherapy received the planned treatment. The 2-year survival of all patients entered on this study is 56%.[27]

A large randomized trial involving 355 stage Ib-IIIa patients, 53% of whom were stage I or II, was reported in preliminary fashion.[28] Induction therapy consisted of 2 cycles of mitomycin, ifosfamide, and cisplatin. Postoperatively, two additional cycles of chemotherapy were given (as well as RT for stage IIIa patients). A trend toward improved survival with induction chemotherapy was seen for the entire group (median survival, 36 versus 26 months; $P = 0.09$). This study had sufficient power to reliably detect only an increase of >15% in median survival. Furthermore, a slight maldistribution of N2 patients favoring the surgery-alone arm occurred (N2 patients, 33% for surgery versus 40% for induction therapy). When corrected for stage using multivariate analysis, induction chemotherapy was found to be a statistically significant independent factor associated with better survival. Although better survival with induction therapy was seen in both the stage Ib-II and IIIa subgroups, subset analysis suggested that the early stage patients (Ib-II) experienced a greater survival benefit (Fig. 19–1).

Results in Stage IIIa,b Non–Small Cell Lung Cancer

The patients who have been included in the prospective phase II trials of induction therapy have generally had relatively extensive stage III lung cancer. Most studies have used surgical staging and have primarily involved patients with histologically proven N2 and N3 disease. There is little doubt that the survival of such patients with surgery alone would be poor. Even in patients with minimal N2 disease detected preoperatively (microscopic nodal involvement or involvement of only one node station), the 5-year survival with surgery alone is only 15% (see Chapter 17). In reality, however, the prospective phase II studies just discussed have included mostly patients with more than minimal N2 disease (eg, patients with bulky N2 disease or N3 involvement), yet the observed 5-year survival after induction therapy and a planned surgical resection is approximately 25% (see Table 19–3). Therefore, the data from phase II trials is highly suggestive of improved survival compared with other series involving surgery alone.

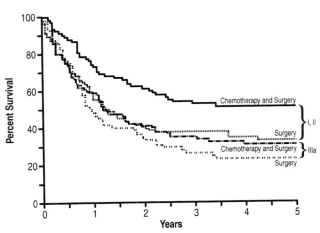

FIGURE 19–1. Survival of patients with stage Ib, IIa,b and IIIa non–small cell lung cancer, randomized to induction chemotherapy and surgery versus surgery alone. (Data from Depierre A, Milleron B, for the French Thoracic Cooperative Group. Phase III trial of neo-adjuvant chemotherapy [NCT] in resectable stage I [except T1N0], II, IIIa non–small cell lung cancer [NSCLC]: the French experience. Proc ASCO. 1999;18:465a.[28])

However, because of the variability in the patient population, it is difficult to be certain from phase II trials that multimodality treatment of patients with IIIa,b NSCLC results in increased survival.

Proof of a benefit to induction therapy compared with surgery alone can come only from randomized phase III trials. Unfortunately, the randomized trials that are available involve only a limited number of patients. Six randomized trials involving at least 50 patients have been reported; the characteristics of the treatment and the patients included are summarized in Table 19–4. Induction therapy has involved two to three cycles of cisplatin-based chemotherapy. In most of the trials, adjuvant therapy has also been given, involving either more chemotherapy, adjuvant RT, or both. The primary surgery arm has generally involved surgery alone, although in a few studies RT was also given, either preoperatively or postoperatively.

In most of the randomized studies, the majority of patients were staged surgically and the majority of patients had N2 nodal involvement. These studies have generally not involved significant numbers of patients with stage IIIb disease. The largest study involved a majority of patients who were stage Ib or IIa,b and was discussed earlier.[28] Only the 167 patients who were stage T1-3N2 or T3N1 are included here. These two TNM groups were evenly proportioned between the study arms, although the total number of IIIa patients was slightly less in the surgery-alone arm compared with the induction arm (75 and 92 patients, respectively).

None of these studies was found to have any statistically significant imbalances in known prognostic factors between the treatment arms. Nevertheless, it is possible that several factors combined may contribute to better survival in one arm, even though there is no statistically significant imbalance in any of the individual prognostic factors. A comprehensive analysis of this issue is not possible because not all prognostic factors have been reported in these studies. The tumor stage, undoubtedly one of the most important factors, has been reported consistently. The distribution of tumor stages shows either no discernible difference or a difference that would be expected to result in better survival in the surgery-alone arm.[29–32] Reported minor differences in PS also tend to favor the surgery arm.[33]

The only nonsignificant factor imbalance that could potentially favor the induction chemotherapy arm was the presence of a K-*ras* genetic mutation in the study reported by Rosell et al.[29] This mutation is generally thought to be a poor prognostic factor in stage I,II patients with NSCLC[34–37] but not in patients with stage III, IV disease.[37,38] However, this factor was analyzed at the time of resection, and no preinduction therapy analysis of K-*ras* positivity was performed. Other studies have found that chemotherapy decreases the expression of this mutation.[30,39] Thus it is unlikely that the minor imbalance of K-*ras* in the Rosell study plays a significant role in the observed survival difference between the two arms.

Survival data from the randomized studies of induction therapy and surgery for IIIa,b NSCLC is shown in Table 19–5. Four of the six trials found better survival in the induction therapy arm, whereas two found no difference. Although these trials were generally small, statistical significance at the $P < 0.05$ level was found in two of four studies that analyzed this. In fact, both of these studies were stopped early when an interim analysis disclosed a highly significant difference ($P < 0.001$ and 0.008).[29,31] Long-term follow-up of both of these studies has shown the difference to be durable.[30,32] Survival curves from these two positive trials are shown in Figure 19–2. Two additional small randomized trials have been reported, involving 26 and 27 patients.[40,41] One of these found a strong trend to better survival with induction therapy (2-year survival, 63% versus 29%; $P = 0.095$),[40] whereas the other found no difference.[41]

Thus, the randomized trials of induction therapy and surgery versus surgery alone have shown mixed results in terms of statistically significant differences. However, these randomized trials of induction therapy have generally involved such small numbers of patients that a negative trial

TABLE 19–4. TREATMENT AND PATIENT CHARACTERISTICS IN RANDOMIZED TRIALS OF INDUCTION CHEMOTHERAPY AND SURGERY VERSUS PRIMARY SURGERY FOR STAGE IIIa,b NON–SMALL CELL LUNG CANCER

STUDY	N	PRIMARY SURGERY ARM Preop Therapy	PRIMARY SURGERY ARM Adjuvant Therapy	INDUCTION ARM Induction Therapy	INDUCTION ARM Adjuvant Therapy	PATIENT CHARACTERISTICS % Surgically Staged[a]	% T3N0	% pN2	% T4/N3
Depierre et al[28b]	167	—	—[c,d]	MIP × 2	Chemo × 2[c,d]	Few	0	73[e]	0
Yoneda et al[49f]	83	—	—[g]	VP × ≥2	RT (50-60 Gy)	—	—	—	53
Roth et al[31,32]	60	—	—[c]	CEP × 3	Chemo × 3[c]	85	23	73	0
Rosell et al[29,30]	60	—	RT (50 Gy)	MIP × 3	RT (50 Gy)	73	22	73	0
Wagner et al[33]	57	RT (44 Gy)	—	MVP × 2	—	100	0	95	14[h]
Elias et al[48]	57	RT (40 Gy)	RT (14-20 Gy)	EP × 2	Chemo × 2/RT (40 Gy)	100	0	100	0

Inclusion criteria: Randomized studies of induction chemotherapy and surgery in ≥50 patients from 1980 to 2000.
[a]Percentage of patients surgically staged (mediastinoscopy or thoracotomy) at the time of entry into trial.
[b]Only stage IIIa patients included here (trial included a majority of patients who were stage I,II).
[c]RT for R$_{1,2}$ patients.
[d]RT for T3 and N2 patients.
[e]Clinical staging.
[f]Only 49% of patients randomized to surgery underwent thoracotomy (and 55% of patients on the induction arm underwent thoracotomy).
[g]RT and chemotherapy for unresected patients.
[h]Only T4.
Chemo, chemotherapy; Ind, induction therapy arm; Preop, preoperative; RT, radiotherapy (dose in Gy); S, surgery arm.
Chemotherapy regimens: CEP = cyclophosphamide, etoposide, cisplatin; EP = etoposide, cisplatin; MIP = mitomycin, ifosfamide, cisplatin; MVP, mitomycin, vincristine, cisplatin; VP = vincristine, cisplatin.

TABLE 19–5. SURVIVAL OUTCOMES IN RANDOMIZED TRIALS OF INDUCTION CHEMOTHERAPY AND SURGERY FOR STAGE IIIa,b NON–SMALL CELL LUNG CANCER

STUDY	n	% T3N0	% pN2	% T4/N3	% Surgically Staged	MST (mo) S	MST (mo) Ind	2 y (%) S	2 y (%) Ind	5 y (%) S	5 y (%) Ind	P
Depierre et al[28a]	167	0	(73)[b]	0	Few	12	14	37	41	22	30	—
Yoneda et al[49c]	83	—	—	53	—	15	14	37	40	—	—	—
Roth et al[31,32]	60	23	73	0	85	14	21	34	50	15	36	0.05[d]
Rosell et al[29,30]	60	22	73	0	73	10	20	10	37	0	17	0.005
Wagner et al[33]	57	0	95	14	100	12	12	—	—	27[e]	27[e]	NS
Elias et al[48]	57	0	100	0	100	23	19	—	—	—	—	NS
Average						**14**	**17**	**30**	**42**	**16**	**28**	

Inclusion criteria: Randomized studies of induction chemotherapy and surgery in ≥50 stage IIIa,b patients from 1980 to 2000.
[a]Only stage IIIa patients included here (trial included a majority of patients who were stage I,II).
[b]In parentheses because clinical staging was used.
[c]Only 49% of patients randomized to surgery underwent thoracotomy (and 55% of patients on the induction arm).
[d]P = 0.056 by log rank; P = 0.048 by Breslow-Gehan-Wilcoxon test.
[e]4-year survival.
Ind, induction chemotherapy arm; MST, median survival time; Surgically staged, staged by mediastinoscopy or thoracotomy on entry in study; S, surgery arm.

only provides evidence that there is not a large improvement in survival (ie, 30% or 40%). Stated differently, a trial involving 60 patients would have only a 50% chance (power) of detecting a survival difference of 15%.

The two positive studies have been criticized because of the inclusion of patients with T3N0,1 tumors. However, inclusion of these patients should have favored the surgery arms because there was a slightly increased proportion (statistically nonsignificant) of T3N0 patients in the surgery arms. Furthermore, it is unclear how many of these patients had T3N0 tumors involving the chest wall. It is this specific group that exhibits good survival with surgery alone (see Chapter 15). The prognosis for patients with central T3 tumors, or T3N1 tumors in any location treated with surgery alone, leads to a survival of only 20% to 25% (see Table 15–4). Furthermore, the remainder of the patients in these two studies, which made up the vast majority of patients, had radiographically enlarged N2 nodes that were all proved by biopsy to truly have malignant involvement.

Another criticism of the study reported by Rosell et al[30] is the fact that survival of the patients in the surgery-alone arm was surprisingly poor, with none alive at 5 years. This is not necessarily surprising for the pN2 patients, who clearly had more than the minimal N2 disease that is usually included in studies of surgical resection alone (see Chapter 17). Nevertheless, the poor survival is unusual, given the fact that 30% of the patients on the surgery-alone arm in the Rosell study had cT3N0 disease. However, the T3N0 patients in this study were staged only radiographically and did not undergo mediastinoscopy.[29] Other studies have suggested that in carefully selected T3N0 patients who are considered good candidates for surgery alone, approximately 25% will have pN2 disease, and in only about 70% will a complete resection be achieved (see Table 15–2). This makes the poor survival of the cT3N0 group in the Rosell study less surprising than if one considers only pT3N0 patients with chest wall involvement.

In summary, the existing data from phase II and phase III studies is suggestive that there may be a benefit to induction chemotherapy before resection in patients with radiographically and histologically detectable N2 disease. However, the data is limited and not entirely consistent. Furthermore, these studies have predominantly involved patients who would be considered poor candidates for a primary surgical approach. Clearly, more research, involving much larger numbers of patients, is necessary. It is unfortunate that this issue is not currently being addressed by any large randomized trials in stage III NSCLC patients.

DATA SUMMARY: SURVIVAL RESULTS WITH INDUCTION THERAPY AND SURGERY

	AMOUNT	QUALITY	CONSISTENCY
The 5-year survival of the selected stage IIIa,b patients treated in phase II studies of induction therapy and planned surgery is 25%	High	High	High
A trend to better intermediate-term (median and 2-year) survival of IIIa is seen in patients treated with induction therapy and surgery compared with surgery alone	**High**	**Mod**	**Mod**
Randomized studies have demonstrated a statistically significant improvement in survival of stage IIIa patients treated with induction therapy and surgery compared with surgery alone	**High**	**Mod**	**Poor**

Type of data rated: Plain text: descriptive statement   *Italics: controlled comparison*   **Bold: randomized comparison**

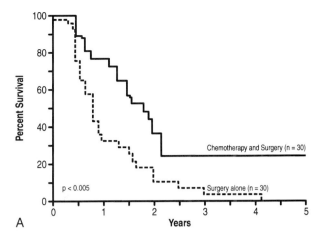

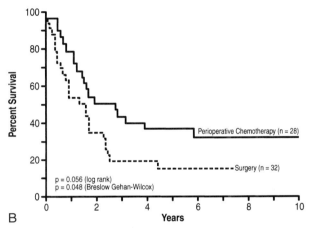

FIGURE 19–2. Survival of patients with stage IIIa NSCLC in randomized trials of induction chemotherapy compared with surgery alone. *A,* 60 patients from Barcelona, Spain, *P* < 0.005. *B,* 60 patients from M.D. Anderson Cancer Center, *P* = 0.008. (*A,* Reprinted from *Lung Cancer,* Vol 47, Rosell R, Gómez-Codina J, Camps C, et al, Presectional chemotherapy in stage IIIA non–small-cell lung cancer: a 7-year assessment of a randomized controlled trial, 7–14, Copyright 1999, with permission from Elsevier Science.[30] *B,* Reprinted from *Lung Cancer,* Vol 21, Roth JA, Atkinson EN, Fossella F, et al, Long-term follow-up of patients enrolled in a randomized trial comparing perioperative chemotherapy and surgery with surgery alone in resectable stage IIIA non–small-cell lung cancer, 1–6, Copyright 1998, with permission from Elsevier Science.[32])

PROGNOSTIC FACTORS

Whether the induction therapy involves chemotherapy alone or chemotherapy and RT does not appear to have a major impact on response or survival (see Table 19–2). The addition of postoperative chemotherapy or RT also has no clear impact. Furthermore, it is difficult to discern differences in outcomes associated with the dose of chemotherapy. For example, of the phase II studies using relatively low doses of cisplatin (≤ 80 mg/m^2 per cycle), two reported median survivals lower than the average,[20,24] one reported median survivals to be the same,[23] and three observed median survivals greater than the average.[3,5,25] However, the number of different agents and schedules used makes comparison difficult.

Table 19–3 groups the phase II studies of patients treated

with induction therapy and surgery according to the proportion of T3N0, T1-3N2,3 and T4/N3 patients included. There are no discernible differences in terms of endpoints such as survival parameters or radiographic or pathologic response rates among studies including many T3N0 patients, only N2 patients, or many IIIb (T4/N3) patients. Even those studies involving careful surgical staging and including nearly 50% stage IIIb patients have shown similar response rates and survival. Those studies relying primarily on radiographic staging have also shown similar response rates and survival, although these series have usually included fewer patients who underwent a complete resection. This suggests that the institutions that were less aggressive about surgical staging were also less aggressive about pursuing resection.

Researchers in some studies have performed univariate analysis to investigate the value of various prognostic factors. In two studies, patients with T3N0 tumors by preoperative staging fared significantly better than those with T1-3N2 tumors.[14,25] In contrast, most studies have found no significant difference in survival of patients with stage IIIa disease compared with patients with stage IIIb disease, although a slight trend favoring the IIIa patients was observed.[1,3,4,23] Only one study found a significant difference by univariate analysis.[5] The ability to carry out a resection following induction therapy has consistently been found to be a highly significant prognostic factor,[4,5,14] whereas the radiographic response rate is only a weak prognostic indicator.[4,14] The ability of induction therapy to downstage the nodal status to yN0,1* has been consistently found to be predictive of better survival in all studies that have examined this (Table 19–6). This difference has been found to be statistically significant in most of these studies. A graph of patient survival taken from one of these studies is shown in Figure 19–3.[2]

It is likely that downstaging is a marker for tumor sensitivity to chemotherapy. However, the disappearance of all tumor (a pCR) is not clearly a prognostic marker. In one of the largest studies, there was no difference in 4-year survival *among patients who were completely resected,* whether residual tumor was present or not (44% versus 46%, *P* = 0.85).[4] Another study found that survival was better among completely resected patients in whom the pathologist judged that the resected tumor contained <10% detectable cancer cells.[6]

Three multivariate analyses of prognostic factors have been performed.[1,2,6] Factors that have consistently been found *not* to be significant include gender, age, histologic type, stage, and radiographic response. When operative findings were included, two studies found that a complete resection was of independent prognostic significance.[2,6] These two studies also found that the pathologic response was independently significant, either assessed as nodal downstaging[2] or as <10% residual cancer cells remaining in the tumor.[6] However, the third multivariate analysis found that a complete resection, a pCR, or downstaging of lymph nodes was not of independent prognostic significance. The only significant variable was the presence of

---

*The prefix *y* refers to repeat staging done after therapy has been administered according to the American Joint Committee on Cancer staging system.[42]

TABLE 19–6. THE IMPACT ON SURVIVAL OF CLEARANCE OF TUMOR FROM MEDIASTINAL NODES BY INDUCTION THERAPY IN IIIa,b NON–SMALL CELL LUNG CANCER

| STUDY | % SURGICALLY STAGED | % N2,3 | % T4/N3 | % DOWN-STAGED[b] | yN0,1[a] | | | PERSISTENT yN2,3 | | | P[c] % |
					N	MST (mo)	4 y (%)	N	MST (mo)	4 y (%)	
Albain et al[1]	100	87	40	53	39	30	33	35	10	11	.003
Eberhardt et al[4]	100	85	42	77	54	30	38	12	18	15	NS
Rice et al[5]	100	98	21	35	14	NR	(83)[d]	31[e]	11	(26)[d]	.005
Rice et al[3]	100	93	45	33	12	NR	(80)[f]	30[e]	18	(27)[f]	(.08)
Sugarbaker et al[21]	100	100[g]	0	16	9	43	43	33	8	16	.01
Choi et al[2]	100	100[g]	0	67	28	NR	60[h]	11	24	18	.04
Average for all[i]				47		34	47		15	15	

Inclusion criteria: Prospective phase II studies of induction chemotherapy in ≥40 patients from 1980 to 2000.
[a]Patients initially N2,3 positive who were yN0,1 after induction therapy (y refers to restaging after induction treatment).
[b]Disappearance of tumor from mediastinal nodes.
[c]Survival of yN0,1 versus yN2,3 by log rank test.
[d]3-year survival.
[e]Includes patients not resected.
[f]2-year survival.
[g]Only N2.
[h]Estimated from reported results for 14 yN0 and 14 yN1 patients (79% and 42%, respectively).
[i]Excluding values in parentheses.
MST, median survival time; NR, not reached; NS, not significant ($P \geq 0.1$).

T4N0 and T1N2 tumors (by pretreatment staging), for which survival was better than that for other tumor TNM subgroups.[1]

MEDIASTINAL RESTAGING

The presence of persistent N2,3 disease after induction therapy and surgery predicts relatively poor survival (see Table 19–6) and suggests that resection in these patients may not be worth the surgical risk and morbidity. However, the presence or absence of nodal disease in these studies has been assessed in *resected specimens*. Whether preoperative restaging of the mediastinum after induction therapy is reliable and can be used to select patients for surgery is

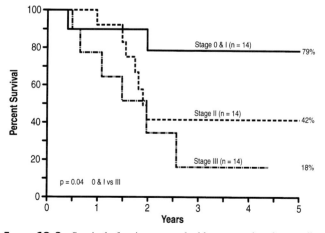

FIGURE 19–3. Survival of patients treated with preoperative chemoradiotherapy by stage of disease, as assessed pathologically following induction treatment at the time of resection. (Data from Choi NC, Carey RW, Daly W, et al. Potential impact on survival of improved tumor downstaging and resection rate by preoperative twice daily radiation and concurrent chemotherapy in stage IIIA non–small-cell lung cancer. J Clin Oncol. 1997;15:712–722.[2])

an important issue. Methods that could potentially be used to assess mediastinal downstaging include assessment of radiographic response, repeat mediastinoscopy, thoracoscopy, and positron-emission tomography (PET) scanning.

Radiographic response appears to correlate poorly with the overall pathologic response (residual tumor at either the primary site or in previously involved nodes), as discussed earlier. The correlation of radiographic response with the status of the mediastinum has received less attention to date. However, it is unlikely that the radiographic response will reliably predict the incidence of downstaging because 9% to 36% of patients with stable disease have been reported to be pathologically yN0,1.[13,21,43,44] Thus, acceptance of a lack of radiographic response alone would deny a resection to a substantial number of patients who have, in fact, been downstaged by the induction treatment.

Repeat mediastinoscopy, following induction chemoradiotherapy and an initial staging mediastinoscopy, was used in one prospective study.[4] This procedure was performed in 63 patients of the 94 entered on the trial and included all patients who had initial N2,3 involvement and were being considered for surgery. Persistent nodal disease by mediastinoscopy was found in 11%, the other 56 patients having been downstaged. At thoracotomy, which included a mediastinal lymphadenectomy, only 2 patients (4%) thought to be negative on repeat mediastinoscopy were found to have N2 disease. In both cases, this involved microscopic foci located in nodes inaccessible to the mediastinoscope. Other series of repeat mediastinoscopy following previous mediastinoscopy (but not in the setting of induction therapy) have also found false negative rates of <10% (see Chapter 5).[45] Although repeat mediastinoscopy has been reported to be safe, it is doubtful that this procedure will be widely accepted, given the reticence of many surgeons to perform primary mediastinoscopy. Mediastinal restaging using thoracoscopy is being investigated prospectively by a Cancer and Leukemia Group B study (CALGB 39803). A small pilot study of PET scanning for mediastinal restaging following induction therapy in nine patients found perfect correlation with pathologic findings.[46]

RECURRENCE PATTERNS AFTER INDUCTION CHEMOTHERAPY

Analysis of recurrence patterns can point out the deficiencies of a therapeutic approach in order to make further improvements. When no therapy whatsoever is used for patients with IIIa,b NSCLC, approximately 75% of patients have been reported to die of local disease.[47] Unfortunately, reports of recurrence patterns after treatment often do not specify whether first sites of recurrence or cumulative recurrences are being reported. In the latter case, it is difficult to compare one study with another if there is variation in the period of follow-up. Furthermore, it is often unclear whether a search for other sites was undertaken at the time a recurrence was first noted. It is likely that subsequent sites of recurrence are underreported after a first site of recurrence is identified. Therefore, an analysis of recurrence patterns must be taken with a grain of salt.

Table 19–7 presents a summary of recurrence patterns as reported in studies of induction therapy and surgery. It has been noted that approximately 60% of patients developed a recurrence. Of these, approximately 60% involved distant sites alone, 15% to 20% both local and distant sites, and approximately 20% to 25% only local sites. The type of recurrence being reported was not specified in these studies, but it is likely that this primarily represented first sites of recurrence. Some variation in the recurrence rates is seen, but there is actually a fair amount of consistency, given the ambiguities of the definition of a recurrence and varying periods of follow-up. These studies suggest that both local disease and distant disease remain an issue. Postinduction surgical resection in these patients with initial mediastinal involvement results in a local recurrence in approximately 25% of all patients. Distant metastases appear to be a greater problem despite the induction chemotherapy, with approximately 50% of all patients experiencing a distant recurrence.

One of the randomized studies of induction therapy offers strong evidence that induction chemotherapy can decrease the rate of distant metastases compared with surgery alone.[28] Actuarial recurrence rates over time revealed that the incidence of distant recurrences was significantly decreased (Fig. 19–4). In this trial, 53% of patients had stage I or II disease, and the recurrence results were not reported separately for patients with stage III versus stage I,II NSCLC. A minimal (nonsignificant) decrease in local recurrence with induction therapy was seen.[28]

ROLE OF RADIATION IN ADDITION TO CHEMOTHERAPY AND SURGERY

Most of the randomized trials of induction therapy in addition to resection have used induction chemotherapy only (see Table 19–4), although routine postoperative radiation was given in some trials[29,48] and selective radiation in many of the rest.[28,31,49] A comparison among phase II trials does not suggest that the addition of RT to induction

chemotherapy (either preoperatively or postoperatively) affects the outcome (see Table 19–2). Only one randomized trial has analyzed whether the addition of radiation to an induction regimen before resection is of benefit. Fleck et al[50] randomized 96 patients with IIIa(N2) and IIIb(T4) NSCLC to induction chemoradiotherapy (cisplatin 100 mg/m² + 5-fluorouracil × 2 cycles 4 weeks apart concurrent with 30 Gy of RT) versus chemotherapy alone (cisplatin 100 mg/m², mitomycin C, vinblastine × 6 cycles every 2 weeks). The response rate was better in the chemoradiotherapy arm (52% versus 31%, $P = 0.03$); and, perhaps as a result of a better response, resection was more commonly achieved in the chemoradiotherapy arm (67% versus 44%, $P = 0.02$). At a median follow-up of 3 years, the disease-free survival was better in the chemoradiation arm (40% versus 21%, $P = 0.04$). An update of this study shows the 5-year survival to be still better (31% versus 15%, $P < 0.05$) (personal communication, G. Giaccone, MD, August 12, 1997). Thus it may be that both chemotherapy and radiation are of benefit before resection. However, given that the data just presented comes from only one study reported only as an abstract, no definite conclusions can be drawn.

RADIOTHERAPY ALONE AS INDUCTION THERAPY BEFORE SURGERY

Preoperative treatment with RT alone has not received much attention since the 1980s. In the 1960s and 1970s, preoperative RT was investigated with the rationale that resection might be easier, that occult local residual disease might be controlled, and that dissemination of viable tumor cells at the time of resection might be reduced.[51] The results of two major randomized trials published in the 1970s involved 331 and 568 operable patients who were randomized to either 40 or 50 Gy of RT preoperatively versus surgery alone.[52,53] The survival curves in each of

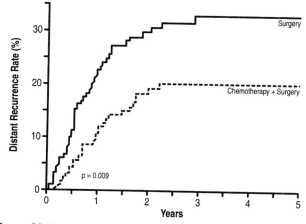

FIGURE 19–4. Rate of distant recurrence in patients with stage Ib, IIa,b, and IIIa non–small cell lung cancer, randomized to either induction chemotherapy and surgery or surgery alone. (Data from Depierre A, Milleron B, for the French Thoracic Cooperative Group. Phase III trial of neo-adjuvant chemotherapy [NCT] in resectable stage I [except T1N0], II, IIIa non–small cell lung cancer [NSCLC]: the French experience. Proc ASCO. 1999;18:465a.[28])

TABLE 19–7. RECURRENCE PATTERNS IN STAGE IIIa,b PATIENTS TREATED WITH INDUCTION THERAPY AND SURGERY

STUDY	N	INDUCTION CHEMO	INDUCTION RT (Gy)	ADJUVANT THERAPY	% pCR/THORACOTOMY[a] N2,3 Nodes	% pCR/THORACOTOMY[a] All Sites	GROUP ANALYZED FOR RECURRENCE	% OF ALL PATIENTS WITH RECURRENCE	DISTRIBUTION OF RECURRENCES (%) L	DISTRIBUTION OF RECURRENCES (%) L/D	DISTRIBUTION OF RECURRENCES (%) D
Martini et al[14]	136	MVP × 2-3	—	Chemo ± RT[b]	—	17	Resected	60	26	—	74
Sugarbaker et al[21]	74	PVb × 2	—	Chemo + 54-60	16	0	R₀	52	8	17	75
Aristu et al[22]	55	MVP × 1-6	—	IORT + 45	—	10	Operated	64	44	38	19
Takita et al[23]	41	PACCO × 2	—	RT[b]	—	—	—	—	—	—	—
Average						9		59	26	—	56
Bonomi et al[25]	128	PF/EPF × 4	c40	—	—	17	—	—	—	—	—
Albain et al[1]	126	EP × 2	c45	—	53	21	All	52	11	28	61
Weiden et al[20]	85	PF × 2	c30	—	—	15	All	71	35	12	53
Weitberg et al[16]	53	EP × 2	c54	Chemo	—	45	Resected	54	8	8	84
Palazzi et al[24]	43	EP × 2	c40[d]	—	—	23	—	—	—	—	—
Strauss et al[18]	41	PFVb × 2	c30	Chemo/c30	—	23	All	63	40	20	40
Average						24		58	24	17	60
Eberhardt et al[4]	94	EP × 3	Ch/cHF45[c]	—	77	26	Resected	36	—28—		72
Thomas et al[6]	54	CbIE × 2	Ch/cHF45	—	—	18	All	59	25	41	34
Pisch et al[19]	47	EPF × 2	cHF40[d]	—	—	0	All	66	29	48	23
Rice et al[5]	45	PT qd	cHF30	Chemo/cHF30	35	13	All	64	12	8	80
Rice et al[3]	42	PEF qd	cHF27	Chemo/cHF27	33	6	All	57	21	17	63
Choi et al[2]	42	PFVb × 2	cHF42[c]	Chemo/cHF18	67	10	All	48	15	10	75
Average						12		53	20	25	58
Average for all					47	16		57	23	22	58

Inclusion criteria: Prospective phase II trials of induction therapy and surgery in ≥40 patients from 1980 to 2000.
[a]Percentage of all patients undergoing thoracotomy who were found to have a pathologic complete response (no tumor remaining) in the mediastinal nodes or at all sites.
[b]Dose not given.
[c]Includes prophylactic cranial irradiation.
[d]Split course RT.

c, concurrent; Chemo, chemotherapy; D, distant recurrence; HF, hyperfractionated; IORT, intraoperative radiotherapy; L, local recurrence; L/D, simultaneous local and distant recurrence; Operated, all patients undergoing thoracotomy; Resected, resected patients; R₀, completely resected patients.

Chemotherapy regimens: CbIE, carboplatin, ifosfamide, etoposide; EP, etoposide, cisplatin; EPF, etoposide, cisplatin, 5-fluorouracil; MVP, mitomycin C, vincristine, cisplatin; PACCO, cisplatin, doxorubicin, cyclophosphamide, CCNU, vincristine; PF, cisplatin, 5-fluorouracil; PFVb, cisplatin, 5-fluorouracil, vinblastine; PT, cisplatin, teniposide; PVb, cisplatin, vinblastine.

these studies were almost identical (5-year survival for preoperative RT [7% and 14%] versus surgery alone [12% and 16%], P = NS).[52,53] There was no difference in the rate of complete resection (52% and 54% versus 55% and 52%) or in the rate or patterns of recurrence.[52,53] One additional randomized study treated 152 patients with marginally operable disease (cT3,4N2,3) with 40 Gy of RT, and then randomized patients to either resection or no further treatment.[53] No difference in survival was found (5-year survival, 8% versus 6%; P = NS).

Each of these trials was carried out in the 1960s and 1970s and reflects the staging studies and RT techniques available at that time. The studies also included 10% to 15% of patients with small cell lung cancer. The suspicion that many of the patients may have had undiagnosed systemic disease is underscored by the fact that 40% to 50% of the patients in each of the arms of these studies were dead within 6 months.[52,53] Although these were large randomized trials that do not suggest any benefit with respect to preoperative RT, their applicability to specific subsets of patients using modern diagnostic and treatment techniques is doubtful. No other randomized trials of preoperative RT involving ≥100 patients have been published. However, given the incidence of systemic recurrences after resection and the advent of active chemotherapy in NSCLC, there is no enthusiasm to re-examine the use of combination therapy using only two local modalities (RT and surgery) in the modern era.

ROLE OF SURGERY IN ADDITION TO CHEMOTHERAPY AND RADIATION

Some form of local treatment is necessary after the use of chemotherapy. Chemotherapy alone has been used only rarely in patients with IIIa,b disease, and no information is available about the rate of local control with this approach. However, residual local tumor has been found at the time

of resection in 80% to 90% of patients after chemotherapy in phase II studies of induction therapy (see Table 19–2). This makes a strong argument that additional local therapy is necessary.

Whether the local therapy used after induction chemotherapy for stage IIIa,b NSCLC should involve surgical resection, RT, or both is an important question. The rates of local control following primary surgery for stage IIIa,b disease (sometimes in combination with RT) are high (see Table 17–5), whereas conventional RT alone achieves local control in only a minority of cases (see Chapter 18). However, these local control rates cannot be compared because the patients selected for surgery are clearly different from the much larger group of patients treated with RT alone. Furthermore, the effectiveness of either surgery or RT in the setting of induction chemotherapy is not necessarily predicted by the local control rates of each modality alone.

Unfortunately, no data is available at this time concerning the role of surgery versus RT in the setting of induction chemotherapy for IIIa,b NSCLC. An Intergroup trial (INT 0139) is underway in the United States that randomizes patients to surgery versus additional RT (15 Gy) after induction concurrent chemoradiotherapy (cisplatin, etoposide, and 30 Gy of RT) (Fig. 19–5). This trial has a target accrual of approximately 600 patients. A similar trial is underway in Europe, randomizing patients to surgery or RT after three cycles of induction chemotherapy (Intergroup study 08941).[54]

EDITORS' COMMENTS

The rationale for multimodality therapy of stage IIIa,b NSCLC is compelling. Chemotherapy, shown to be active in stage IV disease, offers the potential of decreasing the incidence of systemic recurrences, whereas surgery and radiation optimize the chance for local control. Of course, an attractive rationale does not obviate the need to demon-

DATA SUMMARY: PROGNOSTIC FACTORS AND RECURRENCE PATTERNS

	AMOUNT	QUALITY	CONSISTENCY
Response endpoints (objective radiographic response, pathologic complete response rate, median survival) are similar in patients with earlier stage (IIb, IIIa) or later stage (IIIa,b) disease	High	Mod	High
Downstaging of mediastinal nodes predicts significantly better survival after induction therapy and resection	High	Mod	Mod
The 4-year survival of resected *downstaged* patients (negative mediastinal nodes after induction therapy) is 50%	High	High	Mod
The 4-year survival of resected patients with persistent N2 disease after induction therapy is 15%	High	High	High
Mediastinal node downstaging has been found to have occurred in 10% to 30% of patients who show no radiographic response to induction therapy (stable disease)	High	High	Mod
60% of recurrences after induction therapy and surgery involve only distant sites	High	Mod	Mod
40% of recurrences after induction therapy and surgery involve local sites, either alone or in combination with distant sites	High	Mod	Mod

Type of data rated: Plain text: descriptive statement   *Italics: controlled comparison*   **Bold: randomized comparison**

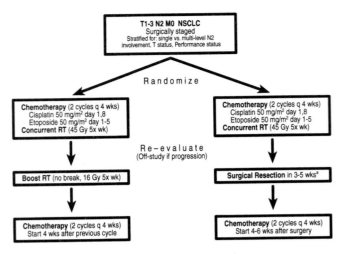

FIGURE 19–5. Schema of Intergroup trial of chemoradiotherapy versus chemoradiotherapy in addition to surgery for stage IIIa non–small cell lung cancer (INT 0139).[54]

strate that the anticipated benefits actually occur. Although many issues remain unresolved, several points regarding induction therapy and surgery for IIIa,b disease are well established.

There is no doubt that the available chemotherapy agents are active, as evidenced by the high radiographic response rate and the ability to achieve mediastinal downstaging and pathologic complete responses with this treatment. Furthermore, the rate of disease progression is low. Such treatment approaches can be used with reasonable morbidity and low mortality rates. This is true despite the use of aggressive regimens involving concurrent chemoradiotherapy and twice-daily radiation. After induction therapy, surgery in these patients with extensive mediastinal disease has been accomplished with no obvious increase in surgical mortality compared with surgery alone in earlier stage disease.

However, some caution is in order when one reads between the lines. There is variability in the rates of complete resection, most likely due to a reluctance in many institutions to attempt resection in patients with extensive local disease. Those centers that have adopted an aggressive attitude have demonstrated that a complete resection can be achieved in the large majority of patients who have not discontinued the planned approach because of intervening events. The patients included in studies of induction therapy and surgery do not appear to have been carefully selected with regard to the extent of locally advanced cancer (T and N stage), but the median age is uniformly young compared with the average population of patients with lung cancer. Although clear data regarding the incidence of comorbidities is not available, it is likely that these patients were carefully selected as being likely to be able to tolerate such treatment with low morbidity and mortality. Furthermore, these studies have been carried out at large centers that have substantial experience in the surgical, radiotherapeutic, and chemotherapeutic treatment of lung cancer. Whether the reported results can be maintained if such treatment is applied more widely to a broader group of patients in a wide variety of institutions is an open question.

The patients included in induction chemotherapy and surgery trials have clearly had extensive local disease. There is no doubt that this group would have fared extremely poorly with surgery alone. The average 5-year survival of 25% is remarkable and strongly suggests a benefit to this approach compared with surgery alone. Unfortunately, the data from randomized studies of induction chemotherapy and surgery versus surgery alone is too limited to clearly define the role of this treatment. Although most studies indicate a trend to better survival, this is statistically significant in only two. Certainly, the possibility of publication bias must be considered. Nevertheless, the fact that two studies of only 60 patients each demonstrated significant differences is amazing and suggests that there may be a substantial benefit.

It appears that relatively few patients with persistent mediastinal nodal disease following induction therapy benefit from resection. Resection in these patients is probably not justified. However, the best method of restaging the mediastinum is unclear at this time. Radiographic staging alone is clearly not reliable. Repeat mediastinoscopy is supported by more data and lower false negative rates than any other technique. However, this data comes from one study, and it is unlikely that this procedure will be widely adopted. The role of PET scanning is also unclear. It is unlikely that a PET scan will be able to detect residual microscopic disease. On the other hand, conversion of a positive PET scan to a negative result may indicate a substantial response and predict a good prognosis, even in the face of residual microscopic disease. Ideally, future studies will provide answers to these questions. Unfortunately, there is a substantial risk that PET scanning will be widely adopted, not because of demonstrated reliability but because it circumvents the reticence to perform mediastinoscopy.

Although the survival results after induction therapy and surgery are provocative, the real issue is whether surgical resection is needed in the face of induction chemotherapy and radiation. Even if mediastinal restaging is found to be reliable in identifying patients who are downstaged and is able to predict a good prognosis in these patients, this does not necessarily indicate that surgical resection itself is of benefit. Although this issue is being addressed by a randomized intergroup study, it will take several years before an answer is available. Furthermore, whether surgical resection is worthwhile in patients with IIIa,b NSCLC will have to be re-examined as improvements in RT are made and more active chemotherapeutic agents are found.

References

1. Albain KS, Rusch VW, Crowley JJ, et al. Concurrent cisplatin/etoposide plus chest radiotherapy followed by surgery for stages IIIA(N2) and IIIB non–small-cell lung cancer: mature results of Southwest Oncology Group Phase II Study 8805. J Clin Oncol. 1995;13:1880–1892.
2. Choi NC, Carey RW, Daly W, et al. Potential impact on survival of improved tumor downstaging and resection rate by preoperative twice-daily radiation and concurrent chemotherapy in stage IIIA non–small-cell lung cancer. J Clin Oncol. 1997;15:712–722.

3. Rice TW, Adelstein DJ, Koka A, et al. Accelerated induction therapy and resection for poor prognosis stage III non–small cell lung cancer. Ann Thorac Surg. 1995;60:586–592.

4. Eberhardt W, Wilke H, Stamatis G, et al. Preoperative chemotherapy followed by concurrent chemoradiation therapy based on hyperfractionated accelerated radiotherapy and definitive surgery in locally advanced non–small-cell lung cancer: mature results of a phase II trial. J Clin Oncol. 1998;16:622–634.

5. Rice TW, Adelstein DJ, Ciezki JP, et al. Short-course induction chemoradiotherapy with paclitaxel for stage III non–small-cell lung cancer. Ann Thorac Surg. 1998;66:1909–1914.

6. Thomas M, Rübe C, Semik M, et al. Impact of preoperative bimodality induction including twice-daily radiation on tumor regression and survival in stage III non–small cell lung cancer. J Clin Oncol. 1999;17:1185–1193.

7. Mathisen DJ, Wain JC, Wright C, et al. Assessment of preoperative accelerated radiotherapy and chemotherapy in stage IIIA (N2) non–small-cell lung cancer. J Thorac Cardiovasc Surg. 1996;111:123–133.

8. Roberts JR, DeVore RF, Carbone DP, et al. Neoadjuvant chemotherapy increases complications in patients undergoing resection for NSCLC [abstract]. Proc ASCO. 1999;18:465a.

9. Deutsch M, Crawford J, Leopold K, et al. Phase II study of neoadjuvant chemotherapy and radiation therapy with thoracotomy in the treatment of clinically staged IIIA non–small cell lung cancer. Cancer. 1994;74:1243–1252.

10. Fowler WC, Langer CJ, Curran WJ Jr, et al. Postoperative complications after combined neoadjuvant treatment of lung cancer. Ann Thorac Surg. 1993;55:986–989.

11. Rusch VW, Benfield JR. Neoadjuvant therapy for lung cancer: a note of caution. Ann Thorac Surg. 1993;55:820–821.

12. Sonett JR, Krasna MJ, Suntharalingam M, et al. Safe pulmonary resection after chemotherapy and high-dose thoracic radiation. Ann Thorac Surg. 1999;68:316–320.

13. Burkes RL, Ginsberg RJ, Shepherd FA, et al. Induction chemotherapy with mitomycin, vindesine, and cisplatin for stage III unresectable non–small-cell lung cancer: results of the Toronto Phase II Trial. J Clin Oncol. 1992;10:580–586.

14. Martini N, Kris MG, Flehinger BJ, et al. Preoperative chemotherapy for stage IIIa (N2) lung cancer: the Sloan-Kettering experience with 136 patients. Ann Thorac Surg. 1993;55:1365–1374.

15. Pujol J-L, Hayot M, Rouanet P, et al. Long-term results of neoadjuvant ifosfamide, cisplatin, and etoposide combination in locally advanced non–small-cell lung cancer. Chest. 1994;106:1451–1455.

16. Weitberg AB, Yashar J, Glicksman AS, et al. Combined-modality therapy for stage IIIA non–small cell carcinoma of the lung. Eur J Cancer. 1993;29A:511–515.

17. Darwish S, Minotti V, Crinò L, et al. A Phase II trial of combined chemotherapy and surgery in stage IIIA non–small cell lung cancer. Lung Cancer. 1995;12(suppl 1):S71–S78.

18. Strauss GM, Herndon JE, Sherman DD, et al. Neoadjuvant chemotherapy and radiotherapy followed by surgery in stage IIIA non–small-cell carcinoma of the lung: report of a Cancer and Leukemia Group B phase II study. J Clin Oncol. 1992;10:1237–1244.

19. Pisch J, Berson AM, Malamud S, et al. Chemoradiation in advanced nonsmall cell lung cancer. Int J Radiat Oncol Biol Phys. 1995;33:183–188.

20. Weiden PL, Piantadosi S, for The Lung Cancer Study Group. Preoperative chemotherapy (cisplatin and fluorouracil) and radiation therapy in stage III non–small-cell lung cancer: a phase II study of the Lung Cancer Study Group. J Natl Cancer Inst. 1991;83:266–272.

21. Sugarbaker DJ, Herndon J, Kohman LJ, et al. Results of Cancer and Leukemia Group B protocol 8935: a multiinstitutional phase II trimodality trial for stage IIIA(N2) non–small-cell lung cancer. J Thorac Cardiovasc Surg. 1995;109:473–485.

22. Aristu J, Rebollo J, Martínez-Monge R, et al. Cisplatin, mitomycin, and vindesine followed by intraoperative and postoperative radiotherapy for stage III non–small cell lung cancer: final results of a phase II study. Am J Clin Oncol. 1997;20:276–281.

23. Takita H, Blumenson LE, Raghavan D. Neoadjuvant chemotherapy of stage III-A and B lung carcinoma using the PACCO regimen. J Surg Oncol. 1995;59:147–150.

24. Palazzi M, Cataldo I, Gramaglia A, et al. Preoperative concomitant cisplatin/VP16 and radiotherapy in stage III non–small cell lung cancer. Int J Radiat Oncol Biol Phys. 1993;27:621–625.

25. Bonomi P, Faber LP. Neoadjuvant chemoradiation therapy in non–small cell lung cancer: the Rush University experience. Lung Cancer. 1993;9:383–390.

26. Weiden PL, Piantadosi S. Preoperative chemotherapy (cisplatin and fluorouracil) and radiation therapy in stage III non–small cell lung cancer: a phase 2 study of the LCSG. Chest. 1994;106(suppl):344S–347S.

27. Pisters KMW, Ginsberg RJ, Giroux DJ, et al, for the Bimodality Lung Oncology Team (BLOT). Induction chemotherapy before surgery for early-stage lung cancer: a novel approach. J Thorac Cardiovasc Surg. 2000;119:429–439.

28. Depierre A, Milleron B, for the French Thoracic Cooperative Group. Phase III trial of neo-adjuvant chemotherapy (NCT) in resectable stage I (except T1N0), II, IIIa non–small cell lung cancer (NSCLC): the French experience. Proc ASCO. 1999;18:465a.

29. Rosell R, Gómez-Codina J, Camps C, et al. A randomized trial comparing preoperative chemotherapy plus surgery with surgery alone in patients with non–small-cell lung cancer. N Engl J Med. 1994;330:153–158.

30. Rosell R, Gómez-Codina J, Camps C, et al. Presectional chemotherapy in stage IIIA non–small-cell lung cancer: a 7-year assessment of a randomized controlled trial. Lung Cancer. 1999;47:7–14.

31. Roth JA, Fossella F, Komaki R, et al. A randomized trial comparing perioperative chemotherapy and surgery with surgery alone in resectable stage IIIA non–small-cell lung cancer. J Natl Cancer Inst. 1994;86:673–680.

32. Roth JA, Atkinson EN, Fossella F, et al. Long-term follow-up of patients enrolled in a randomized trial comparing perioperative chemotherapy and surgery with surgery alone in resectable stage IIIA non–small-cell lung cancer. Lung Cancer. 1998;21:1–6.

33. Wagner H Jr, Piantadosi S, Ruckdeschel JC. Randomized phase II evaluation of preoperative radiation therapy and preoperative chemotherapy with mitomycin, vinblastine, and cisplatin in patients with technically unresectable stage IIIA and IIIB non–small cell cancer of the lung. (Lung Cancer Study Group 881). Chest. 1994;106(suppl):348S–354S.

34. Rosell R, Li S, Skacel Z, et al. Prognostic impact of mutated K-ras gene in surgically resected non–small cell lung cancer patients. Oncogene. 1993;8:2407–2412.

35. Slebos RJC, Kibbelaar RE, Dalesio O, et al. K-ras oncogene activation as a prognostic marker in adenocarcinoma of the lung. N Engl J Med. 1990;323:561–565.

36. Graziano SL. Non–small cell lung cancer: clinical value of new biological predictors. Lung Cancer. 1997;17(suppl 1):S37–S58.

37. Sugio K, Ishida T, Yokoyama H, et al. ras Gene mutations as a prognostic marker in adenocarcinoma of the human lung without lymph node metastasis. Cancer Res 1992;52:2903–2906.

38. Rodenhuis S, Boerrigter L, Top B, et al. Mutational activation of the K-ras oncogene and the effect of chemotherapy in advanced adenocarcinoma of the lung: a prospective study. J Clin Oncol. 1997;15:285–291.

39. Rosell R, Molina F, Moreno I, et al. Mutated K-ras gene analysis in a randomized trial of preoperative chemotherapy plus surgery versus surgery in stage IIIA non–small cell lung cancer. Lung Cancer. 1995;12(suppl):S59–S70.

40. Pass HI, Pogrebniak HW, Steinberg SM, et al. Randomized trial of neoadjuvant therapy for lung cancer: interim analysis. Ann Thorac Surg. 1992;53:992–998.

41. Dautzenberg B, Benichou J, Allard P, et al. Failure of the perioperative PCV neoadjuvant polychemotherapy in resectable bronchogenic non–small cell carcinoma: results from a randomized phase II trial. Cancer. 1990;65:2435–2441.

42. American Joint Committee on Cancer. Cancer Staging Handbook. Philadelphia, Pa: Lippincott-Raven; 1998.

43. Yashar J, Weitberg AB, Glicksman AS, et al. Preoperative chemotherapy and radiation therapy for stage IIIa carcinoma of the lung. Ann Thorac Surg. 1992;53:445–448.

44. Kirn DH, Lynch TJ, Mentzer SJ, et al. Multimodality therapy of patients with stage IIIA, N2 non–small-cell lung cancer: impact of preoperative chemotherapy on resectability and downstaging. J Thorac Cardiovasc Surg. 1993;106:696–702.

45. Meersschaut D, Vermassen F, de la Rivière AB, et al. Repeat mediastinoscopy in the assessment of new and recurrent lung neoplasm. Ann Thorac Surg. 1992;53:120–122.

46. Vansteenkiste JF, Stroobants SG, and the Leuven Lung Cancer Group. Potential use of FDG-PET scan after induction chemotherapy in

surgically staged IIIa-N2 non–small-cell lung cancer: a prospective pilot study. Ann Oncol. 1998;9:1193–1198.

47. Reinfuss M, Skolyszewski J, Kowalska T, et al. Palliative radiotherapy in asymptomatic patients with locally advanced, unresectable, non–small cell lung cancer. Strahlenther Onkol. 1993;169:709–715.

48. Elias AD, Herndon J, Kumar P, et al, for the Cancer and Leukemia Group B. A phase III comparison of "best local-regional therapy" with or without chemotherapy (CT) for stage IIIA Ta-3N2 non–small cell lung cancer (NSCLC): preliminary results [abstract]. Proc ASCO. 1997;16:448a.

49. Yoneda S, Hibino S, Gotoh I, et al. A comparative trial on induction chemoradiotherapy followed by surgery (CRS) or immediate surgery (IS) for stage III non–small call lung cancer (NSCLC) [abstract]. Proc ASCO. 1995;14:367.

50. Fleck J, Camargo J, Godoy D, et al. Chemoradiation therapy (CRT) versus chemotherapy (CT) alone as a neo-adjuvant treatment for stage III non–small cell lung cancer (NSCLC): preliminary report of a phase III prospective randomized trial [abstract]. Proc ASCO. 1993;12:333.

51. Payne DG. Pre-operative radiation therapy in non–small cell cancer of the lung. Lung Cancer. 1991;7:47–56.

52. Shields TW. Preoperative radiation therapy in the treatment of bronchial carcinoma. Cancer. 1972;30:1388–1394.

53. Warram J, for an NCI Collaborative Study. Preoperative irradiation of cancer of the lung: final report of a therapeutic trial (a collaborative study). Cancer. 1975;36:914–925.

54. Splinter TAW, Kirkpatrick A, Darwish S, et al. Randomized trial of surgery versus radiotherapy in patients with stage IIIA non–small cell lung cancer after a response to induction-chemotherapy. Lung Cancer. 1997;18:62–63.

SURGERY FOR STAGE IIIB NON–SMALL CELL LUNG CANCER

Frank C. Detterbeck and David R. Jones

N3 DISEASE

T4 DISEASE

Carina
Other Structures
Induction Therapy

MALIGNANT PLEURAL EFFUSION

EDITORS' COMMENTS

Stage IIIb non–small cell lung cancer (NSCLC) is generally considered to be inoperable, although this does not mean it should be considered incurable. Radiotherapy (RT) has been the traditional treatment of stage IIIb lung cancer, but the new standard of treatment with a combination of chemotherapy and RT now offers a reasonable chance of long-term survival. Such combination treatment without surgery is the subject of Chapter 21.

This chapter reviews the data regarding surgery in the small proportion of patients with IIIb disease who have undergone surgical resection. The focus is on patients for whom surgery constitutes the primary treatment, which primarily involves patients with T4N0,1 disease. This chapter also includes a discussion of those patients (primarily with N3 disease) who are treated with a multimodality approach involving surgical resection as well as chemotherapy and RT and a discussion of resected patients in whom pleural cytology is found to be positive. Significant differences exist within these categories; therefore, this chapter is divided into a discussion of N3 disease, T4 disease on the basis of extension into mediastinal structures, and patients with malignant cells in the pleural fluid.

N3 DISEASE

Naruke[1] reported a remarkable 10% 5-year survival after resection in 88 patients with N3 node involvement. He advocated thoracotomy and attempted resection for practically all patients with disease localized to the chest. He also championed extensive node dissection. Several groups from Japan have extended the concept of radical mediastinal node dissection to include contralateral nodes, which are removed either through a sternotomy or a bilateral thoracotomy.[2–5] These reports have indicated a 2-year survival of 60% in nine patients in one series,[3] and at least one 5-year survivor has been reported.[2] Although these results are intriguing, further studies involving larger numbers of patients and longer follow-up are necessary before this approach can be recommended.

Some investigators have explored the use of surgery for patients with stage IIIb NSCLC after induction chemotherapy or chemoradiotherapy. At least eight phase II or III trials have been reported that have involved ≥20 stage IIIb patients.[6–14] However, some of the studies included many patients with T4N0,1 disease (who appear to have a better prognosis than those with N3 involvement),[6,7,13] and in several of the studies, the staging methods and categories were not specifically reported.[8,9,12] Two studies were reported in which careful surgical staging was done in all patients and which included ≥20 patients with N3 involvement.[6,7]

The first of these included 24 patients with pN3 and 10 patients with pT4N2 disease, all proved by mediastinoscopy.[7] Seventy-two percent of patients had a pathologic complete response in the mediastinal nodes after an aggressive induction regimen (three cycles of etoposide/cisplatin followed by concurrent etoposide/cisplatin and 45 Gy hyperfractionated thoracic RT as well as prophylactic cranial irradiation [PCI]). Fifty-three percent of the 34 patients were taken to thoracotomy, and 72% of these underwent a complete resection. For the entire group of 42 stage pIIIb patients, the median survival was 18 months, and the 5-year survival was 26%.[7] Another study (Southwest Oncology Group [SWOG] 8805) involved 51 stage pIIIb patients, of whom 53% had pN3 disease (proven by mediastinoscopy).[6,15,16] After induction chemoradiotherapy (concurrent etoposide/cisplatin and 45 Gy RT), 63% of the patients underwent thoracotomy and 82% of them had a complete resection. The median survival for all 27 of the N3 patients was 13 months, with a 2-year survival of 25%.[16] Interestingly, this study suggested that survival of patients with supraclavicular N3 disease may be better than that for patients with contralateral N3 disease (2-year survival 35% versus 0%, no *P* value given).[6] In both of these studies, local control was achieved in approximately 80% of all the patients entered on the trial.[6,7]

These results suggest that the categorization of stage IIIb(N3) NSCLC as a nonsurgical disease may need to be re-examined. If chemotherapy becomes effective at controlling microscopic metastatic disease and permits resection with minimal margins (such as is the case with malignant mediastinal nodes), surgery may come to play an important role as consolidative treatment to achieve local control at the sites of initial gross disease. A more detailed discussion of combined modality treatment is found in Chapter 19.

TABLE 20–1. PUBLISHED REPORTS OF CARINAL RESECTIONS FOR LUNG CANCER

STUDY	N	HOSPITAL MORTALITY (%)	SURVIVAL (%) 2-y	SURVIVAL (%) 5-y
Vogt-Moykopf et al[69]	79	17	27	—
Dartevelle[17]	60	7	58	42
Deslauriers et al[20]	38	29	—	13
Mathisen and Grillo[18]	37	18	—	19
Jensik et al[23]	34	29	24	13
Maeda et al[70]	31	19	—	41
Roviaro et al[21]	28	4	(50)[a]	(29)[a,b]
Tsuchiya et al[22]	20	30	59	—
Average[c]		**18**	**42**	**26**

Inclusion criteria: Studies of ≥20 patients undergoing carinal resection from 1980 to 2000.
[a]Crude survival.
[b]4-year survival.
[c]Excluding values in parentheses.

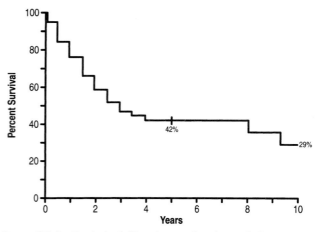

FIGURE 20–1. Survival of 60 patients undergoing carinal pneumonectomy for lung cancer. (Reprinted with permission from the Society of Thoracic Surgeons [*The Annals of Thoracic Surgery,* 1997, Vol 63, 12–19].)[17]

T4 DISEASE

Primary tumor extension into major structures that are not easily resected—trachea or carina, superior vena cava (SVC), aorta, intrapericardial pulmonary artery, esophagus, or vertebral bodies—is classified as T4 disease. Invasion of the recurrent laryngeal nerve is also classified as T4, but phrenic nerve invasion is not. Limited numbers of patients with T4 disease who have not had extensive mediastinal node involvement have been considered for surgical resection, particularly those having involvement of the carina or SVC.

Carina

Table 20–1 presents a summary of all published reports from 1980 to 2000 of carinal resections for lung cancer containing at least 20 patients. These reports encompass 322 patients. The operative mortality is substantial at 18%, and the 5-year survival is roughly the same at about 26%. The best survival, from the Hôpital Marie Lannelongue in France, is shown in Figure 20–1.[17] Most other series have reported 5-year survival rates approximately half that of this series. Table 20–2 shows the nature of complications and causes of mortality in those studies in which this information is available.

Factors influencing the survival of patients undergoing carinal resection have not been well studied. Some authors have stated that patients with N2 disease are not candidates for carinal resection,[18] but others reported long-term survivors in this category.[19,20] Roviaro et al[21] found that 86% of those who were N0, 11% of those who were N1, and none of the five patients who were N2 were alive at the time of their analysis. However, Tsuchiya et al[22] did not find a correlation with nodal status. Indeed, 50% of 10 N2 patients were alive, as was one N3 patient, at the time of their report, but the follow-up period was short (<3 years in all patients). Dartevelle et al[19] did find a correlation between survival and the level of nodal involvement (3-year survival: 43% in 21 N1 patients, 34% in 21 N2

patients with subcarinal node involvement, and 0 in 9 patients with paratracheal node involvement). Thus, although the prognosis may be diminished, the presence of N2 disease in patients with carinal cancers does not necessarily preclude 5-year survival after resection.

RT has been used either preoperatively[21,23] or postoperatively[18,19] with carinal resection. No benefit is apparent from the limited reported data. There is some concern about using RT preoperatively in a procedure that has a relatively high rate of bronchial dehiscence because several reports have suggested a higher rate of airway complications following RT.[24–29]

Other Structures

The largest study of patients undergoing resection for T4 tumors was reported by Tsuchiya et al in 1994.[30] This report encompassed 101 patients, of whom 44 underwent left atrial resection, 32 SVC resection, 28 aortic resection, 13 carinal resection, and 7 resection of the main pulmonary artery. The hospital mortality was 13%, and the overall 5-year survival was also 13%. One-third of the patients

TABLE 20–2. COMPLICATIONS AND MORTALITY RATES FROM PUBLISHED REPORTS OF CARINAL RESECTIONS FOR LUNG CANCER

	COMPLICATION (%)[a]	CAUSE OF DEATH (%)[b]
ARDS/pneumonia	12	8
Bronchial dehiscence	10	6
Empyema	6	
Bronchial stenosis	3	
Hemorrhage	3	
Other	2	3

Inclusion criteria: Studies reporting specific complications in >20 patients undergoing carinal resection from 1980 to 2000.
[a]Major complications, including fatal complications, based on 291 patients. (Data from references 18–23, 69).
[b]Causes of hospital death, based on 243 patients. (Data from references 18–23, 70.)
ARDS, adult respiratory distress syndrome.

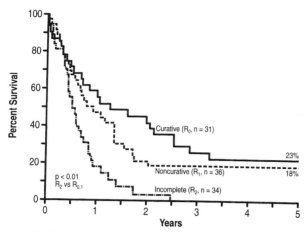

FIGURE 20–2. Survival of 101 patients undergoing extended resections for lung cancer, according to completeness of resection. (Reprinted with permission from the Society of Thoracic Surgeons [*The Annals of Thoracic Surgery,* 1994, Vol 57, 960–965].)[30]

underwent a grossly incomplete resection, one-third were found to have a microscopically positive margin at final pathologic examination, and one-third had a complete resection with clean margins. The median survival for patients undergoing a grossly incomplete resection was 6.5 months, and all of these patients were dead within 3 years. There was no significant difference in the survival of those patients having resection with a positive margin versus those without; these groups together exhibited a median survival of 14 months and a 19% 5-year survival (Fig. 20–2). Multivariate analysis disclosed four prognostic factors for long-term survival: the completeness of the resection, the nodal status, and two factors related to perioperative mortality (postoperative pneumonia and bleeding).

Burt et al[31] reported on 225 patients from Memorial Sloan-Kettering who had either T3 or T4 disease. Survival was not significantly different between 49 patients undergoing complete resection and 33 patients undergoing incomplete resection who were treated with adjuvant brachytherapy (5-year survival, 10% versus 22%). This is in contrast to the 143 patients who were not resected, among whom there were no 5-year survivors regardless of whether or not the patients were treated with brachytherapy. However, the data reported in this study did not separate patients with T3 versus T4 tumors.

Not enough detailed data is available to allow firm conclusions to be drawn about the prognostic implications of involvement of different mediastinal structures. De-

Meester et al[32] found a 5-year survival of 42% in 12 patients with tumor involving the vertebral column. However, only two of these patients had bony destruction that was radiographically obvious preoperatively, and all except one were N0. A five-year survival of 0% to 22% after left atrial resection has been reported (average, 8%) in several series (total of 85 patients).[30,31,33–35] Burt et al[31] found a 14% 5-year survival in seven patients with esophageal involvement. Tsuchiya et al[30] reported that of seven patients undergoing resection of the main pulmonary artery using cardiopulmonary bypass, all were dead within 2½ years.

Resection of involved SVC was reported by several authors (total, 107 patients).[17,30,31,35–41] The intermediate survival appears to be similar to that with other involved mediastinal structures, and an average 5-year survival of 30% has been reported in three series of 14, 25, and 15 patients.[17,35,36] Patency after vena caval reconstruction using Gore-Tex grafts has been excellent.[37,40]

Several authors have suggested a poor prognosis for patients with involvement of the aorta who are not resected.[38,42] Tsuchiya et al's[30] experience in 21 patients suggested that dissecting tumor away from the aorta in a subadventitial plane is not adequate because only 47% were found to have a microscopically negative margin. Full thickness excision of a portion of aorta[30,35,43] and even the aortic arch[38,43] has been reported in 27 patients, with at least three long-term survivors (alive >5 years postresection).[30,35]

Induction Therapy

Several studies have investigated surgical resection of >20 T4N0-2 patients in the context of induction therapy.[10,29] In one of these studies, 73% of patients underwent thoracotomy after induction chemotherapy (mitomycin-C, vinblastine, cisplatin [MVbP] × 3), and 62% of the entire group (36 of 57) could be completely resected.[10] Treatment-related mortality was 2%, and a median survival of 18 months and a 5-year survival of 20% were reported for all patients entered into the study. These results are encouraging, especially given the fact that 60% of the patients had T4N2 cancers as assessed by careful surgical staging. Another study reported a 3-year survival of 54% but included only 23 patients in whom induction therapy and surgical resection could be successfully completed.[29] In this study, 74% of patients were initially staged as T4N0,1.

Because of potential differences in patient selection, it is impossible to compare these results with surgery alone or with chemoradiotherapy without surgery. The SWOG

DATA SUMMARY: SURGERY FOR T4 NON–SMALL CELL LUNG CANCER			
	AMOUNT	**QUALITY**	**CONSISTENCY**
The operative mortality of carinal resection for lung cancer is 20%	High	High	Mod
The 5-year survival following carinal resection for lung cancer is 25%	High	High	Mod
The 5-year survival following resection of non–small cell lung cancer involving other T4 structures is 15%	Mod	Poor	Mod

Type of data rated: Plain text: descriptive statement   *Italics: controlled comparison*   **Bold: randomized comparison**

compared patients with stage IIIb cancers entered onto two consecutive protocols (SWOG 8805 and SWOG 9019) that had identical eligibility criteria: one involved treatment with chemoradiotherapy followed by surgery and the other involved chemoradiotherapy alone. The survival of patients with N3 tumors or T4N2 tumors was similar between the two protocols, but the T4N0,1 patients who were treated on a chemoradiotherapy and surgery protocol exhibited a 2-year survival of 64%, whereas those treated with a chemoradiotherapy protocol had a 2-year survival of 33%.[44] However, because each of these trials involved only 50 patients, of whom <20 had T4N0,1 disease, no definite conclusions were drawn.

MALIGNANT PLEURAL EFFUSION

The presence of a malignant pleural effusion (MPE) is classified as T4 disease, and patients with this condition are widely considered to have a poor prognosis.[45,46] The median survival time in such patients is generally reported as 3 to 6 months, with a negligible 5-year survival.[47–52] However, some data exists that suggests this view may be too simplistic and that certain patients with an MPE may have a better prognosis. In fact, some patients have even been considered candidates for curative treatment including surgery.

The first issue in determining the prognosis of patients with an MPE is whether the diagnosis is secure. Small effusions, not visible on chest radiograph but identified by a computed tomography scan, may well be benign and do not necessarily imply a poor prognosis. Mountain[46] suggested that the mere presence of an effusion was prognostically sufficient and reported finding no difference in the survival of 326 patients whether an effusion was malignant (n = 90), benign (n = 38), or not cytologically examined (n = 198). However, although explicit details about treatment of these patients are not provided, it appears that most, if not all, of the patients in this study were treated only palliatively. The importance of an accurate diagnosis before determining the treatment is demonstrated by a study of 160 resected M0 patients with pleural effusion identified at thoracotomy by Naruke et al,[53] who found that the presence of a benign pleural effusion was of little significance (Fig. 20–3).

The tendency to attribute a poor prognosis to all patients with lung cancer who have an effusion is probably due to the fact that it is not always easy to establish whether the effusion is malignant. The cytologic examination of the pleural fluid by thoracentesis has a false negative rate of 30% to 60%.[49,54,55] The false negative rate can be high (95%) when the fluid is bloody.[49] Although a bloody effusion has a higher likelihood of being due to pleural metastases, not all bloody effusions in patients with lung cancer are malignant. Decker et al[55] reported on 4 patients (of 73) with bloody or exudative effusions who were found not to have pleural metastatic disease and who had excellent long-term survival after resection. Thoracoscopy appears to have a much higher diagnostic accuracy than thoracentesis; Cantó et al[49] found that 97% of lung cancer patients with a pleural effusion were correctly diagnosed by using this modality.

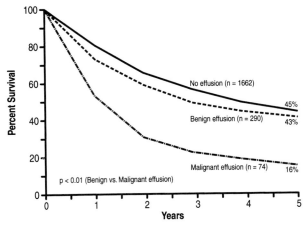

FIGURE 20–3. Survival rates for M0 patients after resection of lung cancer, with pleural effusion determined to be either benign or malignant by cytologic examination. $P < 0.01$ for no effusion versus malignant effusion; $P = NS$ for no effusion versus benign effusion. (From Naruke T, Tsuchiya R, Kondo H, et al. Implications of staging in lung cancer. Chest. 1997;112[suppl]:242S–248S.)[53]

The fact that malignant cells can be identified in the pleural space in a substantial number of early stage patients with lung cancer suggests that the traditional assumption that all patients with an MPE have a poor prognosis may be too simplistic. Numerous studies have consistently found that in approximately 11% of patients (range, 9%–14%) undergoing a resection for lung cancer, a pleural lavage (performed immediately after opening the chest) will demonstrate malignant cells.[56–60] Only one study found a markedly different rate of positive pleural lavage cytology (39%), the reason for which is unclear.[61] The incidence of a positive lavage has consistently been found to be significantly higher in patients with higher T stage tumors (average, 6% versus 19% for T1 versus T2)[57,59] and with tumors that penetrate to or through the pleura (average, 7% for tumors without pleural invasion versus 21% for tumors with pleural invasion).[56–60] Because nodal stage has generally been found not to correlate with the incidence of a malignant lavage,[56–60] the trend to a higher incidence in patients with higher stage tumors[56–58,60,61] appears to be due primarily to the influence of the T stage. It is also likely that the trend toward a higher incidence of a malignant pleural lavage in patients with an adenocarcinoma compared with squamous cell cancers (average, 17% versus 7%)[56–61] may be the result of a more frequent peripheral location of adenocarcinomas. Nevertheless, the mechanism of spread of malignant cells into the pleural space is unclear because 5% to 10% of patients with tumors not invading the pleura will have a malignant pleural lavage. No association has been found with patients who have previously undergone a transthoracic needle aspiration of the tumor.[56,57,62]

The presence of a positive pleural lavage clearly results in a poorer prognosis, with all of the studies examining this demonstrating a consistent trend, which was statistically significant in half.[56–61] The average 3-year survival was 26% (range, 0%–41%) in patients with a malignant lavage compared with 63% (range, 55%–69%) in those with a negative lavage.[57–60] Even when corrected for stage, a malignant lavage was found to be associated with poorer survival[60] and a higher recurrence rate.[57] Furthermore, a multivariate analysis has found malignant lavage to be an independent prognostic factor.[61] Nevertheless, only a minority of resected patients (average, 22%) with a malignant pleural lavage have been found to develop a pleural or pericardial recurrence.[57,58] These results suggest that malignant pleural cytology may involve a spectrum of disease and may not necessarily preclude resection or long-term survival.

A limited number of studies have reported results in patients with an MPE who were treated with curative intent involving a variety of modalities, including surgery. Naruke et al[53] reported on 74 patients with an MPE (presumably found at thoracotomy) in whom a 5-year survival of 16% was achieved after pulmonary resection. Another study of 13 patients who were found at thoracotomy to have a malignant effusion reported an absolute 5-year survival of 31% after resection and intrapleural interleukin-2 treatment.[63] No patients experienced a pleural recurrence.[63] A prospective series of 12 patients with T4N0,1 disease due to an MPE treated with preoperative chemotherapy followed by extrapleural pneumonectomy and RT reported no treatment-related mortality and encouraging intermediate-term survival.[64] The Roswell-Park Institute reported 10 cancer patients with NSCLC and proven MPE who were treated with pleuropneumonectomy and either preoperative (6 patients) or postoperative (4 patients) chemotherapy.[65] Median survival time (including one operative death) was 24 months for chemotherapy followed by surgery and 20 months for primary surgery. Although all patients except 1 have died, survival has extended for up to 57 and 59 months.[65] In a series of 23 patients with malignant pleural involvement who underwent resection and intrapleural mitomycin C, the median survival was 18 months, but all patients died within 4 years (74% had N2 disease).[66] Surgeons in Shanghai, China, treated 32 patients with pleuropneumonectomy and adjuvant intrapleural CCNU chemotherapy.[67] Operative mortality was only 6%, but it appears that survival was relatively poor, with 65% of patients dying within 1 year and only one patient alive after 3 years. Finally, in 38 patients who were found at thoracotomy to have pleural tumor implants without an effusion, a 5-year survival of 19% was observed after resection of the primary tumor and the pleural disease.[68] In fact, the actuarial 5-year survival was 58% in the 11 patients with T4N0 tumors (Fig. 20–4).[68]

These studies cover a variety of treatments and involve patients with malignant pleural involvement with a wide variation in the extent of the primary tumor, nodal involvement, and pleural involvement. In a number of these reports, the majority of patients had N2,3 involvement.[63,65,66,68] The reported survival figures are also widely divergent.

Malignant pleural involvement from lung cancer does not necessarily preclude long-term survival. A better definition of the extent of disease is necessary in order to investigate which patients may benefit from a curative treatment approach.

EDITORS' COMMENTS

Involvement of N3 nodes from NSCLC has been and continues to be a nonsurgical disease. It is important to

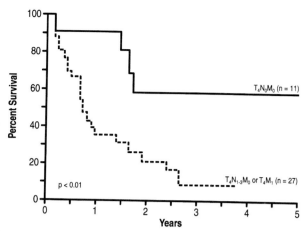

FIGURE 20–4. Survival of 38 patients undergoing resection of lung cancer with pleural dissemination, according to nodal status. (From Shimizu J, Oda M, Morita K, et al. Comparison of pleuropneumonectomy and limited surgery for lung cancer with pleural dissemination. J Surg Oncol. Copyright © 1996, John Wiley & Sons, Inc. Reprinted by permission of Wiley-Liss, Inc., a subsidiary of John Wiley & Sons, Inc.)[68]

maintain an open mind, however, because more effective chemotherapy and radiation may change the oncologic issues and make a local therapy such as surgical resection worthwhile (though it is often incomplete). Currently, however, the data supporting primary surgery for this stage of disease is anecdotal, and the data for resection of N3 disease as part of a multimodality approach is limited and unclear regarding whether the inclusion of surgery is beneficial. Surgery for N3 disease should be considered only as part of a multimodality protocol to explore these issues further.

Resection of NSCLC involving the carina offers a reasonable chance of long-term survival but at the expense of a relatively high operative mortality. Therefore, such patients should generally be referred to a center that has had more than anecdotal experience with such operations. Experience in the technical issues involved in the operation as well as in selection of appropriate patients is undoubtedly important in achieving results that justify employing such an approach. The implications of nodal involvement are not entirely clear, but there is little doubt that it makes the prognosis worse. It is possible that in some instances, involvement of lymph nodes directly adjacent to the primary tumor (perhaps by direct extension) may carry a better prognosis than N2 or N3 involvement from primary lung cancers in other locations. However, given the relatively poor results of carinal resection for lung cancer, one must be extremely cautious about extending the indications to anyone but the best risk patients.

Involvement of other mediastinal T4 structures results in worse survival following surgical treatment than carinal resection. It may be technically feasible to perform such operations, but one must question whether the biologic behavior of these tumors warrants a primarily surgical approach. Although occasionally patients may benefit, such an approach should also be limited only to those patients with the best prognosis.

There is much excitement about the use of induction therapy before surgical resection for patients with IIIa,b

NSCLC. Limited, preliminary data suggests that this approach may prove to be promising, particularly in patients with T4N0,1 disease. However, induction therapy probably reduces the margin for error in the technicalities of performing such resections. This makes meticulous technique and experience all the more important, and physicians should embark on such an approach for T4 NSCLC patients only after careful consideration and with a prospectively planned approach. Ideally, such treatment should be done only in the context of a protocol, but the limited number of patients who present with resectable T4 disease makes this difficult.

An MPE in patients with NSCLC is seen most often in the context of advanced disease, either because of extensive mediastinal tumor invasion or the presence of distant metastases. In such cases, the goal of treatment should be palliative. However, in patients with otherwise limited NSCLC who have a pleural effusion, it is important to consider the possibility that the effusion may be benign. Furthermore, those patients with otherwise early stage disease who are found at thoracotomy to have a small MPE or to have pleural implants may benefit from a curative approach involving surgical resection. The data supporting this is extremely limited, and there are no clear guidelines for patient selection for such an approach. Patients with significant nodal involvement are not likely to benefit, and it is intuitively appealing that the extent of pleural involvement also be important. The data that pleural lavage is positive in a number of patients with early stage tumors not involving the pleura indicates that our current understanding of the implications of an MPE is crude. A system to define the extent of pleural involvement may help promote a better understanding that will lead to appropriate selection of certain of these patients for a curative approach.

References

1. Naruke T. Significance of lymph node metastases in lung cancer. Semin Thorac Cardiovasc Surg. 1993;5:210–218.
2. Naruke T, Goya T, Tsuchiya R, et al. Extended radical operation for N2 left lung cancer through median sternotomy [abstract]. Lung Cancer. 1989;4:A89.
3. Hata E, Hayakawa K, Miyamito H, et al. Incidence and prognosis of the contralateral mediastinal node involvement of the left lung cancer patients who underwent bilateral mediastinal dissection and pulmonary resection through a median sternotomy [abstract]. Lung Cancer. 1988;4(suppl):A87.
4. Nakahara K, Fujii Y, Matsumura A, et al. Role of systematic mediastinal dissection in N2 non–small cell lung cancer patients. Ann Thorac Surg. 1993;56:331–336.
5. Watanabe Y, Ichihashi T, Iwa T. Median sternotomy as an approach to pulmonary surgery. Thorac Cardiovasc Surg. 1988;36:227–231.
6. Albain KS, Rusch VW, Crowley JJ, et al. Concurrent cisplatin/etoposide plus chest radiotherapy followed by surgery for stages IIIA(N2) and IIIB non–small-cell lung cancer: mature results of Southwest Oncology Group Phase II Study 8805. J Clin Oncol. 1995;13:1880–1892.
7. Stamatis G, Eberhardt W, Stüben G, et al. Preoperative chemoradiotherapy and surgery for selected non–small cell lung cancer IIIb subgroups: long-term results. Ann Thorac Surg. 1999;68:1144–1149.
8. Palazzi M, Cataldo I, Gramaglia A, et al. Preoperative concomitant cisplatin/VP16 and radiotherapy in stage III non–small cell lung cancer. Int J Radiat Oncol Biol Phys. 1993;27:621–625.
9. Aristu J, Rebollo J, Martínez-Monge R, et al. Cisplatin, mitomycin, and vindesine followed by intraoperative and postoperative radiother-apy for stage III non–small cell lung cancer: final results of a phase II study. Am J Clin Oncol. 1997;20:276–281.
10. Rendina EA, Venuta F, De Giacomo T, et al. Induction chemotherapy for T4 centrally located non–small cell lung cancer. J Thorac Cardiovasc Surg. 1999;117:225–233.
11. Thomas M, Rübe C, Semik M, et al. Impact of preoperative bimodality induction including twice-daily radiation on tumor regression and survival in stage III non–small cell lung cancer. J Clin Oncol. 1999;17:1185–1193.
12. Takita H, Blumenson LE, Raghavan D. Neoadjuvant chemotherapy of stage III-A and B lung carcinoma using the PACCO regimen. J Surg Oncol. 1995;59:147–150.
13. Grunenwald D, Le Chevalier T, Arriagada R, et al. Results of surgical resection in stage IIIB non–small cell lung cancer (NSCLC) after concomitant induction chemoradiotherapy [abstract]. Lung Cancer. 1997;18:73.
14. Eberhardt W, Wilke H, Stamatis G, et al. Preoperative chemotherapy followed by concurrent chemoradiation therapy based on hyperfractionated accelerated radiotherapy and definitive surgery in locally advanced non–small-cell lung cancer: mature results of a phase II trial. J Clin Oncol. 1998;16:622–634.
15. Rusch VW, Albain KS, Crowley JJ, et al. Surgical resection of stage IIIA and stage IIIB non–small-cell lung cancer after concurrent induction chemoradiotherapy: a Southwest Oncology Group trial. J Thorac Cardiovasc Surg. 1993;105:97–106.
16. Rusch VW, Albain KS, Crowley JJ, et al. Neoadjuvant therapy: a novel and effective treatment for stage IIIb non–small cell lung cancer. Ann Thorac Surg. 1994;58:290–295.
17. Dartevelle PG. Extended operations for the treatment of lung cancer. Ann Thorac Surg. 1997;63:12–19.
18. Mathisen DJ, Grillo HC. Carinal resection for bronchogenic cancer. J Thorac Cardiovasc Surg. 1991;102:16–23.
19. Dartevelle PG, Khalife J, Chapelier A, et al. Tracheal sleeve pneumonectomy for bronchogenic carcinoma: report of 55 cases. Ann Thorac Surg. 1988;46:68–72.
20. Deslauriers J, Beaulieu M, McClish A. Tracheal sleeve pneumonectomy. In: TW S, ed. General Thoracic Surgery. 3rd ed. Philadelphia, Pa: Lea & Febiger; 1989:382–387.
21. Roviaro GC, Varoli F, Rebuffat C. Tracheal sleeve pneumonectomy for bronchogenic carcinoma. J Thorac Cardiovasc Surg. 1994;107:13–18.
22. Tsuchiya R, Goya T, Naruke T, et al. Resection of tracheal carina for lung cancer. J Thorac Cardiovasc Surg. 1990;99:779–787.
23. Jensik RJ, Faber LP, Kittle CF, et al. Survival in patients undergoing tracheal sleeve pneumonectomy for bronchogenic carcinoma. J Thorac Cardiovasc Surg. 1982;84:489–496.
24. Fowler WC, Langer CJ, Curran WJ Jr, et al. Postoperative complications after combined neoadjuvant treatment of lung cancer. Ann Thorac Surg. 1993;55:986–989.
25. Rusch VW, Benfield JR. Neoadjuvant therapy for lung cancer: a note of caution. Ann Thorac Surg. 1993;55:820–821.
26. Linberg E, Cowley R, Bloedorn F, et al. Bronchogenic carcinoma: further experience with preoperative irradiation. Ann Thorac Surg. 1965;1:371–379.
27. Warram J, for an NCI Collaborative Study. Preoperative irradiation of cancer of the lung: preliminary report of a therapeutic trial (a collaborative study). Cancer. 1969;23:419–429.
28. Langer CJ, Curran WJ Jr, Keller SM, et al. Report of phase II trial of concurrent chemoradiotherapy with radical thoracic irradiation (60 Gy), infusional fluorouracil, bolus cisplatin and etoposide for clinical stage IIIB and bulky IIIA non–small cell lung cancer. Int J Radiat Oncol Biol Phys. 1993;26:469–478.
29. Macchiarini P, Chapelier AR, Monnet I, et al. Extended operations after induction therapy for stage IIIb (T4) non–small cell lung cancer. Ann Thorac Surg. 1994;57:966–973.
30. Tsuchiya R, Asamura H, Kondo H, et al. Extended resection of the left atrium, great vessels, or both for lung cancer. Ann Thorac Surg. 1994;57:960–965.
31. Burt ME, Pomerantz AH, Bains MS, et al. Results of surgical treatment of Stage III lung cancer invading the mediastinum. Surg Clin North Am. 1987;67:987–1000.
32. DeMeester TR, Albertucci M, Dawson PJ, et al. Management of tumor adherent to the vertebral column. J Thorac Cardiovasc Surg. 1989;97:373–378.
33. Shirakusa T, Kimura M. Partial atrial resection in advanced lung

carcinoma with and without cardiopulmonary bypass. Thorax. 1991;46:484–487.

34. Sellman M, Henze A, Peterffy A. Extended intrathoracic resection for lung cancer: follow-up of 49 cases. Scand J Thorac Cardiovasc Surg. 1987;21:69–72.

35. Fukuse T, Wada H, Hitomi S. Extended operation for non–small cell lung cancer invading great vessels and left atrium. Eur J Cardiothorac Surg. 1997;11:664–669.

36. Thomas P, Magnan PE, Moulin G, et al. Extended operation for lung cancer invading the superior vena cava. Eur J Cardiothorac Surg. 1994;8:177–182.

37. Spaggiari L, Regnard J-F, Magdeleinat P, et al. Extended resections for bronchogenic carcinoma invading the superior vena cava system. Ann Thorac Surg. 2000;69:233–236.

38. Nakahara K, Ohno K, Mastumura A, et al. Extended operation for lung cancer invading the aortic arch and superior vena cava. J Thorac Cardiovasc Surg. 1989;97:428–433.

39. Inoue H, Shohtsu A, Koide S, et al. Resection of the superior vena cava for primary lung cancer: 5 years' survival. Ann Thorac Surg. 1990;50:661–662.

40. Dartevelle PG, Chapelier AR, Pastorino U, et al. Long-term follow-up after prosthetic replacement of the superior vena cava combined with resection of mediastinal-pulmonary malignant tumors. J Thorac Cardiovasc Surg. 1991;102:259–265.

41. Larsson S, Lepore V. Technical options in reconstruction of large mediastinal veins. Surgery. 1992;111:311–317.

42. Levett J, Darakjian HE, DeMeester TR, et al. Bronchogenic carcinoma located in the aortic window: the importance of the primary lesion as a determinant of survival. J Thorac Cardiovasc Surg. 1982;83:551–562.

43. Klepetko W, Wisser W, Bîrsan T, et al. T4 lung tumors with infiltration of the thoracic aorta: is an operation reasonable? Ann Thorac Surg. 1999;67:340–344.

44. Albain KS, Crowley JJ, Turrisi AT III, et al. Concurrent cisplatin/etoposide plus radiotherapy (PE+RT) for pathologic stage (pathTN) IIIB non–small cell lung cancer (NSCLC): a Southwest Oncology Group (SWOG) phase II study (S9019) [abstract]. Proc ASCO. 1997;16:446a.

45. Mountain CF. A new international staging system for lung cancer. Chest. 1986;89(suppl):225S–233S.

46. Mountain CF. Prognostic implications of the international staging system for lung cancer. Semin Oncol. 1988;15:236–245.

47. Nakahashi H, Yasumoto K, Ishida T, et al. Results of surgical treatment of patients with T3 non–small cell lung cancer. Ann Thorac Surg. 1988;46:178–181.

48. Martini N, McCormack P. Therapy of stage III non-metastatic disease. Semin Surg Oncol. 1993;10:95–110.

49. Cantó A, Ferrer G, Romagosa V, et al. Lung cancer and pleural effusion: clinical significance and study of pleural metastatic locations. Chest. 1985;87:649–652.

50. Martini N, Flehinger BJ, Zaman MB, et al. Prospective study of 445 lung carcinomas with mediastinal lymph node metastases. J Thorac Cardiovasc Surg. 1980;80:390–399.

51. Parker EF. In discussion of Martini et al. Prospective study of 445 lung carcinomas with mediastinal lymph node metastases. J Thorac Cardiovasc Surg. 1980;80:390–399.

52. Naito T, Satoh H, Ishikawa H, et al. Pleural effusion as a significant prognostic factor in non–small cell lung cancer. Anticancer Res. 1997;17:4743–4746.

53. Naruke T, Tsuchiya R, Kondo H, et al. Implications of staging in lung cancer. Chest. 1997;112(suppl):242S–248S.

54. Storey BD, Dines DE, Coles DT. Pleural effusion: a diagnostic dilemma. JAMA. 1976;236:2183–2186.

55. Decker DA, Dines DE, Payne WS, et al. The significance of a cytologically negative pleural effusion in bronchogenic carcinoma. Chest. 1978;74:640–642.

56. Eagen RT, Bernatz PE, Payne WS, et al. Pleural lavage after pulmonary resection for bronchogenic carcinoma. J Thorac Cardiovasc Surg. 1984;88:1000–1003.

57. Okumura M, Ohshima S, Kotake Y, et al. Intraoperative pleural lavage cytology in lung cancer patients. Ann Thorac Surg. 1991;51:599–604.

58. Kondo H, Asamura H, Suemasu K, et al. Prognostic significance of pleural lavage cytology immediately after thoracotomy in patients with lung cancer. J Thorac Cardiovasc Surg. 1993;106:1092–1097.

59. Hillerdal G, Dernevik L, Almgren S-O, et al. Prognostic value of malignant cells in pleural lavage at thoracotomy for bronchial carcinoma. Lung Cancer. 1998;21:47–52.

60. Dresler CM, Fratelli C, Babb J. Prognostic value of positive pleural lavage in patients with lung cancer resection. Ann Thorac Surg. 1999;67:1435–1439.

61. Buhr J, Berghäuser KH, Gonner S, et al. The prognostic significance of tumor cell detection in intraoperative pleural lavage and lung tissue cultures for patients with lung cancer. J Thorac Cardiovasc Surg. 1997;113:683–690.

62. Kjellberg SI, Dresler CM, Goldberg M. Pleural cytologies in lung cancer without pleural effusions. Ann Thorac Surg. 1997;64:941–944.

63. Yasumoto K, Nagashima A, Nakahashi H, et al. Effect of postoperative intrapleural instillations of interleukin-2 in patients with malignant pleurisy due to lung cancer. Biotherapy. 1993;6:133–138.

64. Swanson SJ, Jaklitsch MT, Mentzer SJ, et al. Induction chemotherapy, surgical resection and radiotherapy in patients with malignant pleural effusion, mediastinoscopy negative (stage IIIB) non–small cell lung cancer [abstract]. Proc Am Assn Thorac Surg 1998; p 146.

65. Reyes L, Parvez Z, Regal A-M, et al. Neoadjuvant chemotherapy and operations in the treatment of lung cancer with pleural effusion [letter]. J Thorac Cardiovasc Surg. 1991;101:946–947.

66. Akaogi E, Mitsui K, Onizuka M, et al. Pleural dissemination in non–small cell lung cancer: results of radiological evaluation and surgical treatment. J Surg Oncol. 1994;57:33–39.

67. Wu SF, Huang OL, Wu HS, et al. Critical evaluation of results of extension of indication for surgery for primary bronchogenic carcinoma. Semin Surg Oncol. 1985;1:23–37.

68. Shimizu J, Oda M, Morita K, et al. Comparison of pleuropneumonectomy and limited surgery for lung cancer with pleural dissemination. J Surg Oncol. 1996;61:1–6.

69. Vogt-Moykopf I, Meyer G, Naunheim K, et al. Bronchoplastic techniques for lung resection. In: Baue AE, Geha AS, Hammond GL, et al, eds. Glenn's Thoracic and Cardiovascular Surgery. 5th ed. East Norwalk, Conn: Appleton-Lange; 1991:403–417.

70. Maeda M, Nakamoto K, Tsubota N, et al. Operative approaches for left-sided carinoplasty. Ann Thorac Surg. 1993;56:441–446.

21

CHEMORADIOTHERAPY FOR STAGE IIIA,B NON–SMALL CELL LUNG CANCER

Thomas A. Hensing, Jan S. Halle, and Mark A. Socinski

PATIENT SELECTION

RESPONSE TO
CHEMORADIOTHERAPY

SEQUENTIAL
CHEMORADIOTHERAPY
  Survival Results
  Recurrence Patterns

CONCURRENT
CHEMORADIOTHERAPY
  Survival Results
  Recurrence Patterns

COMPARISON OF SEQUENTIAL
AND CONCURRENT
APPROACHES

TOXICITY

META-ANALYSIS

ROLE OF RADIOTHERAPY

ROLE OF COMBINED-
MODALITY THERAPY IN POOR-
RISK PATIENTS

CURRENT STRATEGIES

EDITORS' COMMENTS

Approximately 30% of patients with non–small cell lung cancer (NSCLC) present with stage III tumors,[1] which are often referred to as *locally advanced disease*. Without any treatment, approximately 75% of these patients will die of the local disease in the chest,[2] with a median survival of approximately 5 to 8 months (see Table 3–4). Treatment with local modalities alone (eg, surgery or radiation) has not had a major impact on survival, although the most common cause of death is not local disease but rather distant metastases (see Tables 17–4 and 17–5). Therefore, these patients represent a challenge in the management of both local and distant disease, and the strategy of combined modality treatment with chemotherapy as well as with a local modality is an attractive concept.

This chapter focuses on the treatment of stage IIIa,b NSCLC patients with a combination of chemotherapy and radiotherapy (RT). Traditionally, patients with preoperatively diagnosed T3,4 or N2,3 tumors have not been treated with surgery. Combined modality treatment including surgical resection is being explored, but this is discussed in Chapter 19 and is not included here. This chapter focuses primarily on data from large (≥100 patients) randomized phase III trials because these trials provide the most accurate data to evaluate the role of chemoradiotherapy in this patient population.

In nonsurgical studies of stage III NSCLC, the stage has been determined radiographically. It is important to remember in this context that the radiographic determination of T3,4 status is difficult at best (see Table 5–3). Furthermore, enlargement of discrete mediastinal lymph nodes (N2,3) has consistently been demonstrated to have approximately a 40% false positive (FP) rate. However,

radiographic evidence of diffuse mediastinal tumor infiltration, which obliterates recognition of discrete lymph nodes and surrounds the major vessels, probably carries a low FP rate, although this has not been studied. The presence of distant metastases is also an issue in patients who are initially thought to have stage IIIa,b disease. There is evidence that approximately 30% of these patients will have detectable systemic disease, even if a history and clinical examination do not disclose signs or symptoms of distant metastases (see Table 6–3). Although these issues must be kept in mind, the randomization process should, at least theoretically, provide equal distribution between treatment arms of such potentially understaged and overstaged patients.

Combined chemotherapy and RT can be given either concurrently or in a sequential manner, usually involving chemotherapy first. There are both theoretical and practical differences between sequential and concurrent sequencing strategies (see Chapter 10). Theoretically, sequential treatment should avoid overlapping toxicities but would prolong the overall treatment time and delay the initiation of radiation. Studies using laboratory models have raised several concerns about the sequential approach, including stimulation of tumor cell repopulation during RT, increasing the probability of cross-resistant tumor cells, and stimulation of distant metastases (see Chapters 9 and 10).[3] These concerns are generally believed to be less of an issue with concurrent scheduling.[3] In addition, the overall treatment time is shorter and the potential for direct interaction between the modalities is increased with concurrent treatment.[3] However, synergistic enhancement of the two modalities may occur in the tumor as well as in the surrounding normal tissues, increasing the likelihood of toxicity and limiting any potential therapeutic gain.

PATIENT SELECTION

Patient selection is an important variable to consider when comparing clinical trials, especially when trying to generalize outcomes to specific patient populations. Despite the revised staging system, stage IIIa,b NSCLC remains a heterogeneous disease. There has been some debate as to whether the substage (IIIa or IIIb) has prognostic implications for patients who are treated nonsurgically. For patients treated with RT alone, the preponderance of data indicates significantly better survival for those with IIIa disease compared with IIIb disease (2-year survival, 27% versus 12%) (see Table 18–3), although one study did not identify a difference.[4] In patients treated with chemotherapy and RT, investigators have identified a significant association between substage and survival.[5–8] These results suggest that it is important to consider the distribution of stage IIIa versus IIIb patients when reviewing treatment outcomes. Performance status (PS) and weight loss have been reported to be associated with response to therapy and survival in patients who have unresectable IIIa,b NSCLC.[5, 7–10] The prognostic value has been more variable for other factors, including age and gender,[5, 8, 10, 11] as well as for selected laboratory parameters (white blood cell count, neutrophil count, and serum calcium level).[8, 10, 11]

The eligibility requirements of the major randomized trials of chemoradiotherapy have been variable. Only six trials required computed tomography (CT) of the chest before enrollment,[5, 12–16] but a chest radiograph and a chest CT scan were probably obtained in most instances in the majority of these trials. Other staging tests, including imaging of the brain, liver, and bones, were required in some of the protocols and were left to the discretion of the investigator in others. A minimum PS was usually specified, but the level was variable. Two of the trials excluded patients who had lost weight,[12, 13] whereas weight loss was not an exclusion criterion in the other protocols.

Table 21–1 lists patient characteristics with respect to prognostic factors in prospective phase III trials involving chemoradiotherapy for stage III NSCLC. The majority of the patients were male (average, 79%), with an average median age of 60 years. Most patients had clinical stage IIIa,b disease, and only a minority of clinical stage I and II patients were included in most trials. Only three trials—reported by Schaake-Koning et al,[15] Johnson et al,[17] and Mattson et al,[18]—involved a relatively high proportion of patients (20%–30%) with cI,II disease. Most patients had minimal symptoms despite radiographic evidence of extensive locally advanced disease. The majority of the patients had a Zubrod PS of 0,1 or a Karnofsky PS of 80–100, with an average of only 13% of patients experiencing weight loss of >10% before enrollment in a trial. Two trials—reported by Jeremic et al,[5] and Mattson et al,[18]—involved a relatively high percentage of patients (>30%) with a poor PS (≥2 or ≤70), whereas three trials—reported by Dillman et al,[12] Sause et al,[13] and Schaake-Koning et al,[15]—involved only highly selected patients.

In general, the characteristics of the patients included in the larger phase III trials of chemoradiotherapy are fairly similar to the characteristics of the general population of patients with locally advanced lung cancer. As discussed

TABLE 21–1. PATIENT CHARACTERISTICS IN PROSPECTIVE PHASE III TRIALS OF CHEMORADIOTHERAPY IN NON–SMALL CELL LUNG CANCER

STUDY	N	MEDIAN AGE (y)	STAGE (%)			% WITH GOOD PS[a]	% WITH WEIGHT LOSS ≥10%
			I/II	IIIa	IIIb		
Sequential (Non–Cisplatin-Based)							
Johnson et al[17]	311	61	28	————72————		79	3
Morton et al[49]	114	63	5	61	34	89	13
Trovo et al[50]	111	62	0	————100————		(79)[b]	21
Sequential (Cisplatin-Based)							
Dillman et al[12]	180	60	7	63	30	100	0
Le Chevalier et al[22]	353	58–59	10	————90————		80	—
Sause et al[13]	452	—	6	45	49	(100)[b]	0
Mattson et al[18]	252	62	19	————65————		69	—
Miller et al[25]	229	61	1	————99————		89	—
Concurrent (Cisplatin-Based)							
Blanke et al[14]	215	60–63	9	50	41	80	—
Jeremic et al[30]	169	59–62	0	50	50	80	(63)[c]
Jeremic et al[5]	131	59	0	47	53	49	(62)[c]
Schaake-Koning et al[15]	331	60	20[d]	————77————		94	(40)[e]
Trovo et al[16]	173	61–62	0	————100————		50	14

Inclusion criteria: Prospective phase III trials of chemotherapy and radiation versus radiation alone in ≥100 patients.
[a]Good performance status = Zubrod 0,1 or Karnofsky 80–100.
[b]PS ≥70.
[c]>5%.
[d]N0,1.
[e]Any weight loss.
PS, performance status; Weight loss, recent loss of ≥10% or ≥10 lb of body weight.

TABLE 21–2. RESPONSE TO CHEMOTHERAPY AND RADIATION COMPARED WITH RADIATION ALONE IN PROSPECTIVE PHASE III TRIALS

STUDY	N	CHEMOTHERAPY	RT (Gy) (BOTH ARMS)	CR + PR (%)		CR (%)		
				RT	Ch/RT	RT	Ch/RT	P
Sequential (Non–Cisplatin-Based)								
Johnson et al[17]	206	Vd	60	30	34	5	2	NS
Morton et al[49]	114	*MACC*	60	41	34	17	14	NS
Trovo et al[50]	111	CAMxPz	45	56	39	10	6	NS
White et al[51a]	54	L	30s	39	38	18	19	NS
White et al[51a]	54	A	30s	39	35	18	12	NS
White et al[51a]	51	LA	30s	39	18	18	7	NS
Average				**41**	**33**	**14**	**10**	
Sequential (Cisplatin-Based)								
Sause et al[13]	454	VbP	63	—	63	—	36	—
Le Chevalier et al[22]	353	VdCPU	65	35	31	20	16	—
Mattson et al[18]	252	CAP	55s	44	49	11	15	NS
Miller et al[25]	229	FVMCAP	58	39	38	13	8	NS
Dillman et al[12]	155	VbP	60	35	46	16	19	NS
Average				**38**	**45**	**15**	**19**	
Concurrent (Cisplatin-Based)								
Blanke et al[14]	215	P every 3 weeks	60–65	38	50	—	—	NS
Schaake-Koning et al[15b]	210	P daily	55	54	63	17	21	—
Schaake-Koning et al[15b]	206	P weekly	55	54	54	17	16	—
Trovo et al[16]	146	P daily	45	59	51	7	7	NS
Jeremic et al[5]	135	CbE daily	69.6 HF	84	92	45	60	NS
Jeremic et al[30c]	117	CbE every 2 weeks	64.8 HF	63	62	25	30	NS
Jeremic et al[30c]	113	CbE weekly	64.8 HF	63	74	25	37	NS
Average				**59**	**64**	**23**	**29**	

Inclusion criteria: Prospective phase III trials of chemotherapy and radiation versus radiation alone in ≥100 patients from 1980 to 2000.
[a]4-arm trial, 107 patients randomized.
[b]3-arm trial, 308 total patients evaluable, 245 total patients evaluable for response.
[c]3-arm trial, 169 total patients evaluable.
Ch, chemotherapy; CR, complete response rate; HF, hyperfractionated; PR, partial response rate; RT, radiotherapy, dose in Gy; s, split-course RT.
Chemotherapy regimens: A, doxorubicin; CAMxPz, cyclophosphamide, doxorubicin, methotrexate, procarbazine; CAP, cyclophosphamide, doxorubicin, cisplatin; CbE, carboplatin, etoposide; FVMCAP, 5-fluorouracil, vincristine, mitomycin C, cyclophosphamide, doxorubicin, cisplatin; L, levamisole; LA, levamisole, doxorubicin; *MACC*, methotrexate, doxorubicin, cyclophosphamide, CCNU; P, cisplatin; VbP, vinblastine, cisplatin; Vd, vindesine; VdCPU, vindesine, cyclophosphamide, cisplatin, CCNU.

in Table 4–2, approximately 80% of patients with limited stage disease and 60% of patients with extensive stage disease in population-based studies had a good PS (0-1 or 80-100). There appears to be a slightly higher proportion of patients with weight loss in the general population of patients with lung cancer (both small cell lung cancer [SCLC] and NSCLC; see Chapter 4). Weight loss is perhaps a more objective parameter than PS, but it may be of lesser prognostic importance.[9,10]

RESPONSE TO CHEMORADIOTHERAPY

Fifteen randomized trials have been conducted comparing chemoradiotherapy with RT alone in ≥100 patients with stage IIIa,b NSCLC. Three of the studies included more than two arms, with the result that 19 pairs of randomized cohorts are available. These trials are divided into those involving sequential non–cisplatin-based chemotherapy, sequential cisplatin-based chemotherapy, and concurrent cisplatin-based chemotherapy regimens. The objective radiographic response rates, using standard definitions (CR, complete response or complete disappearance of all evi-

dence of tumor; PR, partial response or ≥50% reduction in tumor dimensions), are shown in Table 21–2. There were no significant differences in the objective response rates for the chemoradiotherapy arms compared with the RT-alone arms in any of these comparisons.

A slight trend toward better response rates was seen in the patients treated with cisplatin-based chemotherapy compared with RT alone, but this was not statistically significant. A trend toward better response rates with more aggressive treatment is seen when the three groups of trials are compared, perhaps reflecting more aggressive RT. Overall, cisplatin-based chemoradiotherapy resulted in an objective response rate of approximately 50% and a CR rate of approximately 25%. The rate of disease progression during treatment was lower in concurrent chemoradiotherapy trials compared with sequential cisplatin-based trials (5% versus 23%). It is impossible to know whether this is simply a result of earlier assessment (due to a shorter duration of therapy) or reflects a benefit of the concurrent strategy.

Interpretation of radiographic response rates in the setting of chemoradiotherapy for locally advanced disease is difficult, however. RT itself may cause edema or fibrosis, which can be confused with tumor (see Chapter 9). Further-

TABLE 21–3. SURVIVAL OUTCOMES IN RANDOMIZED TRIALS OF SEQUENTIAL CHEMOTHERAPY AND RADIATION (NON-CISPLATIN REGIMENS) IN NON–SMALL CELL LUNG CANCER

STUDY	N	CHEMOTHERAPY	RT (Gy) (BOTH ARMS)	MST (mo)		2-y SURVIVAL (%)		5-y SURVIVAL (%)		P
				RT	Ch/RT	RT	Ch/RT	RT	Ch/RT	
Johnson et al[17]	206	Vd	60	9	9	12	13	1	3	NS
Morton et al[49]	114	MACC	60	10	10	16	21	7	5	NS
Trovo et al[50]	111	CAMxPz	45	12	10	18	16	—	—	NS
White et al[51a]	54	L	30s	13	10	—	—	—	—	NS
White et al[51a]	54	A	30s	13	11	—	—	—	—	NS
White et al[51a]	51	LA	30s	13	6	—	—	—	—	NS
Average				**12**	**9**	**15**	**17**	**4**	**4**	

Inclusion criteria: Prospective phase III trials of chemotherapy (non-cisplatin) and radiation versus radiation alone in ≥100 patients (total) from 1980 to 2000.
[a]4-arm trial, 107 patients evaluable.
Ch, chemotherapy; MST, median survival time; RT, radiotherapy; s, split course RT.
Chemotherapy regimens: A, doxorubicin; CAMxPz, cyclophosphamide, doxorubicin, methotrexate, procarbazine; L, levamisole; LA, levamisole, doxorubicin; MACC, methotrexate, doxorubicin, cyclophosphamide, CCNU; Vd, vindesine.

more, radiographic response rates correlate poorly with pathologic response, as demonstrated in studies involving resection following chemoradiotherapy (see Chapter 19). Finally, radiographic response rates correlate poorly with patient survival, as discussed later in the chapter.[19]

SEQUENTIAL CHEMORADIOTHERAPY

Survival Results

Only one trial has been reported comparing sequential chemotherapy and RT with best supportive care in patients with IIIa,b NSCLC.[20] The treatment arm consisted of three cycles of cisplatin and etoposide and sequential RT (40 Gy), whereas the patients on the control arm were treated with supportive care only. Survival was significantly better on the treatment arm (median survival, 12 versus 9 months; P = 0.05).[20] This is consistent with the experience in randomized trials of supportive care plus chemotherapy

versus supportive care alone in patients with stage IV disease (see Chapter 22) and supports the role of active therapy for this group of patients.

Tables 21–3 and 21–4 list the survival outcomes for patients in randomized trials of sequential chemotherapy and RT compared with RT alone. In Table 21–3, those trials that studied non-cisplatin chemotherapy regimens are considered. The average median survival (12 months) and 5-year survival (4%) for RT alone are consistent with what has been reported in other studies of RT alone (see Chapter 18). None of the trials showed any survival benefit from the addition of chemotherapy. In contrast, four of the six trials using cisplatin regimens (Table 21–4) reported improved survival outcomes with combined-modality therapy,[12,13,18,21,22] with three reaching statistical significance.[12,13,21]

The first trial to demonstrate an improvement in survival with the addition of chemotherapy to RT was reported by Dillman et al[12] and was conducted by the Cancer and Leukemia Group B (CALGB) (Fig. 21–1). In a more recent update, the survival benefit has been shown to persist over

TABLE 21–4. SURVIVAL OUTCOMES IN RANDOMIZED TRIALS OF SEQUENTIAL CHEMOTHERAPY AND RADIOTHERAPY (CISPLATIN REGIMENS) IN NON–SMALL CELL LUNG CANCER

STUDY	N	Ch	RT (Gy) (BOTH ARMS)	MST (mo)		2-y SURVIVAL (%)		5-y SURVIVAL (%)		P
				RT	Ch/RT	RT	Ch/RT	RT	Ch/RT	
Le Chevalier et al[22,21]	353	VdCPU	65	10	12	14	21	(4)[a]	(12)[a]	0.02
Brodin and Noo[26]	330	EP	56	9	9	—	—	—	—	(NS)[b]
Sause et al[24c]	303	VbP	69.6 HF	12	14	24	32	6	8	0.04
Sause et al[24,13c]	300	VbP	63	11	14	19	32	5	8	0.04
Mattson et al[18]	238	CAP	55	10	11	17	19	—	—	(NS)[d]
Miller et al[25]	229	FVMCAP	58	9	9	18	13	3	4	NS
Dillman et al[23,12]	155	VbP	60	10	14	13	26	6	17	0.01
Average				**10**	**12**	**18**	**24**	**5**	**9**	

Inclusion criteria: Prospective phase III trials of sequential chemotherapy (cisplatin-based) and radiation versus radiation alone in ≥100 patients from 1980 to 2000.
[a]3-year survival.
[b]Significant survival advantage (P < 0.05) if poor performance status patients (Zubrod 3) are excluded.
[c]3-arm trial, 452 total patients evaluable.
[d]P <0.05 when analysis restricted to stage III patients.
Ch, chemotherapy; HF, hyperfractionated; MST, median survival time; RT, radiotherapy.
Chemotherapy regimens: CAP, cyclophosphamide, doxorubicin, cisplatin (40 mg/m²); EP, etoposide, cisplatin; FVMCAP, 5-Fluorouracil, vincristine, mitomycin C, cyclophosphamide, doxorubicin, cisplatin; VbP, vinblastine, cisplatin; VdCPU, vindesine, cyclophosphamide, cisplatin, CCNU.

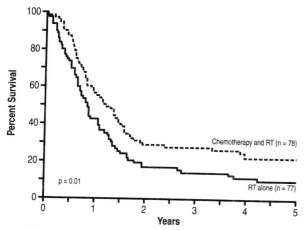

FIGURE 21–1. Survival of patients with stage III non–small cell lung cancer randomized to radiotherapy (RT) alone (60 Gy) versus chemotherapy (cisplatin and vinblastine ×2 cycles) and RT (60 Gy). (From Dillman, RO, Herndon J, Seagren SL, et al. Improved survival in stage III non–small-cell lung cancer: seven year follow-up of Cancer and Leukemia Group B (CALGB) 8433 trial. J Natl Cancer Inst. 1996; 88:1210–1215, by permission of Oxford University Press, Oxford, England.)[23]

7 years of follow-up.[23] The study population consisted of highly selected stage III patients with a PS of 0 to 1, <5% weight loss over the preceding 3 months, and no evidence of supraclavicular lymph node involvement. The patients were well matched with regard to prognostic variables.[6, 12] Two cycles of chemotherapy (cisplatin and vinblastine) before a course of conventional RT (60 Gy in 2-Gy fractions over 6 weeks) resulted in a 4-month improvement in median survival and nearly triple the survival rate at 5 years (17% versus 6%; P = 0.01). Part of the survival difference was attributed to an increased number of early deaths in the RT-alone arm, but the survival difference persisted in an analysis of only those patients who were alive on day 105.[12]

The argument for induction chemotherapy became more compelling when identical results were demonstrated in a confirmatory trial conducted jointly by the Radiation Therapy Oncology Group (RTOG) and the Eastern Cooperative Oncology Group (ECOG).[13] The chemoradiotherapy and conventional RT treatment was identical to that of the CALGB study, and the patients enrolled were also highly selected and well balanced among study arms with respect to prognostic factors. The median and 2-year survival results were almost identical to the CALGB results. The survival benefit has persisted, as reported in a more recent update of this study, although the 5-year survival of the chemoradiotherapy arm was not quite as high as that in the CALGB study (8% and 5%, P = 0.04).[24] This study also involved a third treatment arm consisting of hyperfractionated (HF) RT alone (HF-RT, 69.6 Gy in 1.2-Gy fractions given twice a day over 6 weeks). The survival of this arm was also found to be inferior to the chemoradiotherapy arm.[13] The patient selection criteria were less strict in a multicenter trial in France reported by Le Chevalier et al.[21, 22] Weight loss was not considered, and 20% of patients had a PS ≤70. The survival of patients in both the chemoradiotherapy and the RT-alone arms was slightly worse than that in the previous two trials, but a similar 2- to 3-fold improvement in long-term survival was observed.[21]

Although the consistency of the three trials just discussed is compelling, no statistically significant improvement in survival with combined modality therapy was seen in the remaining three studies.[18, 25, 26] Two of these studies reported a significant survival benefit when only selected patient groups were analyzed.[18, 26] Better survival was found in one trial when patients with a poor PS (≥3) were excluded[26] and in the other trial when only stage III patients were analyzed.[18] Although a secondary analysis using multivariate techniques is reasonable to correct for an imbalance of a known prognostic factor, exclusion of patients after randomization is questionable. In fact, in the trial by Mattson et al,[18] no imbalance of prognostic factors occurred, and multivariate analysis did not show an advantage to treatment with chemoradiotherapy. One of the other negative trials reported no imbalances between the arms,[25] while the other was reported only in abstract form.[26]

Two of the three negative trials used chemotherapy regimens involving cisplatin at a very low dose (40 mg/m²).[18, 25] Furthermore, compliance in at least one of these trials[18] was relatively poor, with only 31% of all randomized patients receiving six of the planned nine cycles of chemotherapy. These factors may have limited any benefit seen with the combined approach. More importantly, it must be noted that a total of 840 patients are needed to demonstrate an improvement in survival from a baseline of 5% to 10% (with an 80% power of detection and P < 0.05) in a randomized trial (see Table 2–1). Thus, the lack of a statistically significant benefit is not unexpected, given the size of the trials. One of the negative trials did suggest a slight trend toward better early survival,[18] and no data is available regarding trends in the others.[25, 26]

Recurrence Patterns

The mechanism for the improvement in survival seen with sequential cisplatin-based chemoradiotherapy appears to be related to a reduction in distant metastases.[22, 27, 28] Two of the three studies that analyzed recurrence patterns found that distant recurrences were significantly reduced by the addition of chemotherapy.[22, 28] In the RTOG/ECOG study,[28] the rate of failure at distant sites (excluding the brain) was significantly lower for the combined-modality arm than for both the conventional RT and HF-RT arms (24% versus 35% and 37%; P < 0.05). First failures within the brain occurred in 12% to 15% of the patients, without any difference related to the treatment strategies.[28] In the French multicenter trial,[22] the actuarial rate of distant metastasis was significantly lower on the combined modality arm (Fig. 21–2), although concern has been raised about the validity of statistical analysis of actuarial recurrence rates.[29] In the third study, a minimal, nonsignificant trend toward fewer distant metastases was seen.[18] The other trials in this group did not perform a detailed analysis of recurrence patterns.[12, 25, 26]

None of the trials of sequential cisplatin-based chemoradiotherapy demonstrated a significant difference in local control. The RTOG/ECOG study reported that the thorax was the first site of progression in 32%, 31%, and 29% of the patients treated with chemoradiotherapy, conventional RT, and HF-RT, respectively.[28] The French multicenter trial

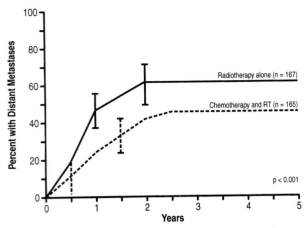

FIGURE 21–2. Rate of appearance of distant metastases in patients with stage III non–small cell lung cancer treated with radiotherapy (RT) alone (65 Gy) versus chemotherapy (cisplatin, vindesine, cyclophosphamide, and CCNU ×3 cycles) before and after RT (65 Gy). (From Le Chevalier T, Arriagada R, Quoix E, et al. Radiotherapy alone versus combined chemotherapy and radiotherapy in nonresectable non–small-cell lung cancer: First analysis of a randomized trial in 353 patients. J Natl Cancer Inst. 1991; 83:417–423, by permission of Oxford University Press, Oxford, England.)[22]

reported that local control at 1 year was 15% with chemoradiotherapy and 17% with RT alone.[22] This study used a rigorous assessment of local control, employing bronchoscopy and biopsy at regular intervals in addition to radiographic imaging, which probably explains the lower local control rate compared with other studies.

CONCURRENT CHEMORADIOTHERAPY

Survival Results

Five trials with ≥100 patients have compared the survival of patients receiving concurrent chemotherapy and radia-

tion with patients receiving definitive RT alone. Two of these trials were three-arm studies, so that there are seven patient cohorts to compare. Table 21–5 lists the survival data from these studies. When considered together, the average median survival for those patients treated with radiation only was 11 months (range, 8–14 months) compared with 14 months for those patients treated on combination arms (range, 10–22 months). In seven of the eight randomized comparisons, better survival with chemotherapy was observed, with the difference being statistically significant in three.

Results from this group of trials suggest that the frequency of delivery of chemotherapy during RT may be important. Of the three trials studying RT with *daily* low dose chemotherapy, two demonstrated a survival benefit, whereas only one of the remaining three trials using less frequent dosing (every 1 to 3 weeks) reported a survival benefit with the combined approach. The effect of the frequency of administration of chemotherapy was addressed directly in a three-arm study conducted by the European Organization for Research and Treatment of Cancer (EORTC).[15] The daily chemotherapy arm was associated with a significant survival benefit ($P = 0.009$), whereas only a nonsignificant trend toward improved survival was seen in the weekly chemoradiotherapy arm compared with RT alone. A benefit to more frequent chemotherapy is also suggested by comparing two different phase III trials conducted by the same investigators, using HF-RT with or without carboplatin and etoposide.[5, 30] The trial using daily chemotherapy during RT demonstrated a significant survival benefit.[5] In a separate study, a significant benefit was also seen in the weekly chemotherapy arm compared with HF-RT alone, but only a nonsignificant trend toward improved survival was observed in an arm using chemotherapy given every 2 weeks.[30] Finally, chemotherapy given every 3 weeks during RT resulted in only minimal improvement in survival in a study reported by Blanke et al.[14]

One randomized study of 146 patients did not demonstrate any benefit to concurrent chemoradiotherapy, even

TABLE 21–5. SURVIVAL OUTCOMES IN RANDOMIZED TRIALS OF CONCURRENT CHEMOTHERAPY AND RADIOTHERAPY (CISPLATIN REGIMENS) IN NON–SMALL CELL LUNG CANCER

STUDY	N	CHEMOTHERAPY	RT (Gy)	MST (mo) RT	MST (mo) Ch/RT	2-y SURVIVAL (%) RT	2-y SURVIVAL (%) Ch/RT	5-y SURVIVAL (%) RT	5-y SURVIVAL (%) Ch/RT	P
Schaake-Koning et al[15a]	210	P daily	55	12	12	13	26	2[b]	10[b]	0.009
Trovo et al[16]	146	P daily	45	10	10	14	14	—	—	NS
Jeremic et al[5]	135	CbE daily	69.6 HF	14	22	26	43	9[b]	23[b]	0.02
Schaake-Koning et al[15a]	206	P weekly	55	12	13	13	19	2[b]	10[b]	NS
Jeremic et al[30c]	113	CbE weekly	64.8 HF	8	18	25	35	5	21	0.003
Jeremic et al[30c]	117	CbE every 2 weeks	64.8 HF	8	13	25	27	5	16	NS
Blanke et al[14]	215	P every 3 weeks	60–65	10	11	13	18	2	5	NS
Average				**11**	**14**	**18**	**26**	**4**	**14**	

Inclusion criteria: Prospective phase III trials of concurrent chemotherapy (cisplatin based) and radiation versus radiation alone in ≥100 patients from 1980 to 2000.
[a]3-arm trial, 308 total evaluable patients.
[b]4-year survival.
[c]3-arm trial, 169 total evaluable patients.
Ch, chemotherapy; HF, hyperfractionated; MST, median survival time (months); RT, radiotherapy, dose in Gy.
Chemotherapy regimens: CbE, carboplatin, etoposide; P, cisplatin.

though it involved daily cisplatin.[16] The only obvious difference between this study and the others involving concurrent chemoradiotherapy was the use of a relatively low dose of RT (45 Gy).[16] It is conceivable that the dose was insufficient to control local disease in either arm, minimizing any potential benefit of combining both modalities. One additional study, not included in Table 21–5 because it involved only 95 patients, also used relatively low dose RT (50 Gy).[31] No significant difference was found in median survival, although a slight trend favoring the chemoradiotherapy arm (weekly cisplatin) was seen (median survival, 16 months versus 11 months; $P = $ NS).[31]

Recurrence Patterns

The major impact of concurrent chemoradiotherapy has been an improvement in local disease control. This was particularly true for those trials using more frequent chemotherapy dosing schedules. Both positive trials of concurrent daily chemotherapy and RT reported a significant improvement in local control.[5, 15] In contrast, only one of the two trials studying RT and weekly chemotherapy reported a trend toward improvement in this outcome,[30] and the remaining trials using less frequent dosing reported no significant difference.[14, 16] In the EORTC study, the time to local recurrence was significantly prolonged when both groups receiving chemotherapy were considered together ($P = 0.015$).[15] This effect was more pronounced in the daily chemotherapy arm compared with the RT-alone arm ($P = 0.003$) and was not statistically significant for the weekly chemotherapy arm ($P = 0.15$), as shown in Figure 21–3. Similarly, in the trial of daily chemotherapy and HF-RT reported by Jeremic et al,[5] the local recurrence-free survival was significantly improved in the chemoradiotherapy arm compared with HF-RT alone ($P = 0.015$).[5]

No improvements in the control of distant metastatic disease were reported in any of the concurrent trials, in contrast to the sequential chemoradiotherapy studies. With

the exception of the trial reported by Blanke et al,[14] which used cisplatin (70 mg/m²) every 3 weeks, the trials of concurrent chemoradiotherapy have used relatively low doses of chemotherapy that would be unlikely to have an impact on distant metastatic disease.

COMPARISON OF SEQUENTIAL AND CONCURRENT APPROACHES

Direct comparisons between sequential and concurrent treatment strategies have been limited. The RTOG has reviewed its phase II and III experience with various chemoradiotherapy schedules in patients with locally advanced NSCLC.[32] The different treatment strategies were divided into three groups: sequential chemotherapy with conventional RT (60 Gy in daily fractions of 2 Gy), combined sequential and concurrent chemotherapy with conventional RT, and concurrent chemotherapy with HF-RT. Significant differences were found in response rates between the first group (63%) and the latter two groups (77% and 79%; $P = 0.03$ and 0.003, respectively). A trend toward improved overall and progression-free survival was seen with concurrent chemotherapy, but the difference was not significant. However, no firm conclusions can be drawn from this analysis because the comparisons were made between studies rather than between randomized cohorts.[32]

One randomized comparison of sequential versus concurrent chemoradiotherapy has been reported.[33] The patients included on this study had stage III disease (23% IIIa, 77% IIIb) with good PS (PS 0-1 in 95% of patients) and minimal weight loss (<10% in 89% of patients). Patients were treated with two cycles of mitomycin C, vindesine, and cisplatin given every 4 weeks either sequentially or concurrently with split-course RT (56 Gy in daily fractions of 2 Gy). Another two cycles of chemotherapy following completion of RT were given to those patients achieving at least a partial response on either arm. The response rate in the concurrent arm was significantly higher (84% versus 66%, $P = 0.0002$), which translated into an improvement in median survival (17 months versus 13 months; $P = 0.04$) and 5-year survival (16% versus 9%) for this group of patients (Fig. 21–4). The treatment arms were well balanced with respect to all known prognostic factors.[33]

Although the concurrent chemotherapy was given every 4 weeks, a trend toward a lower rate of local progression with toward concurrent chemoradiotherapy was seen (33% versus 39%, $P = $ NS). This is somewhat surprising in light of the data in Table 21–6 that suggests that concurrent chemotherapy should be given frequently to be most effective. There was no difference in the overall rate of distant disease progression, although a higher incidence of brain metastasis as the first site of relapse (19% versus 9%; $P = 0.02$) and a lower incidence of supraclavicular lymph node metastasis (2% versus 7%; $P = 0.05$) were seen on the concurrent arm.

These results suggest that concurrent chemoradiotherapy may be better than a sequential approch. However, the two arms did differ in the amount of chemotherapy that was administered, with 59% of patients on the concurrent arm receiving three to four cycles of chemotherapy compared with 25% of patients on the sequential arm ($P = 0.0001$).

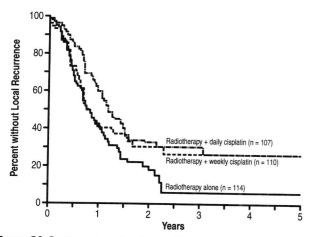

FIGURE 21–3. Percentage of patients with stage III non–small cell lung cancer without local recurrence, by treatment arm. (From Schaake-Koning C, van den Bogaert W, Dalasio O, et al. Effects of concomitant cisplatin and radiotherapy on inoperable non–small-cell lung cancer. N Engl J Med. 1992; 326:524–530. Copyright © 1992 Massachusetts Medical Society. All rights reserved.)[15]

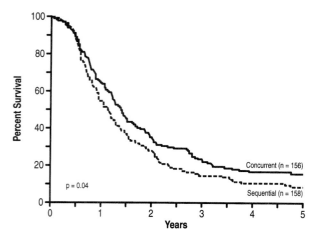

FIGURE 21–4. Survival of patients with stage III non–small cell lung cancer randomized to concurrent versus sequential chemoradiotherapy (mitomycin, cisplatin, vindesine, and 56 Gy). (From Furuse K, et al, for the West Japan Lung Cancer Group. Phase III study of concurrent versus sequential thoracic radiotherapy in combination with mitomycin, vindesine, and cisplatin in unresectable stage III non–small-cell lung cancer. J Clin Oncol. 1999; 17:2692–2699.)[33]

This difference was related entirely to the delivery of postradiation chemotherapy. Whether this difference may partially explain the overall survival benefit is unclear, and the role of such adjuvant chemotherapy has not been investigated. The RTOG has completed accrual to a three-arm study (RTOG 94-10) that includes sequential cisplatin/vinblastine followed by conventional RT, concurrent cisplatin/vinblastine and conventional RT, and concurrent cisplatin/etoposide with HF-RT.[34]

Preliminary results from this trial show that survival is improved with concurrent chemotherapy and conventional RT compared with sequential treatment (median survival, 17 months versus 14.6 months; $P = 0.08$). This is very similar to the results of the randomized trial of concurrent versus sequential chemoradiotherapy reported by Furuse et al.[33] In the RTOG trial, the arm utilizing HF-RT given

concurrently with cisplatin and oral etoposide demonstrated intermediate results (median survival, 15.6 months).[34] Although acute toxicity was worse in the concurrent chemoradiotherapy arms, late toxicity was equivalent.

TOXICITY

Substantial differences have been reported between sequential and concurrent chemoradiotherapy approaches in the pattern of both acute toxicity (within 90 days) and late toxicity (after 90 days). However, the toxicity scoring systems used were frequently different, making specific estimates regarding the severity of toxicity somewhat difficult. The two most commonly used scoring systems are based on the World Health Organization (WHO)[35] or RTOG toxicity scoring criteria.[32] A review of the RTOG experience in phase II and III trials of chemoradiotherapy for stage III NSCLC provides a useful comparison of toxicities and has the advantage of using a single scoring system.[32]

Treatment-related mortality with chemoradiotherapy is rare, averaging 1% to 3% of all patients, and does not differ based on treatment strategy.[5, 14, 15, 22, 32, 36] Acute hematologic toxicity is common with combined chemotherapy and RT but is generally well tolerated. The rates vary depending on the chemotherapy agents and doses, but there is no clear difference based on treatment strategy in making comparisons across studies. In the randomized study of sequential versus concurrent chemoradiotherapy, the incidence of acute grade 3,4 hematologic toxicity was higher on the concurrent arm ($P < 0.0001$), but this may reflect the fact that patients on this arm received significantly more cycles of chemotherapy.[33] The incidence of clinically significant nausea and vomiting is also variable. Although nausea and vomiting are more common with chemoradiotherapy than with RT alone, their development appears to be related primarily to the availability of serotonin receptor antagonists as antiemetic agents rather than to the treatment strategy.

TABLE 21–6. SELECTED PHASE I–II TRIALS EMPLOYING CHEMOTHERAPY AGENTS IN COMBINATION WITH RADIATION IN STAGE III NON–SMALL CELL LUNG CANCER

| | | | CR + PR | | SURVIVAL (%) | |
STUDY	n	TREATMENT	(%)	MST (mo)	1-yr	2-yr
Belani et al[52] a	21	c TxCb/RT (60 Gy)	—	>36	63	54
Choy et al[53]	29	c Tx/RT (60 Gy)	86	20	61	33
Choy et al[54]	39	c TxCb/RT (66 Gy) → TxCb × 3	76	21	56	38
Choy et al[55]	43	c TxCb/RT (69.6 Gy HF) → TxCb × 2	79	—	63	—
Greco et al[56]	33	TxPE × 2 → c TxPE/RT (60 Gy)	82	—	58	—
Langer et al[57]	35	TxCb × 2 → c TxCb/RT (60 Gy)	58	14	62	—
Socinski et al[47]	61	TxCb × 2 → c TxCb/RT (60–74 Gy)[b]	50	26	74	52
Vokes et al[58]	61	GP × 2 → c GP/RT (66 Gy)[c]	58	18[d]	66[d]	—
Vokes et al[58]	64	TxP × 2 → c TxP/RT (66 Gy)[c]	50	18[d]	66[d]	—
Vokes et al[58]	56	NP × 2 → c NP/RT (66 Gy)[c]	55	18[d]	66[d]	—

Inclusion criteria: Selected prospective phase I–II trials of new chemotherapy agents and radiation for patients with stage III non–small cell lung cancer.
[a]Single institution study (the remainder involved multiple institutions).
[b]Three-dimensional computer-assisted radiotherapy planning.
[c]Concurrent therapy given every 3 weeks.
[d]For all three chemotherapy regimens combined.
c, concurrent, given weekly except as indicated; CR + PR = percentage of patients with a complete or a partial response; HF, hyperfractionated; MST, median survival time (months); RT, radiotherapy (dose in Gy).
Chemotherapy abbreviations: GP, gemcitabine and cisplatin; NP, vinorelbine and cisplatin; Tx, paclitaxel; TxCb, paclitaxel and carboplatin; TxP, paclitaxel and cisplatin; TxPE, paclitaxel, cisplatin, and etoposide.

DATA SUMMARY: RESPONSE RATES AND SURVIVAL DATA

	AMOUNT	QUALITY	CONSISTENCY
Objective response rates are not significantly improved with the addition of chemotherapy compared with RT alone	High	High	High
Complete response is seen in approximately 25% of patients with IIIa,b NSCLC treated with RT or chemoradiotherapy	High	High	Mod
Non–cisplatin-based chemoradiotherapy does not improve survival compared with RT alone	High	Mod	High
Sequential cisplatin-based chemoradiotherapy significantly improves survival compared with RT alone	High	High	Mod
The 5-year survival after sequential cisplatin-based chemoradiotherapy is approximately 13%	High	High	High
The rate of distant recurrence is significantly decreased with sequential chemoradiotherapy	Mod	High	Mod
The rate of local control is not altered by the use of sequential chemoradiotherapy	Mod	High	High
Daily or weekly concurrent chemoradiotherapy significantly improves survival compared with RT alone	High	High	Mod
The 5-year survival after concurrent cisplatin-based chemoradiotherapy is approximately 14%	High	High	High
Daily or weekly concurrent chemoradiotherapy significantly improves local control compared with RT alone	High	High	High

Type of data rated: Plain text: descriptive statement   *Italics: controlled comparison*   **Bold: randomized comparison**

The major difference among the various combined modality treatment approaches has been in the incidence of grade 3,4 nonhematologic toxicities.[32] This is true for both acute and late toxicities, as seen in the review of the RTOG experience (Fig. 21–5A,B), but the most pronounced differences have been noted in the rate of acute esophagitis.[32] In trials of sequential cisplatin-based chemotherapy and conventional RT, the incidence of acute grade 3,4 esophagitis is approximately 1% (range, 1%-2%).[12, 13] The range in concurrent trials has been broader, with reported incidence rates between 1% and 16%.[5, 14, 15, 36] In the review

of the RTOG experience, the incidence of acute grade 3 or higher esophageal toxicity was significantly greater in the patients receiving concurrent chemotherapy and HF-RT (1%, 6%, and 34%, respectively; $P = 0.0001$).[32] This did not result in a significant difference in grade 3,4 *late* esophageal toxicity (range, 2%-8%; $P = 0.08$).[32] There was no significant difference in the rates of grade 3,4 acute pulmonary toxicity, but a higher rate of grade 3,4 *late* pulmonary toxicity was seen in both concurrent groups (see Fig. 21–5B).[32] Furthermore, none of the randomized trials found a statistically significant difference in the rate

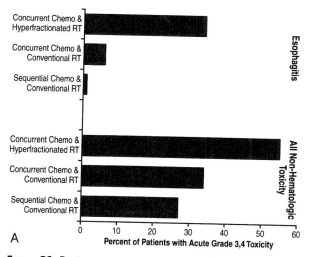

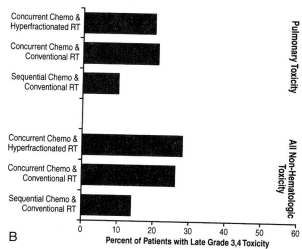

FIGURE 21–5. *A,* Acute toxicity. *B,* Late toxicity of chemoradiotherapy among phase II and phase III RTOG trials for non–small cell lung cancer by treatment with sequential chemotherapy and conventional radiotherapy (RT), concurrent chemotherapy and standard RT, or concurrent chemotherapy and hyperfractionated RT. RTOG, Radiation Therapy Oncology Group. (Data from Byhardt R, Scott C, Sause W, et al. Response, toxicity, failure patterns, and survival in five Radiation Therapy Oncology Group (RTOG) trials of sequential and/or concurrent chemotherapy for locally advanced non–small-cell carcinoma of the lung. Int J Radiat Oncol Biol Phys. 1998; 42:469–478.)[32]

of severe esophagitis or pulmonary toxicity between the chemoradiotherapy arm and the RT-alone arm.[5, 14, 15, 30]

META-ANALYSIS

Three published meta-analyses have evaluated the survival impact of chemotherapy added to definitive RT compared with definitive RT alone.[37–39] Two were based on data from published randomized trials,[37, 38] whereas the third was based on individual patient data from both published and unpublished studies.[39] All three reported a statistically significant modest survival benefit with chemoradiotherapy involving cisplatin-based regimens. The relative risk of death at 2 years was reduced between 13% and 30% in these three meta-analyses, which translated into a mean gain in life expectancy of 2 to 4 months. The issue of schedule was addressed in only one study.[38] There was no apparent difference in the magnitude of benefit when chemotherapy was given either sequentially or concurrently with RT.

These meta-analyses used data that was available before 1994 or 1995. Since then, several additional trials have been published, all of which have shown at least a trend toward better survival with combined chemotherapy and radiotherapy.[5, 14, 24, 30] Therefore, if a meta-analysis were repeated today, it is likely that the statistical significance of a survival benefit would be more pronounced.

ROLE OF RADIOTHERAPY

The poor long-term survival of patients treated with RT as a single modality has raised questions regarding whether RT is essential in the management of unresectable locally advanced NSCLC. Three trials have randomized patients with locally advanced NSCLC to treatment with chemotherapy with or without the addition of RT.[17, 40, 41] The intent in one of these studies was to evaluate the role of RT versus observations, and chemotherapy was used in order to avoid trying to randomize to a no-treatment arm.[17] A response rate of <10% was reported for chemotherapy (single-agent vindesine), and therefore this trial will not be considered further here. The other two studies have treated patients with locally advanced NSCLC with cisplatin-based chemotherapy regimens and then randomized patients either to receive or not to receive RT.[40, 41] However, the design of these trials is somewhat different, making direct comparisons difficult. One trial randomized only patients who had responded to induction chemotherapy to either RT or additional chemotherapy (N = 115),[40] whereas the other trial randomized patients with either responding or stable disease to either RT or observation (N = 63).[41]

Both of these studies found that local recurrences were more common in the arms treated with chemotherapy alone.[40, 41] In the larger study, an improvement in local control was reported for patients on the chemoradiotherapy arm (2-year local control rate, 57% versus 24%; $P = 0.0007$).[40] In the other trial, a local first site of recurrence was seen in 47% of those receiving chemotherapy alone and 16% of those receiving chemoradiotherapy (no P value given).[41] Both trials also found a trend toward poorer sur-

vival with chemotherapy alone (2-year survival, 18% versus 22%[40] and 29% versus 36%.[41]), but this was statistically significant only in the smaller trial ($P = 0.02$). Surprisingly, the smaller trial also reported higher survival rates than the other study, despite the inclusion of nonresponding patients.[41] Although the data regarding survival is somewhat inconsistent, these two studies do suggest that local control is diminished without radiotherapy.[40, 41]

ROLE OF COMBINED-MODALITY THERAPY IN POOR-RISK PATIENTS

The Southwest Oncology Group (SWOG) presented phase II data that supports the ability of poor-risk patients to tolerate concurrent chemotherapy and RT.[42] Poor-risk patients were defined as those with locally advanced disease who would have been excluded from other cisplatin-based chemoradiotherapy trials because of comorbid disease, including at least one of the following: chronic obstructive pulmonary disease (COPD) with a forced expiratory volume in 1 second (FEV_1) of 1 to 2 L, poor renal function with a calculated creatinine clearance of 20 to 50 mL/min, clinically evident hearing loss or peripheral neuropathy, controlled congestive heart failure that might become decompensated as a result of hydration before cisplatin, or a PS of 2 and either a low serum albumin level or a >10% weight loss. Patients were treated with concurrent carboplatin and etoposide and conventional RT. The most common poor-risk feature was moderate-to-severe COPD, followed by a poor PS with either hypoalbuminemia or a >10% weight loss. Myelosuppression was the most frequent toxicity, with an incidence of grade 3,4 leukopenia and thrombocytopenia of 50% and 23%, respectively. Esophageal toxicity was consistent with other concurrent trials (16% grade 3,4 esophagitis). The overall response rate was only 29%. However, a median survival of 13 months and a 2-year survival of 21% were observed, which are consistent with the results seen in combined-modality trials involving better-risk patients.[12, 15] Unfortunately, poor accrual led to the premature closure of a randomized phase III trial comparing this regimen to RT alone in poor-risk patients (RTOG 97-01).

CURRENT STRATEGIES

Given the modest benefits associated with combining chemotherapy and radiation for this patient population, recent effort has focused on optimizing both modalities. As discussed in Chapters 9 and 18, novel radiation strategies, including HF and accelerated RT schedules, as well as conformal three-dimensional planning techniques and higher total doses, offer the potential to improve the therapeutic index of RT. Furthermore, a number of newer third-generation chemotherapy agents have shown superior activity in patients with stage IV NSCLC (see Chapter 22). These include the taxanes, topoisomerase I inhibitors, gemcitabine, and vinorelbine. In stage IV disease, the single-agent objective response rates for these agents have ranged between 20% and 30% (see Table 22–7).[43] When these agents are included in combination regimens with cisplatin

DATA SUMMARY: TOXICITY

	AMOUNT	QUALITY	CONSISTENCY
The addition of chemotherapy to RT has not resulted in increased toxicity compared with RT alone, with the exception of hematologic toxicity and nausea and vomiting	**High**	**Mod**	**Mod**
Concurrent chemoradiotherapy is associated with a rate of grade 3,4 esophagitis of 20%	High	Mod	Poor
Treatment with chemotherapy alone results in an increase in the rate of local failure compared with chemoradiotherapy	Mod	Mod	High

Type of data rated: Plain text: descriptive statement   *Italics: controlled comparison*   **Bold: randomized comparison**

or carboplatin, objective response rates of >50% have been reported.[43]

Table 21–6 lists the results from selected phase I-II trials of chemotherapy and RT that include several of these newer chemotherapy agents, RT techniques, or both. The overall response rates (range, 50%-86%) compare favorably with both the sequential and the concurrent combined-modality arms in the randomized trials shown in Table 21–2. The overall survival data is also quite encouraging. In the phase I–II series included in Table 21–6, the 2-year survival rate ranged from 33% to 54%. By comparison, the 2-year survival rate for this patient population is <10% with best supportive care alone (see Table 3–4), 15% to 20% with conventional RT alone (see Table 18–1), and approximately 25% with either sequential or concurrent cisplatin-based chemoradiotherapy (see Tables 21–4 and 21–5). Although one must be cautious in making comparisons across studies, especially when they involve phase I–II data from single institutions, the data from these studies certainly suggests that further improvements in survival are possible with new treatment strategies.

EDITORS' COMMENTS

The data presented in this chapter clearly defines combined chemoradiotherapy as the standard of care in the curative approach to patients with unresectable stage III NSCLC who have a good PS. This position has also been clearly adopted by the American Society of Clinical Oncology and the National Comprehensive Cancer Network in published clinical guidelines for locally advanced NSCLC.[44, 45] What remains debatable is the optimal strategy to employ in this setting. Many options are currently available with regard to both the selection of chemotherapeutic agents and the ways of integrating chemotherapy with radiation. Likewise, many questions remain regarding the optimal radiotherapeutic strategy when approaching this patient population. It is not possible to define a standard of care with regard to these details in this population.

The two major endpoints one must achieve in curing the patient are control of local macroscopic disease and control of distant microscopic disease. The role of RT is primarily to control macroscopic intrathoracic disease. The role of chemotherapy is likely 2-fold: to control distant occult micrometastatic disease and to improve local control by enhancing the effect of RT. It is also possible that improving local control may reduce the incidence of micrometas-

tatic spread of the disease, as it is not entirely clear when this event occurs. The results of the continuous hyperfractionated accelerated RT (CHART) trial suggest that an improvement in local therapy (three-times-a-day RT) can decrease the rate of systemic metastases compared with once-a-day RT.[46]

The optimal chemotherapeutic approach has not yet been clearly defined. The results of one randomized phase III trial suggested that the concurrent approach is better than sequential treatment.[33] The RTOG has completed a similar study, which also suggests that survival is better with concurrent chemotherapy. When comparing results across trials, the data suggests that the concurrent approach is superior to the sequential approach. Even if it is accepted that concurrent therapy is better, questions remain regarding the optimal way to deliver chemotherapy concurrently, with options ranging from daily or weekly to every 2, 3, or 4 weeks. The total amount of chemotherapy delivered will vary based on the strategy chosen. It appears that more frequent administration of chemotherapy during the course of RT may be superior, but this has not been tested directly in phase III trials. Furthermore, the optimal chemotherapeutic regimen has not been defined. Most of the available phase III trials have been performed with platinum-based regimens. New agents and regimens appear promising, but no phase III data is currently available to define the optimal regimen.

Regarding RT, several issues remain undefined, including optimal dose, fractionation schedule, and the volume to be treated (eg, pre- versus postchemotherapy tumor dimensions or clinically negative nodal stations). Historically, total doses of 60 to 66 Gy have been considered standard but have resulted in poor local control.[27] With the advent of three-dimensional or conformal treatment planning systems, the ability to safely deliver higher doses to the thorax has been demonstrated either alone or with concurrent chemotherapy.[47, 48] Toxicity is reduced by more accurately defining the tumor volume and avoiding excessive dosing to normal surrounding tissue. Whether higher doses will improve survival remains an open question. Future phase III trials will undoubtedly address this issue, but the maximum tolerated dose of thoracic radiotherapy must first be defined. Alternatively, dose-intense delivery of RT by altered fractionation schemes may prove superior, as has been suggested by the results of the CHART trial.[46] Lastly, the principal toxicity of combined modality therapy in this setting is esophagitis, especially with aggressive concurrent treatment. Strategies to reduce the incidence of esophagitis, if successful, would improve the therapeutic index of this potentially curative approach.

Management of the patient with a poor PS has not been addressed adequately. The RTOG failed to complete a well-designed phase III trial in this population of patients because of poor accrual. New treatment strategies with acceptable toxicity profiles are needed for this population of patients. Combined-modality treatment for these patients should be viewed cautiously because the potential for causing substantial toxicity in the absence of a clearly demonstrated survival benefit would violate the dictum of *primum non nocere*. In the absence of a clinical trial, palliative thoracic RT remains the standard of care.

References

1. Bülzebruck H, Bopp R, Drings P, et al. New aspects in the staging of lung cancer: prospective validation of the International Union Against Cancer TNM classification. Cancer. 1992;70:1102–1110.
2. Reinfuss M, Skolyszewski J, Kowalska T, et al. Palliative radiotherapy in asymptomatic patients with locally advanced, unresectable, non–small cell lung cancer. Strahlenther Onkol. 1993;169:709–715.
3. Tannock I. Treatment of cancer with radiation and drugs. J Clin Oncol. 1996;14:3156–3174.
4. Curran WJ Jr, Stafford PM. Lack of apparent difference in outcome between clinically staged IIIA and IIIB non–small cell lung cancer treated with radiation therapy. J Clin Oncol. 1990;8:409–415.
5. Jeremic B, Shibamoto Y, Acimovic L, et al. Hyperfractionated radiation therapy with or without concurrent low-dose daily carboplatin/etoposide for stage III non–small-cell lung cancer: a randomized study. J Clin Oncol. 1996;14:1065–1070.
6. Kreisman H, Lisbona A, Olson L, et al. Effect of radiologic stage III substage on nonsurgical therapy of non–small cell lung cancer. Cancer. 1993;72:1588–1596.
7. Bonomi P, Gale M, Rowland K, et al. Pre-treatment prognostic factors in stage III non–small cell lung cancer patients receiving combined modality treatment. Int J Radiat Oncol Biol Phys. 1990;20:247–252.
8. Sculier JP, Paesmans M, Ninane V, et al. Evaluation of the TN substaging in patients with initially unresectable stage III non–small cell lung cancer treated by induction chemotherapy. Lung Cancer. 1998;22:201–213.
9. Stanley KE. Prognostic factors for survival in patients with inoperable lung cancer. J Natl Cancer Inst. 1980;65:25–32.
10. Paesmans M, Sculier J, Libert P, et al. Prognostic factors for survival in advanced non–small cell lung cancer: univariate and multivariate analyses including recursive partitioning and amalgamation algorithms in 1,052 patients. J Clin Oncol. 1995;13:1221–1230.
11. Buccheri G, Ferrigno D. Prognostic factors in lung cancer: tables and comments. Eur Respir J. 1994;7:1350–1364.
12. Dillman RO, Seagren SL, Propert KJ, et al. A randomized trial of induction chemotherapy plus high-dose radiation versus radiation alone in stage III non–small-cell lung cancer. N Engl J Med. 1990;323:940–945.
13. Sause WT, Scott C, Taylor S, et al. Radiation Therapy Oncology Group (RTOG) 88-08 and Eastern Cooperative Oncology Group (ECOG) 4588: preliminary results of a phase III trial in regionally advanced, unresectable non–small-cell lung cancer. J Natl Cancer Inst. 1995;87:198–205.
14. Blanke C, Ansari CB, Mantravadi R, et al. Phase III trial of thoracic irradiation with or without cisplatin for locally advanced unresectable non–small-cell lung cancer: a Hoosier Oncology Group protocol. J Clin Oncol. 1995;13:1425–1429.
15. Schaake-Koning C, van den Bogaert W, Dalesio O, et al. Effects of concomitant cisplatin and radiotherapy on inoperable non–small-cell lung cancer. N Engl J Med. 1992;326:524–530.
16. Trovo MG, Minatel E, Franchin G, et al. Radiotherapy versus radiotherapy enhanced by cisplatin in stage III non–small cell lung cancer. Int J Radiat Oncol Biol Phys. 1992;24:11–15.
17. Johnson DH, Einhorn LH, Bartolucci A, et al. Thoracic radiotherapy does not prolong survival in patients with locally advanced, unresectable non–small cell lung cancer. Ann Intern Med. 1990;113:33–38.
18. Mattson K, Holsti LR, Holsti P, et al. Inoperable non–small cell lung cancer: radiation with or without chemotherapy. Eur J Cancer Clin Oncol. 1988;24:477–482.
19. Curran W, Scott C, Komaki R, et al. Response to induction chemotherapy does not predict for long term survival among patients with unresected stage III non–small cell lung cancer (NSCLC) receiving sequential chemo-radiation on RTOG 88-04 and 88-08. Int J Radiat Oncol Biol Phys. 1999;32(suppl 1):196.
20. Leung WT, Shiu WCT, Pang JCK, et al. Combined chemotherapy and radiotherapy versus best supportive care in the treatment of inoperable non–small-cell lung cancer. Oncology. 1992;49:321–326.
21. Le Chevalier T, Arriagada R, Tarayre M, et al. Significant effect of adjuvant chemotherapy on survival in locally advanced non–small-cell lung carcinoma. J Natl Cancer Inst. 1992;84:58.
22. Le Chevalier T, Arriagada R, Quoix E, et al. Radiotherapy alone versus combined chemotherapy and radiotherapy in nonresectable non–small-cell lung cancer: first analysis of a randomized trial in 353 patients. J Natl Cancer Inst. 1991;83:417–423.
23. Dillman RO, Herndon J, Seagren SL, et al. Improved survival in stage III non–small-cell lung cancer: seven-year follow-up of Cancer and Leukemia Group B (CALGB) 8433 trial. J Natl Cancer Inst. 1996;88:1210–1215.
24. Sause W, Kolesar P, Taylor S, et al. Five-year results: phase III trial of regionally advanced unresectable non–small cell lung cancer, RTOG 8808, ECOG 4588, SWOG 8992 [abstract]. Proc ASCO. 1998;17:453a.
25. Miller TP, Crowley JJ, Mira J, et al. A randomized trial of chemotherapy and radiotherapy for stage III non–small cell lung cancer. Cancer Therapeutics, 1998;1:229–236.
26. Brodin O, Nou E. Patients with non-resectable squamous cell carcinoma of the lung: a prospective, randomized study. Lung Cancer. 1991;75:165.
27. Arriagada R, Le Chevalier T, Quoix E, et al. ASTRO Plenary: effect of chemotherapy on locally advanced non–small cell lung carcinoma: a randomized study of 353 patients. Int J Radiat Oncol Biol Phys. 1991;20:1183–1190.
28. Komaki R, Scott CB, Sause WT, et al. Induction cisplatin/vinblastine and irradiation vs. irradiation in unresectable squamous cell lung cancer: failure patterns by cell type in RTOG 88-08/ECOG 4588. Int J Radiat Oncol Biol Phys. 1997;39:537–544.
29. Gelman R, Gelber R, Henderson I, et al. Improved methodology for analyzing local and distant recurrence. J Clin Oncol. 1990;8:548–555.
30. Jeremic B, Shibamoto Y, Acimovic L, et al. Randomized trial of hyperfractionated radiation therapy with or without concurrent chemotherapy for stage III non–small-cell lung cancer. J Clin Oncol. 1995;13:452–458.
31. Soresi E, Clerici M, Grilli R, et al. A randomized clinical trial comparing radiation therapy v radiation therapy plus cis-dichlorodiammine platinum (II) in the treatment of locally advanced non-small cell lung cancer. Semin Oncol. 1988;15:20–25.
32. Byhardt R, Scott C, Sause W, et al. Response, toxicity, failure patterns, and survival in five Radiation Therapy Oncology Group (RTOG) trials of sequential and/or concurrent chemotherapy and radiotherapy for locally advanced non–small-cell carcinoma of the lung. Int J Radiat Oncol Bio Phys. 1998;42:469–478.
33. Furuse K, et al, for the West Japan Lung Cancer Group. Phase III study of concurrent versus sequential thoracic radiotherapy in combination with mitomycin, vindesine, and cisplatin in unresectable stage III non–small-cell lung cancer. J Clin Oncol. 1999;17:2692–2699.
34. Curran WJ Jr, Scott C, Langer C, et al. Phase III comparison of sequential vs concurrent chemoradiation for PTS with unresected stage III non–small cell lung cancer (NSCLC): initial report of Radiation Therapy Oncology Group (RTOG) 9410 [abstract]. Proc ASCO. 2000;19:484a.
35. Miller A, Hoogstraten B, Staquet M, et al. Reporting results of cancer treatment. Cancer. 1981;47:207–214.
36. Jeremic B, Jevremovic S, Mijatovic L, et al. Hyperfractionated radiation therapy with and without concurrent chemotherapy for advanced non–small-cell lung cancer. Cancer. 1993;71:3732–3736.
37. Marino P, Preatoni A, Cantoni A. Randomized trials of radiotherapy alone versus combined chemotherapy and radiotherapy in stages IIIa and IIIb nonsmall cell lung cancer: a meta-analysis. Cancer. 1995;76:593–601.
38. Pritchard R, Anthony S. Chemotherapy plus radiotherapy compared

with radiotherapy alone in the treatment of locally advanced, unresectable, non–small-cell lung cancer. Ann Intern Med. 1996;125:723–729.

39. Stewart LA, for the Non-Small Cell Lung Cancer Collaborative Group. Chemotherapy in non–small cell lung cancer: a meta-analysis using updated data on individual patients from 52 randomized clinical trials. BMJ. 1995;311:899–909.

40. Sculier JP, Paesmans M, Lafitte JJ, et al. A randomized phase III trial comparing consolidation treatment with further chemotherapy to chest irradiation in patients with initially unresectable locoregional non–small-cell lung cancer responding to induction chemotherapy. Ann Oncol. 1999;10:295–303.

41. Kubota K, Furuse K, Kawahara M, et al. Role of radiotherapy in combined modality treatment of locally advanced non–small-cell lung cancer. J Clin Oncol. 1994;12:1547–1552.

42. Lau D, Crowley J, Gandara D, et al. Southwest Oncology Group phase II trial of concurrent carboplatin, etoposide, and radiation for poor-risk stage III non–small-cell lung cancer. J Clin Oncol. 1998;16:3078–3081.

43. Carney D. New agents in the management of advanced non–small cell lung cancer. Semin Oncol. 1998;25:83–88.

44. ASCO. Clinical practice guidelines for the treatment of unresectable non–small-cell lung cancer. J Clin Oncol. 1997;15:2996–3018.

45. Ettinger DS, Cox JD, Ginsberg RJ, et al. NCCN non–small-cell lung cancer practice guidelines. Oncology. 1996;10(suppl):81–111.

46. Saunders M, Dische S, Barrett A, et al. Continuous hyperfractionated accelerated radiotherapy (CHART) versus conventional radiotherapy in non–small-cell lung cancer: a randomized multicentre trial. Lancet. 1997;350:161–165.

47. Socinski MA, Halle J, Schell MJ, et al. Induction (I) and concurrent (C) carboplatin/paclitaxel (C/P) with dose-escalated thoracic conformal radiotherapy (TCRT) in stage IIIA/B non–small cell lung cancer (NSCLC): a phase I/II trial [abstract]. Proc ASCO. 2000;19:496a.

48. Hayman JA, Martel MK, Ten Haken RK, et al. Dose escalation in non–small cell lung cancer (NSCLC) using conformal 3-dimensional radiation therapy (C3DRT): update of a phase I trial [abstract]. ASCO. 1999;18:459a.

49. Morton RF, Jett JR, McGinnis WL, et al. Thoracic radiation therapy alone compared with combined chemoradiotherapy for locally unre-

sectable non–small cell lung cancer: a randomized, phase III trial. Ann Intern Med. 1991;115:681–686.

50. Trovo MG, Minatel E, Veronesi A, et al. Combined radiotherapy and chemotherapy versus radiotherapy alone in locally advanced epidermoid bronchogenic carcinoma: a randomized study. Cancer. 1990;65:400–404.

51. White JE, Chen T, Reed R, et al. Limited squamous cell carcinoma of the lung: a Southwest Oncology Group randomized study of radiation with or without doxorubicin chemotherapy and with or without levamisole immunotherapy. Cancer Treat Rep. 1982;66:1113–1120.

52. Belani CP, Aisner J, Ramanathan R, et al. Paclitaxel and carboplatin with simultaneous thoracic irradiation in regionally advanced non–small cell lung cancer. Semin Radiat Oncol. 1997;7(suppl 1):S1–11, S1–14.

53. Choy H, Safran H, Akerley W, et al. Phase II trial of weekly paclitaxel and concurrent radiation therapy for locally advanced non–small cell lung cancer. Clin Cancer Res. 1998;4:1931–1936.

54. Choy H, Akerley W, Safran H, et al. Preliminary analysis of paclitaxel, carboplatin, and concurrent radiation in the treatment of patients with advanced non–small cell lung cancer. J Clin Oncol. 1998;16:3316–3322.

55. Choy H, DeVore RD, Hande KR, et al. Phase II study of paclitaxel, carboplatin, and hyperfractionated radiation therapy for locally advanced inoperable non–small cell lung cancer: a Vanderbilt Cancer Study affiliate network (VCCAN). Proc ASCO. 1998;17:467a.

56. Greco FA, Stroup SL, Gray JR, et al. Paclitaxel in combination chemotherapy with radiotherapy in patients with unresectable stage III non–small-cell lung cancer. J Clin Oncol. 1996;14:1642–1648.

57. Langer CJ, Movsas B, Hudes R, et al. Induction paclitaxel and carboplatin followed by concurrent chemoradiotherapy in patients with unresectable, locally advanced non–small cell lung carcinoma: report of Fox Chase Cancer Center Study 94-001. Semin Oncol. 1997;24(suppl 12):S12–89, S12–S95.

58. Vokes EE, Leopold KA, Herndon JE II, et al. A randomized phase II study of gemcitabine or paclitaxel or vinorelbine with cisplatin as induction chemotherapy (Ind CT) and concomitant chemoradiotherapy (XRT) for unresectable stage III non–small cell lung cancer (NSCLC) (CALGB Study 9431). Proc ASCO. 1999;18:459a.

PART 6

ADVANCED NON–SMALL CELL LUNG CANCER

CHEMOTHERAPY FOR STAGE IV NON–SMALL CELL LUNG CANCER

Mark A. Socinski

SELECTION OF PATIENTS FOR FIRST-LINE TREATMENT

EFFECT OF CHEMOTHERAPY ON SURVIVAL

SYMPTOM PALLIATION AND QUALITY OF LIFE

COST EFFECTIVENESS OF CHEMOTHERAPY IN ADVANCED NON–SMALL CELL LUNG CANCER

CHEMOTHERAPY AGENTS AND REGIMENS
Single Agents
Second-Generation Regimens
Cisplatin With or Without New Agents
Phase III Trials of the Platinums With New Agents

SECOND-LINE CHEMOTHERAPY IN NON–SMALL CELL LUNG CANCER

DURATION OF THERAPY IN ADVANCED NON–SMALL CELL LUNG CANCER

TOXICITY

EDITORS' COMMENTS

Chemotherapy plays a significant role in the management of advanced stage non–small cell lung cancer (NSCLC). This chapter is devoted to the chemotherapeutic management of patients with stage IV NSCLC as well as patients with stage IIIb NSCLC who are not appropriate candidates for combined modality therapy (eg, because of malignant pleural effusion, advanced supraclavicular or contralateral hilar lymphadenopathy). The vast majority of stage IV patients have multiple sites of metastases,[1,2] with the most common sites being bone (33%), brain (18%), contralateral lung (16%), pleura (12%), liver (9%), adrenal glands (6%), and other sites (10%).[3] Radiotherapy may offer a palliative effect for symptoms referable to specific sites (see Chapter 29), which is important because this population of stage IV patients is not curable. It is clear from the literature that chemotherapy offers a survival and palliative benefit to patients with advanced disease and good performance status (PS). This chapter initially focuses on the ability of chemotherapy to improve survival and palliate symptoms, maintain quality of life (QOL), and be delivered in a cost-effective manner. This is followed by a discussion of modern chemotherapeutic agents and regimens and their current role in the management of advanced NSCLC.

SELECTION OF PATIENTS FOR FIRST-LINE TREATMENT

Not all patients with stage IIIb/IV NSCLC should receive chemotherapy. Table 22–1 summarizes prognostic factors in patients with stage IV NSCLC. This data is taken from 10 studies involving a total of 12 419 patients and provides insight into the selection of patients for chemotherapy.[1,4–12] As can be seen, PS is by far the most important assessment in the selection of patients for treatment. Patients who are ambulatory and minimally symptomatic (Eastern Cooperative Oncology Group [ECOG] PS 0,1 or Karnofsky PS 80–100, Table 22–2) are candidates for systemic chemotherapy. It is also clear that patients with a PS of >2 should not be offered chemotherapy because they do not derive a survival or a palliative benefit from treatment and have not been included in randomized clinical trials. The role of systemic chemotherapy for patients with a PS of 2 remains controversial. These patients have notably lower survival rates and greater toxicity than those with a PS of 0,1.[8,9,13] Extent of disease (IIIb versus IV) is also important, although the magnitude of the difference is controversial.[14–17] The proportion of patients with stage IIIb and stage IV NSCLC should always be noted when examining survival results from randomized trials. Other factors such as weight loss, age, lactate dehydrogenase (LDH), and sites of metastases have not been consistently associated with prognosis across all studies or have been examined in only a few studies. Of interest, gender differences exist, with women generally having a better prognosis following treatment than men.

The impact of PS on the benefit of chemotherapy has largely been restricted to studies employing cisplatin-based chemotherapy regimens. These regimens are associated with substantial toxicity, including nausea and vomiting, renal impairment, neuropathy, and myelosuppression. They also require vigorous hydration and antiemetic regimens to prevent morbidity, making patient selection critically important. Some of the newer agents discussed later in this chapter have more favorable toxicity profiles and may be

TABLE 22-1. PROGNOSTIC FACTORS PREDICTING POORER SURVIVAL BY MULTIVARIATE ANALYSIS IN PATIENTS WITH ADVANCED NON–SMALL CELL LUNG CANCER RECEIVING CHEMOTHERAPY

STUDY	YEAR	N	POOR PS	SITE OF DISTANT METASTASES				MALE GENDER	>5% WT LOSS	AGE >65 y	NONSQUAMOUS TYPE	PREVIOUS RT	INCREASED LDH
				Any	Bone	Liver	Brain						
Stan ley[5]	1980	5138	Yes	Yes	—	Yes	—	—	Yes	—	No	No	—
Albain et al[1]	1991	2531	Yes	Yes	—	—	—	Yes	No	Yes	—	—	Yes
Finkelstein et al[7]	1986	893	Yes	Yes	Yes	Yes	No	Yes	Yes	No	Yes	No	—
Bonomi et al[9]	1989	699	Yes	Yes	Yes	Yes	No	No	No	No	—	—	—
Ruckdeschel et al[8]	1986	486	Yes	Yes	Yes	No	No	Yes	No	No	—	—	—
Miller et al[12]	1986	483	Yes	No	No	Yes	Yes	No	—	No	No	No	—
Luedke[11]	1990	435	Yes	Yes	Yes	Yes	Yes	—	Yes	Yes	No	No	—
Lanzotti et al[4]	1977	428	Yes	Yes	Yes	Yes	No	Yes	No	No	Yes	No	Yes
O'Connell et al[6]	1986	378	Yes	Yes	—	No	No	No	No	Yes	No	—	—
Klatersky et al[10]	1989	176	Yes	Yes	—	—	—	No	No	Yes	No	—	—
Estimated prognostic value[a]			**High**	**High**	**Mod**	**Mod**	**Low**	**Mod**	**Mod**	**Low**	**Low**	**Low**	**High**

Inclusion criteria: Studies of ≥100 patients with stage IIIb/IV non–small cell lung cancer reporting multivariate analysis of prognostic factors.
Adapted from Thatcher N, Anderson H, Betticher DC, et al. Symptomatic benefit from gemcitabine and other chemotherapy in advanced non-small-cell lung cancer: changes in performance status and tumour-related symptoms. Anticancer Drugs. 1995; 6(suppl 6): 39–48.[46]
[a]Assessment of proportion of studies in which the factor was prognostic: High, >75%; Mod, 50%–75%; Low, <50%.
LDH, lactate dehydrogenase; No, Factor did not achieve statistical significance; PS, performance status; RT, radiotherapy; WT, weight; Yes, factor achieved statistical significance.

TABLE 22–2. PERFORMANCE STATUS SCALES

ECOG SCALE		KARNOFSKY SCALE	
Status	Scale	Scale	Status
Normal	0	100	Normal, no complaints
Fatigue without significant decrease in activity	1	90	Normal activity, minor signs or symptoms of disease
		80	Normal activity with effort
Fatigue with significant impairment of daily activities or bedrest <50% of waking hours	2	70	Cares for self in daily activities, but unable to carry on normal activity or work
		60	Requires occasional assistance but able to care for most needs
		50	Requires considerable assistance and frequent medical care
Bedrest >50% of waking hours	3	40	Disabled; requires special care and assistance
		30	Severely disabled
		20	Very sick; hospitalization necessary; active supportive treatment necessary
Bedridden or unable to care for self	4	10	Moribund
		0	Dead

ECOG, Eastern Cooperative Oncology Group.
Based on definitions used in phase III trials evaluating the role of chemotherapy in advanced non–small cell lung cancer.

able to be delivered with acceptable toxicity in patients with a poor PS. Substitution of carboplatin for cisplatin is likely to increase the therapeutic index because carboplatin is substantially less toxic than the parent compound, cisplatin. In a study conducted by the ECOG comparing cisplatin/paclitaxel, cisplatin/docetaxel, cisplatin/gemcitabine, and carboplatin/paclitaxel, patients classified as PS 2 had significantly more toxicity when receiving any of the cisplatin-based regimens than when receiving the carboplatin-based regimen.[13] This study highlights the point that chemotherapy regimens with less toxicity may be delivered in patients with poorer PS; however, their impact on survival remains unclear.

EFFECT OF CHEMOTHERAPY ON SURVIVAL

In the pre-cisplatin era, various alkylating agents were used in treating patients with NSCLC. These agents had poor single-agent activity and excessive toxicity in this population of patients. A meta-analysis of this experience suggested that treatment with alkylating agents actually decreased survival as compared with best supportive care (BSC) alone (Table 22–3).[18] All of these trials were carried out before 1980, when chemotherapy and supportive care were in their infancy. Two comparative trials[19,20] conducted in the more modern era of chemotherapy using a non–cisplatin-based combination regimen (*MACC**—methotrexate, doxorubicin, cyclophosphamide, and CCNU) suggested a survival advantage. One of these trials[20] was not randomized but simply compared sequential patient populations, whereas the other trial[19] included only 39 patients and was so strikingly positive as to be almost unbelievable (Table 22–4).

With the introduction of cisplatin, trials comparing combination chemotherapy with BSC demonstrated a survival advantage for patients receiving chemotherapy. As shown in Table 22–4, at least nine randomized trials have been performed in which a cisplatin-containing regimen was compared with BSC.[21–29] The median survival of the treated patients in these trials was always greater than that of the patients receiving BSC alone. In five of these nine trials, the survival advantage was statistically significant. Table 22–4 also shows several randomized trials comparing some of the new "third-generation" single agents with BSC.[30–34] As can be seen, these new third-generation agents have effects on survival similar to those of cisplatin-based combinations.

The trials outlined in Table 22–4 accrued a limited number of patients and therefore lack statistical power to detect real but modest differences. In the meta-analysis performed by the NSCLC Collaborative Group[18] (see Table 22–3), cisplatin-containing chemotherapy was shown to increase 1-year survival by 10% and the median survival by 2 months as compared with BSC alone (Fig. 22–1).

TABLE 22–3. META-ANALYSIS OF CHEMOTHERAPY VERSUS BEST SUPPORTIVE CARE IN ADVANCED NON–SMALL CELL LUNG CANCER

	REGIMEN BASED ON:		
	Alkylating Agents	Etoposide or Vinca Alkaloid	Cisplatin
Total number of patients	226	186	1190
Hazard ratio for death	1.26	0.87	0.73
95% confidence interval	0.96–1.66	0.64–1.20	0.63–0.85
P value	0.095	0.4	< 0.0001
Effect on median survival	−1 mo	+½ mo	+1½ mo
Effect on 1-y survival	−6%	+4%	+10%

Data modified from the Non-Small Cell Lung Cancer Collaborative Group. Chemotherapy in non–small cell lung cancer: a meta-analysis using updated data on individual patients from 52 randomised clinical trials. BMJ. 1995; 311:899–909.[18]

*Italics are used for regimens that are conventionally known by an abbreviation in which the letters used to denote chemotherapeutic agents in the regimen are *different* from the letters commonly used for those agents in other regimens or as single agents.

TABLE 22-4. TRIALS OF CHEMOTHERAPY VERSUS BEST SUPPORTIVE CARE IN ADVANCED NON-SMALL CELL LUNG CANCER

AUTHOR	YEAR	n	CHEMO-THERAPY REGIMEN	MEDIAN SURVIVAL (mo)		P
				Chemo	BSC	
Non-Cisplatin-Based Regimens						
Cormier et al[19]	1982	39	*MACC*	7.0	2.0	0.0005
Buccheri et al[20]	1990	175	*MACC*	7.5	4.6	0.01
Cisplatin-Based Regimens						
Rapp et al[21]	1988	93	CAP	5.7	3.9	0.05
Rapp et al[21]	1988	94	VdP	7.5	3.9	0.01
Quoix et al[22]	1991	49	VdP	6.5	2.4	0.001
Ganz et al[23]	1989	63	VbP	4.7	3.1	NS
Woods et al[24]	1990	201	VdP	6.2	3.9	NS
Cellerino et al[25]	1991	128	CErP↔MxEU	7.9	4.9	NS
Kaasa et al[26]	1991	87	EP	5.0	3.7	NS
Cartei et al[27]	1993	102	MCP	8.5	4.0	0.0001
Thongprasert et al[28]	1999	112	IErP/MVbP	6.0	2.5	0.006
Cullen et al[29]	1999	351	MIP	6.7	4.8	0.03
New Third-Generation Single Agents						
Crawford et al[30] a	1996	216	Vinorelbine	7.0	5.1	0.03
Anderson et al[31]	1997	299	Gemcitabine	6.1	6.0	NS
Thatcher et al[33]	1998	157	Paclitaxel	6.8	4.8	< 0.05
Roszkowski[34]	1999	207	Docetaxel	6.0	4.6	< 0.05
ELVIS[32]	1999	171	Vinorelbine	6.5	4.9	0.03

Inclusion criteria: Randomized studies of chemotherapy versus BSC in advanced non-small cell lung cancer from 1980 to 2000.

aBSC-arm patients were treated with 5-fluorouracil/leucovorin.

BSC, best supportive care; Chemo, chemotherapy; ELVIS, Elderly Lung Cancer Vinorelbine Italian Study.

Chemotherapy regimens: CAP, cyclophosphamide, doxorubicin, cisplatin; CErP-↔MxEU, cyclophosphamide, epirubicin, cisplatin alternating with methotrexate, etoposide, CCNU; EP, etoposide, cisplatin; IErP/MVbP, ifosfamide, epirubicin, cisplatin or mitomycin C, vinblastine, cisplatin; *MACC*, methotrexate, doxorubicin, cyclophosphamide, CCNU; MCP, mitomycin C, cyclophosphamide, cisplatin; MIP, mitomycin C, ifosfamide, cisplatin; VbP, vinblastine, cisplatin; VdP, vindesine, cisplatin.

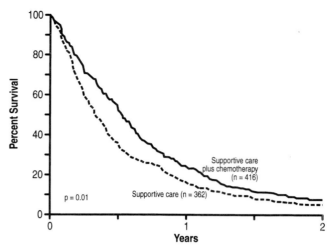

FIGURE 22-1. Meta-analysis of survival of 1190 patients (eight trials) with advanced NSCLC randomized to best supportive care or chemotherapy with a cisplatin-based regimen. (From Stewart LA, for the Non-Small Cell Lung Cancer Collaborative Group. Chemotherapy in non-small cell lung cancer: a meta-analysis using updated data on individual patients from 52 randomised clinical trials. BMJ 1995; 311:899-909.)[18]

SYMPTOM PALLIATION AND QUALITY OF LIFE

The majority of patients with advanced NSCLC are symptomatic at some point as a result of their disease.[39] Symptoms may be either disease specific (cough, hemoptysis, chest pain, dyspnea) or disease nonspecific (weight loss, malaise, declining PS).

At least seven studies have documented palliation of symptoms by chemotherapy in patients with advanced NSCLC (Table 22-5).[40-46] These phase II studies have generally reported percentages of patients with a specific symptom in whom any improvement was noted. A substantial percentage of patients derived symptomatic benefit

Three other meta-analyses of this literature using different analytic methods and study selection criteria have been reported, and all three have shown a survival advantage.[35-37] The survival benefit has been reported in different ways, with one trial focusing on survival at 6 months[36] and the others[35,37] examining the relative risk of death at 3, 6, 9, 12, and 18 months (Fig. 22-2). The latter studies showed that at each time point during the first year, survival was statistically better with chemotherapy, but the advantage was no longer apparent beyond 1 year.

One can conclude from this body of literature that there clearly is a survival benefit with chemotherapy in appropriately selected patients with advanced NSCLC. Figure 22-3A and B shows representative survival curves from the studies by Rapp et al[21] and Cartei et al[27] demonstrating the impact of chemotherapy compared with BSC. As previously noted, the improvement in median and 1-year survival is approximately 2 months and 10%, respectively. Although this is a seemingly modest improvement, it has been estimated that when the median survival is increased by 2 months, approximately one-third of patients will derive a 6-month survival benefit.[38] Given the data presented in Table 22-4 regarding survival with BSC alone, chemotherapy will more than double the survival time of a substantial minority of patients.

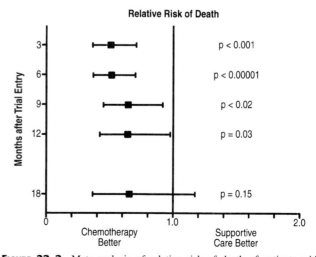

FIGURE 22-2. Meta-analysis of relative risk of death of patients with advanced NSCLC randomized to cisplatin-based chemotherapy or best supportive care. Statistical comparison were made using exact log odds ratio. (From Souquet PJ, Chauvin F, Boissel JP, et al. Polychemotherapy in advanced non-small cell lung cancer: a meta-analysis. Vol 342[8862]:19-21, © by The Lancet, Ltd, 1993.)[35]

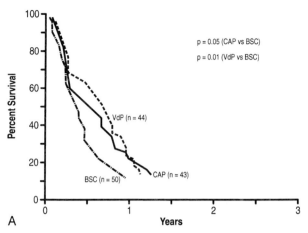

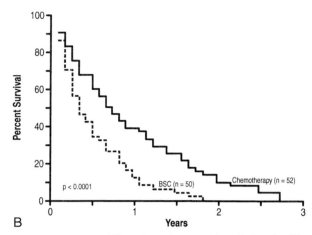

FIGURE 22–3. *A,* Survival of 137 patients with advanced NSCLC randomized to best supportive care (BSC) or chemotherapy with cyclophosphamide, doxorubicin, cisplatin (CAP) or vindesine, cisplatin (VdP) (three-arm trial). *B,* Survival of 102 patients with stage IV NSCLC randomized to best supportive care or chemotherapy (cyclophosphamide, mitomycin, cisplatin). (*A,* From Rapp E, Pater JL, William A, et al. Chemotherapy can prolong survival in patients with advanced non–small-cell lung cancer—report of a Canadian multicenter randomized trial. J Clin Oncol. 1988; 6:633–641.[21] *B,* From Cartei G, Cartei F, Cantone A, et al. Cisplatin-cyclophosphamide-mitomycin combination chemotherapy with supportive care versus supportive care alone for treatment of metastatic non–small-cell lung cancer. J Natl Cancer Inst. 1993; 85:794–800, by permission of Oxford University Press, Oxford, England.[27])

from treatment for both non-specific and organ-specific symptoms. The rate of symptom relief appears to be higher than objective response rates in all the studies reported, suggesting that palliation can be achieved with tumor shrinkage that does not meet the standard criteria for objective responses.

The duration of symptom relief has not been reported consistently. Where reported, typical duration of relief of specific symptoms ranges from 1.5 to 3.5 months.[42,43,45] The review by Thatcher et al,[46] examining the palliative impact of gemcitabine, suggested that some symptoms may be more effectively palliated than others (median relief of 3-5 months for dyspnea, cough, and chest pain; median relief of 2-3 months for anorexia and hemoptysis). When the median duration of symptom relief is compared with the median survival of this population, symptom relief can be achieved for approximately 25% to 50% of the patient's

life span. It is important to provide patients with this information regarding relief of symptoms, which is independent of the survival benefit of chemotherapy.

In addition to symptom relief, the impact of chemotherapy on the patient's overall PS has also been reported. Eight trials involving 770 patients were reported in a review by Thatcher et al.[46] These trials included chemotherapy regimens consisting of platinum combinations and non-platinum single agents and combinations. Almost all trials excluded patients with a PS > 2. Response rates to the chemotherapy regimens ranged from 20% to 59%, and median survival ranged from 5 to 13 months. Approximately one-third of patients experienced an improvement in PS (range, 4%-52%), and another one-third had a stable PS while receiving treatment (range, 30%–67%). Two other trials have confirmed these findings.[23,47] The duration of improvement has not been reported consistently. However,

TABLE 22–5. RELIEF OF SYMPTOMS BY CHEMOTHERAPY IN ADVANCED NON–SMALL CELL LUNG CANCER

AUTHOR	ELLIS ET AL[42]	CULLEN ET AL[44]	OSOBA ET AL[40]	TUMMARELLO ET AL[45]	FERNANDEZ ET AL[41]	HARDY ET AL[43]	THATCHER ET AL[46]
N	120	74	53	46	31	24	NR
Regimen used	MVbP	MIP	BEP	MVbP	PVbMVI	MVbP	Gemcitabine
Objective response rate (%)	32	56	44	33	42	21	20
Median survival (mo)	5.0	9.8	5.0	6.5	—	6	8.1–9.2
Symptom Improvement (%)[a]							
Cough	66	70	68	40	45	71	44
Hemoptysis	—	92	78	100	91	—	63
Pain	60	77	68	39	47	63	32
Dyspnea	59	46	31	66	78	65	26
Weight loss	—	—	44	30	—	—	—
Anorexia	—	58	—	—	50	—	29
Malaise	53	—	53	62	—	—	—

Inclusion criteria: Studies reporting symptom relief with chemotherapy alone in IIIb/IV non–small cell lung cancer.
[a]Percentage of patients with a specific symptom who had relief or improvement in this symptom with treatment.
Chemotherapy regimens: BEP, bleomycin, etoposide, cisplatin; MIP, mitomycin C, ifosfamide, cisplatin; MVbP, mitomycin C, vinblastine, cisplatin; PVbMVI, cisplatin, vinblastine, mitomycin C, vincristine, ifosfamide.

when this has been reported, improvement typically lasted 4 to 6 months.[44,46,47]

A randomized phase III trial comparing gemcitabine with BSC has been reported and highlights the palliative aspect of chemotherapy on disease-related symptoms.[31] Symptom control was the primary endpoint of this study, which involved 299 symptomatic patients with advanced or metastatic NSCLC. Improvements were noted in terms of the need for palliative radiotherapy for progressive symptoms. At 2 months, 42.3% of patients in the BSC arm required radiotherapy compared with 7.3% of patients in the gemcitabine arm. Also, the median time before radiotherapy was needed was 7 months for patients receiving gemcitabine versus 1 month for those receiving BSC ($P < 0.0001$). QOL questionnaires and a patient-assessed symptom scale noted improvements significantly favoring the gemcitabine arm. The overall response rate for gemcitabine was 17%. No difference in survival was noted; however, this was not the endpoint of the study.

QOL is an important aspect of treatment that differs from symptom relief or assessment of PS. QOL attempts to define the patient's perception of how the disease and its treatment affect his or her well-being in all of life's domains (functional, social, psychological, spiritual, disease-related symptoms, and treatment side effects). Several questionnaires have been developed and validated for clinical use.[48,49] These tools are generally patient friendly and easy to administer, requiring only 5 to 10 minutes for patients to complete. Past studies have demonstrated that it is difficult to obtain carefully conducted serial QOL measurements in patients receiving chemotherapy. This may be due to deterioration of the patient's condition and unwillingness or inability to complete the questionnaires.[23,50,51] One of the early QOL instruments developed was the Functional Living Index—Cancer (FLIC).[52] Using this instrument, two reports suggested that initial FLIC QOL scores were more predictive of survival than were other parameters.[53,54] This suggests that QOL measurements could further refine the assessment of PS, as has been suggested in breast cancer patients.[55]

Little data has been reported regarding the longitudinal aspect of QOL while patients are receiving chemotherapy. Three randomized studies all demonstrated improved QOL with chemotherapy compared with BSC.[28,29,32] In one study, single-agent vinorelbine was compared with BSC in patients over the age of 70 years.[32] The QOL instrument used was the European Organization for Research and Treatment of Cancer (EORTC) questionnaire and lung cancer–specific module (QLQ-LC13). Although longitudinal compliance was not optimal, EORTC functional scales were consistently better for the patients receiving vinorelbine than for control patients. Also, symptom improvement scores were clearly better for some lung cancer–specific items (pain and dyspnea). In the other two trials, cisplatin-based combination chemotherapy was compared with BSC.[28,29] QOL assessment showed improvement with combination chemotherapy and deterioration with BSC.

Cella et al[56] suggested that prognosis can be predicted from baseline QOL as well as from early changes in a patient's QOL. Using the Functional Assessment of Cancer Therapy—Lung Cancer (FACT-L), baseline, 6-week, 12-week, and 6-month QOL measurements were obtained for 571 patients. The FACT-L provides subscale scores for physical, functional, emotional, and social well-being; lung cancer symptoms; a total score; and a *trial outcome index* (TOI) that combines physical, functional, and lung cancer scores. The patients were on a three-arm randomized phase III trial comparing cisplatin/etoposide with two different schedules of cisplatin/paclitaxel; the study showed a survival advantage for the paclitaxel-containing arms.[57] There were no differences in any of the QOL scores among the three arms of the study.[56,57] The FACT-L physical well-being emerged second ($P < 0.01$) behind treatment with a paclitaxel regimen ($P < 0.01$) in predicting a response to treatment in a model that considered multiple clinical factors (disease stage, PS, weight loss, comorbidity, presence of symptoms, and FACT-L scores). The baseline TOI correlated highly with survival; but a change from baseline to subsequent assessment proved to be more important.[56] Four groups of patients were identified: (1) those with a high baseline TOI who improved at 6 weeks, (2) those with a high baseline TOI who did not improve at 6 weeks, (3) those with a low baseline TOI who improved at 6 weeks, and (4) those with a low baseline TOI who did not improve at 6 weeks. Median survival for the four groups was 16, 5, 11, and 11 months, respectively. The authors suggested that a change in QOL may be able to predict survival and may aid in decisions made during the course of chemotherapy. Compliance with collection of QOL data was not reported, but one has to wonder how this may have influenced outcome. Although interesting, these findings need corroboration in future studies.

There may be differences in QOL among patients on various treatment regimens. An EORTC study randomized patients with advanced disease to receive either cisplatin/teniposide or cisplatin/paclitaxel.[58] The response rates were 28% for cisplatin/teniposide versus 41% for cisplatin/paclitaxel; however, 1-year survival was the same. Using the EORTC instrument, QOL measurements favored the paclitaxel-containing arm. Despite no survival benefit, the EORTC has subsequently adopted cisplatin/paclitaxel as its new standard regimen, based upon this QOL benefit. In another study comparing cisplatin/etoposide with carboplatin/paclitaxel, the QOL using the FACT-L significantly favored the carboplatin/paclitaxel regimen during the first 6 weeks of treatment.[59] Patients in the carboplatin/paclitaxel arm also had a significantly higher response rate. However, compliance in completing the FACT-L QOL assessment was only 15% after 6 weeks, highlighting the difficulty with longitudinal studies. In two other phase III studies comparing cisplatin/gemcitabine either with mitomycin/ifosfamide/cisplatin or with cisplatin alone, no difference in global QOL was reported between the two arms, despite a significantly higher response rate in the cisplatin/gemcitabine arm in both studies.[60,61]

Baseline QOL appears to be an important prognostic factor, and differences in QOL may occur during treatment with different chemotherapy regimens. More data is needed regarding the longitudinal measurement of QOL during chemotherapy to ascertain how this correlates with baseline PS measurements and response rates.[55] Also, further refinement of QOL instruments will help capture data on the chronic toxicity of chemotherapy and its impact on the patient's QOL.

COST-EFFECTIVENESS OF CHEMOTHERAPY IN ADVANCED NON–SMALL CELL LUNG CANCER

The cost of an intervention is an appropriate concern in our current health care environment. The cost of an intervention must be measured relative to the cost of caring for the patient without this intervention. In this situation, the comparison can be made using absolute cost or incremental cost-effectiveness based on years of life gained by the intervention.

The first study that carefully documented and analyzed cost associated with both BSC and combination chemotherapy was conducted in the Canadian system.[62] This study assessed and analyzed the costs incurred by 61 patients who were enrolled in the Canadian randomized trial reported by Rapp et al.[21] All costs were collected, including drugs, laboratory tests, inpatient and outpatient care, nursing and physician fees, and radiotherapy charges. Personal costs borne by the patients, such as transportation and lost wages, were not included. In this study, cost was defined as actual charges billed to the patients.

The surprising finding of this study[62] was that patients randomized to one of the chemotherapy arms (cyclophosphamide, doxorubicin, and cisplatin, [CAP]) actually incurred lower costs ($950 Canadian dollars less) compared with those patients randomized to BSC. Those randomized to the other chemotherapy arm (vindesine/cisplatin, [VdP]) incurred slightly higher costs ($3637 Canadian dollars more) compared with those patients receiving BSC. These differences were explained by the fact that fewer patients receiving chemotherapy required hospitalization or palliative radiotherapy, or both, and therefore lower hospitalization and radiotherapy costs were incurred. These factors offset the cost of chemotherapy, which was administered primarily on an inpatient basis. Currently, all regimens are delivered on an outpatient basis, which markedly decreases the administration costs and makes the use of chemotherapy even more competitive relative to BSC.

In the trial by Rapp et al,[21] both chemotherapy arms improved survival compared with BSC. The incremental cost of chemotherapy can be calculated relative to BSC on a per-year-of-life gained basis. CAP chemotherapy resulted in a savings of $6172 Canadian dollars per year of life gained, whereas VP chemotherapy resulted in a cost of $14 778 Canadian dollars per year of life gained. A similar study was reported by Smith et al[63] using the survival data from the French vinorelbine study[64] and estimated costs at a United States academic medical center. The authors found that the incremental costs of prolonging survival by using the combination of cisplatin/vinorelbine were approximately $17 700 per year of life gained. To put this in perspective, Table 22–6 shows the incremental cost-effectiveness of several medical interventions that are considered standard medical treatment and are commonly done every day in the United States. As can be seen, the cost of treating patients with advanced NSCLC appears to be acceptable, given the costs of these other interventions.

It seems reasonable to conclude that the cost of chemotherapy is not a major issue. The increased costs of the chemotherapeutic agents appear to be offset by the palliation achieved as well as by the prolongation of survival

TABLE 22–6. COMMON MEDICAL INTERVENTIONS, RANKED BY INCREMENTAL COST-EFFECTIVENESS[a]

INTERVENTION	INCREMENTAL COST-EFFECTIVENESS
Liver transplantation versus medical management	$237 000
Mammography, age <50 years	232 000
Cholestyramine for high cholesterol versus no treatment	178 000
ABMT versus standard chemotherapy for limited metastatic breast cancer	116 000
Captopril versus hydrochlorothiazide for hypertension	82 000
Zidovudine versus no treatment for HIV	8520–88 500
Dialysis versus medical management for renal failure	50 000
Mammography screening for breast cancer, age 50–75 years	20 000–50 000
Drug therapy for moderate hypertension	32 600
Chemotherapy for NSCLC versus best supportive care	**−8400 to + 20 000**
Adjuvant chemotherapy versus no treatment for early-stage breast cancer, 45-year-old woman	4900
CAV + EP versus CAV alone for metastatic SCLC	4600
Smoking cessation counseling	1300

[a]Values are in U.S. dollars, based on estimated charges in 1990–1995.
ABMT, autologous bone marrow transplant.
Chemotherapy regimen: CAV + EP, cyclophosphamide, doxorubicin, vincritine + etoposide, cisplatin.
Modified from Smith TJ, Hillner BE, Neighbors DM, et al. Economic evaluation of a randomized clinical trial comparing vinorelbine, vinorelbine plus cisplatin, and vindesine plus cisplatin for non-small-cell lung cancer. J Clin Oncol. 1995; 13:2166–2173.[63]

and the resultant decreased costs of BSC. There may be differences in costs associated with different agents and combinations; however, a discussion of these issues is beyond the scope of this chapter.[65] The majority of costs incurred in this population are due to hospitalization and the cost of caring for the complications of a progressive and terminal disease.[62]

CHEMOTHERAPY AGENTS AND REGIMENS

Single Agents

Table 22–7 outlines the major chemotherapeutic agents used in the current management of advanced NSCLC, as well as their relative activity based on response and survival rates. Comparison of single-agent response rates is difficult because of the relatively small numbers of patients and the variable patient selection criteria. First-generation agents consisted mainly of alkylating agents, which do not possess significant single-agent activity and are of historical interest only. Second-generation agents possess modest activity (defined as response rates > 10%–15%) and were developed primarily in the 1970s and 1980s. In the 1990s, several new agents (vinorelbine, irinotecan, the taxanes, and the new cytidine analog gemcitabine) were developed and were labeled third-generation agents. In general, response rates for these third-generation agents are superior

TABLE 22–7. ACTIVE SINGLE AGENTS USED IN THE TREATMENT OF ADVANCED NON–SMALL CELL LUNG CANCER

	RESPONSE RATE (%)	MEDIAN SURVIVAL (mo)	1-YEAR SURVIVAL (%)	REFERENCES
Second-Generation Agents				
Cisplatin	9–21	6–9	20–35	61, 66–69, 80
Carboplatin	9–16	7	—	9, 77, 78
Vinblastine	27	—	—	82, 83
Vindesine	16	—	—	82, 83
Mitomycin C	25–30	4	—	84, 85
Etoposide	5–15	—	—	87
Ifosfamide	21	9	—	91
Third-Generation Agents				
Paclitaxel	21–28	6–11	38–55	92
Docetaxel	19–27	8–9	39–71	93–98
Vinorelbine	8–31	5–13	25–32	103–106
Gemcitabine	18–54	6–9	22–40	99
Irinotecan	13–31	9–10	41	71, 102

Inclusion criteria: Selected trials or reviews of single agents in the therapy of non–small cell lung cancer.

to those of the second-generation agents. Each of these agents is discussed briefly in the following sections prior to the discussion of combination regimens.

Cisplatin/Carboplatin

The meta-analysis conducted by the NSCLC Collaborative Group showed that cisplatin-based treatment conclusively prolonged survival in patients with advanced NSCLC.[18] Six phase III trials have used single-agent cisplatin in doses of 75 to 100 mg/m² in the control arm.[10,61,66–69] Response rates ranged from 4% to 19%, median survival from 4 to 9 months, and 1-year survival rates from 20% to 35%. In four of these six trials, the addition of a new agent (etoposide, vinorelbine, gemcitabine, or tirapazamine) in combination with cisplatin significantly improved survival compared with cisplatin alone. Cisplatin has also been added to various single agents, including etoposide, irinotecan, and vinorelbine, in other phase III trials.[64,70–73] The majority of these trials have shown significantly improved response rates and survival attributable to the addition of this agent.

The issue of cisplatin dose intensity has remained controversial since an initial report by Gralla et al[74] suggested a survival benefit when doses to 120 mg/m² were used in combination with vindesine. Although response rates were equivalent, responding patients in the high-dose arm had significantly prolonged survival. Two attempts to repeat this observation have not substantiated this early experience. The Southwest Oncology Group (SWOG) randomized patients to receive either 100 mg/m² of cisplatin on days 1 and 8 every 4 weeks or a dose of 50 mg/m² on days 1 and 8.[75] No difference in response or survival was noted. The EORTC compared low-dose versus high-dose cisplatin in combination with etoposide.[76] Again, no difference in response or survival was noted. Toxicity was increased in all the high-dose arms compared with the low-dose arms. Taken together, these trials suggest no steep dose-response relationship for cisplatin, and standard doses have ranged from 75 to 100 mg/m² delivered every 3 to 4 weeks.

Carboplatin is an analog of cisplatin that induces significantly less nephrotoxicity, ototoxicity, neurotoxicity, and emetogenicity. The drug is excreted renally, and rational dosing schedules have been developed that allow more tailored dosing in individual patients, thereby limiting excessive toxicity. Carboplatin can also be administered without the need for extensive prehydration, making its infusion substantially less involved than that of cisplatin. The single-agent activity of carboplatin is approximately equivalent to that of cisplatin. Three studies using single-agent carboplatin in a total of 208 patients documented an objective response rate of 12% and a median survival of 7 months.[9,77,78] In a randomized phase III trial reported by the ECOG, carboplatin had a median survival superior to that of three cisplatin-containing regimens.[9] At least three randomized trials have compared cisplatin-based chemotherapy with the identical regimen containing carboplatin.[79–81] These trials showed equivalent survival but toxicity profiles favoring the carboplatin-containing regimens. Given this data, it seems justifiable to substitute carboplatin for cisplatin in the treatment of metastatic NSCLC.

The principal toxicities of the platinums include nephrotoxicity, neurotoxicity, nausea and vomiting, myelosuppression, and ototoxicity. Carboplatin has substantially less toxicity in each of these categories, with the exception of myelosuppression.

Vinblastine/Vindesine

Both of these vinca alkaloids are active single agents with response rates ranging from 11% to 28%.[82] Both agents have also been used extensively in combinations, particularly with cisplatin. Their routine use has been supplemented by the new semisynthetic vinca alkaloid, vinorelbine. In a randomized trial, vinorelbine has been shown to have a superior response rate but equivalent survival compared with vindesine.[83] The principal toxicities of the vinca alkaloids include myelosuppression, peripheral neuropathy, abdominal pain, and constipation.

Mitomycin C

Mitomycin C has significant single-agent activity in NSCLC. A review of single agent mitomycin C reported a response rate of 25% in a total of 207 evaluable patients.[84] In addition, a study of 64 patients with metastatic squamous cell carcinoma found a response rate of 30% to mitomycin C.[85] Cumulative myelosuppression is the principal toxicity. Two well known but relatively infrequent complications of mitomycin C include a thrombotic microangiopathic syndrome resembling the hemolytic-uremic syndrome and drug-induced interstitial lung disease.[86]

Etoposide

The single-agent response rate of etoposide in NSCLC, using the standard multiple day administration schedule, ranges from 5% to 15%.[87] As previously noted, the addition of cisplatin to etoposide (or teniposide) has been shown to improve response rates and survival in two different phase III trials.[70,73] Given data for small cell lung cancer suggesting that the response to etoposide may depend on the schedule of administration,[88] long-term oral etoposide has been evaluated in patients with NSCLC. A response rate of 23% was noted in 25 patients treated with 50 mg/m²/ day for 3 weeks;[89] however, a second study of 43 patients showed only a 4% response rate.[90] The principal toxicities of etoposide are myelosuppression, alopecia, and infusional orthostatic hypotension.

Ifosfamide

Ifosfamide has been evaluated extensively in NSCLC. The dose and schedule have varied dramatically. In a review of 326 evaluable patients with NSCLC treated with single-agent ifosfamide, Ettinger[91] reported a pooled response rate of 21% with a median survival of approximately 9 months. The optimal dose and schedule are not known, but no major dose response or schedule response has been suggested thus far. The principal toxicities of ifosfamide are myelosuppression, hemorrhagic cystitis, nausea and vomiting, lethargy, confusion, and alopecia.

Paclitaxel

Paclitaxel was the first identified member of a new class of anticancer drugs known as taxanes. It has significant single-agent activity against a number of solid tumors, including NSCLC. Single-agent paclitaxel has been studied using different schedules and dose levels as first-line treatment.[92] Initial studies based on a 24-hour infusion schedule using doses of 200 to 250 mg/m² resulted in response rates of 21% to 24% with median survival rates of 6 to 9 months and 1-year survival rates of 38% to 42%. The major toxicity when using this schedule was myelosuppression, primarily neutropenia. In subsequent studies based on shorter (3-hour) infusion schedules with doses of 175 to 225 mg/m², single-agent paclitaxel showed an overall response rate of 29% with a median survival of 6 to 11 months and a 1-year survival of 37% to 55%. Similar results were obtained with a 1-hour infusion schedule using doses of 135 to 200 mg/m². A phase III trial comparing single-agent paclitaxel (200 mg/m² given over 3 hours every 3 weeks) with BSC in patients with advanced or metastatic NSCLC showed a survival advantage for the paclitaxel arm versus BSC (median survival, 6.8 versus 4.8 months; $P = 0.045$).[33] The major toxicities with this schedule included neutropenia, neuropathy, and myalgia/arthralgia syndrome.

Docetaxel

At least six phase II trials have been reported documenting the activity of docetaxel in the first-line treatment of NSCLC using doses of 60 mg/m², 75 mg/m², and 100 mg/ m².[93–98] The overall response rate was 27% with a median survival of 9 months and a 1-year survival of 39%. These studies suggest that docetaxel is a highly active agent in stage III/IV NSCLC. A randomized phase III trial has shown improved survival for patients receiving docetaxel compared with those receiving BSC.[34] The principal toxicities of docetaxel include myelosuppression, asthenia, fluid retention, paresthesias, and acute hypersensitivity reaction.

Gemcitabine

Gemcitabine is a novel pyrimidine analog with unique activity against various solid tumors. In a review of phase II trials using gemcitabine as a single agent, patients with advanced NSCLC were treated with doses ranging from 800 to 1250 mg/m² weekly for 3 weeks every 28 days.[99] The overall response rate was 25% (range 18%-54%), with a median survival of 6.6 to 9.4 months and 1-year survival of 22% to 40%. Two small randomized phase II trials[100,101] have compared gemcitabine with cisplatin-etoposide. The overall response rates and survival rates were the same in both studies. Toxicity profiles in both studies favored gemcitabine.

Gemcitabine was compared with BSC in a phase III trial.[31] In this trial, gemcitabine 1000 mg/m² was given days 1, 8, and 15 on a 28-day schedule. The response rate was 17%. No survival advantage was seen compared with BSC, but QOL was superior with gemcitabine. Also, the proportion of patients requiring early intervention with palliative radiotherapy was less on the gemcitabine arm (7%) compared with the BSC arm (42%). The principal toxicities of gemcitabine include neutropenia, thrombocytopenia, nausea and vomiting, fever, and liver function abnormalities.

Irinotecan

Irinotecan is a derivative of camptothecin that inhibits the action of topoisomerase I. Phase II trials employing single-agent irinotecan have reported an overall response rate of 23% (range, 13%–32%).[102] A phase III trial compared cisplatin-vindesine, cisplatin-irinotecan, and irinotecan alone (100 mg/m² on days 1, 8, and 15).[71] The median survival on the irinotecan-alone arm was 11 months with a 1-year survival of 41% and an overall response rate of 21%. The principal toxicities of irinotecan include neutropenia, diarrhea, anemia, fatigue, and nausea and vomiting.

Vinorelbine

Vinorelbine is a semisynthetic vinca alkaloid. Four phase II trials using single-agent vinorelbine at 25 to 30 mg/m² reported an average overall response rate of 24% (range, 8%–31%), with median survival of 5 to 13 months.[103–106] Vinorelbine, at doses of 30 mg/m², has also served as a treatment arm in three phase III trials.[30,32,64] The response rate was 12% to 16%, with a 1-year survival of 25% to 30%. In two trials, single-agent vinorelbine performed as well with regard to survival as the control arms of cisplatin-vindesine[64] and cisplatin-vinorelbine.[72]

Vinorelbine was compared with BSC in elderly patients (age >70 years).[32] The response rate to vinorelbine was 20%. One-year survival with this agent was 32% compared with 14% for BSC. QOL analysis revealed consistently better scores on functional and cancer-related symptom scales for vinorelbine-treated patients compared with patients receiving BSC alone. The principal toxicities of vinorelbine include neutropenia, nausea and vomiting, peripheral neuropathy, and constipation.

Second-Generation Regimens

Prior to the development of the third-generation agents shown in Table 22–7, it was not clear whether combination regimens were superior to single agents. In a meta-analysis done by Lilenbaum et al,[107] combination chemotherapy increased objective response rates almost 2-fold compared with single-agent chemotherapy. However, toxicity was also increased, with a 3.6-fold increase in the risk of treatment-related death. Survival was moderately increased with combination chemotherapy (relative risk of survival at 1 year [RR], 1.22; 95% confidence interval [CI], 1.03-1.45). However, when a platinum analog or vinorelbine was used as a single agent, the survival benefit from combination chemotherapy was no longer significant (RR, 1.10; 95% CI, 0.94-1.43). This data suggests that with more active agents, which possess superior toxicity profiles, benefits in survival may be equivalent whether single-agent or combination chemotherapy is used. Furthermore, combination chemotherapy employing these more active agents may yield superior survival results.

Three large randomized trials were performed in the 1980s comparing both platinum-containing and non–platinum-containing regimens.[8,9,108] In addition, one trial included single-agent carboplatin and iproplatin.[9]

In the first trial, reported in 1986, four combination regimens—CAMxPz (cyclophosphamide, doxorubicin, methotrexate, procarbazine), MVbP (mitomycin C, vinblastine, cisplatin), EP (etoposide, cisplatin), and PVd (cisplatin, vindesine)—were compared in 486 patients.[8] Response rates ranged from 17% to 31%, with MVBP having the highest response rate. Overall median survival was 6 months and was not significantly different among treatments. The overall 1-year survival was 19%, with the MVbP arm having a significantly lower 1-year survival (12%) compared with the other arms (P = 0.003). In the second trial, MVbP was compared with PVb (cisplatin, vinblastine) and MVbP alternating with CAMxPz, as well as with single-agent carboplatin and iproplatin in 699 patients.[9] Response rates ranged from 6% to 20%, with MVbP once again having the highest response rate. However, single-agent carboplatin had the highest median survival, 7 months, which was significantly better than any of the other arms (P = 0.006). In the third trial, the SWOG compared EP, EP plus methylguazone (EPMg), PVb, PVb alternating with vinblastine and mitomycin C, and FVM/CAP (5-fluorouracil, vincristine, mitomycin C/cyclophosphamide, doxorubicin, cisplatin) in 680 patients.[108] Response rates ranged from 10% for FVM/CAP to 33% for EPMg. However, there was no difference in survival between the arms, and the overall median survival was 5 to 6 months.

In summary, these three large phase III randomized trials performed in the 1980s suggested that (1) there was no standard regimen, (2) response rates did not correlate with survival, (3) single agents may be equivalent to combination regimens, and (4) alternating strategies using second-generation agents provided no benefit.

Cisplatin With or Without New Agents

Before 1990, most medical oncologists used regimens consisting of cisplatin plus an epiphyllotoxin (etoposide, also known as VP-16) or vinca alkaloid (vindesine or vinblastine), despite evidence that there was no clear survival advantage for these combinations in individual trials.[109] These regimens were considered the standard of care based on survival endpoints and not necessarily on response rates. Subset analysis of collective ECOG studies from the 1980s revealed that the combination of cisplatin/etoposide yielded the highest 1-year survival rate (~25%) of all regimens tested.[110] Two trials randomized patients to cisplatin versus cisplatin/etoposide.[10,66] Although response rates were higher with cisplatin/etoposide in both studies, a survival advantage for this regimen was observed in only one study (Table 22–8).

Since 1990, several new agents with substantial activity against NSCLC and novel mechanisms of action or more favorable toxicity profiles have been developed (see Table 22–7). Many of these agents have been combined successfully with cisplatin and have been compared with cisplatin alone (see Table 22–8). All of the studies showed improved response rates, and most showed improved survival with the addition of the new agent to cisplatin alone. These studies suggest that combination therapy is superior to single-agent cisplatin therapy in advanced NSCLC. However, comparison of a platinum-based regimen that included one of the newer, more active single agents compared with the newer single agent alone has yielded conflicting results.[64,71,72]

Phase III Trials of the Platinums With New Agents

Given the number of new agents, several treatment options are currently available, with no combination regimen being

TABLE 22–8. PHASE III TRIALS OF CISPLATIN PLUS OR MINUS ETOPOSIDE OR A THIRD-GENERATION AGENT IN ADVANCED NON–SMALL CELL LUNG CANCER

STUDY	YEAR	N	NEW AGENT	RESPONSE RATE (%) Cisplatin Alone	Plus New Agent	MEDIAN SURVIVAL (mo) Cisplatin Alone	Plus New Agent	1-YEAR SURVIVAL (%) Cisplatin Alone	Plus New Agent	P
Klatersky et al[10]	1989	162	Etoposide	19	26	6.0	5.1	25	25	NS
Crino et al[66]	1990	156	Etoposide	4	30	4.2	8.5	—	—	0.001
Sandler et al[61]	2000	520	Gemcitabine	11	30	7.6	9.1	26	39	0.004
Gatzemeier et al[68]	1998	414	Paclitaxel	17	26	8.6	8.1	35	30	NS
von Pawel et al[69]	2000	446	Tirapazamine	4	28	6.4	8.0	21	33	0.008
Wozniak et al[67]	1998	415	Vinorelbine	12	26	6.0	8.0	20	36	0.0018
Average				**11**	**28**	**6.4**	**7.8**	**25**	**33**	

Inclusion criteria: Trials comparing cisplatin alone in the control arm with cisplatin plus etoposide or plus a third-generation agent.

TABLE 22–9. RANDOMIZED PHASE III TRIALS INVOLVING THIRD-GENERATION AGENTS IN COMBINATION REGIMENS IN ADVANCED NON–SMALL CELL LUNG CANCER

AUTHOR	YEAR	N	REGIMEN		RESPONSE RATE (%)		MEDIAN SURVIVAL (mo)		1-y SURVIVAL (%)		P
			Control	Invest	Control	Invest	Control	Invest	Control	Invest	
Le Chevalier et al[64][a]	1994	612[a]	PVd	PN	19	30	7.4	9.3	27	35	0.04
Le Chevalier et al[64][a]	1994	612[a]	PVd	N	19	14	7.4	7.2	27	30	NS
Depierre et al[72]	1994	365	PN	N	43	16	7.7	7.4	26	22	NS
Kelly et al[111]	1999	408	PN	CbTx	27	27	8.0	8.0	33	36	NS
Belani et al[59]	1998	369	EP	CbTx	14	22	8.0	8.2	37	32	NS
Bonomi et al[57][a]	2000	560[a]	EP	PTx	13	25	7.6	9.5	32	37	< 0.05[b]
Bonomi et al[57][a]	2000	560[a]	EP	PTx + GCSF	13	28	7.6	10.1	32	40	< 0.05[b]
Giaccone et al[58]	1998	312	PT	PTx	28	41	9.9	9.7	41	43	NS
Cardenal et al[115]	1999	135	PE	PG	22	41	7.2	8.7	25	32	NS
Crinò et al[60][a]	1999	307	PIM	PG	26	38	9.6	8.6	—	—	NS
Masuda et al[71][a]	1999	398[a]	PVd	PIr	31	43	11.0	11.7	40	49	NS
Masuda et al[71][a]	1999	398[a]	PVd	Ir	31	21	11.0	10.8	40	44	NS
Niho et al[116]	1999	210	PVd	PIr	22	29	11.5	10.6	—	—	NS

Inclusion criteria: Randomized phase III trials reported in which a third-generation agent was included in the control or investigational arm of the study.
[a]3-arm trial.
[b]For both PTx arms considered together versus EP.
Control, control or standard arm of the trial; GCSF, granulocyte colony-stimulating factor; Invest, new or investigational arm of the study.
Chemotherapy regimens: CbTx, carboplatin, paclitaxel; Ir, irinotecan; N, vinorelbine; PE, cisplatin, etoposide; PG, cisplatin, gemcitabine; PIM, cisplatin, ifosfamide, mitomycin C; PIr, cisplatin, irinotecan; PN, cisplatin, vinorelbine; PT, cisplatin, teniposide; PTx, cisplatin, paclitaxel; PVd, cisplatin, vindesine.

clearly superior to another. Current phase III data shows that one combination regimen is often superior to another based on at least one endpoint of interest (ie, response rate, toxicity, QOL, or survival).

Vinorelbine was the first new agent to demonstrate improved activity against NSCLC, both alone and combined with cisplatin (Table 22–9). Six major phase III trials using this agent have been reported. Two trials compared vinorelbine with either BSC[32] or ineffective chemotherapy[30] and showed a survival advantage for vinorelbine. Two trials used vinorelbine alone versus cisplatin/vinorelbine,[64,72] one of which included a third arm using cisplatin/vindesine.[64] The addition of vinorelbine to cisplatin improved response rates compared with vinorelbine alone, but survival results were mixed. Of importance, vinorelbine alone was equivalent to cisplatin/vindesine; however, both regimens were inferior to cisplatin/vinorelbine. This finding again suggests that the new agents offer superior survival results, either alone or combined with a platinum. A SWOG study found that the regimen of cisplatin/vinorelbine was equivalent to carboplatin/paclitaxel with regard to response rate and survival.[111] Finally, the addition of vinorelbine to cisplatin improved survival compared with cisplatin alone.[67]

Several phase III trials have evaluated the effect of paclitaxel in combination with either cisplatin or carboplatin (see Table 22–9). Only one trial showed clearly positive results regarding a survival benefit.[57] However, three trials showed significantly improved response rates when paclitaxel combined with either cisplatin or carboplatin was compared with second-generation regimens.[57–59] The SWOG study just mentioned revealed equivalent response and survival rates with carboplatin/paclitaxel and cisplatin/vinorelbine.[111] Two trials showed improved QOL scores for those patients receiving the paclitaxel-containing regimens.[58,59] The one trial that showed a survival benefit[57] used paclitaxel as a 24-hour infusion, whereas all others used the 3-hour infusion schedule. The

optimal infusion schedule for paclitaxel is not known, and all infusion schedules appear active in the phase II trials reported to date.[92] However, a breast cancer study demonstrated that infusion duration does have an impact on response rates.[112] Whether this is also true in lung cancer and whether or not it could have an impact on survival are not known.

In addition to infusion schedules, the issue of dose is also in question. The ECOG trial did not show a difference in survival when paclitaxel was given at 135 mg/m[2] and at 250 mg/m[2] on the 24-hour infusion schedule.[57] Both of these arms were superior to the cisplatin/etoposide control arm. In contrast, a Greek trial comparing a paclitaxel dose of 225 mg/m[2] with a dose of 175 mg/m[2] on the 3-hour infusion schedule (in combination with carboplatin) showed improved median time to progression (4.3 months versus 6.4 months; $P = 0.044$) and median survival (9.5 months versus 11.4 months; $P = 0.16$) for the 225 mg/m[2] dose.[113] Although it is difficult to interpret this data, it is clear that more studies are needed to determine the optimal dose and schedule of paclitaxel. This is particularly evident when one looks at studies using weekly dose-dense schedules of paclitaxel,[114] which show response and survival rates superior to what has been reported with the traditional every-3-week administration schedule.

These trials have also raised the issue of second-line treatment having an impact on survival. The ECOG trial was carried out before the commercial availability of paclitaxel; therefore, patients on the control arm could not be crossed over to paclitaxel or any other taxane.[57] The other trials were carried out after paclitaxel became commercially available, and second-line treatment with a taxane has been raised as an issue that may have obscured a survival difference in the analysis of the impact of first-line treatment. In one trial, there was a clear suggestion that patients who received a second-line taxane after receiving cisplatin/etoposide as first-line treatment had improved survival compared with patients who did not receive a second-line taxane.[59] Also, the 1-year survival (37%) of the cisplatin/etoposide arm of that study was the best 1-year survival ever reported for that regimen. None of these studies was initially designed to address the impact of second-line treatment, and this confounding variable therefore remains conjectural.

Gemcitabine was initially studied in two randomized phase II trials comparing gemcitabine with the combination of cisplatin/etoposide.[100,101] In both trials, single-agent gemcitabine appeared equivalent to the combination of cisplatin/etoposide with regard to response and survival rates. However, the randomized phase II format prohibited direct comparison between the arms, and both of these trials enrolled very small numbers of patients (53 in one, 146 in the other). In a subsequent phase III trial, the combination of cisplatin/gemcitabine proved superior to cisplatin/etoposide based on the response rate, which was the main endpoint of this study, although overall survival was similar.[115] In another phase III trial, the combination of cisplatin/gemcitabine did not appear to improve survival compared with the combination of mitomycin C, ifosfamide, and cisplatin.[60] The only other phase III comparison of the combination of cisplatin/gemcitabine has been with cisplatin alone (see Table 22–8), which demonstrated that the addition of gemcitabine to cisplatin proved superior to cisplatin alone.[61]

Only two trials have been reported to date examining the impact of irinotecan in the phase III setting. In one trial, irinotecan alone was compared with cisplatin/irinotecan and cisplatin/vindesine.[71] The trial design was similar to the design used in the vinorelbine trial reported by Le Chevalier et al.[64] In fact, the results were also similar. The response rate to cisplatin/irinotecan was 43% versus 20% for single-agent irinotecan and 31% for cisplatin/vindesine. However, survival on all three arms was good, with 1-year survival of 49%, 44%, and 40% for cisplatin/irinotecan, single-agent irinotecan, and cisplatin/vindesine, respectively. A second phase III trial found no difference in survival between cisplatin/vindesine and cisplatin/irinotecan.[116]

What should one conclude from the available phase III trial data regarding the optimal chemotherapy regimen for treatment of advanced NSCLC? The obvious conclusion is that there is not one clearly superior regimen. In general, the new third-generation agents (see Table 22–7) in combination with cisplatin improve response rates compared with cisplatin alone or cisplatin plus an older agent (etoposide, vindesine, ifosfamide). Although the response rate may not be the most important endpoint, it still is important because responders are likely to survive longer, experience relief of disease-related symptoms, and presumably have improved QOL.[58,59] It is not always clear that the new agents in combination with cisplatin improve survival when compared with older regimens. Some studies suggest they do[57,64,71]; however, several other trials have failed to show this finding.[58–60,72,115]

SECOND-LINE CHEMOTHERAPY IN NON–SMALL CELL LUNG CANCER

The concept of second-line chemotherapy has only recently been tested in phase III trials. Before these reports, the overall role of second-line treatment of patients with NSCLC whose disease progressed after first-line treatment was unclear. Probably most telling of the experiences of the 1980s was the ECOG trial, which randomized patients with advanced NSCLC to either three cisplatin-containing combination regimens, single-agent carboplatin, or single-agent iproplatin.[9] In the design of that trial, patients treated with single-agent carboplatin who developed progressive disease were supposed to receive the combination regimen of mitomycin C, vinblastine, and cisplatin (MVP). Only 50% of the patients whose disease progressed after first-line carboplatin received MVP as second-line treatment. The explanation for this was not given, but many of the patients undoubtedly had a worsening PS that precluded further treatment. The response rate to second-line MVP was 6% versus 20% when MVP was used as first-line therapy in that same study. This underscores the refractory nature of NSCLC once it has progressed after first-line treatment. Finally, survival of patients on the single-agent carboplatin arm of the study was the same regardless of whether or not patients received second-line MVP.

One of the difficulties in interpreting data regarding the impact of second-line treatment in advanced NSCLC is the lack of sufficient information on the population of patients entered onto these trials. It is also not clear what proportion of patients whose disease progresses after first-line treatment receive second-line treatment. In a recent phase III trial, only 18% to 27% of patients received second-line treatment after failing first-line treatment.[61] As noted earlier in this chapter, a number of prognostic factors for first-line chemotherapy have been defined. However, prognostic factors in the second-line setting are not necessarily known. It seems intuitive that the major prognostic factor (performance status) in the first-line setting would also be important in the second-line setting. What is often lacking is first-line response information because disease sensitivity in the first-line setting may well predict a second-line response.[117] The duration of the first-line response is also usually not reported. It would also seem intuitive that patients who have a prolonged progression-free interval (>3 months) after first-line treatment would more likely benefit from second-line treatment, as is true in patients with small cell lung cancer.[118] It is also not clear what proportion of patients are truly cisplatin refractory versus cisplatin exposed when they receive second-line treatment.

Almost all of the new agents have been studied in the second-line setting as single agents.[119,120] The population of patients entered onto these phase II studies has varied, and many of the issues just discussed are apparent when reviewing this literature. From these studies, it appears that certain agents (docetaxel, gemcitabine, and paclitaxel) have notable activity in the second-line setting,[117,119–122] whereas other agents (vinorelbine, ifosfamide) have less encouraging activity. However, one cannot draw firm conclusions about the impact of second-line treatment from phase II studies.

Two phase III trials have suggested a benefit to second-line treatment (Table 22–10).[123,124] One trial randomized patients with recurrent NSCLC to one of two dose levels of docetaxel (75 mg/m² or 100 mg/m²) versus either ifosfamide or vinorelbine (investigator's choice).[123] All patients had received prior cisplatin-based chemotherapy, and ap-

TABLE 22–10. RANDOMIZED PHASE III TRIALS OF SECOND LINE CHEMOTHERAPY IN ADVANCED NON–SMALL CELL LUNG CANCER

	FOSSELLA ET AL[95]			SHEPHERD ET AL[124]		
	Docetaxel (100 mg/m²)	Docetaxel (75 mg/m²)	Vinorelbine or Ifosfamide	Docetaxel (100 mg/m²)	Docetaxel (75 mg/m²)	BSC
N	125	125	123[a]	49	55	100
Median age	60	59	60	61	61	61
ECOG PS 0,1 (%)	83	82	85	78	74	76
Stage IV (%)	86	90	91	82	73	81
Response rate (%)	12[b]	7.5[c]	1	6.3	5.5	—
Median survival (mo)	5.5	5.7	5.6	5.9	7.5[e]	4.6
1-y survival (%)	21	32[d]	19	19	37[f]	19

Inclusion criteria: Randomized phase III trials addressing the value of second-line chemotherapy in advanced NSCLC.
[a] 89 treated with vinorelbine, 34 with ifosfamide.
[b] $P = 0.001$ versus vinorelbine/ifosfamide, using Fisher's Exact test.
[c] $P = 0.036$ versus vinorelbine/ifosfamide, using Fisher's Exact test.
[d] $P = 0.025$ versus vinorelbine/ifosfamide, chi-square test.
[e] $P = 0.01$ for docetaxel 75 mg/m² versus BSC, chi-square test.
[f] $P = 0.003$ for docetaxel 75 mg/m² versus BSC, log rank test.
BSC, best supportive care; ECOG PS, Eastern Cooperative Oncology Group performance status.

proximately one-third of patients had received a prior taxane. The response rate for docetaxel in the second-line setting was 7% to 12%, notably lower than the activity of this agent in the first-line setting (see Table 22–7). Early results suggested a modest survival benefit that was observed only on the lower dose arm of docetaxel (75 mg/m²). In the analysis of that study, patients were censored at the time of third-line treatment, and it was suggested that survival may have been influenced by third-line chemotherapy. Also, survival was not affected by prior taxane exposure. The fact that nearly all taxane-exposed patients had received paclitaxel as their previous taxane suggests some degree of cross-resistance, but insufficient data is provided regarding the first-line paclitaxel response and subsequent response to second-line docetaxel.

In the second trial, patients who failed to benefit from prior platinum-based chemotherapy and were taxane naive were initially randomized to receive 100 mg/m² of docetaxel or BSC alone.[124] That dose of docetaxel was too toxic, and patients received a median of only two cycles. The study was amended by decreasing the docetaxel dose to 75 mg/m². At 75 mg/m², a median of four cycles was delivered. Analysis of all patients failed to show a significant survival benefit for docetaxel. However, when only the patients treated with docetaxel at 75 mg/m² were compared with patients receiving BSC, a significant survival advantage was noted with docetaxel. Both of these trials measured QOL in the second-line setting, and both analyses suggested improved QOL with docetaxel.[125,126]

Taken together, these two phase III trials provide insight into the second-line treatment of recurrent NSCLC. Both trials suggest a modest survival benefit that appears statistically significant. They also highlight the fact that some chemotherapy agents (ifosfamide, vinorelbine) and even effective agents used at intolerable doses (docetaxel at 100 mg/m²) do not benefit patients in the second-line setting. Given the effect of second-line treatment, trials using survival as an endpoint for first-line treatment must now control for or at least report what second-line treatment is given to the patients entered into these studies. It also

leaves open the fact that recently reported negative trials may have been influenced by this variable, particularly those trials in which first-line treatment included a nontaxane arm followed by possible crossover to a taxane-containing second-line regimen.

DURATION OF THERAPY IN ADVANCED NON–SMALL CELL LUNG CANCER

The optimal duration of therapy in patients with advanced NSCLC has not been defined. The palliative effect of treatment (ie, prolongation of survival, relief of symptoms, and improved QOL) is offset by toxicity; however, the number of chemotherapy courses that maximizes the impact of chemotherapy on these endpoints has not been studied adequately. In more recent trials of combination chemotherapy, the typical median number of cisplatin- or carboplatin-based chemotherapy cycles delivered is approximately three to four.[59,60,64,111] The reasons that patients do not continue on therapy are not typically reported. Potential reasons for discontinuing therapy include progression of disease, intolerable toxicity, attainment of what is believed to be a maximum response, and patient refusal or death. Now that it is known that second-line treatment may have an impact on survival, the role of subsequent treatment and its impact on survival and palliation of symptoms must be accounted for when defining the optimal duration of therapy.

Surprisingly, few studies have addressed the issue of duration in the palliative treatment of patients with advanced NSLCL. Buccheri et al[127] reported a trial involving 74 patients with advanced NSCLC who had stable disease following two to three cycles of non–cisplatin-based chemotherapy. These patients were subsequently randomized to continue chemotherapy with *MACC* (methotrexate, doxorubicin, cyclophosphamide, CCNU) or to stop treatment. The median survival of patients randomized to continued chemotherapy arm was improved by 50% compared with the observation arm (11 versus 7 months). However, this was not statistically significant because of the small number of patients.

After observing that the major palliative effort of chemotherapy on disease-related symptoms occurred during the first three cycles of treatment, Smith et al[128] randomized patients with advanced NSCLC to either three or six cycles of mitomycin C, vinblastine, and cisplatin (MVbP).[128] There did not appear to be any benefit to delivering six rather than three cycles of MVbP. The overall objective response rates (32% for three cycles versus 37% for six cycles) and symptomatic response rates (65% for three cycles versus 75% for six cycles) were equivalent. The median survival for patients receiving three cycles was 6.8 months versus 7.0 months for those receiving six cycles. The 1-year survival was 23% in both arms of the study.

These two studies do not provide conclusive evidence to make a firm recommendation regarding the optimal duration of treatment in advanced NSCLC. From this data, it does appear that a prolonged duration of treatment is not warranted. However, these studies do not address the potential benefit to the select subset of patients who may have continued evidence of tumor shrinkage or stabilization and exceptional tolerance to therapy. This is the focus of an ongoing randomized phase III trial in which patients with advanced NSCLC are randomized to receive either four cycles of carboplatin/paclitaxel or continued treatment with carboplatin/paclitaxel until objective tumor progression or intolerable toxicity occurs (Fig. 22–4). The primary endpoints of this trial are survival and QOL. Completion of the trial will add further information about the optimal duration of treatment in this setting. For now, it seems reasonable to recommend four to six cycles of treatment in the first-line setting as standard therapy. However, the recommendation is empiric, and insufficient data exists to firmly define the optimal duration of therapy. In their practice guidelines, the American Society of Clinical Oncology notes this lack of sufficient data and recommends no more than eight cycles in the first-line setting.[129]

TOXICITY

The impact of chemotherapy on survival and palliation of symptoms in patients with stage IV NSCLC is potentially

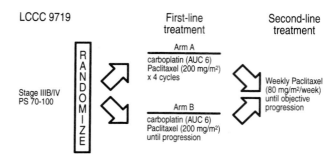

FIGURE 22–4. Schema of Lineberger Comprehensive Cancer Center trial 9719.

offset by its toxicity. The reporting of toxicity is usually divided into hematologic and nonhematologic categories and graded by one of several grading systems (see Chapter 10). Some toxicities are relatively objective, relying mainly on the results of a laboratory test (eg, complete blood count), whereas others are more subjective, relying on a patient's report of how severe particular symptoms are (eg, nausea, vomiting, or both). The impact that these toxicities have on a particular patient as experienced by the patient theoretically should be captured on QOL measurements. As discussed earlier in this chapter, QOL is generally improved as a result of chemotherapy, suggesting that the benefits of chemotherapy generally outweigh the toxicity.[29,32,58]

Table 22–11 summarizes toxicity reporting from several of the more recent phase III trials. The trials included in this table utilized regimens that are considered standard, including cisplatin/paclitaxel,[58] carboplatin/paclitaxel,[59] cisplatin/vinorelbine,[64] and cisplatin/gemcitabine.[60,61] The major types of toxicity are neutropenia and thrombocytopenia. Despite this, sepsis and febrile neutropenia occur in only a small percentage of patients. Serious nonhematologic toxicity occurs in only a minority of patients. Toxicity is responsible for treatment discontinuation in 8% to 30% of patients.[64,111] Treatment-related death occurs in 1% to 4% of patients and is related mainly to sepsis in the setting of neutropenia.[58–60,64]

DATA SUMMARY: ROLE OF CHEMOTHERAPY IN STAGE IV NON–SMALL CELL LUNG CANCER	AMOUNT	QUALITY	CONSISTENCY
Chemotherapy prolongs survival in patients with stage IV NSCLC	**High**	**High**	**High**
Performance status is the most important prognostic factor for survival	High	High	High
Chemotherapy can effectively palliate symptoms and improve QOL in patients with advanced NSCLC	Mod	Mod	High
Delivery of chemotherapy in patients with advanced NSCLC is cost effective	Mod	High	High
Cisplatin plus a third generation agent improves survival compared with cisplatin alone	**High**	**High**	**High**
Survival is not substantially improved with third-generation agents versus second-generation agents	**High**	**High**	**Mod**
Chemotherapy can improve survival and QOL as second-line treatment for advanced NSCLC	**Mod**	**Mod**	**High**

Type of data rated: Plain text: descriptive statement   *Italics: controlled comparison*   **Bold: randomized comparison**

TABLE 22–11. INCIDENCE OF GRADE 3,4 TOXICITY OF CHEMOTHERAPY IN ADVANCED NON–SMALL CELL LUNG CANCER[a]

TOXICITY	LE CHEVALIER ET AL[64]		CRINÒ ET AL[60]		BELANI ET AL[59]		GIACONNE ET AL[58]	SANDLER ET AL[61]	
	NP	N	GP	MIP	EP	CbTx	PTx	P	GP
Neutropenia	79	53	50	34	29	23	55	5	57
Thrombocytopenia	3	0	64	28	—	—	2	4	50
Sepsis/febrile neutropenia	4	3	1	0	8	4	3	1	5
Neuropathy	7	9	1	1	1	16	9	8	17
Nausea/vomiting	58	12	18	22	10	4	—	40	50
Diarrhea	11	4	1	0	3	1	—	1	4
Alopecia	32	14	12	34	—	—	>50[b]	—	—
Renal	6	0	1	1	—	—	—	2	5
Hepatic	1	1	2	2	—	—	—	2	5

Inclusion criteria: Recent phase III trials reporting toxicity of commonly used regimens in advanced non–small cell lung cancer.
[a]Numbers represent percentage of patients experiencing grade 3 or 4 toxicity.
[b]Reported as occurring in the "majority of patients."
Chemotherapy regimens: CbTx, carboplatin, paclitaxel; EP, etoposide, cisplatin; GP, gemcitabine, cisplatin; MIP, mitomycin C, ifosfamide, cisplatin; N, vinorelbine; NP, vinorelbine, cisplatin; PTx, cisplatin, paclitaxel.

EDITORS' COMMENTS

The available data discussed in this chapter shows that chemotherapy has a positive impact on the course of stage IV NSCLC. The impact is manifested by prolongation of survival and palliation of symptoms, which presumably improve the patient's overall QOL. The benefit is restricted to patients who have a good PS (ie, ambulatory, minimally symptomatic patients). Selection of patients for chemotherapy is still the most important aspect in the overall impact of treatment of stage IV NSCLC. This allows one to avoid treating patients with a poor PS who do not benefit from treatment and are more likely to suffer toxicity. It is hoped that, in the future, prognostic factors will be refined and individual predictors of response to specific therapies will be identified, allowing better selection of therapies for individual patients.

It also seems evident that the progress made has reached a plateau. In all the trials discussed, the median survival ranges from 8 to 10 months. The questions that seem appropriate at this time are:

1. Is there a standard of care?
2. Are the platinums still necessary?
3. Are active single agents as effective as combination regimens?
4. Are non-platinum doublets superior to platinum doublets?
5. Should triplet regimens be explored (platinum-based or non–platinum-based)?
6. How will the next generation of "fourth-generation" agents be integrated into the management of stage IV NSCLC?
7. What duration of therapy optimizes its impact on survival and QOL?
8. Can we expand the population of patients we treat by using less toxic single agents in patients with a poor PS?
9. Will alternating or sequential strategies with third-generation agents improve survival?
10. What is the optimal strategy now that the data suggests that second-line therapy can alter survival?

At this time, there is no one standard regimen. Current phase III data suggests that a platinum (cisplatin or carboplatin) in combination with one of the new agents (paclitaxel, gemcitabine, vinorelbine, irinotecan) represents a reasonable standard in the care of these patients. All of these regimens have been tested in the phase III setting and have been shown to be superior on the basis of either response rate, QOL assessment, toxicity profile, or survival. Ongoing phase III trials will continue to refine the standard of care and identify regimens that should be compared in future trials.

As noted in this chapter, cisplatin was the first agent to conclusively prolong survival in patients with this disease. Although direct comparative data is relatively scant, carboplatin appears equivalent to cisplatin in treating stage IV NSCLC, but has a much superior toxicity profile. Because the platinums have been so important in treating this disease, we must have data from appropriately designed phase III trials that documents that non-platinum treatment regimens yield equivalent survival results before we can omit the platinums from standard treatment regimens. Such trials are ongoing, and data regarding the role of the platinums will become available in the next 2 to 3 years.

The reason why the role of the platinums is even being addressed is that several new agents with substantial single-agent activity have been developed and integrated into the care of patients. Given this, some investigators have explored single agents in the management of stage IV NSCLC. The Cancer and Leukemia Group B (CALGB) is comparing the combination of carboplatin/paclitaxel versus paclitaxel alone. The primary outcomes of interest in this study are survival and QOL. In this trial, the single agent paclitaxel is being delivered on a conventional every-3-week administration schedule. However, this may not be the most active schedule. Akerley et al[114] have reported a single-agent response rate of 40% for weekly dose-dense paclitaxel. The use of single agents that have toxicity profiles superior to the platinums may allow therapy to be delivered to populations of patients who do not benefit from platinum-based therapies. This would include patients with a marginal PS in whom cytotoxic therapy could be of benefit either by enhancing survival or by simply palliating symptoms. Non-platinum doublets are also reasonable regimens to be tested. Initial phase II trials suggest activity and survival results at least equivalent to traditional platinum-based regimens.[130] Triplet regimens, either platinum or non–platinum based, have also shown impressive results in phase I/II trials thus far.[131,132] However, concerns about excessive toxicity are real and should be addressed in randomized phase III trials.

Although the data is limited, there is a suggestion that second-line treatment may have an impact on survival and QOL. This raises issues regarding the optimal strategy in managing this incurable stage of the disease. With the goal of prolonging survival and improving overall QOL, the initial duration of therapy that optimizes this goal remains uncertain, particularly when many patients may be eligible for second-line therapies. Ongoing clinical trials will help define this issue (see Fig. 22–4). More research is needed to determine the impact of second-line therapies and to define which patients benefit from which therapies, as well as how previous treatments predict benefit from subsequent treatments.

Several new "fourth-generation" classes of agents with novel mechanisms of action are being developed. These include antiangiogenic agents, farnesyl transferase inhibitors, matrix metalloproteinase inhibitors, proteosome inhibitors, and antigrowth factor monoclonal antibodies. These agents are undergoing clinical development and will be studied in patients with NSCLC. The appropriate endpoints for these studies need to be defined because none of these new agents is likely to cure the disease and many exert only a cytostatic effect. Whether these new agents will be added to conventional chemotherapy regimens or used as adjunctive therapy needs to be defined. Thoughtful questions based on preclinical data should be addressed in appropriately designed phase III trials. For instance, preclinical data suggests that a combination of cisplatin and gemcitabine may be more active against NSCLC tumors that overexpress $p185^{neu}$, the protein product of *HER2/neu*.[133] The possibility that the combination of cisplatin/gemcitabine with trastuzumab is superior to cisplatin/gemcitabine alone would be a rational trial design, based on this preclinical data. Without a logical approach, the possibilities for study are endless. However, our resources are not, and we must move the field forward with intelligent concepts that address clinically relevant issues.

References

1. Albain KS, Crowley JJ, LeBlanc M, et al. Survival determinants in extensive-stage non–small-cell lung cancer: the Southwest Oncology Group Experience. J Clin Oncol. 1991;9:1618–1626.
2. Luketich JD, Martini N, Ginsberg RJ, et al. Successful treatment of solitary extracranial metastases from non–small cell lung cancer. Ann Thorac Surg. 1995;60:1609–1611.
3. Ferguson MK. Diagnosing and staging of non–small cell lung cancer. Hematol Oncol Clin North Am. 1990;4:1053–1068.
4. Lanzotti VJ, Thomas DR, Boyle LE, et al. Survival with inoperable lung cancer: an integration of prognostic variables based on simple clinical criteria. Cancer. 1977;39:303–313.
5. Stanley KE. Prognostic factors for survival in patients with inoperable lung cancer. J Natl Cancer Inst. 1980;65:25–32.
6. O'Connell JP, Kris MG, Gralla RJ, et al. Frequency and prognostic importance of pretreatment clinical characteristics in patients with advanced non–small-cell lung cancer treated with combination chemotherapy. J Clin Oncol. 1986;4:1604–1614.
7. Finkelstein DM, Ettinger DS, Ruckdeschel JC. Long-term survivors in metastatic non–small-cell lung cancer: an Eastern Cooperative Oncology Group study. J Clin Oncol. 1986;4:702–709.
8. Ruckdeschel JC, Finkelstein DM, Ettinger DS, et al. A randomized trial of the four most active regimens for metastatic non–small-cell lung cancer. J Clin Oncol. 1986;4:14–22.
9. Bonomi PD, Finkelstein DM, Ruckdeschel JC, et al. Combination chemotherapy versus single agents followed by combination chemotherapy in stage IV non–small-cell lung cancer: a study of the Eastern Cooperative Oncology Group. J Clin Oncol. 1989;7:1602–1613.
10. Klastersky J, Sculier JP, Bureau G, et al. Cisplatin versus cisplatin plus etoposide in the treatment of advanced non–small-cell lung cancer. J Clin Oncol. 1989;7:1087–1092.
11. Luedke DW, Einhorn L, Omura GA, et al. Randomized comparison of two combination regimens versus minimal chemotherapy in non-small-cell lung cancer: a Southeastern Cancer Study Group Trial. J Clin Oncol. 1990;8:886–891.
12. Miller TP, Chen TT, Coltman CA, et al. Effect of alternating combination chemotherapy on survival of ambulatory patients with metastatic large cell and adenocarcinoma of the lung: a Southwest Oncology Group Study. J Clin Oncol. 1986;4:502–508.
13. Johnson DH, Zhu J, Schiller J, et al. E1594—a randomized phase III trial in metastatic non–small cell lung cancer (NSCLC): outcome of PS 2 patients (Pts). An Eastern Cooperative Group Trial (ECOG) [abstract]. Proc ASCO. 1999;18:461a.
14. Livingston RB. Treatment of advanced non–small cell lung cancer: the Southwest Oncology Group experience. Semin Oncol. 1988;15(suppl):37–41.
15. Livingston RB. Current management of unresectable non–small cell lung cancer. Semin Oncol. 1994;21:4–13.
16. Donnadieu N, Paesmans M, Sculier J-P. Chemotherapy of non–small cell lung cancer according to disease extent: a meta-analysis of the literature. Lung Cancer. 1991;7:243–252.
17. Bonomi P, Kim C, Kugler K, et al. Results of a phase III trial comparing taxol-cisplatin (TC) regimens to etoposide-cisplatin (EC) in non–small cell lung cancer (NSCLC) [abstract]. Lung Cancer. 1997;18(suppl):10.
18. The Non-Small Cell Lung Cancer Collaborative Group. Chemotherapy in non–small cell lung cancer: a meta-analysis using updated data on individual patients from 52 randomised clinical trials. BMJ. 1995;311:899–909.
19. Cormier Y, Bergeron D, La Forge J, et al. Benefits of polychemotherapy in advanced non–small-cell bronchogenic carcinoma. Cancer. 1982;50:845–849.
20. Buccheri G, Ferrigno D, Rosso A, et al. Further evidence in favour of chemotherapy for inoperable non–small cell lung cancer. Lung Cancer. 1990;6:87–98.
21. Rapp E, Pater JL, Willan A, et al. Chemotherapy can prolong survival in patients with advanced non–small-cell lung cancer—report of a Canadian multicenter randomized trial. J Clin Oncol. 1988;6:633–641.
22. Quoix E, Dietemann A, Charbonneau J, et al. La chimiothérapie comportant du cisplatine est elle utile dans le cancer bronchique non microcellulaire au stade IV? Resultats d'une étude randomisée. Bull Cancer. 1991;78:341–346.
23. Ganz PA, Figlin RA, Haskell CM, et al. Supportive care versus supportive care and combination chemotherapy in metastatic non–small cell lung cancer. Cancer. 1989;63:1271–1278.
24. Woods RL, Williams CJ, Levi J, et al. A randomised trial of cisplatin and vindesine versus supportive care only in advanced non–small cell lung cancer. Br J Cancer. 1990;61:608–611.
25. Cellerino R, Tummarello D, Guidi F, et al. A randomized trial of alternating chemotherapy versus best supportive care in advanced non–small-cell lung cancer. J Clin Oncol. 1991;9:1453–1461.
26. Kaasa S, Lund E, Thorud E, et al. Symptomatic treatment versus combination chemotherapy for patients with extensive non–small cell lung cancer. Cancer. 1991;67:2443–2447.
27. Cartei G, Cartei F, Cantone A, et al. Cisplatin-cyclophosphamide-mitomycin combination chemotherapy with supportive care versus supportive care alone for treatment of metastatic non–small-cell lung cancer. J Natl Cancer Inst. 1993;85:794–800.
28. Thongprasert S, Sanguanmitra P, Juthapan N, et al. Relationship between quality of life and clinical outcomes in advanced non–small cell lung cancer: best supportive care (BSC) versus BSC plus chemotherapy. Lung Cancer. 1999;24:17–24.

29. Cullen MH, Billingham LJ, Woodroffe CM, et al. Mitomycin, ifosfamide, and cisplatin in unresectable non–small-cell lung cancer: effects on survival and quality of life. J Clin Oncol. 1999;17:3188–3194.

30. Crawford J, O'Rourke M, Schiller JH, et al. Randomized trial of vinorelbine compared with fluorouracil plus leucovorin in patients with stage IV non–small-cell lung cancer. J Clin Oncol. 1996;14:2774–2784.

31. Anderson H, Cottier B, Nicolson M, et al. Phase III study of gemcitabine (Gemzar) versus best supportive care (BSC) in advanced non–small cell lung cancer (NSCLC) [abstract]. Lung Cancer. 1997;18(suppl 1):9.

32. The Elderly Lung Cancer Vinorelbine Italian Study (ELVIS) Group. Effects of vinorelbine on quality of life and survival in elderly patients with advanced non–small-cell lung cancer. J Natl Cancer Inst. 1999;91:66–72.

33. Thatcher N, Ranson M, Anderson H, et al. Phase III study of paclitaxel (Taxol)(T) versus best supportive care (BSC) in inoperable non–small cell lung cancer (NSCLC) [abstract]. Ann Oncol. 1998;9(suppl 4):1.

34. Roszkowski K, Pluzanska A, Krzakowski M, et al. A multicenter, randomized phase III study of docetaxel plus best supportive care versus best supportive care in chemotherapy-naive patients with metastatic or non-resectable localized non–small cell lung cancer (NSCLC). Lung Cancer. 2000;27:145–157.

35. Souquet PJ, Chauvin F, Boissel JP, et al. Polychemotherapy in advanced non–small cell lung cancer: a meta-analysis. Lancet. 1993;342:19–21.

36. Marino P, Pampallona S, Preatoni A, et al. Chemotherapy vs supportive care in advanced non–small-cell lung cancer: results of a meta-analysis of the literature. Chest. 1994;106:861–865.

37. Grilli R, Oxman AD, Julian JA. Chemotherapy for advanced non–small-cell lung cancer: how much benefit is enough? J Clin Oncol. 1993;11:1866–1872.

38. Le Chevalier T. Chemotherapy for advanced NSCLC: will meta-analysis provide the answer? Chest. 1996;109:107S–109S.

39. Hollen PJ, Gralla RJ, Kris MG, et al. Quality of life assessment in individuals with lung cancer: testing the Lung Cancer Symptom Scale (LCSS). Eur J Cancer. 1993;29A(suppl 1):S51–S58.

40. Osoba D, Rusthoven JJ, Turnbull KA, et al. Combination chemotherapy with bleomycin, etoposide, and cisplatin in metastatic non–small-cell lung cancer. J Clin Oncol. 1985;3:1478–1485.

41. Fernandez C, Rosell R, Abad-Esteve A, et al. Quality of life during chemotherapy in non–small cell lung cancer patients. Acta Oncol. 1989;28:29–33.

42. Ellis PA, Smith IE, Hardy JR, et al. Symptom relief with MVP (mitomycin C, vinblastine and cisplatin) chemotherapy in advanced non–small-cell lung cancer. Br J Cancer. 1995;71:366–370.

43. Hardy JR, Noble T, Smith IE. Symptom relief with moderate dose chemotherapy (mitomycin-C, vinblastine and cisplatin) in advanced non–small-cell lung cancer. Br J Cancer. 1989;60:764–766.

44. Cullen MH, Joshi R, Chetiyawardana AD, et al. Mitomycin, ifosfamide and cis-platin in non–small cell lung cancer: treatment good enough to compare. Br J Cancer. 1988;58:359–361.

45. Tummarello D, Graziano F, Isidori P, et al. Symptomatic, stage IV, non–small-cell lung cancer (NSCLC): response, toxicity, performance status change and symptom relief in patients treated with cisplatin, vinblastine and mitomycin-C. Cancer Chemother Pharmacol. 1995;35:249–253.

46. Thatcher N, Anderson H, Betticher DC, et al. Symptomatic benefit from gemcitabine and other chemotherapy in advanced non–small cell lung cancer: changes in performance status and tumour-related symptoms. Anticancer Drugs. 1995;6(suppl 6):39–48.

47. Vinante O, Bari M, Segati R, et al. The combination of mitomycin, vinblastine and cisplatin is active in the palliation of stage IIIB-IV non–small-cell lung cancer. Oncology. 1993;50:1–4.

48. Montazeri A, Gillis CR, McEwen J. Quality of life in patients with lung cancer: a review of literature from 1970 to 1995. Chest. 1998;113:467–481.

49. Cella DF, Tulsky DS, Gray G, et al. The functional assessment of cancer therapy scale: development and validation of the general measure. J Clin Oncol. 1993;11:570–579.

50. Finkelstein DM, Cassileth BR, Bonomi PD, et al. A pilot study of the functional living index—cancer (FLIC) scale for the assessment of quality of life for metastatic lung cancer patients: an Eastern Cooperative Oncology Group study. Am J Clin Oncol. 1988;11:630–633.

51. Bonomi P. Non–small cell lung cancer chemotherapy. In: Pass HI, Mitchell JB, eds. Lung Cancer: Principles and Practice. Philadelphia, Pa: Lippincott-Raven; 1996:811–823.

52. Schipper H, Clinch J, McMurray A, et al. Measuring the quality of life of cancer patients: the Functional Living Index—Cancer (FLIC): development and validation. J Clin Oncol. 1984;2:472–478.

53. Ganz PA, Lee JJ, Sian J. Quality of life assessment: an independent prognostic variable for survival in lung cancer. Cancer. 1991;67:3131–3139.

54. Ruckdeschel JC, Piantadosi S. Assessment of quality of life by Functional Living Index—Cancer (FLIC) is superior to performance status for prediction of survival in patients with lung cancer. Proc ASCO. 1989;8:311.

55. Weeks J. Quality-of-life assessment: performance status upstaged? J Clin Oncol. 1992;10:1827–1829.

56. Cella D, Fairclough DL, Bonomi PB, et al. Quality of life (QOL) in advanced non–small cell lung cancer (NSCLC): results from Eastern Cooperative Oncology Group (ECOG) study E5592 [abstract]. Proc ASCO. 1997;16:2a.

57. Bonomi P, Kim KM, Fairclough D, et al. Comparison of survival and quality of life in advanced non–small-cell lung cancer patients treated with two dose levels of paclitaxel combined with cisplatin versus etoposide with cisplatin: results of an Eastern Cooperative Oncology Group trial. J Clin Oncol. 2000;18:623–631.

58. Giaccone G, Splinter TAW, Debruyne C, et al. Randomized study of paclitaxel-cisplatin versus cisplatin-teniposide in patients with advanced non–small-cell lung cancer. J Clin Oncol. 1998;16:2133–2141.

59. Belani CP, Natale RB, Lee JS, et al. Randomized phase III trial comparing cisplatin/etoposide versus carboplatin/paclitaxel in advanced and metastatic non–small cell lung cancer (NSCLC) [abstract]. Proc ASCO. 1998;17:455a.

60. Crinò L, Scaglotti GV, Ricci S, et al. Gemcitabine and cisplatin versus mitomycin, ifosfamide, and cisplatin in advanced non–small-cell lung cancer: a randomized phase III study of the Italian Lung Cancer Project. J Clin Oncol. 1999;17:3522–3530.

61. Sandler AB, Nemunaitis J, Denham C, et al. Phase III trial of gemcitabine plus cisplatin versus cisplatin alone in patients with locally advanced or metastatic non–small-cell lung cancer. J Clin Oncol. 2000;18:122–130.

62. Jaakkimainen L, Goodwin PJ, Pater J, et al. Counting the costs of chemotherapy in a National Cancer Institute of Canada randomized trial in nonsmall-cell lung cancer. J Clin Oncol. 1990;8:1301–1309.

63. Smith TJ, Hillner BE, Neighbors DM, et al. Economic evaluation of a randomized clinical trial comparing vinorelbine, vinorelbine plus cisplatin, and vindesine plus cisplatin for non–small-cell lung cancer. J Clin Oncol. 1995;13:2166–2173.

64. Le Chevalier T, Brisgand D, Douillard J-Y, et al. Randomized study of vinorelbine and cisplatin versus vindesine and cisplatin versus vinorelbine alone in advanced non–small-cell lung cancer: results of a European multicenter trial including 612 patients. J Clin Oncol. 1994;12:360–367.

65. Mather D, Sullivan SD, Parasuraman TV. Beyond survival: economic analyses of chemotherapy in advanced, inoperable NSCLC. Oncology. 1998;12:199–209.

66. Crino L, Tonato M, Darwish S, et al. A randomized trial of three cisplatin-containing regimens in advanced non–small-cell lung cancer (NSCLC): a study of the Umbrian Lung Cancer Group. Cancer Chemother Pharmacol. 1990;26:52–56.

67. Wozniak AJ, Crowley JJ, Balcerzak SP, et al. Randomized trial comparing cisplatin with cisplatin plus vinorelbine in the treatment of advanced non–small-cell lung cancer: a Southwest Oncology Group Study. J Clin Oncol. 1998;16:2459–2465.

68. Gatzemeier U, von Pawel J, Gottfried M, et al. Phase III comparative study of high-dose cisplatin (HD-CIS) versus a combination of paclitaxel (TAX) and cisplatin (CIS) in patients with advanced non–small cell lung cancer (NSCLC) [abstract]. Proc ASCO. 1998;17:454a.

69. von Pawel J, von Roemeling R, Gatzemeier V, et al. Tirapazamine plus cisplatin versus cisplatin in advanced non–small-cell lung cancer: a report of the international CATAPULT I Study Group. Cisplatin and tirapazamine in subjects with advanced previously untreated non–small-cell lung tumors. J Clin Oncol. 2000;18:1351–1359.

70. Rosso R, Salvati F, Ardizzoni A, et al. Etoposide versus etoposide plus high-dose cisplatin in the management of advanced non–small cell lung cancer: results of a prospective randomized FONICAP trial. Cancer. 1990;66:130–134.

71. Masuda N, Fukuoka M, Negoro S, et al. Randomized trial comparing cisplatin (CDDP) and irinotecan (CPT-11) versus CDDP and vindesine (VDS) versus CPT-11 alone in advanced non–small cell lung cancer (NSCLC), a multicenter phase III study [abstract]. Proc ASCO. 1999;18:459a.

72. Depierre A, Chastang CI, Quoix E, et al. Vinorelbine versus vinorelbine plus cisplatin in advanced non–small cell lung cancer: a randomized trial. Ann Oncol. 1994;5:37–42.

73. Splinter TA, Sahmoud T, Festen J, et al. Two schedules of teniposide with or without cisplatin in advanced non–small-cell lung cancer: a randomized study of the European Organization for Research and Treatment of Cancer Lung Cancer Cooperative Group. J Clin Oncol. 1996;14:127–134.

74. Gralla RJ, Casper ES, Kelsen DP, et al. Cisplatin and vindesine combination chemotherapy for advanced carcinoma of the lung: a randomized trial investigating two dosage schedules. Ann Intern Med. 1981;95:414–420.

75. Gandara DR, Crowley J, Livingston RB, et al. Evaluation of cisplatin intensity in metastatic non–small cell lung cancer: a phase III study of the Southwest Oncology Group. J Clin Oncol. 1993;11:873–878.

76. Klastersky J, Sculier JP, Ravez P, et al. A randomized study comparing a high and a standard dose of cisplatin in combination with etoposide in the treatment of advanced non–small-cell lung carcinoma. J Clin Oncol. 1986;4:1780–1786.

77. Kreisman H, Ginsberg S, Propert KJ, et al. Carboplatin or iproplatin in advanced non–small cell lung cancer: a Cancer and Leukemia Group B study. Cancer Treat Rep. 1987;71:1049–1052.

78. Kramer BS, Birch R, Greco A, et al. Randomized phase II evaluation of iproplatin (CHIP) and carboplatin (CBDCA) in lung cancer: a Southeastern Cancer Study Group trial. Am J Clin Oncol. 1988;11:643–645.

79. Gatzemeier U, Rosell R, Betticher D, et al. Randomized pan-European trial comparing paclitaxel/carboplatin versus paclitaxel/cisplatin in advanced non–small-cell lung cancer [abstract]. Eur J Cancer. 1999;35(suppl 4):246.

80. Klastersky J, Sculier JP, Lacroix H, et al. A randomized study comparing cisplatin or carboplatin with etoposide in patients with advanced non–small-cell lung cancer: European Organization for Research and Treatment of Cancer Protocol 07861. J Clin Oncol. 1990;8:1556–1562.

81. Jelic S, Radosavjelic D, Elezar E. Survival advantage for carboplatin 500 mg/m² substituting cisplatin 120 mg/m² in combination with vindesine and mitomycin C in patients with stage IIIB and IV squamous-cell bronchogenic carcinoma: a randomized phase III study in 221 patients. Lung Cancer. 1997;18(suppl 1):14.

82. Sorensen JB, Osterlind K, Hansen HH. Vinca alkaloids in the treatment of non–small cell lung cancer. Cancer Treat Rev. 1987;14:29–41.

83. Furuse K, Fukuoka M, Kuba M, et al. Randomized study of vinorelbine versus vindesine in previously untreated stage IIIB or IV non–small-cell lung cancer. Ann Oncol. 1996;7:815–820.

84. Spain RC. The case for mitomycin in non–small cell lung cancer. Oncology. 1993;50(suppl 1):35–52.

85. Veeder MH, Jett JR, Su J, et al. A phase III trial of mitomycin C alone versus mitomycin C, vinblastine and cisplatin for metastatic squamous cell lung carcinoma. Cancer. 1992;70:2281–2287.

86. Rivera MP, Kris MA, Gralla MJ, et al. Syndrome of acute dyspnea related to combined mitomycin plus vinca alkaloid chemotherapy. Am J Clin Oncol. 1995;18:245–250.

87. Ruckdeschel JC. Etoposide in the management of non–small cell lung cancer. Cancer. 1991;67(suppl):250–253.

88. Slevin ML, Clark PJ, Joel SP, et al. A randomized trial to evaluate the effect of schedule on the activity of etoposide in small cell lung cancer. J Clin Oncol. 1989;7:1333–1340.

89. Waits TM, Johnson DH, Hainsworth JD, et al. Prolonged administration of oral etoposide in non–small cell lung cancer: a phase II trial. J Clin Oncol. 1992;10:292–296.

90. Saxman S, Loehrer PJ Sr, Logie K, et al. Phase II trial of daily oral etoposide in patients with advanced non–small cell lung cancer. Invest New Drugs. 1991;9:253–256.

91. Ettinger DS. Ifosfamide in the treatment of non–small cell lung cancer. Semin Oncol. 1989;16(suppl 3):31–38.

92. Socinski MA. Single-agent paclitaxel in the treatment of advanced non–small cell lung cancer. Oncologist. 1999;4:408–416.

93. Burris H, Eckardt J, Fields S, et al. Phase II trial of Taxotere in patients with non–small cell lung cancer [abstract]. Proc ASCO. 1993;12:335.

94. Cerny T, Kaplan S, Pavlidis N, et al. Docetaxel (Taxotere) is active in non–small-cell lung cancer: a phase II trial of the EORTC early clinical trials group (ECTG). Br J Cancer. 1994;70:384–387.

95. Fossella FV, Lee JS, Murphy WK, et al. Phase II study of docetaxel for recurrent or metastatic non–small-cell lung cancer. J Clin Oncol. 1994;12:1238–1244.

96. Francis PA, Rigas JR, Kris MG, et al. Phase II trial of docetaxel in patients with stage III and IV non–small-cell lung cancer. J Clin Oncol. 1994;12:1232–1237.

97. Kunitoh H, Watanabe K, Onoshi T, et al. Phase II trial of docetaxel in previously untreated advanced non–small cell lung cancer: a Japanese Cooperative Study. J Clin Oncol. 1996;14:1649–1655.

98. Miller VA, Rigas JR, Francis PA, et al. Phase II trial of a 75-mg/m² dose of docetaxel with prednisone premedication for patients with advanced non–small cell lung cancer. Cancer. 1995;75:968–972.

99. Sandler A, Ettinger DS. Gemcitabine: single-agent and combination therapy in non–small cell lung cancer. Oncologist. 1999;4:241–251.

100. Perng R-P, Chen Y-M, Ming-Liu J, et al. Gemcitabine versus the combination of cisplatin and etoposide in patients with inoperable non–small-cell lung cancer in a phase II randomized study. J Clin Oncol. 1997;15:2097–2102.

101. Manegold C, Bergman B, Chemaissani A, et al. Single-agent gemcitabine versus cisplatin-etoposide: early results of a randomised phase II study in locally advanced or metastatic non–small-cell lung cancer. Ann Oncol. 1997;8:525–529.

102. Bunn PA Jr, Kelly K. New chemotherapeutic agents prolong survival and improve quality of life in non–small cell lung cancer: a review of the literature and future directions [abstract]. Clin Cancer Res. 1998;4:1087–1100.

103. Gridelli C, Perrone F, Gallo C, et al. Vinorelbine is well tolerated and active in the treatment of elderly patients with advanced non–small cell lung cancer: a two-stage phase II study. Eur J Cancer. 1997;33:392–397.

104. Veronesi A, Crivellari D, Magri MD, et al. Vinorelbine treatment of advanced non–small cell lung cancer with special emphasis on elderly patients. Eur J Cancer. 1996;32A:1809–1811.

105. Furuse K, Kubota K, Kawahara M, et al. A phase II study of vinorelbine, a new derivative of vinca alkaloid, for previously untreated advanced non–small cell lung cancer. Lung Cancer. 1994;11:385–391.

106. Carrato A, Rosell R, Camps C, et al. Modified weekly regimen with vinorelbine as a single agent in unresectable non–small cell lung cancer. Lung Cancer. 1997;17:261–266.

107. Lilenbaum RC, Langenberg P, Dickersin K. Single agent versus combination chemotherapy in patients with advanced nonsmall cell lung carcinoma: a meta-analysis of response, toxicity, and survival. Cancer. 1998;82:116–126.

108. Weick JK, Crowley J, Natale RB, et al. A randomized trial of five cisplatin-containing treatments in patients with metastatic non–small-cell lung cancer: a Southwest Oncology Group study. J Clin Oncol. 1991;9:1157–1162.

109. Johnson DH. Treatment strategies for metastatic non–small-cell lung cancer. Clin Lung Cancer. 1999;1:34–41.

110. Bonomi P. Eastern Cooperative Oncology Group experience with chemotherapy in advanced non–small cell lung cancer. Chest. 1998;113(suppl):13S–16S.

111. Kelly K, Crowley J, Bunn PA, et al. A randomized phase III trial of paclitaxel plus carboplatin (PC) versus vinorelbine plus cisplatin (VC) in untreated advanced non–small cell lung cancer (NSCLC): a Southwest Oncology Group (SWOG) trial. Proc ASCO. 1999;18:461a.

112. Mamounas E, Brown A, Smith R, et al. Effect of Taxol duration of infusion in advanced breast cancer (ABC): results of NSABP B-26 trial comparing 3- to 24-hr infusion of high dose Taxol [abstract]. Proc ASCO. 1998;17:101a.

113. Kosmidis PA, Mylonakis N, Skarlos D. A multicenter randomized trial of paclitaxel (175 mg/m²) plus carboplatin (6AUC) versus paclitaxel (225 mg/m²) plus carboplatin (6AUC) in advanced non–small cell lung cancer (NSCLC). Proc ASCO. 1999;18:463a.

114. Akerley W, Herndon J, Egorin MJ, et al. CALGB 9731: Phase II trial of weekly paclitaxel for advanced non–small cell lung cancer (NSCLC). Proc ASCO. 1999;18:462a.
115. Cardenal F, Lopez-Cabrerizo M, Anton A, et al. Randomized phase III study of gemcitabine-cisplatin versus etoposide-cisplatin in the treatment of locally advanced or metastatic non–small-cell lung cancer. J Clin Oncol. 1999;17:12–18.
116. Niho S, Nagao K, Nishiwaki Y, et al. Randomized multicenter phase III trial of irinotecan (CPT-11) and cisplatin (CDDP) versus CDDP and vindesine (VDS) in patients with advanced non–small cell lung cancer (NSCLC). Proc ASCO. 1999;18:492a.
117. Crinò L, Mosconi AM, Scagliotti G, et al. Gemcitabine as second-line treatment for advanced non–small-cell lung cancer: a phase II trial. J Clin Oncol. 1999;17:2081–2085.
118. Brahmer JR, Ettinger DS. The role of topotecan in the treatment of small cell lung cancer. Oncologist. 1998;3:11–14.
119. Belani CP. Single agents in the second-line treatment of non–small cell lung cancer. Semin Oncol. 1998;25(suppl 8):10–14.
120. Socinski MA, Steagall A, Gillenwater H. Second-line chemotherapy with 96-hour infusional paclitaxel in refractory non–small cell lung cancer: report of a phase II trial. Cancer Invest. 1999;17:181–188.
121. Fossella FV, Lee JS, Shin DM, et al. Phase II study of docetaxel for advanced or metastatic platinum-refractory non–small-cell lung cancer. J Clin Oncol. 1995;13:645–651.
122. Gandara DR, Vokes E, Green M, et al. Activity of docetaxel in platinum-treated non–small-cell lung cancer: results of a phase II multicenter trial. J Clin Oncol. 2000;18:131–135.
123. Fossella FV, DeVore R, Kerr J, et al. Phase III trial of docetaxel 100 mg/m² or 75 mg/m² vs vinorelbine/ifosfamide for non–small-cell lung cancer previously treated with platinum-based chemotherapy [abstract]. Proc ASCO. 1999;18:460.
124. Shepherd FA, Dancey J, Ramlau R, et al. Prospective randomized trial of docetaxel versus best supportive care in patients with non–small-cell lung cancer previously treated with platinum-based chemotherapy. J Clin Oncol. 2000;18:2095–2103.
125. Miller VA, Fossella FV, DeVore R, et al. Docetaxel (D) benefits lung cancer symptoms and quality of life (QOL) in a randomized phase III study of non–small cell lung cancer (NSCLC) patients previously treated with platinum-based therapy [abstract]. Proc ASCO. 1999;18:491a.
126. Dancey J, Shepherd F, Ramlau R, et al. Quality of life (QOL) assessment in a randomized study of taxotere (TAX) versus best supportive care (BSC) in non–small cell lung cancer (NSCLC) patients (pts) previously treated with platinum-based chemotherapy [abstract]. Proc ASCO. 1999;18:491a.
127. Buccheri GF, Ferrigno D, Curcio A, et al. Continuation of chemotherapy versus supportive care alone in patients with inoperable non–small cell lung cancer and stable disease after two or three cycles of MACC. Cancer. 1989;63:428–432.
128. Smith I, O'Brien M, Norton A, et al. Duration of chemotherapy for advanced non–small-cell lung cancer (NSCLC): a phase III randomised trial of 3 versus 6 courses of mitomycin, vinblastine, cisplatin (MVP) [abstract]. Proc ASCO. 1998;17:457a.
129. American Society of Clinical Oncology. Clinical practice guidelines for the treatment of unresectable non–small-cell lung cancer. J Clin Oncol. 1997;15:2996–3018.
130. Georgoulias V, Papadakis E, Alexopoulos A. Docetaxel plus cisplatin versus docetaxel plus gemcitabine chemotherapy in advanced non–small cell lung cancer: a preliminary analysis of a multicenter randomized phase II trial. Proc ASCO. 1999;18:461a.
131. Socinski MA, Sandler AB, Miller LL, et al. Phase I/II trial of irinotecan (CPT-11), paclitaxel (P), and carboplatin (C) in advanced or metastatic non–small cell lung cancer (NSCLC) [abstract]. Cancer Invest. 1999;18(suppl 1):89.
132. Frasci G, Panza N, Comella G, et al. Is there any impact of new drugs on the outcome of advanced NSCLC? An overview of the Southern Italy Cooperative Oncology Group Trials. Oncologist. 1999;4:379–385.
133. Tsai CM, Chang KT, Chen JY, et al. Cytotoxic effects of gemcitabine-containing regimens against human non–small cell lung cancer cell lines which express different levels of p185^{neu}. Cancer Res. 1996;56:794–801.

SURGICAL TREATMENT OF STAGE IV NON–SMALL CELL LUNG CANCER

Frank C. Detterbeck, Mark S. Bleiweis, and Matthew G. Ewend

Patients with stage IV non–small cell lung cancer (NSCLC) are generally regarded as having widespread metastases, and the usual treatment is systemic chemotherapy and supportive care. Thus far, this approach has not resulted in many 5-year survivors among these patients. However, some patients with stage IV NSCLC present with a solitary metastatic focus or only a limited number of metastases and are said to have oligometastatic disease.[1] In some of these patients, a definitive local therapy has been used in an attempt to eradicate all known disease or to destroy a life-threatening lesion, such as a brain metastasis. Stage IV patients who are treated with such local therapy are the focus of this chapter.

Definitive local therapy for stage IV NSCLC has primarily involved surgical resection of the primary tumor and the metastatic sites. Stereotactic radiosurgery (RS) is also being used increasingly to destroy metastatic foci in the brain. Despite the name, this technique does not involve any surgery but rather precisely focused radiotherapy (RT). Because RS is a type of definitive local treatment as well, it is also included in this chapter.

Treatment that is given with curative intent does not always result in cure of the patient, especially in stage IV NSCLC. However, even when cure is not achieved, the treatment may result in a palliative benefit for the patient. This is especially true in the case of brain metastases, which are rapidly fatal when not treated, but may also be true with adrenal metastases. The palliative benefits of definitive local therapy of metastases are also reviewed in this chapter. Palliative treatment that does not involve surgery or RS is discussed in Chapter 29.

BRAIN METASTASIS

Patients with NSCLC who are found to have a brain metastasis may be approached in several ways. At one extreme, patients may be given only supportive care. At the other extreme, patients may be treated with curative intent. This latter approach makes sense only in patients without other sites of metastases in whom a curative treatment of the primary and the brain metastasis is possible. When a curative approach is not feasible, palliation may be pursued in an aggressive manner with resection or RS destruction of the brain metastasis or in a nonaggressive manner involving steroids and whole brain RT (WBRT).

Incidence

Patients with NSCLC that has metastasized to the brain are not uncommon. In autopsy series of patients with lung cancer, the incidence of brain metastases ranges from 25% to 55%.[2–6] Furthermore, most clinical series of metastatic intracranial tumors report that approximately half of these are caused by lung cancers.[7–16] Approximately 25% of patients who have stage IV NSCLC at initial presentation have brain metastases (see Table 6–1). In addition, the brain is the most common site of first recurrence among resected patients with NSCLC, accounting for 17% to 18% of all first recurrences.[2,17] The magnitude of this problem is illustrated by the observation that the annual incidence of NSCLC patients with brain metastases is comparable to the incidence of new primary cancers of the rectum, pancreas, or stomach.[18,19]

The risk of developing a brain metastasis among resected patients with adenocarcinoma is approximately 10%, whereas in patients with squamous cell cancers it has been reported to be approximately 3%.[2,17] The risk of a brain metastasis is 2% to 6% in resected stage I and II patients but has been found to be 6% to 21% in resected stage IIIa patients.[2,17] Between 60% and 90% of such brain recurrences occur within 12 months of resection of the primary lung cancer.[2,17,20] This raises the question of whether aggressive surveillance of the brain during the first year is beneficial,[17] although it is not known whether earlier detection of a metastasis might result in better survival.

It is unclear how many patients with NSCLC involving the brain are potential candidates for aggressive therapy. Two studies have reported that >90% of previously resected patients who develop a brain metastasis as a recurrence (*metachronous cases*) have no other sites of disease, but it is unclear how diligently other potential sites of disease were investigated in these studies.[2,17] Among patients who present with lung cancer involving the brain (*synchronous cases*), 59% to 65% are found to have no other sites of metastases, but once again, it is not clear to what extent other sites were evaluated.[11,20,21] Brain metastases are preferentially located in the superficial distal arterial fields (watershed areas), and 90% are supratentorial.[12] A number of studies have reported that only a single brain metastasis (on the basis of computed tomography [CT]) is found in an average of 45% of cases of NSCLC involving the brain (range, 28%-62%).[11,12,17,22–25] It may be that the relatively high rates of finding isolated and single lesions in patients who present with a brain metastasis are primarily a reflection of a limited ability to detect other sites of disease. Unfortunately, little follow-up data is available. The proportion of all brain metastases that are resectable in NSCLC ranges from 14% to 44%[23,25,26] and was found to be 36% in a prospective study of patients who underwent resection of an early stage NSCLC.[17] Furthermore, most brain metastases that are thought to be unresectable are amenable to RS.[16,27]

Nonaggressive Palliative Therapy

The natural history of patients with isolated cranial metastases who might be candidates for a curative approach has not been studied specifically. However, it is probably similar to the natural history of patients with brain metastases in general because the effects of untreated brain metastases are so devastating that other patient characteristics become relatively unimportant. In studies from the 1960s, patients with untreated brain metastasis experienced rapid neurologic deterioration, with a median survival of approximately 1 month, but it is unclear whether this data is applicable to patients who are diagnosed with a brain metastasis today, using modern scans and facilities.[28,29] Corticosteroids alone increase survival to approximately 2 months.[30,31] Whole brain irradiation results in a median survival of 3 to 6 months.[10,22,32,33] These treatments are covered in more detail in Chapter 29.

Survival After Potentially Curative Resection

Although stage IV NSCLC is usually incurable, it is a well established fact that an aggressive approach can sometimes result in a cure, particularly in cases involving brain metastases. Such an approach can be considered only when no other metastases are present and curative treatment of both the primary site and the intracranial metastasis is feasible. This section examines data involving NSCLC patients with brain metastases in whom all of the known tumor is treated in a definitive manner (with surgery or RS). Approximately two-thirds of such cases of a curative approach involve previously resected patients in whom a brain metastasis is subsequently discovered (metachronous cases).[34–37] The remainder of cases involve a synchronous presentation of a primary lung cancer and an intracranial metastasis.

Reports involving at least 20 patients who underwent resection of brain metastases with curative intent (both synchronous and metachronous cases) are shown in Table 23–1. The operative mortality is low, averaging 2%. The resection of the brain metastasis was reported to be complete in almost all cases, and the primary cancer could also be completely resected in most instances when this had not already been accomplished previously. The 5-year survival for all patients treated with curative intent averages 14%, with little variation between studies (range, 8%-21%).

TABLE 23–1. RESULTS OF SURGICAL RESECTION OF BRAIN METASTASES IN PATIENTS WITH NON–SMALL CELL LUNG CANCER WITH INTENT TO CURE

STUDY	N ALL	% OP MORT	% R₀ BRAIN	% R₀ LUNG	SURVIVAL (ALL PATIENTS)			N R₀	SURVIVAL (R₀ PATIENTS)		
					MST	2 y (%)	5 y (%)		MST	2 y (%)	5 y (%)
Wronski et al[34]	231	3	94	78	11	24	13	144	14	34	18
Nakagawa et al[26]	51	—	—	67	9	14	12	—	—	—	—
Mussi et al[35]	45	0	100	100	—	—	—	45	19	31	16
Magilligan et al[38]	41	2	95	—	13	31	21	—	—	—	—
Rossi et al[40]	40	2	—	—	—	25	13	—	—	—	—
Ehrenhaft[96]	40	1	—	—	—	25	13	—	—	—	—
Macchiarini et al[37]	37	0	100	100	—	—	—	37	27	58	30
Read et al[36]	35	0	94	77	12	40	20	—	—	—	—
Saitoh et al[99]	24	8	—	84	7	—	8	—	—	—	—
Torre et al[41]	21	0	—	—	13	35	10	—	—	—	—
Average		**2**	**97**	**84**	**11**	**28**	**14**		**20**	**41**	**21**

Inclusion criteria: Studies from 1980 to 2000 of ≥20 patients who underwent resection of the lung cancer primary as well as an isolated brain metastasis.
MST, median survival time in months; op mort, 30-day mortality for the thoracotomy and craniotomy combined; R₀, complete resection with no residual disease.

Relief of neurologic symptoms is achieved in 78% to 91% of patients.[35,36,38]

Recurrence patterns have been reported in one study and involved the brain in 22% of patients, a local recurrence within the chest in 39%, and diffuse systemic metastases in 39%.[35] Most of the systemic recurrences occurred within 2 to 3 months of resection of all tumor. The high rate of local thoracic recurrences despite a complete resection reported in this study is unusual among surgical series and may reflect poor nodal staging. The cause of death was reported in two studies and was found to be recurrent intracranial cancer in 33% to 50%, systemic recurrence in 29% to 37%, local thoracic recurrence in 7% to 10%, and a nononcologic cause in 6% to 29% of patients.[36,38]

Patient Selection for Curative Treatment

The patients reported in Table 23–1 undoubtedly represent a select group, but given the potential for cure, it is important that these patients be identified and treated. As recently as 1989, Read et al[36] found that more than one-third of patients with solitary brain metastases and resectable intrathoracic disease were not even referred for consideration of surgery. The difficulty, of course, lies in defining selection criteria that predict a reasonable chance of long-term survival. This is made more difficult by the number of factors that are likely to have an impact and the fact that most series have involved only a small number of patients.

A multivariate analysis of prognostic factors has been carried out in a large series of patients from Memorial Sloan-Kettering Cancer Center. Most patients (80%) underwent both craniotomy and thoracotomy and were presumably treated with curative intent.[34] Five factors demonstrated independent prognostic value at a level of statistical significance of $P = 0.05$ (Table 23–2). The most important factor was complete resection of the primary tumor, as can also be seen in Figure 23–1. Complete resection of the brain metastasis was not a statistically significant factor, although none of the patients who underwent an incomplete

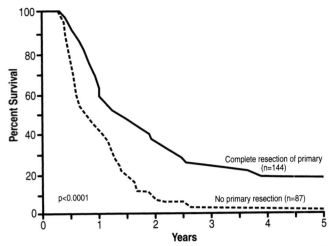

FIGURE 23–1. Survival from the time of craniotomy in 231 patients with brain metastases from lung cancer by surgical management of primary lung disease, that is, complete resection versus incomplete and no resection ($P < 0.0001$ by log-rank test). (From Wronski M, Arbit E, Burt M, et al. Survival after surgical treatment of brain metastases from lung cancer: a follow-up study of 231 patients treated between 1976 and 1991. J Neurosurg. 1995;83:605–616.[34])

resection of the brain metastasis was alive at 2 years. This may be because of the small number of patients (n = 13) who underwent incomplete resection of the brain lesion (as defined by postoperative CT).

Several additional factors that were not found to have multivariate prognostic significance are worthy of discussion. Although patients with multiple brain metastases exhibited poorer survival (median survival, 9 months versus 11 months; univariate $P = 0.02$), this difference was not found to be significant by multivariate analysis.[34] A preoperative performance status (PS) ≤2 was also found to be significant by univariate analysis but not by multivariate analysis. No difference was found in survival among histologic subtypes of NSCLC (univariate, $P = 0.34$).[34] Among patients with synchronous presentation, no difference was found in survival according to the stage of the primary lesion (excluding the brain metastasis), as can be seen in Figure 23–2. Other authors, in much smaller studies, have generally reported poor survival in patients with mediastinal node involvement and univariate P values < 0.05,[35,39–41] although some have found no difference.[37] Among patients with metachronous presentation, better survival was found in one study when the interval between the two lesions was >14 months (median survival, 34 months versus 12 months; $P = 0.04$).[35]

What criteria, then, should be used to select patients for potentially curative resection of both the primary tumor and the metastasis (synchronous cases)? It seems clear that a thorough search for other metastatic sites should be undertaken and that patients with extracranial metastases be excluded from a resection with curative intent. Patients should be considered for resection only if all of the tumor (at both the primary and any metastatic sites) can be completely resected. The presence of more than one brain metastasis is probably not significant, provided the number of metastases is small (i.e., ≤3) and provided all metastases can be completely resected with confidence and with ac-

TABLE 23–2. NEGATIVE PROGNOSTIC FACTORS BY COX MULTIVARIATE ANALYSIS IN 231 PATIENTS[a]

FACTOR	P
Incomplete resection of primary tumor	.0002
Presence of systemic metastases	.0083
Male gender	.0088
Age ≥60 y	.0398
Infratentorial lesion	.0497
Large brain tumor (≥3 cm)	.0530
Persistence after previous WBRT	.0572
N2,3 node involvement	.0872
No en bloc resection of brain metastasis	.1025
Incomplete resection of brain metastasis	.1025
No postoperative WBRT	.1187

[a]All patients underwent craniotomy, and 80% underwent thoracotomy with intent to resect both sites of cancer.
WBRT, whole brain radiotherapy.
Data from Wronski M, Arbit E, Burt M, et al. Survival after surgical treatment of brain metastases from lung cancer: a follow-up study of 231 patients treated between 1976 and 1991. J Neurosurg. 1995; 83:605–616.[34]

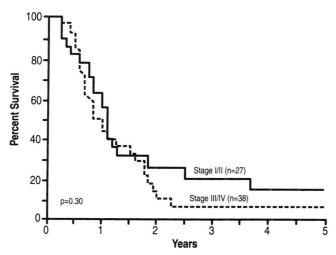

FIGURE 23–2. Survival of patients undergoing resection of brain metastases for non–small cell lung cancer by stage of locoregional primary cancer (ie, excluding brain metastasis). The trend toward a difference did not reach significance (P = 0.30). (From Burt M, Wronski M, Arbit E, et al. Resection of brain metastases from non–small-cell lung carcinoma: results of therapy. J Thorac Cardiovasc Surg. 1992;103:399–411.[18])

ceptable morbidity. The patient must also be fit enough to tolerate both operations. The histologic subtype is not important. A preoperative mediastinoscopy should be carried out to rule out N2,3 node involvement, although the data supporting the fact that the presence of mediastinal node involvement precludes a good outcome is unclear. However, because patients with preoperatively demonstrated mediastinal node involvement are not generally candidates for surgical resection, it is hard to argue that such patients should undergo thoracic surgical resection simply because they also have a brain metastasis.

The outlook is likely to be more optimistic for patients who are younger and female and have a metachronous presentation. The outlook may also be better in patients with supratentorial lesions and those with brain metastases <3 cm. However, these considerations are relative and should not necessarily exclude patients who are otherwise fit and in whom a complete resection is likely to be achieved.

Palliative Resection of Brain Metastases

The ability to control the devastating effects of intracranial metastases in some patients suggests that aggressive treatment (resection or RS) of brain metastases may be of palliative benefit, even when a cure is not achieved.[23,42] The patients selected for aggressive treatment are likely to have a more favorable prognosis simply because of the process of selection and not necessarily as a result of the treatment. Fortunately, three randomized studies assessed the palliative benefit of resection followed by RT compared with RT alone in patients with resectable single brain metastases.[9,10,13] All of these studies included patients with a variety of cancers, but patients with NSCLC accounted for the majority of cases in each of the studies.

Two of these randomized studies found better survival

after surgery and RT,[9,10] whereas the third study found no difference.[13] Each of the studies involved similar numbers of patients (N = 48, 63, and 84 patients) and patient groups that were well matched relative to major prognostic factors. Overall survival curves from the two positive studies are shown in Figure 23–3. In these two studies, median survival was 9 and 10 months in the surgery plus RT arms, compared with 3 and 6 months in the RT-alone arms.[9,10] In the third study, median survival was 6 months in both arms. The duration of functional independence was also significantly prolonged in the first two studies (9 months versus 2 months, P < 0.005; and 8 versus 4 months, P = 0.06)[9,10] but not in the third.[13]

The first study included only patients with a PS ≥70, and the average PS was 90.[10] The latter two studies also included patients with a PS as low as 2 (World Health Organization scale) or 50 to 60 (Karnofsky scale), accounting for 27% and 22% of the patients in these latter studies.[9,13] This may be significant because the second study found that better survival was seen in the entire group and in the patients with stable extracranial disease, whereas there was no benefit to resection in patients with uncontrolled extracranial disease.[9] An association between the extent of extracranial disease and PS was not evaluated, but it is likely that the patients with uncontrolled extracranial disease had a poor PS. However, it is not clear that the inclusion of patients with a poor PS or disseminated disease accounts for the lack of a benefit with surgery in the third study,[13] although there is some data suggesting that patients with extracranial disease may not benefit from resection of the brain metastasis.

Radiosurgery

Stereotactic RS uses multiple well-collimated beams of ionizing radiation that are focused precisely on an intracranial lesion using stereotaxy. The hallmark of this tech-

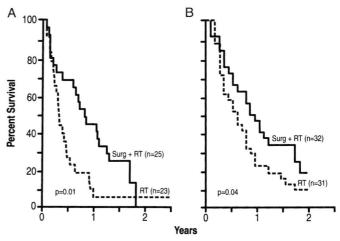

FIGURE 23–3. Survival of patients with brain metastases randomized to surgery plus RT versus RT alone. *A*, Survival in 48 patients from the University of Kentucky (P = 0.01). *B*, Survival in 63 patients in a multi-institutional study from the Netherlands (P = 0.04). RT, radiotherapy. (*A*, Data from Patchel RA, Tibbs PA, Walsh JW, et al. A randomized trial of surgery in the treatment of single metastases to the brain. N Engl J Med. 1990;322:494–500.[10] *B*, Data from Vecht CJ, Haaxma-Reiche H, Noordijk EM, et al. Treatment of single brain metastasis: radiotherapy alone or combined with neurosurgery? Ann Neurol. 1993;33:583–590.[9])

nique is the steep dose fall-off outside of the target area and the use of a single, ablative dose of radiation. This allows tumors to be destroyed much as if they were surgically resected, hence the name *radiosurgery*. The two most commonly used techniques employ a linear accelerator (LINAC) or multiple beams of gamma radiation using multiple cobalt-60 sources (Gamma knife). The differences in outcomes between these two techniques are minor, and there are no major differences in either efficacy or safety.[27] Usually, a dose of approximately 16 to 20 Gy is given in a single outpatient treatment. RS can be used to treat both single and multiple lesions and has the advantage of being able to be used to treat lesions virtually anywhere in the brain, including deep-seated lesions and brain stem tumors.[16,27]

RS has been shown to have low rates of acute and chronic complications. The 30-day mortality was 2% in a large series, with none of the deaths being due to the RS treatment. Minor acute morbidity was seen in 13% of patients and involved mostly self-limited nausea (especially in posterior fossa lesions) or seizure (especially in patients with a known seizure disorder).[43] Approximately 7% of patients eventually undergo craniotomy, usually because of mass effect from radiation necrosis or intratumor hemorrhage.[43,44]

The results of the larger published series of RS for brain metastases are summarized in Table 23–3. The studies generally included patients with a variety of solid tumors, but lung cancer is the largest group and generally accounts for 30% to 50% of the cases. Furthermore, the larger series have found that the primary tumor type was not a significant predictor of outcome,[15,16,43,45,46] with the exception of two studies reporting results that were in conflict with one another.[44,47] Therefore, these studies provide a reasonable

assessment of the results of RS for lung cancer metastases, even though few studies have focused specifically on the results in patients with lung cancer.

The median survival of patients with brain metastases treated with RS has been just under 1 year, and 2-year survival is approximately 20% (see Table 23–3). Many studies have reported crude local control rates of 80% to 90%,[16,43–45,48,49] but these are difficult to interpret unless the duration of follow-up is taken into account. Local control expressed as actuarial freedom from progression at the treated site was reported in several studies and is approximately 70% at 2 years (see Table 23–3). Local freedom from progression does not necessarily imply complete disappearance of the intracranial lesion. Instead, it means that the lesion remained radiographically (and symptomatically) stable or decreased in size. CT or magnetic resonance imaging scans were obtained every 3 months in each of these studies. New brain metastases that were separate from a treated lesion were not counted as local failure.

The cause of death was reported to be neurologic in 25% and 41% of deaths in two studies of RS.[15,43] The majority of deaths are due to systemic progression of cancer, which provides good evidence that the most imminent cause of death in patients with brain metastases is effectively eliminated by RS in the majority of cases. This finding argues strongly that aggressive treatment of brain metastases is of palliative benefit.

Comparison of Radiosurgery and Surgery

A review of Table 23–3 suggests that the palliative benefit of surgical resection and RS treatment of brain metastases

TABLE 23–3. OUTCOMES OF SURGERY OR RADIOSURGERY AS AGGRESSIVE PALLIATIVE CARE[a] FOR BRAIN METASTASES

STUDY	N	TREAT-MENT	% WITH LUNG CANCER	% WITH SYSTEMIC DISEASE	% PS < 70	OVERALL SURVIVAL (%)			LOCAL FAIL (%)	
						MST	1 y	2 y	1 y	2 y
Moriarty et al[16]	353	RS	48	37[b]	0	11	44	22	12	25
Auchter et al[15]	122	RS	48	69	0	13	53	30	15	23
Shu et al[46]	116	RS	34	53	—	10	40	15	24	—
Flickinger et al[44]	116	RS	35	—	—	11	48	21	27	33
Young et al[45]	107	RS	43	—	—	8	37	—	—	—
Shiau et al[62]	100	RS	39	—	7	11	46	23	23	30
Average		**RS**				11	45	22	20	28
Wronski et al[34]	231	S	100	20[b]	6[c]	11	46	24	—	—
Sundaresan et al[20]	125	S	40	50	20[d]	12	50	25	—	—
White et al[97]	122	S	31	5	—	7	28	15	—	—
Ferrara et al[98]	100	S	51	—	—	13	52	10	—	—
Average		**S**				11	44	19	—	—

Inclusion criteria: Studies of ≥100 patients undergoing surgery or radiosurgery as aggressive palliative care of brain metastases.
[a]Aggressive palliative care involves definitive treatment of a brain metastasis by surgery or radiosurgery, although the primary tumor and other systemic metastases may be present and not necessarily treated.
[b]Only *active* systemic disease.
[c]PS < 60.
[d]Neurologic functional status of ≥2.
Local fail, local failure, meaning any increase in size of >25% of a treated lesion or new neurologic symptoms attributable to a treated lesion; MST, median survival time in months; PS, Karnofsky performance status; RS, radiosurgery; S, surgery.

is similar. There is little difference in survival rates, and there is no obvious difference in selection factors, at least insofar as the presence of extracranial disease and PS is concerned. It is likely that surgical series have included few patients with more than one brain metastasis, but this has been shown not to affect the outcome with either treatment. Several studies have shown equal survival among patients treated with RS who had either a single or several metastases.[43,44,48] Furthermore, in one study, the survival of patients with multiple brain metastases (two to three lesions in 26 patients) who underwent complete resection was the same as that of a matched group of patients who had a single metastasis.[50]

It is difficult to compare local control in patients undergoing surgery and RS because of differences in how local control is measured, but the results appear to be similar. Studies of RS have defined *local control* as freedom from progression at a treated site as measured by periodic follow-up imaging studies. In the surgical series, brain imaging at regular intervals has not been carried out, and *local control* is defined as stability of the neurologic examination. Crude freedom from local progression rates of 80% to 90% are reported following RS,[15,43–45,48,49] whereas recurrences at the site of a resected metastasis are reported in 20% to 33% of surgically resected cases.[10,20,23,34,51] Recurrences in the brain, both at treated sites and new metastases, are involved as the cause of death in 25% to 41% of all deaths after RS[15,43] and in 28% to 50% after surgical resection.[9,13,34,51] Therefore, it is probably best to conclude that local control is similar, given the differences in assessment and perhaps patient populations.

A randomized trial of surgery versus RS for single brain metastases was initiated in 1983 but was stopped due to poor accrual.[52] A retrospective comparison of these treatments has been carried out in 93 patients who were matched according to a large number of prognostic factors (including extent of systemic disease, PS, interval between diagnosis of cancer and appearance of brain metastases, number of brain metastases, age, gender, and primary tumor type).[53] The median survival was significantly better in patients treated with surgery and was due entirely to a lower rate of local recurrences at the site of treated brain lesions. The rate of progression of systemic disease was the same.[53] Yet another comparison of similar patients suggested that the results of surgery and RS are comparable and that there may be a slight trend favoring RS.[15] This latter analysis included only patients with single brain metastases who were surgically resectable.[15] The patients were required to satisfy the same inclusion and exclusion criteria as in the randomized trial of surgery versus WBRT reported by Patchell et al,[10] and as a result, the patients included in these two trials were similar. The median survival after RS was 13 months compared with 9 months after surgery.[10,15]

The morbidity and mortality rates of both treatments are low. RS is done on an outpatient basis, resulting in costs approximately 25% lower than those for surgery.[43,54] However, the median hospital stay for resection of a brain metastasis is currently only 4 days,[50] and neurologic improvement is faster following surgery.[55] The survival is similar, as is the rate of local control. In summary, surgery and RS are comparable methods of treatment for brain metastases.

Surgery and RS for brain metastases should best be viewed as complementary rather than competitive modalities, and technical issues are likely to be the determining factors in selecting the most appropriate treatment. The location of lesions in functionally critical areas of the brain makes surgery a less desirable choice. On the other hand, lesions >3 cm in diameter are difficult to treat with RS.[55] Lesions that require immediate decompression or that threaten to obstruct the flow of cerebrospinal fluid are generally best treated by surgery.[27] In some instances, surgical resection is indicated because there is a need to make a histologic diagnosis of a brain lesion.

Selection of Patients for Palliative Resection of Brain Metastases

It is clear that appropriate selection of patients for definitive treatment of brain metastases is important, but consensus has not been reached about which selection criteria are most appropriate. Although many studies have examined a variety of prognostic factors, interpretation is hampered by the fact that different studies have focused on different factors. Many of the factors may be related, such as the presence of uncontrolled systemic disease and poor PS. Using multivariate analysis is the best way to cull out factors that have independent prognostic value. However, even among series involving multivariate analysis of large patient cohorts, not all studies have examined the same factors, which may account for some of the inconsistencies in the reported results.

A summary of the results of studies reporting multivariate analyses of prognostic factors for survival after definitive treatment of brain metastases in at least 50 patients is shown in Table 23–4. Most of these studies involved patients treated with RS. The presence of extracranial metastases and poor PS (usually defined as PS ≤ 60) are strong predictors of poor survival. Older age (>60-65 years) and larger brain lesions (usually defined as >3 cm) are probably also negative prognostic factors, although the impact of these factors appears to be weaker and less consistent. The negative prognostic impact of male gender and infratentorial lesions is questionable. The type of cancer and a synchronous versus a metachronous presentation do not seem to be of independent prognostic value. The presence of multiple lesions also does not have independent prognostic significance, but the data is limited to patients who had only a small number of metastases. Furthermore, patients treated by surgery or RS because prior WBRT failed to control the intracranial disease were not found to have significantly different survival than other patients.[34,44] It is interesting that similar prognostic factors were identified in a recursive partitioning analysis of 1200 patients treated nonaggressively with WBRT alone (see Fig. 29–1).[56] This study identified a PS < 70, an uncontrolled primary tumor, the presence of other extracranial metastases, and age >65 years as the major factors predicting worse survival.[56]

Which patients should be selected for aggressive palliative treatment of brain metastases? The analysis just noted suggests that patients with uncontrolled extracranial disease and those with a PS < 70 will probably not benefit from such therapy. This conclusion is further supported by the

TABLE 23–4. FAVORABLE PROGNOSTIC FACTORS FOR AGGRESSIVE PALLIATIVE TREATMENT[a] OF BRAIN METASTASES[b]

STUDY	N	TREAT-MENT	ABSENT SYS DIS	HIGH PS	SMALL SIZE	AGE <60–65	SEX F>M	SUPRA-TENTORIAL	CANCER TYPE	SINGLE/ MULT	SYNCH/ METACH
Moriarty et al[16]	353	RS	.0001	—	—	.007	NS	—	NS	NS	—
Auchter et al[15]	122	RS	.001	.0001	—	NS	NS	NS	NS	—	NS
Shu et al[46]	116	RS	.006	.009	.0005[c]	.04	NS	NS	—	NS	—
Flickinger et al[44]	116	RS	—	—	NS	NS	—	—	.0002[d]	—	—
Young et al[45]	107	RS	—	<.05	—	(<.05)[e]	NS	—	NS	NS	—
Kim et al[48 d]	77	RS	.00001[g]	NS	.009	NS	NS	NS	—	NS	NS
Wronski et al[34f,h]	231	S	.008	NS	(.05)[i]	.04	.009	.05	—	NS	NS
Smalley et al[47]	229	S	NS	.005[j]	NS	NS	.02	.001	.001[k]	.002	NS[l]
Prognostic importance			**High**	**High**	**Mod**	**Mod**	**?**	**?**	**—**	**—**	**—**

Inclusion criteria: Studies reporting prognostic factors for survival using multivariate analysis for >50 patients undergoing surgery or radiosurgery as palliative treatment of brain metastases.

[a]Aggressive palliative treatment involves definitive treatment of a brain metastasis by surgery or radiosurgery, although the primary tumor and other systemic metastases may be present and not necessarily treated.

[b]Values shown are P values by multivariate analysis.

[c]Total tumor volume for all lesions.

[d]Better survival for breast cancer.

[e]Older patients exhibited better survival.

[f]All non–small cell lung cancer; no difference between histologic subtypes.

[g]Inactive (not necessarily absent) systemic disease.

[h]80% of patients also underwent resection of all other sites of disease (primary tumor).

[i]$P = 0.053$.

[j]Moderate or severe neurologic deficit.

[k]Worse survival for breast cancer and melanoma.

[l]$P = 0.001$ for interval ≥ or <36 months between diagnosis of primary cancer and brain metastasis.

NS, not significant ($p > 0.05$); PS, performance status; RS, radiosurgery; S, surgery; Single/mult, single versus multiple brain metastases; Small size, brain metastases <3–4 cm; Supratentorial, supratentorial versus infratentorial brain metastasis; Synch/metach, synchronous versus metachronous diagnosis of primary cancer and brain metastasis; Sys dis, systemic (extracranial) disease.

randomized data reported by Vecht et al,[9] in which only the patients with stable extracranial disease experienced better survival after surgery compared with WBRT. However, what is meant by stable extrathoracic disease is not defined in any of the studies, and in fact, most of the multivariate analyses have found that the presence of *any* extrathoracic disease is of major importance.[15,34,43,46] Therefore, although uncontrolled extracranial disease is a clear contraindication to an aggressive approach, stable extrathoracic disease should probably be only a relative contraindication to an aggressive approach and should not necessarily be used to exclude patients with this condition. Older age (>65 years) also represents a relative contraindication to aggressive therapy. Brain metastases >3 cm in diameter are somewhat of a conundrum. Although the survival of such patients after aggressive treatment may be worse than survival of patients with smaller tumors (especially with RS), such large tumors are more likely to cause significant mass effect, which may make resection more appealing.

Recurrent Brain Metastases

Between 28% and 48% of patients develop recurrent brain metastases after undergoing a previous resection of an intracranial metastasis.[10,20,23,34,51] Approximately half involve a local recurrence at the site of a previous lesion and half involve new brain metastases.[10,20,23,34,51] Some of the patients have multiple brain lesions or other extracranial metastases at the time a recurrence is found, and, as a result, only about one third are candidates for a repeat craniotomy.[57] A study of 214 patients who had undergone craniotomy for lung cancer metastatic to the brain found no factors that correlated with an increased risk of a brain relapse (including the stage of the primary lesion, histologic type, PS at the first operation, number of lesions, and whether initial presentation of a brain metastasis was synchronous or metachronous with the diagnosis of lung cancer).[57]

The results of a repeat craniotomy for recurrence of brain metastases are good. In studies involving ≥20 such patients (with all cancer types), the 1-year survival has been found to be 50% to 63%, the 2-year survival 22% to 26%, and the 5-year survival 16% to 17% from the time of the second craniotomy.[57–59] Approximately half of these patients had extrathoracic metastases at the time of the second craniotomy.[58,59] Whether the recurrence was local (at the site of a previous resection) or at a new intracranial site does not affect survival.[58] However, the absence of extracranial disease, a PS ≥ 80, an interval of ≥4 months between resections, and younger age (<40 years) were all significant favorable prognostic factors in a study of 48 such cases involving various types of cancer.[58] Patients who did not have at least two of these factors had poor survival despite repeat resection.[58] Although RS can also be used to treat recurrent brain metastases, no report has analyzed the outcome separately for those patients undergoing this treatment.

Adjuvant Whole Brain Radiotherapy

In many institutions, WBRT is used in an adjuvant fashion following aggressive treatment of brain metastases by surgery or RS, although this approach has been based primarily on theoretical considerations rather than on data. The rationale for WBRT is to reduce the incidence of new intracranial metastases by eradicating additional microscopic metastases that are radiographically occult. Although improved survival is the goal, the rate of recurrent brain metastases is likely to be a more sensitive measure of the impact of WBRT.

Overall survival has generally been shown to be unaffected by the use of WBRT following surgery or RS for brain metastases. The only prospective randomized study found no difference in survival in 95 completely resected patients, of whom 64% had extracranial sites of disease.[51] No difference in survival was found whether or not WBRT was given in a study of 64 patients who were carefully matched according to all significant prognostic factors (including extent of extracranial disease, PS, intrathoracic stage, age, gender, number of brain metastases, synchronous versus metachronous presentation, and extent of intracranial resection).[60] Of three multivariate analyses (involving 231, 116, and 229 patients), two found no survival difference,[34,44] whereas one found a benefit ($P < 0.001$) to WBRT.[47] Closer analysis in this latter study revealed that the survival benefit was seen only in patients without extracranial disease (Fig. 23–4). In contrast, a study from Memorial Sloan-Kettering Cancer Center involving 185 patients, most of whom (62%) also had no extracranial disease, demonstrated no survival benefit to WBRT (Fig. 23–5).[18] Univariate analyses from all other studies involving at least 50 patients have shown no survival benefit to WBRT.[16,45,46]

Studies of the effect of adjuvant WBRT on the rate of recurrent brain metastases have shown conflicting results. A study involving patients who were carefully matched relative to all significant prognostic factors found no difference in the rate of brain relapses.[60] On the other hand, two studies employing multivariate analysis found significantly lower brain relapse rates with WBRT.[44,61] Other studies using univariate analysis in ≥50 patients have generally

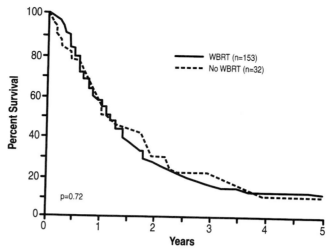

FIGURE 23–5. Retrospective analysis of survival of 185 patients undergoing resection of brain metastases from non–small cell lung cancer according to whether adjuvant whole-brain radiation therapy (WBRT) was used. Most patients (62%) had no extracranial sites of disease, and 94% underwent complete resection of all brain metastases. (From Burt M, Wronski M, Arbit E, et al. Resection of brain metastases from non–small-cell lung carcinoma: results of therapy. J Thorac Cardiovasc Surg. 1992;103:399–411.[18])

shown no difference.[45,62] A benefit was suggested by one study, but patients were clearly mismatched, favoring the WBRT group.[63] However, the only randomized study of WBRT (after surgical resection) found the rate of brain recurrences to be significantly lower (18% versus 70%, $P < 0.001$) after WBRT in 95 well-matched patients.[51] This was true both for recurrences at the site of resection and for recurrences elsewhere in the brain.[51]

In conclusion, the benefit of WBRT following surgery or RS is unclear. The only randomized study found a decrease in the rate of intracranial recurrences but no survival benefit with WBRT in resected patients, most of whom had extracranial sites of disease. Retrospective studies have found mixed results with respect to intracranial recurrence and no survival benefit, at least in patients with extracranial disease. It is logical that a benefit may occur only in patients who have no extracranial disease. This is supported by the results reported by Smalley et al[47] (see Fig. 23–4). An analogy can be made to prophylactic cranial irradiation for patients with small cell cancer. The benefit of prophylactic cranial irradiation in this population has been controversial since the early 1980s, but more recently consensus is mounting that there is a small survival benefit in patients who have a complete response after induction chemoradiotherapy (see Fig. 24–3). The benefit of WBRT must be balanced against the risk of late toxicity. Although the overall risk is low, some data suggests that among patients who survive >1 year, there may be a 10% risk of significant toxicity (Chapter 29).[63,64]

ADRENAL METASTASES

Autopsy studies of patients with advanced stage lung cancer have shown that approximately one-third harbor adrenal metastases.[65,66] Isolated adrenal metastases occur in 2% to

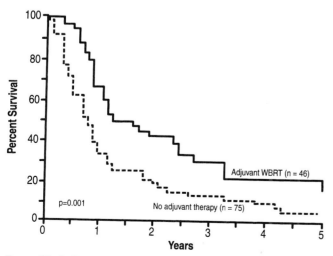

FIGURE 23–4. Retrospective analysis of survival of 121 patients with no systemic disease who underwent complete resection of a brain metastasis according to whether adjuvant whole brain radiotherapy was used (log rank, $P = 0.001$). (From Smalley SR, Laws ER Jr, O'Fallon JR, et al. Resection for solitary brain metastasis. J Neurosurg. 1992;77:531–540.[47])

DATA SUMMARY: RESECTION OF BRAIN METASTASES

	AMOUNT	QUALITY	CONSISTENCY
The operative mortality of resection of a brain metastasis is 2%	High	High	High
The 5-year survival of patients with non–small cell lung cancer who undergo resection of both the primary tumor and an isolated brain metastasis is 15%	High	High	High
Palliative resection of a brain metastasis results in prolongation of survival	**Mod**	**Mod**	**Mod**
The 2-year survival after palliative resection (surgery or radiosurgery) of a brain metastasis is 20%	High	High	High
Favorable prognostic factors with palliative resection include the absence of systemic disease and a PS ≥ 70	High	High	Mod
Repeat resection (surgery or radiosurgery) of a recurrent isolated brain metastasis results in a 5-year survival of 15%	Mod	Mod	High
Adjuvant whole brain radiotherapy following resection of a brain metastasis decreases the intracranial recurrence rate, but does not improve survival	**Poor**	**High**	—

Type of data rated: Plain text: descriptive statement   *Italics: controlled comparison*   **Bold: randomized comparison**

4% of NSCLC patients (see Chapter 6).[67] Through the end of 1998, 75 patients with NSCLC who underwent resection of an adrenal metastasis with curative intent were reported[68–78] (and M. Higashiyama, MD, personal communication, July 7, 1998). Three additional reported patients were not included because the intent of their treatment was not to cure.[71,73] Of the 75 patients with NSCLC and adrenal metastases, 42 were reported as part of three series of adrenal resections for a variety of cancers.[74–76] Few details are available from these latter studies, but the authors reported median survival figures of 14, 13, and 18 months for all patients.[74–76]

Details are available about 31 patients with adrenal metastases who were treated curatively. Most of these patients (77%) had adenocarcinoma, and 58% presented with synchronous adrenal metastases. The median interval between detection of the tumors in metachronous cases was 13 months (range, 8-24 months). Approximately half of the adrenal metastases (46%) were ipsilateral to the primary cancer. No association was found between ipsilateral and contralateral metastasis and the stage of the primary tumor. The primary tumor was classified as stage I in 22%, stage II in 34%, and stage IIIa,b in the remainder (disregarding the metastasis). Approximately one-third of the patients were given chemotherapy, usually in an adjuvant fashion.

Survival for the entire group of 31 patients at 2 years was approximately 45% and at 5 years was 23%. Figure 23–6 shows the survival relative to the stage of the primary tumor. Patients with stage pI,II tumors (disregarding the adrenal metastases) demonstrated 55% actuarial survival at 5 years. A trend toward worse survival was seen in pIIIa,b patients. Although this was not statistically significant, the average follow-up in these patients was only 16 months, and the longest follow-up was 28 months. Other factors, such as synchronous versus metachronous metastases, ipsilateral versus contralateral metastases, histology, and the use of adjuvant therapy, did not show any correlation with the chance of survival.

Some authors have suggested that adrenal metastases may occur via lymphatic connections through the dia-

phragm as opposed to hematogenous spread,[79] although this remains controversial.[80] The combined experience presented here does not suggest a difference based on whether the adrenal metastasis is ipsilateral versus contralateral to the primary tumor. Indeed, there is no clinical data suggesting that adrenal metastases arise through local lymphatic spread.

Two studies have suggested that in addition to the potential for a long-term cure, resection of an isolated adrenal metastasis may have a palliative benefit.[73,81] The first study analyzed all patients over a 5-year span who had a resectable primary lung cancer, a good PS, and an isolated adrenal metastasis and compared the patients who underwent surgical resection with those treated with chemotherapy alone.[81] No difference was found in the patients' age, histologic type, stage of the primary tumor, or size of the adrenal metastasis; in fact, a trend was seen toward a greater proportion of stage III primary tumors in the surgi-

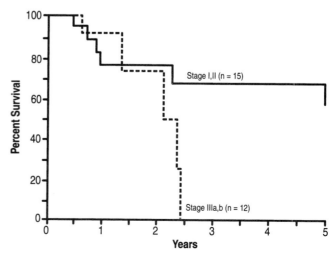

FIGURE 23–6. Survival of patients with adrenal metastases undergoing curative resection, according to stage of the primary lesion (excluding the adrenal metastasis) (P = NS by log rank). (Data from references 68–73, 77, and 78.)

cal group. The median survival was significantly longer in the patients who were resected (31 versus 9 months, $P = 0.03$).[81] The second study examined all resected patients over a 12-year period who subsequently developed an isolated adrenal metastasis and compared those undergoing adrenalectomy with those receiving either chemotherapy or RT to the adrenal metastasis.[73] This study also found that the median survival was longer in resected patients (20 versus 3 months, no P value given).[73] Although both of these studies were retrospective and involved small numbers of patients (N = 14 and 9), the lack of a difference in clinical characteristics between the resected and nonresected patients does suggest a possible palliative benefit to adrenalectomy for isolated adrenal metastases.[73,81]

PULMONARY METASTASES

The staging classification of pulmonary metastases has undergone several changes. The 1997 system classifies a satellite nodule of cancer that is within the same lobe as the primary tumor as T4 (stage IIIb) and additional foci of cancer in different lobes as M1 (stage IV).[82] In a clarification reported in 1993, the 1986 staging system classified pulmonary metastasis as T2 or T3 when located in the same lobe, as T4 when located in an ipsilateral different lobe, and as M1 when the second focus of cancer was contralateral to the primary lung cancer.[83] However, none of these classifications has been universally accepted, and different authors have used a variety of definitions when reporting on patients with a second pulmonary focus of a primary lung cancer.

The classification of pulmonary metastases is difficult because of the existence of several factors that appear to influence patient outcomes and that probably represent different mechanisms of spread. Patients with bronchioloalveolar cancers (BACs) have a high propensity for intrapulmonary spread. A fair amount of evidence suggests that the behavior of these tumors, and perhaps the mechanism of spread, is distinct from that of other NSCLCs (see Chapter 27), and these patients probably should be considered separately. Furthermore, patients with same-lobe satellite nodules (SLSN) appear to have markedly improved survival compared with those who have additional foci in other lobes (see Chapter 30). Some evidence suggests that SLSNs may occur through a local mechanism of spread rather than via hematogenous spread, and these patients probably should be considered separately as well (Chapter 30). However, the data regarding BACs and SLSN is not completely clear, and separate consideration of these tumors is not universally accepted.

Several studies have reported on patients with stage IV NSCLC involving pulmonary metastases who were resected (Table 23–5). The reported 5-year survival is generally good, at approximately 20%. How many of these patients had BAC is not reported, but in most of the studies, the majority of tumors were adenocarcinomas (which leaves open the possibility that many were BACs). Closer analysis of these studies reveals that most of the patients had SLSNs. Little data exists specifically addressing the survival of only those patients with pulmonary metastases in a different lobe. Five-year survivals of 0%

TABLE 23–5. SURVIVAL FOLLOWING RESECTION OF A PRIMARY LUNG CANCER AND A PULMONARY METASTASIS

STUDY	N	% ADENO	% BAC	% SLSN	% 5-YEAR SURVIVAL
Naruke et al[87]	146	68	—	61	(8)[a]
Deslauriers et al[91]	84	25	5	81	22
Nakajima et al[92]	50	84	58	94	30
Watanabe et al[93]	49	56[b]	—	—	22
Yano et al[84]	47	62	—	83	33[c]
Suzuki et al[94]	46	100	Most	100	36
Yoshino et al[95]	42	74	—	—	24[b]
Shimizu et al[85]	42	67	—	88	26
Fukuse et al[86]	41	66	—	49	26

Inclusion criteria: Studies reporting survival of ≥20 patients undergoing resection of a primary lung cancer and a pulmonary metastasis.
[a]For all resected M1 patients (N = 258).
[b]Estimated.
[c]For SLSN; 0 for metastasis in different lobe.
Adeno, adenocarcinoma; BAC, bronchioloalveolar cancer; SLSN, same-lobe satellite nodule (occurring in same lobe as primary cancer).

and 20% were reported in two studies involving eight and five patients[84,85] and a 3-year survival of 21% in 21 patients was reported in another study,[86] and only 3 long-term survivors were found in 57 patients in a fourth study.[87] The survival of resected patients with isolated pulmonary metastases therefore depends on whether a broad or a narrow definition of pulmonary metastases is used. If SLSNs and BACs are included, the survival is fairly good, whereas limited data suggests that the survival is poor if these patients are excluded.

OTHER SITES

Few patients have been reported who have undergone an attempt at curative treatment of isolated metastases from NSCLC involving sites other than the brain or the adrenal gland. The largest series included 14 cases of resected patients who subsequently developed isolated metastases, collected over a 10-year period at the Memorial Sloan-Kettering Cancer Center.[88] These sites included extrathoracic lymph nodes,[6] skeletal muscle,[4] bone,[3] and small bowel[1] and involved resection in 12 cases and curative radiation in 2 cases. The 10-year actuarial survival was an astounding 86% (median follow-up, 8.4 years). Another study reported on three patients who underwent resection of the primary lung cancer and an adrenal metastasis, as well as resection of other abdominal metastases.[73] Two of these patients were alive without evidence of cancer at 24 and 40 months. Resection of an esophageal metastasis has been reported.[89] Although this metastasis presented 5 years after pulmonary resection of the primary tumor, it was classified as a metastasis because of the histologic appearance and the lack of mucosal involvement of the esophagus. In addition, Yokoi et al[90] reported a patient who had survived more than 5 years after resection of an subcutaneous metastasis in the thoracotomy incision performed 9 months earlier to remove a T3N1 adenocarcinoma. These patients are undoubtedly highly selected, and there can be little doubt that many other cases with poor survival have not been reported due to publication bias. Nevertheless, these studies are provocative and suggest that there is a role for curative local therapy for extracranial, extraadrenal metastases from NSCLC in some instances.

EDITORS' COMMENTS

A substantial number of patients with stage IV NSCLC are candidates for surgical or RS treatment of brain metastases, and, in fact, cure is possible in some of these patients. However, they are frequently not identified and referred for such definitive local therapy of metastatic disease, despite multiple reports documenting long-term cures in some patients and randomized trials showing a palliative benefit in others. Of course, not all patients are candidates for such aggressive treatment, and appropriate patient selection is crucial.

The published data is clear that appropriate selection of patients for potentially curative treatment of stage IV NSCLC is based primarily on the ability to achieve complete resection of all known disease. This includes resection of the primary site, as well as definitive treatment of all metastatic foci. Whether this involves single or multiple brain metastases does not appear to be important, provided a complete resection of all lesions can be achieved. However, it must be recognized that this has been applied only to patients with a small number (two to four) of metastatic cranial foci and cannot necessarily be extrapolated to other situations. Most often, resection of a brain metastasis for cure involves patients who have previously been resected and who present with an isolated cranial recurrence. The chance of cure may be somewhat higher in younger patients, female patients, and those with supratentorial lesions. In patients who present with an isolated brain metastasis and a potentially resectable primary lesion, mediastinal node metastases should be excluded by mediastinoscopy, although clear data regarding this issue is lacking.

Aggressive treatment of brain metastases with surgery or RS offers a significant palliative benefit, at least in patients with stable extracranial disease. This has been clearly demonstrated in two randomized studies. Patients with progressing, uncontrolled extracranial sites of disease probably do not derive a benefit from such aggressive treatment. The results for surgery and RS are similar in terms of median survival, improvement in neurologic symptoms, and chance of maintaining functional independence. Various technical factors favor one approach versus another, and the most appropriate treatment should be selected on an individual basis.

Aggressive palliative treatment of brain metastases with surgery or RS is warranted in patients with a good PS and stable extracranial disease. However, the definition of stable disease is not clear. Those patients with no sites of extracranial disease should be considered for a curative approach. We propose that patients should be selected for aggressive palliative treatment if there is documentation of stability of extracranial disease for a period of at least 2 months or, alternatively, if there are only small extracranial foci of cancer that can be controlled or are judged to be not likely to cause clinical symptoms within the next 4 months. A PS ≥ 70 is essential. Older age (>60-65) is a relative exclusion criterion. In previously treated patients who develop recurrent brain metastases, aggressive retreatment results in reasonable survival. This approach is appropriate in patients with a good PS, no systemic disease, and an interval between brain tumors of at least 4 months.

Adjuvant WBRT after definitive treatment with surgery or RS is controversial. In many instances, it does not provide any benefit, and a number of studies have found no improvement in survival. However, in patients who are treated with curative intent, adjuvant WBRT may be of benefit in decreasing the incidence of recurrent brain metastases.

The data regarding curative resection of adrenal metastases is limited. However, the reported 5-year survival of >40% is provocative. Clearly, patients undergoing resection of an adrenal metastasis are highly selected. If such an approach were adopted more widely, it is likely that the 5-year survival would decrease. The data regarding the survival of patients undergoing resection of a true isolated pulmonary metastasis is even more limited, if one excludes patients with satellite nodules in the same lobe (SLSN) as the primary tumor. The long-term survival appears to be 10% to 15%, similar to that of patients with isolated brain metastases.

Taken together, the ability to achieve cure through local treatment in stage IV NSCLC clearly supports the concept that oligometastatic disease occurs in some patients. The difficulty, of course, lies in defining criteria that consistently identify these patients. A prolonged observation period is not practical, given the median survival of only 4 to 6 months for patients with stage IV NSCLC. Furthermore, an aggressive curative approach makes sense only in patients with a good PS. Because such patients are good candidates for systemic chemotherapy, this should be the initial treatment. Those patients who do not develop new metastatic sites during treatment may be candidates for resection of their metastatic disease, although it is difficult to know how to interpret a lack of progression in the face of systemic treatment.

It is possible that whole body positron-emission tomography scanning may be useful in identifying patients with oligometastatic disease. Immunohistochemical markers to define occult micrometastases in bone marrow may also be useful. It may be most appropriate to explore the possibility of curative local therapy in patients with a good PS who demonstrate persistence of only isolated sites of disease after several cycles of chemotherapy. Many advances in the treatment of NSCLC are occurring, and we should give careful consideration to such novel ideas that may provide a chance of cure for some patients.

References

1. Hellman S, Weichselbaum RR. Oligometastases. J Clin Oncol. 1995;13:8–10.
2. Figlin RA, Piantadosi S, Feld R, et al. Intracranial recurrence of carcinoma after complete surgical resection of stage I, II, and III non–small-cell lung cancer. N Engl J Med. 1988;318:1300–1305.
3. Cox JD, Yesner RA. Adenocarcinoma of the lung: recent results from the Veterans Administration Lung Group. Am Rev Respir Dis. 1979;120:1025–1029.
4. Galluzzi S, Payne PM. Brain metastases from primary bronchial

carcinoma: a statistical study of 741 necropsies. Br J Cancer. 1956;10:408–414.

5. Knights EM Jr. The increasing importance of lung cancer as related to metastatic brain tumors. J Neurosurg. 1954;11:306.

6. Posner JB, Chernik NL. Intracranial metastases from systemic cancer. Adv Neurol. 1978;19:579–592.

7. Kurtz JM, Gelber R, Brady LW, et al. The palliation of brain metastases in a favorable patient population: a randomized clinical trial by the Radiation Therapy Oncology Group. Int J Radiat Oncol Biol Phys. 1981;7:891–895.

8. Gelber RD, Larson M, Borgelt BB, et al. Equivalence of radiation schedules for the palliative treatment of brain metastases in patients with favorable prognosis. Cancer. 1981;48:1749–1753.

9. Vecht CJ, Haaxma-Reiche H, Noordijk EM, et al. Treatment of single brain metastasis: radiotherapy alone or combined with neurosurgery? Ann Neurol. 1993;33:583–590.

10. Patchell RA, Tibbs PA, Walsh JW, et al. A randomized trial of surgery in the treatment of single metastases to the brain. N Engl J Med. 1990;322:494–500.

11. Zimm S, Wampler GL, Stablein D, et al. Intracerebral metastases in solid-tumor patients: natural history and results of treatment. Cancer. 1981;48:384–394.

12. Delattre JY, Krol G, Thaler HT, et al. Distribution of brain metastases. Arch Neurol. 1988;45:741–744.

13. Mintz AH, Kestle J, Rathbone MP, et al. A randomized trial to assess the efficacy of surgery in addition to radiotherapy in patients with a single cerebral metastasis. Cancer. 1996;78:1470–1476.

14. Sundaresan N, Galicich JH. Surgical treatment of brain metastases: clinical and computerized tomography evaluation of the results of treatment. Cancer. 1985;55:1382–1388.

15. Auchter RM, Lamond JP, Alexander E III, et al. A multiinstitutional outcome and prognostic factor analysis of radiosurgery for resectable single brain metastasis. Int J Radiat Oncol Biol Phys. 1996;35:27–35.

16. Moriarty TM, Loeffler JS, Black PM, et al. Long-term follow-up of patients treated with stereotactic radiosurgery for single or multiple brain metastases. Radiosurgery. 1996;1:83–91.

17. Yokoi K, Miyazawa N, Arai T. Brain metastasis in resected lung cancer: value of intensive follow-up with computed tomography. Ann Thorac Surg. 1996;61:546–551.

18. Burt M, Wronski M, Arbit E, et al. Resection of brain metastases from non–small-cell lung carcinoma: results of therapy. J Thorac Cardiovasc Surg. 1992;103:399–411.

19. Wingo PA, Tong T, Bolden S. Cancer statistics, 1995. CA Cancer J Clin. 1995;45:8–30.

20. Sundaresan N, Galicich JH. Surgical treatment of single brain metastases from non–small-cell lung cancer. Cancer Invest. 1985;3:107–113.

21. Borgelt B, Gelber R, Kramer S, et al. The palliation of brain metastases: final results of the first two studies by the Radiation Therapy Oncology Group. Int J Radiat Oncol Biol Phys. 1980;6:1–9.

22. Newman SJ, Hansen HH. Frequency, diagnosis, and treatment of brain metastases in 247 consecutive patients with bronchogenic carcinoma. Cancer. 1974;33:492.

23. Patchell RA, Cirrincione C, Thaler HT, et al. Single brain metastases: surgery plus radiation or radiation alone. Neurology. 1986;36:447–453.

24. Cairncross JG, Kim J-H, Posner JB. Radiation therapy for brain metastases. Ann Neurol. 1980;7:529–541.

25. Chang D-B, Yang P-C, Luh K-T, et al. Late survival of non–small cell lung cancer patients with brain metastases: influence of treatment. Chest. 1992;101:1293–1297.

26. Nakagawa H, Miyawaki Y, Fujita T, et al. Surgical treatment of brain metastases of lung cancer: retrospective analysis of 89 cases. J Neurol Neurosurg Psychiatry. 1994;57:950–956.

27. Young RF. Radiosurgery for the treatment of brain metastases. Semin Surg Oncol. 1998;14:70–78.

28. Richards P, McKissock W. Intracranial metastases. BMJ. 1963;1:15–18.

29. Stoier M. Metastatic tumors of the brain. Acta Neurol Scand. 1965;41:262–268.

30. Martini N. Rationale for surgical treatment of brain metastasis in non–small cell lung cancer. Ann Thorac Surg. 1986;42:357–358.

31. Ruderman NB, Hall TC. Use of glucocorticoids in the palliative treatment of metastatic brain tumors. Cancer. 1965;18:298–306.

32. Deeley TJ, Rice Edwards JM. Radiotherapy in the management of cerebral secondaries from bronchial carcinoma. Lancet. 1968;1:1209–1213.

33. Montana GS, Meacham WF, Caldwell WL. Brain irradiation for metastatic disease of lung origin. Cancer. 1972;29:1477–1480.

34. Wronski M, Arbit E, Burt M, et al. Survival after surgical treatment of brain metastases from lung cancer: a follow-up study of 231 patients treated between 1976 and 1991. J Neurosurg. 1995;83:605–616.

35. Mussi A, Pistolesi M, Lucchi M, et al. Resection of single brain metastasis in non–small-cell lung cancer: prognostic factors. J Thorac Cardiovasc Surg. 1996;112:146–153.

36. Read RC, Boop WC, Yoder G, et al. Management of nonsmall cell lung carcinoma with solitary brain metastasis. J Thorac Cardiovasc Surg. 1989;98:884–891.

37. Macchiarini P, Buonaguidi R, Hardin M, et al. Results and prognostic factors of surgery in the management of non–small cell lung cancer with solitary brain metastasis. Cancer. 1991;68:300–304.

38. Magilligan DJ Jr, Duvernoy C, Malik G, et al. Surgical approach to lung cancer with solitary cerebral metastasis: twenty-five years' experience. Ann Thorac Surg. 1986;42:360–364.

39. Hankins JR, Miller JE, Salcman M, et al. Surgical management of lung cancer with solitary cerebral metastasis. Ann Thorac Surg. 1988;46:24–28.

40. Rossi NP, Zavala DC, VanGilder JC. A combined surgical approach to non–oat-cell pulmonary carcinoma with single cerebral metastasis. Respiration. 1987;51:170–178.

41. Torre M, Quaini E, Chiesa G, et al. Synchronous brain metastasis from lung cancer: result of surgical treatment in combined resection. J Thorac Cardiovasc Surg. 1988;95:994–997.

42. Mandell L, Hilaris B, Sullivan M, et al. The treatment of single brain metastasis from non–oat cell carcinoma: surgery and radiation versus radiation therapy alone. Cancer. 1986;58:641–649.

43. Alexander E III, Moriarty TM, Davis RB, et al. Stereotactic radiosurgery for the definitive, noninvasive treatment of brain metastases. J Natl Cancer Inst. 1995;87:34–40.

44. Flickinger JC, Kondziolka D, Lunsford LD, et al. A multi-institutional experience with stereotactic radiosurgery for solitaty brain metastasis. Int J Radiat Oncol Biol Phys. 1994;28:797–802.

45. Young RF, Jacques DB, Duma C, et al. Gamma knife radiosurgery for treatment of multiple brain metastases: a comparison of patients with single versus multiple lesions. Radiosurgery. 1996;1:92–101.

46. Shu H-KG, Sneed PK, Shiau C-Y, et al. Factors influencing survival after gamma knife radiosurgery for patients with single and multiple brain metastases. Cancer J Sci Am. 1996;2:235–242.

47. Smalley SR, Laws ER Jr, O'Fallon JR, et al. Resection for solitary brain metastasis. J Neurosurg. 1992;77:531–540.

48. Kim YS, Kondziolka D, Flickinger JC, et al. Stereotactic radiosurgery for patients with nonsmall cell lung carcinoma metastatic to the brain. Cancer. 1997;80:2075–2083.

49. Shirato H, Takamura A, Tomita M, et al. Stereotactic irradiation without whole-brain irradiation for single brain metastasis. Int J Radiat Oncol Biol Phys. 1997;37:385–391.

50. Bindal RK, Sawaya R, Leavens ME, et al. Surgical treatment of multiple brain metastases. J Neurosurg. 1993;79:210–216.

51. Patchell RA, Tibbs PA, Regine WF, et al. Postoperative radiotherapy in the treatment of single metastases to the brain: a randomized trial. JAMA. 1998;280:1485–1489.

52. Sause WT, Crowley JJ, Morantz R, et al. Solitary brain metastasis: results of an RTOG/SWOG protocol evaluation surgery + RT versus RT alone. Am J Clin Oncol. 1990;13:427–432.

53. Bindal AK, Bindal RK, Hess KR, et al. Surgery versus radiosurgery in the treatment of brain metastasis. J Neurosurg. 1996;84:748–754.

54. Mehta M, Noyes W, Craig B, et al. A cost-effectiveness and cost-utility analysis of radiosurgery vs. resection for single-brain metastases. Int J Radiat Oncol Biol Phys. 1997;39:445–454.

55. Lang FF, Sawaya R. Surgical treatment of metastatic brain tumors. Semin Surg Oncol. 1998;14:53–63.

56. Gaspar L, Scott C, Rotman M, et al. Recursive partitioning analysis (RPA) of prognostic factors in three Radiation Therapy Oncology Group (RTOG) brain metastases trials. Int J Radiat Oncol Biol Phys. 1997;37:745–751.

57. Arbit E, Wronski M, Burt M, et al. The treatment of patients with recurrent brain metastases: a retrospective analysis of 109 patients with nonsmall cell lung cancer. Cancer. 1995;76:765–773.

58. Bindal RK, Sawaya R, Leavens ME, et al. Reoperation for recurrent metastatic brain tumors. J Neurosurg. 1995;83:600–604.

59. Sundaresan N, Sachdev VP, DiGiacinto GV, et al. Reoperation for brain metastases. J Clin Oncol. 1988;6:1625–1629.

60. Armstrong JG, Wronski M, Galicich J, et al. Postoperative radiation for lung cancer metastatic to the brain. J Clin Oncol. 1994;12:2340–2344.

61. Smalley SR, Schray MF, Laws ER Jr, et al. Adjuvant radiation therapy after surgical resection of solitary brain metastasis: association with pattern of failure and survival. Int J Radiat Oncol Biol Phys. 1987;13:1611–1616.

62. Shiau C-Y, Sneed PK, Shu H-KG, et al. Radiosurgery for brain metastases: relationship of dose and pattern of enhancement to local control. Int J Radiat Oncol Biol Phys. 1997;37:375–383.

63. DeAngelis LM, Mandell LR, Thaler HT, et al. The role of postoperative radiotherapy after resection of single brain metastases. Neurosurgery. 1989;24:798–805.

64. Crossen JR, Garwood D, Glatstein E, et al. Neurobehavioral sequelae of cranial irradiation in adults: a review of radiation-induced encephalopathy. J Clin Oncol. 1994;12:627–642.

65. Luketich JD, Van Raemdonck DE, Ginsberg RJ. Extended resection for higher-stage non–small-cell lung cancer. World J Surg. 1993;17:719–728.

66. Engelman RM, McNamara WL. Bronchogenic carcinoma: a statistical review of two hundred and thirty-four autopsies. J Thorac Surg. 1954;27:227–237.

67. Oliver TW Jr, Bernardino ME, Miller JI, et al. Isolated adrenal masses in nonsmall-cell bronchogenic carcinoma. Radiology. 1984;153:217–218.

68. Twomey P, Montgomery C. Successful treatment of adrenal metastases from large-cell carcinoma of the lung. JAMA. 1982;248:581–583.

69. Urschel JD, Finley RK, Takita H. Long-term survival after bilateral adrenalectomy for metastatic lung cancer: a case report. Chest. 1997;112:848–850.

70. Reyes L, Parvez Z, Nemoto T, et al. Adrenalectomy for adrenal metastasis from lung carcinoma. J Surg Oncol. 1990;44:32–34.

71. Raviv G, Klein E, Yellin A, et al. Surgical treatment of solitary adrenal metastasis from lung carcinoma. J Surg Oncol. 1990;43:123–124.

72. Ayabe H, Tsuji H, Hara S, et al. Surgical management of adrenal metastasis from brochogenic carcinoma. J Surg Oncol. 1995;58:149–154.

73. Higashiyama M, Doi O, Kodama K, et al. Surgical treatment of adrenal metastasis following pulmonary resection for lung cancer: comparison of adrenalectomy with palliative therapy. Int Surg. 1994;79:124–129.

74. Wade TP, Longo WE, Virgo KS, et al. A comparison of adrenalectomy with other resections for metastatic cancers. Am J Surg. 1998;175:183–186.

75. Lo CY, van Heerden JA, Soreide JA, et al. Adrenalectomy for metastatic disease to the adrenal glands. Br J Surg. 1996;83:528–531.

76. Kim SH, Brennan MF, Russo P, et al. The role of surgery in the treatment of clinically isolated adrenal metastasis. Cancer. 1998;82:389–394.

77. Porte HL, Roumilhac D, Graziana J-P, et al. Adrenalectomy for a solitary adrenal metastasis from lung cancer. Ann Thorac Surg. 1998;65:331–335.

78. Kirsch AJ, Oz MC, Stoopler M, et al. Operative management of adrenal metastases from lung carcinoma. Urology. 1993;42:716–719.

79. Károlyi P. Do adrenal metastases from lung cancer develop by lymphogenous or hematogenous route? J Surg Oncol. 1990;43:154–156.

80. Beitler AL, Urschel JD, Velagapudi SRC, et al. Surgical management of adrenal metastases from lung cancer. J Surg Oncol. 1998;69:54–57.

81. Luketich JD, Burt ME. Does resection of adrenal metastases from non–small cell lung cancer improve survival? Ann Thorac Surg. 1996;62:1614–1616.

82. Mountain CF. Revisions in the International System for Staging Lung Cancer. Chest. 1997;111:1710–1717.

83. Beahrs OH, Henson DE, Hutter RVP, et al. Handbook for Staging of Cancer. Philadelphia, Pa: JB Lippincott; 1993.

84. Yano M, Arai T, Inagaki K, et al. Intrapulmonary satellite nodule of lung cancer as a T factor. Chest. 1998;114:1305–1308.

85. Shimizu N, Ando A, Date H, et al. Prognosis of undetected intrapulmonary metastases in resected lung cancer. Cancer. 1993;71:3868–3872.

86. Fukuse T, Hirata T, Tanaka F, et al. Prognosis of ipsilateral intrapulmonary metastases in resected nonsmall cell lung cancer. Eur J Cardiothorac Surg. 1997;12:218–223.

87. Naruke T, Tomoyuki G, Tsuchiya R, et al. Prognosis and survival in resected lung carcinoma based on the new international staging system. J Thorac Cardiovasc Surg. 1988;96:440–447.

88. Luketich JD, Martini N, Ginsberg RJ, et al. Successful treatment of solitary extracranial metastases from non–small cell lung cancer. Ann Thorac Surg. 1995;60:1609–1611.

89. Oka T, Ayabe H, Kawahara K, et al. Esophagectomy for metastatic carcinoma of the esophagus from lung cancer. Cancer. 1993;71:2958–2961.

90. Yokoi K, Miyazawa N, Imura G. Isolated incisional recurrence after curative resection for primary lung cancer. Ann Thorac Surg. 1996;61:1236–1237.

91. Deslauriers J, Brisson J, Cartier R, et al. Carcinoma of the lung: evaluation of satellite nodules as a factor influencing prognosis after resection. J Thorac Cardiovasc Surg. 1989;97:504–512.

92. Nakajima J, Furuse A, Oka T, et al. Excellent survival in a subgroup of patients with intrapulmonary metastasis of lung cancer. Ann Thorac Surg. 1996;61:158–163.

93. Watanabe Y, Shimizu J, Oda M, et al. Proposals regarding some deficiencies in the new international staging system for non–small cell lung cancer. Jpn J Clin Oncol. 1991;21:160–168.

94. Suzuki K, Nagai K, Yoshida J, et al. The prognosis of resected lung carcinoma associated with atypical adenomatous hyperplasia: a comparison of the prognosis of well-differentiated adenocarcinoma associated with atypical adenomatous hyperplasia and intrapulmonary metastasis. Cancer. 1997;79:1521–1526.

95. Yoshino I, Nakanishi R, Osaki T, et al. Postoperative prognosis in patients with non–small cell lung cancer with synchronous ipsilateral intrapulmonary metastasis. Ann Thorac Surg. 1997;64:809–813.

96. Ehrenhaft JL, in Discussion of Magilligan DJ Jr, Duvernoy C, Malik G, et al. Surgical approach to lung cancer with solitary cerebral metastasis: twenty-five years' experience. Ann Thorac Surg. 1986;42:360–364.

97. White KT, Fleming TR, Laws ER Jr. Single metastasis to the brain: surgical treatment in 122 consecutive patients. Mayo Clin Proc. 1981;56:424–428.

98. Ferrara M, Bizzozzero L, Talamonti G, et al. Surgical treatment of 100 single brain metastases: analysis of the results. J Neurosurg Sci. 1990;34:303–308.

99. Saitoh Y, Minami K, Tokunou M, et al. Results of surgery for bronchogenic carcinoma located in the aortic window. Lung Cancer. 1997;18:47–56.

PART 7

SMALL CELL LUNG CANCER

LIMITED STAGE SMALL CELL LUNG CANCER

David E. Morris, Mark A. Socinski, and Frank C. Detterbeck

Approximately 20% of all lung cancers are small cell lung cancers (SCLC) (see Table 3–6), although the percentage may be decreasing. Approximately 40% of these are classified as limited stage small cell lung cancers (see Table 6–1). Although limited stage small cell lung cancer (LS SCLC), by definition, involves gross disease that is still localized to the chest, it is likely that most patients with this disease actually harbor occult systemic micrometastases. Nevertheless, there are important differences in the issues presented by LS SCLC and extended stage (ES) SCLC. For example, in LS SCLC, all of the gross tumor can be treated by chest radiotherapy (RT) in addition to chemotherapy. The use of both treatment modalities may be important if the tumor in the chest harbors drug-resistant cells. Furthermore, the effect of chemotherapy on microscopic distant metastatic deposits in patients with LS SCLC may be different from the effect on gross systemic metastases in patients with ES SCLC. Therefore, this chapter focuses specifically on patients with LS SCLC, whereas ES SCLC is discussed in Chapter 25.

DEFINITIONS/STAGING

In practice, the distinction between LS and ES SCLC is usually fairly clear, although there is no definition that is universally agreed upon. The most commonly used definition is that limited stage involves disease that can be encompassed by a reasonable single radiation port. A "reasonable" port usually means that the disease is localized to one hemithorax and the mediastinum. Despite general agreement about most patients who are classified as having

LS SCLC, several controversial areas exist (Fig. 24–1). For example, there is disagreement about whether patients with contralateral, or even ipsilateral, supraclavicular lymphadenopathy should be classified as having limited stage or extensive stage disease.[1,2] Similar disagreements exist regarding patients with contralateral hilar lymphade-

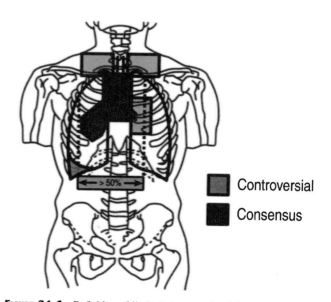

FIGURE 24–1. Definition of limited stage small cell lung cancer. Darkly shaded areas represent tumors that are widely agreed upon as being limited stage. There is controversy about whether tumors involving areas shaded lightly should be classified as limited stage or extensive stage.

nopathy and isolated ipsilateral pleural effusions, based on reports that the prognosis of such patients is similar to that of patients with more clearly defined limited intrathoracic disease.[3]

The Radiation Therapy Oncology Group (RTOG) and the Eastern Cooperative Oncology Group (ECOG) define limited stage disease as disease confined to one hemithorax and exclude patients with a malignant pleural effusion, contralateral hilar lymphadenopathy, or contralateral supraclavicular lymphadenopathy. The European Organization for Research and Treatment of Cancer (EORTC) defines limited stage disease as involving <50% of the maximum transverse diameter of the thorax on a posteroanterior radiograph before chemotherapy.[4] The National Cancer Institute of Canada (NCIC) Clinical Trials Group considers limited stage disease to be limited to one lung, the mediastinum, and the ipsilateral supraclavicular lymph nodes.[5] No cooperative group is currently enrolling patients who have isolated ipsilateral malignant pleural effusions in clinical trials for LS SCLC, which suggests these patients should be classified as having ES SCLC. Furthermore, the American Joint Committee on Cancer staging system applies the TNM system to SCLC, although this practice has not gained routine clinical acceptance.[6] Intrathoracic and extrathoracic staging of SCLC is discussed in Chapters 5 and 6.

NATURAL HISTORY

Limited data exists regarding the natural history of (untreated) SCLC. The Veterans Administration Lung Study Group (VALSG) reported that the median survival of 108 untreated extensive stage patients was 5 weeks, and the median survival of 38 untreated limited stage patients was 12 weeks.[7] A natural history of 8 to 12 weeks was reported in a prospective trial that randomized patients with ES SCLC between chemotherapy and best supportive care.[8] Another trial, involving 31 patients with LS SCLC who received only best supportive care, found a median survival of 18 weeks and a 1-year survival of 7%.[9] All of these studies predate the availability of computed tomography (CT), which means that a number of the LS SCLC patients may have been understaged.

PROGNOSTIC FACTORS

Almost all studies that have assessed prognostic factors have combined limited and extensive stage patients. Multivariate analysis usually finds that limited stage disease is a good prognostic feature. After the stage is taken into account, other prognostic factors (eg, patient characteristics, extent of measurable disease, laboratory parameters, serologic markers, and presence or absence of paraneoplastic syndromes) are often no longer predictive of survival.[10] However, one study of 264 patients with LS SCLC found that the absence of mediastinal lymph node involvement (by either CT or mediastinoscopy) predicted better survival (median survival, 15 months versus 12 months; $P = 0.02$).[11] Because data about prognostic factors primarily involves extensive stage patients, individual prognostic factors are discussed in the chapter on ES SCLC (Chapter 25).

EPIDEMIOLOGY AND PATHOLOGIC CLASSIFICATION

Approximately 180 000 new cases of lung cancer occur in the United States each year, and more than 160 000 deaths from lung cancer are reported annually. SCLC constitutes approximately 20% of these cancers, approximately 40% of which are limited stage disease. The primary risk factor for SCLC worldwide is tobacco consumption.[12] In fact, the occurrence of SCLC in a nonsmoker is so rare (0%-3%) that one must question the diagnosis of SCLC in a patient who is a lifelong nonsmoker.[13–17] Additional risk factors include exposure to asbestos, radon, uranium mining, and bis-chloromethyl ether.[18]

The most commonly used histopathologic classification of SCLC is that proposed by the International Association for the Study of Lung Cancer in 1988[19] (see Table 3–5). The pure small cell type accounts for approximately 95% of cases, and the other types of SCLC are uncommon. Moreover, no prognostic or therapeutic implications of the morphologic types of SCLC have been defined.[20,21]

CLINICAL PRESENTATION AND DIAGNOSIS

Signs and symptoms of SCLC relate to the bulk of disease and anatomic location of the tumor. In a population-based retrospective review of presenting symptoms, cough, weight loss, dyspnea, and chest pain were each present in approximately one-third of patients with LS SCLC.[22] Hemoptysis and hoarseness also occur frequently. Regional and mediastinal lymphadenopathy are present in the majority of patients (see Table 5–2). Various paraneoplastic syndromes have been reported with SCLC.[23] These include the syndrome of inappropriate antidiuretic hormone (SIADH), hyponatremia, ectopic ACTH production, and Eaton-Lambert syndrome (see Chapter 25).

The diagnosis is typically suspected when a chest radiograph shows evidence of a pulmonary infiltrate and associated hilar and mediastinal lymphadenopathy. A pleural effusion or atelectasis may also be present (Table 4–5). SCLCs tend to be located more centrally than their non–small cell counterparts, but they occasionally present as peripheral nodules. However, histologic and cytologic confirmation is necessary because small cell carcinoma cannot reliably be distinguished from non–small cell carcinoma on the basis of radiographic findings. A cytologic diagnosis can usually be obtained from sputum, bronchoscopic brushings and washings, or transthoracic fine needle aspiration. The sensitivity rates for diagnosis of SCLC have been reported to be 50% for sputum, 69% for bronchial brushings, and 64% for bronchial washings.[24] Histologic specimens can be obtained from core needle biopsy, bronchoscopic biopsy, mediastinoscopy, thoracoscopy, or thoracotomy. In a prospective study comparing cytologic examination of fine needle aspirate specimens with histologic examinations of core needle biopsies for thoracic tumors, diagnostic reliability was significantly enhanced with core needle biopsy (97% versus 59%).[25] However, some institutions have reported that the diagnostic yield of a transthoracic needle aspirate can be as high as 80%[26] to

95% (when done with fluoroscopic guidance).[27] Overall, fiberoptic bronchoscopy with either cytologic or histologic specimens provided a correct diagnosis in 93% of patients in a study of 180 patients with SCLC.[28] Mediastinoscopy, thoracoscopy, and thoracotomy are reserved for patients in whom other techniques have failed to obtain a diagnosis.

CHEMOTHERAPY

Single Agent and Combination Chemotherapy

Several older randomized trials have compared chemotherapy or surgery with RT alone. Although most of the results are only of historical interest today, a consistent and important finding has been that 95% of patients treated with RT alone die of their disease, usually because of systemic metastases.[29–31] Furthermore, in an autopsy series of 19 patients who died of postoperative complications within 30 days of a "curative" resection of LS SCLC, 70% had identifiable metastatic disease.[32] These results point to a need for effective systemic therapy. In prospective phase II trials, at least 16 chemotherapeutic agents have been shown to have activity against SCLC, with response rates >20% (Table 24–1). However, none of these agents, used alone, consistently produced response rates >50%, and there were few documented complete responses. These findings led naturally to the study of multi-agent chemotherapy.

Treatment with combination chemotherapy regimens has yielded better response rates than those seen in the single-agent studies. There is little doubt that combination chemotherapy represents better treatment, despite the fact that there are few randomized trials directly comparing combination with single-agent chemotherapy. A randomized trial comparing initial treatment using cyclophosphamide with

a regimen of cyclophosphamide, doxorubicin, and dacarbazine (DTIC) was reported by Lowenbraun et al.[33] Two hundred eighty-eight patients were enrolled and stratified according to extent of disease, prior RT, and performance status (PS). Only the first 68 patients (12 LS, 56 ES) of a target of 288 patients were randomized because a statistically significant difference in response rate was found favoring combination therapy (12% versus 59%; $P < 0.005$), and the randomization was discontinued. For the total group, the combination therapy also demonstrated a statistically significant benefit in median survival time (31 weeks versus 18 weeks; $P = 0.01$). Another randomized trial compared oral etoposide with intravenous cyclophosphamide, doxorubicin, and vincristine (CAV) in 339 patients with SCLC and poor PS.[34] The combination chemotherapy arm had better overall response (51% versus 45%; $P = 0.03$), median survival time (6 months versus 4 months; $P = 0.03$), and 6-month survival (49% versus 35%; $P = 0.03$). These studies, in conjunction with a series of phase II single-agent studies, have demonstrated that combination chemotherapy is superior to single-agent treatment.

The most effective combination chemotherapy regimen remains the subject of investigation. However, a few combinations have become fairly standard. In this regard, two frequently cited phase II trials are particularly important because of the influence they have had on current standard treatment. The Southwest Oncology Group (SWOG) treated 108 patients with limited stage disease with CAV followed by radiation to the primary tumor and the brain.[35] A 41% complete response rate and a 75% complete and partial response rate were observed, as well as a 52-week median survival. In a second trial, involving 28 patients treated with etoposide and cisplatin (EP), Evans et al[36] demonstrated a 43% complete response (CR) rate and an additional 43% partial response (PR) rate. Of the 11 patients with limited stage disease, the median duration of response was 9 months and the median survival time was 16 months. Partly because of these results, CAV and EP, with minor variations, were adopted as the most commonly used chemotherapy regimens throughout the 1990s.

In summary, combination chemotherapy appears to be superior to single-agent therapy, based on multiple phase II trials and on two phase III trials. Although the randomized trials may not always have used the best single agent for comparison, the differences in responses with combination therapy have been sufficient to justify combination therapy as the standard of care. The optimal combination regimen has not yet been determined. Commonly used regimens include either cyclophosphamide, doxorubicin, vincristine (CAV) or etoposide, cisplatin (EP). Because of less myelotoxicity with the EP combination and the risk of toxicity when doxorubicin is combined with radiation, the EP combination has been favored when it is delivered concurrently with radiation.

Alternating Versus Sequential Chemotherapy

Multiple studies have been performed to determine the appropriate timing and delivery of chemotherapy. Based on a mathematical model that they developed, Goldie and

TABLE 24–1. CHEMOTHERAPEUTIC AGENTS DEMONSTRATING SINGLE-AGENT ACTIVITY IN SMALL CELL LUNG CANCER

AGENT	N STUDIES	CR/PR RATE (%)	REFERENCES
Etoposide	6	23–81	122–127
Teniposide	5	28–90	128–132
Cisplatin	1	22	133
Carboplatin	1	41	134
Nimustine	1	47	135
Cyclophosphamide	2	22–70	136, 137
Ifosfamide	1	49	138
Doxorubicin	1	23	139
Epirubicin	2	48	140, 141
Vincristine	1	42	142
Vindesine	2	21–27	143, 144
Docetaxel	1	23	145
Paclitaxel	2	29–34	146, 147
Topotecan	3	22–39	148–150
Gemcitabine	1	25	151
Hexamethylmelamine	1	42	152

Inclusion criteria: Studies involving >20 patients with either limited stage or extensive stage small cell lung cancer from 1975 to 2000 reporting single agent response rates; agents not reported to have at least a 20% response rate as single agents have been excluded.

CR/PR, complete or partial response.

Coldman[37] proposed that non–cross-resistant combinations be delivered in as rapid a sequence as possible to maximize the chances of tumor eradication (see Chapter 10). Because of overlapping toxic effects of the drugs, alternating chemotherapy combinations that are non–cross-resistant appeared to be a logical and attractive hypothesis to test. The 10 randomized studies involving at least 100 patients with LS SCLC are summarized in Table 24–2. The studies that used either CAV or EP are discussed in the following paragraphs.

Fukuoka et al[38] randomized 288 patients with limited stage disease to receive CAV, EP, or alternating delivery of these two drug combinations. Thoracic radiation was included after chemotherapy. Complete response rates were similar in all three groups (16%, 18%, 22%), but the overall response rate was higher in the alternating regimen and the EP group compared with the CAV group (88% versus 77% versus 51%; $P < 0.01$). The median survival time with the alternating regimen was significantly superior to that seen with the other two regimens (17 months versus 12 months and 12 months; $P = 0.02$).

A SWOG study randomized patients with LS disease to an alternating regimen of CAV and EP or concurrent cyclophosphamide, doxorubicin, vincristine, and etoposide (CAVE).[39] With 400 patients randomized, no statistical difference was seen in either the complete response rate or the median survival time. This study did not specifically test the Goldie–Coldman hypothesis because it did not test the alternating regimen against one of its single combinations, but the study did have sufficient power to state that there is no apparent difference between a four-drug regimen and an alternating regimen using five different drugs.

The National Cancer Institute of Canada (NCIC) performed a randomized trial involving 300 patients with LS disease to study whether alternating CAV with EP was better than sequential administration of the two drug combinations.[40] A trend toward a higher CR rate was found with the alternating regimen (52% versus 40%; $P = 0.2$),

but there was no significant difference in disease-free or overall survival. The authors concluded that either the study had insufficient power or that EP is a superior regimen and that exposure to these two drugs early in treatment improves results.

Wolf et al[41] randomized 134 patients with limited stage disease either to alternating treatment with ifosfamide/etoposide (IE) and CAV, rigidly alternating with each cycle, or to response-oriented therapy with IE until maximal response was observed, followed by CAV. With a minimum of 2 years of follow-up, the study demonstrated no difference in response, median survival time, or 2-year survival. These investigators concluded that there was no advantage to alternating therapies.

In summary, most randomized trials of alternating chemotherapy in patients with LS SCLC have found no difference with respect to survival or response rates. Some differences have been seen in the regimens used and in the duration of treatment. The design of some trials involving alternating chemotherapy arms did not clearly address the Goldie–Coldman hypothesis. However, taken together, these trials provide a strong argument that alternating chemotherapy does not have a major effect on survival in patients with LS SCLC. The additional complexity of alternating treatment does not appear to be worthwhile.

Dose Intensity, Drug Delivery, and Late Consolidation

Dose intensity in chemotherapy has been defined as the amount of drug delivered in a given period of time and is usually standardized to body surface area (eg, $mg/m^2/day$). Increased dose intensity has been correlated with improved outcomes in other types of cancers.[42,43] Klasa et al[44] performed a meta-analysis to determine whether a relationship between dose intensity and outcome exists in SCLC and which commonly used agents in combination have desir-

TABLE 24–2. RANDOMIZED TRIALS OF STANDARD VERSUS ALTERNATING CHEMOTHERAPY REGIMENS FOR LIMITED STAGE SMALL CELL LUNG CANCER

STUDY	N[b]	STANDARD REGIMEN	ALTERNATING REGIMEN	MST (mo)[a] Standard	MST (mo)[a] Alternating	2-y SURVIVAL (%)[a] Standard	2-y SURVIVAL (%)[a] Alternating	P
Urban et al[153]	394	CAEU	CUE↔PEVd	13	10	25	10	0.01
Goodman et al[39]	388	CAVE	EP↔CAV	15	17	20	25	NS
Wolf et al[41]	321	IE→CAV	IE↔CAV	12	12	21	18	NS
Havemann et al[154]	302	CAV	EVdI↔PAVd↔CMxU	11	13	11	14	0.05
Feld et al[40]	300	CAV→EP	CAV↔EP	13	13	18	18	NS
Fukuoka et al[38c]	191	CAV	CAV↔EP	12	17	11	31	0.01
Fukuoka et al[38c]	191	EP	CAV↔EP	12	17	21	31	0.02
Daniels et al[155]	132	CUVPz	AEMx↔CUVPz[d]	10	16	25	25	NS
Ueoka et al[156]	129	CAV→EP	CAV↔EP	21	18	30	30	NS
Aisner et al[157]	109	CAE	CAE↔MxUVPz	16	12	25	25	NS
Average				**14**	**15**	**21**	**23**	

Inclusion criteria: Randomized trials from 1980 to 2000 involving >100 patients total, reporting survival for limited stage small cell lung cancer exclusively.
[a]Survival results are for limited stage patients only.
[b]Total number of patients in study (both extensive-stage and limited-stage small cell lung cancer).
[c]Three-arm study.
[d]Alternating treatment began after initial AEMx × 3.
Chemotherapy regimens: AEMx, doxorubicin, etoposide, methotrexate; CAE, cyclophosphamide, doxorubicin, etoposide; CAEU, cyclophosphamide, doxorubicin, etoposide, CCNU; CAV, cyclophosphamide, doxorubicin, vincristine; CAVE, cyclophosphamide, doxorubicin, vincristine, etoposide; CMxU, cyclophosphamide, methotrexate, CCNU; CUE, cyclophosphamide, CCNU, etoposide; CUVPz, cyclophosphamide, CCNU, vincristine, procarbazine; EP, etoposide, cisplatin; EVdI, etoposide, vindesine, ifosfamide; IE, ifosfamide, etoposide; MxUVPz, methotrexate, CCNU, vincristine, procarbazine; PAVd, cisplatin, doxorubicin, vindesine; PEVd, cisplatin, etoposide, vindesine.
MST, median survival time; →, sequential; ↔, alternating with.

able dose-intensity outcome characteristics. They reviewed 60 studies and performed the analysis on the *intended* dose intensity as specified in the protocols. Dose intensity was evaluated in relation to objective response (CR + PR), complete response, and median survival time. Thirty-five studies used only limited stage patients. Sixteen of these used CAV, 11 used cyclophosphamide, doxorubicin, and etoposide (CAE) with or without vincristine, and 8 used EP. No statistically significant relationship could be demonstrated between dose intensity and outcome.

Whereas the meta-analysis evaluated intended dose intensity, Arriagada et al[45] performed a randomized trial evaluating the effect of the *delivered* dose intensity of cisplatin and cyclophosphamide in patients with LS SCLC. One hundred and five patients were randomized to a first cycle of "dose-escalated" versus "standard" chemotherapy. The two regimens were 300 mg/m² of cyclophosphamide day 1 to 4 and 100 mg/m² of cisplatin versus 225 mg/m² of cyclophosphamide day 1 to 4 and 80 mg/m² of cisplatin, in conjunction with the same doses of doxorubicin, etoposide, and radiation in both arms. All patients received the prescribed dose during the first cycle of chemotherapy. An improvement was found in the 6-month CR rate (67% versus 54%; $P = 0.02$) and a trend toward increased median duration of CR in the dose-escalated arm (18 months versus 12 months, $P = 0.06$). At 30 months of follow-up, overall survival was improved in the dose-escalated arm (28% versus 11%; $P = 0.02$), and 2-year disease-free survival was better (28% versus 8%; $P = 0.02$). There was a trend toward increased toxicity with the dose-escalated arm, characterized primarily by an increased rate of severe granulocytopenia (39% versus 23%; $P = 0.09$). No additional toxicity was seen, and no difference was found in the ability to deliver the remaining cycles of chemotherapy.

Testing the mode of drug delivery, the North Central Cancer Treatment Group (NCCTG) evaluated different sequencing effects and administration schedules of EP.[46] This study randomized 188 patients with LS SCLC among four different intravenous regimens: (1) bolus cisplatin at 30 mg/m² followed by bolus etoposide at 130 mg/m²; (2) bolus etoposide at 130 mg/m² followed by bolus cisplatin at 30 mg/m²; (3) etoposide, 130 mg/m² by 24-hour infusion, followed by bolus cisplatin at 30 mg/m²; and (4) etoposide, 130 mg/m² by 24-hour infusion, followed by cisplatin, 45 mg/m² by 24-hour infusion. Subsequent therapy was the same for all arms, with four cycles of CAV at 4-week intervals. Two-year and median survival were better on arm 1 (42%, 20 months) than on arm 2 (25%, 13 months) but not significantly better than arm 3 (33%, 17 months) and arm 4 (34%, 20 months). These results suggest that bolus administration of cisplatin followed by etoposide may be the most effective regimen. They also suggest that the timing and duration of administration may be significant.

In an attempt to evaluate the benefit of consolidation treatment, the Southeastern Cancer Study Group randomized 148 evaluable patients who had responded to CAV (with or without radiation) to either consolidation with two cycles of EP or no further therapy.[47] There was significant improvement in terms of median survival (23 months versus 16 months, $P = 0.009$) and median duration of remis-

sion (11 months versus 6 months, $P = 0.0008$) in patients receiving EP. Another randomized trial evaluated whether late intensification chemotherapy followed by autologous bone marrow transplantation could increase remission and survival rates.[48] Of 101 patients who received initial treatment, only 45 were eligible for randomization to consolidation with myeloablative doses or conventional doses of cyclophosphamide, BCNU, and etoposide. There was an improvement in median relapse-free survival (6 months versus 2 months, $P = 0.002$) and a trend toward an improvement in median overall survival (16 months versus 13 months) for the myeloablative arm, but this was not statistically significant in this small study. Primary site relapses were common.

In conclusion, dose intensification and late consolidation thus far have not clearly demonstrated improved survival or response. Many of the studies did not have sufficient power to determine a statistically significant difference, but the negative findings of the meta-analysis for all drug regimens do not provide much incentive for further studies using current drug regimens. However, it is important to note that the majority of studies addressed intended dose rather than actual dose delivered, and thus the issue of whether delivered dose intensity has an effect on survival remains unclear. The one published randomized study is suggestive that delivered dose intensity does make a difference.[45] Furthermore, the mode of delivery also appears to have an effect on survival.

Maintenance Chemotherapy and Immunotherapy

During the 1970s, maintenance chemotherapy for responding patients with limited stage disease was based primarily on the results of the treatment of other chemotherapy-responsive malignancies. Nine randomized trials that included LS SCLC patients have been performed using various chemotherapy regimens, and those involving ≥100 patients are shown in Table 24–3.[49–57] All but one of these trials demonstrated no significant difference and no consistent trend in survival. Therefore, maintenance chemotherapy beyond the initial four to six cycles is not routinely recommended. A review in 1998 of this issue also concluded that no benefit had been demonstrated with maintenance chemotherapy, but that the size and quality of the trials were poor and a small benefit could not be conclusively ruled out.[58]

Two randomized trials of ≥100 patients have evaluated the role of maintenance interferon therapy; neither study found a benefit.[59,60] Kelly et al[59] randomized 132 patients with LS SCLC who demonstrated an objective response to induction chemotherapy to receive either recombinant interferon-α for 2 years or observation.[59] No difference was seen in progression-free survival (9 months versus 10 months; $P = 0.7$) or median survival (16 months versus 13 months; $P = 0.8$). Forty-three of 64 patients discontinued treatment because of intolerable side effects. The NCCTG randomized 100 patients (78 with LS SCLC) who had a CR to chemotherapy, radiation, and PCI to receive recombinant interferon-γ for 6 months or observation.[60] No difference was seen in progression-free survival (7 months versus 8

TABLE 24–3. RANDOMIZED TRIALS OF MAINTENANCE CHEMOTHERAPY VERSUS OBSERVATION IN LIMITED STAGE SMALL CELL LUNG CANCER

STUDY	N	ELIGIBILITY CRITERIA	CHEMO	NO. OF CYCLES		MST[a] (mo)		2-y SURVIVAL[a] (%)		P
				Ind	Maint	Control	Maint	Control	Maint	
Spiro et al[54]	610	All	CVE	4	4	9	10	9	8	NS
Giaccone et al[55]	434	CR, PR, SD	CAE	5	7	4	6	10	11	NS
Bleehen et al[49]	309	All	CMxVE	3	3	7	9	7	8	NS
MRC[50]	265	CR, PR	CMxVE	6	6	7	6	(<10)	(<10)	NS
Mattson et al[51]	146	CR, PR	CVE[b]	3–6	6[b]	10	11	(<10)	0	NS
Average[c]						7	8	9	7	

Inclusion criteria: Randomized trials involving limited stage small cell lung cancer patients from 1980 to 2000, with >100 patients total.
[a]Survival results are for limited stage only.
[b]Maintenance chemotherapy with CAP.
[c]Excluding values in parentheses.
All, all patients, randomized at entry on trial; Chemo, chemotherapy; Control, control arm receiving induction chemotherapy cycles only; CR, complete response; Ind, induction therapy (given to both arms); Maint, maintenance chemotherapy; MST, median survival time; PR, partial response; SD, stable disease.
Chemotherapy regimens: CAE, cyclophosphamide, doxorubicin, etoposide; CMxVE, cyclophosphamide, methotrexate, vincristine, etoposide; CVE, cyclophosphamide, vincristine, etoposide.

months; $P = 0.5$) or median survival (13 months versus 19 months; $P = 0.4$). In summary, interferon therapy has not been demonstrated to be of benefit as maintenance therapy.

COMBINED CHEMOTHERAPY AND RADIATION

Thirteen randomized trials have been performed addressing the effect of the addition of RT to improve both local control and survival, 11 of which have been published.[61–71] Table 24–4 presents the results from the individual published studies involving ≥100 patients with LS SCLC. The results of the individual studies have been conflicting, with almost half being considered negative studies. However, almost all of the negative studies had insufficient power to demonstrate a 5% to 10% survival benefit. Five of the studies[61–65] in Table 24–4 found a clear trend toward better 2-year survival with combination chemoradiotherapy, whereas one study[72] found only a minimal trend and one[66] found a trend toward worse survival. Overall, the studies involving ≥100 patients with LS SCLC, shown in Table 24–4, have suggested a modest survival benefit, with an improvement in median survival of approximately 1 month and an improvement in 2-year survival of 6%.

Besides median and overall survival, the issue of local control has been addressed in 11 published studies.[61–71] All of these studies showed a statistically significant improvement in local control. The manner in which each study reported the results was defined differently by different investigators. For example, some studies included only initial sites of failure, whereas others reported any in-field failure. When only the initial site of failure is reported, the local control rate is likely to have been overestimated. Other studies considered radiographic partial responses as local failures. This is not justified, however, because more than one-third of patients with radiographic partial responses are long-term survivors.[73] Nevertheless, treatment with RT appears to at least double the local control rate in patients with limited stage disease.[61–71]

Two meta-analyses have been performed in an attempt to elucidate whether thoracic radiation confers a survival benefit. Warde and Payne[74] analyzed the results of 11 published randomized trials that addressed this issue. By odds ratio, there was a 53% greater likelihood of surviving 2 years with the addition of radiation. This result translates into an absolute 2-year survival benefit of 5.4%. There was also an absolute improvement in intrathoracic tumor control of 25%. This overall improvement in local control and survival was not without increased risk, however, and there was an increase of 1.2% in treatment-related mortality.

DATA SUMMARY: CHEMOTHERAPY ISSUES IN LIMITED STAGE SMALL CELL LUNG CANCER			
	AMOUNT	QUALITY	CONSISTENCY
Treatment with alternating chemotherapy regimens has not resulted in better median or 2-year survival	High	High	Mod
Modifications of planned dose intensity have not resulted in improved survival	High	Mod	Mod
Late consolidation treatment improves survival	Poor	Mod	—
Maintenance chemotherapy beyond the initial four to six cycles does not improve survival	High	High	High

Type of data rated: Plain text: descriptive statement   *Italics: controlled comparison*   **Bold: randomized comparison**

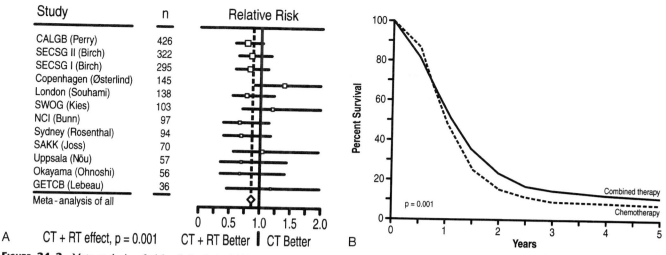

FIGURE 24–2. Meta-analysis of risk of death in 2103 patients with small cell lung cancer (83% LS, 17% ES) treated with chemotherapy and radiotherapy compared with chemotherapy alone in randomized trials. *A,* Result of individual studies. The horizontal lines represent 95% confidence intervals, and the pooled confidence interval is shown by the diamond. *B,* Pooled overall survival. (From Pignon J-P, Arriagada R, Ihde DC. A meta-analysis of thoracic radiotherapy for small-cell lung cancer. N Engl J Med. 1992;327:1618–1624. Copyright © 1992 Massachusetts Medical Society. All rights reserved.[75])

The meta-analysis by Pignon et al[75] of 13 published and unpublished randomized trials confirmed these findings of a modest survival advantage, as shown in Figure 24–2A,B.

In conclusion, for patients who are able to tolerate combined modality treatment, the data is convincing for a small but significant survival advantage of chemotherapy and thoracic RT compared with chemotherapy alone. Local control is clearly improved. The precise timing, dose, and volume to be irradiated cannot be determined by these studies or by meta-analyses.

RADIATION DOSES AND FRACTIONATION SCHEMES

In various prospective and retrospective studies involving RT, local control has ranged from 0% to 64% (using doses of 30 to 65 Gy and daily fractionation schemes of 1.8 to 3.0 Gy). Given such poor local control, maximizing RT in order to improve local control seems logical. A total dose of 70 Gy in 2-Gy daily fractions, delivered concurrently with chemotherapy (the fourth cycle of cyclophosphamide, cisplatin, and etoposide [CPE]), was found to be tolerable in a phase I trial conducted by the Cancer and Leukemia Group B (CALGB).[76] Although two of six patients developed grade 4 esophagitis, dose-limiting toxicity was not reached even at a total dose of 70 Gy. This trial also investigated hyperfractionated RT and found the maximum tolerated dose (given concurrently with chemotherapy) to be 45 Gy (1.5 Gy twice daily [bid]). Two of five patients treated with 50 Gy (1.25 Gy bid) developed grade 4 esophagitis.[76] No clinically significant pulmonary toxicity was observed in either group. Other prospective studies have found slightly higher doses to be well tolerated (48 Gy bid or 54 Gy bid given concurrently with chemotherapy).[77,78]

TABLE 24–4. RANDOMIZED STUDIES OF CHEMOTHERAPY VERSUS COMBINATION CHEMOTHERAPY AND RADIATION IN LIMITED STAGE SMALL CELL LUNG CANCER

STUDY	N	CHEMO	RT DOSE TOTAL/Fx	TIMING OF RT (wk)[a]	MST (mo) Chemo	MST (mo) Chemo/RT	2-y SURVIVAL (%) Chemo	2-y SURVIVAL (%) Chemo/RT	P
Johnson et al[61]	369	CAV ± EP	45/3	1, 7[b]	13	14	23	33	(0.08)
Creech et al[62]	310	CMxU	50/2	7	14	17	13	19	0.003
Birch et al[63]	291	CAV	40/2.9	5, 8, 11[b]	11	13	16	24	0.04
Perry et al[64,65]	274	CAVE	c50/2	9	14	15	7	21	0.002
Perry et al[64,65]	254	CAVE	c50/2	1	14	13	7	17	(0.08)
Østerlind et al[66]	145	CMxVU	c40/2	6, 10[b]	12	11	12	5	NS
Souhami et al[72c]	130	AV/CMx	40/2	13	12	13	12	14	NS
Average					**13**	**14**	**13**	**19**	

Inclusion criteria: Randomized studies of chemotherapy versus combination chemotherapy and radiation in ≥100 patients with limited stage small cell lung cancer.
[a]Week from initiation of therapy to start of RT.
[b]Split-course RT.
[c]Includes extensive stage patients.

c, concurrent RT and chemotherapy; Chemo, chemotherapy; Chemo/RT, combination chemotherapy and RT; Fx, fraction (dose in Gy); MST, median survival time; RT, radiotherapy.

Chemotherapy regimens: AV, doxorubicin, vincristine; CAV, cyclophosphamide, doxorubicin, vincristine; CAVE, cyclophosphamide, doxorubicin, vincristine, etoposide; CMx, cyclophosphamide, methotrexate; CMxU, cyclophosphamide, methotrexate, CCNU; CMxVU, cyclophosphamide, methotrexate, vincristine, CCNU; EP, etoposide, cisplatin.

Only one randomized trial has addressed whether there is a dose response to RT with regard to local control and survival. Coy et al[79] randomized 168 chemotherapy-responsive patients (demonstrating either a complete or a partial response) to receive either 25 Gy in 10 fractions or 37.5 Gy in 15 fractions. The overall response rate was 94%, with no significant difference in the CR rate between the two groups (69% versus 65%). Patients in the high-dose arm had an improvement in median local disease-free progression (11 months versus 9 months; $P = 0.03$) and actuarial 2-year local disease-free progression (80% versus 69%; $P = 0.03$). However, the crude in-field local failure rate was reported as 65% and 60% in the high and low dose arms, respectively. No difference was seen in overall survival. With regard to toxicity, the high dose arm had a higher rate of dysphagia (49% versus 26%, $P = 0.002$). This study suggests a local control benefit with higher doses of radiation; however, the fractionation schemes and total doses are different from those routinely used in the United States.

To assess whether hyperfractionated RT could improve local control and survival, Turrisi et al[80] randomized 417 patients to receive either 45 Gy of twice-daily radiation (1.5 Gy fractions) or daily radiation (1.8 Gy fractions) with concurrent cisplatin and etoposide. The radiation was administered concurrently with the first cycle of chemotherapy. With a minimum follow-up of almost 5 years, a statistically significant difference was seen in median survival (22 months versus 19 months; $P = 0.04$), 2-year survival (47% versus 41%; $P = 0.02$), and 5-year survival (26% versus 16%; $P = 0.03$) in patients receiving hyperfractionated RT. Local failure remained a persistent problem, with a documented local recurrence in 75% of the complete responders on the daily fractionation arm and 42% of the complete responders on the hyperfractionated arm. In another study addressing the role of hyperfractionated RT, no advantage to twice-daily RT was observed.[78] However, the hyperfractionated RT in this study was de-layed until the fourth cycle of chemotherapy and delivered as a split course with a 2.5-week delay, which may explain the discrepancy in the results. In conclusion, although there is some data suggesting that more aggressive RT can improve the survival of patients with LS SCLC, the optimal dose and schedule of RT remains an area of controversy that needs further study.

TIMING OF CHEMOTHERAPY AND RADIATION

RT can be given before, after, or during chemotherapy. Furthermore, if delivered during chemotherapy, it can be administered concurrently or in an alternating "sandwiched" fashion (eg, one cycle of chemotherapy followed by 3 weeks of radiation followed by additional chemotherapy). There are endless ways in which chemotherapy and radiation can be used. Table 24–5 summarizes the results of randomized trials with thoracic radiation that have focused on the impact of the timing of the radiation. The studies randomized either between early versus delayed thoracic radiation or between alternating chemotherapy and radiation versus sequential delivery of these therapies. Because each of these studies has a different radiation regimen, the studies are difficult to compare with each other and are discussed separately.

Gregor et al[4] enrolled 335 patients in a randomized trial to determine whether alternating RT would be better than sequential therapy. Patients were randomized to receive either alternating chemoradiotherapy (CAE and 50 Gy of RT; five monthly cycles of chemotherapy on day 1 and RT day 21-26) versus sequential chemotherapy (CAE for five cycles every 3 weeks) followed by RT (50 Gy in 20 daily fractions over 4 weeks). No statistically significant differences in median survival (14 months versus 15 months) or 2-year survival (26% versus 23%) were observed.

TABLE 24–5. TIMING OF RADIOTHERAPY IN COMBINED CHEMORADIOTHERAPY TREATMENT OF LIMITED STAGE SMALL CELL LUNG CANCER

STUDY	N	RT TIMING (wk) Early	RT TIMING (wk) Late	MST (mo) Early	MST (mo) Late	2-y SURVIVAL (%) Early	2-y SURVIVAL (%) Late	5-y SURVIVAL (%) Early	5-y SURVIVAL (%) Late	P
Gregor et al[4a]	335	7[b]	15	14[b]	15	26[b]	23	4[b]	10	NS
Murray et al[5]	308	3	15	21	16	40	34	20	11	0.008
Perry et al[64,65]	270	1	9	13	15	17	21	7	10	NS
Work et al[81]	199	1/4[c]	18/21[c]	11	12	20	19	11	12	NS
Jeremic et al[77d]	103	1	6	34	26	71	53	30	15	0.05
Average				**19**	**17**	**35**	**30**	**14**	**12**	

Inclusion criteria: Randomized studies of ≥100 patients.
[a]Alternating chemotherapy and RT with each 4-week cycle versus sequential RT after chemotherapy completed.
[b]Alternating arm
[c]Split-course RT.
[d]Hyperfractionated RT.
MST, median survival time; RT, radiotherapy; RT Timing, week from initiation of therapy to start of RT.
Chemotherapy drugs; radiotherapy regimen (total dose/dose per fraction):
Gregor et al, CAE; 50/2.
Murray et al, CAV/EP (alternating with each cycle); 40–2.7.
Perry et al, CAVE; 50/2.
Work et al, EP/CAV (EP used whenever RT also given); 40 to 45/2 split course.
Jeremic et al, EP; 54/1.5 hyperfractionated.
CAE, cyclophosphamide, doxorubicin, etoposide; CAV, cyclophosphamide, doxorubicin, vincristine; CAVE, cyclophosphamide, doxorubicin, vincristine, etoposide; EP, etoposide, cisplatin.

Murray et al[5] randomized 308 patients with LS SCLC to receive early thoracic radiation during the first chemotherapy cycle (week 3) versus late thoracic radiation during the last cycle of chemotherapy (week 15). An alternating chemotherapy schedule of CAV with EP every 3 weeks was used. The early arm had a planned 1-week delay in the third cycle of chemotherapy to decrease the interaction of radiation with doxorubicin. A dose of 40 Gy in 15 daily fractions was delivered in 3 weeks. PCI was delivered to all responding patients (25 Gy in 10 fractions). The delivered chemotherapy doses on each arm were similar. The response rates were not significantly different between the arms, but the progression-free survival significantly favored the early thoracic radiation arm at 3 years (26% versus 19%; $P = 0.05$), with a minimum follow-up of 32 months for all evaluable patients in the study. There was also a benefit in median survival (21 months versus 16 months; $P = 0.008$) and 5-year overall survival (20% versus 11%; $P = 0.006$). Neutropenia was common in patients in both arms of the study, but infectious complications requiring hospitalization occured in <5% of the patients. Anemia, esophagitis, and dermatitis were worse in patients randomized to the early thoracic radiation arm.

Perry et al[64] reported the results from CALGB Study 8083, which randomized 399 patients to either chemotherapy with no thoracic radiation or concurrent chemotherapy and thoracic radiation during either the first or the fourth cycle of chemotherapy (cyclophosphamide, etoposide, vincristine, and later doxorubicin). Thoracic radiation involved 40 Gy to the gross tumor and the mediastinum, with a boost to the gross tumor volume of an additional 10 Gy. PCI of 30 Gy was delivered to all patients. Although there was a statistically significant difference between the chemotherapy-alone arm and the other two arms of the trial in favor of RT, there was no statistically significant difference between the two RT arms with regard to median survival (13 months versus 15 months) or median time to clinical failure (11 months versus 11 months).

Work et al[81] published the results of the Aarhus Lung Cancer Group with 199 consecutive patients randomized to receive early or late thoracic radiation delivered sequentially with alternating EP (three cycles) and CAV (six cycles). The thoracic radiation was delivered using two courses of 20 to 22.5 Gy given in 11 daily fractions with a 21-day break between courses. Early thoracic irradiation

was initiated before the start of chemotherapy, and late irradiation was started during week 18 of therapy. CT scans of the chest or head were not required. PCI was delivered to all patients who received early thoracic irradiation and to 58% of the patients receiving late irradiation. There was no statistical difference with regard to median survival time (11 months versus 12 months, early versus late) or 2-year overall survival. In-field recurrences remained a persistent problem, with 72% versus 68% of patients receiving early versus late thoracic irradiation, respectively, developing local recurrence within 2 years of treatment.

Jeremic et al[77] randomized 107 patients to receive either early hyperfractionated radiation or late hyperfractionated radiation (54 Gy bid in 1.5 Gy fractions) given concurrently with daily EP (30 mg daily of each drug). Patients on the early arm received initial concurrent chemoradiotherapy followed by four cycles of EP after completion of the radiation. Patients on the late arm received an initial two cycles of EP followed by the same accelerated hyperfractionated radiation, and then two additional cycles of EP. All patients were to receive PCI of 25 Gy in 10 fractions. The survival was significantly better for the early arm (median survival, 34 months versus 26 months; 5-year survival, 30% versus 15%; $P = 0.03$)

In summary, the data from the randomized trials is conflicting with regard to the most appropriate timing of thoracic radiation because of the lack of consistent comparisons. There is a suggestion that early radiation and concurrent chemotherapy may be better than delayed radiation or sequential therapy. The two studies with positive results were the only studies that required staging with CT scans of the head, chest, and upper abdomen, and a bone scan.[5,77] As a consequence, it is possible that a proportion of the patients in the other studies were understaged and actually had gross distant metastases and a more significant tumor burden. The higher percentage of patients alive at 2 years in both arms of these two positive studies also supports this hypothesis.

ROLE OF PROPHYLACTIC CRANIAL IRRADIATION

Central nervous system (CNS) failure rates have been reported to be between 13% and 67% in prospective studies

DATA SUMMARY: RADIOTHERAPY ISSUES IN LIMITED STAGE SMALL CELL LUNG CANCER	AMOUNT	QUALITY	CONSISTENCY
The addition of thoracic radiation to the treatment of LS SCLC patients results in improved survival (~5% at 2 years)	High	High	High
The addition of thoracic radiation to the treatment of LS SCLC patients results in significantly improved rates of local control	High	High	High
Hyperfractionated RT results in better local control and better survival in LS SCLC patients	Poor	High	—
Early RT has not resulted in improved survival compared with late RT.	High	Mod	Poor

Type of data rated: Plain text: descriptive statement   *Italics: controlled comparison*   **Bold: randomized comparison**

TABLE 24–6. ROLE OF PROPHYLACTIC CRANIAL IRRADIATION IN LIMITED STAGE SMALL CELL LUNG CANCER

STUDY	N	PCI DOSE (Gy) Total	Fx	% CR OF ALL	% CNS FAILURE[a] PCI	Control	P	MST (mo) PCI	Control	2-y SURVIVAL (%) PCI	Control	P
Gregor et al[84]	314	8–36	2–8	100	38	54	0.02	10	10	25	19	NS
Seydel et al[158]	219	30	3	100	(5)[b]	(20)[b]	0.0008	10	10	—	—	NS
Laplanche et al[159c]	211	24–30	3	100	44	51	NS	10	10	22	16	NS
Maurer et al[1c]	163	30	3	~30	(4)[b]	(18)[b]	0.009	8	9	8	14	NS
Arriagada et al[83c]	145	24	3	100	40	67	0.0001	14	12	29	22	NS
Hansen et al[82]	109	30	2	—	(9)[b]	(13)[b]	NS	9	10	11	17	NS
Average[d]					**41**	**57**		**10**	**10**	**19**	**18**	

Inclusion criteria: Randomized studies of PCI involving ≥100 SCLC patients.
[a]Actuarial rate with ≥2 years observation, unless otherwise indicated.
[b]Crude incidence.
[c]Includes approximately 20% to 30% extensive stage patients.
[d]Excluding values in parentheses.
CNS, central nervous system; Control, control arm, not receiving PCI; CR, complete response; Fx, fraction; PCI, prophylactic cranial irradiation.

in which no CNS-directed treatment was administered.[82,83] During the 1970s and 1980s, a series of randomized trials were designed to address what effect PCI had on survival and brain recurrences (Table 24–6). These studies consistently demonstrated a reduction in the rate of brain recurrences with PCI but failed to demonstrate a survival benefit. The lack of a survival benefit may partly be due to insufficient power (most studies involved <100 patients) and patient selection (many studies included patients with residual disease after the initial treatment). Total radiation doses ranged from 20 Gy to 40 Gy, and dose per fraction ranged from 2 to 4 Gy. Unfortunately, rates of brain relapses have not been reported consistently and are sometimes reported as crude rates rather than acturial rates. In addition, the authors of these studies often did not state whether the results were crude or actuarial, making comparisons difficult.

Two studies[83,84] have prospectively addressed the role of PCI in patients with complete remission and warrant further discussion because they evaluated neurocognitive function in a prospective manner. Arriagada et al[83] randomized 300 patients (163 with LS SCLC) who had a complete remission to receive either no treatment or PCI (24 Gy in 8 fractions). Serial neuropsychologic examinations were also performed. Ninety-eight percent of the patients with brain metastases developed these lesions in the first 2 years, and the actuarial rate of isolated brain metastases at 2 years was 45% in the control group and 19% in the treatment group. The actuarial rate of all brain metastases at 2 years was 67% in the control group and 40% in the treatment group. No significant differences were seen between the two groups with regard to neuropsychologic function, nor was a significant difference observed in the 2-year overall survival rate (22% versus 29%; P = 0.14).

Gregor et al[84] reported the results of a randomized trial comparing various dose levels of PCI with a control of no radiation in patients with LS disease who had a complete remission. Initially, the study was designed as a three-arm study of 36 Gy in 18 fractions, 24 Gy in 12 fractions, and no radiation. Because of slow accural, the study was changed to two arms and allowed the treating physician to determine the dose fractionation schedule. At 2-year fol-

low-up, patients in the radiation arm had a decreased actuarial brain failure rate (52% versus 29%; P < 0.0002). Patients initially treated with 24 Gy in 12 fractions had brain rate failure similar to patients in the control arm. No statistically significant neurocognitive deficits could be attributed to PCI. There was also no statistically significant difference in survival, although this trial had insufficient power to detect a 5% to 7% difference in survival.

In an attempt to clarify the role of PCI in patients with CRs, the Prophylactic Cranial Irradiation Overview Collaborative Group performed a meta-analysis using individual patient data from the seven randomized trials that included patients with complete remissions.[85,86] A total of 987 patients were included in the study and were evaluated on an intent-to-treat basis. This group found a statistically significant difference in the relative risk of death with the addition of PCI, as shown in Figure 24–3. With a median

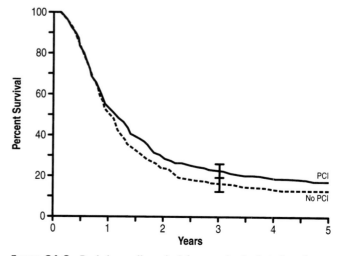

FIGURE 24–3. Pooled overall survival from randomized studies of prophylactic cranial irradiation (PCI) in patients with small cell lung cancer in complete remission. (From Aupérin A, Arriagada R, Pignon J-P et al. Prophylactic cranial irradiation for patients with small cell lung cancer in complete remission. N Engl J Med. 1999;341:476–480. Copyright © 1999 Massachusetts Medical Society. All rights reserved.[85])

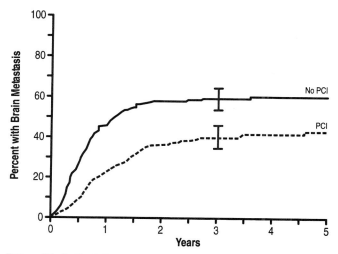

FIGURE 24–4. Pooled cumulative incidence of brain metastasis from randomized studies of prophylactic cranial irradiation (PCI) in patients with small cell lung cancer in complete remission. (From Aupérin A, Arriagada R, Pignon J-P, et al. Prophylactic cranial irradiation for patients with small cell lung cancer in complete remission. N Engl J Med. 1999;341:476–480. Copyright © 1999 Massachusetts Medical Society. All rights reserved.[85])

follow-up of 5.9 years, there was a reduction of 16% in mortality and a 5.4% absolute increase in the 3-year survival rate (15.3% versus 20.7%). PCI also increased the disease-free survival and reduced the incidence of subsequent brain metastases, as shown in Figure 24–4. When higher total doses were used, there was a trend toward a decreased rate of brain metastases (relative risk of brain metastases 0.76, 0.52, 0.34, and 0.27 for total doses of 8, 24, 30, and 36-40 Gy PCI, respectively; $P = 0.01$).

In summary, the randomized data has been limited by insufficient power to demonstrate statistical significance for a small survival benefit, but the meta-analysis suggests an improvement in survival for patients receiving PCI. There is convincing evidence that PCI reduces the rate of brain metastases and that, in the short term, no statistically significant difference can be seen with regard to neurocognitive function. The lack of a difference in neurocognitive function is confounded by the bias of increasing attrition due to both intracranial and extracranial relapses.[87] Further follow-up is necessary to determine whether clinically sig-

nificant neurocognitive deficits will develop in the long-term survivors. Although there is no clear indication of an optimal dose, there is a suggestion that higher doses are better for local control.

SURGERY

Surgery has generally been viewed as having no role in the treatment of patients with LS SCLC since a study conducted by the British Medical Research Council was published in 1973.[31] This study randomized 144 "operable" patients who had no evidence of extrathoracic metastases to receive either surgery or RT, with crossover and other treatments being allowed. The absolute survival at 5 years was 1% in the surgery arm and 4% in the RT arm. The median survival was significantly longer in the RT group (10 months versus 7 months; $P = 0.04$). To date, this is the only randomized trial involving surgery as the primary treatment modality. This study has been criticized because patients needed to have a positive bronchoscopic biopsy in order to be eligible. As a consequence, the study was limited to patients with more central or locally advanced disease who would be less likely to be able to undergo resection.[88] Only 48% of patients in the surgery arm underwent resection. This study does not rule out the possibility of a role for surgery in other subsets of patients or in the context of multimodality treatment, especially when the advances in radiographic imaging, diagnostic techniques, and therapeutic modalities are considered.

The high local failure rate and the low cure rates of combined chemotherapy and RT have led to a re-evaluation of the role of surgery. Surgery may be used in the treatment of SCLC in a variety of clinical contexts. Resection may be undertaken in patients who were not suspected preoperatively of having SCLC, or it may be done as a planned intervention in patients who have clinical stage I or II SCLC (as evidenced by CT or a negative mediastinoscopy). Surgery may be considered as an adjuvant modality after primary treatment with chemotherapy has been administered either instead of or in addition to RT. Finally, surgery may be considered as a salvage treatment in patients who have relapsed or failed to respond to primary treatment involving chemotherapy and RT.

No study has focused exclusively on the results of sur-

DATA SUMMARY: PROPHYLACTIC CRANIAL IRRADIATION			
	AMOUNT	**QUALITY**	**CONSISTENCY**
Prophylactic cranial irradiation (PCI) for all patients with LS SCLC has resulted in a lower rate of brain recurrences	High	Mod	High
PCI for all patients with LS SCLC has not improved survival	**High**	**Mod**	**High**
Individual studies restricted to patients with a complete response after induction therapy have not shown PCI to result in improved survival	**Mod**	**High**	**High**
Meta-analysis of those patients *from all* randomized studies of PCI who have a complete response after induction therapy has demonstrated a survival benefit for PCI	**High**	**High**	**Mod**

Type of data rated: Plain text: descriptive statement   *Italics: controlled comparison*   **Bold: randomized comparison**

TABLE 24–7. THE ROLE OF SURGERY IN LIMITED STAGE SMALL CELL LUNG CANCER

STUDY	N RESECTED	TREATMENT[a]	% INCIDENTAL SCLC[b]	% pCR	% R$_0$	SURVIVAL (ALL PATIENTS) MST (mo)	% 2 y	% 5 y	5-y SURVIVAL (%) pI	pII	pIIIa[c]	ANY LOCAL RECURRENCE (%)
Merkle et al[98]	170	Various	—	—	—	—	—	18	20	—	—	—
Rea et al[160]	104	Various	—	—	—	28	—	32	52	30	15	24
Prasad et al[161]	97	Various	27	—	—	12	37	17	35	23	0	—
Maassen et al[162]	94	Various	—	—	86	—	35	(15)[d]	(34)[d,e]	(21)[d,e]	(11)[d,e]	—
Hage et al[96]	74	Various	43	—	—	17	35	25	39	8	(17)	—
Davis et al[90]	118	S	—	—	—	18	39	20	—	—	—	—
Sørensen[163]	71	S	—	—	—	—	—	(12)[d]	—	—	—	—
Shore et al[89]	40	S	57	—	—	—	—	27	—	—	—	20
Shah et al[164]	28	S	36	—	93	34	55	43	57	0	(56)[f]	—
Shields et al[165g]	132	S→Chemo-RT	58	—	—	11	33	23	37[h]	15[h]	4	(11)[j]
Karrer et al[92]	112	S→Chemo[i]	31	—	99	37	60	(51)[e]	(62)[e]	(50)[e]	(41)[e]	16
Lucchi et al[166]	92	S→Chemo	64	—	90	24	50	32	46	15	9	11
Shepherd et al[93]	63	S→Chemo-RT[i]	—	—	38	19	45	31	45	25	24	—
Østerlind et al[102]	52	S→Chemo	—	—	—	—	—	(25)[k]	—	—	—	—
Lad et al[104]	70	Chemo→S-RT[i]	—	19	77	15	20	10	72	—	—	—
Shepherd et al[94]	38	Chemo→S-RT[i]	—	8	87	21	47	36	72	38	18	18
Eberhardt et al[167]	32	Chemo-RT→S	—	34	72	36	—	46	—	—	—	—
Holoye et al[168]	22	Chemo→S	—	19	—	25	54	33	67	0	0	14
Williams et al[99]	21	Chemo→S[i]	—	16	84	—	—	—	—	—	—	28
Shepherd et al[91]	28	Salvage[l]	—	—	82	24	48	23	—	—	—	—
Average [m]	**81**		—	—		**22**	**44**	**28**	47	17	11	19

Inclusion criteria: The five largest studies in each category of treatment strategy (involving ≥20 patients) from 1980 to 2000.

[a]Predominant (≥80%) treatment regimen.
[b]Percentage of patients in whom SCLC was not diagnosed preoperatively.
[c]Includes >75% N2 except where indicated.
[d]Absolute survival.
[e]3-year survival.
[f]Only 18% N2.
[g]4% to 11% operative mortality excluded from survival figures.
[h]Estimated using a weighted average of individual TNM groups.
[i]Plus PCI (prophylactic cranial irradiation).
[j]As cause of death
[k]3.5-year survival.
[l]Salvage therapy, consisting of resection of patients who had persistent or locally recurrent disease after chemotherapy (±RT).
[m]Excluding values in parentheses.

Chemo, chemotherapy; MST, median survival time; pCR, pathologic complete response; % Any local recur, percentage of all patients who experience a local recurrence, either as an isolated event or in combination with distant recurrence; % R$_0$, percentage of patients undergoing thoracotomy in whom a complete resection is achieved; RT, radiotherapy; S, surgery; →, followed by; SCLC, small cell lung cancer.

gery in patients who were not suspected of having SCLC preoperatively. However, in studies involving surgery as the primary treatment, approximately half of the patients were not diagnosed with SCLC preoperatively. Only about 10% of all patients with SCLC have been included in such studies using primary surgical treatment,[89,90] and the vast majority of patients have had cI or cII disease. The median survival in these studies is approximately 2 years, with an average 5-year survival of 26% (Table 24–7). The variability in the reported results is probably due to inclusion of varying numbers of patients with more advanced disease (although all are limited stage). An examination of the results by TNM stage suggests that the 5-year survival of resected patients with SCLC is only slightly worse than that of patients with NSCLC.

After a resection has been carried out in patients with SCLC, a decision must be made about whether to give adjuvant (postoperative) chemotherapy. Most experts in this field believe strongly that adjuvant chemotherapy should be given, although there is little direct data on which to base this.[88,91,92] The results in Table 24–7 do not show an obvious difference in this regard. The argument to give adjuvant therapy is based on the historically poor survival of patients treated with surgery alone (in studies in the 1960s and 1970s), the frequent presence of systemic metastases in SCLC, and the responsiveness of the disease to chemotherapy.[91,92] Furthermore, the correlation between preoperative clinical stage and postoperative pathologic stage has consistently been found to be poor, with most patients (20%-60%) having a higher pathologic stage and few patients (<10%) having a lower stage.[92–96] Even mediastinoscopy appears to have a high false-negative rate in patients with SCLC.[93,97,98] These observations support the argument that even patients thought to be N0 should be given postoperative chemotherapy.

Primary chemotherapy followed by surgical resection as adjuvant treatment in patients with SCLC has been investigated in a number of prospective phase II studies (see Table 24–7). Although the phase II nature of these studies does not permit a definite answer regarding a survival benefit, a number of observations can be made. Although these studies have selected only those LS SCLC patients considered "operable," they have not focused only on patients with stage I,II cancer; in fact, approximately half of the patients had stage IIIa disease. Approximately 50% of all patients with LS disease have been considered eligible for adjuvant resection in studies explicitly reporting this data (range 30%-64%),[99–102] and other studies corroborate this.[103,104] Surgical resection was undertaken in patients who demonstrated a complete or partial response (CR or PR) to the induction treatment, which consisted of active regimens described earlier in this chapter. Approximately 80% of patients entered in studies of adjuvant surgical resection have undergone surgery, and a complete resection (R_0) was achieved in approximately 90% of these (see Table 24–7).

In approximately 20% of patients undergoing surgery, no viable tumor was found in the resected specimen, but there appears to be little correlation between the radiographic response and the pathologic absence of tumor. One study found viable tumor remaining in 79% of patients with a radiographic PR and 75% of those with a radio-

graphic CR.[99] Some authors have suggested that resection is not necessary if a thoracotomy is done and no obvious tumor is found.[105] However, a local recurrence rate of 71% (five of seven patients) was observed in those patients who did not undergo resection because intraoperative exploration and biopsies were negative.[105] These observations suggest that the extent of resection should be based primarily on the pretreatment CT scan, rather than on a posttreatment scan or intraoperative findings.

The timing of chemotherapy in the context of combined modality treatment involving surgery (usually also including thoracic RT and PCI) was examined in a retrospective study of 119 patients.[91] No difference was found in survival between patients undergoing primary surgery and adjuvant chemotherapy compared with those being treated with primary chemotherapy followed by surgery. However, the primary surgery group included many patients not suspected of having SCLC, and included more clinical stage I patients (73% versus 28%) and fewer clinical stage III patients (8% versus 43%). Similar differences were found when comparing the pathologic stages in the two groups. The fact that the survival curves were similar despite the more advanced stage distribution in the cohort receiving primary chemotherapy suggests that the use of chemotherapy as the initial treatment may be the preferred approach when surgery is being considered.[91] An advantage to preoperative chemotherapy was also suggested by a retrospective (uncontrolled) study of 46 patients by Wada et al.[95] However, a small prospective randomized study of only 16 patients found significantly higher survival in patients receiving adjuvant chemotherapy compared with preoperative chemotherapy.[106]

The resurgence of interest in surgical resection as part of a multimodality approach stems in part from the high local recurrence rate after chemoradiotherapy alone. In studies involving surgery, approximately 15% of all resected patients have experienced a local recurrence. When this data is analyzed in terms of the distribution among only those patients experiencing a recurrence, an average of 20% of first sites of recurrence are reported as local only, 15% as local plus distant, and 65% as distant.[93,94,104,105] There is no difference in the recurrence pattern relative to the timing of surgery in conjunction with other treatments. It is inappropriate to compare the local failure rate in these surgical series, which involved selected patients with LS disease, with the local failure rate in LS SCLC patients treated with chemoradiotherapy alone.

Surgery does not seem to improve the survival of patients when used in combined modality programs. The survival rates shown in Table 24–7 for chemotherapy and surgery are better than those reported for chemoradiotherapy, but such a comparison is not valid because the series involving chemotherapy and adjuvant surgery undoubtedly represent a subgroup of patients with less advanced disease.

Only one randomized trial has addressed the role of adjuvant surgery after primary chemotherapy with subsequent thoracic RT and PCI in all patients.[104] This study found no difference in the 2-year survival, and the median survival was 15 months for the surgical arm and 19 months for the nonsurgical arm. Furthermore, no difference in local control was observed. This study involved 146 randomized patients (70 surgery, 76 no surgery) who responded appro-

TABLE 24–8. INCIDENCE OF NON–SMALL CELL LUNG CANCER AND MIXED HISTOLOGY IN PATIENTS WITH SMALL CELL LUNG CANCER[a]

STUDY	N	TREATMENT SETTING	% PURE SCLC	% MIXED HISTOLOGY	% PURE NSCLC
Radice et al[111]	156	Chemo/RT[b]	88	12	—[c]
Shepherd et al[91]	79	S→Chemo	82	18	—[c]
Davis et al[97]	35	S→Chemo	91	9	—[c]
Lad et al[104]	57	Chemo→S	86	4	10
Shepherd et al[91]	40	Chemo→S	83	8	8
Johnson et al[105]	23	Chemo→S	100	0	0
Holoye et al[168]	26	Chemo→S[d]	71	29	
Shepherd et al[109]	28	Salvage[e]	64	14	21
Abeloff[110]	40	Autopsy[f]	72	15	13

Inclusion criteria: Studies of ≥20 SCLC patients reporting incidence of mixed histologic tumors.
[a]As diagnosed in resected specimens (except as noted).
[b]Diagnosed by biopsy at time of presentation.
[c]Excluded by definition.
[d]Only patients with a partial response; patients with a complete response were excluded.
[e]Surgery performed because of nonresponse or relapse after chemoradiation.
[f]After (failed) chemoradiation.
→, sequential treatment; Chemo, chemotherapy; NSCLC, non–small cell lung cancer; RT, radiotherapy; S, surgery; SCLC, small cell lung cancer.

priately to the primary chemotherapy, out of 328 patients who were initially enrolled.[104] All patients in this study had SCLC that was proven by a bronchoscopic biopsy. An additional retrospective study of 79 SCLC patients who met defined criteria for having operable tumors found no survival difference between patients who did in fact undergo surgery and those who did not.[107]

Surgical resection provides an opportunity to study the histology of the resected tumors. At initial presentation, approximately 15% of patients with SCLC are found to have a mixed tumor, with both an SCLC and an NSCLC component (Table 24–8). In patients who have received preoperative chemotherapy, approximately 5% have a mixed tumor, and approximately 10% are found to have a pure NSCLC tumor at the time of resection.[91,105,108] Most often, there are characteristics that suggest that this latter group was not initially misdiagnosed, but rather that a mixed histology tumor was present initially, with the induction chemotherapy having left only the NSCLC compo-

nent.[91,105,108] In patients who experience a failure after chemotherapy, the proportion having NSCLC appears to be increased.[109,110] It has been suggested that surgical resection may be appropriate for patients with mixed histology tumors[109] because they are less responsive to chemotherapy.[111]

One study has investigated the role of surgery as a *salvage* treatment when the planned treatment of chemoradiotherapy without surgery has failed (either because of a lack of radiographic response or because of a local relapse after an initial response).[109] This study involved 28 patients, of whom 82% were able to be completely resected. The median survival of this select group was 31 months, with a 5-year survival of 32%. Thirty-six percent of these patients were found to have either a pure NSCLC or a tumor of mixed histology. This data suggests that surgery may have a role as salvage treatment in those patients with resectable limited stage disease who fail chemoradiotherapy alone.

DATA SUMMARY: SURGERY FOR LIMITED STAGE SMALL CELL LUNG CANCER	AMOUNT	QUALITY	CONSISTENCY
Half of the reported patients with SCLC who were treated with surgery as the primary modality were not diagnosed as having SCLC preoperatively	High	Mod	Mod
The 5-year survival of stage pI patients with SCLC treated with surgery as the primary modality is approximately 50%	High	Mod	Mod
Adjuvant chemotherapy should be given after resection of an SCLC	Poor	—	—
Preoperative chemotherapy may result in better survival than postoperative chemotherapy in SCLC patients treated with surgery	*Mod*	*Poor*	*Mod*
Limited stage SCLC patients treated with combined modality therapy have similar survival whether or not surgery is included in the approach	**Poor**	**High**	—
10% to 15% of patients have mixed SCLC/NSCLC tumors	High	Poor	High

Type of data rated: Plain text: descriptive statement   *Italics: controlled comparison*   **Bold: randomized comparison**

SECOND PRIMARY MALIGNANCIES

Several studies have reported a high rate of new primary malignancies in long-term survivors of SCLC.[112–116] The incidence of new primary cancers has been estimated to be 5% to 10% per year and is approximately 30% at 5 years.[113–119] The risk of a new primary malignancy is higher than the risk of recurrence after approximately 3 years.[112–114,116] On average, a new lung cancer has accounted for 50% (range, 21%-86%) of the second cancers, leukemia (probably related to alkylating agent chemotherapy) has accounted for 8% (range, 0%-23%), and an average of 11% (range, 0%-35%) of secondary malignancies involve the genitourinary system.[112–119] These results raise questions about a possible acquired genetic predisposition to the development of a malignancy, but an association with thoracic radiation and alkylating chemotherapy has also been suggested.[112,115,116] At any rate, close follow-up of patients with SCLC appears to be warranted, and a new abnormality occurring late after the original diagnosis of SCLC should be investigated and should not necessarily be assumed to be a recurrence of SCLC. Cessation of smoking appears to substantially reduce the risk of a new primary malignancy in patients with SCLC.[115,118,119]

EDITORS' COMMENTS

LS SCLC is a potentially curable disease, with clinical trials suggesting that cure can be attained in one of every four or five patients. However, the optimal curative strategy is not entirely clear. The data reviewed in this chapter strongly suggests that combination chemotherapy with concurrent early thoracic RT is the standard of care, and PCI should be given to patients who have a CR to chemotherapy. However, the details of how to optimize each of these modalities are not clear.

The chemotherapy regimen of etoposide and cisplatin (EP) is the standard of care. A chemotherapy regimen that results in clearly better outcomes has not been identified. There is not enough data about substituting carboplatin for cisplatin in patients with LS SCLC to recommend using carboplatin in a curative setting. Many new agents and novel combinations are in development, and early results suggest substantial activity and excellent tolerability in both limited and extensive stage disease. Clinical trials will be combining these new agents and regimens with thoracic RT in an attempt to improve both local and distant control.

The data regarding dose intensity in patients with LS SCLC is confusing. The trial by Arriagada et al[45] suggests a dose-response effect and is the only randomized trial employing first-cycle dose intensity in LS SCLC. The initial dose-intensity issue has not been settled in patients with LS SCLC, and the results of phase II studies suggest two areas that deserve further investigation: (1) early dose-intense treatment in complete responders[120] and (2) initial dose intensity using peripheral blood progenitor cells and growth factor support.[121]

There are many variables regarding thoracic RT that need clarification. The optimal dose and fractionation schedule are not entirely clear and, overall, the total dose employed has been relatively conservative. Ongoing studies are exploring use of higher doses of thoracic RT delivered on a traditional once-a-day schedule. It remains to be shown whether higher doses of once-daily RT result in the same improvement in survival achieved with lower doses of twice-daily RT. Furthermore, issues regarding the RT treatment volume have not been addressed. In general, volumes have typically included the gross tumor volume and the upper mediastinum and subcarinal region. In addition, if thoracic RT is not given on the first day of chemotherapy, the issue of treating the pre- versus the postchemotherapy volume has not been addressed.

None of the randomized studies exploring PCI has shown a significant survival advantage, but all have suggested a reduction in the recurrence rate in the brain. A meta-analysis has shown that PCI increases 3-year survival by 5%. This benefit is similar to the benefit gained by adding thoracic RT to chemotherapy. We believe that PCI should be given to patients with LS SCLC who are in or near a complete remission after primary therapy. What is not clear is the optimal dose and appropriate timing of PCI. Ongoing studies will help clarify these important issues. Long-term survivors of SCLC are at significant risk of developing subsequent lung cancers. The appropriate follow-up and potential role for screening in this population have not been addressed.

The role of surgery in LS SCLC is restricted to patients in whom the diagnosis is either unknown or in doubt, as well as to patients who have failed nonsurgical treatment but remain resectable. If the accuracy of a diagnosis of SCLC is in doubt, there should be no hesitation in proceeding with resection. On the other hand, if the diagnosis is secure, there is little role for surgery in general. Those select patients who fail to respond to chemoradiotherapy or who experience a relapse but have resectable tumors should undergo surgery. There is a high probability that these patients have an NSCLC component to their tumor, and there is compelling, albeit limited, data suggesting that a substantial number of these patients can be cured by resection.

References

1. Maurer LH, Tulloh M, Weiss RB, et al. A randomized combined modality trail in small cell carcinoma of the lung: comparison of combination chemotherapy-radiation therapy vs. cyclophosphamide radiation therapy: effects of maintenance chemotherapy and prophylactic whole brain irradiation. Cancer. 1980;45:30–39.
2. Urban T, Chastang C, Vaylet F, et al. Prognostic significance of supraclavicular lymph nodes in small cell lung cancer: a study from four consecutive clinical trials, including 1,370 patients. Chest. 1998;114:1538–1541.
3. Livingston RB, McCracken JD, Trauth CJ, et al. Isolated pleural effusion in small cell lung carcinoma: favorable prognosis. A review of the Southwest Oncology Group experience. Chest. 1982;81:208–211.
4. Gregor A, Drings P, Burghouts P, et al. Randomized trial of alternating versus sequential radiotherapy/chemotherapy in limited-disease patients with small-cell lung cancer: a European Organization for Research and Treatment of Cancer Lung Cancer Cooperative Group study. J Clin Oncol. 1997;15:2840–2849.
5. Murray N, Coy P, Pater JL, et al. Importance of timing for thoracic irradiation in the combined modality treatment of limited-stage small-cell lung cancer. J Clin Oncol. 1993;11:336–344.
6. American Joint Committee on Cancer. AJCC Cancer Staging Man-

ual. 5th ed. Chicago, Ill: American Joint Committee on Cancer; 1997.

7. Zelen M. Keynote address on biostatistics and data retrieval. Cancer Chemother Rep. 1973;4:31–42.

8. Green RA, Humphrey E, Close H. Alkylating agents in bronchogenic carcinoma. Am J Med. 1969;46:516–525.

9. Roswit B, Patno ME, Rapp R, et al. The survival of patients with inoperable lung cancer: a large-scale randomized study of radiation therapy versus placebo. Radiology. 1968;90:688–697.

10. Sagman U, Maki E, Evans WK, et al. Small-cell carcinoma of the lung: derivation of a prognostic staging system. J. Clin Oncol. 1991;9:1639–1649.

11. Shepherd FA, Ginsberg RJ, Haddad R, et al. Importance of clinical staging in limited small-cell lung cancer: a valuable system to separate prognostic subgroups. J Clin Oncol. 1993;11:1592–1597.

12. Parkin DM, Sankaranarayanan R. Overview on small-cell lung cancer in the world. Anticancer Res. 1994;14:277–282.

13. Barbone F, Bovenzi M, Cavallieri F, et al. Cigarette smoking and histologic type of lung cancer in men. Chest. 1997;112:1474–1479.

14. Damber LA, Larsson L-G. Smoking and lung cancer with special regard to type of smoking and type of cancer: a case-control study in north Sweden. Br J Cancer. 1986;53:673–681.

15. Morabia A, Wynder EL. Cigarette smoking and lung cancer cell types. Cancer. 1991;68:2074–2078.

16. Auerbach O, Garfinkel L. The changing pattern of lung carcinoma. Cancer. 1991;68:1973–1977.

17. Vincent RG, Pickren JW, Lane WW, et al. The changing histopathology of lung cancer: a review of 1682 cases. Cancer. 1977;39:1647–1655.

18. Steenland K, Loomis D, Shy C, et al. Review of occupational lung carcinogens. Am J Ind Med. 1996;29:474–490.

19. Hirsch FR, Matthews MJ, Aisner S, et al. Histopathologic classification of small-cell lung cancer: changing concepts and terminology. Cancer. 1988;62:973–977.

20. Hirsch FR, Osterlind K, Hansen HH. The prognostic significance of histopathologic subtyping of small cell carcinoma of the lung according to the classification of the World Health Organization: a study of 375 consecutive patients. Cancer. 1983;52:2144–2150.

21. Carney DN, Matthews MJ, Ihde DC, et al. Influence of histologic subtype of small carcinoma of the lung on clinical presentation, response to therapy, and survival. J Natl Cancer Inst. 1980;65:1225–1230.

22. Chute CG, Greenberg ER, Baron J, et al. Presenting conditions of 1539 population-based lung cancer patients by cell type and stage in New Hampshire and Vermont. Cancer. 1985;56:2107–2111.

23. Patel AM, Davila DG, Peters SG. Paraneoplastic syndromes associated with lung cancer. Mayo Clin Proc. 1993;68:278–287.

24. Truong LD, Underwood RD, Greenberg SD, et al. Diagnosis and typing of lung carcinomas by cytopathologic methods: a review of 108 cases. Acta Cytol. 1985;29:379–384.

25. Yang PC, Lee YC, Yu CJ, et al. Ultrasonographically guided biopsy of thoracic tumors. Cancer. 1992;69:2553–2560.

26. Shepherd FA. Screening, diagnosis, and staging of lung cancer. Curr Opin Oncol. 1993;5:310–322.

27. Karsell PR, McDougall JC. Diagnostic tests for lung cancer. Mayo Clin Proc. 1993;68:288–296.

28. Arriagada R, Le Chevalier T. Therapeutic approaches to small cell lung cancer. In: Aisner J, Arriagada R, Green MR, et al (eds). Comprehensive Textbook of Thoracic Oncology. 1st ed. Baltimore, Md: Williams & Wilkins; 1996;459–460.

29. Bergsagel DE, Jenkin RD, Pringle JF, et al. Lung cancer: clinical trial of radiotherapy alone vs. radiotherapy plus cyclophosphamide. Cancer. 1972;30:621–627.

30. Anonymous. Radiotherapy alone or with chemotherapy in the treatment of small-cell carcinoma of the lung: the results at 36 months. 2nd report to the Medical Research Council on the 2nd small-cell study. Br J Cancer. 1981;44:611–617.

31. Fox W, Scadding JG. Medical Research Council comparative trial of surgery and radiotherapy for primary treatment of small-celled or oat-celled carcinoma of bronchus: ten-year follow-up. Lancet. 1973;2:63–65.

32. Matthews MJ, Kanhouwa S, Pickren J, et al. Frequency of residual and metastatic tumor in patients undergoing curative surgical resection for lung cancer. Cancer Chemother Rep. 1973;4:63–67.

33. Lowenbraun S, Bartolucci A, Smalley RV, et al. The superiority of combination chemotherapy over single agent chemotherapy in small cell lung carcinoma. Cancer. 1979;44:406–413.

34. Girling DJ. Comparison of oral etoposide and standard intravenous multidrug chemotherapy for small cell lung cancer: a stopped multicentre randomised trial (Medical Research Council Lung Cancer Working Party). Lancet. 1996;348:563–566.

35. Livingston RB, Moore TN, Heilbrun L, et al. Small-cell carcinoma of the lung combined chemotherapy and radiation. A Southwest Oncology Group study. Ann Intern Med. 1978;88:194–199.

36. Evans WK, Shepherd FA, Feld R, et al. VP-16 and cisplatin as first-line therapy for small-cell lung cancer. J Clin Oncol. 1985;3:1471–1477.

37. Goldie JH, Coldman AJ. A mathematical model for relating the drug sensitivity of tumors to their spontaneous mutation rate. Cancer Treat Rep. 1979;63:1727–1733.

38. Fukuoka M, Furuse K, Saijo N, et al. Randomized trial of cyclophosphamide, doxorubicin, and vincristine versus cisplatin and etoposide versus alternation of these regimens in small-cell lung cancer. J Natl Cancer Inst. 1991;83:855–861.

39. Goodman GE, Crowley JJ, Blasko JC, et al. Treatment of limited small-cell lung cancer with etoposide and cisplatin alternating with vincristine, doxorubicin, and cyclophosphamide versus concurrent etoposide, vincristine, doxorubicin, and cyclophosphamide and chest radiotherapy: a Southwest Oncology Group study. J Clin Oncol. 1990;8:39–47.

40. Feld R, Evans WK, Coy P, et al. Canadian Multicenter Randomized Trial comparing sequential and alternating administration of two non-cross-resistant chemotherapy combinations in patients with limited small-cell carcinoma of the lung. J Clin Oncol. 1987;5:1401–1409.

41. Wolf M, Pritsch M, Drings P, et al. Cyclic-alternating versus response-oriented chemotherapy in small-cell lung cancer: a German Multicenter Randomized Trial of 324 patients. J Clin Oncol. 1991;9:614–624.

42. Attal M, Harousseau JL, Stoppa AM, et al. A prospective, randomized trial of autologous bone marrow transplantation and chemotherapy in multiple myeloma (Intergroupe Francais du Myelome). N Engl J Med. 1996;335:91–97.

43. Gianni AM, Bregni M, Siena S, et al. High-dose chemotherapy and autologous bone marrow transplantation compared with MACOP-B in aggressive B-cell lymphoma. N Engl J Med. 1997;336:1290–1297.

44. Klasa RJ, Murray N, Coldman AJ. Dose-intensity meta-analysis of chemotherapy regimens in small-cell carcinoma of the lung. J Clin Oncol. 1991;9:499–508.

45. Arriagada R, Le Chevalier T, Pignon JP, et al. Initial chemotherapeutic doses and survival in patients with limited small-cell lung cancer. N Engl J Med. 1993;329:1848–1852.

46. Maksymiuk AW, Jett JR, Earle JD, et al. Sequencing and schedule effects of cisplatin plus etoposide in small-cell lung cancer: results of a North Central Cancer Treatment Group randomized clinical trial. J Clin Oncol. 1994;12:70–76.

47. Einhorn LH, Crawford J, Birch R, et al. Cisplatin plus etoposide consolidation following cyclophosphamide, doxorubicin, and vincristine in limited small-cell lung cancer. J Clin Oncol. 1988;6:451–456.

48. Humblet Y, Symann M, Bosly A, et al. Late intensification chemotherapy with autologous bone marrow transplantation in selected small-cell carcinoma of the lung: a randomized study. J Clin Oncol. 1987;5:1864–1873.

49. Bleehen NM, Girling DJ, Machin D, et al. A randomized trial of three or six courses of etoposide, cyclophosphamide, methotrexate and vincristine or six courses of etoposide and ifosfamide in small cell lung cancer. I—Survival and prognostic factors (Medical Research Council Lung Cancer Working Party). Br J Cancer. 1993;68:1150–1156.

50. Lung Cancer Working Party. Controlled trial of twelve versus six courses of chemotherapy in the treatment of small-cell lung cancer. Report to the Medical Research Council. Br J Cancer. 1989;59:584–590.

51. Mattson K, Niiranen A, Pryhönen S, et al. Natural interferon alfa as maintenance therapy for small cell lung cancer. Eur J Cancer. 1992;28A:1387–1391.

52. Sculier JP, Paesmans M, Bureau G, et al. Randomized trial comparing induction chemotherapy versus induction chemotherapy followed

53. LeBeau B, Chastang CL, Allard P, et al. Six vs. twelve cycles for complete responders to chemotherapy in small cell lung cancer: definitive results of a randomized clinical trial. Eur Respir J. 1992;5:286–290.

54. Spiro SG, Souhami RL, Geddes DM, et al. Duration of chemotherapy in small cell lung cancer: a Cancer Research Campaign trial. Br J Cancer. 1989;59:578–583.

55. Giaccone G, Dalesio O, McVie GJ, et al. Maintenance chemotherapy in small-cell lung cancer: long-term results of a randomized trial. J Clin Oncol. 1993;11:1230–1240.

56. Cullen M, Morgan D, Gregory W, et al. Maintenance chemotherapy for anaplastic small cell carcinoma of the bronchus: a randomized, controlled trial. Cancer Chemother Pharmacol. 1986;17:157–160.

57. Byrne MJ, Van Hazel G, Trotter J, et al. Maintenance chemotherapy in limited small cell lung cancer: a randomized controlled clinical trial. Br J Cancer. 1989;60:413–418.

58. Sculier JP, Berghmans T, Castaigne C, et al. Maintenance chemotherapy for small cell lung cancer: a critical review of the literature. Lung Cancer. 1998;19:141–151.

59. Kelly K, Crowley JJ, Bunn PA Jr. Role of recombinant interferon alfa-2 maintenance in patients with limited-stage small-cell lung cancer responding to concurrent chemoradiation: a Southwest Oncology Group study. J Clin Oncol. 1995;13:2924–2930.

60. Jett JR, Maksymiuk AW, Su JQ. Phase III trial of recombinant interferon gamma in complete responders with small cell lung cancer. J Clin Oncol. 1994;12:2321–2326.

61. Johnson DH, Bass D, Einhorn LH, et al. Combination chemotherapy with or without thoracic radiotherapy in limited-stage small-cell lung cancer: a randomized trial of the Southeastern Cancer Study Group. J Clin Oncol. 1993;11:1223–1229.

62. Creech R, Richter M, Finkelstein D. Combination chemotherapy with or without consolidation radiation therapy (RT) for regional small cell carcinoma of the lung [abstract]. Proc ASCO. 1988;7:196.

63. Birch R, Omura G, Greco FM, et al. Patterns of failure in combined chemotherapy and radiotherapy for limited small-cell lung cancer: South Eastern Chemotherapy Group experience. Monogr Natl Cancer Inst. 1988;6:265–270.

64. Perry M, Herndon JE, Eaton WL, et al. Thoracic radiation therapy added to chemotherapy for small-cell lung cancer: an update of Cancer and Leukemia Group B Study 8083. J Clin Oncol. 1998;16:2466–2467.

65. Perry MC, Eaton WL, Propert KJ, et al. Chemotherapy with or without radiation therapy in limited small-cell carcinoma of the lung. N Engl J Med 1987;316:912–918.

66. Østerlind K, Hansen HH, Hansen HS, et al. Chemotherapy *versus* chemotherapy plus irradiation in limited small cell lung cancer: results of a controlled trial with 5 years follow-up. Br J Cancer. 1986;54:7–17.

67. Bunn PA Jr, Lichter AS, Makuch RW, et al. Chemotherapy alone or chemotherapy with chest radiation therapy in limited stage small cell lung cancer: a prospective randomized trial. Ann Intern Med. 1987;106:655–662.

68. Kies MS, Mira JG, Crowley JJ, et al. Multimodality therapy for limited small-cell lung cancer: a randomized study of induction combination chemotherapy with or without thoracic radiation in complete responders; and with wide-field versus reduced-field radiation in partial responders: a Southwest Oncology Group study. J Clin Oncol. 1987;5:592–600.

69. Rosenthal MA, Tattersall MHN, Fox RM, et al. Adjuvant thoracic radiotherapy in small cell lung cancer: ten-year follow-up of a randomized study. Lung Cancer. 1991;7:235–241.

70. Nõu E, Brodin O, Bergh J. A randomized study of radiation treatment in small cell bronchial carcinoma treated with two types of four-drug chemotherapy regimens. Cancer. 1988;62:1079–1090.

71. Carlson RW, Sikic BI, Gandara DR, et al. Late consolidative radiation therapy in the treatment of limited-stage small cell lung cancer. Cancer. 1991;68:948–958.

72. Souhami RL, Geddes DM, Spiro SG, et al. Radiotherapy in small cell cancer of the lung treated with combination chemotherapy: a controlled trial. BMJ. 1984;288:1643–1646.

73. Turrisi AT, Kim K, Sause W, et al. Observations after 5 year follow up of Intergroup Trial 0096: four cycles of cis-platin, etoposide and concurrent 45 Gy thoracic radiotherapy given in daily or twice daily fractions followed by 25 Gy PCI. Survival differences and patterns of failure. Proc ASCO. 1998;17:457a.

74. Warde P, Payne D. Does thoracic irradiation improve survival and local control in limited-stage small cell carcinoma of the lung? A meta-analysis. J Clin Oncol. 1992;10:890–895.

75. Pignon JP, Arriagada R, Ihde DC. A meta-analysis of thoracic radiotherapy for small-cell lung cancer. N Engl J Med. 1992; 327:1618–1624.

76. Choi N, Herndon J, Rosenman J, et al. Phase I study to determine the maximum tolerated dose of radiation in standard daily and hyperfractionated-accelerated twice-daily radiation schedules with concurrent chemotherapy for limited-stage small-cell lung cancer. J Clin Oncol. 1998;16:3528–3536.

77. Jeremic B, Shibamoto Y, Acimovic L, et al. Initial versus delayed accelerated hyperfractionated radiation therapy and concurrent chemotherapy in limited small-cell lung cancer: a randomized study. J Clin Oncol. 1997;15:893–900.

78. Bonner JA, Sloan JA, Shanahan TG, et al. Phase III comparison of twice-daily split-course irradiation versus once-daily irradiation for patients with limited stage small-cell lung carcinoma. J Clin Oncol. 1999;17:2681–2691.

79. Coy P, Hodson I, Payne DG, et al. The effect of dose of thoracic irradiation on recurrence in patients with limited stage small cell lung cancer: initial results of a Canadian multicenter randomized trial. Int J Radiat Oncol Biol Phys. 1988;14:219–226.

80. Turrisi A, Kim K, Blum R, et al. Twice-daily compared with once-daily thoracic radiotherapy in limited small-cell lung cancer treated concurrently with cisplatin and etoposide. N Engl J Med. 1999;340:265–271.

81. Work E, Nielsen O, Bentzen S, et al. Randomized study of initial versus late chest irradiation combined with chemotherapy in limited stage small-cell lung cancer. J Clin Oncol. 1997;15:3030–3037.

82. Hansen HH, Dombernowsky P, Hirsch FR, et al. Prophylactic irradiation in bronchogenic small cell anaplastic carcinoma: a comparative trial of localized versus extensive radiotherapy including prophylactic brain irradiation in patients receiving combination chemotherapy. Cancer. 1980;46:279–284.

83. Arriagada R, Le Chevalier T, Borie F, et al. Prophylactic cranial irradiation for patients with small-cell lung cancer in complete remission. J Natl Cancer Inst. 1995;87:183–190.

84. Gregor A, Cull A, Stephens RJ, et al. Prophylactic cranial irradiation is indicated following complete response to induction therapy in small cell lung cancer: results of a multicentre randomised trial. United Kingdom Coordinating Committee for Cancer Research (UKCCCR) and the European Organization for Research and Treatment of Cancer (EORTC). Eur J Cancer. 1997;33:1717–1719.

85. Aupérin A, Arriagada R, Pignon JP, et al. Prophylactic cranial irradiation for patients with small-cell lung cancer in complete remission. N Engl J Med. 1999;341:476–484.

86. Arriagada R, Aupérin A, Pignon JP, et al. Prophylactic cranial irradiation overview (PCIO) in patients with small cell lung cancer (SCLC) in complete remission (CR) [abstract]. Proc ASCO. 1998;17:457a.

87. Souhami R, Law K. Longevity in small cell lung cancer: a report to the Lung Cancer Subcommittee of the UK Coordinating Committee for Cancer Research. Br J Cancer. 1990;61:584–589.

88. Deslauriers J. Surgery for small cell lung cancer. Lung Cancer. 1997;17(suppl):S91–S98.

89. Shore DF, Paneth M. Survival after resection of small cell carcinoma of the bronchus. Thorax. 1980;35:819–822.

90. Davis S, Wright PW, Schulman SF, et al. Long-term survival in small-cell carcinoma of the lung: a population experience. J Clin Oncol. 1985;3:80–91.

91. Shepherd FA, Ginsberg RJ, Feld R, et al. Surgical treatment for limited small-cell lung cancer: the University of Toronto Lung Oncology Group experience. J Thorac Cardiovasc Surg. 1991; 101:385–393.

92. Karrer K, Shields TW, Denck H, et al. The importance of surgical and multimodality treatment for small cell bronchial carcinoma. J Thorac Cardiovasc Surg. 1989;97:168–176.

93. Shepherd FA, Evans WK, Feld R, et al. Adjuvant chemotherapy following surgical resection for small-cell carcinoma of the lung. J Clin Oncol. 1988;6:832–838.

94. Shepherd FA, Ginsberg RJ, Patterson GA, et al. A prospective study of adjuvant surgical resection after chemotherapy for limited small

cell lung cancer: a University of Toronto Lung Oncology Group study. J Thorac Cardiovasc Surg. 1989;97:177–186.

95. Wada H, Yokomise H, Tanaka F, et al. Surgical treatment of small cell carcinoma of the lung: advantage of preoperative chemotherapy. Lung Cancer. 1995;13:45–56.

96. Hage R, Elbers JRJ, Brutel de la Rivière A, et al. Surgery for combined type small cell lung carcinoma. Thorax. 1998;53:450–453.

97. Davis S, Crino L. Tonato M, et al. A prospective analysis of chemotherapy following surgical resection of clinical Stage I-II small-cell lung cancer. Am J Clin Oncol. 1993;16:93–95.

98. Merkle NM, Mickisch GH, Kayser K, et al. Surgical resection and adjuvant chemotherapy for small cell carcinoma. Thorac Cardiovasc Surg. 1986;34:39–42.

99. Williams CJ, McMillan I, Lea R, et al. Surgery after initial chemotherapy for localized small-cell carcinoma of the lung. J Clin Oncol. 1987;5:1579–1588.

100. Zatopek NK, Holoye PY, Ellerbroek NA, et al. Resectability of small-cell lung cancer following induction chemotherapy in patients with limited disease (stage II-IIIb). Am J Clin Oncol. 1991;14:427–432.

101. Müller LC, Salzer GM, Huber H, et al. Multimodal therapy of small cell lung cancer in TNM stages I through IIIa. Ann Thorac Surg. 1992;54:493–497.

102. Østerlind K, Hansen M, Hansen HH, et al. Influence of surgical resection prior to chemotherapy on the long-term results in small cell lung cancer: a study of 150 operable patients. Eur J Cancer Clin Oncol. 1986;22:589–593.

103. Fujimori K, Yokoyama A, Kurita Y, et al. A pilot phase 2 study of surgical treatment after induction chemotherapy for resectable stage I to IIIA small cell lung cancer. Chest. 1997;111:1089–1093.

104. Lad T, Piantadosi S, Thomas P, et al. A prospective randomized trial to determine the benefit of surgical resection of residual disease following response of small cell lung cancer to combination chemotherapy. Chest. 1994;106(suppl):320S–323S.

105. Johnson DH, Einhorn LH, Mandelbaum I, et al. Postchemotherapy resection of residual tumor in limited stage small cell lung cancer. Chest. 1987;92:241–246.

106. Macchiarini P, Mussi A, Basolo F, et al. Optimal treatment for T1-3N0M0 small cell lung cancer: surgery plus adjuvant chemotherapy. Anticancer Res. 1989;9:1623–1626.

107. Østerlind K, Hansen M, Hansen HH, et al. Treatment policy of surgery in small cell carcinoma of the lung: retrospective analysis of a series of 874 consecutive patients. Thorax. 1985;40:272–277.

108. Baker RR, Ettinger DS, Ruckdeschel JD, et al. The role of surgery in the management of selected patients with small-cell carcinoma of the lung. J Clin Oncol. 1987;5:697–702.

109. Shepherd FA, Ginsberg R, Patterson GA, et al. Is there ever a role for salvage operations in limited small-cell lung cancer? J Thorac Cardiovasc Surg. 1991;101:196–200.

110. Abeloff MD, Eggleston JC, Mendelsohn G, et al. Changes in morphologic and biochemical characteristics of small cell carcinoma of the lung: a clinicopathologic study. Am J Med. 1979;66:757–764.

111. Radice PA, Matthews MJ, Ihde DC, et al. The clinical behavior of "mixed" small cell/large cell bronchogenic carcinoma compared to "pure" small cell subtypes. Cancer. 1982;50:2894–2902.

112. Sagman U, Lishner M, Maki E, et al. Second primary malignancies following diagnosis of small-cell lung cancer. J Clin Oncol. 1992;10:1525–1533.

113. Johnson BE, Ihde DC, Matthews MJ, et al. Non–small-cell lung cancer: major cause of late mortality in patients with small cell lung cancer. Am J Med. 1986;80:1103–1110.

114. Østerlind K, Hansen HH, Hansen M, et al. Mortality and morbidity in long-term surviving patients treated with chemotherapy with or without irradiation for small-cell lung cancer. J Clin Oncol. 1986;4:1044–1052.

115. Tucker MA, Murray N, Shaw EG, et al. Second primary cancers related to smoking and treatment of small-cell lung cancer. J Natl Cancer Inst. 1997;89:1782–1788.

116. Heyne KH, Lippman SM, Lee JJ, et al. The incidence of second primary tumors in long-term survivors of small-cell lung cancer. J Clin Oncol. 1992;10:1519–1524.

117. Jacoulet P, Depierre A, Moro D, et al. Long-term survivors of small-cell lung cancer (SCLC): a French multicenter study. Ann Oncol. 1997;8:1009–1014.

118. Johnson BE, Linnoila RI, Williams JP, et al. Risk of second aerodi-

119. Kawahara M, Ushijima S, Kamimori T, et al. Second primary tumours in more than 2-year disease-free survivors of small-cell lung cancer in Japan: the role of smoking cessation. Br J Cancer. 1998;78:409–412.

120. Elias A, Ibrahim J, Skarin AT, et al. Dose-intensive therapy for limited-stage small-cell lung cancer: long-term outcome. J Clin Oncol. 1999;17:1175.

121. Leyvraz S, Perey L, Rosti G, et al. Multiple courses of high-dose ifosfamide, carboplatin, and etoposide with peripheral-blood progenitor cells and filgrastin in small cell lung cancer: a feasibility study by the European Group for Blood and Marrow Transplantation. J Clin Oncol. 1999;17:3531–3539.

122. Tucker RD, Ferguson A, Van Wyk C, et al. Chemotherapy of small cell carcinoma of the lung with VP-16-213. Cancer. 1978;41:1710–1714.

123. Hansen M, Hirsch F, Dombernowsky P, et al. Treatment of small cell anaplastic carcinoma of the lung with the oral solution of VP-16-213. Cancer. 1977;40:633–637.

124. Cavelli F, Sonntag RW, Jungi F, et al. VP-16-213 monotherapy for remission induction of small cell lung cancer: a randomized trial using three dosage schedules. Cancer Treat Rep. 1978;62:473–475.

125. Postmus PE, Haaxma-Reiche H, Sleijer DT, et al. High dose etoposide for brain metastases of small cell lung cancer: a phase II study. The EORTC Lung Cancer Cooperative Group. Br J Cancer. 1989;59:254–256.

126. Einhorn LH, Pennington K, McClean J. Phase II trial of daily oral VP-16 in refractory small cell lung cancer: a Hoosier Oncology Group study. Semin Oncol. 1990;17(suppl 2):32–35.

127. Carney DN, Grogan L, Smit EF, et al. Single-agent oral etoposide for elderly small cell lung cancer patients. Semin Oncol. 1990;17(suppl 1):49–53.

128. Woods RL, Fox RM, Tattersall MH. Treatment of small cell bronchogenic carcinoma with VM-26. Cancer Treat Rep. 1979;63:2011–2013.

129. Pedersen AG, Bork E, Østerlind K, et al. Phase II study of teniposide in small cell carcinoma of the lung. Cancer Treat Rep. 1984;68:1289–1291.

130. Cerny T, Pedrazzini A, Joss RA, et al. Unexpected high toxicity in a phase II study of teniposide (VM-26) in elderly patients with untreated small cell lung cancer (SCLC). Eur J Cancer Clin Oncol. 1988;24:1791–1794.

131. Bork E, Hansen M, Dombernowsky P, et al. Teniposide (VM-26), an overlooked highly active agent in small-cell lung cancer: results of a phase II trial in untreated patients. J Clin Oncol. 1986;4:524–527.

132. Giaccone G, Donadio M, Bonardi G, et al. Teniposide in the treatment of small-cell lung cancer: the influence of prior chemotherapy. J Clin Oncol. 1988;6:1264–1270.

133. Cavelli F, Goldhirsch K, Siegaltthaler P, et al. Phase II study with cis-dichlorodiamineplatinum in small cell anaplastic bronchogenic carcinoma. Eur J Cancer. 1980;16:617–621.

134. Smith IE, Harland SJ, Robinson BA, et al. Carboplatin: a very active new cisplatin analog in the treatment of small cell lung cancer. Cancer Treat Rep. 1985;69:43–46.

135. Saijo N, Niitani H. Experimental and clinical effect of ACNU in Japan, with emphasis on small-cell carcinoma of the lung. Cancer Chemother Pharmacol. 1980;4:165–171.

136. Edmonson JH, Lagakos SW, Selawry OS, et al. Cyclophosphamide and CCNU in the treatment of inoperable small cell carcinoma of the lung. Cancer Treat Rep. 1976;60:925–932.

137. Ettinger DS, Karp JE, Abeloff MD. Intermittent high-dose cyclophosphamide chemotherapy for small cell carcinoma of the lung. Cancer Treat Rep. 1978;62:413–424.

138. Ettinger DS, Finkelstein DM, Ritch P, et al. Randomized trial of single agents vs. combination chemotherapy in extensive stage small cell lung cancer (SCLC) [abstract]. Proc ASCO. 1992;11:295.

139. Knight EW, Lagakos S, Stolbach L, et al. Adriamycin in the treatment of far-advanced lung cancer. Cancer Treat Rep. 1976;60:939–941.

140. Blackstein M, Eisenhauer EA, Weirzbicki R, et al. Epirubicin in extensive small-cell lung cancer: a phase II study in previously untreated patients: a National Cancer Institute of Canada Clinical Trials Group study. J Clin Oncol. 1990;8:385–389.

141. Eckhardt S, Kolaric K, Vukas D, et al. Phase II study of 4'-epi-doxorubicin in patients with untreated, extensive small cell lung cancer. Med Oncol Tumor Pharmacother. 1990;7:19–23.

142. Dombernowsky P, Hansen HH, Sorenson PG, et al. Vincristine (NSC-67574) in the treatment of small-cell anaplastic carcinoma of the lung. Cancer Treat Rep. 1976;60:239–240.

143. Østerlind K, Dombernowsky P, Sorenson PG, et al. Vindesine in the treatment of small cell anaplastic bronchogenic carcinoma. Cancer Treat Rep. 1981;65:245–248.

144. Natale RB, Gralla RJ, Wittes RE. Phase II trial of vindesine in patients with small cell lung carcinoma. Cancer Treat Rep. 1981;65:129–131.

145. Hesketh PJ, Crowley JJ, Burris HA, et al. Evaluation of docetaxel in previously untreated extensive-stage small cell lung cancer: a Southwest Oncology Group Phase II trial. Cancer J Sci Am. 1999;5:237–241.

146. Ettinger DS, Finkelstein DM, Sarma RP, et al. Phase II study of paclitaxel in patients with extensive-disease small-cell lung cancer: an Eastern Cooperative Oncology Group study. J. Clin Oncol. 1995;13:1430–1435.

147. Smit EF, Fokkema E, Biesma B, et al. A phase II study of paclitaxel in heavily pretreated patients with small-cell lung cancer. Br J Cancer. 1998;77:347–351.

148. Schiller JH, Kim K, Hutson P, et al. Phase II study of topotecan in patients with extensive-stage small-cell carcinoma of the lung: an Eastern Cooperative Oncology Group Trial. J Clin Oncol. 1996;14:2345–2352.

149. Ardizzoni A, Hansen H, Dombernowsky P, et al. Topotecan, a new active drug in the second-line treatment of small-cell lung cancer: a phase II study in patients with refractory and sensitive disease. The European Organization for Research and Treatment of Cancer Early Clinical Studies Group and New Drug Development Office, and the Lung Cancer Cooperative Group. J Clin Oncol. 1997;15:2090–2096.

150. von Pawel J, Schiller JH, Shepherd FA, et al. Topotecan versus cyclophosphamide, doxorubicin, and vincristine for the treatment of recurrent small-cell lung cancer. J Clin Oncol. 1999;17:658–667.

151. Cormier Y, Eisenhauer E, Muldal A, et al. Gemcitabine is an active new agent in previously untreated extensive small cell lung cancer (SCLC): a study of the National Cancer Institute of Canada Clinical Trials Group. Ann Oncol. 1994;5:283–285.

152. Goldsweig HG, Edgerton F, Redden CS, et al. Hexamethylmelamine as a single agent in the treatment of small-cell carcinoma of the lung. Am J Clin Oncol. 1982;5:267–272.

153. Urban T, Baleyte T, Chastang CL, et al. Standard combination versus alternating chemotherapy in small cell lung cancer: a randomized clinical trial including 394 patients. Lung Cancer. 1999;25:105–113.

154. Havemann K, Wolf M, Holle R, et al. Alternating versus sequential chemotherapy in small cell lung cancer: a randomized German multicenter trial. Cancer. 1987;59:1072–1082.

155. Daniels JR, Chak LY, Sikic BI, et al. Chemotherapy of small-cell carcinoma of lung: a randomized comparison of alternating and sequential combination chemotherapy programs. J Clin Oncol. 1984;2:1192–1199.

156. Ueoka H, Kiura K, Tabata M, et al. A randomized trial of hybrid administration of cyclophosphamide, doxorubicin, and vincristine (CAV)/cisplatin and etoposide (PVP) versus sequential administration of CAV-PVP for the treatment of patients with small cell lung carcinoma: results of long-term follow-up. Cancer. 1998;83:283–290.

157. Aisner J, Whitacre M, Van Echo DA, et al. Doxorubicin, cyclophosphamide, and VP16-213 (ACE) in the treatment of small cell lung cancer. Cancer Chemother Pharmacol. 1982;7:187–193.

158. Seydel HG, Creech R, Pagano M, et al. Prophylactic versus no brain irradiation in regional small cell lung carcinoma. Am J Clin Oncol. 1985;8:218–223.

159. Laplanche A, Monnet I, Santos-Miranda JA, et al. Controlled clinical trial of prophylactic cranial irradiation for patients with small-cell lung cancer in complete remission. Lung Cancer. 1998;21:193–201.

160. Rea F, Callegaro D, Favaretto A, et al. Long-term results of surgery and chemotherapy in small cell lung cancer. Eur J Cardio-thorac Surg. 1998;14:398–402.

161. Prasad US, Naylor AR, Walker WS, et al. Long-term survival after pulmonary resection for small cell carcinoma of the lung. Thorax. 1989;44:784–787.

162. Maassen W, Greschuchna D. Small cell carcinoma of the lung—to operate or not? Surgical experience and results. Thorac Cardiovasc Surg. 1986;34:71–76.

163. Sørensen HR. Survival in small cell lung carcinoma after surgery. Thorax. 1986;41:479–482.

164. Shah SS, Thompson J, Goldstraw P. Results of operation without adjuvant therapy in the treatment of small cell lung cancer. Ann Thorac Surg. 1992;54:498–501.

165. Shields TW, Higgins GA Jr, Matthews MJ, et al. Surgical resection in the management of small cell carcinoma of the lung. J Thorac Cardiovasc Surg. 1982;84:481–488.

166. Lucchi M, Mussi A, Chella A, et al. Surgery in the management of small cell lung cancer. Eur J Cardiothorac Surg. 1997;12:689–693.

167. Eberhardt W, Stamatis G, Stuschke M, et al. Aggressive trimodality treatment including chemoradiation induction and surgery (S) in LD-small-cell lung cancer (LD-SCLC) (stages I-IIIB)—long-term results [abstract]. Proc ASCO. 1998;17:450a.

168. Holoye PY, McMurtrey MJ, Mountain CF, et al. The role of adjuvant surgery in the combined modality therapy of small-cell bronchogenic carcinoma after a chemotherapy-induced partial remission. J Clin Oncol. 1990;8:416–422.

EXTENSIVE STAGE SMALL CELL LUNG CANCER

Heidi H. Gillenwater and Mark A. Socinski

Small cell lung cancer (SCLC) accounts for between 17% and 25% of all lung cancers, with approximately 60% of patients with SCLC presenting with extensive stage disease (Chapter 6).[1,2] About 25 000 Americans were diagnosed with this disease in 1999.[3] SCLC is staged as either limited stage (LS) or extensive stage (ES) based on the two-stage system of the Veterans Administration (VA) Lung Cancer Study Group. *Limited stage disease* is defined as disease that is confined to a hemithorax and regional lymph nodes and that can be encompassed into a reasonable radiation port, whereas *extensive stage disease* is defined as disease that exists beyond these limits. There is controversy as to whether patients with contralateral mediastinal and hilar lymph nodes or contralateral supraclavicular nodes should be included as limited or extensive stage (Chapter 24). In general, patients with ipsilateral pleural effusions thought to be malignant are considered to have ES SCLC.

The staging workup for SCLC should include a chest and abdominal computed tomography (CT) scan, a magnetic resonance imaging (MRI) or a CT scan of the brain, and a bone scan (Chapter 6). Bilateral bone marrow biopsies were formerly a routine part of the staging workup for patients with SCLC; however, <5% of patients with no other sites of metastatic disease and a normal complete blood count (CBC) have bone marrow involvement.[4] Therefore, routine bone marrow biopsies are not currently recommended as a part of the standard workup. The most common sites of extrathoracic disease include bone, liver, bone marrow, brain, lymph nodes, and soft tissue.[5]

PARANEOPLASTIC SYNDROMES

The remote effects of cancer not related to the direct effect of either the primary tumor or metastatic foci are generally termed *paraneoplastic*. SCLC is the solid tumor that is most likely to be associated with paraneoplastic syndromes. The most common paraneoplastic syndromes associated with SCLC include the syndrome of inappropriate secretion of antidiuretic hormone (SIADH), Cushing syndrome, and neurologic syndromes such as Lambert-Eaton syndrome and limbic encephalitis (Table 25–1).

SCLC is the most common tumor to be associatd with SIADH.[6,7] SIADH was found to occur in 11% of 350 patients with SCLC (both limited and extensive stage) in one study.[8] The median sodium in this patient population was 117 mEq/L, but only 27% of these patients were symptomatic as a result of hyponatremia. In the majority of patients, the hyponatremia resolved within 3 weeks of initiating combination chemotherapy. No correlation was found between the occurrence of SIADH and the stage of disease, the distribution of metastatic sites, or the prognosis.

Approximately 15% to 20% of cases of Cushing syndrome are caused by ectopic adrenocorticotropic hormone (ACTH) or corticotropin-releasing hormone production.[9] SCLC accounts for most of these cases.[10,11] A retrospective review of 545 patients with SCLC seen at Toronto General Hospital between 1980 and 1990 identified 23 patients (4.2%) with Cushing syndrome and ectopic ACTH production.[12] Eighty-seven percent of these patients had extensive stage disease at the time of diagnosis of Cushing syndrome, and their response rate was 46%. The median survival of 3.6 months was substantially less than expected for patients with ES SCLC. Only two of these patients had complete resolution of Cushing disease after treatment with chemotherapy. Collichio et al[13] also reviewed the association of Cushing syndrome with SCLC. They identified 10 of 345 patients (2.8%) with SCLC treated at two hospitals

TABLE 25–1. PARANEOPLASTIC SYNDROMES COMMONLY SEEN IN SMALL CELL LUNG CANCER

SYNDROME	% SCLC	DIAGNOSTIC TESTS	TREATMENT[a]	PROGNOSIS[b]
SIADH	10	↓ Na, exclude other causes of hyponatremia	Fluid restriction, ± demeclocycline	Unchanged
Cushing	2–5	↓ K, ↑ ACTH, ↑ cortisol, lack of suppression with dexamethasone, ↑ 24-h urinary free cortisol level	Ketaconazole	Poor
Lambert-Eaton	3	Electrophysiologic testing	3,4-Diaminopyridine, immunosuppression	Possibly more indolent
Limbic encephalitis	3	Anti-Hu antibodies present	Immunosuppression	Possibly more indolent

Inclusion criteria: Most common paraneoplastic syndromes.
[a]In addition to chemotherapy for the SCLC.
[b]Relative to SCLC patients in general.
ACTH, adrenocorticotropic hormone; K, potassium; Na, sodium; SCLC, small cell lung cancer; SIADH, syndrome of inappropriate secretion of antidiuretic hormone.
Data from references 8, 12, 14, 17, 20.

from 1979 to 1990. They also found these patients to have a poor prognosis. Dimopoulos et al[14] also found Cushing disease associated with SCLC to be a poor prognostic sign. However, in patients whose hypercortisolism can be controlled with chemotherapy combined with treatment to inhibit cortisol biosynthesis, effective palliation can be achieved.[13]

Lambert-Eaton syndrome is rare and is caused by impaired release of acetylcholine from the nerve terminals at the neuromuscular junction due to antibodies that are directed against the voltage-gated calcium channels of peripheral nerve terminals.[15,16] This paraneoplastic syndrome affects approximately 3% of patients with SCLC and may occur 2 to 4 years before the diagnosis of SCLC is made.[17] This syndrome is manifested by muscle weakness (especially in the proximal muscles of the lower extremities), hyporeflexia, and autonomic dysfunction. Cranial nerve involvement may also occur manifested by dysarthria, dysphagia, diplopia, and ptosis. Electrophysiologic findings are diagnostic. Criteria for making the diagnosis include nerve conduction studies that demonstrate a decrement of >10% during repetitive stimulation at 2 Hz and facilitation of more than 200% after 10 seconds of exercise in two different nerve-muscle combinations without evidence of other nerve or muscle disease.[18] Successful treatment of the tumor can result in remission of Lambert-Eaton syndrome.[19]

Limbic encephalitis is characterized by cognitive dysfunction, memory impairment, seizures, and psychiatric features such as depression, anxiety, and hallucinations.[20] Anti-Hu antibodies, also known as type 1 antineuronal nuclear auto antibodies (ANNA 1), are associated with this syndrome and were seen in 50% of patients with limbic encephalitis in a small retrospective study.[21] Another study examined clinical characteristics and tumor type in 162 patients who were found to be seropositive for ANNA 1.[22] SCLC was found in 87% of these patients. Interestingly, only 62% of these patients were found to have SCLC at initial workup; the remainder were found to have the disease only after a more aggressive search with MRI, bronchoscopy, mediastinoscopy, or thoracotomy.

OVERALL RESULTS WITH TREATMENT OF EXTENSIVE STAGE SMALL CELL LUNG CANCER

Survival

Untreated SCLC is a lethal disease. The ES median survival of patients with untreated ES SCLC is between 5 and

12 weeks.[23,24] With active treatment, median survival is dramatically improved to 7 to 10 months.[25] The median time to progression is approximately 4 to 6 months, whereas the median duration of response in responding patients is approximately 7 months.[26–28] Representative survival curves of patients with ES SCLC from three large studies conducted during the 1980s by the Southwest Oncology Group (SWOG) are shown in Figure 25–1. The average survival in these studies was 24% at 1 year and 5% at 2 years. These studies have also reported a small percentage of patients with ES SCLC who are 5-year survivors. These findings are consistent with other large studies.[26,27,29–33]

Quality of Life

Although there is a general perception that treatment of ES SCLC results in an improvement in the quality of life (QOL), this has not been studied extensively. The majority of patients with SCLC are symptomatic at the time of presentation, with one large study of 458 patients reporting cough in 84%, fatigue in 81%, anorexia in 51%, chest pain in 47%, and hemoptysis in 31%.[34] In general, approximately

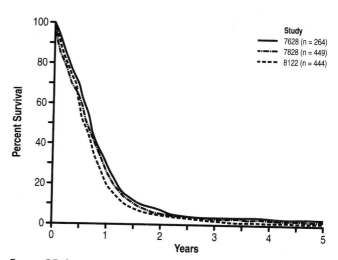

FIGURE 25–1. Overall survival of patients with extensive stage small cell lung cancer from three large studies (1157 patients total). (From Albain KS, Crowley JJ, LeBlanc M, et al. Determinants of improved outcome in small-cell lung cancer: an analysis of the 2,580-patient Southwest Oncology Group data base. J Clin Oncol. 1990;8:1563–1574.[39])

half of those with specific symptoms reported mild symptoms, with the other half reporting moderate or severe symptoms.[34] Treatment with chemotherapy resulted in palliation of the major symptoms in 63% of patients in this study, in which careful diaries of symptoms were kept. Palliation was achieved in 79% with cough, 50% with fatigue, 78% with anorexia, 85% with chest pain, and 89% with hemoptysis. The symptoms disappeared completely in approximately 90% of the patients reporting palliation. Furthermore, the average duration of palliation lasted for 63% of the patient's survival.[34]

QOL has not been studied extensively in SCLC. One of the largest studies examining this issue involved 406 patients treated as part of a phase III trial comparing different sequencing schedules of two chemotherapy regimens, using a European Organization for Research and Treatment of Cancer (EORTC)-QOL tool.[35] The QOL questionnaires were completed by just over 50% of patients with each cycle, but no significant differences in biomedical data were found between those who completed the questionnaires and those who did not. Among the patients reporting data at multiple time points, overall QOL was found to improve over baseline with treatment, as shown in Figure 25–2. Most of the improvement was seen with the first cycle and was sustained throughout the treatment period. An improvement in QOL was seen in patients with both LS and ES SCLC and in patients with good and with poor performance status (PS). In fact, the patients with a poor PS experienced a greater improvement in QOL compared with those with a good PS.[35]

Trends Over Time

Several studies have examined survival of SCLC patients in the 1970s, 1980s, and 1990s.[2,25,36] The reported overall response rates improved from 1960 to 1980, although the complete response (CR) rates remained relatively low.[2] Since 1980, the CR rates have improved from 10% to between 20% and 40%.[2] Short-term survival has improved as well, as evidenced by median survival rates improving from 5 to 6 months in the 1970s to 8 to 9 months in the 1990s in population-based studies in both Europe and the United States.[25,36] There is some evidence to suggest that stage migration may play a role in this change,[37] but the more important factor appears to be treatment of a larger proportion of patients with chemotherapy.[36] The improvement in median survival also appears to be related to how aggressive the treatment approach is, as shown in Figure 25–3. However, there has been little overall improvement in long-term survival in patients with ES SCLC.[36]

PROGNOSTIC FACTORS

Multiple retrospective studies have assessed patient demographics, tumor characteristics, and laboratory values and their impact on the prognosis of patients with SCLC.[37–41] The results of studies performing multivariate analysis of prognostic factors are summarized in Table 25–2. Although not all studies have analyzed the same factors, a number of conclusions can be drawn. A poor PS and elevated

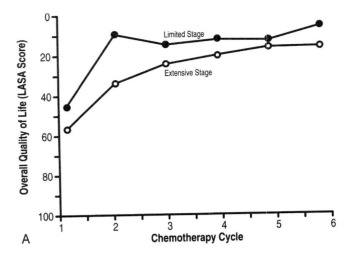

A

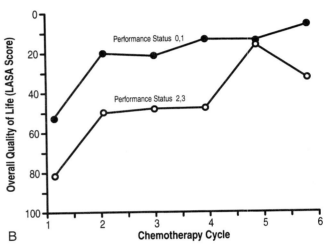

B

FIGURE 25–2. Overall quality of life before each cycle of chemotherapy in 407 patients with small cell lung cancer. *A,* Initial disease stage. *B,* Initial performance status. Quality of life is measured by the linear analog self-assessment (LASA) score of the European Organization for Research and Treatment of Cancer Quality of Life questionnaire, with a worse quality of life indicated by a higher score. (From Bernhard J, Hurny C, Bacch M, et al. Initial prognostic factors in small-cell lung cancer patients predicting quality of life during chemotherapy. Swiss Group for Clinical Cancer Research [SAKK]. Br J Cancer. 1996;74:1660–1667.[35])

lactose dehydrogenase (LDH) levels are consistently associated with poor survival. Male gender and multiple sites of metastatic disease were also found to be independent predictors of poor survival in the majority of studies. It is interesting that disease stage (limited versus extensive) was an independent prognostic factor in only four of seven studies when other factors such as LDH and PS were included. The prognostic significance of low serum sodium, elevated alkaline phosphatase, and older age is less clear. The few studies that have analyzed prognostic factors separately for limited and extensive stage disease have reported results similar to those that have analyzed all patients with SCLC together.

The prognostic value of PS and LDH is demonstrated clearly by the consistency of studies examining these fac-

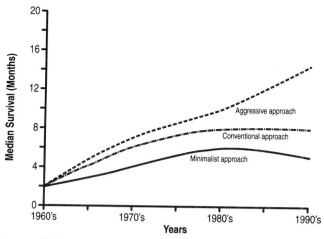

FIGURE 25–3. Trends in median survival over time in reported trials of extensive stage small cell lung cancer. (From Aisner J. Extensive-disease small-cell lung cancer: the thrill of victory, the agony of defeat. J Clin Oncol. 1996;14:658–665.[2])

found that the most consistent and important prognostic factors are disease stage, PS, and a laboratory measurement of liver involvement.[40] In this study, the latter test most often involved alkaline phosphatase because LDH was not assessed in the vast majority of patients in the United Kingdom during this time.

Many other factors have been examined by only a few multivariate studies, often with inconsistent results. A poor prognosis was associated with a low hemoglobin in one of three studies[30,39,42] and with a low platelet count (<150) in one of three studies, as well.[29,30,42] An elevated white blood cell count (WBC) was not of independent prognostic value in three studies.[39,42,43] A low serum albumin level was a marker of a poor prognosis in two studies,[30,43] but weight loss was not.[42,43] Two studies examining the prognostic significance of mediastinal nodal involvement reported conflicting results.[29,30] The presence of a brain metastasis was associated with a worse prognosis in one of three studies,[29,37,42] as was the presence of bone metastases.[29,30,37] The presence of liver metastases was an independent predictor of a poor prognosis in two studies.[30,37]

The data presented in the previous paragraphs does not clearly define how to select patients with SCLC for treatment. Patients with a poor PS or with elevated LDH can be expected to have a shorter survival, but these patients often experience palliation of symptoms and better QOL with treatment. Treatment is also likely to extend the life of these patients markedly, even though their survival is shorter than that of patients with good prognostic factors. On the other hand, the risk of toxicity with treatment appears to be higher in patients with a poor PS, although this is not well defined, making the optimal selection of patients a matter of judgment. Unfortunately, there is little explicit data to serve as a guide in this matter.

tors. This is further corroborated by two studies that analyzed prognostic factors in a slightly different way.[39,40] The first is an analysis using recursive partitioning analysis (RPA) of 2580 patients with SCLC from the SWOG experience.[39] This analysis found the stage of disease to be the most important split, followed by the LDH level (for both limited and extensive stage disease). In patients with LS SCLC and a normal LDH, additional prognostic factors included the presence of a pleural effusion, age >70 years, and female gender. The results of this RPA are corroborated by a comprehensive review of prognostic factors from six large patient cohorts from the United Kingdom, which

TABLE 25–2. PROGNOSTIC FACTORS FOR POOR SURVIVAL BY MULTIVARIATE ANALYSIS IN PATIENTS WITH SMALL CELL LUNG CANCER[a]

STUDY	N	% LS	PS ≤ 2	↑LDH	EXTENSIVE STAGE	MALE GENDER	NO. OF METASTASES	↑ALK PHOS	↓Na	AGE >60 y
Rawson and Peto[40 b]	1960	41	<.001	—	<.001	<.001	—	<.001	<.001	<.001
Østerlind and Andersen[42]	778	51	<.001	<.001	.001	<.01	NS	NS	<.01	.001
Sagman et al[29]	614	46	.0002	<.05	NS	NS	.004	NS	NS	NS
Dearing et al[37]	411	34	<.0001	.0003	NS	.03	NS	.002	—	NS
Cerny et al[184]	407	58	.01[c]	<.0001	.0001	NS	—	.02	.0009	NS
Souhami et al[43]	371	?	<.0001[c]	—	.006	NS	—	.0002	.01	NS
Vincent et al[30]	333	?	.04	—	NS	NS	—	NS	NS	NS
Albain et al[39]	1217	0	.02	.00005	—	.004	NS	NS	NS	NS[d]
Spiegelman et al[41]	697	0	.001	—	—	.02	.01	—	—	NS
Sagman et al[29]	328	0	.0009	NS	—	NS	—	NS	NS	NS
Albain et al[39]	1363	100	.00005	NS	—	.0001	—	NS	NS	.00005[d]
Spiegelman et al[41]	782	100	.001	—	—	.01	—	—	—	.008
Sagman et al[29]	286	100	NS	.0008	—	NS	—	NS	NS	NS
Prognostic importance[e]			**High**	**High**	**Mod**	**Mod**	**Mod**	**Low**	**Low**	**Low**

Inclusion criteria: Studies performing Cox multivariate analysis of prognostic factors in ≥250 patients with small cell lung cancer from 1980 to 2000. Prognostic factors that were analyzed by <5 studies are omitted from the table.
[a]Values shown are P values by multivariate analysis.
[b]Includes patients also included in studies by Cerny, Vincent, and Souhami.
[c]Karnofsky PS < 60.
[d]Age >70 y.
[e]High if 75%–100%, moderate if 50%–74%, low if 25%–29% of studies found factors to be independently significant.
Alk phos, alkaline phosphatase; LDH, lactose dehydrogenase; LS, limited stage; Na, serum sodium; NS, not significant; PS, performance status by Eastern Cooperative Oncology Group scale; ?, unknown.

CHOICE OF CHEMOTHERAPY AGENTS

Conventional Chemotherapeutic Agents

The importance of systemic chemotherapy in the treatment of SCLC became apparent after a randomized study by the VA Lung Cancer Study Group demonstrated a doubling of the median survival in patients with SCLC who were treated with cyclophosphamide compared with placebo.[24] Following publication of that study, a flurry of phase II trials testing single agents were performed to identify active agents in this disease: 141 trials evaluating 57 agents were performed between 1970 and 1990.[44] The 11 agents found to have significant single-agent activity—defined as having response rates of at least 20% in previously untreated and 10% in previously treated patients—were carboplatin, cisplatin, cyclophosphamide, doxorubicin, etoposide, epirubicin, hexamethylenamine, nimustine, teniposide, vincristine, and vindesine (Table 25-3). Ifosfamide, which was determined in this review to have been inadequately tested but to have possible activity, has subsequently been shown to have significant activity in SCLC.[45] It is of interest that cisplatin has not been adequately tested in previously untreated patients and had only a 9% response rate in previously treated patients. Despite this, cisplatin in combination with etoposide has become a standard of care in ES SCLC.

Combination chemotherapy tends to yield higher response rates and survival rates in patients with SCLC.[2,46] Among the older agents, carboplatin, cisplatin, cyclophosphamide, doxorubicin, etoposide, and vincristine have been the agents used most commonly in combination. Trials in the 1970s focused on cyclophosphamide-based regimens. The addition or substitution of etoposide in cyclophosphamide-based regimens was tested extensively in the 1980s. Platinum-based regimens were then tested in the 1980s and 1990s. Today, the combination of cisplatin or carboplatin and etoposide is the most commonly used regimen, based on its activity and favorable toxicity profile.

Cyclophosphamide-Based Combinations

Cyclophosphamide was the first chemotherapeutic agent to show significant activity in SCLC.[24] Cyclophosphamide, doxorubicin, and vincristine (CAV) was the most commonly used regimen during the 1980s and, until recently, was the standard against which new combinations were compared. Other cyclophosphamide-based regimens that have been tested include CAV plus etoposide (CAVE); cyclophosphamide, doxorubicin, and etoposide (CAE); and cyclophosphamide, etoposide, and vincristine (CEV) (Table 25-4). In seven randomized phase III trials in which CAV was used in one of the treatment arms, the mean CR rate was 14% (range, 6%-27%), and the mean overall response rate was 52% (range, 40%-60%).[27,28,47-51] Average median survival in these trials was 8 months (range, 7-10 months).

A randomized study comparing CAVE to CAV found a trend to higher overall response rates with CAVE (55% versus 35%, P = NS) and a trend to better survival for the 43 patients in this study with extensive stage disease (7.8 versus 4.6 months, P = NS).[52] Hematologic toxicity was more frequent for the etoposide-containing arm (grade 3-4 leukopenia, 56% versus 41%, no P value given). Another randomized trial comparing these two regimens in 116 patients with ES SCLC observed a significantly better response rate for the etoposide-containing regimen (70% versus 46%, P = 0.008); however, no difference in survival was observed (9.4 versus 7.8 months, P = 0.08).[53] Again, hematologic toxicity was greater in the etoposide-containing regimen (grade 3-4 leukopenia, 54% versus 27%, P = 0.002). In summary, the addition of etoposide to CAV resulted in a higher response rate, and both studies found a trend toward improved survival but also greater toxicity. The lack of statistical significance for the survival difference is inconclusive, however, because of the small size of these studies.

CAV, CEV, and cyclophosphamide and vincristine (CV) were compared in a three-arm randomized phase III trial involving 353 patients with both LS and ES SCLC.[47] Because early evidence showed that the three-drug regimens were superior to CV, accrual to this arm was closed. The CR rate in extensive stage patients was 49% for CEV, 47% for CAV, and 40% for CV (P = NS). The overall response

TABLE 25-3. SINGLE AGENT ACTIVITY OF ACTIVE CONVENTIONAL CHEMOTHERAPY AGENTS IN SMALL CELL LUNG CANCER

AGENT	NO. OF TRIALS	NO. OF PATIENTS	% PREVIOUSLY TREATED	RESPONSE RATE[a] (%) Average	Range
Etoposide	18	651	67	23	0-81
Teniposide	9	223	62	31	0-90
Vincristine	2	42	57	21	0-42
Vindesine	6	110	92	28	0-50
Doxorubicin	6	56	48	44	21-67
Epirubicin	3	139	0	48	33-50
Nimustine	2	69	57	29	11-47
Cisplatin	8	124	78	9	0-31
Carboplatin	5	124	61	28	6-79
Cyclophosphamide	7	204	0	22	0-70
Ifosfamide	6	262	68	47	6-77
Hexamethylenamine	3	49	71	37	0-42

Inclusion criteria: Single-agent response data for chemotherapeutic agents conventionally considered active in small cell lung cancer, taken from recent reviews.[44,45]
[a]Objective response rate as conventionally defined (partial response + complete response).

TABLE 25–4. ACTIVITY OF COMMONLY USED REGIMENS IN SMALL CELL LUNG CANCER

REGIMEN	CR (RANGE) (%)	CR+PR (RANGE) (%)	MST (mo)
Cyclophosphamide Based			
CAV	14 (6-27)	52 (40-66)	8
CAVE	32 (29-35)	63 (55-70)	9
CAE	14	—	10
CEV	14	42	9
Platinum Based			
EP	15 (8-21)	69 (53-79)	9
ECb	9	61 (58-64)	8
VIP	21	73	9
ICE	23	83	8

Inclusion criteria: Representative phase III studies of commonly used regimens in small cell lung cancer.
CR, complete response; MST, median survival time; PR, partial response.
Chemotherapy regimens: CAE, cyclophosphamide, doxorubicin, etoposide[54]; CAV, cyclophosphamide, doxorubicin, vincristine[27,28,47–51]; CAVE, cyclophosphamide, doxorubicin, vincristine, etoposide[52,53]; CEV, cyclophosphamide, etoposide, vincristine[47]; EP, etoposide, cisplatin[27,69–71]; ECb, etoposide, carboplatin[84–86]; ICE, ifosfamide, carboplatin, etoposide[91]; VIP, etoposide, ifosfamide, cisplatin.[69]

rate for patients with extensive stage disease was better for CEV (42% versus 32%, $P = 0.002$). Median survival was superior for extensive stage patients treated with CEV versus CAV/CV (9.0 versus 7.1 months, $P = 0.01$).[47]

Experience with the CAE combination over 10 years was reported by Aisner et al,[54] who used this regimen to treat 119 patients with ES SCLC. They reported a CR rate of 43% and a median survival of 9.5 months in this series.

Platinum-Based Combinations

Cisplatin (P) was the first platinum compound to show substantial activity in SCLC, initially in patients with refractory disease.[55–60] Etoposide was also documented to have significant single activity in this disease.[61–65] Because in vitro data suggested that the combination of etoposide and cisplatin (EP) would be synergistic, several phase II trials using this combination were performed.[66] In two phase II trials in which this regimen was tested in chemonaive patients, CR rates were 29% and 34%, with an overall response rate of 88% in both trials for patients with extensive stage disease.[67,68] The median survivals in these two trials were 9.0 and 9.7 months for this group of patients. In four phase III trials in which EP was one of the arms, the mean CR rate was 15% (8%-21%) and the mean overall response rate was 69% (53%-79%).[27,69–71] The average median survival in these trials was 9 months (range, 7-10 months).

Two studies have compared CAV to EP.[27,71] Fukuoka et al[71] randomized patients to receive CAV versus EP versus alternation of these regimens (CAV↔EP). The CR rates for patients with ES disease were similar for all groups: 13% for CAV, 10% for EP, and 9% for CAV↔EP. The overall response rates were significantly higher for the EP-containing regimens and were 59% for CAV compared with 78% for EP and 63% for CAV↔EP ($P = 0.05$). The median survival for patients with extensive stage disease treated with CAV, EP, or CAV↔EP was 8.7, 8.3, and 9 months, respectively, and the differences were not statistically significant. Grade 3-4 leukopenia was more common in the CAV-containing arms (78% for CAV, 46% for EP, and 72% for CAV↔EP; $P < 0.001$). No statistically significant difference was reported in other parameters of hematologic toxicity or nonhematologic toxicity.

Roth et al[27] conducted the other study comparing EP and CAV. They also randomized patients to CAV versus EP versus CAV↔EP. There was no difference in CR rate (7%, 10%, and 7%, respectively) or overall response rate (51%, 61%, and 59%). Median survival was similar in all groups, as well (8.3 months, 8.6 months, and 8.1 months, respectively). Patients in this study received crossover second-line treatment at the time of progression, and the second line response to EP was better than the response to CAV (28% versus 14% in patients who had initially responded to the first-line treatment, and 15% versus 8% in patients who were refractory to the first-line treatment). This trial also reported a higher incidence of grade 3 and 4 leukopenia for the patients treated with CAV ($P = 0.001$). There was no reported difference in nonhematologic toxicity. Lastly, Evans et al[48] randomized patients to CAV versus alternating CAV↔EP. Both the response rate and survival were superior in the alternating arm. This is likely due to the inclusion of EP in the alternating arm rather than to the combination of the two regimens. In summary, the EP-containing regimens trended toward higher response rates, produced less hematologic toxicity compared with CAV, and resulted in similar survival rates.

Carboplatin (Cb) is a platinum compound that is different from cisplatin in its toxicity profile. Myelosuppression, especially thrombocytopenia, is dose limiting and is more pronounced than that seen with cisplatin.[72] However, carboplatin is associated with substantially less nephrotoxicity, ototoxicity, neurotoxicity, and emetogenic potential than cisplatin.[73,74] It has shown significant activity in SCLC as a single agent, with response rates ranging from 10% to 79%, depending on whether previously treated patients were included in the studies.[75–79]

The question remains whether carboplatin is equally efficacious when compared with cisplatin for the treatment of SCLC. In germ cell tumors, carboplatin has been shown to be inferior when compared with cisplatin in four trials.[80–83] Only one randomized phase III study has been conducted comparing ECb with EP in SCLC (147 patients).[84] No difference was found in response rates for ECb versus EP (86% versus 76% for limited stage, 67% versus 60% for extensive stage) or in median survival (11.8 versus 12.5 months for all patients). However, this trial did not have sufficient power to detect a small but clinically meaningful difference in outcome. Two other trials have compared regimens containing either cisplatin or carboplatin, and neither found a significant difference in response rates or survival.[85,86] At this time, further study is necessary to compare the efficacy of these agents in the treatment of SCLC. Given the paucity of comparative data, one has to consider cisplatin the standard platinum, especially for limited stage disease. However, because the goal of treatment in patients with ES SCLC is palliation, carboplatin offers an option with less nonhematologic toxicity.

Ifosfamide-Based Combinations

Ifosfamide has been tested extensively as a single agent in the phase II setting to treat SCLC.[45,87–89] Response rates are reported to be between 6% and 43% for previously treated patients and between 44% and 58% for chemonaive patients. This agent has also been studied in combination with either EP (*VIP*,* where V stands for VP-16, which is another name for etoposide) or carboplatin and etoposide (*ICE*).[69,90,91]

Wolff et al[91] performed a phase II study that examined the combination of ifosfamide, carboplatin, and oral etoposide (*ICE*) in patients with extensive stage disease. Ifosfamide 5g/m^2 by continuous intravenous (IV) infusion with mesna on day 1, carboplatin 300 mg/m^2 IV on day 1, and etoposide 50 mg/m^2 orally on days 1 through 21 were given to 18 patients with ES SCLC. Because of severe hematologic toxicity, the subsequent 17 patients received a reduction of the ifosfamide to 3.75 g/m^2 on day 1 and a decrease in the duration of etoposide to 14 days instead of 21. The CR rate for this combination for all patients in the study was 23%, with an overall response rate of 83%. The median survival was 8.3 months, and 2-year survival was impressive at 14%. Myelotoxicity was the most significant toxicity of this regimen, and 89% of the patients on the first schedule had grade 3-4 neutropenia after cycle 1. At the reduced dose schedule, grade 3-4 neutropenia was reduced to 43%. Because this regimen lacks significant nonhematologic toxicity, it has been examined in dose-intense regimens to treat SCLC. Other investigators have used similar combinations of *ICE* with similar results.[92,93]

At least four trials have evaluated the triplet combination of cisplatin, etoposide, and ifosfamide (*VIP*).[94–97] The overall response rates have ranged from 74% to 100%, with CR rates of 27% to 43%. Median survival has been reported in the 10 to 12 month range. Based on this data, the Hoosier Oncology Group performed a randomized phase III study comparing EP with *VIP* in 171 patients with extensive stage disease.[69] Patients were treated with EP (100 mg/m^2 and 20 mg/m^2, both IV day 1-4) or *VIP* (75 mg/m^2, 1.2 g/m^2, and 20 mg/m^2, all given IV day 1-4). A statistically significant improvement in the 2-year survival was seen with *VIP* (13% versus 5%, $P < 0.05$). There was a nonsignificant trend toward better median survival (9 versus 7.3 months) and response rate (73% versus 67%) with *VIP*. This came at the price of more frequent hematologic and nonhematologic toxicities in the *VIP* arm.

---

*Italics are used for regimens that are conventionally known by an abbreviation in which the letters used to denote chemotherapeutic agents in this regimen are *different* than the letters commonly used for these agents in other regimens or as a single agent.

TABLE 25–5. NEW AGENTS IN SMALL CELL LUNG CANCER

	FIRST LINE RESPONSE RATE[a] (%)	SECOND LINE RESPONSE RATE[a] (%)
Topotecan	39[99]	6-38[149, 150]
Irinotecan	—	47[154]
Gemcitabine	27[110]	—
Paclitaxel	34-53[102, 103]	29[155]
Docetaxel	—	20[157]
Vinorelbine	5[112]	13[158]

Inclusion criteria: Studies of single agent activity of selected new chemotherapeutic agents in ≥20 patients with small cell lung cancer.
[a]Objective response (partial response + complete response).

Another phase III randomized study compared the standard EP to ifosfamide and etoposide (IE) in patients with LS and ES SCLC.[90] At the time of progression, patients were treated with CAV. The CR rate for patients with extensive stage disease (n = 87) was 22% for EP and 18% for IE, with overall response rates of 55% and 61%, respectively. The median survival for patients with ES disease was 8.9 versus 7.5 months, but the 2-year survival was 5% and 9% for EP versus IE (*P* value not given).

New Chemotherapeutic Agents

In the 1990s, a number of new agents became available that are being tested in phase II and III trials. These include topotecan, irinotecan, gemcitabine, paclitaxel, docetaxel, and vinorelbine (Table 25–5). Topotecan, paclitaxel, gemcitabine, and vinorelbine have been tested in the first-line setting, whereas docetaxel, irinotecan, and vinorelbine have been studied as second-line treatment and are discussed in the section entitled Second-Line Therapy.

Topotecan, a new campotothecin analog, is a topoisomerase I inhibitor that has been found to have activity in a number of tumor types in addition to SCLC.[98] A study conducted by the Eastern Cooperative Oncology Group (ECOG) examined topotecan as a single agent for patients with ES SCLC.[99] Forty-eight patients were treated with 2.0 mg/m^2 of topotecan daily for 5 days. The overall response rate was 39%. Median survival was 10 months, and 1-year survival was 39%. The first 13 patients in this study were treated without colony-stimulating factor support, and 92% of these patients experienced grade 3 or 4 neutropenia. Grade 3-4 neutropenia was decreased to 29% when granulocyte colony–stimulating factor (G-CSF) was added to the regimen. Nonhematologic toxicity was minimal. Topotecan is also currently undergoing investigation in combination with other agents such as paclitaxel, carboplatin, and etoposide in first-line treatment of SCLC. The initial experience with these combinations has been encouraging.[100]

Paclitaxel promotes stabilization of microtubules, which results in inhibition of cell division.[101] Two phase II studies that looked at paclitaxel in previously untreated patients reported response rates of 34%[102] and 53%.[103] The median survival for both studies was approximately 7 months. The combination of paclitaxel, etoposide and carboplatin or cisplatin for ES SCLC has been evaluated in five phase II studies.[104–108] The schedules and doses of the component drugs have varied somewhat, and several of the studies[105–107] used growth factors to ameliorate myelosuppression. Also, some of the studies used oral etoposide,[104,106] whereas others used IV etoposide.[105,107,108] A total of 149 patients have been studied on these trials. Overall response rates with these combinations have ranged from 65% to 100%, with complete responses seen in 12% to 25%. Median survival rates range from 7 to 11 months, with a 1-year survival rate of approximately 40%. Grade 4 neutropenia was significant and was seen in up to 73% of patients. Treatment-related death rates ranged from 0 to 5%. Because of this impressive activity, the triplet regimen of cisplatin, etoposide, and paclitaxel is being compared with cisplatin/etoposide in a randomized phase III trial in the United States.

Gemcitabine is a pyrimidine analog that is activated intracellularly by deoxycytidine kinase to the active form of the drug.[109] Gemcitabine has been studied in the first-line setting and has been shown to have a response rate of 27%, all partial responses.[110] The median survival in this study was 12 months. The treatment was well tolerated, and only moderate myelosuppression was seen. Vinorelbine is a semisynthetic vinca alkaloid that inhibits microtubule assembly.[111] Higano et al[112] studied this single agent in previously untreated patients with ES SCLC and had only 1 of 22 patients with a partial response lasting more than 4 weeks.

In summary, there are several newer agents that have shown single-agent response rates of 20% to 40% for patients with ES SCLC. Before these agents can be widely accepted for standard use in the treatment of ES SCLC, further phase II testing of these agents in combination regimens followed by randomized phase III testing of the most promising combinations must be done.

DOSE-INTENSIVE CHEMOTHERAPY

Both preclinical and clinical evidence exists to support the use of maximum dose intensity in chemosensitive tumors to improve response rates and survival.[113–115] Dose intensity can be increased by increasing the dose or decreasing the interval of standard chemotherapy with or without

hematopoietic growth factor support, or by using autologous bone marrow or peripheral blood stem cell support. These methods of increasing dose intensity have been investigated in patients with SCLC and, for the most part, results have been discouraging. In general, the dose-intensive regimens have shown increased toxicity and no improvement in survival when dose intensity has been increased.

A meta-analysis retrospectively examined the effect of dose intensity in SCLC in 60 trials involving treatment with cyclophosphamide, doxorubicin, vincristine, etoposide, and cisplatin.[116] It should be noted that this meta-analysis examined the question based on intended dose intensity rather than actual dose intensity. Despite this, no statistically significant relationship was found between dose intensity and outcome (either in response rate or survival) for CAV or EP. With CAE and CAVE, there was a statistically significant improvement in median survival for patients with ES disease ($P < 0.05$).

Six phase III randomized trials have compared dose-intensive regimens without hematopoietic growth factor support to standard chemotherapy in SCLC (Table 25–6),[28,33,117–120] but two of these trials involved <50 patients total.[119,120] None of these trials showed a survival advantage for the dose-intensive arm, and the dose-intensive regimen often resulted in greater toxicity. In addition, a majority of these trials failed to deliver the intended dose intensity in the high-dose arms. In order to diminish the toxicity of increased dose-intensive regimens, several trials have used growth factor support (Table 25–7).[32,121–124] With one exception,[124] these trials have also failed to demonstrate improved survival with more dose-intensive therapy.

The use of stem cell support to allow increased dose intensity for patients with SCLC has been studied.[125–127] These trials, which included both LS and ES SCLC patients, are all small, ranging from 10 to 100 patients. The available data does not allow any meaningful conclusions to be drawn regarding the use of high dose chemotherapy with stem cell support in ES SCLC. Dose-intensive strategies employing high dose chemotherapy supported by stem cell or bone marrow are difficult to use in this population, where the median age of patients with SCLC is 60 to 65 years.[128] Also, these patients frequently have associated

TABLE 25–6. RANDOMIZED TRIALS OF DOSE INTENSITY WITHOUT GRANULOCYTE COLONY–STIMULATING FACTOR IN SMALL CELL LUNG CANCER

REFERENCE	n	CHEMOTHERAPY REGIMEN	AGENTS WITH A DIFFERENCE IN DOSE INTENSITY	RELATIVE DOSE INTENSITY[a]	RESPONSE RATE (%)			MST (mo)		
					Dose Intensive Arm	Control Arm	P	Dose Intensive Arm	Control Arm	P
Souhami et al[33]	438[b]	IA↔EP/CAV↔EP[c]	E,P,A(I/C,V)[c]	1.6,1.3,1.3[c]	82	81	NS	10.8	10.7	NS
Johnson et al[28]	298	CAV	C,A	1.2,1.8	63	53	NS	6.7	7.8	NS
Figueredo et al[118]	105[d]	CAV	C,A	1.5,1.2	71	61	NS	14	12	NS
Ihde et al[117]	90	EP	E,P	1.4,1.7	86	83	NS	11.4	10.7	NS

Inclusion criteria: Randomized trials of dose intensity without growth factor support ≥50 patients with small cell lung cancer from 1980 to 2000.
[a] Dose intensive versus control regimen for the agents listed in previous column.
[b] 63% Limited stage.
[c] Certain agents given to only one group (Dose intensive/Control).
[d] 34% Limited stage.
Agents with a difference in dose intensity, chemotherapy agents with a difference in the dose intensity between arms (agents used only in one arm listed in parentheses); MST, median survival time; NS, not significant.
Chemotherapy abbreviations: A, doxorubicin; C, cyclophosphamide; E, etoposide; I, ifosfamide; P, cisplatin; V, vincristine; ↔, alternating schedule.

TABLE 25–7. RANDOMIZED TRIALS OF DOSE INTENSIVE THERAPY WITH GRANULOCYTE COLONY–STIMULATING FACTOR OR GRANULOCYTE-MACROPHAGE COLONY-STIMULATING FACTOR IN SMALL CELL LUNG CANCER

REFERENCE	n	CHEMOTHERAPY REGIMEN[a]	AGENTS WITH A DIFFERENCE IN DOSE INTENSITY	RELATIVE DOSE INTENSITY[b]	RESPONSE RATE (%) Dose Intensive Arm	Control Arm	P	MST (mo) Dose Intensive Arm	Control Arm	P
Steward et al[124c]	300	V-*ICE*	V,I,Cb,E	1.33 for all	83	83	NS	14.6	11.5	.0014
Pujol et al[121]	298	CErEP	C,Er,E,P	1.5,1.5,1.5,1.2	87	75	.09	8.9	10.8	.0005
Furuse et al[32]	227	*CODE*/CAV↔EP[d]	E,P,A,V(C)[d]	2.4,1.9,7.2,1.9[d]	84	77	NS	11.6	10.9	NS
Woll et al[123e]	65	V-*ICE*	Sched. freq. PRN	1.06 for all	94	95	NS	15.9	15.0	NS

Inclusion criteria: Randomized trials of dose intensity with growth factor support ≥50 patients with small cell lung cancer from 1980 to 2000.
[a]Dose intensive arms all given GCSF or GMCSF.
[b]Dose intensive versus control regimen for the agents listed in previous column.
[c]Approximately 65% LS.
[d]Certain agents given to only one group (DI/Cont).
[e]92% LS.
Agents with a difference in dose intensity, chemotherapy agents with a difference in the dose intensity between arms (agents used in only one arm listed in parentheses); MST, median survival time; NS, not significant, Sched. freq. PRN, the dose was the same in both arms without dose modification, but schedule frequency was left to the discretion of the treating physician.
Chemotherapy abbreviations: A, doxorubicin; C, cyclophosphamide; Cb, carboplatin; *CODE*, cisplatin, vincristine, doxorubicin, etoposide; E, etoposide; Er, epirubicin; I, ifosfamide; *ICE*, ifosfamide, carboplatin, etoposide; P, cisplatin; V, vincristine.

comorbid illness as a result of tobacco abuse that precludes aggressive treatment.[129]

MAINTENANCE CHEMOTHERAPY

The role of maintenance chemotherapy in the treatment of SCLC has been controversial. The 13 randomized trials that have investigated this subject have reported mostly negative results.[31,49,130–140] Three of these studies included only patients with limited stage disease,[131,132,135] 9 investigated patients with either extensive or limited stage disease,[31,130,133,134,136–140] and only 1 exclusively studied patients with extensive stage disease.[49] However, 1 of the trials that included both extensive and limited stage patients analyzed survival separately based on extent of disease.[31] The results of trials involving patients with limited stage disease are discussed in Chapter 24.

In the trial involving only patients with ES SCLC, 577 patients were initially randomized to an induction regimen of either CAV or CAV alternating with hexamethylenamine, etoposide, and methotrexate (CAV↔HmEMx).[49] The 86 patients who had a CR to either induction regimen were then randomized to observation versus maintenance therapy with their induction regimen. All of these patients also received prophylactic cranial irradiation (PCI). Only 5 patients remained free of relapse, 3 of whom were in the control group and 2 of whom were in the maintenance group. Maintenance chemotherapy did not result in a significant improvement in survival in either the CAV or the CAV↔HmEMx arm.

The other trial reporting specifically on patients with extensive stage disease randomized 61 patients with a CR or a good response (only minor residual abnormalities on staging studies) after six cycles of CAV to either observation or maintenance chemotherapy with CAV.[31] Patients with extensive stage disease who were randomized to maintenance chemotherapy showed a significant survival advantage (median survival, 12 versus 8.5 months, P = 0.006).

However, although there is some conflicting data regarding the benefit of maintenance chemotherapy in ES SCLC, the trials involving patients with LS SCLC have not shown a benefit (see Table 24–3). Patients with ES SCLC who had responded to four cycles of EP were randomized to observation versus four cycles of topotecan in an ECOG study.[141] Progression-free survival was significantly better for the patients randomized to topotecan compared with the observation arm (3.4 versus 2.3 mo, P = 0.0001), but there was no difference in overall survival.

TREATMENT OF THE ELDERLY OR PATIENTS WITH POOR PERFORMANCE STATUS

The numbers of patients >65 years of age or with a poor PS who are diagnosed with SCLC are difficult to determine because most cooperative groups exclude these patients from clinical trials. It has been estimated that almost half of all lung cancers diagnosed are in patients >65.[128] Population-based studies have shown that among patients with extensive stage lung cancer (both SCLC and non–small cell lung cancer), 20% are PS 2 and approximately 20% are PS 3,4 (Table 4–2). One population-based study reporting specifically on SCLC found that 23% of patients with ES SCLC had a poor PS (Karnofsky <60), and 52% had weight loss of >10 pounds.[142]

Many physicians believe that the potential toxicities of chemotherapy in the elderly outweigh the potential benefits and that chemotherapy should be withheld from this group of patients.[143,144] Two retrospective studies question this policy. The first is a study by Shepherd et al[145] that retrospectively studied 123 patients with SCLC who were ≥70 years of age. Of these patients, 10% were >80 years of age and 80% had comorbid illnesses. Sixty-three percent of these patients were treated with combination chemotherapy, 16% received radiation therapy alone, and 20% received best supportive care (BSC). The median survival was 1.1

months for those treated with BSC, 7.8 months for those treated with radiation therapy, and up to 11 months for those receiving at least four cycles of chemotherapy. Fifty percent of patients treated with chemotherapy had dose reductions for either myelotoxicity or gastrointestinal toxicity. The median nadir WBC was $2.8 \times 10^9/L$, and eight episodes of febrile neutropenia occurred. Nonhematologic toxicities were mild. Of the patients treated with BSC, 3 had refused treatment and 22 were placed in that arm on the basis of physician decision. Further analysis of those receiving only BSC revealed that PS was the only factor that was different compared with patients who were offered chemotherapy (PS 3,4 in 62% versus 34%, respectively). Given this, it is difficult to assess the true impact of chemotherapy in this population.

The second retrospective study, by Dajczman et al,[146] reviewed 312 patients with SCLC, of whom 81 were ≥70 years of age. Twenty-two percent of the patients >70 years had a poor PS (ECOG PS 3,4) compared with 10% of the patients who were ≤60 years, and more of them had comorbid illnesses (75% versus 48%). Neither the response rates nor the survival was different for younger patients compared with older patients. Of course, these encouraging results in older or poor PS patients treated with chemotherapy cannot be readily extrapolated to all SCLC patients with increased age or poor PS because patient selection undoubtedly played a role in these retrospective studies.

Oral etoposide as a single agent has been used extensively as palliative therapy for elderly patients or patients with a poor PS. However, two randomized studies have found significantly better survival in this patient population for those treated with combination IV chemotherapy compared with oral etoposide. In fact, both of these studies were stopped early when an interim analysis found significant differences in survival. The first study, performed by the Medical Research Council Lung Cancer Working Party,[147] involved 339 patients treated with oral etoposide 50 mg twice daily for 10 days or IV etoposide and vincristine or IV CAV. There was a significant survival advantage for the patients receiving IV chemotherapy (median survival, 6.1 versus 4.3 months, $P = 0.03$). A second study, by Souhami et al,[148] involved 155 patients randomized between oral etoposide 100 mg twice daily for 5 days and alternating CAVE and cisplatin. Survival was better for those receiving IV therapy (median survival, 5.9 versus 4.8 months; 1-year survival, 19% versus 10%; $P = 0.05$). The toxicity was similar in the two groups with the exception of nausea and vomiting, which was more common in patients receiving IV chemotherapy. QOL, as measured by the Rotterdam Symptom Checklist and daily diary card, was the same in the two groups. Based on the results of these two randomized trials, oral etoposide should not be used as a single agent as palliative treatment for patients with SCLC who are elderly or have a poor PS. These studies emphasize that even for elderly or poor PS patients, combination chemotherapy is superior to a single agent.

SECOND-LINE THERAPY

The majority of patients with ES SCLC eventually die of progressive disease. Many of these patients still have a

TABLE 25–8. SECOND-LINE THERAPY IN SMALL CELL LUNG CANCER: SINGLE AGENTS

REFERENCE	n	CHEMOTHERAPY	RESPONSE RATE (%)	MST (mo)
von Pawel et al[150]	107	Topotecan	24	5.8
Ardizzoni et al[149]	45[a]	Topotecan	38[a]	6.9[a]
Ardizzoni et al[149]	47[b]	Topotecan	6[b]	4.7[b]
Einhorn et al[151]	26	Oral etoposide	23	4.2
Johnson et al[152]	22	Oral etoposide	46	3.5
Smit et al[155]	24	Paclitaxel	29	3.2
Smyth et al[157]	34	Docetaxel	20	—
Furuse et al[158]	24	Vinorelbine	13	4.7

Inclusion criteria: Studies of second-line chemotherapy regimens in ≥20 patients with small cell lung cancer.
[a]Sensitive patients who responded to first-line therapy.
[b]Refractory patients who did not respond to first-line therapy.
MST, median survival time; Response rate, partial response + complete response.

good PS and desire further treatment if it will be of benefit. The chance that patients will respond to second-line therapy is highly dependent on whether they responded to first-line therapy and the duration of time between best response and progression. Those who responded to first-line therapy and have had at least a 3-month progression-free interval are the patients most likely to have a meaningful response to second-line therapy. A number of single agents and combinations have been studied in this setting.[27,149–159] Overall response rates range from 6% to 46% for single agents and from 18% to 72% for combinations. The median survival rate after the start of second-line therapy is approximately 4 to 6 months (Tables 25–8 and 25–9).

A recently published randomized phase III study was conducted to compare topotecan and a single agent with CAV as second-line therapy for patients with sensitive disease, based on the same definition used in the earlier study.[150] Patients were randomized to receive either topotecan 1.5 mg/m² as a 30-minute infusion day 1 to 5 every 21 days or cyclophosphamide 1000 mg/m², doxorubicin 45 mg/m² on day 1, and vincristine 2 mg/m² IV on day 1 every 21 days. The overall response rates were similar for patients treated with topotecan versus CAV (24% versus 18%, $P = $ NS), as was the median survival (5.8 versus 5.7 months, $P = $ NS). However, a greater proportion of patients treated with topotecan experienced an improvement

TABLE 25–9. SECOND-LINE THERAPY IN SMALL CELL LUNG CANCER: COMBINATION REGIMENS

REFERENCE	n	CHEMOTHERAPY REGIMEN	RESPONSE RATE (%)	MST (mo)
von Pawel et al[150]	104	CAV	18	5.7
Roth et al[27]	41	CAV	12	4.3
Groen et al[156]	35	CbTx	74	7.2
Roth et al[27]	59	EP	22	5.1
Faylona et al[159]	46	VIP	55	6.7

Inclusion critera: Studies of second-line chemotherapy regimens for small cell lung cancer in ≥20 patients.
MST, median survival time; Response rate, partial responses + complete response.
Chemotherapy abbreviations: A, doxorubicin; C, cyclophosphamide; Cb, carboplatin; E, etoposide; P, cisplatin; Tx, paclitaxel; V, vincristine; VIP, etoposide, ifosfamide, cisplatin.

in disease-related symptoms including dyspnea, anorexia, hoarseness, and fatigue compared with those who received CAV ($P \leq 0.043$). Based on this study, topotecan has recently been approved by the FDA for the treatment of SCLC in the second-line setting.

RADIATION THERAPY

SCLC is a radiosensitive disease, and it is clear that the addition of thoracic radiotherapy improves the survival rate in patients with LS SCLC (Chapter 24). However, randomized studies in the late 1970s and early 1980s found no difference in survival when thoracic radiation was given with curative intent to patients with ES SCLC,[160–163] and thoracic radiation is not recommended as standard initial therapy for these patients. Other small randomized trials looking at the addition of radiation to all sites of disease also failed to show a survival advantage in this group of patients.[164,165]

A recent study by Jeremic et al[166] gives reason to re-examine the role of thoracic radiotherapy in ES SCLC. This study treated 210 patients with three cycles of EP. Patients who had a CR at distant sites and either a partial or complete response at local sites were randomized to receive an additional four cycles of EP versus hyperfractionated accelerated radiation therapy (HART) to the chest (54 Gy in 36 fractions over 18 days) concurrent with daily ECb, followed by two cycles of EP. All patients with a CR at distant sites received PCI. A total of 109 of 210 patients achieved a CR at distant sites with either a CR or PR in the chest and were randomized (55 to HART plus concurrent chemotherapy and 54 to additional chemotherapy alone). Median survival was 17 months for the group randomized to receive HART and concurrent chemotherapy and 11 months for the chemotherapy-alone group. The 5-year survival rates were 9% and 4%, respectively ($P = 0.04$).

There are several possible reasons why this trial was positive, whereas many trials in the past have been negative for the use of thoracic radiation in ES SCLC. First, this trial selected patients who had a CR at distant sites and were most likely to benefit from the addition of radiation therapy, whereas the older trials did not select for responding patients. Second, the radiation was given in a hyperfractionated accelerated fashion, whereas the older studies used less modern radiotherapy techniques. Finally, the chemotherapy used was modern chemotherapy, which can be more easily combined with radiotherapy. Although the results of this study suggest that the addition of thoracic radiotherapy may produce a survival advantage for a very select group of patients with ES SCLC, the small number of patients does not allow firm conclusions to be drawn from this study.

PCI has not been studied extensively in ES SCLC.[167–169] Because the central nervous system is a pharmacologic sanctuary for many diseases, including SCLC, PCI attempts to treat microscopic disease in this area. A recently published meta-analysis found a survival advantage with PCI in patients with SCLC in complete remission.[170] The relative risk of death in the PCI group compared with the control group was 0.84 (95% confidence interval, 0.73 to 0.97; $P = 0.01$). The 3-year survival rate was 21% in the PCI group compared with 15% in the control group. However, of the 987 patients with a CR who were included, only 14% had ES SCLC at the time of diagnosis. The small number of patients with ES SCLC included in this meta-analysis precludes making firm recommendations regarding the routine use of PCI in patients with ES SCLC who achieve a CR.

Radiotherapy is frequently used for palliation of patients with ES SCLC. The most common conditions for which palliative radiotherapy is used in ES SCLC include brain metastasis, spinal cord compression, and painful bone metastasis. Brain metastasis occurs in 25% to 35% of patients with SCLC.[171] The median survival for patients with brain metastasis is 1 to 2 months without treatment and 4 to 6 months with whole brain radiation therapy.[172,173] Spinal cord compression is a medical emergency that should be suspected in patients with a history of ES SCLC who present with back pain. The goal of treatment is to preserve neurologic function; therefore, it is paramount that the diagnosis be made before neurologic deterioration. Only approximately 16% of patients who present with paraplegia are ambulatory after treatment.[174–178] Bone metastases occur frequently in patients with SCLC and are often painful. Radiation to these lesions can provide pain relief in 80% to 90% of patients.[179,180] Palliative treatment for the conditions listed above is discussed in more detail in Chapter 29.

EDITORS' COMMENTS

ES SCLC remains a major challenge to physicians who manage this disease. Chemotherapy has made a major impact in ES SCLC, with the majority of patients experiencing a response and a substantial minority achieving a complete remission. Despite this, the median survival for ES SCLC has reached a plateau of approximately 9 to 11 months, and fewer than 10% of patients survive 2 years from the time of diagnosis. Although more aggressive regimens result in higher response and median survival rates (see Fig. 25–3), they do not offer patients an improved chance of cure. In a disease in which a more dose-intensive approach would seem logical, the results of multiple trials have been disappointing.[181] Clearly, new strategies are needed if substantial improvements in survival are to be realized.

On the basis of activity and toxicity profiles, the standard of care in ES SCLC remains a platinum (cisplatin or carboplatin) in combination with etoposide. As noted in this chapter, several new agents with substantial single-agent activity in SCLC have been developed. Whether they will have an impact in this disease remains to be seen. Based on the historical experience with this disease, we are unlikely to see major improvements as a result of these new agents. Having said that, small benefits that are clinically meaningful may be seen. The two drugs of most interest are paclitaxel and topotecan. Both of these agents are being studied in different capacities. Based on the phase I and II experience with the triplet regimen of cisplatin/etoposide/paclitaxel,[106,108] this regimen is being compared with the standard of cisplatin/etoposide in a randomized phase III fashion in the United States. The Eastern Cooperative Oncology Group has completed a trial in which

DATA SUMMARY: EXTENSIVE STAGE SMALL CELL LUNG CANCER

	AMOUNT	QUALITY	CONSISTENCY
The natural history of untreated ES SCLC is approximately 1 to 2 months	Mod	Mod	Mod
Combination chemotherapy has resulted in a median survival of 7 to 10 months for patients with ES SCLC	High	High	High
Combination chemotherapy improves the quality of life of the majority of patients with ES SCLC	Mod	Mod	High
A poor performance status and elevated LDH are the most important prognostic factors in ES SCLC	High	High	High
EP-based chemotherapy results in response rates and survival similar to those for CAV but with less toxicity	*Mod*	*Mod*	*High*
Dose-intensive regimens have not significantly altered the prognosis for patients with ES SCLC	**High**	**High**	**Mod**
Maintenance chemotherapy offers no benefit to patients with ES SCLC	**Mod**	**Mod**	**Mod**
Second-line chemotherapy can palliate approximately one-fourth of relapsing patients, especially those who were initially sensitive to treatment	High	High	High
Definitive thoracic radiotherapy improves survival in patients with ES SCLC who achieve a CR at distant sites	**Poor**	**Mod**	—

Type of data rated: Plain text: descriptive statement   *Italics: controlled comparison*   **Bold: randomized comparison**

patients with ES SCLC who have responded to cisplatin and etoposide are subsequently randomized to receive topotecan versus observation alone. Both of these studies will help define the role of these two new agents in the management of ES SCLC.

Given the limitations of standard chemotherapy regimens in ES SCLC, it seems logical that a promising avenue of research is to pursue strategies that exploit the biology of SCLC. A number of new classes of agents offer a degree of optimism in the continuing struggle to treat ES SCLC. Combination therapy using the optimal chemotherapy regimen with antiangiogenic agents hold promise for the future. Also, molecular abnormalities in genes such as *p53, Rb,* and *bcl-2* are common in SCLC and should serve as the focus of targeted innovative therapies in ES SCLC. Antisense strategies targeting *bcl-2* in SCLC have shown promising results in vitro[182] and are being tested in vivo. Overexpression of ganglioside antigens has led investigators to study immunotherapeutic strategies in this disease,[183] with very encouraging results. Based on this phase II experience, a multicenter randomized phase III trial of chemotherapy plus or minus a ganglioside-directed vaccine is planned. Active basic and clinical research exploiting the biology of SCLC should be pursued vigorously.

The role of radiotherapy in ES SCLC remains controversial. A limited number of patients with ES SCLC were included in the meta-analysis of PCI that suggested a benefit in survival. Continued study of PCI in ES SCLC is needed to expand the database on which we make therapeutic recommendations in this setting. Likewise, the benefit of radiating a limited number of sites after a complete response in ES SCLC remains unproven. We must continue to study the role of radiation therapy in ES SCLC by designing, implementing, and completing appropriate stud-

ies in well-defined patient populations that address clinically relevant questions.

Whether the approach is with standard chemotherapeutic agents, novel therapeutics, or the incorporation of radiation therapy in new ways, carefully designed trials must be conducted to guide in the continued effort to improve our therapeutic approach to the patient with ES SCLC. This effort requires the commitment of both physicians and patients to the clinical trial process.

References

1. Osterlind K, Ihde DC, Ettinger DS, et al. Staging and prognostic factors in small cell carcinoma of the lung. Cancer Treat Rep. 1983;67:3–9.
2. Aisner J. Extensive-disease small-cell lung cancer: the thrill of victory; the agony of defeat. J Clin Oncol. 1996;14:658–665.
3. Landis SH, Murray T, Bolden S, et al. Cancer statistics, 1999. CA Cancer J Clin. 1999;49:8–31.
4. Campling B, Quirt I, DeBoer G, et al. Is bone marrow examination in small-cell lung cancer really necessary? Ann Intern Med. 1986;105:508–512.
5. Abrams J, Doyle LA, Aisner J. Staging, prognostic factors, and special considerations in small cell lung cancer. Semin Oncol. 1988;15:261–277.
6. De Troyer A, Demanet JC. Clinical, biological and pathogenic features of the syndrome of inappropriate secretion of antidiuretic hormone: a review of 26 cases with marked hyponatraemia. Q J Med. 1976;45:521–531.
7. Sorensen JB, Andersen MK, Hansen HH. Syndrome of inappropriate secretion of antidiuretic hormone (SIADH) in malignant disease [review]. J Intern Med. 1995;238:97–110.
8. List AF, Hainsworth JD, Davis BW, et al. The syndrome of inappropriate secretion of antidiuretic hormone (SIADH) in small-cell lung cancer. J Clin Oncol. 1986;4:1191–1198.
9. Orth DN. Cushing's syndrome. N Engl J Med. 1995;332:791–803.
10. Liddle GW, Nicholson WE, Island DP, et al. Clinical and laboratory

studies of ectopic humoral syndromes. Recent Prog Horm Res. 1969;25:283–314.

11. Orth DN. Ectopic hormone production. In: Felig P, Baxter JD, Broadus AE, et al, eds. Endocrinology and Metabolism. 2nd ed. New York, NY: McGraw-Hill; 1987:1692–1735.

12. Shepherd FA, Laskey J, Evans WK, et al. Cushing's syndrome associated with ectopic corticotropin production and small-cell lung cancer. J Clin Oncol. 1992;10:21–27.

13. Collichio FA, Woolf PD, Brower M. Management of patients with small cell carcinoma and the syndrome of ectopic corticotropin secretion. Cancer. 1994;73:1361–1367.

14. Dimopoulos MA, Fernandez JF, Samaan NA, et al. Paraneoplastic Cushing's syndrome as an adverse prognostic factor in patients who die early with small cell lung cancer. Cancer. 1992;69:66–71.

15. McEvoy K, Windebank A, Daube J, et al. 3,4-Diaminopyridine in the treatment of Lambert-Eaton myasthenic syndrome. N Engl J Med. 1998;321:1567–1571.

16. McEvoy K. Diagnosis and treatment of Lambert-Eaton myasthenic syndrome. Neurol Clin. 1994;12:387–399.

17. Elrington GM, Murray NM, Spiro SG, et al. Neurological paraneoplastic syndromes in patients with small cell lung cancer. A prospective survey of 150 patients. J Neurol Neurosurg Psychiatry. 1991;54:764–767.

18. Kimura J. Electrodiagnosis in Diseases of Nerve and Muscle: Principles and Practice. Philadelphia; PA: FA Davis; 1983:193.

19. Chalk CH, Murray NM, Newsom-Davis J, et al. Response of the Lambert-Eaton myasthenic syndrome to treatment of associated small-cell lung carcinoma. Neurology. 1990;40:1552–1556.

20. Bakheit AM, Kennedy PG, Behan PO. Paraneoplastic limbic encephalitis: clinicopathological correlations. J Neurol Neurosurg Psychiatry. 1990;53:1084–1088.

21. Alamowitch S, Graus F, Uchuya M, et al. Limbic encephalitis and small cell lung cancer: clinical and immunological features. Brain. 1997;120:923–928.

22. Lucchinetti CF, Kimmel DW, Lennon VA. Paraneoplastic and oncologic profiles of patients seropositive for type 1 antineuronal nuclear autoantibodies. Neurology. 1998;50:652–657.

23. Zelen M. Panel report: Interdisciplinary Group on Clinical Trials. Cancer Chemother Rep. 1973;4(pt3):317–319.

24. Green RA, Humphrey E, Close H, et al. Alkylating agents in bronchogenic carcinoma. Am J Med. 1969;46:516–525.

25. Chute JP, Chen T, Feigal E, et al. Twenty years of phase III trials for patients with extensive-stage small-cell lung cancer: perceptible progress. J Clin Oncol. 1999;17:1794–1801.

26. Postmus PE, Scagliotti G, Groen HJ, et al. Standard versus alternating non–cross-resistant chemotherapy in extensive small cell lung cancer: an EORTC phase III trial. Eur J Cancer. 1996;32A:1498–1503.

27. Roth BJ, Johnson DH, Einhorn LH, et al. Randomized study of cyclophosphamide, doxorubicin, and vincristine versus etoposide and cisplatin versus alternation of these two regimens in extensive small-cell lung cancer: a phase III trial of the Southeastern Cancer Study Group. J Clin Oncol. 1992;10:282–291.

28. Johnson DH, Einhorn LH, Birch R, et al. A randomized comparison of high-dose versus conventional-dose cyclophosphamide, doxorubicin, and vincristine for extensive-stage small-cell lung cancer: a phase III trial of the Southeastern Cancer Study Group. J Clin Oncol. 1987;5:1731–1738.

29. Sagman U, Maki E, Evans WK, et al. Small-cell carcinoma of the lung: derivation of a prognostic staging system. J Clin Oncol. 1991;9:1639–1649.

30. Vincent MD, Ashley SE, Smith IE. Prognostic factors in small cell lung cancer: a simple prognostic index is better than conventional staging. Eur J Cancer Clin Oncol. 1987;23:1589–1599.

31. Cullen M, Morgan D, Gregory W, et al. Maintenance chemotherapy for anaplastic small cell carcinoma of the bronchus: a randomized, controlled trial. Cancer Chemother Pharmacol. 1986;17:157–160.

32. Furuse K, Fukuoka M, Nishiwaki Y, et al. Phase III study of intensive weekly chemotherapy with recombinant human granulocyte colony-stimulating factor versus standard chemotherapy in extensive-disease small-cell lung cancer. The Japan Clinical Oncology Group. J Clin Oncol. 1998;16:2126–2132.

33. Souhami RL, Rudd R, Ruiz de Elvira MC, et al. Randomized trial comparing weekly versus 3-week chemotherapy in small-cell lung cancer: a Cancer Research Campaign trial. J Clin Oncol. 1994;12:1806–1813.

34. Bleehen NM, Girling DJ, Machin D, et al. A randomised trial of three or six courses of etoposide cyclophosphamide methotrexate and vincristine or six courses of etoposide and ifosfamide in small cell lung cancer (SCLC), II: quality of life. Medical Research Council Lung Cancer Working Party. Br J Cancer. 1993;68:1157–1166.

35. Bernhard J, Hurny C, Bacchi M, et al. Initial prognostic factors in small-cell lung cancer patients predicting quality of life during chemotherapy. Swiss Group for Clinical Cancer Research (SAKK). Br J Cancer. 1996;74:1660–1667.

36. Janssen-Heijnen MLG, Schipper RM, Klinkhamer PJJM, et al. Improvement and plateau in survival of small-cell lung cancer since 1975: a population-based study. Ann Oncol. 1998;9:543–547.

37. Dearing MP, Steinberg SM, Phelps R, et al. Outcome of patients with small-cell lung cancer: effect of changes in staging procedures and imaging technology on prognostic factors over 14 years. J Clin Oncol. 1990;8:1042–1049.

38. Sagman U, Feld R, Evans WK, et al. The prognostic significance of pretreatment serum lactate dehydrogenase in patients with small-cell lung cancer. J Clin Oncol. 1991;9:954–961.

39. Albain KS, Crowley JJ, LeBlanc M, et al. Determinants of improved outcome in small-cell lung cancer: an analysis of the 2,580-patient Southwest Oncology Group data base. J Clin Oncol. 1990;8:1563–1574.

40. Rawson NS, Peto J. An overview of prognostic factors in small cell lung cancer: a report from the Subcommittee for the Management of Lung Cancer of the United Kingdom Coordination Committee on Cancer Research. Br J Cancer. 1990;61:597–604.

41. Spiegelman D, Maurer LH, Ware JH, et al. Prognostic factors in small-cell carcinoma of the lung: an analysis of 1,521 patients. J Clin Oncol. 1989;7:344–354.

42. Osterlind K, Andersen PK. Prognostic factors in small cell lung cancer: multivariate model based on 778 patients treated with chemotherapy with or without irradiation. Cancer Res. 1986;46:4189–4194.

43. Souhami RL, Bradbury I, Geddes DM, et al. Prognostic significance of laboratory parameters measured at diagnosis in small cell carcinoma of the lung. Cancer Res. 1985;45:2878–2882.

44. Grant SC, Gralla RJ, Kris MG, et al. Single-agent chemotherapy trials in small-cell lung cancer, 1970 to 1990: the case for studies in previously treated patients. J Clin Oncol. 1992;10:484–498.

45. Ettinger DS. The place of ifosfamide in chemotherapy of small cell lung cancer: the Eastern Cooperative Oncology Group experience and a selected literature update. Semin Oncol. 1995;22(suppl 2):23–27.

46. Lowenbraun S, Bartolucci A, Smalley R, et al. The superiority of combination chemotherapy over single agent chemotherapy in small cell lung carcinoma. Cancer. 1979;44:406–413.

47. Hong WK, Nicaise C, Lawson R, et al. Etoposide combined with cyclophosphamide plus vincristine compared with doxorubicin plus cyclophosphamide plus vincristine and with high-dose cyclophosphamide plus vincristine in the treatment of small-cell carcinoma of the lung: a randomized trial of the Bristol Lung Cancer Study Group. J Clin Oncol. 1989;7:450–456.

48. Evans WK, Feld R, Murray N, et al. Superiority of alternating non–cross-resistant chemotherapy in extensive small cell lung cancer: a multicenter, randomized clinical trial by the National Cancer Institute of Canada. Ann Intern Med. 1987;107:451–458.

49. Ettinger DS, Finkelstein DM, Abeloff MD, et al. A randomized comparison of standard chemotherapy versus alternating chemotherapy and maintenance versus no maintenance therapy for extensive-stage small-cell lung cancer: a phase III study of the Eastern Cooperative Oncology Group. J Clin Oncol. 1990;8:230–240.

50. Livingston RB, Schulman S, Mira JG, et al. Combined alkylators and multiple-site irradiation for extensive small cell lung cancer: a Southwest Oncology Group Study. Cancer Treat Rep. 1986;70:1395–1401.

51. Ettinger DS, Finkelstein DM, Abeloff MD, et al. Justification for evaluating new anticancer drugs in selected untreated patients with extensive-stage small-cell lung cancer: an Eastern Cooperative Oncology Group randomized study [see comments]. J Natl Cancer Inst. 1992;84:1077–1084.

52. Messeih AA, Schweitzer JM, Lipton A, et al. Addition of etoposide to cyclophosphamide, doxorubicin, and vincristine for remission induction and survival in patients with small cell lung cancer. Cancer Treat Rep. 1987;71:61–66.

53. Jackson DV Jr, Case LD, Zekan PJ, et al. Improvement of long-term survival in extensive small-cell lung cancer. J Clin Oncol. 1988;6:1161–1169.

54. Aisner J, Whitacre M, Abrams J, et al. Doxorubicin, cyclophosphamide, etoposide and platinum, doxorubicin, cyclophosphamide and etoposide for small-cell carcinoma of the lung. Semin Oncol. 1986;13:54–62.

55. Bhuchar VK, Lanzotti VJ. High-dose cisplatin for lung cancer. Cancer Treat Rep. 1982;66:375–376.

56. Rossof AH, Bearden JD, Coltman CA Jr. Phase II evaluation of cis-diamminedichloroplatinum (II) in lung cancer. Cancer Treat Rep. 1976;60:1679–1680.

57. Levenson RM Jr, Ihde DC, Huberman MS, et al. Phase II trial of cisplatin in small cell carcinoma of the lung. Cancer Treat Rep. 1981;65:905–907.

58. Dombernowsky P, Sorenson S, Aisner J, et al. cis-Dichlorodiammineplatinum (II) in small cell anaplastic bronchogenic carcinoma: a phase II study. Cancer Treat Rep. 1979;63:543–545.

59. De Jager R, Longeval E, Klastersky J. High-dose cisplatin with fluid and mannitol-induced diuresis in advanced lung cancer: a phase II clinical trial of the EORTC Lung Cancer Working Party (Belgium). Cancer Treat Rep. 1980;64:1341–1346.

60. Cavalli F, Goldhirsch A, Siegenthaler P, et al. Phase-II study with cis-dichlorodiammineplatinum (II) in small cell anaplastic bronchogenic carcinoma. Eur J Cancer. 1980;16:617–621.

61. Tucker RD, Ferguson A, Van Wyk C, et al. Chemotherapy of small cell carcinoma of the lung with V.P. 16–213. Cancer. 1978;41:1710–1714.

62. Tempero M, Kessinger A, Lemon HM. VP-16–213 therapy in patients with small-cell carcinoma of the lung after failure on combination chemotherapy. Cancer Clin Trials. 1981;4:155–157.

63. Hansen M, Hirsch F, Dombernowsky P, et al. Treatment of small cell anaplastic carcinoma of the lung with the oral solution of VP-16–213 (NSC 141540, 4′-demethylepipodophyllotoxin 9-(4,6-O-ethylidene-beta-D-glucopyranoside). Cancer. 1977;40:633–637.

64. Falkson G, van Dyk JJ, van Eden EB, et al. A clinical trial of the oral form of 4′-demethyl-epipodophyllotoxin-beta-D ethylidene glucoside (NSC 141540) VP 16–213. Cancer. 1975;35:1141–1144.

65. Cohen MH, Broder LE, Fossieck BE, et al. Phase II clinical trial of weekly administration of VP-16–213 in small cell bronchogenic carcinoma. Cancer Treat Rep. 1977;61:489–490.

66. Schabel FM Jr., Trader MW, Laster WR Jr, et al. cis-Dichlorodiammineplatinum (II): combination chemotherapy and cross-resistance studies with tumors of mice. Cancer Treat Rep. 1979;63:1459–1473.

67. Evans W, Shepherd F, Feld R, et al. VP-16 and cisplatin as first-line therapy for small-cell lung cancer. J Clin Oncol. 1985;3:1471–1477.

68. Boni C, Cocconi G, Bisagni G, et al. Cisplatin and etoposide (VP-16) as a single regimen for small cell lung cancer. Cancer. 1989;63:638–642.

69. Loehrer PJ Sr, Ansari R, Gonin R, et al. Cisplatin plus etoposide with and without ifosfamide in extensive small-cell lung cancer: a Hoosier Oncology Group study. J Clin Oncol. 1995;13:2594–2599.

70. Rowland KM Jr, Loprinzi CL, Shaw EG, et al. Randomized double-blind placebo-controlled trial of cisplatin and etoposide plus megestrol acetate/placebo in extensive-stage small-cell lung cancer: a North Central Cancer Treatment Group study. J Clin Oncol. 1996;14:135–141.

71. Fukuoka M, Furuse K, Saijo N, et al. Randomized trial of cyclophosphamide, doxorubicin and vincristine versus cisplatin and etoposide versus alternation of these regimens in small-cell lung cancer. J Natl Cancer Inst. 1991;83:855–861.

72. Go RS, Adjei AA. Review of the comparative pharmacology and clinical activity of cisplatin and carboplatin. J Clin Oncol. 1999;17:409–422.

73. Canetta R, Rozencweig M, Carter S. Carboplatin: the clinical spectrum to date. Cancer Treat Rev. 1985;12:125–136.

74. Rozencweig M, Nicaise C, Beer M, et al. Phase I study of carboplatin given on a five-day intravenous schedule. J Clin Oncol. 1983;1:621–626.

75. Kramer B, Birch R, Greco A, et al. Randomized phase II evaluation of iproplatin (CHIP) and carboplatin (CBDCA) in lung cancer. a Southeastern Cancer Study Group trial. Am J Clin Oncol. 1988;11:643–645.

76. Jacobs R, Bitran J, Deutsch M, et al. Phase II study of carboplatin in previously treated patients with metastatic small cell lung carcinoma. Cancer Treat Rep. 1987;71:311–312.

77. Tamura T, Saijo N, Shinkai T, et al. Phase II study of carboplatin in small cell lung cancer. Jpn J Clin Oncol. 1988;18:27–32.

78. Dimitrovsky E, Seifter E, Gazdar A, et al. A phase II study of carboplatin (CBDCA) in small-cell and non–small cell lung cancer: correlation to in vitro analysis of cytotoxicity. Am J Clin Oncol. 1990;13:285–289.

79. Smith I, Harland S, Robinson B, et al. Carboplatin: a very active new cisplatin analog in the treatment of small cell lung cancer. Cancer Treat Rep. 1985;69:43–46.

80. Tjulandin SA, Garin AM, Mescheryakov AA, et al. Cisplatin-etoposide and carboplatin-etoposide induction chemotherapy for good-risk patients with germ cell tumors. Ann Oncol. 1993;4:663–667.

81. Bajorin DF, Sarosdy MF, Pfister DG, et al. Randomized trial of etoposide and cisplatin versus etoposide and carboplatin in patients with good-risk germ cell tumors: a multiinstitutional study [see comments]. J Clin Oncol. 1993;11:598–606.

82. Bokemeyer C, Kohrmann O, Tischler J, et al. A randomized trial of cisplatin, etoposide and bleomycin (PEB) versus carboplatin, etoposide and bleomycin (CEB) for patients with "good-risk" metastatic non–seminomatous germ cell tumors. Ann Oncol. 1996;7:1015–1021.

83. Horwich A, Sleijfer DT, Fossa SD, et al. Randomized trial of bleomycin, etoposide, and cisplatin compared with bleomycin, etoposide, and carboplatin in good-prognosis metastatic nonseminomatous germ cell cancer: a Multiinstitutional Medical Research Council/European Organization for Research and Treatment of Cancer Trial. J Clin Oncol. 1997;15:1844–1852.

84. Skarlos DV, Samantas E, Kosmidis P, et al. Randomized comparison of etoposide-cisplatin vs. etoposide-carboplatin and irradiation in small-cell lung cancer: a Hellenic Co-Operative Oncology Group study. Ann Oncol. 1994;5:601–607.

85. Lassen U, Kristjansen PE, Osterlind K, et al. Superiority of cisplatin or carboplatin in combination with teniposide and vincristine in the induction chemotherapy of small-cell lung cancer: a randomized trial with 5 years follow up. Ann Oncol. 1996;7:365–371.

86. Bunn P, Canetta R, Ozols R, et al, eds. Carboplatin (JM-8): Current Perspectives and Future Directions. Philadelphia, PA: WB Saunders; 1990.

87. Morgan LR, Posey LE, Rainey J, et al. Ifosfamide: a weekly dose fractionated schedule in bronchogenic carcinoma. Cancer Treat Rep. 1981;65:693–695.

88. Loehrer PJ Sr, Birch R, Kramer BS, et al. Ifosfamide plus N-acetylcysteine in the treatment of small cell and non–small cell carcinoma of the lung: a Southeastern Cancer Study Group Trial. Cancer Treat Rep. 1986;70:919–920.

89. Cantwell BM, Bozzino JM, Corris P, et al. The multidrug resistant phenotype in clinical practice; evaluation of cross resistance to ifosfamide and mesna after VP16–213, doxorubicin and vincristine (VPAV) for small cell lung cancer. Eur J Cancer Clin Oncol. 1988;24:123–129.

90. Wolf M, Havemann K, Holle R, et al. Cisplatin/etoposide versus ifosfamide/etoposide combination chemotherapy in small-cell lung cancer: a multicenter German randomized trial. J Clin Oncol. 1987;5:1880–1889.

91. Wolff AC, Ettinger DS, Neuberg D, et al. Phase II study of ifosfamide, carboplatin, and oral etoposide chemotherapy for extensive-disease small-cell lung cancer: an Eastern Cooperative Oncology Group pilot study. J Clin Oncol. 1995;13:1615–1622.

92. Thatcher N, Lind M, Stout R, et al. Carboplatin, ifosfamide, and etoposide with mid-course vincristine and thoracic radiotherapy for "limited" stage small cell carcinoma of the bronchus. Br J Cancer. 1989;60:98–101.

93. Smith IE, Perren TJ, Ashley SA, et al. Carboplatin, etoposide, and ifosfamide as intensive chemotherapy for small-cell lung cancer. J Clin Oncol. 1990;8:899–905.

94. Evans WK, Stewart DJ, Shepherd FA, et al. VP-16, ifosfamide and cisplatin (VIP) for extensive small cell lung cancer. Eur J Cancer. 1994;30A:299–303.

95. Loehrer PJ, Rynard S, Ansari R, et al. Etoposide, ifosfamide, and cisplatin in extensive small cell lung cancer. Cancer. 1992;69:669–673.

96. Munoz MA, Arrivi A, Guaraz R, et al. VP-16, ifosfamide and cisplatin (VIP) as treatment of small cell lung cancer: a preliminary report. Proceedings of the Fourth European Conference on Clinical Oncology and Cancer Nursing, Madrid, Spain, November 1987. London, England, Medical Tribune Group, 1988.

97. Carney DM, Grogan L. Phase II study of VP-16, ifosfamide and cisplatin (VIP) in small cell and non–small cell lung cancer [abstract]. Proc ASCO. 1990;9:244.

98. Kingsbury W, Boehm J, Jakas D, et al. Synthesis of water-soluble (aminoalkyl) camptothecin analogues: inhibition of topoisomerase I and antitumor activity. J Med Chem. 1991;34:98–107.

99. Schiller JH, Kim K, Hutson P, et al. Phase II study of topotecan in patients with extensive-stage small-cell carcinoma of the lung: an Eastern Cooperative Oncology Group Trial. J Clin Oncol. 1996;14:2345–2352.

100. Jett J, Day R, Levitt M, et al. Topotecan and paclitaxel in extensive stage small cell lung cancer (ED-SCLC) patients without prior therapy [abstract]. Lung Cancer. 1997;18:13a.

101. Rowinsky EK, Cazenave LA, Donehower RC. Taxol: a novel investigational antimicrotubule agent. J Natl Cancer Inst. 1990;82:1247–1259.

102. Ettinger D, Finkelstein D, Sarma R, et al. Phase II study of paclitaxel in patients with extensive disease small cell lung cancer: an Eastern Cooperative Oncology Group study. J Clin Oncol. 1995;13:1430–1435.

103. Kirschling RJ, Grill JP, Marks RS, et al. Paclitaxel and G-CSF in previously untreated patients with extensive stage small-cell lung cancer: a phase II study of the North Central Cancer Treatment Group. Am J Clin Oncol. 1999;22:517–522.

104. Hainsworth JD, Gray JR, Stroup SL, et al. Paclitaxel, carboplatin, and extended-schedule etoposide in the treatment of small-cell lung cancer: comparison of sequential phase II trials using different dose-intensities. J Clin Oncol. 1997;15:3464–3470.

105. Levitan N, McKenney J, Tahsildar H, et al. Results of a phase I dose escalation trial of paclitaxel, etoposide, and cisplatin followed by filgrastim in the treatment of patients with extensive stage small cell lung cancer [abstract]. Proc ASCO. 1995;14:379.

106. Kelly K, Wood ME, Bunn PA. A phase I study of cisplatin, etoposide and paclitaxel in extensive stage small cell lung cancer [abstract]. Proc ASCO. 1996;15:400.

107. Hainsworth JD, Niell HB. Taxol (paclitaxel) injection, carboplatin, and etoposide in the management of small cell lung cancer: clinical update. Princeton, NJ: Squibb; 1999.

108. Glisson BS, Kurie JM, Perez-Solar R, et al. Cisplatin, etoposide, and paclitaxel in the treatment of patients with extensive small-cell lung carcinoma. J Clin Oncol. 1999;17:2309–2315.

109. Abbruzzese JL, Grunewald R, Weeks EA, et al. A phase I clinical, plasma, and cellular pharmacology study of gemcitabine. J Clin Oncol. 1991;9:491–498.

110. Cormier Y, Eisenhauer E, Muldal A, et al. Gemcitabine is an active new agent in previously untreated extensive small cell lung cancer (SCLC): a study of the National Cancer Institute of Canada Clinical Trials Group. Ann Oncol. 1994;5:283–285.

111. Bore P, Rahmani R, van Cantfort J, et al. Pharmacokinetics of a new anticancer drug, Navelbine, in patients: comparative study of radioimmunologic and radioactive determination methods. Cancer Chemother Pharmacol. 1989;23:247–251.

112. Higano CS, Crowley JJ, Veith RV, et al. A phase II trial of intravenous vinorelbine in previously untreated patients with extensive small cell lung cancer: a Southwest Oncology Group study. Invest New Drugs. 1997;15:153–156.

113. Frei ED. Antitumor agents—dose response curve: clinical and experimental considerations. Exp Hematol. 1979;7(suppl 5):262–264.

114. Frei ED, Canellos GP. Dose: a critical factor in cancer chemotherapy. Am J Med. 1980;69:585–594.

115. Frei ED. Dose response for adjuvant chemotherapy of breast cancer: experimental and clinical considerations. Recent Results Cancer Res. 1989;115:25–27.

116. Klasa RJ, Murray N, Coldman AJ. Dose-intensity meta-analysis of chemotherapy regimens in small-cell carcinoma of the lung. J Clin Oncol. 1991;9:499–508.

117. Ihde DC, Mulshine JL, Kramer BS, et al. Prospective randomized comparison of high-dose and standard-dose etoposide and cisplatin chemotherapy in patients with extensive-stage small-cell lung cancer. J Clin Oncol. 1994;12:2022–2034.

118. Figueredo AT, Hryniuk WM, Strautmanis I, et al. Co-trimoxazole prophylaxis during high-dose chemotherapy of small-cell lung cancer. J Clin Oncol. 1985;3:54–64.

119. Hande KR, Oldham RK, Fer MF, et al. Randomized study of high-dose versus low-dose methotrexate in the treatment of extensive small cell lung cancer. Am J Med. 1982;73:413–419.

120. Murray N, Livingston RB, Shepherd FA, et al. Randomized study of CODE versus alternating CAV/EP for extensive-stage small-cell lung cancer: an intergroup study of the National Cancer Institute of Canada Clinical Trials Group and the Southwest Oncology Group. J Clin Oncol. 1999;17:2300–2308.

121. Pujol J-L, Douillard J-Y, Riviere A, et al. Dose-intensity of a four-drug chemotherapy regimen with or without recombinant human granulocyte-macrophage colony-stimulating factor in extensive-stage small-cell lung cancer: a multicenter randomized phase III study. J Clin Oncol. 1997;15:2082–2089.

122. Miles DW, Fogarty O, Ash CM, et al. Received dose-intensity: a randomized trial of weekly chemotherapy with and without granulocyte colony-stimulating factor in small-cell lung cancer. J Clin Oncol. 1994;12:77–82.

123. Woll PJ, Hodgetts J, Lomax L, et al. Can cytotoxic dose-intensity be increased by using granulocyte colony-stimulating factor? A randomized controlled trial of lenograstim in small-cell lung cancer. J Clin Oncol. 1995;13:652–659.

124. Steward WP, von Pawel J, Gatzemeier U, et al. Effects of granulocyte-macrophage colony-stimulating factor and dose intensification of V-ICE chemotherapy in small-cell lung cancer: a prospective randomized study of 300 patients. J Clin Oncol. 1998;16:642–650.

125. Humblet Y, Symann M, Bosly A, et al. Late intensification chemotherapy with autologous bone marrow transplantation in selected small-cell carcinoma of the lung: a randomized study. J Clin Oncol. 1987;5:1864–1873.

126. Pettengell R, Woll PJ, Thatcher N, et al. Multicyclic, dose-intensive chemotherapy supported by sequential reinfusion of hematopoietic progenitors in whole blood. J Clin Oncol. 1995;13:148–156.

127. Stewart P, Buckner CD, Thomas ED, et al. Intensive chemoradiotherapy with autologous marrow transplantation for small cell carcinoma of the lung. Cancer Treat Rep. 1983;67:1055–1059.

128. O'Rourke M, Crawford J. Lung cancer in the elderly. Clin Geriatr Med. 1987;3:595–623.

129. Clamon GH, Audeh MW, Pinnick S. Small cell lung carcinoma in the elderly. J Am Geriatr Soc. 1982;30:299–302.

130. Maurer L, Tulloh M, Weiss R, et al. A randomized combined modality trial in small cell carcinoma of the lung. Cancer. 1979;45:30–39.

131. Einhorn L, Crawford J, Birch R, et al. Cisplatin plus etoposide consolidation following cyclophosphamide, doxorubicin and vincristine in limited small-cell lung cancer. J Clin Oncol. 1988;6:451–456.

132. Johnson DH, Bass D, Einhorn LH, et al. Combination chemotherapy with or without thoracic radiotherapy in limited-stage small-cell lung cancer: a randomized trial of the Southeastern Cancer Study Group [see comments]. J Clin Oncol. 1993;11:1223–1229.

133. Bleehen N, Fayers P, Girling D, et al. Controlled trial of twelve versus six courses of chemotherapy in the treatment of small-cell lung cancer. Br J Cancer. 1989;59:584–590.

134. Spiro S, Souhami R, Geddes D, et al. Duration of chemotherapy in small cell lung cancer: a Cancer Research Campaign trial. Br J Cancer. 1989;59:578–583.

135. Byrne M, van Hazel G, Trotter J, et al. Maintenance chemotherapy in limited small cell lung cancer: a randomized controlled clinical trial. Br J Cancer. 1989;60:413–418.

136. Mattson K, Niiranen A, Pyrhonen S, et al. Natural interferon alfa as maintenance therapy for small cell lung cancer. Eur J Cancer. 1992;28A:1387–1391.

137. Lebeau B, Chastang C, Allard P, et al. Six vs twelve cycles for complete responders to chemotherapy in small cell lung cancer: definitive results of a randomized trial. Eur Respir J. 1992;5:286–290.

138. Giaccone G, Dalesio O, McVie G, et al. Maintenance chemotherapy in small-cell lung cancer: long-term results of a randomized trial. J Clin Oncol. 1993;11:1230–1240.

139. Bleehen NM, Girling DJ, Machin D, et al. A randomised trial of three or six courses of etoposide cyclophosphamide methotrexate and vincristine or six courses of etoposide and ifosfamide in small cell lung cancer (SCLC), I: survival and prognostic factors. Medical Research Council Working Party. Br J Cancer. 1993;68:1150–1156.

140. Beith J, Clarke S, Woods R, et al. Long-term follow-up of a randomized trial of combined chemoradiotherapy induction treatment, with and without maintenance chemotherapy in patients with small cell carcinoma of the lung. Eur J Cancer. 1996;32A:438–443.

141. Johnson DH, Adak S, Cella DF, et al: Topotecan (T) vs. observation

(OB) following cisplatin (P) plus etoposide (E) in extensive-stage small cell lung cancer (ES SCLC) (E7593): a phase III trial of the Eastern Cooperative Oncology Group (ECOG) [abstract]. Proc Am Soc Clin Oncol. 2000;19:482a.

142. Chute CG, Greenberg ER, Baron J, et al. Presenting conditions of 1539 population-based lung cancer patients by cell type and stage in New Hampshire and Vermont. Cancer. 1985;56:2107–2111.

143. Samet J, Hunt W, Key C, et al. Choice of cancer therapy varies with age of patient. JAMA. 1986;255:3385–3390.

144. Godwin J, Hunt W, Humble C, et al. Cancer treatment protocols: who gets chosen? Arch Intern Med. 1988;148:2258–2260.

145. Shepherd FA, Amdemichael E, Evans WK, et al. Treatment of small cell lung cancer in the elderly. J Am Geriatr Soc. 1994;42:64–70.

146. Dajczman E, Fu L, Small D, et al. Treatment of small cell lung carcinoma in the elderly. Cancer. 1996;77:2032–2038.

147. Medical Research Council Lung Cancer Working Party. Comparison of oral etoposide and standard intravenous multidrug chemotherapy for small-cell lung cancer: a stopped multicentre randomized trial. Lancet. 1996;348:563–566.

148. Souhami RL, Spiro SG, Rudd RM, et al. Five-day oral etoposide treatment for advanced small-cell lung cancer: randomized comparison with intravenous chemotherapy. J Natl Cancer Inst. 1997;89:577–580.

149. Ardizzoni A, Hansen H, Dombernowsky P, et al. Topotecan, a new active drug in the second-line treatment of small-cell lung cancer: a phase II study in patients with refractory and sensitive disease. J Clin Oncol. 1997;15:2090–2096.

150. von Pawel J, Schiller JH, Shepherd FA, et al. Topotecan versus cyclophosphamide, doxorubicin, and vincristine for the treatment of recurrent small-cell lung cancer. J Clin Oncol. 1999;17:658–667.

151. Einhorn LH, Pennington K, McClean J. Phase II trial of daily oral VP-16 in refractory small cell lung cancer: a Hoosier Oncology Group study. Semin Oncol. 1990;17:32–35.

152. Johnson DH, Greco FA, Strupp J, et al. Prolonged administration of oral etoposide in patients with relapsed or refractory small-cell lung cancer: a phase II trial. J Clin Oncol. 1990;8:1613–1617.

153. Hsiang Y-H, Liu LF, Wall ME, et al. DNA topoisomerase I-mediated DNA cleavage and cytotoxicity of camptothecin analogues. Cancer Res. 1989;49:4385–4389.

154. Masuda N, Fukuoka M, Kusunoki Y, et al. CPT-11: a new derivative of camptothecin for the treatment of refractory or relapsed small-cell lung cancer. J Clin Oncol. 1992;10:1225–1229.

155. Smit EF, Fokkema E, Biesma B, et al. A phase II study of paclitaxel in heavily pretreated patients with small-cell lung cancer. Br J Cancer. 1998;77:347–351.

156. Groen HJM, Fokkema E, Biesma B, et al. Paclitaxel and carboplatin in the treatment of small-cell lung cancer patients resistant to cyclophosphamide, doxorubicin, and etoposide: a non–cross-resistant schedule. J Clin Oncol. 1999;17:927–932.

157. Smyth JF, Smith IE, Sessa C, et al. Activity of docetaxel (Taxotere) in small cell lung cancer. The Early Clinical Trials Group of the EORTC. Eur J Cancer. 1994;30A:1058–1060.

158. Furuse K, Kubota K, Kawahara M, et al. Phase II study of vinorelbine in heavily previously treated small cell lung cancer. Japan Lung Cancer Vinorelbine Study Group. Oncology. 1996;53:169–172.

159. Faylona EA, Loehrer PJ, Ansari R, et al. Phase II study of daily oral etoposide plus ifosfamide plus cisplatin for previously treated recurrent small-cell lung cancer: a Hoosier Oncology Group trial. J Clin Oncol. 1995;13:1209–1214.

160. Williams C, Alexander M, Glatstein EJ, et al. Role of radiation therapy in combination with chemotherapy in extensive oat cell cancer of the lung: a randomized study. Cancer Treat Rep. 1977;61:1427–1431.

161. Chahinian AP, Comis RL, Maurer LH, et al. Small cell anaplastic carcinoma of the lung: the Cancer and Leukemia Group B experience. Bull Cancer. 1982;69:79–82.

162. Mira JG, Livingston RB, Moore TN, et al. Influence of chest radiotherapy in frequency and patterns of chest relapse in disseminated small cell lung carcinoma. A Southwest Oncology Group study. Cancer. 1982;50:1266–1272.

163. Livingston RB, Moore TN, Heilbrun L, et al. Small-cell carcinoma

of the lung: combined chemotherapy and radiation: a Southwest Oncology Group study. Ann Intern Med. 1978;88:194–199.

164. Alexander M, Glatstein EJ, Gordon DS, et al. Combined modality treatment for oat cell carcinoma of the lung: a randomized trial 1,2,3. Cancer Treat Rep. 1977;61:1–6.

165. Wilson HE, Stanley K, Vincent RG, et al. Comparison of chemotherapy alone versus chemotherapy and radiation therapy of extensive small cell carcinoma of the lung. J Surg Oncol. 1983;23:181–184.

166. Jeremic B, Shibamoto Y, Nikolic N, et al. Role of radiation therapy in the combined-modality treatment of patients with extensive disease small-cell lung cancer: a randomized study [abstract]. J Clin Oncol. 1999;17:2092.

167. Jackson D, Richards F, Cooper M, et al. Prophylactic cranial irradiation in small cell carcinoma of the lung. JAMA. 1977;237:2730–2733.

168. Hansen H, Dombernowsky P, Hirsch F. Prophylactic irradiation in bronchogenic small cell anaplastic carcinoma: a comparative trial of localized versus extensive radiotherapy including prophylactic irradiation in patients receiving combination chemotherapy. Cancer. 1980;46:279–284.

169. Beiler D, Kane R, Bernath A, et al. Low dose elective brain irradiation in small cell carcinoma of the lung. Int J Radiat Oncol Biol Phys. 1979;5:944–945.

170. Auperin A, Arriagada R, Pignon JP, et al. Prophylactic cranial irradiation for patients with small-cell lung cancer in complete remission: Prophylactic Cranial Irradiation Overview Collaborative Group [see comments]. N Engl J Med. 1999;341:476–484.

171. Nugent JL, Bunn PA Jr, Matthews MJ, et al. CNS metastases in small cell bronchogenic carcinoma: increasing frequency and changing pattern with lengthening survival. Cancer. 1979;44:1885–1893.

172. Veslemes M, Polyzos A, Latsi P, et al. Outcome of patients with brain metastases after combined modality therapy in small cell lung cancer (SCLC): a retrospective study. J Chemother. 1995;7:460–462.

173. Nussbaum ES, Djalilian HR, Cho KH, et al. Brain metastases. Histology, multiplicity, surgery, and survival. Cancer. 1996;78:1781–1788.

174. Findlay GF. Adverse effects of the management of malignant spinal cord compression. J Neurol Neurosurg Psychiatry. 1984;47:761–768.

175. Findlay GF. The role of vertebral body collapse in the management of malignant spinal cord compression. J Neurol Neurosurg Psychiatry. 1987;50:151–154.

176. Leviov M, Dale J, Stein M, et al. The management of metastatic spinal cord compression: a radiotherapeutic success ceiling. Int J Radiat Oncol Biol Phys. 1993;27:231–234.

177. Sorensen S, Borgesen SE, Rohde K, et al. Metastatic epidural spinal cord compression: results of treatment and survival. Cancer. 1990;65:1502–1508.

178. Kim RY, Smith JW, Spencer SA, et al. Malignant epidural spinal cord compression associated with a paravertebral mass: its radiotherapeutic outcome on radiosensitivity. Int J Radiat Oncol Biol Phys. 1993;27:1079–1083.

179. Price P, Hoskin PJ, Easton D, et al. Prospective randomised trial of single and multifraction radiotherapy schedules in the treatment of painful bony metastases. Radiother Oncol. 1986;6:247–255.

180. Tong D, Gillick L, Hendrickson FR. The palliation of symptomatic osseous metastases: final results of the study by the Radiation Therapy Oncology Group. Cancer. 1982;50:893–899.

181. Johnson DH, Carbone DP. Increased dose-intensity in small-cell lung cancer: a failed strategy? J Clin Oncol. 1999;17:2297–2299.

182. Ziegler A, Luedke GH, Fabbro D, et al. Induction of apoptosis in small-cell lung cancer cells by an antisense oligodeoxynucleotide targeting the Bcl-2 coding sequence. J Natl Cancer Inst. 1997;89:1027–1036.

183. Grant SC, Kris MG, Houghton AW, et al. Long survival of patients with small cell lung cancer after adjuvant treatment with the anti-idiotypic antibody BEC2 plus Bacillus Calmette-Guerin. Clin Cancer Res. 1999;5:1319–1323.

184. Cerny T, Blair V, Anderson H, et al. Pretreatment prognostic factors and scoring system in 407 small-cell lung cancer patients. Int J Cancer. 1987;39:146–149.

PART 8

OTHER TYPES OF LUNG CANCER

26

CARCINOID AND MUCOEPIDERMOID TUMORS

Andy C. Kiser and Frank C. Detterbeck

CARCINOID TUMORS
  Definitions
  Clinical Presentation
  Diagnosis
  Treatment

  Treatment Outcomes
MUCOEPIDERMOID TUMORS
  Incidence
  Clinical Presentation

  Diagnosis
  Treatment

EDITORS' COMMENTS

CARCINOID TUMORS

Definitions

Carcinoid tumors constitute a relatively uncommon group of pulmonary neoplasms, being responsible for only 0.4% to 3% of resected lung cancers.[1–5] The lung is the second most common site of origin for carcinoid tumors (after the gastrointestinal tract).[6] For many years it was uncertain as to whether to classify these tumors as benign or malignant, hence the ambiguous term *carcinoid.* Until the early 1970s, carcinoid tumors were also known as *bronchial adenomas,* implying a benign nature. In 1972, a subgroup known as *atypical* carcinoid tumors was described that had a more malignant histologic appearance (frequent mitotic figures) and demonstrated more aggressive clinical behavior (frequent lymph node and systemic metastases).[7] This led to the recognition that even typical carcinoid tumors have the capacity to metastasize, although they do so only rarely. All carcinoid tumors are therefore appropriately classified as malignant. The staging of carcinoid tumors follows the same TNM system that is used for other lung cancers.

Carcinoid tumors are currently classified as neuroendocrine tumors and are thought to arise from Kulchitsky cells of the bronchus, which are part of the poorly understood amine precursor uptake decarboxylation (APUD) system.[8] Kulchitsky cells, bronchial carcinoid tumors, and small cell lung cancer (SCLC) all contain neurosecretory granules, and several authors have suggested that typical carcinoids, atypical carcinoids, and SCLC represent a spectrum of disease.[8–10] Typical carcinoid tumors, also known as Kulchitsky cell class I tumors (KCC-I), exhibit only very low grade malignant behavior. Atypical carcinoids (KCC-II) are more aggressive, and metastases and lymph node involvement are not uncommon. SCLC (KCC-III) is the most aggressive cell type.[8–10] Large cell neuroendocrine carcinomas have been included as a fourth type of neuroendocrine tumor by some authors; these tumors exhibit behavior intermediate between atypical carcinoid tumors and SCLC.[11]

The distinction between typical and atypical carcinoid tumors is determined by their histologic appearance and is based on the extent of architectural disorganization and the number of mitotic figures.[8] Typical carcinoid tumors are defined as groups of neuroendocrine cells that have an alveolar or glandular appearance. The cells are orderly and rather small, with small nuclei and a fine chromatin network. Mitoses are rare. An atypical carcinoid tumor is recognized by the presence of one or more of the following histologic features: 1) a recognizable carcinoid pattern with increased mitotic activity, 2) pleomorphic or irregular nuclei with nuclear prominence and hyperchromatism, 3) areas of increased cellularity with disorganized architecture, and 4) areas of tumor necrosis. These features may be focal; therefore, adequate tumor sampling is imperative.[7] Furthermore, some of these criteria are subjective or vague, and the diagnosis of an atypical carcinoid is only moderately reproducible among different pathologists.[12] A detailed analysis of this issue has led to a new definition, in which an atypical carcinoid tumor is defined as a neuroendocrine tumor with 2 to 10 mitoses per 10 high-power fields or with a focus of necrosis.[11]

Pulmonary tumorlets bear some similarity to carcinoid tumors, but they are not discussed in this chapter because the association is controversial and malignant behavior of these lesions has not been demonstrated. Tumorlets are microscopic nodules of neuroendocrine cells that are well differentiated and lack atypia and mitotic figures.[13] They are usually located in the periphery of the lung and are usually discovered as an incidental finding during a resection for other reasons. Tumorlets have been associated most commonly with chronic inflammation (eg, bronchiectasis) or occasionally with larger carcinoid tumors.[14] No clear prognostic meaning for isolated tumorlets has been defined.[13]

Clinical Presentation

Symptoms

Patients with pulmonary carcinoid tumors have a wide age distribution, with reports of these tumors occurring in patients as young as 9 years and as old as 86 years.[15] The average median age of patients with pulmonary carcinoid tumors is 47 years (range of reported median age, 39–55 years),[2,16–26] which is nearly 20 years younger than the median age of patients with lung cancer in general (see Fig. 4–2). Among studies reporting on ≥50 patients with both typical and atypical carcinoids, the average percentage of women is 52% (range, 42%–66%).[2,7,8,17–21,24–28] Unlike bronchogenic carcinoma in general, no risk factors have been identified that predispose individuals to the development of carcinoid tumors. In series reporting carcinoid tumors, the proportion of smokers is similar to that of the general population.[8,29]

There is a bimodal age distribution, with one peak at approximately 35 years of age and another at about 55 years of age (Fig. 26–1).[8,17–19,27,28] The reason for this is not entirely clear. Part of the late peak can be attributed to an increasing incidence of atypical carcinoid tumors, which do not have a bimodal age distribution and have a peak incidence at approximately age 55 years.[7,16,29,30] In a patient suspected of having a carcinoid tumor, the chance that this is an atypical carcinoid is approximately 25% in patients over 50 years of age and <10% in patients under 30 years of age.[8,17,19] For all ages combined, atypical carcinoids constitute 13% of all carcinoid tumors in studies of ≥50 patients reporting this data.[2,17,19,21,23,27,28,30]

The presentation of a patient with a carcinoid tumor of the lung is largely dependent upon the location of the tumor. Patients with peripheral carcinoid tumors are usually asymptomatic, and the tumor is discovered incidentally on a routine chest radiograph (CXR). Centrally located tumors are more often symptomatic. Patients with these tumors may present with cough, hemoptysis, recurrent pneumonia, wheezing, and sometimes pain and dyspnea (Table 26–1). An analysis of 1447 patients with both typical and atypical

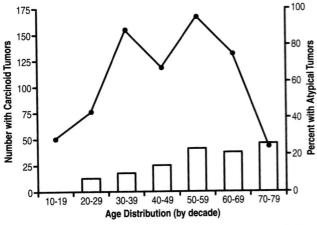

Figure 26–1. Age distribution of patients with bronchial carcinoid tumors (line graph) and percentage of carcinoid tumors that are atypical by decades of age (bar graph). Data for overall age distribution from references 8, 17–19, 27, and 28. Data for percentage of atypical carcinoids from references 8, 17, and 19.

TABLE 26–1. CLINICAL PRESENTATION OF 1447 PATIENTS WITH CARCINOID TUMORS (BOTH TYPICAL AND ATYPICAL)

SYMPTOM	N	% OF PATIENTS WITH SYMPTOMS[a]
Cough	315	30
Hemoptysis	303	29
Recurrent pneumonia	271	26
Pain	67	6
Wheezing	41	4
Dyspnea	44	4
Asymptomatic	406	(32)[b]

Inclusion criteria: Studies reporting data on clinical presentation of ≥100 patients with carcinoid tumors.
[a]Patients may have more than one symptom.
[b]Percentage of all patients.
Data from references 2, 7, 16, 20, 23, 24, 27, and 28.

pulmonary carcinoid tumors showed that one-third were asymptomatic on presentation (see Table 26–1). Of those patients who were symptomatic, the vast majority presented with cough, recurrent pneumonia, and hemoptysis (see Table 26–1). Similar findings were reported in a review of 1875 patients with bronchopulmonary carcinoids.[26]

The diagnosis of a carcinoid tumor is often delayed, even in symptomatic patients. Although 99% of patients in one study (n = 91) saw a physician within 1 year of symptom onset, only 71% were diagnosed within 1 year of the clinical presentation (onset of symptoms or radiographic detection in asymptomatic patients).[18] In fact, 13% were not diagnosed until >5 years after the initial presentation.[18] The fact that many patients are relatively young and may lack risk factors for lung cancer probably contributes to the delay in diagnosis. Many patients with a carcinoid tumor are treated for respiratory tract infections or asthma before the correct diagnosis is made.

Paraneoplastic Syndromes

The incidence of carcinoid syndrome at presentation in patients with bronchial carcinoid tumors is 0.7% (9 of 1250 patients) in reports of >50 patients that provided this data.[2,17–19,21,23,24,27,28,31,32] During follow-up, an additional 2% to 5% of patients develop this syndrome, which consists of episodic flushing and diarrhea.[19,21,24,33] An increased urinary level of the serotonin metabolite 5-hydroxyindoleacetic acid (5-HIAA) is almost always found in such patients.[13,24,26] In patients with pulmonary carcinoid tumors, the carcinoid syndrome is associated with the presence of liver metastases in approximately 90% of cases.[34] The incidence of this syndrome may be higher (5%-10%) in patients with atypical carcinoids, consistent with the greater propensity of these tumors to metastasize.[30] Although the classic carcinoid syndrome is rare, one study of 126 patients noted complaints of flushing in 12% of patients, diarrhea in 10%, and elevated 5-HIAA levels in 25%,[20] suggesting that milder forms of the syndrome may be more frequent than is commonly thought. A review in 1999[26] of 1875 patients with bronchopulmonary carcinoid tumors found a similar incidence of flushing (11%) and diarrhea (10%). However, elevated serotonin levels were found in

TABLE 26–2. CHEST RADIOGRAPH FINDINGS IN PATIENTS WITH CARCINOID TUMORS

STUDY	N	NORMAL CHEST RADIOGRAPH (%)	ATELECTASIS (%)	CENTRAL MASS (%)	PERIPHERAL MASS (%)
Okike et al[23a]	199	11	22	50	18
Ducrocq et al[16a]	139	9	43	48	
Vadasz et al[2]	120	6	37		
Mårtensson et al[18]	91	1	20	15	43
Chughtai et al[32]	86	7	16	49	30
Bertelsen et al[19]	82	4	87	—	—
Hurt and Bates[17]	79	3	72	7	0
Marty-Ané et al[30]	79	0	56	25	44
Average (%)		**5**	**42**	**30**	**27**

Inclusion criteria: Studies reporting radiographic findings of ≥50 patients with carcinoid tumors (typical and atypical).
[a]Typical carcinoid tumors only.

47%, and 8% of all patients were reported to have carcinoid syndrome.

Cushing's syndrome occurs in approximately 1% to 6% of patients with pulmonary carcinoid tumors,[13,16,26,28,29,35] and bronchial carcinoids represent the most common source of ectopic production of corticotropin (ACTH).[13] This syndrome may be more common in patients with atypical carcinoid tumors.[30] In contrast to patients with the carcinoid syndrome, approximately 80% of patients with Cushing's syndrome have localized disease.[35] In a review of this subject, the tumor could not be seen on a CXR in two-thirds of patients with a carcinoid tumor and Cushing's syndrome, although a lesion was demonstrated by computed tomography (CT) in most patients.[35] The syndrome resolves after resection in most patients.[28,30,35] Nearly 60% of these patients have lymph node involvement, and approximately 80% are typical carcinoid tumors.[36,37]

Other syndromes associated with pulmonary carcinoid tumors have been reported very rarely.[13] Several cases of acromegaly have been reported as a result of secretion of growth hormone by the tumor (all of which resolved after resection),[13,38–40] and secretion of parathyroid hormone by a pulmonary carcinoid tumor has been documented in a patient with metastases.[41] Valvular disease of the right side of the heart has been noted rarely with pulmonary carcinoid tumors.[34] Carcinoid crisis, a life-threatening complication of carcinoid syndrome, may occasionally be precipitated by diagnostic or therapeutic interventions, including initia-

tion of chemotherapy.[13] This is manifested by prolonged flushing, confusion, coma, and either hypotension or hypertension. It can be treated by administration of somatostatin.[13,42]

Radiographic Appearance

Chest radiograph findings in patients with carcinoid tumors are usually nonspecific, the most common being atelectasis. Table 26–2 presents a summary of the radiographic findings in 875 patients with carcinoid tumors. Ninety-five percent of the patients had an abnormal finding, usually a mass or atelectasis. In light of this, it is remarkable that 32% of patients were asymptomatic, the lesion having been detected incidentally on a routine CXR. The data in Table 26–2 shows that approximately 25% of patients have a peripheral lesion, and approximately 70% have radiographic evidence of a central lesion (either atelectasis or a hilar mass). There is some variability in the reported data, most likely due to differences in the definition of a mass versus atelectasis.

A consistent difference in the radiographic appearance of typical carcinoid tumors compared with atypical tumors has not been reported. One study of 124 patients reported that carcinoid tumors ≥3 cm had a higher chance of being atypical.[24] However, other studies have noted minimal differences in size between the two types of carcinoid tumors.[7,10,43] Furthermore, a large review found no difference in the proportion of typical and atypical carcinoids among

TABLE 26–3. LOCATION OF CARCINOID TUMORS

STUDY	N	DISTRIBUTION (%) OF CARCINOID TUMORS								
		LUL	LLL	RUL	RML	RLL	BI	RMSB	LMSB	Tr
Okike et al[23]	203	14	20	14	12	23	5	3	8	0
Ducrocq et al[16 a]	139	18	22	18	12	19	7	1	2	0
McCaughan et al[24]	124	24	18	11	18	14	4	6	6	0
Schreurs et al[22 a]	93	20	12	23	13	15	3	6	6	1
Mårtensson et al[18]	91	12	26	17	23	17	1	1	2	0
Chughtai et al[32]	86	26	21	11	14	24	2	0	1	0
Bertelsen et al[19]	82	23	22	9	17	12	11	1	5	0
Average (%)		**20**	**20**	**15**	**16**	**18**	**5**	**3**	**4**	**0.1**

Inclusion criteria: Studies providing information on location of carcinoid tumors (both typical and atypical) in ≥50 patients.
[a]Excluding one patient with bilateral tumors.
BI, bronchus intermedius; LLL, left lower lobe; LMSB, left mainstem bronchus; LUL, left upper lobe; RLL, right lower lobe; RML, right middle lobe; RMSB, right mainstem bronchus; RUL, right upper lobe; Tr, trachea.

tumors of various sizes, with the exception of a slightly higher incidence of atypical carcinoids among tumors > 5 cm.[26]

Tumor Location

Although carcinoid tumors may occur in any location throughout the tracheobronchial tree or lung parenchyma, there is a significant propensity for these tumors to occur in a central location. Studies of the anatomic location of carcinoid tumors have found that 75% occur within a major or segmental bronchus (see Diagnosis section). The remaining 25% occur in the peripheral lung tissue and are not associated with an airway. This is identical to the reported distribution based on radiographic data. The exact location of carcinoid tumors is presented in Table 26–3. Fifty-six percent of carcinoid tumors occur on the right side. The distribution among the lobes of the lungs is fairly uniform and approximately parallels the proportion of bronchial segments per lobe. Although the majority of carcinoid tumors are central, only 12% occur in the main-stem bronchi or trachea. In summary, although most carci-noid tumors occur in a central location, most involve lobar or segmental bronchi rather than the main airways.

The locations of typical and atypical carcinoid tumors are slightly different. An average of 75% of typical carci-noid tumors were found to be central (range, 65-96) in studies of >50 patients reporting such data.[8,16,19,22,26,28–30] On average, only 53% of atypical tumors were reported to be central in these studies, but there was considerable variability among studies (range, 32%-83%).[8,16,19,22,26,28–30] The high variability among atypical tumors in the propor-tion of central tumors may be related to varying definitions of central tumors (especially given the propensity of these tumors for hilar lymph node metastases), as well as to the smaller numbers of patients.

Data regarding the probability of a typical versus an atypical tumor in a specific location (central or peripheral) is shown in Table 26–4. A central tumor has consistently been found to have an 80% chance of being a typical carcinoid (range, 71%–93%) in studies of ≥50 patients reporting carcinoid type–specific data. This is important,

TABLE 26–4. PROBABILITY OF TYPE OF CARCINOID TUMOR BY ANATOMIC LOCATION[a]

STUDY	CENTRAL TUMORS			PERIPHERAL TUMORS		
	N	Typ %	Atyp %	N	Typ %	Atyp %
Soga et al[26]	753	91	9	447	73	27
Wilkins et al[28]	193	93	7	18	39	61
Paladugu et al[8]	116	71	29	40	83	17
Bertelsen et al[19]	65	82	18	17	71	29
Warren et al[29]	50	80	20	42	26	74
Marty-Ané et al[30]	44	77	23	35	51	49
Average (%)		82	18		57	43

Inclusion criteria: Studies reporting on ≥50 patients with carcinoid tumors that specified tumor location by tumor type.
[a]Anatomic location as interpreted (but not explicitly defined) by the individual study authors. It is especially unclear how a peripheral primary with a hilar nodal mass was classified.
Atyp, atypical carcinoid tumor; Typ, typical carcinoid tumor.

TABLE 26–5. STAGE OF CARCINOID TUMORS AT PRESENTATION

STUDY	N	CARCINOID TYPE	PATIENTS (%)		
			N0[a]	N1	N2
Okike et al[23]	203	Typical	95	—5—	
Ducrocq et al[16]	139	Typical	91	8	1
Paladugu et al[8b]	115	Typical	96	4	0
Vadasz et al[2]	109	Typical	94	—6—	
Wilkins et al[28]	100	Typical	95	—5—	
Schreurs et al[22]	93	Typical	90	10	0
McCaughan et al[24]	72	Typical	89	—11—	
Bertelsen et al[19]	65	Typical	97	—3—	
Warren et al[29]	52	Typical	88	8	4
Marty-Ané et al[30]	52	Typical	96	4	0
Average (%)			92	7	1
Warren et al[29]	37	Atypical	73	11	16
Paladugu et al[8b]	34	Atypical	65	21	15
Marty-Ané et al[30]	27	Atypical	58	26	22
McCaughan et al[24]	23	Atypical	52	—48—	
Ceresoli et al[44b]	20	Atypical	75	10	15
Rea et al[21]	18	Atypical	72	—28—	
Stamatis et al[27]	17	Atypical	59	18	24[c]
Bertelsen et al[19]	16	Atypical	44	—56—	
Average (%)			62	17	18

Inclusion criteria: Studies of resected patients involving ≥50 typical or ≥15 atypical carcinoid tumors.
[a]Includes T1, T2, and T3.
[b]Patients with M1 disease excluded in these percentages in this table.
[c]One patient had N3 involvement.

because patients with central lesions are more likely to be diagnosed preoperatively as having a carcinoid tumor (ei-ther by bronchoscopic appearance alone or by biopsy) and are more likely to be considered for a conservative resec-tion. A peripheral lesion, on the other hand, has approxi-mately a 50:50 chance of being a typical versus an atypical carcinoid. However, this observation must be interpreted with caution, because there is so much variability in the reported results and because many other diagnoses, in addi-tion to carcinoid tumor, are possible in patients with periph-eral masses. Thus, the location of a tumor, coupled with the bronchoscopic findings and the age of the patient, may allow a reasonable prediction of the type of carcinoid to be made preoperatively.

Stage at Presentation

The stage at presentation is markedly different for typical and atypical carcinoid tumors. In series based on pathology records or tumor registries, 10% to 30% of patients with atypical tumors present with distant metastases, whereas this is found in <5% of patients with typical carcinoid tumors.[8,20,24,44] However, most reported series have involved patients who had undergone resection and have excluded patients with stage IV disease. The incidence of lymph node involvement in surgical series is shown in Table 26–5. Typical carcinoid tumors rarely spread to lymph nodes, especially mediastinal lymph nodes, whereas the rate of N1 or N2 lymph node involvement with atypical tumors is approximately 40%. Some authors have suggested an association between the presence of nodal involvement and either larger or more central tumors,[20,24] but this is controversial.[16] However, the data in Table 26–5 provides

DATA SUMMARY: CLINICAL PRESENTATION OF CARCINOID TUMORS

	AMOUNT	QUALITY	CONSISTENCY
The mean age of patients with carcinoid tumors is 45	High	High	High
The mean age of patients with atypical carcinoid tumors is 55	High	High	High
Tracheal, mainstem, or bronchus intermedius lesions constitute 13% of carcinoid tumors	Mod	High	High
Central lesions constitute 75% of carcinoid tumors	High	Mod	Mod
80% of central carcinoid tumors are of the typical type	High	High	High
50% of peripheral carcinoid tumors are of the atypical type	High	Poor	Poor
Lymph node involvement is seen in 5% of resected typical carcinoid tumors	High	High	High
Lymph node involvement is seen in 40% of resected atypical carcinoid tumors	High	High	Mod

Type of data rated: Plain text: descriptive statement   *Italics: controlled comparison*   **Bold: randomized comparison**

convincing evidence of a consistent association between nodal involvement and the histologic type of carcinoid tumor, which has itself been associated with tumor size and location.

Diagnosis

In many patients, a presumptive diagnosis of a carcinoid tumor can be made based on the history and clinical presentation. A young patient who has never smoked and who presents with recurrent infections or radiographic evidence of central obstruction should be suspected of having a carcinoid tumor. Similar patients who present with a well-circumscribed peripheral nodule also suggest the diagnosis of a carcinoid tumor. In either situation, however, further investigation is necessary to rule out other possible diagnoses.

Bronchoscopy is clearly indicated for patients who pre-

sent with evidence of central obstruction. An endobronchial tumor could be visualized in the main, lobar, or segmental bronchi in an average of 74% of patients undergoing bronchoscopy in studies of ≥50 patients (range, 58%–89%).[16–19, 23,25,27,29,30] A smooth or lobulated, fleshy appearing intraluminal mass is characteristic of a carcinoid tumor as seen by bronchoscopy. Visualization of such a tumor effectively excludes many other possibilities such as a foreign body, central bronchiectasis, or conventional lung cancer (which invariably appears irregular and friable). Benign endobronchial growths are much less common than carcinoid tumors (see Chapter 28). Therefore, a typical endobronchial appearance in a patient with an appropriate history is highly suggestive of a carcinoid tumor. For patients with peripheral masses, however, there are no radiographic characteristics that can strongly confirm a suspicion (based on clinical presentation) of a carcinoid tumor.

A summary of data regarding bronchoscopy in 1315 patients with carcinoid tumors is provided in Table 26–6.

TABLE 26–6. RESULTS OF BRONCHOSCOPY IN PATIENTS WITH CARCINOID TUMORS

STUDY	N PATIENTS	N BRONCH	N BIOPSY	N BLEEDING	N MAJOR BLEEDING	% DIAG ACHIEVED
Stamatis et al[27]	227	—	190	—	4	82
Okike et al[23]	203	140	124	—	—	97
Ducrocq et al[16]	139	139	102	2	0	—
McCaughan et al[24]	124	—	25	3	0	96
Schreurs et al[22]	93	—	65	—	—	82
Mårtensson et al[18]	91	83	50	—	—	82
Bertelsen et al[19]	82	78	60	2	0	80
Hurt and Bates[17]	79	79	61	2	0	—
Marty-Ané et al[30]	79	78	37	0	0	41
Francioni et al[25]	69	69	48	4	0	85
Todd et al[31]	69	35	23	6	0	—
Rea et al[21]	60	60	27	0	0	67
Total	1315	>761	812	19	4	
Total (%)[a]				5	1	79[b]

Inclusion criteria: Studies of ≥50 patients from 1975 to 2000 reporting results of bronchoscopy.
[a]Percentage of patients undergoing biopsy for whom the respective data is reported.
[b]Average of percentages (of patients undergoing biopsy).
N Biopsy, number of patients undergoing biopsy; N Bleeding, number of patients who had bleeding reported after biopsy; N Bronch, number of patients undergoing bronchoscopy; N Major bleeding, number of patients who required operative treatment or blood products because of bleeding after biopsy; % Diag achieved, percentage of patients undergoing biopsy in whom a diagnosis was achieved.

DATA SUMMARY: DIAGNOSIS OF CARCINOID TUMORS

	AMOUNT	QUALITY	CONSISTENCY
The tumor can be seen in 75% of patients with a carcinoid tumor who undergo bronchoscopy	High	High	High
Endobronchial biopsy is able to diagnose a carcinoid tumor in 80% of the patients in whom it is done	High	High	High
The risk of major bleeding from endobronchial biopsy is 1%	High	High	High
Distinguishing a typical from an atypical carcinoid tumor by preoperative biopsy (including intraoperative frozen section) is difficult	Mod	Mod	High

Type of data rated: Plain text: descriptive statement   *Italics: controlled comparison*   **Bold: randomized comparison**

More than 80% of all patients underwent bronchoscopy, and an endoscopic biopsy was performed in 62% of all patients. A diagnosis of a carcinoid tumor was made in approximately 80% of those patients undergoing biopsy. Historically, however, many authors have strongly discouraged endobronchial biopsy of a suspected carcinoid tumor because of concerns of a significant risk of uncontrollable hemorrhage.[45,46] If a biopsy is deemed necessary, some authors recommend that it should be done in an operating room with a rigid bronchoscope,[27] but others recommend a flexible bronchoscope because of a lower perceived risk of bleeding.[24,29] However, among 812 patients in Table 26–6 who underwent endobronchial biopsy (mostly with flexible bronchoscopy), bleeding occurred in only 5%, and only four patients (1%) required operative management via thoracotomy to control the postbiopsy bleeding. All four of these patients, reported in a single study,[27] had atypical carcinoid tumors that were cherry red in bronchoscopic appearance. No deaths related to endobronchial biopsy of a carcinoid tumor have been reported. Thus, the data supports the ability to biopsy carcinoid tumors with a flexible or rigid bronchoscope without significant risk of hemorrhage.

Cytologic study of bronchoscopic brushings or washings or of expectorated sputum is rarely useful in establishing the diagnosis of carcinoid tumor.[23,24,29,32] In one study, a diagnosis of malignancy was obtained in only 18% of 68 patients, and a diagnosis of a carcinoid tumor could not be made in any patients.[24] Because many carcinoid tumors are covered by normal bronchial mucosa, biopsy specimens may appear normal even when tumors are actually present.[22] Furthermore, practically all studies report an appreciable error rate among endobronchial biopsies that are read as *positive* for some type of cancer.[2,16,17,21,22,25] Among larger series of patients with carcinoid tumors, the average error rate is 8% (range, 1%–22%) and mostly involves confusion of carcinoid tumors with small cell or squamous cell carcinomas. Moreover, in several series of patients with *atypical* carcinoid tumors, the error rate was found to be 40% to 80%.[27,29,30]

It has been difficult to accurately differentiate between typical and atypical carcinoid tumors preoperatively. Part of the difficulty is that there is a spectrum in the progression from typical to atypical and to small cell carcinomas in the number of mitoses, nuclear pleomorphism, nuclear to cytoplasmic ratio, and nuclear DNA content, which may be confusing to the pathologist.[8,17] Fine needle aspirations and bronchial brushings are notoriously inaccurate in differentiating typical from atypical carcinoids because important differentiating criteria such as cellular patterns and tissue necrosis cannot easily be obtained by these techniques.[7,8,30] Even by bronchoscopic biopsy, an accuracy of only 20% has been reported in differentiating between atypical and typical carcinoid tumors.[30] Furthermore, frozen section diagnoses are also notoriously inaccurate. McCaughan et al[24] reported a 60% success rate in accurately diagnosing typical or atypical carcinoid tumors by frozen section. Because of difficulty in obtaining a reliable

TABLE 26–7. DISTRIBUTION OF PROCEDURES PERFORMED TO RESECT CARCINOID TUMORS (%)[a]

STUDY	N TOTAL	WEDGE/ SEGMENT	LOBEC- TOMY	BILOBEC- TOMY	PNEUMONEC- TOMY	SLEEVE LOBEC- TOMY	BRONCH RESEC- TION	ENDOBRONCH RESECTION
Stamatis et al[27]	227	16	40	9	14	14	5	1
Okike et al[23]	203	4	—————65—————		27	2	2	—
Ducrocq et al[16]	139	4	62	9	5	14	5	0
Vadasz et al[2]	118	14	53	6	8	10	8	0
Wilkins et al[28]	111	14	37	16	22	5	5	1
Harpole et al[20]	106	21	51	—	14	8	0	6
McCaughan et al[24]	101	15	51	9	14	5	0	6
Total (%)		**13**	**49**	**10**	**15**	**8**	**4**	**2**

Inclusion criteria: Studies of ≥100 patients with carcinoid tumors (typical and atypical) (total, 1005 procedures).
[a]Values shown are percentage of all procedures for each study (except total number of patients).
Bronch resection, bronchial resection; endobronch resection, endobronchial resection; wedge/segment, wedge resection or segmentectomy.

preoperative histologic diagnosis of a typical versus an atypical carcinoid tumor, the presumptive clinical diagnosis should weigh heavily in treatment planning. If the clinical presentation strongly favors one tumor type rather than the other, it may be appropriate to base treatment decisions on this, despite an ambiguous or conflicting biopsy result.

Treatment

The mainstay of treatment of carcinoid tumors is surgical resection. These tumors are generally considered to be resistant to radiation,[13] although a few long-term survivors have been reported who were treated with radiotherapy (RT) alone.[47] There may be a role for palliative RT of symptomatic metastatic lesions.[13] Furthermore, atypical carcinoid tumors, which appear to have more rapid cell division, may be more radiosensitive than typical tumors. A limited experience exists in treating such tumors (not all of bronchial origin) with chemotherapy. Regimens similar to those used in SCLC have been reported to have a good response rate (67%) in patients with atypical carcinoid tumors, whereas the response rate in patients with typical carcinoid tumors is only 7%.[13,48] The rarity of these tumors hampers attempts to accumulate ample data, but it appears to be a reasonable extrapolation to treat atypical carcinoid tumors with chemotherapy when resection is not possible.

Surgical Resection

A wide variety of surgical procedures have been used to treat carcinoid tumors, ranging from endobronchial removal to sleeve pneumonectomy. The procedures that have been used in the larger series reported from 1980 to 2000 are summarized in Table 26–7. Although the location of the tumor is the primary determinant of which procedure to use, many secondary issues are less clear. For example, a peripheral stage I tumor can be removed by wedge resection or by lobectomy, and a central tumor can be removed by a pneumonectomy, sleeve lobectomy, or resection of the involved airway without removing any lung parenchyma (bronchial sleeve resection). The data in Table 26–7, together with the fact that approximately 25% of carcinoid tumors arise as peripheral lesions, suggests that about half of the peripheral tumors have been resected by a wedge or segmentectomy rather than a lobectomy. Most of the central tumors are resected using conventional procedures such as lobectomy, bilobectomy, or pneumonectomy. The relatively infrequent use of a sleeve lobectomy or a bronchial resection without an associated pulmonary resection is consistent with the observation that relatively few tumors are located in the mainstem bronchi.

The percentage of patients undergoing pneumonectomy in the studies shown in Table 26–7 varies from 5% to 27%. A range of 2% to 14% is also seen in the percentage of patients undergoing sleeve lobectomy. Studies reporting a low rate of sleeve lobectomy show a correspondingly higher rate of pneumonectomy. Similarly, studies that involved few resections by a wedge or segmentectomy had a correspondingly higher rate of resection by a lobectomy. These observations demonstrate that institutions vary in the use of limited resections as well as lung-sparing bronchoplastic techniques.

There is some evidence that the use of resection techniques that preserve more lung tissue has become more frequent over time.[22,25,28] One study reported that the use of segmental resections for patients with peripheral tumors had increased from 26% to 60% since 1980, and the percentage of patients undergoing bronchoplastic or bronchial sleeve resections for central tumors had increased from 40% to 65%.[22] This raises issues regarding the success rate of lung-sparing procedures in eradicating the tumor and how much normal bronchial tissue beyond the edge of a carcinoid tumor must be removed in order to obtain an adequate margin. Complicating matters is the fact that identification of a tumor as a typical or an atypical carcinoid often cannot be established reliably until after resection. These specific surgical issues are discussed later.

Treatment Outcomes

Typical Carcinoid Tumors

Numerous studies have reported treatment results in patients with typical carcinoid tumors; these are summarized in Table 26–8. Long-term survival has been consistently found to be good, with 5- and 10-year survival rates of $\geq$90%. The results are even more impressive considering that only 10% of the deaths that occur are due to recurrence of carcinoid tumor. In fact, the crude recurrence rate is only 3% in patients undergoing resection of a typical carcinoid tumor. The consistency among studies for each of these findings is remarkable.

Atypical Carcinoid Tumors

Less data is available about the outcomes of patients with atypical carcinoid tumors than of patients with typical tumors because atypical tumors occur much less commonly. The data from studies including at least 15 patients is shown in Table 26–8. The 5- and 10-year survival rates of these patients are approximately 60%. One-third of the patients experience a recurrence, and 70% of the deaths are due to cancer. There is some variation in the reported results, but this is to be expected because of the small size of the studies. Nevertheless, the survival of patients with an atypical carcinoid is clearly worse than that of patients with a typical tumor, suggesting a more aggressive biologic behavior of the atypical cell type. On the other hand, more patients with atypical carcinoid tumors present with lymph node involvement, so that the stage of disease at presentation is already less favorable in these patients. Representative survival curves for patients with atypical and typical carcinoid tumors from one of the larger studies is shown in Figure 26–2A.

N1,2 Involvement

Little data is available regarding the survival of resected patients with lymph node involvement by a carcinoid tumor. Such nodal disease is rare in patients with typical tumors, and although it is much more frequent in patients with atypical tumors, the much lower incidence of atypical carcinoid tumors limits the number of patients available for analysis. The largest study involved 37 N1,2 patients (both typical and atypical carcinoid tumors) and reported 5- and 10-year survival rates of 37% and 22%.[20] However,

TABLE 26-8. SURVIVAL OF RESECTED PATIENTS WITH TYPICAL AND ATYPICAL CARCINOID TUMORS

STUDY	N	CARCINOID TYPE	% SURVIVAL			CAUSE OF DEATH (%)		% WITH RECUR[a]
			5 y	10 y	15 y	Other	Recur	
Soga et al[26]	947	Typical	93	82	—	—	—	—
Stamatis et al[27]	210	Typical	98	98	—	100	0	0
Okike et al[23]	169	Typical	94	87	76[b]	—	—	2
Ducrocq et al[16]	139	Typical	92	88	76	82	18	4
Schreurs et al[22]	93	Typical	(100)[c]	(100)[c]	(100)[c]	87	13	2
Harpole et al[20] [d]	80	Typical	96	92	—	—	—	—
Hurt and Bates[17]	78	Typical	96	94	80	—	—	3
McCaughan et al[24]	72	Typical	100	87	—	—	—	—
Chughtai et al[32]	72	Typical	(97)[c]	(95)[c]	—	—	—	3
Bertelsen et al[19]	65	Typical	—	—	—	78	22	3
Marty-Ané et al[30]	52	Typical	90	—	—	100	0	—
Warren et al[29]	52	Typical	—	84	—	91	9	4
Average[e] (%)			**95**	**89**	**77**	**90**	**10**	**3**
Soga et al[26]	132	Atypical	69	59	—	—	—	—
Harpole et al[20]	41	Atypical	(40)[f]	(31)[f]	—	—	—	—
Warren et al[29]	37	Atypical	—	—	—	—	—	33
Marty-Ané et al[30]	27	Atypical	82	49	—	43	57	19
McCaughan et al[24]	23	Atypical	69	52	—	—	—	—
Rea et al[21]	18	Atypical	66	60	—	44	56	28
Stamatis et al[27]	17	Atypical	41	—	—	29	71	29
Bertelsen et al[19]	16	Atypical	—	—	—	0	100	50
Average[e] (%)			**65**	**55**		**29**	**71**	**32**

Inclusion criteria: Studies of resected patients (≥50 typical or ≥15 atypical carcinoid tumors).
[a]Percentage of all patients who experienced a recurrence (any recurrence at any time).
[b]20-year survival.
[c]Disease-free survival.
[d]Some patients did not undergo resection.
[e]Excluding values in parentheses.
[f]Many patients did not undergo resection.
Other, other, unrelated causes; Recur, recurrence of carcinoid tumor.

many of these patients did not undergo resection, making interpretation of the results difficult. Furthermore, given the differences in the biologic behavior of the two histologic types of carcinoid, reporting both types together greatly hampers analysis.

Those few studies reporting outcomes in patients with nodal involvement separately for typical and atypical carcinoid tumors are summarized in Table 26-9. Nodal involvement in patients with typical tumors does not affect survival greatly at 5 years, but decreases survival somewhat at 10 years. The early survival may be misleading, consid-

TABLE 26-9. SURVIVAL OF CARCINOID PATIENTS WITH LYMPH NODE INVOLVEMENT WHO UNDERWENT RESECTION[a]

STUDY	N	CARCINOID TYPE	% SURVIVAL	
			5 y	10 y
Ducrocq et al[16]	13	Typical	100	—
Martini et al[43]	12	Typical	92	76
Okike et al[23]	11	Typical	71	—
Average			**88**	**76**
Martini et al[43]	13	Atypical	60	24

Inclusion criteria: Studies of ≥10 patients with nodal involvement from carcinoid tumors.
[a]Either N1 or N2 involvement.

ering the indolent growth of these tumors, as will be discussed later. The available data regarding nodal involvement in patients with atypical carcinoid tumors also suggests that survival is minimally decreased at 5 years, but is clearly affected at 10 years. These observations are corroborated by comparing the survival curves of patients with nodal involvement from one of the studies (Fig. 26-2B) with the survival curves in Figure 26-2A. In both histologic types, however, the outcome is good enough to justify resection, even in patients with nodal involvement.

Lymph node disease primarily involves N1 nodes in patients with typical tumors, whereas nodal involvement is split evenly between N1 and N2 sites in patients with atypical tumors. The only study to report specifically on the survival of patients with N1 versus N2 disease found that survival in patients with N1 involvement is similar to that of patients with typical carcinoid tumors and positive lymph nodes (5- and 10-year survival, 90% and 75%), whereas survival in patients with N2 disease was remarkably similar to that of patients with atypical tumors and positive lymph nodes (5- and 10-year survival, 65% and 31%).[43] This study grouped typical and atypical carcinoid tumors together in reporting the data for N1 and N2 disease and did not report the proportion of tumor types in each category. Thus, it is unclear whether the survival rate in patients with positive lymph node involvement is determined primarily by the histologic tumor type or by the nodal stage. The histologic appearance of atypical carcinoid

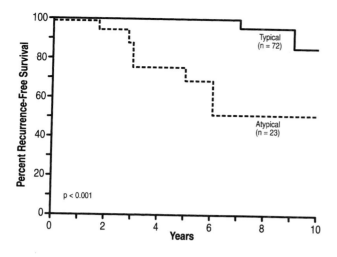

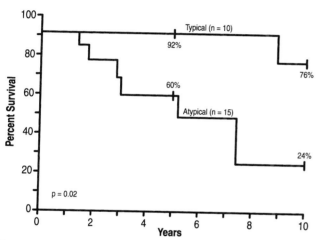

FIGURE 26–2. *A,* Recurrence-free survival of 95 patients who underwent resection of a carcinoid tumor by histologic type (*P*<0.001). (From McCaughan BC, Martini N, Bains MS. Bronchial carcinoids: review of 124 cases. J Thorac Cardiovasc Surg. 1985;89:8–17.[24]) *B,* Survival of 25 patients who underwent resection of a carcinoid tumor involving lymph nodes (either N1 or N2) by histologic type (*P*=0.02). (From Martini N, Zaman MB, Bains MS, et al. Treatment and prognosis in bronchial carcinoids involving regional lymph nodes. J Thorac Cardiovasc Surg. 1994;107:1–7.[43])

tumors, with frequent mitotic figures and similarities to SCLC, coupled with the observation that the stage at presentation is more advanced, suggests that these tumors have a more aggressive behavior than typical carcinoid tumors. However, a stage-by-stage comparison of the two types of carcinoid tumors has never been published.

Specific Surgical Issues

The technique of simple removal of a carcinoid tumor from the airway has shown almost uniformly poor results. Endoluminal tumor removal can be accomplished through a bronchoscope, with a laser, or with an open technique via an incision in the overlying bronchial wall. This treatment approach has been used infrequently and is often reserved for patients who cannot tolerate a thoracotomy.[24] Recurrence has been seen in 87% of 30 reported cases of endo-

luminal tumor removal that included follow-up.[19,22–24,27] Recurrence is seen after endoluminal tumor removal in the majority of patients with typical carcinoids,[19] although the histologic type is often not reported. It is likely that most of the reported patients have had typical carcinoid tumors, given the tumors' greater propensity for a central location. Persistent tumor was also found in eight of nine patients who underwent endobronchial tumor removal with a laser before an open resection.[22] In another report of laser endobronchial resection, 5 of 6 patients who underwent subsequent surgery had residual disease, and the follow-up period in the remaining 13 patients was short (average, 26 months).[49] Thus, endoluminal removal of a carcinoid tumor does not result in an adequate resection, even when histologic findings show a typical tumor or when using modern bronchoscopic techniques.

As a palliative procedure, however, endoluminal removal of carcinoid tumors may be very worthwhile. Intervals ranging from 1 to 18 years in 14 patients have been reported from the time of the first treatment to treatment of a recurrence (which usually involved a resection). At least three patients had an interval of ≥12 years.[19,23,27] One reported case involved a woman who could not tolerate a formal resection and underwent endoluminal tumor removal 41 times over 15 years before she died of unrelated causes.[24]

Most patients undergo a complete resection of the carcinoid tumor via a thoracotomy, although this may involve a limited resection or a bronchoplastic resection in order to preserve functioning lung tissue. There is little data regarding the outcome of patients with peripheral tumors in whom a limited resection was performed. Studies involving primarily patients with typical tumors (34 patients) have reported good 5-year survival and a recurrence rate of approximately 10%.[22–24] Several authors have found that limited resection of an atypical carcinoid tumor resulted in recurrence in the majority of patients,[24,28,30] but these studies involved small numbers of patients. This data suggests that although a limited resection may be appropriate for patients with a peripheral typical carcinoid tumor, this approach may be associated with a high recurrence rate in the case of an atypical carcinoid tumor.

The scant direct data just noted regarding the appropriateness of a limited resection in patients with a peripheral typical versus an atypical carcinoid tumor can be corroborated by theoretical considerations. Considering the rate of spread of typical tumors, a wedge or segmentectomy would seem appropriate for a typical carcinoid tumor with no evidence of nodal involvement, provided an adequate margin is obtained. However, the propensity of atypical carcinoid tumors to spread appears similar to that of non–small cell lung cancer (NSCLC) in general, for which a randomized study has shown that limited resection results in poorer survival and a higher local recurrence rate (see Fig. 11–3).[50,51] Furthermore, there is a high incidence of atypical tumors in patients with peripheral lesions, and intraoperative frozen section has frequently been reported to be misleading.[24] These findings suggest using caution when considering a limited resection for patients with peripheral carcinoid tumors.

In patients with central carcinoid tumors, the available indirect and direct data suggest that a lung-sparing operation is equivalent to a larger resection. In NSCLC, a sleeve resection offers results similar to those for lobectomy or pneumonectomy (see Table 12–4). An uncontrolled retrospective review of published literature up to 1980, involving both typical and atypical carcinoid tumors, found that survival was similar up to 15 years, although at 20 years it was better for patients who underwent lobectomy compared with limited resection.[52] A detailed multivariate analysis of 203 patients with typical carcinoid tumors treated at the Mayo Clinic found no difference in survival at 5, 10, or 15 years for patients who underwent limited resection compared with lobectomy or pneumonectomy.[16] Other studies have reported good long-term survival in patients with typical tumors treated by sleeve resection.[22,23] Overall, most of the available data suggests that lung-sparing procedures are a reasonable alternative, at least in patients with typical carcinoid tumors.

There is little data from which to determine the minimal bronchial margin necessary to achieve an adequate resection. The bronchial margin is defined as the distance from the gross tumor to the cut end of the resected bronchus. Data from patients with NSCLC suggests that the margin will be microscopically positive in 30% of patients, with a gross margin of 2 to 5 mm (see Chapter 14).[53] This rate may be lower in patients with carcinoid tumors, and the low rate of local recurrence among such patients (see recurrence patterns) suggests that the surgeon's judgment of "adequate" was accurate in most cases. Most authors recommend only a clear surgical margin by frozen section.[27,30] One author reported no recurrences of carcinoid tumor with a margin of ≥5 mm, but provided no information on the number of patients or the length of follow-up.[29] A few patients have been reported who were found to have a microscopically positive margin with no sign of recurrence during follow-up periods of 1 to 10 years.[22,31]

In conclusion, what constitutes an adequate margin has not been defined, but 5 mm seems to be a reasonable, albeit somewhat arbitrary, estimate.

Recurrence Patterns

Because of the good survival of patients with carcinoid tumors, little data has been reported regarding recurrence patterns. The data that has been reported, however, clearly demonstrates that distant recurrences are involved in the overwhelming majority of patients (Table 26–10). There is no difference in the recurrence patterns for typical and atypical carcinoid tumors. The data shown in Table 26–10 involves recurrences noted at any time, rather than only the first site of recurrence. Approximately 7% of patients experience only a local recurrence, and an additional 11% initially manifest a local recurrence but are subsequently found to have systemic metastases as well. It is likely that the converse (initial systemic recurrence, followed by recurrent local disease) may be underreported.

Systemic metastases are seen in the liver, bone, and brain, as well as other sites.[8,17,29] Several authors have reported data that suggests that the liver is the most common site of metastatic disease from bronchial carcinoid tumors.[16,17,25,29,33] This would represent a distinctly different pattern from what is seen with other forms of lung cancer. Patients with pulmonary carcinoid tumors who have liver metastases often manifest carcinoid syndrome. It is possible that this leads to better recognition of systemic disease when the liver is involved, and that other sites of distant disease are underreported.

Carcinoid tumors clearly can exhibit indolent growth, and prolonged survival has been observed even in patients with systemic metastases. Two authors have reported regional recurrences in patients 27 and 32 years after resection of the primary tumor.[2,54] Many others have reported

DATA SUMMARY: TREATMENT OF CARCINOID TUMORS	AMOUNT	QUALITY	CONSISTENCY
The 10-year survival of resected patients with typical tumors is 90%	High	High	High
Only 10% of late deaths in resected patients with typical tumors are due to recurrence	High	High	High
The 10-year survival of resected patients with atypical tumors is 55%	Mod	High	High
70% of late deaths in resected patients with atypical tumors are due to recurrence	High	High	Mod
The 5-year survival of N1,2 patients is similar to that of N0 patients (within 10% for both typical and atypical types)	High	High	Mod
The 10-year survival of resected patients with N1,2 typical carcinoid tumors is 75%	Poor	High	—
The 10-year survival of resected patients with N1,2 atypical carcinoid tumors is 20%	Poor	High	—
Endobronchial tumor removal has a recurrence rate of 90%	Mod	High	High
Bronchoplastic resection of central typical carcinoid tumors results in survival equivalent to larger resections	Mod	Poor	High
The recurrence pattern for both typical and atypical tumors is 10% local, 10% combined, and 80% systemic	Poor	Poor	High

Type of data rated: Plain text: descriptive statement   *Italics: controlled comparison*   **Bold: randomized comparison**

TABLE 26–10. RECURRENCE PATTERNS FOR RESECTED PATIENTS WITH CARCINOID TUMORS[a]

STUDY	N	CARCINOID TYPE	RECURRENCE (N)		
			L	L&D	D
Vadasz et al[2]	10	Both	1	—	9
McCaughan et al[24]	10	Both	1	—	9
Subtotal (%)			**10%**	**—**	**90%**
Ducrocq et al[16]	5	Typical	1	1	3
Okike et al[23]	4	Typical	0	—	4
Hurt and Bates[17]	2	Typical	0	1[b]	1
Schreurs et al[22]	2	Typical	0	1[b]	1
Bertelsen et al[19]	2	Typical	0	0	2
Warren et al[29]	2	Typical	0	0	2
Subtotal (%)			**6%**	**18%**	**76%**
Bertelsen et al[19]	8	Atypical	0	2[b]	6
Marty-Ané et al[30]	5	Atypical	1	1	3
Warren et al[29]	5	Atypical	0	0	5
Subtotal (%)			**6%**	**17%**	**78%**
Total (%)			**7%**	**11%**	**82%**

Inclusion criteria: Studies of ≥50 patients total with carcinoid tumors reporting specific recurrence patterns.
[a]Recurrence defined as cumulative recurrence at any time.
[b]Initially local, but after repeat resection, distant metastases eventually became apparent.
Both, typical and atypical; D, distant; L, locoregional; L&D, both locoregional and distant.

recurrences well over 10 years after initial resection.[17,24,25,27,29] A local recurrence may sometimes be able to be treated successfully with reoperation.[2,27] In addition, several authors have reported patients who are alive and well despite histologically proven metastatic disease for periods of 3 to 8 years. These observations suggest that patients with carcinoid tumors should be followed closely for their entire life and that the appearance of systemic disease does not necessarily imply short survival.

MUCOEPIDERMOID TUMORS

Incidence

Tracheobronchial mucoepidermoid tumor (MET), also called *mucoepidermoid carcinoma,* was first described in 1952 by Smetana et al[55] and Liebow.[56] The term *mucoepidermoid* arose from the similarity of these tumors to mucoepidermoid carcinomas of the salivary glands.[55] These tumors are thought to arise from minor salivary glands of the tracheobronchial tree and have historically been classified as a type of bronchial adenoma, together with carcinoid tumors and adenoid cystic carcinoma.[57] Although the term *adenoma* suggests a benign condition and although an indolent course is often seen, all of these lesions, including MET, are currently recognized as malignancies. Mucoepidermoid tumors are uncommon. These tumors constitute only 0.2% of all lung cancers[45,58–61] and only 5% of all bronchial adenomas.[59,61,62] Fewer than 200 patients with MET of the lung have been reported in the literature.

A thorough understanding of tracheobronchial METs is hampered by the rarity of these lesions. The biologic behavior of tracheobronchial METs was controversial until it was recognized that both low-grade and high-grade types exist, similar to salivary mucoepidermoid carcinoma.[63,64] The histologic distinction between low- and high-grade MET is based on increased mitotic activity, high levels of cellular necrosis, and a higher incidence of nuclear pleomorphism in high-grade tumors.[57,59] Although in general the histologic appearance has correlated with the biologic behavior, sporadic cases of seemingly low-grade tumors that exhibit aggressive behavior have been reported.[57,65]

Partly because of the rarity of METs, it may be difficult for a pathologist to differentiate between low- and high-grade METs, mucus-secreting bronchogenic carcinoma, and adenosquamous carcinoma, especially when provided with only a small biopsy specimen.[45,57] The diagnosis of MET is supported by cells with a uniform bland appearance, with no areas of keratinization and with no evidence of carcinoma in situ, although these criteria are less well defined in high-grade METs.[66] High-grade mucoepidermoid carcinomas are histologically similar to adenosquamous carcinomas,[57] and some authors believe that these are the same entity.[59,67] The term *mucoepidermoid carcinoma* is used for tumors that occur in the proximal airways (the location of 100% of reported cases), whereas adenosquamous carcinomas occur peripherally (in 96% of reported cases).[68]

Clinical Presentation

METs tend to occur in a younger population than other types of NSCLC. There are several reports of METs occurring in children,[57,62,64,65,69] and a 1997 review found 51 reported cases in patients <16 years of age (96% low-grade tumors).[70] The mean age at diagnosis is approximately 35 years, but there is a wide range extending from 3 months to 78 years.[57,71] Low-grade METs, in particular, are seen frequently in young patients (Table 26–11). The largest study, from the Armed Forces Institute of Pathology, reported that 51% of patients with low-grade METs were <30 years of age.[57] The average age of patients with high-grade METs in this study was 10 years older (45 years), and nearly 40% of high-grade tumors occurred in patients >60 years of age.[57] In contrast, the average age of patients with adenosquamous carcinoma is 62 years, and approximately two-thirds of patients are men.[67,68,72,73]

A slight difference in gender distribution may exist between patients with low- and high-grade METs (see Table 26–11). Women may be more likely to have a low-grade tumor, whereas men may be more likely to have a high-grade tumor.[57,74] Thus, in a woman <30 years old the likelihood is high that an MET is low-grade. On the other hand, because approximately 80% of METs are low grade,[57,59] a MET in a man >50 years of age is still more likely to be low grade than high grade. No risk factors for the development of MET have been identified. The incidence of smoking in two series was found to be 22%.[57,59]

The presenting symptoms of patients with a MET are primarily a result of the location of the tumor. All reported METs have been located in the major airways and are

TABLE 26–11. DEMOGRAPHIC AND SURVIVAL DATA FOR PATIENTS WITH MUCOEPIDERMOID CARCINOMAS

STUDY	N	MET TYPE	MEAN AGE (y)	% FEMALE	N R_0 RESECT	% N1,2 POS	% DIED OF MET	MEAN F/U (mo)
Breyer et al[64] [a]	67	Both	—	—	42	7	7	—
Kim et al[74]	12	Both	36	58	—	0	0	30
Yousem and Hochholzer[57]	45	Low	35	60	45	2	0	88
Heitmiller et al[59]	15	Low	36	—	12	—	0	56
Conlan et al[62]	9	Low[b]	39[c]	71[c]	8	0	0	112
Yousem and Hochholzer[57]	13	High	45	54	12	17	17[d]	49
Turnbull et al[60]	12	High	59	25	4	—	100	0–18
Heitmiller et al[59]	3	High	40	—	0	—	—	—
Conlan et al[62]	1	High	67	(0)	0	—	—	—

Inclusion criteria: Studies reporting on ≥10 patients (total) with mucoepidermoid carcinoma.
[a] Collective review of MET through 1980.
[b] Grade 1 and 2 tumors as defined by study author.
[c] Based on seven patients for whom data is available.
[d] One additional patient experienced a local recurrence that could be successfully resected.
    Both, both high-grade and low-grade MET; Mean F/U, mean follow-up period (in months) of patients who underwent complete resection; MET type, low grade or high grade mucoepidermoid tumor; N R_0 Resect, number of patients who underwent a complete resection with no residual cancer (R_0); % Died of MET, percentage of completely resected patients who died of MET; % N1,2 POS, percentage of patients undergoing a complete resection who were found to have N1,2 nodal involvement.

thus prone to producing symptoms of obstruction such as recurrent pneumonia, hemoptysis, cough, wheezing, and dyspnea (in order of decreasing frequency).[57] However, the most common symptom is chest pain, probably because of infection.[57] Only approximately 20% of patients are asymptomatic.[57,59,74] Patients with MET can have a prolonged duration of symptoms. The average duration of symptoms was 5.5 years (range, 1 week-30 years) in a review of 29 patients reported in 1966.[63]

It is unclear how many patients have disseminated disease at the time of diagnosis because most reports are based on series of patients who have undergone resection. In a collected review of 67 patients, 27% were found to have either metastatic disease or inoperable locally advanced cancers.[64] Another series of only patients with high-grade tumors found that 42% had stage IV disease.[60] Both reports primarily involved cases that were diagnosed between 1950 and 1970 and may reflect a delay in diagnosis that is not as prevalent today. Nevertheless, the proportion of patients with advanced disease should leave no doubt about the malignant nature of MET.

Diagnosis

Because of the frequency of symptoms of obstruction, most patients with MET undergo a bronchoscopic examination. On bronchoscopy, a MET appears as a gray, exophytic, polypoid lesion covered by smooth mucosa.[57] Ten percent are located in the trachea, 15% in the mainstem bronchi, nearly 75% in a lobar or segmental bronchus.[64,74] There is discrepancy in whether MET occurs more commonly in lobar or segmental bronchi.[64,74] The differential diagnosis includes a carcinoid tumor, an adenoid cystic carcinoma, a benign tracheobronchial neoplasm, and a bronchogenic carcinoma with an unusual appearance. The patient's age, smoking history, and duration of symptoms may make a diagnosis of bronchogenic carcinoma less likely. An irregular, friable, or superficially ulcerated mass is suggestive of an adenoid cystic or a squamous cell carcinoma. A smooth

endobronchial mass located in the more proximal airways favors a mucoepidermoid carcinoma, whereas a reddish-brown smooth endoluminal tumor occurring in a segmental bronchus favors the diagnosis of a carcinoid tumor. Because adenosquamous carcinomas present as peripheral masses, it is unlikely that a diagnosis of these rare tumors will be made preoperatively. Although the histologic appearance of adenosquamous carcinoma and MET is similar, the clinical presentation of adenosquamous carcinoma precludes any confusion with mucoepidermoid carcinomas. Furthermore, the behavior of adenosquamous carcinoma suggests that these tumors should be approached in a manner similar to that of other NSCLC,[67,68,73] which makes preoperative recognition of this tumor type less important.

Endobronchial biopsy has been reported to be very useful in establishing the diagnosis of MET.[59,64] However, some authors have suggested that it may be difficult to differentiate low-grade and high-grade tumors because many high-grade tumors have areas of low-grade growth.[57] Distinguishing between these two types preoperatively may influence which staging studies are performed and may alter the operative approach, given the marked difference in propensity for malignant spread (see the following section). Serious complications during bronchoscopy have not been reported.[59,62,64]

Treatment

The mainstay of treatment of METs is surgical resection. All reported patients treated nonoperatively died of their cancer.[57,59,64] In contrast, none of the patients with a low-grade MET who underwent a complete resection died of cancer, and mean follow-up periods ranged from nearly 5 to >9 years (see Table 26–11). The only reported patient with lymph node involvement from a low-grade MET was lost to follow-up.[57] Four patients with low-grade tumors have been reported who were found to have a positive resection margin.[59,61] Two of these patients experienced a local recurrence after 2 and 9 years, and the other two patients had been followed for only 6 and 15 months.[59,61]

Data regarding the survival of patients with a high-grade MET is limited, but there is little doubt that their survival is poorer than that of patients with low-grade tumors. Many patients with high-grade tumors are found to be unresectable or can be resected only with a positive margin. All patients who were not completely resected died of cancer within 18 months, despite the use of other treatment modalities.[59,60,62] In the largest series of completely resected patients with high-grade tumors, 25% (3 of 12) experienced a recurrence.[57] The two patients with distant recurrences died, and the one patient with a local recurrence after 4 years was able to undergo a repeat resection and had no evidence of disease 7 years after the second procedure.[57] The two reported patients with a resected high-grade MET that had nodal involvement have both died of distant metastases.[57]

EDITORS' COMMENTS

Typical carcinoid tumors are clearly a distinct type of lung cancer. These tumors are definitely malignant and have the ability to metastasize and be fatal if not treated properly. However, they exhibit slow growth and are truly a low-grade type of malignancy. Whether atypical carcinoid tumors should be viewed as anything other than an NSCLC is unclear. The stage at presentation of atypical carcinoid tumors is very similar to that of NSCLC, and the outcome after resection also appears to be similar, although the data is limited. Typical and atypical carcinoid tumors may have a different etiology, as suggested by the different age distribution. Not enough research has been done regarding other demographic features of atypical carcinoid tumors to comment on similarities or differences as compared with NSCLC.

Bronchoscopy is imperative in patients who present with signs of a central mass or obstruction because it can rule out other causes of obstruction. The typical bronchoscopic appearance of a carcinoid tumor, given the appropriate clinical setting, establishes the clinical diagnosis of a carcinoid tumor quite reliably. A biopsy is safe and is able to confirm the clinical diagnosis in 80% of patients. However, because of the 20% false-negative rate and the poor ability

to differentiate a typical from an atypical carcinoid, a biopsy is unlikely to provide information that will change the management. Mediastinoscopy is indicated in patients with mediastinal lymph node enlargement, but it is not clear how the findings should affect management.

In patients with a peripheral lesion suspected of being a carcinoid tumor, a wedge resection may be appropriate to confirm the diagnosis, but definitive treatment should entail a lobectomy. A limited resection of an atypical carcinoid is likely to result in a higher recurrence rate. A limited resection may have acceptable results in patients with typical carcinoid tumors, but the error rate of frozen section examination is too high to justify not proceeding with a complete resection. Furthermore, these patients are usually young and able to tolerate a lobectomy without difficulty. There is little reason to take a chance on compromising the long-term outcome in these patients.

Central tumors can be treated with a lobectomy, sleeve lobectomy, pneumonectomy, or bronchial resection, as dictated by the location of the tumor. A margin of ≥ 5 mm should be obtained, although a larger margin may be more appropriate in the unlikely case of a central atypical tumor.

In our opinion, any resection of a carcinoid tumor, whether central or peripheral, typical or atypical, should include mediastinal lymph node dissection. Although there is no data to substantiate this approach in patients with NSCLC, a therapeutic benefit might be derived in patients with typical carcinoid tumors because of the indolent nature of these tumors. The late local recurrences, which have caused compression of airways or the superior vena cava, might be prevented by this approach. For patients with atypical tumors, better staging may allow patients to be considered for adjuvant therapy, although the benefit of such an approach remains largely speculative at present.

Surgical resection of a carcinoid tumor should be undertaken even if mediastinal lymph node involvement is present. Although the indolent nature of these tumors may result in a prolonged survival even without surgery, resection results in a number of apparent "cures." In these patients, who are mostly young, the focus should be on cure, if possible, rather than on palliative treatment. Adjuvant or neoadjuvant therapy, such as that being explored extensively in NSCLC, is reasonable in patients who have

DATA SUMMARY: MUCOEPIDERMOID TUMORS

	AMOUNT	QUALITY	CONSISTENCY
Mucoepidermoid tumor is a rare cancer that occurs in the larger airways	High	High	High
Approximately 80% of MET are low grade	Mod	Mod	High
Low-grade MET occurs in young patients, with an average age of 35 years	High	High	High
Approximately 30% of patients with MET have advanced disease at presentation	Mod	Poor	High
Complete resection of low-grade MET results in long-term survival without recurrence	Mod	Mod	High
Complete resection of high-grade MET results in survival without recurrence in most patients	Poor	Mod	—

Type of data rated: Plain text: descriptive statement   *Italics: controlled comparison*   **Bold: randomized comparison**

atypical tumors with N2 involvement. It may also be appropriate to follow patients with atypical carcinoids closely, particularly for evidence of hepatic metastases. There may be instances in which early institution of a local therapy for a metastasis (eg, cryotherapy) may result in a therapeutic or palliative benefit, although only limited data is currently available regarding such an approach.

MET is a rare tumor and is distinguished by the fact that it is located in the larger airways (trachea, mainstem bronchi, or lobar bronchi). The low-grade type of MET is more common and is likely to be present in young patients and patients in whom there is no evidence of nodal or systemic spread. In such patients, a limited resection involving a sleeve lobectomy or a bronchial (or tracheal) resection without loss of lung parenchyma is the best treatment. It is important to obtain a negative margin, but a wide margin of normal tissue is probably not necessary. Patients with a high-grade MET should be approached much the same as patients with NSCLC. There should be a low threshold for investigating possible systemic or mediastinal spread of the tumor. In patients with localized disease, resection offers the only demonstrated chance of cure, although the data is limited.

References

1. Conley YD, Cafoncelli AR, Khan JH, et al. Bronchial carcinoid tumor: experience over 20 years. Am Surg. 1992;58:670–672.
2. Vadasz P, Palffy G, Egervary M, et al. Diagnosis and treatment of bronchial carcinoid tumors: clinical and pathological review of 120 operated patients. Eur J Cardiothorac Surg. 1993;7:8–11.
3. World Health Organization. The World Health Organization histological typing of lung tumours (2nd ed). Am J Clin Pathol. 1982;77:123–136.
4. Rosai J. Ackerman's surgical pathology. 6th ed. St. Louis, Mo: CV Mosby; 1981.
5. Carter D, Eggleston JC. Tumors of the lower respiratory tract. Washington, DC: Armed Forces Institute of Pathology; 1980.
6. Godwin JD II. Carcinoid tumors: an analysis of 2837 cases. Cancer. 1975;36:560–569.
7. Arrigoni MG, Woolner LB, Bernatz PE. Atypical carcinoid tumors of the lung. J Thorac Cardiovasc Surg. 1972;64:413–421.
8. Paladugu RR, Benfield JR, Pak HY, et al. Bronchopulmonary Kulchitzky cell carcinomas: a new classification scheme for typical and atypical carcinoids. Cancer. 1985;55:1301–1311.
9. Mills S, Walker AN, Cooper PH, et al. Atypical carcinoid tumor of the lung: a clinicopathologic study of 17 cases. Am J Surg Pathol. 1982;6:643–654.
10. DeCaro LF, Paladugu R, Benfield JR, et al. Typical and atypical carcinoids within the pulmonary APUD tumor spectrum. J Thorac Cardiovasc Surg. 1983;86:528–536.
11. Travis WD, Rush W, Flieder DB, et al. Survival analysis of 200 pulmonary neuroendocrine tumors with clarification of criteria for atypical carcinoid and its separation from typical carcinoid. Am J Surg Pathol. 1998;22:934–944.
12. Travis WD, Gal AA, Colby TV. Reproducibility of neuroendocrine lung tumor classification. Hum Pathol. 1998;29:272–279.
13. Davila DG, Dunn WF, Tazelaar HD, et al. Bronchial carcinoid tumors. Mayo Clin Proc. 1993;68:795–803.
14. Whitwell F. Tumourlets of the lung. J Pathol Bacteriol. 1955;70:529–541.
15. Brandt B III, Heintz SE, Rose EF, et al. Bronchial carcinoid tumors. Ann Thorac Surg. 1984;38:63–65.
16. Ducrocq X, Thomas P, Massard G, et al. Operative risk and prognostic factors of typical bronchial carcinoid tumors. Ann Thorac Surg. 1998;65:1410–1414.
17. Hurt R, Bates M. Carcinoid tumours of the bronchus: a 33 year experience. Thorax. 1984;39:617–623.
18. Mårtensson H, Böttcher G, Hambraeus G, et al. Bronchial carcinoids: an analysis of 91 cases. World J Surg. 1987;11:356–364.
19. Bertelsen S, Aasted A, Lund C, et al. Bronchial carcinoid tumours: a clinicopathologic study of 82 cases. Scand J Thorac Cardiovasc Surg. 1985;19:105–111.
20. Harpole DH Jr, Feldman JM, Buchanan S, et al. Bronchial carcinoid tumors: a retrospective analysis of 126 patients. Ann Thorac Surg. 1992;54:50–55.
21. Rea F, Binda R, Spreafico G, et al. Bronchial carcinoids: a review of 60 patients. Ann Thorac Surg. 1989;47:412–414.
22. Schreurs JM, Westermann CJJ, van den Bosch JMM, et al. A twenty-five-year follow-up of ninety-three resected typical carcinoid tumors of the lung. J Thorac Cardiovasc Surg. 1992;104:1470–1475.
23. Okike N, Bernatz PE, Woolner LB. Carcinoid tumors of the lung. Ann Thorac Surg. 1976;22:270–277.
24. McCaughan BC, Martini N, Bains MS. Bronchial carcinoids: review of 124 cases. J Thorac Cardiovasc Surg. 1985;89:8–17.
25. Francioni E, Rendina EA, Venuta F, et al. Low grade neuroendocrine tumours of the lung (bronchial carcinoids): 25 years experience. Eur J Cardiothorac Surg. 1990;4:472–476.
26. Soga J, Yakuwa Y. Bronchopulmonary carcinoids: an analysis of 1875 reported cases with special reference to a comparison between typical carcinoids and atypical varieties. Ann Thorac Cardiovasc Surg. 1999;5:211–219.
27. Stamatis G, Freitag L, Greschuchna D. Limited and radical resection for tracheal and bronchopulmonary carcinoid tumour: report on 227 cases. Eur J Cardiothorac Surg. 1990;4:527–533.
28. Wilkins EW Jr, Grillo HC, Moncure AC, et al. Changing times in surgical management of bronchopulmonary carcinoid tumor. Ann Thorac Surg. 1984;38:339–344.
29. Warren WH, Faber LP, Gould VE. Neuroendocrine neoplasms of the lung. J Thorac Cardiovasc Surg. 1989;98:321–332.
30. Marty-Ané C-H, Costes V, Pujol J-L, et al. Carcinoid tumors of the lung: do atypical features require aggressive management? Ann Thorac Surg. 1995;59:78–83.
31. Todd TR, Cooper JD, Weissberg D, et al. Bronchial carcinoid tumors: twenty years' experience. J Thorac Cardiovasc Surg. 1980;79:532–536.
32. Chughtai TS, Morin JE, Sheiner NM, et al. Bronchial carcinoid—twenty years' experience defines a selective surgical approach. Surgery. 1997;122:801–808.
33. Attar S, Miller JE, Hankins J, et al. Bronchial adenoma: a review of 51 patients. Ann Thorac Surg. 1985;40:126–132.
34. Ricci C, Patrassi N, Massa R, et al. Carcinoid syndrome in bronchial adenoma. Am J Surg. 1973;126:671–677.
35. Limper AH, Carpenter PC, Scheithauer B, et al. The Cushing syndrome induced by bronchial carcinoid tumors. Ann Intern Med. 1992;117:209–214.
36. Pass HI, Doppman JL, Nieman L, et al. Management of the ectopic ACTH syndrome due to thoracic carcinoids. Ann Thorac Surg. 1990;50:52–57.
37. Shrager JB, Wright CD, Wain JC, et al. Bronchopulmonary carcinoid tumors associated with Cushing's syndrome: a more aggressive variant of typical carcinoid. J Thorac Cardiovasc Surg. 1997;114:367–375.
38. Garcia-Luna PP, Leal-Cerro A, Montero C, et al. A rare cause of acromegaly: ectopic production of growth hormone-releasing factor by a bronchial carcinoid tumor. Surg Neurol. 1987;27:563–568.
39. Carroll DG, Delahunt JW, Teague CA, et al. Resolution of acromegaly after removal of a bronchial carcinoid shown to secrete growth hormone releasing factor. Aust N Z J Med. 1987;17:63–67.
40. Sönksen PH, Ayres AB, Braimbridge M, et al. Acromegaly caused by pulmonary carcinoid tumours. Clin Endocrinol. 1976;5:503–513.
41. Docherty HM, Heath DA. Multiple forms of parathyroid hormone-like proteins in a human tumour. J Molec Endocrinol. 1989;2:11–20.
42. Marsh HM, Martin JK, Kvols LK, et al. Carcinoid crisis during anesthesia: successful treatment with a somatostatin analogue. Anesthesiology. 1987;66:89–91.
43. Martini N, Zaman MB, Bains MS, et al. Treatment and prognosis in bronchial carcinoids involving regional lymph nodes. J Thorac Cardiovasc Surg. 1994;107:1–7.
44. Ceresoli G, Panucci MG, Reni M, et al. Atypical bronchial carcinoid tumor (ABCT): retrospective analysis of a single-institution series of 22 cases [abstract]. Lung Cancer. 1998;21(suppl 1):S40.
45. Wilkins EW Jr, Darling RC, Soutter L, et al. A continuing clinical

survey of adenomas of the trachea and bronchus in a general hospital. J Thorac Cardiovasc Surg. 1963;46:279–289.

46. Rozenman J, Pausner R, Lieberman Y, et al. Bronchial adenoma. Chest. 1987;92:145–147.

47. Turnbull AD, Huvos AG, Goodner JT, et al. The malignant potential of bronchial adenoma. Ann Thorac Surg. 1972;14:453–464.

48. Moertel CG, Kvols LK, O'Connell MJ, et al. Treatment of neuroendocrine carcinomas with combined etoposide and cisplatin: evidence of major therapeutic activity in the anaplastic variants of these neoplasms. Cancer. 1991;68:227–232.

49. van Boxem TJ, Venmans BJ, van Mourik JC, et al. Bronchoscopic treatment of intraluminal typical carcinoid: a pilot study. J Thorac Cardiovasc Surg 1998;116:402–406.

50. Ginsberg RJ, Rubinstein LV, for the Lung Cancer Study Group. Randomized trial of lobectomy versus limited resection for T1 N0 non-small cell lung cancer. Ann Thorac Surg. 1995;60:615–623.

51. Rubinstein LV, Ginsberg RJ. Reply to "Randomized trial of lobectomy versus limited resection for T1 N0 non-small cell lung cancer," 1995 article by the Lung Cancer Study Group. Ann Thorac Surg. 1996;62:1249–1250.

52. Åberg T, Blöndal T, Nõu E, et al. The choice of operation for bronchial carcinoids. Ann Thorac Surg. 1981;32:19–22.

53. Kayser K, Anyanwu E, Bauer H-G, et al. Tumor presence at resection boundaries and lymph-node metastasis in bronchial carcinoma patients. Thorac Cardiovasc Surg. 1993;41:308–311.

54. Kirschner PA Discussion of Okike N, Bernatz PE, Wodner LB. Carcinoid tumors of the lung. Ann Thorac Surg. 1976;22:270–277.

55. Smetana HF, Iverson L, Swan LL. Bronchogenic carcinoma: analysis of 100 autopsy cases. Milit Surg. 1952;3:335.

56. Liebow AA. Tumors of the lower respiratory tract. In: Atlas of Tumor Pathology. Washington, DC: Armed Forces Institute of Pathology; 1952:26–53.

57. Yousem SA, Hochholzer L. Mucoepidermoid tumors of the lung. Cancer. 1987;60:1346–1352.

58. Axelsson C, Burcharth F, Johansen A. Mucoepidermoid lung tumors. J Thorac Cardiovasc Surg. 1973;65:902–908.

59. Heitmiller RF, Mathisen DJ, Ferry JA, et al. Mucoepidermoid lung tumors. Ann Thorac Surg. 1989;47:394–399.

60. Turnbull AD, Huvos AG, Goodner JT, et al. Mucoepidermoid tumors of bronchial glands. Cancer. 1971;28:539–544.

61. Leonardi HK, Jung-Legg Y, Legg MA, et al. Tracheobronchial mucoepidermoid carcinoma: clinicopathological features and results of treatment. J Thorac Cardiovasc Surg. 1978;76:431–438.

62. Conlan AA, Payne WS, Woolner LB, et al. Adenoid cystic carcinoma (cylindroma) and mucoepidermoid carcinoma of the bronchus: factors affecting survival. J Thorac Cardiovasc Surg. 1978;76:369–377.

63. Reichle FA, Rosemond GP. Mucoepidermoid tumors of the bronchus. J Thorac Cardiovasc Surg. 1966;51:443–448.

64. Breyer RH, Dainauskas JR, Jensik RJ, et al. Mucoepidermoid carcinoma of the trachea and bronchus: the case for conservative resection. Ann Thorac Surg. 1980;29:198–204.

65. Seo S, Warren J, Mirkin D, et al. Mucoepidermoid carcinoma of the bronchus in a 4-year-old child. Cancer. 1984;53:1600–1604.

66. Klacsmann PG, Olson JL, Eggleston JC. Mucoepidermoid carcinoma of the bronchus: an electron microscopic study of the low grade and the high grade variants. Cancer. 1979;43:1720–1733.

67. Takamori S, Noguchi M, Morinaga S, et al. Clinicopathologic characteristics of adenosquamous carcinoma of the lung. Cancer. 1991;67:649–654.

68. Shimizu J, Oda M, Hayashi Y, et al. A clinicopathologic study of resected cases of adenosquamous carcinoma of the lung. Chest. 1996;109:989–994.

69. Noda S, Sundaresan S, Mendeloff EN. Tracheal mucoepidermoid carcinoma in a 7-year-old child. Ann Thorac Surg. 1998;66:928–929.

70. Granata C, Battistini E, Toma P, et al. Mucoepidermoid carcinoma of the bronchus: a case report and review of the literature. Pediatr Pulmonol. 1997;23:226–232.

71. Lack EE, Harris CBG, Eraklis AJ, et al. Primary bronchial tumors in childhood: a clinicopathologic study of six cases. Cancer. 1983;51:492–497.

72. Sridhar KS, Bounassi MJ, Raub W Jr, et al. Clinical features of adenosquamous lung carcinoma in 127 patients. Am Rev Resp Dis. 1990;142:19–23.

73. Naunheim KS, Taylor JR, Skosey C, et al. Adenosquamous lung carcinoma: clinical characteristics, treatment, and prognosis. Ann Thorac Surg. 1987;44:462–466.

74. Kim TS, Lee KS, Han J, et al. Mucoepidermoid carcinoma of the tracheobronchial tree: radiographic and CT findings in 12 patients. Radiology. 1999;212:643–648.

BRONCHIOLOALVEOLAR CARCINOMA

Frank C. Detterbeck, David R. Jones, and William K. Funkhouser, Jr.

Bronchioloalveolar cancer (BAC), also known as *alveolar cell cancer,* is classified as a subtype of adenocarcinoma. However, this entity has several unique features that justify discussion as a special type of lung cancer. There is evidence that the incidence has been increasing, and BAC may have an etiology that is different from other lung cancers. The clinical presentation is different, in that nodal metastases and distant metastases are less common than in other types of non–small cell lung cancer (NSCLC). Furthermore, the radiographic presentation of disease in the chest is varied. It may present as a solitary pulmonary nodule, a lobar infiltrate, multiple nodules, or diffuse bilateral pulmonary involvement. Because of this, it has been suggested that this cancer may be able to spread throughout the lung via aerogenous dissemination.

INCIDENCE

Although there are no studies directly addressing the actual incidence of BAC, the reported proportion of BAC varies between 2% and 37% of all lung cancers.[1,2] Most of the available reports from 1980 to 2000 are summarized in Table 27–1, where they have been arranged chronologically. Whether the series were based on local pathology records or surgical series of patients having resections does not seem to matter. Similarly, whether or not a pathologic review was performed to ensure that cases were appropriately classified seems to have had little influence.

In general, there appears to be a significant increase in the proportion of BAC. Indeed, most of the increased incidence of adenocarcinoma has been reported to be due to an increased occurrence of BAC.[3,4] It is difficult to dismiss this increase as being due completely to changing definitions because, in most of these series, all cases were retrospectively reviewed and classified according to standard World Health Organization (WHO) definitions.[5] It is

also not possible to simply ascribe the increased proportion of BAC to the experience of one institution because it has been reported by several investigators, including the Lung Cancer Study Group. However, a few studies have failed to find an increasing occurrence.[1,6,7] It may be that no increase in BAC was found in these studies because they extended back to an earlier time when the incidence of BAC was still lower[7] or because they focused on the four major histologic types of lung cancer and did not provide truly accurate data on histologic subtypes, such as BAC.[1,6] In conclusion, although there is conflicting data, the majority of studies supports an increased proportion of BAC among lung cancers.

HISTOLOGIC DEFINITION

Criteria for classification of a tumor as a BAC have been established and are used consistently.[5,8] These criteria follow:

1. No extrathoracic primary adenocarcinoma
2. Not a central bronchogenic cancer
3. Peripheral location
4. No distortion of lung interstitium
5. Neoplastic cells growing along alveolar spaces.

Nevertheless, some difficulties still exist in interpretation of these criteria.[9–11] Many adenocarcinomas may exhibit a bronchioloalveolar type of pattern at the periphery of the tumor.[12] Some authors have included *mixed tumors* (adenocarcinoma and BAC) as BAC if the predominant pattern was that of BAC.[13–16] It has been suggested that tumors be classified as BAC only if the entire neoplasm meets WHO criteria, excluding those with foci of poorly differentiated adenocarcinoma.[12] Many pathologists have adopted this policy, but there is potential for institutional biases toward more liberal criteria. Unfortunately, most papers do not

TABLE 27-1. OVERALL INCIDENCE OF BRONCHIOLOALVEOLAR CANCER

STUDY	YEARS	N WITH BAC	TYPE OF SERIES	PATH REVIEW[a]	INCIDENCE (%)
Devesa et al[1]	1969-1971	479	Registry	No	3
Barsky et al[15 b,c]	1971-1975	21	Pathologic	Yes	8
Rossing[94]	1955-1978	241	Pathologic	No	4
Auerbach and Garfinkel[4 c]	1973-1978	8	Pathologic	No	9
Greco et al[19]	1969-1983	122	Pathologic	No	4
Heikkila[13 b]	1961-1983	92	Surgical	Yes	4
Daly et al[18]	1976-1983	140	Surgical	Yes	3
Harpole[46]	1970-1985	205	Pathologic	No	3
Ikeda[49]	1982-1985	36	Pathologic	No	15[d]
Devesa et al[1]	1984-1986	675	Registry	No	2
Grover et al[8]	1977-1988	235	Surgical	Yes	15
Auerbach and Garfinkel[4]	1973-1989	74	Pathologic	No	15
Barsky et al[15 b]	1955-1990	184	Pathologic	Yes	12
Linnoila et al[2 e]	1984-1989	92	—	Yes	37
Auerbach and Garfinkel[4 c,e]	1986-1989	25	Pathologic	No	20
Barsky et al[15 b,c,e]	1986-1990	66	Pathologic	Yes	24
Dumont et al[7]	1975-1993	105	Surgical	No	4

Inclusion criteria: Studies reporting on the proportion of BAC among NSCLC patients and including ≥20 patients with BAC.
[a] All cases of BAC and adenocarcinoma reviewed to ensure appropriate classification.
[b] Included tumors with foci of adenocarcinoma.
[c] Based on a subset of the entire group.
[d] Only nonmucinous BAC.
[e] Includes both BAC and papillary adenocarcinoma.
[f] NSCLC only.
BAC, bronchioloalveolar cancer; NSCLC, non–small cell lung cancer; Pathologic, series based on review of pathology records or registries; Registry, series based on records from a regional or national registry; Surgical, surgical series (all patients underwent surgery).

provide details on how stringent or liberal their classification policy is. Some authors have specifically included tumors with nuclear pleomorphism[15] or areas of solid adenocarcinoma,[13-17] but most simply state that standard WHO criteria were used.[7,8,18,19]

In one study addressing the accuracy of a pathologic diagnosis of BAC, 29% of BAC cases were reclassified as adenocarcinoma on pathologic review, whereas 17% of adenocarcinomas were reclassified as BAC.[11] A blinded study of consistency of classification of lung cancer among five pathologists found the least agreement in BAC.[10] Agreement of at least four of five pathologists occurred in only 53% of cases, although at least three of five agreed in 97%.[10]

BAC has been divided into *mucinous* and *nonmucinous*

subtypes.[9,14,18,20] In addition, some authors also distinguish a *sclerotic* subtype.[9,15] The distinction between the mucinous and nonmucinous types is reasonably clear, although some reports include a group of mixed tumors that exhibit both mucinous and nonmucinous characteristics.[14,18] The nonmucinous subtype is seen in approximately 50% of cases, whereas the mucinous type is seen in 33% (Table 27-2). The definition of tumors as sclerotic is more difficult. Sclerotic tumors are similar to nonmucinous BAC, but they contain a central area of sclerosis.[9,12] However, many BACs contain some foci of scar.[9,14,17,21] As a result, many authors have not classified any of the BACs as sclerotic. At any rate, this does not appear to be a common subtype.

A more consistent observation is that approximately 25%

TABLE 27-2. DISTRIBUTION OF HISTOLOGIC SUBTYPES OF BRONCHIOLOALVEOLAR CANCER (%)

STUDY	N	MUCINOUS	NONMUCINOUS	SCLEROTIC	MIXED	POORLY DIFFERENTIATED
Daly et al[18]	134	41	45	—	14	—
Barsky et al[15]	122	42	48	12	—	20
Okubo et al[17]	119	22	69	—	9	—
Elson et al[95]	115	44	56	—	—	—
Dumont et al[7]	97	43	57	—	—	—
Tao et al[16]	85	35[a]	65[a]	—	—	29
Clayton[9]	72	22	39	39	—	—
Régnard et al[48]	70	51	24	11	13	—
Albertine et al[47]	54	19	61	—	20	—
Manning et al[14]	42	21	60	—	19	29[b]
Average		**34**	**52**	**—**	**15**	**26**

Inclusion criteria: Studies of ≥40 patients with bronchioloalveolar cancer reporting histologic subtypes.
[a] Mucinous-nonmucinous classification excluded poorly differentiated cases.
[b] Cases that contained a focus of adenocarcinoma.

of BACs show areas of poorly differentiated tumor.[14–16,18] This finding was significantly more common in the sclerotic subtype (42% sclerotic, 27% mucinous, 10% nonmucinous; $P < 0.05$) in the study by Barsky et al,[15] more commonly associated with the mucinous subtype (36% mucinous, 13% nonmucinous and mixed, P not reported) in the study by Daly et al,[18] and more frequently associated with nonmucinous tumors (40% versus 22%, $P = $ NS) in the study by Manning et al.[14] It has been suggested that these tumors with areas of poor differentiation portend a poor prognosis.[15,16] However, it may be most appropriate to classify these tumors as adenocarcinoma and not as BAC, as discussed earlier.[12]

The cell of origin of BAC has been debated. It appears likely that the mucinous type arises from bronchial mucous cells, whereas the nonmucinous type exhibits morphologic similarities to Clara cells or, less commonly, type II pneumocytes.[21–23] However, this classification can be difficult and furthermore does not appear to be of any prognostic or clinical significance.

ETIOLOGY

Although the etiology of BAC is unclear, several interesting hypotheses have been put forth. This tumor bears a striking resemblance to a disease known as *jaagsiekte* or pulmonary adenomatosis in sheep.[24] This is a diffuse pulmonary disease that has an appearance identical to human BAC by histology and ultrastructure analysis.[24] In later stages, the sheep develop copious watery bronchorrhea and distant organ metastases. This disease is mediated by a retrovirus and can easily be passed from one sheep to another or passed by pulmonary inoculation with infected sputum.[24] However, only two cases have been reported of BAC arising in human beings exposed to affected sheep.[25,26] Although intranuclear inclusions can be seen in some human BACs, these may be more consistent with type II cell differentiation than viral components,[12] and no virus has ever been isolated from human beings.[23]

Anecdotal reports of familial clusters of BAC have been reported.[27–29] Similarly, there have been anecdotal reports of BAC in association with congenital cystic adenomatoid malformation.[30–32] The youngest reported patient is a 7-year-old girl who developed bilateral BAC following chemotherapy and radiation for Hodgkin's disease.[33] Other anecdotal reports following chemotherapy or immunosuppression would seem to corroborate the possibility of a viral etiology.[23,34]

BAC has also been postulated to represent malignant degeneration of a similar-appearing benign lesion known as *atypical adenomatous hyperplasia* (AAH).[35–37] These are small (<5 mm) nodules found incidentally in patients with lung cancer.[35,38] These lesions are found in few patients with squamous cancer (3%-7%), in a moderate number of patients with adenocarcinomas (10%-35%), and in a higher number of patients with BAC (18%).[35,38,39] Many of these lesions show significant cellular atypia, particularly with increasing size.[35,37,38] A detailed morphometric and immunohistochemical study suggested a continuum of changes from benign typical alveolar epithelial hyperplasia to AAH and eventually to overt BAC.[37] Several other investigators came to remarkably similar conclusions through somewhat different lines of research.[36,38,40] These findings provide a moderate amount of evidence that AAH may represent a premalignant lesion.

The concept of cancer arising from a pulmonary scar is an old one, but proponents of this concept persist.[4,13] In fact, the incidence of scar carcinomas may be increasing,[41] and sclerosing BAC may account for a large proportion of these scar carcinomas.[12,13,22,23] Debate continues regarding whether the fibrosis is induced by the tumor or whether the scar somehow causes malignant degeneration.[23] Some laboratory data suggests that the scar is due to newly formed (rather than pre-existing) collagen.[42,43] An analysis of the size and morphology of the scar in both the primary tumor and metastases also suggests that the scar is a desmoplastic response to the tumor.[44]

EPIDEMIOLOGY

BAC has been reported to occur in patients ranging in age from 7 to 89 years.[33,45] The average age at the time of diagnosis is approximately 60 years (range, 58-65 years).[7,13,15,17–19,21,46–48] There does not appear to be a striking age difference relative to other lung cancers, although the average age of patients with BAC was found to be slightly younger in the only study that analyzed this (59.2 versus 64; $P < 0.05$).[15] Much more impressive is the widely consistent finding that BAC presents more commonly in women (male to female ratio, 1:1 to 1.4:1) than other lung cancers, which have a strong male preponderance.[8,15,19,21,46,47] Three studies found a male to female ratio of approximately 2:1,[13,17,48] whereas only one found a ratio similar to that seen in other NSCLCs (6:1).[7]

The role of smoking in the development of BAC is unclear. It is often stated that smoking is not as commonly associated with BAC as with other cancers.[8,11,15,19,22,23,48,49] The Lung Cancer Study Group found that patients with BAC are more likely to have no history of smoking relative to patients with a non-BAC adenocarcinoma ($P < .001$).[8] On the other hand, although many patients with BAC are nonsmokers, it appears that smoking increases the risk of developing BAC. In two epidemiologic case control studies, smoking increased the risk of BAC in a dose- and duration-dependent fashion.[50,51]

BAC has been reported to be more common in people employed in construction, motor freight occupations, wood and paper mill industries, and sugar cane farming.[23] This was corroborated in a case control series involving 21 patients with definite BAC and 101 controls matched by age, gender, and location of residence.[50] The risk was most marked for people involved in motor freight occupations for 10 or more years (odds ratio, 4.4). However, for each of the occupations analyzed (motor freight, construction, mechanics, petroleum refining, and sugar cane farming), the confidence intervals of the odds ratios were wide and had a lower limit of <1, indicating a lack of statistical significance for the associations noted in this relatively small series.[50]

NATURAL HISTORY

Little information is available about the natural history of untreated patients with BAC. Fitzpatrick et al[52] reported on

DATA SUMMARY: BRONCHIOLOALVEOLAR CANCER—EPIDEMIOLOGIC ASPECTS

	AMOUNT	QUALITY	CONSISTENCY
The incidence of BAC may be increasing	High	High	Mod
The male to female ratio for BAC is ~1 : 1	High	High	Mod
BAC occurs in younger patients more than other NSCLCs	Poor	Poor	—
BAC is less associated with smoking than other NSCLCs	Poor	High	—
~50% of BACs are nonmucinous	High	High	Mod
~33% of BACs are mucinous	High	High	Mod

Type of data rated: Plain text: descriptive statement   *Italics: controlled comparison*   **Bold: randomized comparison**

20 patients with solitary BAC who had not undergone resection (3 patients had radiotherapy [RT]). Most of these patients had had radiographic evidence of a lesion for several years before a histologic diagnosis was made. Starting from the time the lesion was noted radiographically, the (absolute) survival was 50% at 1 year, 33% at 3 years, and 8% at both 5 and 10 years.[52] The reports of patients who have been followed for long periods (11-15 years) certainly corroborate that a protracted natural history can be seen occasionally.[53–55] It is interesting that this natural history data closely parallels data about indolent growth in the small percentage of patients who exhibit a long interval from first radiographic diagnosis to pathologic confirmation.[56]

In contrast, patients with diffuse disease had an average survival of 4 months, and there were no 3-year survivors in a report of 31 patients who were not curatively resected (10 received radiation).[57] Another report of 16 patients with unresected diffuse disease (9 received chemotherapy or radiation) found no 2-year survivors.[58] Nearly 50% of those with diffuse disease die of respiratory failure.[59] The site of distant metastases in advanced disease involves the opposite lung in >50% of patients.[60,61]

CLINICAL PRESENTATION

A relatively consistent finding in reports from 1980 to 2000 was that 50% to 60% of patients are asymptomatic at the time of presentation (Table 27–3).[7,13,14,17–19,48] Cough is the most common symptom, occurring in ~33% of patients, although sputum production is seen in only ~25% of patients. Constitutional symptoms suggesting advanced disease, such as fatigue and weight loss, are rarely seen. Several authors have indicated that symptomatic patients have a poorer prognosis compared with asymptomatic patients (5-year survival: 0% versus 70%,[13] 19% versus 37%,[46] 23% versus 56%[19]; no *P* values reported; 14% versus 55%, *P* < .001[48]). This is not surprising because symptoms (either local or constitutional) have been associated with advanced stage disease.[19,46] In one study, 70% of asymptomatic patients were stage I, as opposed to 29% of symptomatic patients.[19] In another study, univariate analysis disclosed that the presence of practically any symptom was associated with advanced stage disease with a high degree of statistical significance.[46]

On rare occasions, BAC can present with some highly unusual symptoms. The amount of frothy bronchorrhea experienced by some patients can be striking. Sputum

production of up to 3 to 4 L per day has been described and can be severe enough to lead to dehydration and protein and electrolyte imbalances.[23,45,62–65] In an earlier review, which contained more patients with advanced disease than what is seen in current series, 27% of patients were found to have at least moderate amounts of bronchorrhea (>90 mL/day).[45] However, in a more recent review of 272 cases in which data about symptoms was specifically mentioned, the incidence of significant bronchorrhea was only 7%.[66] This review also noted that significant bronchorrhea is generally a sign of advanced disease and carries a poor prognosis.[66] Attempts to treat this problem symptomatically with steroids,[62,65,68] atropine,[65,68] adrenocorticotropic hormone, stellate ganglion blocks,[22] or inhaled indomethacin[67] have been partially successful. Chemotherapy has been unsuccessful.[62,65,68] Palliative radiation (~20 Gy) dramatically reduced bronchorrhea in two cases,[54,63] but others suggested no benefit.[69]

At least three cases have been described in which areas of lobar consolidation from BAC resulted in severe hypoxemia due to a physiologic shunt.[64,70,71] In these carefully documented cases, the degree of hypoxemia was striking and resolved instantaneously in two patients during balloon occlusion of the pulmonary artery.[70,71] Surgical resection in each of these patients resulted in dramatic resolution of the hypoxemia.[64,70,71]

RADIOGRAPHIC PRESENTATION

An interesting feature of BAC is that the radiographic presentation is varied. The tumor can present as a well

TABLE 27–3. SYMPTOMS AT PRESENTATION (%)

REFERENCE	18	19	48	14	13[a]	61[b]
Number of Patients	134	122	70	42	33	25
Asymptomatic	68	58	46	50	48	4
Cough	22	35	20	31	42	60
Sputum production	17	24	11	5	36	68
Dyspnea	4	15	9	24	—	56
Chest pain	10	7	9	2	15	40
Fever	3	8	—	—	21	—
Hemoptysis	4	11	9	2	6	16
Fatigue	3	—	—	—	21	84[c]
Weight loss	4	13	9	—	6	56
Other	4	24	19	—	15	24

Inclusion criteria: Studies reporting symptoms in ≥20 patients with BAC.
[a]Only patients with typical BAC.
[b]All patients with metastatic disease.
[c]Performance status >0.
BAC, bronchioloalveolar cancer.

TABLE 27–4. DISTRIBUTION OF RADIOGRAPHIC PRESENTATION OF BRONCHIOLOALVEOLAR CANCER (%)

STUDY	TYPE OF SERIES	N	SOLITARY NODULE	LOCALIZED INFILTRATE	MULTIFOCAL NODULES	DIFFUSE OR BILATERAL DISEASE
Harpole et al[46]	Pathologic	205	58[a]	28	—	14
Barsky et al[15 b]	Pathologic	122	38	37[c]	22	3
Greco et al[19]	Pathologic	122	(88)[d]	(3)[d]	—	9
Clayton[21]	Pathologic	45	29	33[d]	29	9
Daly et al[318 e]	Surgical	134	69[a,c]	31[a,c]	10	7
Okubo et al[17]	Surgical	119	67	13	8	12
Heikkila[13 b]	Surgical	92	86[a]	14	—	0[f]
Régnard et al[48]	Surgical	70	60	30	—	10
Albertine et al[47]	Surgical	54	70	19	7	4
Average[g]			**60**	**26**	**15**	**8**
Edgerton et al[66]	Historical[h]	650	—63—		16	21
Storey et al[45]	Historical[h]	153	29	37	11	23

Inclusion criteria: Studies including ≥50 patients with bronchioloalveolar cancer and reporting radiographic data.
[a]Mostly solitary lesions, but may have included some multiple nodules.
[b]Includes tumors with focal adenocarcinoma.
[c]Mostly solitary lesions, but may have included some bilateral cases.
[d]Vague definitions.
[e]Values do not add up to 100 because values given for solitary nodule included multiple nodules and bilateral disease.
[f]Not explicitly stated, but implied.
[g]Excluding values in parentheses
[h]Historical review of cases from 20 to 50 years ago.
Diffuse or bilateral disease, includes infiltrates or multiple nodules; Localized infiltrate, infiltrate or consolidation with indistinct borders confined to one lobe or one lung (may occasionally not be strictly solitary, but lobulated or multifocal); Multifocal nodules, discrete nodules confined to one lobe or lung; Solitary nodule, discrete single nodule or mass.

circumscribed solitary nodule or mass. It can also appear as an infiltrate involving a portion of a lobe, an entire lobe, or even an entire lung. It can present as multiple nodules within one lobe, within one lung, or bilaterally. Finally, the disease can also present as a diffuse bilateral infiltrate. In this chapter (Table 27–4), these different radiographic presentations have been grouped into categories that are likely to be viewed differently from a clinical standpoint: a solitary pulmonary nodule, a localized infiltrate or consolidation, multifocal nodules localized to one lobe, and bilateral disease (either widely scattered nodules or a diffuse infiltrate).

The solitary nodular form is the most common, occurring in approximately 60% of patients. The next most common is an infiltrate localized to a single lobe or portion of one lung. This is true not only in surgical series, which would likely be biased toward solitary, resectable lesions, but also in pathologic series. Multifocal nodules localized in one lobe or lung, and especially bilateral or diffuse forms, are not as common. However, two earlier reviews showed that at least 20% of patients presented with a diffuse, bilateral form.[45,66] It seems likely that these earlier reports included more patients with advanced disease.[45,66]

Approximately 60% of solitary BAC occurs in the upper lobes.[18,72,73] The infiltrative lobar form may not have a predilection for a particular location.[69,74] An air bronchogram is seen on plain chest radiograph (CXR) in approximately 20% of patients, and a tail extending to the pleura is seen in approximately 20% also.[11,19,55] These findings are seen in <5% of other lung cancers.[11] Cavitation is seen in about 10% of BAC cases,[11,19,55] and a pleural effusion is present in 30%.[55]

By computed tomography (CT) scan, solitary nodular BAC has been found to have the following characteristics: peripheral location (69%–91%), spiculation (44%–78%), pleural tags (50%–77%), and pseudocavitation or low at-tenuation (19%–60%).[74–76] One study of 22 patients with solitary BAC found air bronchograms by CT in 95%.[76] The following CT characteristics have been noted with the infiltrative lobar form: low attenuation or cystic areas (50%–88%), CT angiogram sign (30%–33%), fissural bulging (25%–63%), and air bronchograms (39%–100%).[74,76,77] However, studies have reported conflicting results regarding the predictive power of any of these findings, and the suspicion of BAC on the basis of radiographic appearance remains very subjective.[76–79] In a blinded study, radiologists were able to identify BAC in only 75% of cases, and the false positive rate of a high probability ranking for BAC was approximately 60%.[75] Positron emission tomography (PET) scan has limited utility in patients suspected of having BAC because it has been found to be negative in many patients with BAC.[80,81]

It is frequently mentioned in earlier series that BAC may present with indolent growth and may have been visible for years on CXR.[22] In contemporary series, however, this is not noted, probably because pulmonary lesions are generally not followed in the current era. The fact that so many patients in contemporary series present with an asymptomatic lesion on CXR provides a circumstantial argument that there may be a long period of indolent growth that provides enough time for an incidental CXR to have been taken.[13,14,18,19] Indeed, many older series, and those in which some patients were followed, report patients with nodules that were either stable or enlarged only slightly over 2 to 13 years.[7,52–54,72,82] Hawkins et al analyzed 17 cases of BAC in which a prior film was available and found that the lesion had been visible for ≥2 years in >50% of the cases, and ≥5 years in 25% of the cases.[56]

DIAGNOSIS

The ability to diagnose BAC without subjecting the patient to a thoracotomy is <50% in most series of patients with

TABLE 27–5. METHODS OF DIAGNOSIS

| STUDY | N | % WITH POSITIVE RESULT | | | PREOPERATIVE DIAGNOSIS (%) |
		Sputum	Bronchoscopy	FNA	
Edgerton et al[66]	650	33	26	—	51
Harpole et al[46]	205	19	26	74	—
Daly et al[18]	134	18	43[a]	50[b]	31
Greco et al[19]	122	28	14	61	23
Elson et al[95] c	116	45	27	83	60
Tao et al[16] c	101	38	25	95	66
Heikkila[13] c	92	21	13	83	43
Average		**29**	**25**	**75**	**46**

Inclusion criteria: Studies including ≥50 patients with bronchioloalveolar cancer and reporting method of diagnosis.
[a]51% with transbronchial biopsy; 27% with washings alone.
[b]Only 4 patients.
[c]Includes tumors with focal adenocarcinoma.
FNA, fine needle aspiration.

solitary pulmonary nodules (Table 27–5). Transbronchial biopsy appears to be somewhat more effective than sputum analysis and bronchoscopic washings alone.[18] Fine needle aspiration, which is probably used primarily for patients with discrete masses, has shown a somewhat better yield. However, for those patients with diffuse involvement, the rate of diagnosis with sputum cytology is approximately 80%.[16] A high rate of establishing a diagnosis by sputum or bronchoscopic cytology in cases of diffuse disease has also been noted by others.[7,18,19,46]

CLINICAL STAGING

It is important to know which tests (head CT, bone scan, mediastinoscopy) are indicated for a patient with a suspected BAC. In actual practice, however, these patients will likely be approached as any patient suspected of having NSCLC would be, because in the majority of cases, a histologic diagnosis of BAC will not be available. Nevertheless, for those patients for whom a diagnosis of BAC is available or strongly suspected, it is useful to consider which staging tests are appropriate.

Most patients with BAC present with early stage disease (stage I, II), as shown in Table 27–6. Indeed, approximately 50% of all BAC patients present with stage I disease, as opposed to only 15% of patients with other types of NSCLC.[83] Stage III or IV disease is relatively uncommon in surgical series, but is present in approximately 40% in pathologic series. Therefore, although many patients with BAC present with early stage disease, presentation with stage IV disease is frequent enough to make it reasonable to perform a metastatic workup, at least where there is a suspicion of advanced stage disease.

Given the association of symptoms with higher stage disease, it seems prudent to undertake a metastatic workup in symptomatic patients. This should include patients with local symptoms, as well as patients with constitutional symptoms.[46] A careful univariate analysis found that the following factors were significantly correlated with stage III or IV disease: anorexia, weight loss, any symptom, weakness, dyspnea, male gender, copious sputum production, and chest pain.[46] However, by multivariate analysis, only weight loss and profound dyspnea were independent predictors of stage III or stage IV disease.[46] No information is available about the relative incidence of distant metastases with the different radiographic presentations.

The diagnosis of BAC is probably an argument against doing routine mediastinoscopy in that patient. A radiographically suspicious lymph node, however, should be

DATA SUMMARY: BRONCHIOLOALVEOLAR CANCER—CLINICAL PRESENTATION

	AMOUNT	QUALITY	CONSISTENCY
Some cases of BAC exhibit indolent growth (visible for >2 years on chest radiograph)	High	Mod	*High*
50%–60% of patients are asymptomatic	High	High	High
Symptoms correlate with advanced stage	Mod	High	High
The majority of patients have a solitary nodule	High	High	Mod
50% of patients present with stage I disease	High	Mod	Mod
Bilateral disease is seen in 10%	High	High	High
In most patients, a preoperative diagnosis cannot be established	High	High	Mod
In patients with diffuse disease, diagnosis by bronchoscopy/sputum is highly successful	High	Mod	High

Type of data rated: Plain text: descriptive statement   *Italics: controlled comparison*   **Bold: randomized comparison**

TABLE 27–6. DISTRIBUTION OF STAGE AT PRESENTATION (%)

STUDY	TYPE OF SERIES	N	Ia	Ib	II	IIIa,b	IV
Grover et al[8]	Surgical	235	64	20	6	8	—
Daly et al[18]	Surgical	134	43	29	3	5	17
Okubo et al[17]	Surgical	105	52	25	7	4	1
Heikkila[13]	Surgical	92	——77——		10	——13——	
Régnard et al[48]	Surgical	70	24	29	8	40	—
Albertine et al[47]	Surgical	53	——70——		15	15	—
Harpole et al[46]	Pathologic	205	——39——		20	19	20
Hsu et al[84]	Pathologic	50	12	28	8	28	24
Greco et al[19]	Pathologic	78	——53——		6	——41——	

Inclusion criteria: Studies including ≥50 patients with bronchioloalveolar cancer and reporting stage at presentation.

confirmed by mediastinoscopy, just as is done for other NSCLC patients, although there is no data specifically addressing this issue in BAC. The more relevant question is whether mediastinoscopy should be carried out in the face of a negative chest CT in BAC. Table 27–6 shows that the incidence of nodal metastases is much lower in BAC than in other lung cancers, at least for solitary lesions. Although this data is not correlated with CT scan results, it suggests that the rate of finding a positive node in the face of a negative mediastinum on CT scan must be low, and that it may not be worth performing a mediastinoscopy in patients with BAC with a solitary pulmonary nodule.

There is no data available about the incidence of mediastinal node involvement for patients who present with a localized infiltrate or multifocal localized nodules. However, given the poor survival of patients with a localized infiltrate or multifocal localized nodules, it seems prudent to perform mediastinoscopy in the face of a negative CT scan before undertaking a resection in such patients. The patients who present with bilateral disease have a relatively high incidence of positive nodes. Although it is likely that this latter group of patients would probably not be approached surgically, there are probably some patients with limited bilateral disease for whom surgery is considered (eg, patients with two to three nodules). In fact, in all of the major series, such patients with bilateral disease who have been resected are reported, although they were probably highly selected.[18,19,46] If resection is contemplated in a patient with bilateral disease, it seems reasonable to perform mediastinoscopy even in the face of a negative CT scan.

SURGICAL TREATMENT

The treatment of BAC has been mainly surgical. The majority of patients present with either a solitary pulmonary nodule or a localized infiltrate, which certainly seem amenable to surgical resection. Furthermore, nodal involvement and distant metastases are relatively uncommon. Most authors report data for the entire group of resected patients (ie, those with solitary nodules, localized infiltrates, multifocal nodules, or bilateral disease). However, it is more clinically useful to define the outlook for a patient with a particular radiographic type of disease. We have attempted to consider the ability to achieve a curative resection and the survival for each of these particular presentations. This material is summarized in Table 26–7.

For patients with a solitary pulmonary nodule, it appears that the ability to achieve a curative resection (R_0) is 90% or greater. Most of the patients with a solitary pulmonary nodule present with N0 disease, have nonmucinous histology, and achieve a 5-year survival of approximately 60%. Limited data is available relating to resectability of patients with a localized infiltrate. No data is available on the incidence of nodal metastases or stage for this group of patients. The histology is mixed between mucinous and nonmucinous, and the 5-year survival is 25%. Even less data is available for the group with multifocal (localized) nodules. Daly et al[18] reported a resectability rate of 86% in 14 patients in a surgical series. There is no data available on the incidence of nodal metastases. Various histologic subtypes are seen, and survival is similar to that for a localized infiltrative pattern. Patients with bilateral disease generally do not undergo resection, although resection rates of 22%, 55%, and 57% have been reported.[16,18,48] It appears that a large number of patients with bilateral disease have nodal metastases. Although the selected patients who are resected have been reported not to have had nodal metastases,[18] there have been no reported 5-year survivors in this group.

Prognostic Factors

It is useful to ascertain whether there are particular characteristics of the tumor that can help predict the prognosis. Although such prognostic factors are available, they cannot be correlated with a specific radiographic presentation and will be discussed only for the entire group of patients. Because most of these factors are pathologic, this data pertains primarily to surgically resected patients. Extrapolation of this data to nonresected patients may not be accurate.

Cell Type

Many authors have commented on the prognostic significance of the histologic subtypes of BAC. Unfortunately, the data supporting this contention is rather limited. Table 27–7 shows that there is some correlation of histology to radiographic presentation, in that the nonmucinous cell

TABLE 27-7. SURVIVAL BY RADIOGRAPHIC CLASSIFICATION

STUDY	N	CLASSIFICATION	% CURATIVE RESECTION	INCIDENCE (%) Muc	INCIDENCE (%) Non	INCIDENCE (%) N0	N1	N2	5-y SURVIVAL (%)
Harpole et al[46]	115	Sol nodule	—	—	—	—	—	—	34
Daly et al[18]	111	Sol nodule	91[a]	—	—	87	4	8	64[b]
Okubo et al[c17]	93	Sol nodule	—	—	—	—	—	—	70
Dumont et al[7]	85	Sol nodule	92[c]	42	58	75	15	8	51
Heikkila[13]	79	Sol nodule	98[c,d]	—	—	77[c]	10[c]	13[c]	67
Barsky et al[15]	47	Sol nodule	—	26	74	—	—	—	—
Hsu et al[84]	40	Sol nodule	83	—	—	—	—	—	35
Régnard et al[48]	38	Sol nodule	90	52	38	66	13	21	39
Albertine et al[47]	37	Sol nodule	—	32	68	81	11	8	(68)[e]
Clayton[9]	36	Sol nodule	—	22	78	77[f]	23[f]	0[f]	(58)[e]
Harpole et al[46]	56	Loc infiltrate	—	—	—	—	—	—	12
Barsky et al[15]	45	Loc infiltrate	—	65	35	—	—	—	—
Daly et al[18]	30	Loc infiltrate	91[a]	67	33	—	—	—	(~25)[g]
Régnard et al[48]	19	Loc infiltrate	90	57	29	42	0	58	26
Okubo et al[17]	14	Loc infiltrate	—	—	—	—	—	—	40
Heikkila[13]	13	Loc infiltrate	—	—	—	—	—	—	0
Dumont et al[7]	12	Loc infiltrate	92[a]	50	50	58	8	33	25
Barsky et al[15]	30	Multifocal	—	54	46	—	—	—	—
Daly et al[18]	14	Multifocal	86	—	—	—	—	—	36
Harpole et al[46]	28	Bilateral	—	—	—	—	—	—	0
Daly et al[18]	9	Bilateral	22	—	—	—	—	—	0
Régnard et al[48]	7	Bilateral	57	29	43	—	—	—	0
Clayton[9]	38	Infil/Diffuse	—	50	50	—	—	—	(5)[e]
Albertine et al[47]	16	Infil/Diffuse	—	34	56	44	25	31	(31)[e]
Hsu et al[84]	10	Infil/Diffuse	30	—	—	—	—	—	10[h]

Inclusion criteria: Studies from 1980 to 2000 reporting data by radiographic presentation on survival, histologic subtype, or nodal status in ≥50 patients (total) with bronchioloalveolar cancer.
[a]For entire study group.
[b]N0 patients only.
[c]For entire group, but >85% solitary pulmonary nodule.
[d]Resection rate (? all curative).
[e]Absolute survival.
[f]Excludes the mucinous patients (14%).
[g]Estimated from other survival data reported.
[h]4-year survival.
Bilateral, diffuse or bilateral disease; Infil/Diffuse, infiltrate, multiple nodules or bilateral disease; Loc infiltrate, infiltrate or consolidation localized to one lobe or lung; Muc, mucinous; Multifocal, multiple nodules confined to one lobe or lung; Non, nonmucinous; resec, resection; Sol nodule, solitary pulmonary nodule.

type is the predominant type in patients with solitary pulmonary nodules and in those with diffuse bilateral disease. A different arrangement of this data, which correlates histologic type with survival, is shown in Table 27–8, although such survival data by cell type is limited. Patients with a nonmucinous cell type appear to have slightly better survival, but this may well be due to the fact that more of these patients had solitary pulmonary nodules and no lymph node involvement than patients with the other cell types.

Closer scrutiny of the studies that suggested nonmucinous BAC patients have a better prognosis also supports the conclusion that the stage of disease and the radiographic presentation are of primary importance, rather than the histology. Daly et al[18] reported that for the entire group of patients with BAC, the nonmucinous cell type was associated with a better survival (median survival, 10 years versus 5 years; $P < 0.02$). However, when only patients with a particular stage, such as stage I, were considered, no difference in survival was seen according to the cell type.[18] Similarly, Clayton[21] reported that patients with mu-

cinous BAC had a poor prognosis. However, 89% of these patients with mucinous BAC had diffuse disease. In fact, their prognosis was similar to that of patients with diffuse nonmucinous BAC and was different only when compared with nonmucinous *solitary* tumors. The conclusion that histologic cell type has no prognostic significance as opposed to stage and radiographic presentation is also supported by an analysis of 54 patients by Albertine et al.[47]

Other histologic factors, such as poor differentiation or the presence of scar, have been suggested to be of prognostic importance, but there is little data to support this contention. Although there is some suggestion that patients with poorly differentiated tumors are likely to have nodal metastases,[16] no data is available about the survival of such patients. One author found that mixed tumors (BAC and adenocarcinoma) have worse survival,[13] but these patients should probably not be included as patients with BAC.[12] No data exists on the survival of patients with the sclerotic type of BAC. However, the presence of scar in the lesion was found to be a good prognostic factor by Daly et al,[18] both for the entire group and for only those patients with

TABLE 27–8. SURVIVAL BY HISTOLOGIC CLASSIFICATION

STUDY	N	CLASSIFICATION	% CURATIVE RESECTION	INCIDENCE (%)		5-y SURVIVAL (%)
				N0	Sol Nod	
Daly et al[18]	55	Mucinous	91a	—	—	50
Barsky et al[15]	51	Mucinous	—	—	22	—
Dumont et al[7]	42	Mucinous	92a	—	86	59
Régnard et al[48 b]	35	Mucinous	97	—	—	44
Albertine et al[47]	19	Mucinous	—	67	63	(55)c
Clayton[9]	16	Mucinous	—	—	31	(19)c
Daly et al[18]	60	Nonmucinous	91a	—	—	(72)d
Barsky et al[15 e]	59	Nonmucinous	—	—	56	—
Dumont et al[7]	55	Nonmucinous	92a	—	89	54
Albertine et al[47]	35	Nonmucinous	—	71	74	(57)c
Clayton[9 e]	29	Nonmucinous	—	—	62	(52)c
Régnard et al[48 b]	21	Nonmucinous	84	—	—	22
Clayton[9]	29	Sclerotic	—	—	45	(14)c
Barsky et al[15]	12	Sclerotic	—	—	25	—

Inclusion criteria: Studies from 1980 to 2000 reporting data by histologic subtype on survival or resectability in ≥50 patients with bronchioloalveolar cancer.
aFor all patients in the study.
bExcludes 13%–19% of cases with mixed histology.
cAbsolute survival.
dEstimated from median survival.
eExcludes sclerotic.

stage I disease (median survival, 13.5 years with scar versus 3.6 years without scar; $P < .001$). Okubo et al[17] found that tumors with sclerosis or scar had a worse prognosis, although this was not true when multivariate analysis was performed. In summary, it must be concluded that there is no clear data that tumor histology is of prognostic significance in BAC.

Stage

The survival of patients by stage of disease is shown in Table 27–9. Patients with stage I disease have a survival of approximately 70%. Particularly those with T1N0 disease exhibit good survival, as high as 91% in the series reported by Daly et al.[18] The data reported by Harpole et al[46] is not quite as optimistic, probably because the study extends back to an earlier period (1970) and is a pathologic series in which not all patients were resected. The survival difference between T1N0 and T2N0 is quite marked in the studies by Daly et al,[18] Grover et al,[8] and Hsu et al[84] and was found to be statistically significant ($P < 0.0001$) in the analysis by Daly et al.[18]

Overall, the survival of patients with BAC is similar, stage for stage, to that of patients with other types of NSCLC. Univariate analysis of the Lung Cancer Study Group data found that patients with BAC had better survival rates than those with other types of adenocarcinoma ($P = 0.008$); in fact, it was the cell type with the best survival curve of all.[8] However, when the data was adjusted for T and N status, weight loss, age, and gender, the difference was only marginally significant ($P = 0.089$).[8]

TABLE 27–9. SURVIVAL BY STAGE

STUDY	TYPE OF SERIES	N	5-y SURVIVAL (%)				
			Ia	Ib	IIa,b	IIIa,b	IV
Grover et al[8]	Surgical	235	69a	54a,b	————13————		—
Daly et al[18]	Surgical	134	91	55	(~50)c	(~30)c	—
Dumont et al[7]	Surgical	97	————65————		16	19d	—
Régnard et al[48]	Surgical	58	————56————		—	8	—
Harpole et al[46]	Pathologic	205	————52————		20	—	—
Greco et al[19]	Pathologic	78	————(75)c————		(66)c	————(10)c————	
Hsu et al[84]	Pathologic	50	83	51	25	20d	—
Averagef			**81**	**53**	**20**	**16**	**—**

Inclusion criteria: Studies including ≥50 patients with bronchioloalveolar cancer and reporting survival by TNM stage (adapted to 1997 staging system).
aEstimated from Hazard rate.
bIncludes 10% T1N1 patients.
cEstimated from median survival.
dIIIa only.
eAbsolute survival.
fExcluding values in parentheses.

In summary, BAC presents with early stage disease more commonly than other NSCLC and exhibits survival that is similar, stage for stage, (or arguably slightly better) relative to other NSCLCs.

Extent of Resection

The majority of resections performed have been lobectomies. Three authors have noted no difference in survival whether a limited resection (wedge or segmentectomy) or lobectomy was performed, as long as a complete resection (R_0) was accomplished.[17,18,46] In addition, one of these authors found a *lower* local recurrence rate after limited resection (24% versus 34%, *P* not reported).[46] The only other author who remarked on the value of a limited resection stated that a limited resection should not be done, but provided little data.[19] This author reported that several patients who underwent segmentectomy developed recurrence along the plane of the initial resection, but he did not report whether these had been complete resections. This finding suggests that perhaps the limited resection was not as much an issue as was a positive margin. An incomplete resection has been clearly shown by others to result in statistically significant worse survival compared with a complete resection.[17,18,48]

RADIOTHERAPY

RT has been reported to have been used to treat BAC in approximately 30 patients.[52,54,57,60,63,69,85] Most of these reports are not from a contemporary time period, and no details about the degree of localization of the cancer or field size is given. Doses used, where reported, ranged from 20 to 70 Gy. No 5-year survivors were reported,[52,57,60,69,85] but it is often unclear whether the goal of treatment was cure or palliation. Radiation was of clear palliative benefit, however, in two patients with copious bronchorrhea.[54,63]

CHEMOTHERAPY

Although many series mention having treated unresectable patients with chemotherapy, no data about response or survival was presented in most of these reports. A review in 1981 noted that no responses to chemotherapy had been seen in any previous reports.[66] Only three reports addressed this question more recently.[61,86,87] In one report, stage III and IV BAC was found to have an increased response rate compared with other subtypes of adenocarcinoma, although survival was only slightly prolonged.[86] A second report[61] involved 25 patients with stage IV BAC and 223 patients with metastatic adenocarcinoma treated during the same period at the Mayo Clinic, who were well matched in terms of age, gender, weight loss, performance status, and presence of distant metastases, and all chemotherapy regimens used were cisplatin based. The partial response rate in patients with BAC was identical to that in patients with other types of adenocarcinomas (32%), and there were no complete responses.[61] The median duration of response (4–5 months) and the 2-year survival (8–8.5 months) were almost identical in both groups. Another study reported a lower response rate to chemotherapy in patients with stage IIIb, IV BAC compared with other types of NSCLC, yet better survival.[87] Thus it appears that, in general, patients with BAC are no less responsive to chemotherapy than patients with other forms of adenocarcinoma.

RECURRENCE PATTERNS

Recurrent BAC after resection is seen most often in the lung. Studies containing data on recurrence patterns are summarized in Table 27–10. Approximately one-third to two-thirds of patients experience a recurrence, although the reported median time to recurrence after surgery is relatively long, 21 to 30 months.[18,48] When a local recurrence occurs, it is usually in the lung and often initially solitary.[18,48] Heikkila et al[13] also reported a high incidence of local recurrence in the lung in patients with typical BAC. In this report, another larger group of patients with mixed histology (BAC with adenocarcinoma) exhibited a recurrence pattern more reminiscent of adenocarcinoma than of BAC (82% distant).[13] Daly et al[18] found that the risk of recurrence was increased with higher stage disease: stage Ia, 17%; Ib, 47%; IIa,b, 75%; IIIa, 71%.

The risk of recurrence also appears to be influenced by

DATA SUMMARY: BRONCHIOLOALVEOLAR CANCER—TREATMENT			
	AMOUNT	**QUALITY**	**CONSISTENCY**
90% of patients with solitary nodule can be resected	High	Mod	High
75% of patients with solitary nodule are N0	High	High	High
The 5-year survival of resected patients with a solitary nodule is >50%	High	Mod	Mod
The 5-year survival of resected patients with a localized infiltrate is ≤25%	Mod	Mod	High
The 5-year survival of resected patients with bilateral or diffuse disease is ≤10%	Mod	Poor	High
Limited resection yields results similar to those for lobectomy	*Mod*	*Mod*	*High*
The majority of recurrences of bronchioloalveolar cancer after resection are in the lung	High	High	Mod

Type of data rated: Plain text: descriptive statement   *Italics: controlled comparison*   **Bold: randomized comparison**

TABLE 27–10. RECURRENCE PATTERNS

STUDY	N	SELECTION CRITERIA	% OF ALL PATIENTS	% OF ALL RECURRENCES			% OF ALL PATIENTS		
				Lung	L+D	D	L	L+D	D
Grover et al[8][a]	235	Resected	32	30[b]	——70——		10	——23——	
Daly et al[18]	134	Resected	38	80[c]	—	16	31	—	7
Harpole et al[46]	80	Resected[d]	31	—	—	—	—	—	—
Régnard et al[48]	61	Resected	59	67	10[e]	23	—	—	—
Breathnach et al[96]	36	Resected[d]	36	75	17	8	27	6	3
Heikkila[13]	33	Typical BAC	61	65	—	35	39	—	21
Marcq and Galy[82]	21	All patients	71	60	13	27	42	10	19
Average				**63**	**13**	**22**	**30**	**—**	**13**

Inclusion criteria: Studies including >20 patients with BAC and reporting recurrence data.
[a]Assuming definition of local and distant is the same as that used in other Lung Cancer Study Group reports.
[b]Not specified as lung recurrence, only as local.
[c]Evenly spread among ipsilateral, contralateral, and bilateral; most often was new solitary lesion.
[d]Stage I only.
[e]10% recurrence in mediastinal nodes.
BAC, bronchioloalveolar cancer; D, distant; L, local (within chest); Lung, within lung parenchyma.

the radiographic presentation. Daly et al[18] found that patients who had multiple nodules at the time of presentation had a recurrence rate of 95%. Régnard et al[48] also found that patients with localized infiltrative presentations or with bilateral disease had recurrence rates of 75% and 79% versus 47% in those with solitary nodules ($P < 0.05$). There does not appear to be a difference in the recurrence rates or recurrence patterns with respect to the histologic subtypes.[48]

METHOD OF METASTATIC SPREAD

Clearly, BAC can spread by lymphatic and hematogenous routes. Lymphatic spread to N1, N2, and N3 lymph nodes is well documented, even though nodal involvement is not common at the time of presentation (see Table 27–6). Extrathoracic, hematogenously spread metastases are also well documented and have an organ distribution similar to that of other NSCLCs.[60,61] However, a striking characteristic of BAC is the high incidence of intrapulmonary metastases (see Table 27–10). Furthermore, in nearly 50% of patients who underwent autopsy, no extrapulmonary metastases were found, even in the event of extensive pulmonary involvement that was fatal.[45] Others also observed that intrapulmonary metastases are often not associated with other sites of distant disease.[13,18,61,82,87] Aerogenous spread throughout the lung was postulated as a mechanism that would explain the frequent initial presentation of diffuse bilateral disease and the high rate of pulmonary metastases without distant metastases.[45] The possibility of aerogenous spread of BAC has been debated extensively since the 1950s, and the debate continues today.[23]

An alternative hypothesis to explain the frequent diffuse presentation and the high rate of pulmonary metastases without distant metastases is the occurrence of multiple synchronous foci of primary cancer throughout the lung. Until the 1950s, most authors believed this to be true and thought BAC was not amenable to a local therapy such as surgery,[45] probably because so many patients in early series presented with diffuse disease.[45,60,88] The possibility of a viral etiology (jaagsiekte) is also consistent with this hy-

pothesis. However, later investigators realized that BAC could present as a solitary lesion.[56,88,89] The fact that these patients frequently experience good long-term survival after resection is a strong argument against the occurrence of multiple primary cancers.

The preponderance of evidence supports the conclusion that progression of a solitary nodule to either a more diffuse infiltrate or multiple nodules is not only well documented but in fact appears to be characteristic of BAC. Numerous studies have documented a solitary BAC that later became multifocal and, finally, diffuse.[26,54,55,64,69,88,90,91] Many more references document this in addition to the ones cited here. This type of intrapulmonary progression has been observed for both a solitary nodule[55,90] and for lesions that are initially apparent as a localized infiltrate.[64,69,91] This progression has been investigated most carefully by Hill, who studied 46 patients for whom serial radiographs were available.[55] In each of these patients, progression to increasing numbers of nodules, increasing consolidation, or diffuse disease was observed. A solitary nodule was more likely to progress to multiple nodules or masses and a localized infiltrate to diffuse consolidation, but some crossover between patterns occurred in both directions (solitary nodule to infiltrate in 25% of cases; localized infiltrate to multiple nodules in 11% of cases).[55] Only one report suggested that a solitary nodule of BAC does not progress to diffuse pulmonary involvement over time if not resected.[58] These authors based this statement on observation of 7 (out of 43) patients who were observed for 1 to 8 years. The fact that progression of a solitary BAC to diffuse disease has been widely documented, and the finding that surgical resection often seems to interrupt this natural history, are arguments supportive of aerogenous dissemination.

A frequent finding in BAC is the presence of tumor cells that appear loose and unattached in the smaller airways on histologic sectioning.[12] Three cases have been reported that lend strong support for aerogenous dissemination of BAC.[90–92] In two of these cases, pulmonary secretions from the involved lobe were spilled to other areas of the lung and were suctioned out. Later, recurrent BAC was found to occur in these areas and eventually led to diffuse disease.[90,91] In the third case, expectorated tumor cells were documented histologically.[92] Several months later, tumor involvement in the upper respiratory tract was found. At autopsy, this was clearly shown to be BAC lining alveolar walls that had implanted in the mucosa of the nose and the ear. This was a mucinous BAC with histology identical to that of the lung primary.[92]

Some authors have stated that the mucinous subtype of BAC is more likely than other subtypes to exhibit aerogenous dissemination.[14,23,92] Unfortunately, the cell type is not documented in the vast majority of cases in which aerogenous dissemination appears to have occurred.[26,54,55,64,69,90,91] However, most authors have shown that mucinous BAC is less likely to appear as solitary nodules at the time of presentation (see Table 27–8),[14,15,21] with only one exception (no difference).[16] An immunohistochemical study found that mucinous BAC has increased type IV collagenase expression and decreased α-2 integrin receptor expression, which may make mucinous BAC more likely to detach from the underlying basement membrane.[93] In contrast, sclerotic BAC showed much more disruption of the basement membrane, similar to that found in adenocarcinomas, which may make it more likely to disseminate by lymphatic spread.[93] Indeed, Clayton[9] found that the sclerotic subtype is more likely to involve lymphatic spread.

Thus, a fair amount of observational evidence supports aerogenous dissemination as a mechanism of metastatic spread. Furthermore, the fact that resected solitary lesions exhibit good 5-year survival in most cases is a strong argument against the alternative hypothesis of multifocal primary tumors as the mechanism for the development of multinodular or diffuse BAC. This is countered by the evidence suggesting a viral etiology for BAC and the possible relationship of BAC to atypical adenomatous hyperplasia. Furthermore, Barsky et al[3] have provided some limited data supporting multiclonality (separate primary tumors) in multifocal BAC. This finding was based on analysis of only three patients with multifocal disease in which two to four foci per patient were studied. If this finding can be corroborated, the debate about the mechanism of intrapulmonary spread will continue.

EDITORS' COMMENTS

There are clearly situations in which a pulmonary nodule that has been stable for several years can be confidently viewed as benign and not followed any further. On the other hand, because it has been clearly demonstrated that BAC has the propensity to remain stable for many years, it is generally best to continue to evaluate a seemingly chronic nodule with regular radiographs. If there is any suspicion that this could be a BAC, based on the appearance of the lesion, then resection should be carried out. Furthermore, any unusual appearing mass or infiltrate that cannot be diagnosed by bronchoscopy should be resected.

For any patient with a suspected BAC who has symptoms, even local symptoms such as a cough, distant organ scanning and mediastinoscopy are indicated. Furthermore, distant organ scanning and mediastinoscopy should be carried out in patients with multiple localized nodules or infiltrates. However, asymptomatic patients with a solitary nodule or mass and a radiographically negative chest CT scan probably do not need to undergo further staging tests. Because the success rate of bronchoscopy and sputum analysis is relatively low with localized lesions, it may not be worthwhile trying to establish a diagnosis preoperatively in such cases.

All solitary nodules of BAC should be resected. A wedge resection with a reasonable margin ($\geq$2 cm) is probably adequate. A localized infiltrative BAC, as well as multiple localized nodules, should also be approached surgically. However, such patients must be carefully scrutinized to rule out nodal metastases, distant metastases, or involvement of other areas in the lung. Patients with intermediate stage lesions (stage Ib-IIIa) should be considered for adjuvant studies in the same manner as any other patients with NSCLC. The role of radiation in the treatment of this disease is limited to rare attempts at palliation of copious bronchorrhea in patients with diffuse involvement. Patients with extensive disease (stage IIIa-IV) should be considered for treatment with chemotherapy, just as other patients with NSCLC would be.

References

1. Devesa SS, Shaw GL, Blot WJ. Changing patterns of lung cancer incidence by histological type. Cancer Epidemiol Biomarkers Prev. 1991;1:29–34.
2. Linnoila RI, Jensen SM, Steinberg SM, et al. Peripheral airway cell marker expression in non–small cell lung carcinoma: association with distinct clinicopathologic features. Am J Clin Pathol. 1992;97:233–243.
3. Barsky SH, Grossman DA, Ho J, et al. The multifocality of bronchioloalveolar lung carcinoma: evidence and implications of a multifocal origin. Mod Pathol. 1994;7:633–640.
4. Auerbach O, Garfinkel L. The changing pattern of lung carcinoma. Cancer. 1991;68:1973–1977.
5. World Health Organization. The World Health Organization histological typing of lung tumours. 2nd ed. Am J Clin Pathol. 1982;77:123–136.
6. Quinn D, Gianlupi A, Broste S. The changing radiographic presentation of bronchogenic carcinoma with reference to cell types. Chest. 1996;110:1474–1479.
7. Dumont P, Gasser B, Rougé C, et al. Bronchoalveolar carcinoma: histopathologic study of evolution in a series of 105 surgically treated patients. Chest. 1998;113:391–395.
8. Grover FL, Pianiadosi S, and the Lung Cancer Study Group. Recurrence and survival following resection of bronchioloalveolar carcinoma of the lung—the Lung Cancer Study Group experience. Ann Surg. 1989;209:779–790.
9. Clayton F. The spectrum and significance of bronchioloalveolar carcinomas. Pathol Annu. 1988;23:361–394.
10. Roggli VL, Vollmer RT, Greenberg SD, et al. Lung cancer heterogeneity: a blinded and randomized study of 100 consecutive cases. Hum Pathol. 1985;16:569–579.
11. Schraufnagel D, Peloquin A, Paré JAP, et al. Differentiating bronchioloalveolar carcinoma from adenocarcinoma. Am Rev Respir Dis. 1982;125:74–79.
12. Colby TV, Koss MN, Travis WD. Bronchioloalveolar carcinoma. In: AFIP Atlas of Tumor Pathology. Series 3, Fascicle 13: Tumors of the Lower Respiratory Tract. Washington, D.C.: Armed Forces Institute of Pathology; 1994:203–234.
13. Heikkila L. Results of surgical treatment in bronchioloalveolar carcinoma. Ann Chir Gynaecol. 1986;75:183–191.
14. Manning JT Jr, Spjut HJ, Tschen JA. Bronchioloalveolar carcinoma: the significance of two histopathologic types. Cancer. 1984;54:525–534.
15. Barsky SH, Cameron R, Osann KE, et al. Rising incidence of bronchioloalveolar lung carcinoma and its unique clinicopathologic features. Cancer. 1994;73:1163–1170.

16. Tao LC, Delarue NC, Sanders D, et al. Bronchiolo-alveolar carcinoma: a correlative clinical and cytologic study. Cancer. 1978;42:2759–2767.

17. Okubo K, Mark EJ, Flieder D, et al. Bronchioloalveolar carcinoma: clinical, radiological, pathological factors and survival. J Thorac Cardiovasc Surg. 1999;118:702–709.

18. Daly RC, Trastek VF, Pairolero PC, et al. Bronchoalveolar carcinoma: factors affecting survival. Ann Thorac Surg. 1991;51:368–377.

19. Greco RJ, Steiner RM, Goldman S, et al. Bronchoalveolar cell carcinoma of the lung. Ann Thorac Surg. 1986;41:652–656.

20. Greenberg SD, Smith MN, Spjut HJ. Bronchiolo-alveolar carcinoma—cell of origin. Am J Clin Pathol. 1975;63:153–167.

21. Clayton F. Bronchioloalveolar carcinomas: cell types, patterns of growth, and prognostic correlates. Cancer. 1986;57:1555–1564.

22. Edwards CW. Alveolar carcinoma: a review. Thorax. 1984;39:166–174.

23. Barkley JE, Green MR. Bronchioloalveolar carcinoma. J Clin Oncol. 1996;14:2377–2386.

24. Perk K, Hod I. Sheep lung carcinoma: an endemic analogue of a sporadic human neoplasm [guest editorial]. J Natl Cancer Inst. 1982;69:747–749.

25. Heimann HL, Samuel E. Pulmonary adenomatosis: case report. S Afr Med J. 1953;27:934–935.

26. Shipman SJ, Stephens HB, Binkley FM. Pulmonary alveolar adenomatosis. Am Rev Tuberc. 1949;60:788–793.

27. Beaumont F, Jansen HM, Elema JD, et al. Simultaneous occurrence of pulmonary interstitial fibrosis and alveolar cell carcinoma in one family. Thorax. 1981;36:252–258.

28. Paul SM, Bacharach B, Goepp C. A genetic influence on alveolar cell carcinoma. J Surg Oncol. 1987;36:249–252.

29. Joishy SK, Cooper RA, Rowley PT. Alveolar cell carcinoma in identical twins: similarity in time of onset, histochemistry, and site of metastasis. Ann Intern Med. 1977;87:447–450.

30. Kaslovsky RA, Purdy S, Dangman BC, et al. Bronchioloalveolar carcinoma in a child with congenital cystic adenomatoid malformation. Chest. 1997;112:548–551.

31. Ribet ME, Copin M-C, Soots JG, et al. Bronchioloalveolar carcinoma and congenital cystic adenomatoid malformation. Ann Thorac Surg. 1995;60:1126–1128.

32. Benjamin DR, Cahill JL. Bronchioloalveolar carcinoma of the lung and congenital cystic adenomatoid malformation. Am J Clin Pathol. 1991;95:889–892.

33. Kowalski P, Rodziewicz R, Pejcz J. Bilateral bronchioloalveolar carcinoma of the lungs in a 7 year old girl treated for Hodgkin's disease. Tumori. 1989;75:449–451.

34. Travis WD, Linnoila RI, Horowitz M, et al. Pulmonary nodules resembling bronchioloalveolar carcinoma in adolescent cancer patients. Mod Pathol. 1988;1:372–377.

35. Miller RR. Bronchioloalveolar cell adenomas. Am J Surg Pathol. 1990;14:904–912.

36. Kodama T, Biyajima S, Watanabe S, et al. Morphometric study of adenocarcinomas and hyperplastic epithelial lesions in the peripheral lung. Am J Clin Pathol. 1986;85:146–151.

37. Kitamura H, Kameda Y, Nakamura N, et al. Atypical adenomatous hyperplasia and bronchoalveolar lung carcinoma: analysis by morphometry and the expressions of p53 and carcinoembryonic antigen. Am J Surg Pathol. 1996;20:553–562.

38. Nakanishi K, Hiroi S, Kawai T, et al. Argyrophilic nucleolar-organizer region counts and DNA status in bronchioloalveolar epithelial hyperplasia and adenocarcinoma of the lung. Hum Pathol. 1998;29:235–239.

39. Logan PM, Miller RR, Evans K, et al. Bronchogenic carcinoma and coexistent bronchioalveolar cell adenomas: assessment of radiologic detection and follow-up in 28 patients. Chest. 1996;109:713–717.

40. Mori M, Chiba R, Takahashi T. Atypical adenomatous hyperplasia of the lung and its differentiation from adenocarcinoma. Cancer. 1993;72:2331–2340.

41. Auerbach O, Garfinkel L, Parks VR. Scar cancer of the lung: increase over a 21 year period. Cancer. 1979;43:636–642.

42. Madri JA, Carter D. Scar cancers of the lung: origin and significance. Hum Pathol. 1984;15:625–631.

43. Barsky SH, Huang SJ, Bhuta S. The extracellular matrix of pulmonary scar carcinomas is suggestive of a desmoplastic origin. Am J Pathol. 1986;124:412–419.

44. Shimosato Y, Hashimoto T, Kodama T, et al. Prognostic implications of fibrotic focus (scar) in small peripheral lung cancers. Am J Surg Pathol. 1980;4:365–373.

45. Storey CF, Knudtson KP, Lawrence BJ. Bronchiolar ("alveolar cell") carcinoma of the lung. J Thorac Surg. 1953;26:331–406.

46. Harpole DH, Bigelow C, Young WG Jr, et al. Alveolar cell carcinoma of the lung: a retrospective analysis of 205 patients. Ann Thorac Surg. 1988;46:502–507.

47. Albertine KH, Steiner RM, Radack DM, et al. Analysis of cell type and radiographic presentation as predictors of the clinical course of patients with bronchioloalveolar cell carcinoma. Chest. 1998;113:997–1006.

48. Régnard JF, Santelmo N, Romdhani N, et al. Bronchioloalveolar lung carcinoma: results of surgical treatment and prognostic factors. Chest. 1998;114:45–50.

49. Ikeda T, Kurita Y, Inutsuka S, et al. The changing pattern of lung cancer by histological type—a review of 1151 cases from a university hospital in Japan, 1970–1989. Lung Cancer. 1991;7:157–164.

50. Falk RT, Pickle LW, Fontham ETH, et al. Epidemiology of bronchioloalveolar carcinoma. Cancer Epidemiol Biomarkers Prev. 1992;1:339–344.

51. Morabia A, Wynder EL. Relation of bronchioloalveolar carcinoma to tobacco. BMJ. 1992;304:541–543.

52. Fitzpatrick HF, Miller RE, Edgar MS Jr, et al. Bronchiolar carcinoma of the lung: a review of 33 patients. J Thorac Cardiovasc Surg. 1961;42:310–326.

53. Arany LS. Bronchiolar (alveolar cell) carcinoma: failure to cause symptoms for more than twelve years. Am Rev Tuberc. 1958;78:632–636.

54. White JN, Madding GF, Hershberger LR. Alveolar cell tumor of the lung. Dis Chest. 1952;21:655–662.

55. Hill CA. Bronchioloalveolar carcinoma: a review. Radiology. 1984;150:15–20.

56. Hawkins JA, Hansen JE, Howbert J. A clinical study of bronchiolar carcinoma: a clue to unicentricity or multicentricity. Am Rev Respir Dis. 1963;88:1–5.

57. Delarue NC, Anderson W, Sanders D, et al. Bronchiolo-alveolar carcinoma: a reappraisal after 24 years. Cancer. 1972;29:90–97.

58. Miller WT, Husted J, Freiman D, et al. Bronchioloalveolar carcinoma: two clinical entities with one pathologic diagnosis. AJR Am J Roentgenol. 1978;130:905–912.

59. James EC, Schuchmann GF, Hall RV, et al. Preferred surgical treatment for alveolar cell carcinoma. Ann Thorac Surg. 1976;22:157–162.

60. Watson WL, Farpour A. Terminal bronchiolar or "alveolar cell" cancer of the lung: two hundred sixty-five cases. Cancer. 1966;19:776–780.

61. Feldman ER, Eagan RT, Schaid DJ. Metastatic bronchioloalveolar carcinoma and metastatic adenocarcinoma of the lung: comparison of clinical manifestations, chemotherapeutic responses, and prognosis. Mayo Clin Proc. 1992;67:27–32.

62. Homma H, Kira S, Takahashi Y, et al. A case of alveolar cell carcinoma accompanied by fluid and electrolyte depletion through production of voluminous amounts of lung liquid. Am Rev Respir Dis. 1975;111:857–862.

63. Levinsky WJ, Kern RA. Fluid, electrolyte, and protein depletion secondary to the bronchorrhea of pulmonary adenomatosis: a complication heretofore unreported. Am J Med Sci. 1952;223:512–521.

64. Fishman HC, Danon J, Koopot N, et al. Massive intrapulmonaty venoarterial shunting in alveolar cell carcinoma. Am Rev Respir Dis. 1974;109:124–128.

65. Hidaka N, Nagao K. Bronchioloalveolar carcinoma accompanied by severe bronchorrhea. Chest. 1996;110:281–282.

66. Edgerton F, Rao U, Takita H, et al. Bronchio-alveolar carcinoma: a clinical overview and bibliography. Oncology. 1981;38:269–273.

67. Homma H, Kawabata M, Kishi K, et al. Successful treatment of refractory bronchorrhea by inhaled indomethacin in two patients with bronchioloalveolar carcinoma. Chest. 1999;115:1465–1468.

68. Spiro SG, Lopez-Vidriero M-T, Charman J, et al. Bronchorrhea in a case of alveolar cell carcinoma. J Clin Pathol. 1975;28:60–65.

69. Epstein DM, Gefter WB, Miller WT. Lobar bronchioloalveolar cell carcinoma. Am J Radiol. 1982;139:463–466.

70. Sarlin RF, Schillaci RF, Georges TN, et al. Focal increased lung perfusion and intrapulmonary veno-arterial shunting in bronchioloalveolar cell carcinoma. Am J Med. 1980;68:618–623.

71. Chetty KG, Dick C, McGovern J, et al. Refractory hypoxemia due to intrapulmonary shunting associated with bronchioloalveolar carcinoma. Chest. 1997;111:1120–1121.

72. McNamara JJ, Kingsley WB, Paulson DL, et al. Alveolar cell (bronchiolar) carcinoma of the lung. J Thorac Cardiovasc Surg. 1969;57:648–656.

73. Shapiro R, Wilson GL, Yesner R, et al. A useful roentgen sign in the diagnosis of localized bronchioloalveolar carcinoma. Am J Radiol. 1972;114:516–524.

74. Trigaux J-P, Gevenois PA, Goncette L, et al. Bronchioloalveolar carcinoma: computed tomography findings. Eur Respir J. 1996;9:11–16.

75. Kuhlman JE, Fishman EK, Kuhajda FP, et al. Solitary bronchioloalveolar carcinoma: CT criteria. Radiology. 1988;167:379–382.

76. Akata S, Fukushima A, Kakizaki D, et al. CT scanning of bronchioloalveolar carcinoma: specific appearances. Lung Cancer. 1995;12:221–230.

77. Aquino S, Chiles C, Halford P. Distinction of consolidative bronchioloalveolar carcinoma from pneumonia: do CT criteria work? Am J Roentgenol. 1998;171:359–363.

78. Akira M, Atagi S, Kawahara M, et al. High-resolution CT findings of diffuse bronchioloalveolar carcinoma in 38 patients. Am J Roentgenol. 1999;173:1623–1629.

79. Im J-G, Han MC, Yu EJ, et al. Lobar bronchioloalveolar carcinoma: "angiogram sign" on CT scans. Radiology. 1990;176:749–753.

80. Kim B-T, Kim Y, Lee KS, et al. Localized form of bronchioloalveolar carcinoma: FDG PET findings. Am J Roentgenol. 1998;170:935–939.

81. Higashi K, Ueda Y, Seki H, et al. Fluorine-18–FDG PET imaging is negative in bronchioloalveolar lung carcinoma. J Nucl Med. 1998;39:1016–1020.

82. Marcq M, Galy P. Bronchioloalveolar carcinoma: clinicopathologic relationships, natural history, and prognosis in 29 cases. Am Rev Respir Dis. 1973;107:621–629.

83. Bülzebruck H, Bopp R, Drings P, et al. New aspects in the staging of lung cancer: prospective validation of the International Union Against Cancer TNM classification. Cancer. 1992;70:1102–1110.

84. Hsu C-P, Chen C-Y, Hsu N-Y. Bronchioloalveolar carcinoma. J Thorac Cardiovasc Surg. 1995;110:374–381.

85. Ludington LG, Verska JJ, Howard T, et al. Bronchiolar carcinoma (alveolar cell), another great imitator; a review of 41 cases. Chest. 1972;61:622–628.

86. Sorensen JB, Hirsch FR, Olsen J. The prognostic implication of histopathologic subtyping of pulmonary adenocarcinoma according to the classification of the World Health Organization: an analysis of 259 consecutive patients with advanced disease. Cancer. 1988;62:361–367.

87. Breathnach OS, Ishibe N, Williams J, et al. Clinical features of patients with stage IIIB and IV bronchioloalveolar carcinoma of the lung. Cancer. 1999;86:1165–1173.

88. Liebow AA. Bronchiolo-alveolar carcinoma. Adv Intern Med. 1960;10:329–358.

89. Munnell ER, Dilling E, Grantham RN, et al. Reappraisal of solitary bronchiolar (alveolar cell) carcinoma of the lung. Ann Thorac Surg. 1978;25:289–297.

90. Donovan WD, Yankelevitz DF, Henschke CI, et al. Endobronchial spread of bronchioloalveolar carcinoma. Chest. 1993;104:951–953.

91. Ferraro L, Solis R, Khan MA. Endobronchial spread of bronchoalveolar cell carcinoma [letter]. Chest. 1994;105:1627–1628.

92. Hidaka N, Hidaka Y, Tajima Y, et al. Bronchioloalveolar carcinoma presenting aerogenous metastasis to the upper airway. Eur J Cancer. 1996;32A:1261–1262.

93. Ohori NP, Yousem SA, Griffin J, et al. Comparison of extracellular matrix antigens in subtypes of bronchioloalveolar carcinoma and conventional pulmonary adenocarcinoma: an immunohistochemical study. Am J Surg Pathol. 1992;16:675–686.

94. Rossing TH, Rossing RG. Survival in lung cancer: an analysis of the effects of age, sex, resectability, and histopathologic type. Am Rev Respir Dis. 1982;126:771–777.

95. Elson CE, Moore SP, Johnston WW. Morphologic and immunocytochemical studies of bronchioloalveolar carcinoma at Duke University Medical Center, 1968-1986. Anal Quant Cytol Histol. 1989;11:261–274.

96. Breathnach OS, Kwiatkowski DJ, Godleski JJ, et al. Bronchioloalveolar carcinoma of the lung: recurrences and survival in patients with stage I disease. Proc Am Soc Clin Oncol. 2000;19:502a. [Abstract.]

28

TRACHEAL CANCERS

David R. Jones, Frank C. Detterbeck, and David E. Morris

Malignant tumors of the trachea are uncommon. For this reason, most physicians will diagnose and treat these lesions only once or twice in their careers. Because of the rarity of these tumors, only a few major academic centers worldwide have any significant clinical experience with these neoplasms. Despite these observations, it is important for physicians involved in the treatment of thoracic malignancies to be able to diagnose and formulate a treatment strategy for a patient suspected of having a tracheal malignancy. This chapter focuses on the two most common malignant tracheal neoplasms: squamous cell and adenoid cystic carcinoma. Mucoepidermoid and carcinoid tumors are reviewed in Chapter 26.

INCIDENCE AND HISTOLOGY

Primary malignant neoplasms of the trachea account for 0.2% (0.1%–0.3%) of all malignancies.[1-3] The incidence of these tumors is <0.2 per 100 000 persons per year, with a prevalence of 1 per 15 000 autopsies.[1-3] This extremely low incidence explains the relative paucity of substantial clinical experience with these malignancies.

Clinically, it is important to differentiate between benign and malignant tracheal tumors. The vast majority (86%-91%) of tracheal lesions in adults are malignant,[4-6] whereas >90% of tracheal tumors in children are benign.[7] Although more than 20 different histologic types of cancer have been reported in adults, >80% of these are either adenoid cystic (43%) or squamous cell (40%) carcinoma.[5,6] Carcinoid (9%) and mucoepidermoid tumors (3%) account for most of the remainder among surgical series involving >100 patients.[5-7] However, series based on patients receiving primary radiation, as well as pathologic and tumor registry studies, have found squamous cell carcinoma to account for approximately 70% and adenoid cystic carcinoma for 10% of all tracheal tumors.[2,3,8-11]

Adenoid cystic carcinoma (formerly known as *cylindroma*) originates in the epithelium of mucous glands.[4,6,7,12]

Of adenoid cystic tumors that present in the respiratory tract over 90% are located in the trachea,[13] and approximately 50% are in the upper third of the trachea, arising from the anterior and lateral tracheal wall.[11,14] On gross examination, adenoid cystic carcinoma is a well circumscribed tumor of firm consistency, usually without ulceration.[7,13] Adenoid cystic carcinoma spreads most commonly by direct extension, often by submucosal or perineural invasion.[7,12] Therefore, the actual extension of this tumor is often greater than suggested by bronchoscopy or by intraoperative palpation. These tumors are known to grow slowly and may be large at the time of presentation. Adenoid cystic carcinomas metastasize most commonly to the lungs but can also spread to the brain, bone, kidneys, or liver.[7]

Squamous cell carcinomas of the trachea usually originate in the posterior or lateral tracheal wall, are frequently exophytic and ulcerative, and also grow slowly.[7,11] Approximately 50% of these squamous cell carcinomas occur in the lower third of the trachea.[2,9,11] Differentiation between a primary tracheal or an esophageal squamous cell carcinoma is important; therefore, esophagoscopy is mandatory before initiating treatment.

CLINICAL PRESENTATION

Squamous cell carcinoma occurs predominantly in patients in their 50s and 60s, and 75% to 92% of the patients are men.[2,5,6,11] This neoplasm is distinctly uncommon in patients <50 years of age[3,6] and is strongly associated with a history of tobacco use.[2,5,9,10] In addition, 40% of patients who undergo resection of a tracheal squamous cell carcinoma have had a history, a concurrent finding, or a later occurrence of a second primary tobacco-related cancer (in the lungs, larynx, oropharynx, esophagus, or bladder).[5,6,8]

In contrast to squamous cell carcinoma, adenoid cystic carcinoma predominates in patients in their 40s, but 36% of patients are diagnosed before age 40.[6] In patients <40 years of age with a tracheal tumor, only 3% were found to have a squamous cell carcinoma, 46% had an adenoid cystic carcinoma, and 51% had various other types of tumors, most of which were benign or typical carcinoid tumors in one large series.[6] The male to female ratio for adenoid cystic carcinomas is 1:1, and a significant smoking history has never been found to be a risk factor for the development of these tumors.[2,5,6,13]

Because of the rarity of tracheal tumors, it can be difficult to make a diagnosis in a timely fashion. This is supported by the fact that the mean duration of symptoms before diagnosis is relatively long (4–17 months).[5,13,14] The most common presenting symptom is dyspnea, which occurs in approximately 40% of patients.[5,11,13–16] Dyspnea secondary to tracheal obstruction from neoplasms is inspiratory in most instances, contrary to dyspnea in asthma or emphysema, which is expiratory.[7] Symptoms of dyspnea, wheezing, or both do not occur until more than half of the cross-sectional area of the airway is obstructed.[7,15] Because the chest radiograph is normal in ≥75% of patients,[3,15,17] these patients are often treated for asthma or chronic obstructive pulmonary disease, thus delaying the diagnosis. Other presenting symptoms include hemoptysis, coughing, hoarseness, wheezing, pneumonia, stridor, and chest pain. Less than 5% of patients with tracheal neoplasms are asymptomatic at the time of presentation.[9,15] Symptomatic distant metastases from primary tracheal cancers are relatively rare, probably because of the early development of local symptoms.[7]

PATIENT EVALUATION

Radiographic Evaluation

The trachea in adults is 10 to 11 cm long, of which half is in the middle mediastinum and half is above the thoracic inlet. Because the trachea is intimately surrounded by vital structures in both the neck and the mediastinum, tumors of the trachea can and do involve structures such as the esophagus, innominate artery and vein, pulmonary artery, aorta, superior vena cava, thyroid gland, and larynx. Thus, an accurate radiographic assessment of the trachea and surrounding structures is paramount as the first diagnostic study in a patient suspected of having tracheal cancer.

Initial radiographic evaluation of a patient with symptoms or signs of a tracheal tumor includes an anteroposterior overpenetrated (high kilovolt) view of the larynx and trachea to the level of the carina.[7] Lateral views of the extended neck may also be helpful. Fluoroscopy of the trachea with spot films (with or without specific opacification of the esophagus with barium) may also be indicated if recurrent laryngeal nerve or esophageal involvement is suspected.[7] Computed tomography (CT), with or without three-dimensional reconstruction, is generally performed in every patient and provides important information about the extraluminal extent of the tumor, the presence of enlarged mediastinal lymph nodes, and metastatic disease to the lungs, liver, or adrenal glands. No study has compared CT with magnetic resonance imaging in patients with tracheal cancers. Magnetic resonance angiography has been useful in evaluating vascular involvement of the innominate ar-

tery, aorta, or superior vena cava, although conventional angiography is also useful.[18]

Endoscopic Evaluation

No radiographic assessment can evaluate the trachea as well as a bronchoscopic examination. Bronchoscopy permits the surgeon to accurately record the length of trachea involved by the malignancy and, therefore, how much trachea will be left for reconstruction. Bronchoscopy is also useful in establishing a histologic diagnosis, although differentiating between an adenoid cystic carcinoma, a carcinoid tumor, or an adenocarcinoma from a biopsy fragment alone may occasionally be difficult.[7]

The timing and method of bronchoscopy and the indication for bronchoscopic biopsy of the lesion require judgment on the part of the endoscopist. Patients with clinically and radiographically smaller tumors can undergo flexible bronchoscopy in an outpatient setting. Lesions that appear to have a significant vascular component should not be biopsied with a flexible bronchoscope in an outpatient setting. In patients with larger tumors, the flexible bronchoscope should be passed proximal to the tumor only, because manipulation of the tumor may result in fragmentation with distal emboli or airway swelling, either of which may cause severe respiratory distress.

If the patient has a clinically or radiographically larger tumor, rigid bronchoscopy under general anesthesia is the preferred approach. This may be done days before a planned surgical resection of the tumor or immediately before the operation. Use of the rigid bronchoscope permits better airway management for larger tracheal tumors, as well as control of any bleeding associated with "coring out" or biopsy of the tumor. Additionally, it may be necessary to use a rigid bronchoscope to mechanically debride a larger tracheal tumor preoperatively. This can facilitate management of the airway at the time of the planned curative resection.

STAGING

There is no staging system for tracheal cancer in common use. The TNM system includes a specific designation of T1 for tumors arising within the wall of the central airways but does not address the vast majority of tracheal tumors that have penetrated the tracheal wall or involve paratracheal lymph nodes.[19] An alternative staging system for tracheal tumors based on the depth of tumor penetration has been proposed but has not been used thus far.[7] Furthermore, the same extent of tumor involving either an adenoid cystic or a squamous cell carcinoma has different implications because of the markedly different biologic behavior of these two tumor types.

An assessment of the extent of a tracheal malignancy must primarily address the question of whether the tumor is resectable. The most important staging study is bronchoscopic evaluation of the tracheobronchial tree. Important information obtained at bronchoscopy includes the length of the trachea from the vocal cords to the carina, tumor length, distance from the vocal cords to the top of the tumor, and distance from the bottom of the tumor to the carina. One-half of the trachea is the maximal length that can safely be resected and reconstructed. Thus, if a tumor is more than 5 or 6 cm in length, the patient is not a surgical candidate because the amount of trachea that must be resected precludes safe reconstruction of the airway.

Invasion of surrounding structures or involvement of paratracheal lymph nodes may be suggested by a CT scan. No information is available to assess the false positive (FP) or false negative (FN) rate of CT results in this regard. The FN rate in patients with a tracheal squamous cell carcinoma is likely to be relatively high because the FN rate of CT for "central" non–small cell lung cancer located in the lung parenchyma is approximately 20% to 25% (see Fig. 5–7). Mediastinoscopy can be used to evaluate enlarged mediastinal lymph nodes identified on CT and to assess locoregional invasion by the primary tumor. Histologically positive lymph nodes at multiple levels (particularly for squamous cell carcinoma) or a "frozen" mediastinum due to extensive tumor invasion has been used as a criterion of unresectability.[15] Locoregional staging of the tumor involves esophagoscopy when the tracheal tumor is close to the esophagus. Esophagectomy and partial esophageal wall excision have been performed concomitantly with tracheal resection, but only in highly selected patients.[13,15]

The likelihood of systemic metastases in relation to the clinical examination has not been reported for tracheal cancers. For patients with adenoid cystic carcinoma, distant metastases most commonly involve the lung and therefore would probably be apparent on a chest CT scan. Other scans are not likely to be helpful. However, local tumor control by resection may sometimes be justified in patients with adenoid cystic carcinomas, even in the presence of distant metastases.[13,17] The metastatic behavior of tracheal squamous cell carcinomas is similar to that of other bronchogenic squamous cell carcinomas. Given the lack of data, the rarity of these tumors, and the potential risks of tracheal resection, it may be appropriate to perform imaging studies to rule out distant metastases in most of these patients.

TREATMENT

Surgery With or Without Radiotherapy

In most reported series, surgery is the primary treatment modality for the majority of patients diagnosed with a tracheal malignancy, but this may in part be a reflection of referral patterns to the institutions involved in these series.[4–6,13,14,20,21] As noted previously, contraindications to surgery include >50% of tracheal length involved by tumor, extensive locoregional tumor extension, poor patient performance status, and multiple positive nodal stations or distant metastasis (although a palliative resection may sometimes still be indicated in patients with adenoid cystic carcinoma).[7,13,17] Despite these considerations, approximately 75% of patients with a histologically proven tracheal malignancy are surgical candidates,[6,7,13] and, among these, there is a 66% resectability rate.[6]

It is beyond the scope of this chapter to discuss the operative management of tracheal carcinomas. It is, however, important to realize that the location and extent of the tumor dictate the surgical approach, magnitude of the procedure, and perioperative morbidity and mortality.[5] For example, patients with tumors requiring carinal resection with or without concomitant pulmonary resection have increased perioperative morbidity and mortality compared with patients whose tumors require cervical tracheal resection alone. Despite surgical and anesthetic innovations, the operative mortality for resection of a malignant tracheal tumor in the hands of experienced thoracic surgeons is 10% (Tables 28–1 and 28–2).

Adenoid cystic carcinoma has a propensity for submucosal and perineural extension beyond the visible borders of the tumor.[5,6,12,13] No data is available regarding the average distance of this extension, but the use of frozen section examination in encouraged.[13] However, the surgeon must frequently sacrifice complete resection of an adenoid cystic tumor in order to be able to safely accomplish tracheal reconstruction, although this violates a basic surgical oncologic principle. Surgical resection margins are histologically positive in 40% to 50% of patients undergoing adenoid cystic carcinoma resection.[5,6,13,14] Several studies have found no significant survival difference between patients who have had complete and incomplete resections (Fig. 28–1).[5,6,13,14,22] However, a nonsignificant trend toward poorer survival after incomplete resection has been seen in the larger studies (10-year survival, 64% and 69% for R_0 patients versus 30% and 45% for $R_{1,2}$ patients).[5,13] In addition, the incidence of suture line recurrence is low (≤ 10%) in all patients undergoing resection of an adenoid cystic carcinoma (usually with adjuvant radiotherapy [RT]).[5,6,13]

Survival following resection of adenoid cystic carcinoma is good, with 5- and 10-year survival rates of 75% and

TABLE 28–1. RESULTS OF SURGERY FOR ADENOID CYSTIC CARCINOMA OF THE TRACHEA[a]

STUDY	N	% OF ALL PATIENTS SEEN	POSITIVE NODES (%)	POSITIVE SURGICAL MARGIN (%)	OPERATIVE DEATH (%)	OVERALL SURVIVAL (%) 5 y	OVERALL SURVIVAL (%) 10 y
Régnard et al[5]	63	—	9	38	6	73	57
Grillo and Mathisen[6]	60	80	42	42	13	—	—
Perelman et al[7]	56	—	—	—	14	66	56
Maziak et al[13]	32	84	16	50	9	79	51
Average					**11**	**73**	**55**

Inclusion criteria: Studies with ≥20 patients.
[a]The majority of patients had induction or adjuvant radiotherapy.

TABLE 28–2. RESULTS OF SURGERY FOR SQUAMOUS CELL CARCINOMA OF THE TRACHEA[a]

STUDY	N	% OF ALL PATIENTS SEEN	POSITIVE NODES (%)	POSITIVE SURGICAL MARGIN (%)	OPERATIVE DEATH (%)	OVERALL SURVIVAL (%)	
						5 y	10 y
Régnard et al[5]	94	—	31	26	14	47	36
Grillo and Mathisen[6]	44	63	23	31	7	—	—
Perelman et al[7][b]	20	—	—	—	—	13	13

Inclusion criteria: Studies with ≥20 patients.
[a]The majority of patients had induction or adjuvant radiotherapy.
[b]Only 5 of 20 patients had adjuvant radiotherapy.

55% (see Table 28–1). Two studies have not found a survival difference between patients with or without lymph node involvement.[5,13] All of the studies in Table 28–1 have >20 years of follow-up. It is important to have long follow-up of patients with these tumors because these neoplasms typically demonstrate indolent growth. This is evidenced by the frequent finding of a long period (average, 1-2 years) of symptoms before a diagnosis is made[5,13,14] and survival of several patients for 5 to 16 years even after the appearance of distant metastases.[12,13] Several authors have reported late recurrences, appearing up to 27 years after the original resection.[6,23]

The majority of patients who underwent resection for adenoid cystic carcinoma also received RT, especially if there was a positive surgical margin or lymph node involvement.[5,6,12,13] It is possible that the addition of RT has contributed to the good survival rate of these patients after resection. Although the two largest series found no survival advantage with adjuvant RT, the studies had insufficient power to demonstrate a modest survival advantage.[5,13] It is striking that all centers with experience in treating this disease recommend RT for all patients in the belief that this will decrease the recurrence rate.[4–6,12,13]

Survival of patients undergoing surgery and adjuvant RT for squamous cell carcinoma is approximately 45% at 5

years and 35% at 10 years (see Table 28–2). Both lymph node involvement and positive surgical margins are frequently found, each occurring in approximately 30% of patients (see Table 28–2). Although one study has suggested poorer survival in patients with lymph node involvement,[6] a larger retrospective study found no difference in survival (5-year survival, 46% versus 47%).[5] Incomplete resection ($R_{1,2}$) has been found to result) in poorer survival (5-year survival, 25% versus 55%; $P < 0.02$),[5] a finding that is supported by others as well.[6] In a retrospective analysis, adjuvant RT in a small number of patients with positive surgical margins was associated with improved survival (Fig. 28–2),[5] although RT was of no clear benefit in completely resected patients (Fig. 28–3).

Radiotherapy Alone

Patients who have contraindications to resection of a tracheal malignancy are most commonly managed with external beam RT as the primary treatment modality. The majority of studies of RT as single modality therapy involve patients with squamous cell carcinoma of the trachea.[3,9,24–29] No large series of patients receiving RT alone for adenoid cystic carcinoma have been reported. The majority of pa-

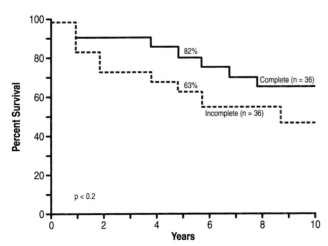

FIGURE 28–1. Survival of patients with adenoid cystic carcinomas according to completeness of resection. (From Régnard JF, Fourquier P, Levasseur P, et al. Results and prognostic factors in resections of primary tracheal tumors: a multicenter retrospective study. J Thorac Cardiovasc Surg. 1996;111:808–814.[5])

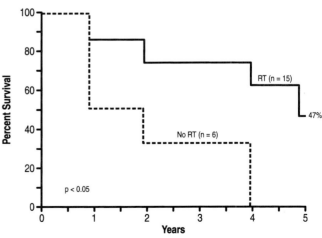

FIGURE 28–2. Survival of incompletely resected patients with squamous cell carcinoma according to whether adjuvant radiotherapy was used. (From Régnard JF, Fourquier P, Levasseur P, et al. Results and prognostic factors in resections of primary tracheal tumors: a multicenter retrospective study. J Thorac Cardiovasc Surg. 1996;111:808–814.[5])

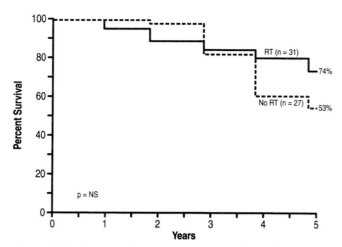

FIGURE 28–3. Survival of completely resected patients with squamous cell carcinoma according to whether adjuvant radiotherapy was given. (From Régnard JF, Fourquier P, Levasseur P, et al. Results and prognostic factors in resections of primary tracheal tumors: a multicenter retrospective study. J Thorac Cardiovasc Surg. 1996;111:808–814.[5])

tients who undergo RT alone for a tracheal squamous cell carcinoma are considered to be unresectable or have distant metastases. Typically, patients undergoing RT for a tracheal squamous cell carcinoma have a performance status ≥2 and are clinically symptomatic.[10,24,26,28]

Radiation doses used for patients with tracheal cancers range from 10 to >70 Gy.[10,26] The average median survival of patients treated with RT alone is approximately 8 months, but ranges from 6 to 24 months (Table 28–3). There is a wide variation in the rate of complete response and local control. The variability of the results should come as no surprise if the mixture of patient characteristics, treatment goals (curative versus palliative), and RT doses is considered. Data for patients treated with curative intent (or those treated with RT doses >50 Gy, which presumably implies curative intent) shows that the 5-year survival is

24%. The 5-year survival of palliatively treated patients (or those treated with <50 Gy) has been reported by several authors to be poor (0%-5%).[9,24–26]

Two studies employing multivariate analysis have found poor performance status (≥2)[26] and weight loss (>10%)[9] to be negative prognostic indicators. Other authors, using univariate analysis, have reported increasing age (>63 years),[26] larger tumor size (>3 cm),[26] mediastinal lymph node involvement,[9,10] and squamous cell tumor histology[24] to be associated with a poorer prognosis in patients undergoing RT for a tracheal malignancy.[10,24,26] Two studies involving small numbers of patients with adenoid cystic carcinoma reported better response rates and survival for these patients compared with patients with squamous cell carcinoma.[24,28]

A higher RT dose (>50 Gy) was found by univariate analysis to be predictive of improved survival in the Australian experience,[9] but multivariate analysis in these 32 patients suggested this was due entirely to selection of patients with a better prognosis (weight loss <10%, absence of lymph node involvement).[9] In contrast, in a larger multivariate analysis involving 84 patients, Mornex et al[26] found a higher RT dose (≥56 Gy) and a better performance status (<2) to be *independent* predictors of improved survival. This is supported by the good survival reported by Jeremic et al[10] in 22 patients, all of whom received 60 to 70 Gy of RT (median survival, 24 months; 5-year survival, 27%). Furthermore, most of the radiographic complete responses have been seen in patients given ≥50 Gy of RT. Based on these retrospective analyses, most authors recommend a dose of ≥60 Gy for patients treated with curative intent.[24–29]

RT is successful in palliating dyspnea in approximately 50% of patients with tracheal malignancies (24%-58%).[10,24,25] Other methods of palliation (eg, endobronchial tumor removal, stent placement, laser therapy, cryotherapy) are also likely to be of significant palliative benefit in these patients, as discussed in Chapter 29.

TABLE 28–3. RADIOTHERAPY ALONE AS THE PRIMARY TREATMENT MODALITY FOR TRACHEAL CANCER

STUDY	N	% SQUAMOUS CELL CARCINOMA	% ADENOID CYSTIC CARCINOMA	% CURATIVE INTENT[a]	% CR	% LOCAL CONTROL[b]	SYMPTOMATIC RELIEF (%)	ALL PATIENTS MST (mo)	ALL PATIENTS 5-y Survival (%)	CURATIVE PATIENTS[a] 5-y Survival (%)
Mornex et al[26]	84	83	0	48[c,d]	51	—	—	8	8	12
Manninen et al[2]	44	100	0	65	52[e]	50	—	10	—	(9)[f]
Chao et al[9]	42	67	7	26[c]	10[e]	19	—	6	6	30
Makarewicz et al[24]	23	56	30	35	26[e]	33	56[g]	10	—	25
Jeremic et al[10]	22	100	0	100	36[e]	45	48	(24)[h]	—	27
Average[i]								**8**	**7**	**24**

Inclusion criteria: Studies from 1980 to 2000 with ≥20 patients treated with primary radiotherapy.
[a]Patients treated explicitly with intent to cure, or arbitrarily defined as those treated with ≥50 Gy as indicated.
[b]No definition provided in studies reporting this.
[c]Defined by radiation dose.
[d]≥56 Gy.
[e]All CR patients received ≥50 Gy.
[f]Only CR patients.
[g]Dyspnea.
[h]All patients treated with curative intent.
[i]Excluding values in parentheses.
CR, complete response; Curative patients, patients treated with curative intent; MST, median survival time.

Brachytherapy

Intraluminal tracheobronchial brachytherapy is used either as a boost after primary RT or as an adjunct to manage local recurrence. Schraube et al[30] reported on five patients with tracheal cancer in whom 3 or 4 fractions of 5 Gy each were delivered following external beam RT of 46 to 50 Gy. One patient developed a necrotizing tracheitis that resulted in tracheal stenosis requiring stent placement. Makarewicz and Mross[24] used 6 to 7.5 Gy in 2 to 3 fractions in 16 of 23 patients treated with external beam RT of 20 to 60 Gy. In another study,[31] a complete response was achieved in 5 of 7 patients treated with brachytherapy (3–5 Gy in 3–5 fractions) after external beam RT of 50 Gy. The median survival was 34 months, but 2 patients developed tracheal stenosis, and chondromalacia and chronic tracheitis developed in 2 additional patients.[31] Other authors have used brachytherapy to help manage local recurrence after primary RT years earlier.[32,33] However, given the limited experience, the role of brachytherapy in tracheal malignancies is unclear at present. It may be useful in managing local recurrences or as adjuvant therapy after surgery when there is microscopic disease at the surgical margin.

Chemotherapy

There are only anecdotal reports of chemotherapy in the treatment of patients with tracheal malignancies.[26,28] Manninen et al[28] treated 21 patients with recurrent or metastatic squamous cell carcinoma with varying combinations of cyclophosphamide, vincristine, bleomycin, and doxorubicin. The authors concluded that these tumors were resistant to chemotherapy. However, because second- and third-generation chemotherapy agents have shown much better activity in squamous cell carcinoma of the lung than the agents just noted, the newer agents may have a role in treating tracheal squamous cell carcinoma. Furthermore, no studies have addressed the radiosensitizing properties of certain chemotherapy agents in patients with tracheal malignancies, although intuitively this approach has appeal, given the success in other tumors.

INCIDENCE AND TREATMENT OF RECURRENCES

The vast majority of distant recurrences after resection and adjuvant RT for adenoid cystic carcinoma are pulmonary, although brain, liver, and bone metastases have also been reported.[5,6,12–14,17] Régnard et al[5] reported that 18% of 65 patients developed distant metastases (all pulmonary) at a mean interval of 4 years postoperatively. Maziak et al[13] reported a 45% incidence of metachronous distant metastases, of which 76% were pulmonary, after a mean interval of 8 years (range, 1-25 years). The presence of pulmonary metastases does not connote the impending death of the patient because the mean survival after diagnosis is 37 months (range, 4 months-7 years),[13] and survival for up to 16 years has been reported.[12]

Local recurrences after resection with or without RT for adenoid cystic carcinomas develop in 14% to 25% of patients and can occur synchronously with distant metastases.[5,13,17] The incidence of local recurrences has not been correlated with the presence of histologically positive surgical margins or lymph nodes. Adenoid cystic carcinomas have a propensity for late recurrences (up to 27 years after

DATA SUMMARY: TRACHEAL CANCERS	AMOUNT	QUALITY	CONSISTENCY
Approximately 80% of tracheal cancers are either squamous cell or adenoid cystic carcinomas	High	High	High
Squamous cell carcinomas occur predominantly in male smokers >60 years of age	High	High	High
Adenoid cystic carcinomas occur over a wide age range without any gender predilection	Mod	High	High
Adenoid cystic carcinomas extend submucosally beyond the visible border of the tumor	High	High	High
Resection of adenoid cystic carcinoma results in a positive surgical margin in 40% of patients	Mod	High	High
Survival after incomplete resection of adenoid cystic carcinoma and postoperative RT is only slightly worse (~15%) than after complete resection	*Mod*	*Mod*	*High*
5-year survival for patients with squamous cell carcinoma treated by resection with or without RT is approximately 25%	Mod	Mod	Mod
RT alone given with curative intent in patients with squamous cell carcinoma results in a 5-year survival of 25%	Mod	Poor	Mod
RT alone provides local control of tracheal cancer in 40% of patients	High	Poor	Mod
RT doses >50 Gy are associated with improved survival	Mod	Mod	High

Type of data rated: Plain text: descriptive statement   *Italics: controlled comparison*   **Bold: randomized comparison**

resection),[23] and lifelong follow-up, which should include bronchoscopy, is therefore recommended.[5,6,13]

Treatment for local recurrences of an adenoid cystic carcinoma may be a second resection if resection and reconstruction are feasible. More commonly, endoscopic palliation (with or without stent placement or brachytherapy, or both) is used. External beam RT may be a good option if this was not part of the initial treatment. Pulmonary metastases are frequently asymptomatic.[5,13] Metastectomy, after appropriate intra- and extrathoracic staging, has been reported.[5,7,17] The role of chemotherapy for distant metastases remains anecdotal and unproved.[13,14,28]

In patients with squamous cell carcinoma, distant recurrence occurred in 12% of those who had resection and adjuvant RT, and the local recurrence rate was 28% in the series reported by Régnard et al.[5] These recurrences occurred after a mean disease-free interval of 18 months, far less than that of adenoid cystic carcinomas. Importantly, approximately 20% of patients with squamous cell carcinoma developed a second primary cancer (mainly lung or head and neck cancers) during follow-up.[5,6,8]

EDITORS' COMMENTS

Tracheal cancers are rare and commonly involve either adenoid cystic carcinoma or squamous cell carcinoma. Differentiation between these two should not be difficult. Adenoid cystic carcinoma should be suspected because of a typical bronchoscopic appearance or because the patient is <40 years old and is a nonsmoker. The possibility of a benign lesion must also be considered, especially in the younger age groups. A biopsy to firmly establish the diagnosis is essential in most patients. Squamous cell carcinomas are more commonly seen in older men who smoke; these tumors have an irregular, ulcerated appearance on bronchoscopy.

Adenoid cystic carcinomas should be managed by resection whenever possible. Because of the well known extension of these tumors beyond the visible borders, strong consideration should be given to referral to one of the few centers worldwide that have accumulated experience in treating this cancer. A center with experience in tracheal resection and reconstruction has a better basis for judging how much trachea to resect in order to be able to achieve a safe reconstruction. Having said this, although an incomplete resection leads to poorer survival, it does not imply a dismal prognosis, at least if adjuvant RT is given. An accurate assessment of the role of adjuvant RT cannot be made because there is no controlled data; nevertheless, radiation for patients with positive surgical margins is difficult to argue against. Whether adjuvant RT should be given to patients who have undergone a complete resection with negative surgical margins is even more unclear. However, all of the centers having experience with tracheal adenoid cystic carcinomas advocate postoperative RT for all patients, regardless of tumor histology or margins. Because of the propensity to develop a late recurrence, patients with an adenoid cystic carcinoma should be followed closely for life.

Patients with primary squamous cell carcinomas of the trachea are less likely than those with adenoid cystic carcinomas to be candidates for surgery. Many of these tumors involve mediastinal lymph nodes and other mediastinal structures and sometimes also have distant metastases. Significant palliation for unresectable patients can be achieved using a variety of techniques to relieve airway obstruction. Before undertaking treatment of a patient with squamous cell carcinoma, a careful search for other smoking-related cancers should be made because these are common. Surgery should be considered for those patients who present with an early stage, localized lesion. A complete resection must be achieved whenever possible. Involvement of lymph nodes that are directly adjacent to the tumor is probably not as important as the ability to achieve a complete resection. Although some retrospective data suggests that adjuvant RT after an incomplete resection may result in reasonable survival, RT has not been demonstrated to salvage patients after incomplete resection of non–small cell lung cancer in other locations.

Primary RT for squamous cell carcinoma offers some hope for long-term survival in selected patients. However, the data regarding this is limited because most of the patients treated with RT have had extensive disease or were poor-risk patients. Definitive treatment of squamous cell carcinoma by RT has resulted in similar survival compared with resection, but this has not been as well documented in patients treated with RT as in patients undergoing surgery. Combined modality treatment with chemotherapy and RT is likely to be a good way to treat many patients with tracheal squamous cell carcinoma. Too few patients with adenoid cystic carcinoma have been treated with primary RT to allow any conclusions regarding this modality to be made with confidence.

References

1. Ranke EJ, Presley SS, Holinger PH. Tracheogenic carcinoma. JAMA. 1962;182:121–124.
2. Manninen MP, Antila PJ, Pukander JS, et al. Occurrence of tracheal carcinoma in Finland. Acta Otolaryngol (Stockh). 1991;111:1162–1169.
3. Rostom AY, Morgan RL. Results of treating primary tumors of the trachea by irradiation. Thorax. 1978;33:387–393.
4. Refaely Y, Weissberg D. Surgical management of tracheal tumors. Ann Thorac Surg. 1997;64:1429–1433.
5. Régnard JF, Fourquier P, Levasseur P, et al. Results and prognostic factors in resections of primary tracheal tumors: a multicenter retrospective study. J Thorac Cardiovasc Surg. 1996;111:808–814.
6. Grillo HC, Mathisen DJ. Primary tracheal tumors: treatment and results. Ann Thorac Surg. 1990;49:69–77.
7. Perelman MI, Koroleva NS. Primary tumors of the trachea. In: Grillo HC, Eschapasse H, eds. International Trends in General Thoracic Surgery. Vol. 2. Philadelphia: WB Saunders; 1987:91–106.
8. Hajdu SI, Huvos AG, Goodner JT, et al. Carcinoma of the trachea: clinicopathologic study of 41 cases. Cancer. 1970;25:1448–1456.
9. Chao MWT, Smith JG, Laidlaw C, et al. Results of treating primary tumors of the trachea with radiotherapy. Int J Radiat Oncol Biol Phys. 1998;41:779–785.
10. Jeremic B, Shibamoto Y, Acimovic L, et al. Radiotherapy for primary squamous cell carcinoma of the trachea. Radiother Oncol. 1996;41:135–138.
11. Yang K-Y, Chen Y-M, Huang M-H, et al. Revisit of primary malignant neoplasms of the trachea: clinical characteristics and survival analysis. Jpn J Clin Oncol. 1997;27:305–309.
12. Pearson FG, Todd TRJ, Cooper JD. Experience with primary neo-

plasms of the trachea and carina. J Thorac Cardiovasc Surg. 1984;88:511–518.

13. Maziak DE, Todd TRJ, Keshavjee SH, et al. Adenoid cystic carcinoma of the airway: thirty-two-year experience. J Thorac Cardiovasc Surg. 1996;112:1522–1532.

14. Azar T, Abdul-Karim FW, Tucker HM. Adenoid cystic carcinoma of the trachea. Laryngoscope. 1998;108:1297–1300.

15. Meyers BF, Mathisen DJ. Management of tracheal neoplasms. Oncologist. 1997;2:245–253.

16. Lee C-H, Lin H-C. Descriptive study of prognostic factors influencing survival of patients with primary tracheal tumors. Chang Gung Med J. 1995;18:224–230.

17. Prommegger R, Salzer GM. Long-term results of surgery for adenoid cystic carcinoma of the trachea and bronchi. Eur J Surg Oncol. 1998;24:440–444.

18. Mathisen DJ. Tracheal tumors. Chest Surg Clin North Am. 1996;6:875–898.

19. Mountain CF. Revisions in the International System for Staging Lung Cancer. Chest. 1997;111:1710–1717.

20. Perelman MI, Koroleva N, Birjukov J, et al. Primary tracheal tumors. Semin Thorac Cardiovasc Surg. 1996;8:400–402.

21. Le-Tian X, Zhen-Fu S, Ze-Jian L, et al. Tracheobronchial tumors: an eighteen-year series from Capital Hospital, Peking, China. Ann Thorac Surg. 1983;35:590–596.

22. Gelder CM, Hetzel MR. Primary tracheal tumours: a national survey. Thorax. 1993;48:688–692.

23. Pearson FG. In discussion of Régnard JF, Fourquier P, Levasseur P, et al. Results and prognostic factors in resections of primary tracheal tumors: a multicenter retrospective study. J Thorac Cardiovasc Surg. 1996;111:808–814.

24. Makarewicz R, Mross M. Radiation therapy alone in the treatment of tumours of the trachea. Lung Cancer. 1998;20:169–174.

25. Cheung AYC. Radiotherapy for primary carcinoma of the trachea. Radiother Oncol. 1989;14:279–285.

26. Mornex F, Coquard R, Danhier S, et al. Role of radiation therapy in the treatment of primary tracheal carcinoma. Int J Radiat Oncol Biol Phys. 1998;41:299–305.

27. Chow DC, Komaki R, Libshitz HI, et al. Treatment of primary neoplasms of the trachea: the role of radiation therapy. Cancer. 1993;71:2946–2952.

28. Manninen MP, Pukander JS, Flander MK, et al. Treatment of primary tracheal carcinoma in Finland in 1967-1985. Acta Oncologica. 1993;3:277–282.

29. Fields JN, Rigaud G, Emami BN. Primary tumors of the trachea: results of radiation therapy. Cancer. 1989;63:2429–2433.

30. Schraube P, Latz D, Wannenmacher M. Treatment of primary squamous cell carcinoma of the trachea: the role of radiation therapy. Radiother Oncol. 1994;33:254–258.

31. Harms W, Latz D, Becker H, et al. HDR-brachytherapy boost for residual tumour after external beam radiotherapy in patients with tracheal malignancies. Radiother Oncol. 1999;52:251–255.

32. Percapio B, Price JC, Murphy P. Endotracheal irradiation of adenoid cystic carcinoma of the trachea. Radiology. 1978;128:209–210.

33. Boedker A, Hald A, Kristensen D. A method for selective endobronchial and endotracheal irradiation. J Thorac Cardiovasc Surg. 1982;84:59–61.

PART 9

MISCELLANEOUS ISSUES

PALLIATIVE TREATMENT OF LUNG CANCER

Frank C. Detterbeck, David R. Jones, and David E. Morris

NEUROLOGIC SYMPTOMS
 Brain Metastases
 Spinal Cord Compression

BONE METASTASES

LOCAL THORACIC SYMPTOMS
 General Aspects
 Nonobstructive Airway Symptoms
 Obstructive Airway Symptoms

MALIGNANT PLEURAL EFFUSION

EDITORS' COMMENTS

Palliation of symptoms caused by lung cancer is frequently possible, even when curative treatments are futile. Palliative treatment may involve general basic supportive care measures, such as narcotics for pain control, or specific measures, such as the use of steroids to decrease cerebral edema associated with brain metastases. In addition, palliative treatment may involve therapy that actively treats the cancer, such as radiation or chemotherapy. Both specific supportive care and active treatment measures given with the intent of palliation are included in this chapter. Curative therapies are discussed in other chapters. The focus of this chapter is the palliation of specific intrathoracic and extrathoracic symptoms that are commonly caused by lung cancer; treatment of systemic symptoms such as fatigue, anorexia, and weight loss is not included. The effect of systemic treatment on such generalized constitutional symptoms is discussed in Chapters 22 and 25.

NEUROLOGIC SYMPTOMS

Brain Metastases

Brain metastases occur frequently in patients with lung cancer and have a profound effect on both quality of life and survival. Headaches (40%), motor deficits (36%), seizures (27%), disorientation (24%), and lethargy (16%) account for the vast majority of presenting symptoms.[1,2] In the absence of any treatment, the survival of patients with brain metastases is commonly cited as 1 to 2 months.[1] This figure has been passed down from historical series,[3,4] and no natural history data is available from studies published between 1980 and 2000. Most of the studies of brain metastases involve patients with a variety of types of cancer, but lung cancer accounts for the majority.[5–8] Furthermore, no difference in survival has been noted among

patients with different primary cancers in most studies,[8–11] although some researchers have found better survival in patients with breast cancer.[5]

Steroids are commonly used to palliate symptoms caused by brain metastases by decreasing the surrounding edema. This results in moderate relief of symptoms in approximately 40% and a major improvement in approximately 20% of patients.[12] Complications from steroid treatment are seen in approximately 30% of patients.[12,13] The median survival with steroids alone is approximately 1 to 2 months.[1,13,14] Typically, 8 to 24 mg of dexamethasone per day is given in several divided doses. However, a randomized study of 97 patients found no difference in improvement of symptoms among patients given 4, 8, or 16 mg of dexamethasone per day.[12] Although the serum half-life of dexamethasone is approximately 4 to 6 hours, the half-life of the clinical effect has been reported to be approximately 36 to 54 hours,[12,15] suggesting that lower and less frequent dosing may be more appropriate, at least in patients without severe symptoms. Approximately 20% of patients with brain metastases develop seizures.[1,16] However, retrospective analyses have concluded that prophylactic administration of anticonvulsants is not beneficial.[16]

Whole brain radiotherapy (WBRT) has been commonly used in order to provide improved palliation over what can be achieved by steroids alone. In the United States, this typically involves 30 Gy of radiation delivered in 10 fractions over 2 weeks. Approximately 50% of patients have shown improvement after 2 weeks, and approximately 75% are improved by the end of 4 weeks.[5] Relief of specific neurologic symptoms follows a similar pattern. The cumulative rate of relief or significant improvement in specific symptoms is approximately 80% (range, 60%–100%).[5,7] However, uncontrolled brain metastases remain the cause of death in approximately 40% of patients receiving WBRT (range, 31%–49%).[5,6,8,9,17]

TABLE 29–1. SURVIVAL OF PATIENTS TREATED WITH PALLIATIVE WHOLE BRAIN RADIOTHERAPY[a]

STUDY	N	TREATMENT PARAMETERS Total Dose	Fx Dose	No. of Fx	Duration (wk)	MST (mo)
Murray et al[18]	213	54 AH	1.6 AH	34	2	5.0
Kurtz et al[6]	125	50	2.5	20	4	3.9
Borgelt et al[5]	227	40	2	20	4	3.7
Borgelt et al[5]	227	40	2.6	15	3	4.2
Borgelt et al[5]	233	40	2.6	15	3	4.2
Haie-Meder et al[10]	106	18 + 25[b]	6/2.5[b]	3 + 10[b]	0.5 + 2[b]	5.3
Borgelt et al[5]	217	30	2	15	3	4.2
Komarnicky et al[8]	436	30	5	6	3	3.6
Borgelt et al[5]	233	30	3	10	2	4.8
Borgelt et al[5]	228	30	3	10	2	3.5
Murray et al[18]	216	30	3	10	2	5.0
Kurtz et al[6]	130	30	3	10	2	4.2
Komarnicky et al[8]	423	30	3	10	2	4.2
Priestman et al[7]	263	30	3	10	2	2.8[c]
Borgelt et al[5]	447	20	4	5	1	3.5
Haie-Meder et al[10]	110	18	6	3	0.5	4.2
Priestman et al[7]	270	12	6	2	0.3	2.5[c]

Inclusion criteria: Randomized studies of whole brain radiotherapy from 1980 to 2000 with ≥100 patients per arm.
[a]None of the survival results was statistically different from the other arms in these randomized studies, except as indicated.
[b]Split course.
[c]$P < 0.05$.
AH, accelerated hyperfractionated (twice daily); Fx, fraction; MST, median survival time; N, number of evaluable patients.

The median survival of patients with brain metastases who undergo WBRT has been consistently reported to be approximately 4 months (range, 2.5–5.3 months).[5–8,10,18] This data is taken from randomized phase III studies involving WBRT with at least 100 patients per arm. The dose or fractionation of WBRT has been shown in a large number of randomized studies not to have an effect on the duration of survival (Table 29–1). The doses investigated have ranged from 12 Gy to 54 Gy, with fractions ranging from 1.6 to 6 Gy. None of these studies found a survival difference between the treatment arms, with one exception.[7] In this study, which compared 12 Gy given in two fractions with 30 Gy given in 10 fractions, a P value of 0.04 was found, although the median survival was 2.5 versus 2.8 months, the 1-year survival was 5% versus 10%, and the 2-year survival was virtually identical.[7] The authors of this study did not believe that the apparent survival difference was clinically significant.[7] The most aggressive regimen, involving 54 Gy of accelerated (17 days) hyperfractionated radiotherapy (RT) (twice daily for the first 10 days) found no survival benefit, even in the most favorable subgroup.[18] It must be concluded, then, that the data currently available indicates that alterations in dose or fractionation have no clear influence on the length of survival in patients receiving WBRT for brain metastases (see Table 29–1). Furthermore, alterations in total dose or fractionation have been shown to have no influence on the promptness, extent, or duration of neurologic improvement.[5]

Prognostic factors have been analyzed using multivariate analysis (1200 patients) or recursive partitioning analysis (780 patients) in two studies, although there was some overlap in the patients involved in these analyses.[11,19] Both studies found a performance status (PS) ≥ 70, a controlled primary site, age <60 or 65 years, and no other extracranial sites of disease to be favorable prognostic indicators. The larger study identified three patient groups.[11] The most favorable group had a PS ≥ 70, an age <65 years, and no

extracranial sites of disease, and the patients were found to have a median survival of 7.1 months. Any patient with a PS ≥ 70 but with either older age or extracranial sites of cancer did not fare as well, with a median survival of 4.2 months. Finally, those patients with a PS < 70 exhibited a median survival of only 2.3 months (Fig. 29–1).[11]

Patients with a poor PS have a limited life expectancy. If WBRT is to be used in these patients, it seems that a

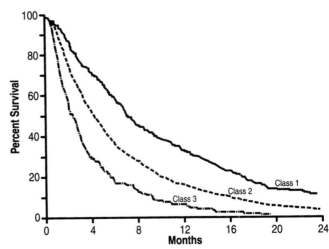

FIGURE 29–1. Survival of three prognostically distinct groups of patients with brain metastases from various primary cancers treated with whole brain radiotherapy, as defined by recursive partitioning analysis of patients from three multi-institutional studies. Class 1, patients with performance status (PS) ≥ 70, age <65 years, and no extracranial sites of cancer; Class 2, patients with PS ≥ 70, age >65 years, and an uncontrolled primary cancer site or other sites of extracranial disease; Class 3, patients with PS < 70. (Reprinted from *International Journal of Radiation Oncology, Biology, Physics,* Vol 37, Gasper L, Scott C, Rotman M, et al, Recursive partitioning analysis [RPA] of prognostic factors in three Radiation Therapy Oncology Group [RTOG] brain metastases trials, 745–751, Copyright 1997, with permission from Elsevier Science.[11])

limited course of RT involving a small number of fractions should be used in order to minimize the treatment time. Furthermore, the limited life expectancy means that concerns about late toxicity from a higher dose per fraction are irrelevant. Those patients with a good PS and no extracranial sites of disease exhibit much better survival with WBRT. However, these are the patients who should be considered for a more aggressive, potentially curative approach (see Chapter 23). Those patients falling in between may achieve some benefit from WBRT, although minimizing the treatment time in these patients is logical, given that their life expectancy is limited.

The potential late neurotoxicity of WBRT has been the subject of controversy.[20,21] In general, the studies that have measured the incidence of late toxicity in all patients, regardless of length of survival, have not found this to be a significant problem. However, an extensive literature review has found that dementia occurs in approximately 10% of patients who survive >1 year.[21] There is a suggestion that this is seen more frequently with larger radiation doses per fraction.[21,22] However, the details of late radiation toxicity in long-term survivors are poorly defined and warrant further study in a prospective fashion.

It has generally been assumed that chemotherapy is ineffective in treating brain metastases because the drugs do not effectively cross the blood-brain barrier. More recent data suggests that the blood-brain barrier is disrupted by metastatic tumor foci.[23] Several reports involving only limited numbers of patients have found that the response rates of brain metastases to chemotherapy, in both small cell lung cancer (SCLC) and non–small cell lung cancer (NSCLC), are the same as the response rates of such tumors elsewhere in the body.[23,24]

Spinal Cord Compression

Spinal cord compression is an oncologic emergency that requires urgent intervention to prevent further decline in neurologic function. Neurologic impairment can have significant effects on quality of life that include difficulty with ambulation, loss of bowel and bladder function, loss of sexual function, and sensory loss. Spinal cord compression can occur from intramedullary (within the spinal cord) or epidural compression. Intramedullary involvement is rarely seen and is not discussed further. Spinal cord compression from epidural metastases can occur from bony metastatic involvement of the vertebral body (~85%), paravertebral metastases with invasion through the intravertebral foramen (~10%–15%), or, rarely, from involvement of the epidural space itself.[25,26] In almost all patients (96%) with cord compression, the initial symptom is pain. At the time of diagnosis, approximately three-quarters of the patients experience weakness, and slightly more than half will have autonomic dysfunction or sensory loss.[25]

Focusing specifically on patients with lung cancer, a study of all 102 such patients with spinal cord compression admitted to an oncology, neurology, or neurosurgery service in Eastern Denmark found that SCLC was most commonly involved (40%), followed by adenocarcinoma (26%), squamous cell cancer (18%), and large cell cancer (9%).[27] The majority of patients experienced pain (77%),

sensory disturbances (90%), loss of motor function (paraplegia, 63%; mild deficit, 33%), and sphincter disturbances (71%). The majority (74%) of the epidural metastases were located in the thoracic region, 18% were in the lumbar region, and 5% were in the cervical region. After treatment with laminectomy, radiation, or both, 15% of patients with SCLC and 22% of patients with NSCLC regained the ability to walk. All patients with SCLC who were ambulatory retained the ability to walk, whereas 5% of NSCLC patients lost this ability. There was no significant effect on reversing sphincter dysfunction. Only 9% of patients survived longer than 12 months, and the median survival was approximately 2 months. The patient's pretreatment neurologic status appears to be the best predictor of outcome. In a smaller series of 29 patients with SCLC, surgery or RT was also able to prevent progression but failed to significantly benefit patients with pre-existing neurologic impairment.[28]

The diagnostic evaluation involves both a careful neurologic examination and imaging. Radiographically, 74% of bony abnormalities consistent with metastatic epidural compression can be visualized on a plain radiograph in patients with lung cancer.[29] Bone scans are sensitive in detecting metastatic bone disease and are also specific for evaluating cord compression in areas where plain radiographs are negative. In cancer patients with negative plain radiographs and negative bone scans, the risk of epidural disease was found to be 0.1% in one study.[30] Magnetic resonance imaging is the preferred imaging study at most centers for detecting spinal cord compression because it demonstrates the extent of vertebral and paravertebral metastases better and has equivalent sensitivity in detecting cord compression compared with myelography.[31,32]

Therapy should be initiated rapidly once a diagnosis of cord compression is confirmed. In general, primary treatment is oral or intravenous corticosteroids and radiation to the area involved. The optimal dose of steroids is unknown, but the doses commonly used are similar to those used in the management of brain metastases.[33] Higher doses have been tried, but no apparent benefit in neurologic outcome has been observed.[34] Radiation therapy delivered in a short course with large fractions remains the standard of care. Total doses between 20 Gy and 40 Gy with daily fraction sizes ranging from 2 Gy to 4 Gy are commonly used.[25]

The role of surgical intervention remains less clear. In a retrospective series of 25 patients with spinal cord compression from metastatic lung cancer who underwent surgical decompression, stabilization, or both, 89% remained ambulatory after surgery and 67% maintained their ambulatory status for more than 6 months.[35] One prospective randomized trial evaluated the role of laminectomy before radiation compared with radiation alone.[36] No significant difference was observed in motor performance, sphincter function, or pain relief, and there were also no significant differences in complications. However, only 29 patients were enrolled in the study, and there was insufficient statistical power to determine the role of laminectomy. Although the role of surgery in the initial management of spinal cord compression is unclear, it should be considered for patients who received previous irradiation to the area, for patients who experience progressive neurologic deterioration while receiving radiation, and for patients with symptomatic spinal instability or bone fragments causing compression.[26]

BONE METASTASES

Bone metastases typically present as painful lesions, and in a minority of cases, pathologic fractures occur. Little data specifically addresses bone metastases from lung cancer. Most investigators have not found the primary cancer type to affect the outcome of patients with bone metastases,[37-39] whereas some have found less frequent palliation in patients with lung cancer compared with those with breast or prostate cancer.[40] RT is commonly used to treat painful bone metastases. In studies involving all types of cancer, at least partial relief of pain is experienced by approximately 80% of patients, and approximately 30% to 50% have complete relief of their pain.[37,40-43] Approximately 30% to 50% of all patients experience some relief within 2 weeks, and approximately 75% within 4 weeks.[37-39,41,42] The average duration of pain relief is 9 months.[41,42] Retreatment of previously radiated sites, on recurrence of pain, has been found to result in the same rate of response as a first treatment in 105 patients.[44]

Alterations in the total dose or fractionation have been shown not to affect the overall rate of response.[37,40] In several randomized studies with at least 100 patients per arm, no differences in response (rapidity, duration, or amount of pain relief) were found among 12 different schedules ranging from 8 Gy given as a single fraction to 40.5 Gy given over 3 weeks.[37,38,40,43,45] Two additional randomized trials (≥100 patients per arm) that compared a single dose of 4 Gy with 8 Gy found that the response rate was lower when 4 Gy was used.[39,42] Because of the limited life expectancy of these patients, it seems best to keep the treatment time short.

Patients sometimes have widespread painful bony metastases requiring palliation. The Radiation Therapy Oncology Group (RTOG) performed a randomized trial comparing localized radiation treatment of 30 Gy in 10 fractions with localized treatment with the addition of hemibody irradiation (8 Gy).[46] With 450 evaluable patients, there was a statistically significant delay in the progression of disease (13 versus 6 months, $P = 0.03$) and a decreased likelihood of requiring additional therapy (24% versus 40% at 1 year, $P = 0.003$). This treatment has a limited role in a select group of patients.

The role of surgical intervention for bony metastases has been primarily to prevent or rectify pathologic fractures and their clinical consequences. No prospective trials have evaluated the risk for impending fractures, and the data has been based primarily on retrospective studies. No uniform criteria exist regarding the role of surgery for vertebral fractures. However, if there is a mechanical problem of displaced bone impinging on the spinal cord or nerve roots, surgical intervention may be indicated to improve stability, relieve cord compression, and relieve pain. Prophylactic internal fixation should be considered for long bone metastases in ambulatory patients who have >50% cortical involvement or subtrochanteric, intertrochanteric, or femoral neck involvement.

LOCAL THORACIC SYMPTOMS

General Aspects

The majority of patients with lung cancer develop symptoms related to the tumor mass within the chest. These local thoracic symptoms can be distressing and fatal in some instances. Therefore, palliative treatment can be of significant benefit, even though survival may remain short due to other aspects of an incurable disease. Clearly, the most common symptom is cough. In prospective series of patients treated for palliation, cough was present in approximately 90% to 95% of patients, although it was classified as moderate or severe in only 50%.[47,48] Hemoptysis is reported by approximately 40% of patients, and it is moderate or severe in nearly 20%.[47-49] In addition, approximately half of the patients report chest pain and dyspnea.[47-49]

The most commonly used palliative treatment for thoracic symptoms in patients with lung cancer is RT. Indeed, this has represented the primary therapy for inoperable

DATA SUMMARY: PALLIATIVE TREATMENT OF BRAIN AND BONE METASTASES	AMOUNT	QUALITY	CONSISTENCY
The median survival of patients with brain metastases who are untreated or given steroids alone is ≤2 months	Mod	Poor	High
WBRT results in palliation in 75% of patients with brain metastases	Mod	Mod	High
Median survival of patients with brain metastases treated with WBRT is 4 months	High	High	High
Alterations in dose or fractionation in palliative WBRT of brain metastases do not alter survival	**High**	**High**	**High**
RT results in palliation (at least partial relief) in 80% of patients with symptomatic bone metastases	Mod	Mod	High
Alterations in dose or fractionation in palliative RT for bone metastases do not affect symptom relief	**High**	**Mod**	**High**

Type of data rated: Plain text: descriptive statement   *Italics: controlled comparison*   **Bold: randomized comparison**

patients for several decades. In the United States, a palliative RT regimen typically involves 30 to 60 Gy of radiation delivered in daily fractions over 2 to 6 weeks. However, a wide variety of treatment regimens have been used, particularly in Britain, Australia, and Europe. Randomized trials comparing different radiation schedules have shown no difference in survival, tumor response rates, palliation rates, or toxicity.[47–51] Three of these trials, conducted by the Medical Research Council in Britain, carefully documented symptoms over the course of 1 year in 374, 235, and 509 patients.[47,48,50] No differences were seen in patients randomized to receive either 10 Gy delivered as a single fraction, 17 Gy delivered in two fractions 1 week apart, or conventional RT involving 27 to 30 Gy delivered in 6 to 10 fractions, but palliation was slightly poorer in patients treated with 39 Gy in 13 fractions. Another trial, conducted by the RTOG in North America, compared 40 Gy given as a split course (20 fractions), 40 Gy given as a continuous course (20 fractions), and 30 Gy given as a continuous course (10 fractions) in 409 patients.[49] No differences in outcomes were seen in this three-arm trial. Thus it appears that when palliation is the goal, equal results can be achieved with a simple one- or two-dose hypofractionated regimen as with conventionally fractionated regimens.

Overall, RT has resulted in complete relief of symptoms in approximately 40% of patients (range, 25%–29%) in carefully documented prospective, randomized trials of palliative treatment. Significant palliation of symptoms was seen in 67% of patients (range, 59%–72%).[47–51] The average median duration of symptom relief has been reported to be 2 to 3 months.[47,48] Although this may seem like a short time, it constitutes 50% to 60% of the patient's remaining survival time.[47,48]

Does thoracic RT result in a palliative prolongation of survival in patients with lung cancer who have incurable disease? Randomized studies are necessary to examine this question, and comparison of median survival time addresses this issue most clearly. There are few randomized studies of radiation versus observation, and they have involved radiation given with curative intent. In an early Veterans Administration study, 554 stage III lung cancer patients (NSCLC and SCLC) were randomized to 40 Gy versus observation alone. The median survival of the patients treated with RT was 30 days longer than the observation arm (142 days versus 112 days).[52] Although the survival difference was reported to be statistically significant, it is doubtful that the difference is clinically significant or that this difference would be significant using actuarial survival curves and current statistical analyses. Furthermore, because approximately 90% of patients received orthovoltage treatment, the applicability of this study to current patients is limited at best. Another older study involving 125 patients randomized to 40 Gy or observation found no difference in mean survival (8.3 versus 8.4 months).[53] A more recent trial randomized 212 inoperable stage I-III NSCLC patients to 60 Gy of radiation versus single-agent low dose vincristine.[54] The latter arm was intended as a placebo arm, and indeed, this agent was found not to be effective. However, RT was also not effective, and no difference was found in median survival.[54]

Does prophylactic thoracic RT in asymptomatic patients result in a palliative benefit by preventing the later occurrence of local intrathoracic symptoms? Although this question has not been addressed directly, several studies suggest that approximately 50% of patients with inoperable lung cancer who are initially asymptomatic do not subsequently develop symptoms that warrant RT (range, 46%–59%).[53–55] Whether prophylactic radiation of asymptomatic patients lowers the rate of development of symptoms to <50% has not been reported. However, it seems likely that even among the prophylactically treated patients, a proportion would develop symptoms before death, considering that the median duration of symptom relief is only 2 to 3 months in symptomatic patients who are treated with radiation. Thus there is no data demonstrating that prophylactic palliative RT is beneficial in asymptomatic patients, and several indirect pieces of data suggest that any benefit would be limited to a minority of the patients treated. However, there may be some patients (eg, patients with tumor encasing a main stem bronchus and impending obstruction) for whom a reasonable argument for prophylactic treatment can be made.

Nonobstructive Airway Symptoms

Cough is an extremely common symptom in patients with lung cancer. This may result from endobronchial tumor or extrinsic airway irritation from either the primary tumor or associated lymph nodes. External beam RT results in palliation in an average of 59% of patients (range, 52%–64%).[47–49,51,56] Endoluminal radiation delivered by brachytherapy techniques has also been reported to result in palliation in an average of 62% of patients (range, 24%–85%) in studies involving at least 20 patients with this symptom.[57–63] The wide range of response rates to brachytherapy may result from the varying definitions, relatively small patient cohorts, or inclusion of different patient populations. In fact, a majority of patients in most series of brachytherapy had already received prior external beam RT, but despite this, brachytherapy retained the ability to palliate cough fairly well. It is interesting that chemotherapy alone has also been reported to palliate cough in approximately 60% of patients with NSCLC in several studies (range, 45%–68%).[61,64–66]

Although hemoptysis can be a distressing symptom to patients, it responds well to treatment. In prospective trials of palliative external beam RT, relief of hemoptysis was seen in an average of 84% of patients (range, 74%–97%).[47–49,51,56] Brachytherapy also resulted in palliation of hemoptysis in an average of 87% of patients (range, 77%–99%) in studies involving at least 20 patients with this symptom,[57,58,60,67–69] despite the fact that most of the patients had previously received external beam RT. Other modalities also appear to be effective, although the data is limited. Neodymium:yttrium-argon-garnet (Nd:YAG) laser treatment was reported to be successful in 67% of patients (16 of 24).[70] Cryotherapy resulted in a 94% rate of palliation among 62 patients with hemoptysis.[71] Even chemotherapy has been reported to relieve hemoptysis in 75% of NSCLC patients (range, 63%–91%).[61,64,66]

Other symptoms also appear to be relatively well relieved by external beam RT. Hoarseness is reported to respond in 60% of patients.[49] Chest pain is relieved in approximately 71% of patients (range, 50%–88%).[47–49,51] A lower rate of response is seen using more objective response measures such as re-expansion of atelectatic lung (23%) or relief of vocal cord paralysis (6%).[72]

A limited amount of data is available regarding the use of re-irradiation with external beam RT for carcinoma of the lung. Four studies involving a total of 104 patients for whom initial therapy consisted of a median dose between 53 and 60 Gy have been published.[73–76] Median retreatment doses ranged between 30 and 35 Gy, with an overall rate of symptomatic improvement after the retreatment of 65%. Complications were noted in 5% and consisted of pneumonitis, rib fracture, and myelopathy.

In conclusion, external beam RT is able to palliate a wide variety of symptoms caused by intrathoracic tumor in approximately two-thirds of the patients with lung cancer and has been the primary palliative therapy used for nonobstructive airway symptoms. Other local therapies also have been found to be effective.

Obstructive Airway Symptoms

The most distressing intrathoracic symptom of lung cancer is undoubtedly progressive airway obstruction. This can be caused by central endobronchial tumors or hilar or mediastinal nodal disease. Palliation of associated symptoms, such as dyspnea or obstructive pneumonia, can be of major benefit to such patients and can prolong survival even when a cure is not possible. A variety of techniques are available to treat airway obstruction, including bronchoscopic or laser resection, photodynamic therapy, cryotherapy, endoluminal brachytherapy, and placement of stents, as well as external beam RT. Although a large number of retrospective series of patients treated by each of these techniques has been published, there are very few prospective or comparative series. Because the patients selected for a particular treatment may not be the same as those treated by another method, it is difficult to compare one treatment modality with another, and no one treatment has been identified as clearly superior in all situations.

The approach taken in this section is to first examine the results of "optimally selected" patients treated with a particular modality. The characteristics of the patients selected for a particular mode of treatment are also examined. Furthermore, an assessment is made of which patients exhibited the best response to a particular type of treatment. This must be viewed as a general approximation because most of the patients also underwent another type of treatment either before or subsequent to the treatment that was the subject of each study. Finally, an attempt is made to rate the advantages and disadvantages of each treatment modality relative to specific clinical situations in order to provide a way of selecting a treatment for a particular patient.

Rigid Bronchoscopy

Probably the most straightforward palliative treatment of airway obstruction is rigid bronchoscopy and mechanical removal of the obstructing tumor. Although this technique has been practiced for >40 years, little published data exists providing a detailed assessment of patient outcomes. The largest study reports a 91% overall success rate in

56 patients.[77] The success rate was only 38% in patients presenting with lobar obstruction, whereas it was well over 90% in patients with tracheal or main stem bronchial lesions. There were no intraoperative deaths, but 7% of the patients died within 2 weeks (most commonly of pneumonia and debilitation). Complications occurred in 20% of the patients and included pneumonia (10%), hemorrhage (5%), and pneumothorax (4%). Only 4% of patients required an additional treatment by the same method within 2 months, and the median survival time of patients with unresectable tumors was 6 months (range, 2–82 months).

Although reportedly only two patients were rejected for treatment by rigid bronchoscopy during the study period, these patients are clearly selected. Sixty-two percent of the patients were treated electively, and the rest required either urgent or emergent treatment. Eighty-six percent of the patients had tumors involving the trachea, carina, or main stem bronchi, and most had endoluminal tumors. Almost all of these patients went on to receive further treatment, which included open surgical resection in 28% and RT in 60%. The high percentage of patients who underwent open resection suggests that this may be an unusual cohort of patients who were selectively referred because of this institution's reputation for resection of tracheal lesions.

Laser Treatment
The data encompassing the largest number of patients treated for bronchial obstruction involves the use of endobronchial lasers. Historically, the CO_2 laser was used first to treat airway lesions. Although tissue vaporization is rapid, treatment with the CO_2 laser suffers from a limited ability to coagulate bleeding and the fact that the laser beam can be transmitted only in a straight line. The CO_2 laser is now rarely used for endobronchial tumors, and most of the published data involves use of the Nd:YAG laser. The Nd:YAG laser can be transmitted through flexible fiberoptic quartz fibers, has a tissue penetration of 3 to 6 mm, and has excellent coagulative properties. However, this modality involves an initial outlay of approximately $150 000 and an expense of approximately $500 for each use.[78]

Although the Nd:YAG laser can be used with a flexible bronchoscope, all of the centers with a large amount of experience with the laser currently use it with a rigid bronchoscope under general anesthesia.[58,79,80] These centers all initially performed laser resections with the flexible bronchoscope but changed their practice because of better safety and efficacy with the rigid scope. The rigid bronchoscope allows better aspiration of blood, even simultaneously with firing of the laser, and general anesthesia provides better control of coughing and breathing.[79] In addition, the rigid bronchoscope allows mechanical debridement to be done more effectively and prevents the risk (albeit low) of igniting the flexible bronchoscope or endotracheal tube.[79]

The success rate of Nd:YAG laser in the palliation of bronchial obstruction is approximately 80% in several large series (Table 29–2). Several studies report success rates of 40% to 60% in patients with lobar obstruction, whereas the success rate is 70% to 95% in patients with more central lesions[58,70,81] (Fig. 29–2). Complete occlusion of the airway makes the procedure more difficult, with the success rate being lower (57%).[81] Approximately 85% to 90% of these

TABLE 29–2. PALLIATION OF AIRWAY OBSTRUCTION

STUDY	N	INTERVENTION	RELIEF[a] (%)	HOW ASSESSED?	MST (mo)	MORTALITY (%)[b]
Mathisen et al[77]	56	Rigid Bronch	91	Bronch, symp	6	7[c]
Cavaliere et al[58]	1838	Laser	93	Bronch	(6)	0.4
Personne et al[80]	700	Laser	—	—	>6	3
Brutinel et al[81]	116	Laser	80	Bronch	5	3
Hetzel et al[70]	100	Laser	68	Symp	3	2
Cavaliere et al[58]	306	Stent	98	Symp	4	0
Wilson et al[83]	56	Stent[d]	77	Symp	3[e,f]	7
Hauck et al[82]	51	Stent[d]	98	?	4[f]	0
McCaughan and Williams[87]	175	PDT	—	—	5[g]	4[h]
Hayata[86]	67	PDT	60	?	—	—
Marasso et al[71]	183	Cryo	68	CXR	—	—
Maiwand[91]	153	Cryo	65	PFT	13	—
Maiwand[90]	75	Cryo	67	Symp	—	0
Gollins et al[154]	406	Brachy	59	CXR	6	—
Speiser and Spratling[95]	342	Brachy	86	Symp	5	—
Taulelle et al[94]	189	Brachy	79	Bronch	7	—
Ornadel et al[59]	117	Brachy	50	Symp	12	3[h]
Mehta et al[67]	97	Brachy	80	CXR	5	—
Huber et al[93]	93	Brachy	45	Bronch	4	—
Cavaliere et al[58]	66	Brachy	79	Symp	—	0
Aygun et al[155]	62	Brachy[i]	—	—	13	—
Macha et al[164]	56	Brachy	7	Various	—	0
Kabarowski et al[156]	52	Brachy	85	Various	—	—
Trédaniel et al[60]	51	Brachy	55	Symp	5	—
Burt et al[68]	50	Brachy	46	CXR	4	—
Slawson and Scott[72]	330	External RT	23	?	—	—
Simpson et al[49]	316	External RT	37	?	6	—
Collins et al[56]	96	External RT[j]	53	?	9	4[h]
Mantravadi et al[102]	94	External RT	46	?	—	—
Chetty et al[103]	57	External RT	21	CXR	—	—

Inclusion criteria: Studies reporting data on palliation of airway obstruction from malignant tumors in ≥50 patients.

[a]Relief of dyspnea or bronchial obstruction. Response is assessed by the most objective means reported.
[b]Early (1-wk) mortality, regardless of cause.
[c]2-week mortality.
[d]Uncovered stents.
[e]For patients who died.
[f]Mean survival.
[g]For III,IV patients.
[h]1-month mortality.
[i]In addition to external beam radiotherapy in all patients.
[j]18–48 Gy.

Bronch, bronchoscopy; Brachy, brachytherapy; Cryo, cryotherapy; CXR, chest radiograph; External RT, external beam radiotherapy; MST, median survival time; PDT, photodynamic therapy; PFT, pulmonary function tests; Symp, symptomatic assessment; ?, unknown.

patients have had tracheal, carinal, or main stem bronchial tumors, and almost all of the patients have had endoluminal lesions. Although not clearly defined quantitatively, patients with extrinsic compression have generally been excluded from this treatment modality.

Approximately 50% to 60% of the patients have required retreatment, with an average interval of 3 to 4 months.[58,81] The mortality of the procedure is low (0.4%–3%).[58,70,79–81] Complications have been reported to occur in 3% of patients and involve hemorrhage in approximately half of these cases.[58,59] The reported median survival is approximately 6 months.

Stents

A number of airway stents are available. These include Silastic stents for the trachea or main stem bronchi, as well as Silastic Y stents for use at the carinal level. In addition, expandable wire stents, with or without a plastic covering,

are available. Use of uncovered wire stents for malignant obstruction is rarely indicated because of rapid regrowth of tumor through the interstices of the stent (in 67% in 2 months).[82] The advantage of covered wire stents is that they can be placed with a flexible bronchoscope under fluoroscopic guidance. However, if they are malpositioned, removal is difficult, even with rigid bronchoscopy. Furthermore, use of these stents is usually combined with prior debridement with a rigid bronchoscope or treatment with an Nd:YAG laser. Thus it is generally most practical to place them in an operating room setting, with the patient under anesthesia.

The success rate of endoluminal stents is approximately 90%. The mortality rate is relatively low (0–7%). Approximately 10% to 20% of patients have early complications.[58,83,84] Early complications primarily involve stent migration and mucus retention. Retreatment with another stent is not commonly reported, but additional bronchoscopy or

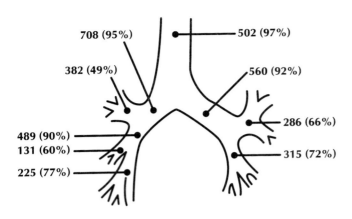

708 (95%)   502 (97%)

382 (49%)   560 (92%)

286 (66%)

489 (90%)

131 (60%)   315 (72%)

225 (77%)

FIGURE 29–2. Immediate results after neodymium:YAG laser resection of obstructing bronchogenic carcinoma in 1838 patients. Site and number of treatments are indicated, and the percentage of successful relief of obstruction is given in parentheses. (From Cavaliere S, Venuta F, Foccoli P, et al. Endoscopic treatment of malignant airway obstructions in 2,008 patients. *CHEST.* 1996;110:1536–1542.[58])

treatment with another modality (radiation) is frequent. From 90% to 95% of patients undergoing stent placement have had central tumors, and many of these patients have had severe obstruction. In one series, 53% of patients had >90% obstruction.[83] Stents placed at a lobar level appear to be successful much less frequently (45%) than those placed for central lesions.[82] Stent placement has been used both in patients with endoluminal obstruction and in patients with extrinsic compression.

Photodynamic Therapy

Photodynamic therapy (PDT) involves the intravenous administration of a photosensitizer (dihematoporphyrin ether), which is preferentially retained in tumor cells. When illuminated with the appropriate wavelength of light, the photosensitizer produces singlet oxygen, which therefore preferentially destroys the tumor cells. PDT requires specialized equipment, and patients must minimize exposure to sunlight for 1 month after injection of the photosensitizer. However, tracheobronchial lesions are ideal tumors to treat with this type of therapy.

Because the light from PDT is reported to penetrate to a depth of 5 to 10 mm, there is potential to treat tumor outside of the airway. However, in a small study the success rate was 80% with tumors that were strictly endoluminal, 40% with mixed tumors, and 0% with tumors that were completely extrinsic.[85] No information is available regarding the relative success of treating central versus lobar tumors.

The success rate of PDT in the palliation of obstructive symptoms is approximately 60%.[85,86] A 4% 1-month mortality rate and a 2% risk of major hemorrhage has been reported in a prospective, multi-institutional study.[87] Survival in unresectable (stage III,IV patients) is approximately 5 months. Most patients have required retreatment, with an average of 2.8 procedures per patient at an average interval of 2 to 5 months.[85,87]

Cryotherapy

Cryotherapy involves rapid freezing of tissues, which destroys the cells. Probes are available that can be used through either rigid or flexible bronchoscopes. The cost of this equipment is <$10 000, and the cost per application is minimal.[78] Although endobronchial cryotherapy has been used since the 1970s, the published data is limited mostly to small series of patients.[78,88,89] The rate of palliation has

been reported to be approximately 60% to 70%.[71,78,88–91] It is higher in central lesions (60%) than in lobar lesions (35%).[71] The success rate is poor (29%) in patients with extrinsic tumor.[90] The procedure requires that several bronchoscopic procedures be performed in the week following cryotherapy to debride necrotic obstructing tissue.[71] Although cells below the surface can be destroyed, no data regarding the durability of this treatment has been reported.

Brachytherapy

Brachytherapy involves the delivery of radiation from an endobronchial source. Brachytherapy requires placement of a hollow catheter across the lesion to be treated, using flexible bronchoscopy. The catheter is then loaded in the RT treatment suite with an appropriate radiation source that remains in place for the length of time needed to deliver the prescribed dose of radiation. Although the radiation penetrates tissues for a short distance (1–2 cm), a rapid dropoff occurs in the amount of radiation delivered at an increasing depth (hence the name *brachytherapy*). Because the delivery of radiation is relatively localized, brachytherapy has been used even after prior external beam RT.

Currently, a typical dose of brachytherapy involves 7 to 8 Gy of radiation (calculated at 1 cm from the source) delivered in three treatments, each approximately 2 weeks apart.[60,62,92,93] There appears to be no difference in outcomes when larger[59] or smaller[93] doses per treatment are used. The radiation source most commonly used at this time is high activity Iridium[192]. Use of high dose rate radiation sources allows the treatment to be completed within minutes, as opposed to low dose rate treatment, where the radiation source is left in place for 1 to 2 days.[67] A comparison of high dose rate with low dose rate brachytherapy treatment has revealed no difference in response rates, duration of palliation, or complications.[67]

Brachytherapy has resulted in the palliation of airway obstruction in 50% to 80% of patients, as assessed by symptoms, response on chest radiograph (CXR), or bronchoscopy (see Table 29–2). In the few studies that have analyzed predictors of a good outcome, no difference is seen between patients with only endobronchial obstruction and those with extrinsic obstruction,[60,62] with the exception of one study that found a better response in patients with no extrinsic disease, but included patients with small early stage endobronchial tumors.[94] There is no clear difference between central lesions and lobar lesions; in fact, lobar lesions appear to respond slightly more often.[62] Although repeat brachytherapy can be administered, no data is available on how often this is done. In most centers, a treatment course involves two to four treatment sessions, although some have used a single treatment.[59,68] The duration of symptom relief has been reported to be 4 to 5 months in one of the larger series.[59] The reported survival following brachytherapy for palliative treatment has generally been on the order of 4 to 5 months, although much better survival is seen in patients who have a relatively small tumor involving primarily an endobronchial component.[60]

The 1-month mortality in patients treated with brachytherapy is approximately 3% to 5%.[59,92] A mild to moderate radiation bronchitis occurs in approximately 10% of patients following brachytherapy,[95] and some fibrosis and narrowing is seen in 50% of patients after more than 6 months.[96] A subject of much concern has been the incidence of massive hemoptysis as a cause of late death. This concern was prompted primarily by a small study (12 patients) that found that 50% of patients died of massive hemoptysis 1 to 7 months after brachytherapy.[97] Two additional studies of brachytherapy in patients who had previously received external beam RT both reported fatal hemoptysis in 32% of patients.[98,99] However, many other studies have reported low rates of major hemoptysis, and extensive reviews of the published literature as well as a large series of 406 patients have found that the overall rate of late fatal hemoptysis following brachytherapy is between 7% and 8%.[95,96,100] It is unlikely that this complication is related to the brachytherapy treatment. The risk of fatal hemoptysis in patients with lung cancer, regardless of treatment received, has been reported to be 13% in patients with central airway tumors and 3% in patients with lobar tumors in a large autopsy study of 877 patients.[101] This rate is similar to that seen in patients treated with brachytherapy, most of whom have central tumors.

External Radiotherapy

Although external beam RT is clearly the most commonly used palliative treatment modality, surprisingly little data exists on how often symptoms of obstruction are relieved. Relief of obstruction was found to occur in only 20% to 50% of patients in five series reporting on more than 50 patients (see Table 29–2).[49,56,72,102,103] There is a suggestion that the response may be somewhat better when doses over 50 Gy are used.[103,104] In one study of 57 patients, the response rate was found to be 31% for patients with lobar obstruction versus 8% for patients with main stem bronchial obstruction.[103]

Comparison of Palliative Treatment Modalities

It is extremely difficult to compare the relative value of one palliative treatment for obstruction with another from the published data. In all reports, many (if not most) patients received more than one type of treatment. Data regarding specific combinations of treatment (eg, laser and stent placement) is even more sparse and difficult to interpret than the reports involving one modality, shown in Table 29–2. All patients reported in this table received one type of treatment, although many also received various

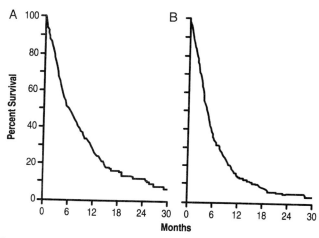

FIGURE 29–3. *A,* Survival from time of first laser treatment to death in 333 patients with lung cancer. *B,* Survival from the start of brachytherapy in 406 patients with lung cancer. (*A,* From Cavaliere S, Foccoli P, Farina PL. Nd:YAG laser bronchoscopy: a five-year experience with 1,396 applications in 1,000 patients. *CHEST.* 1988;94:15–21.[153] *B,* Reprinted from *Radiotherapy and Oncology,* Vol 33, Gollins SW, Burt PA, Barber PV, et al, High dose rate intraluminal radiotherapy for carcinoma of the bronchus: outcome of treatment of 406 patients, 31–40,[154] Copyright 1994, with permission from Elsevier Science.)

other types of treatment either before or after the modality being reported.

Several definite conclusions can be reached regarding the treatment of malignant airway obstruction. The acute mortality seen with these various treatments is similar, at 0 to 5%. The overall median survival also appears to be relatively similar. Furthermore, a median survival of 4 to 6 months is probably adequate to make palliative treatment worthwhile for those patients who suffer from severe dyspnea because of airway obstruction (Fig. 29–3A,B). There appears to be a difference in the rate of palliation among treatment approaches: lowest for external beam RT and brachytherapy and somewhat higher for the other interventions. However, such a comparison is not justified because the patients selected for the various treatments are not necessarily the same.

What is the best therapy for a particular patient who presents with dyspnea from airway obstruction? The factors guiding treatment selection can be divided into patient-related and technical issues. Patient-related issues include where the obstruction is located along the tracheobronchial tree; whether the obstruction is primarily endoluminal or extrinsic; and whether the degree of respiratory compromise demands an emergent (within 1–2 days), an urgent (within 1 week), or an elective intervention. Technical issues include the need for specialized equipment and knowledge, patient tolerance of the procedure, and the durability of the results.

An assessment of the value of each of the treatments with regard to the patient-related and technical factors just cited is shown in Table 29–3. Patients with life-threatening conditions are probably best treated by rigid bronchoscopy or laser resection. Patients with extrinsic compression are more amenable to treatment with stents or external beam RT, and patients with lobar obstruction are more appropriately treated with RT techniques. Certainly other factors,

TABLE 29–3. PARAMETERS INFLUENCING THE OPTIMAL PALLIATIVE TREATMENT MODALITY FOR PATIENTS WITH AIRWAY OBSTRUCTION

PARAMETER	RIGID BRONCH	LASER	STENT	PDT	CRYO	BRACHY	EXTERN RT
Patient Characteristics							
Location of Obstruction							
Trachea	+ + + +	+ + + +	+ + + +	+ + + +	+ + + +	+ + + +	+ +
MSB, BI	+ + +	+ + + +	+ + + +	+ + + +	+ + + +	+ + + +	+ + +
Lobar, segmental	+	+ +	+	+ + +	+ +	+ + +	+ + + +
Nature of Obstruction							
Endoluminal	+ + + +	+ + + +	+ +	+ + +	+ + +	+ + +	+ +
Mixed	+ +	+ +	+ + +	+ + +	+ + +	+ + +	+ + +
Extrinsic	0	0	+ + + +	+	+	+ + +	+ + + +
How Life-Threatening?							
Emergent (1 dª)	+ + + +	+ +	+ +	0	0	0	0
Urgent (1 wkª)	+ + +	+ + +	+ + +	+	+	+	0
Elective (1 moª)	+ +	+ + +	+ + +	+ + + +	+ + + +	+ + + +	+ + + +
Technical Issues							
Ease for Patient	+ +	+ +	+ +	0	+ + +	+ + +	+ + + +
Durability	0	+	+ + +	+ + +	+ + +	+ + +	+ + +
Availabilityᵇ	+ + +	+	+ +	0	+ +	+ +	+ + + +
Penetrationᶜ (mm)	0	3	0	5	10	15	50

Inclusion criteria/rating method: This table represents the authors' and editors' consensus judgment of the value of various treatments based on the published literature and personal experience. 0, no utility; increasing numbers of + signs indicates greater utility.
ªExpected survival without treatment.
ᵇAvailability and ease of acquisition of both necessary equipment and expertise.
ᶜDepth of penetration of treatment into tissue (mm).
BI, bronchus intermedius; Brachy, brachytherapy; Bronch, bronchoscopy; Cryo, cryotherapy; Extern RT, conventional external beam radiotherapy; MSB, main stem bronchus; PDT, photodynamic therapy.

such as prior treatment, the availability of different interventions, and risk of anesthesia, play a role. It is probably best to consider the treatment of airway obstruction in two different phases. The need for an acute intervention to more rapidly reestablish airway patency should be assessed first. Once this has been accomplished (and in patients in whom an acute intervention is not necessary), consideration should be given to whether additional therapy should be used in order to improve the durability of the results.

An evidence-based assessment of the durability of the results is not possible because of the limited amount of published data. Much of the assessment noted in Table 29–3 is based on intuitive judgment. For example, it stands to reason that simple mechanical removal of endoluminal tumor by rigid bronchoscopy does nothing to prevent tumor regrowth, whereas stent placement is likely to result in a durable relief, although hard data demonstrating this is not available. The authors of the largest published series of laser interventions state that, in their opinion, laser treatment of the airway wall results in a more durable response (median duration of relief, 102 days) than was seen in their early experience with simple mechanical debridement alone (median duration of relief, 29 days in 33 patients).[58] Assessment of the durability of PDT and cryotherapy is strictly inferred from the reported depth of treatment. Finally, although RT would, in theory, provide the most thorough treatment of the tumor mass, the published data regarding the rate of relief of obstruction and the durability of this response suggests that the ability of this modality to control obstructing tumors is somewhat limited. However, a small randomized study of 29 patients found the duration

of progression-free survival to be significantly improved with the use of brachytherapy after initial Nd:YAG laser treatment (7.5 versus 2.2 months, $P < 0.05$).[105]

In summary, malignant airway obstruction is a distressing symptom that can often be life-threatening. Fortunately, it can be palliated by a variety of treatment modalities. Acute relief of obstruction is best achieved by rigid bronchoscopy, laser resection, and perhaps also stent placement. The durability of the relief may be prolonged by additional interventions (brachytherapy, photodynamic therapy, or cryotherapy), but clear data addressing this is not available. Lobar obstruction is probably best treated with RT (external beam or brachytherapy). The choice of therapy will likely be influenced by the availability of treatment modalities. Although an argument can be made for major treatment centers to have more than one modality in their armamentarium, there is little reason to aspire to being able to provide most or all of the treatment options.

MALIGNANT PLEURAL EFFUSION

A large review of 1669 patients with pleural effusions found that almost half (45%) were due to malignancy.[106] Lung cancer and breast cancer account for approximately 60% of cases of malignant pleural effusion (MPE), with lymphoma and adenocarcinoma of unknown primary site making up most of the remainder (Table 29–4). However, any type of cancer can cause a pleural effusion. Usually, an MPE is a manifestation of widespread disease and portends a poor life expectancy. Treatment of this condition

DATA SUMMARY: THORACIC SYMPTOMS

	AMOUNT	QUALITY	CONSISTENCY
Thoracic RT results in palliation in 67% of patients	Mod	Mod	High
Alterations in dose or fractionation in palliative thoracic RT does not alter survival or response rates	**Mod**	**Mod**	**High**
Prophylactic thoracic RT in asymptomatic patients does not prolong survival	Mod	Poor	Mod
External beam RT results in palliation of cough in 60% of patients	High	Mod	High
External beam RT results in palliation of hemoptysis in 80% of patients	High	Mod	High
Brachytherapy results in palliation of hemoptysis in 90% of patients	High	Mod	High
Median survival time in treated patients with symptomatic bronchial obstruction is approximately 5 months	High	Mod	Poor
Palliation in appropriately selected patients with central bronchial obstruction is seen in 70% of patients treated with a variety of techniques (rigid bronchoscopy, laser, stent, photodynamic therapy, cryotherapy, brachytherapy)	High	Mod	Poor

Type of data rated: Plain text: descriptive statement   *Italics: controlled comparison*   **Bold: randomized comparison**

has a major palliative impact because most patients have marked dyspnea, but it must be considered in the context of a limited life expectancy.

It is often difficult to achieve a definite diagnosis of an MPE. Estimation of the false negative rate of cytologic examination of pleural fluid in patients who are suspected of having an MPE is not available from published studies. However, the sensitivity of pleural fluid cytology in confirming the diagnosis of cancer in patients who do, in fact, have an MPE has been widely reported to be 50% to 60%.[107–109] The sensitivity of a second or third thoracentesis in patients in whom the first thoracentesis was negative is diminished (35%–48%).[107,108] The sensitivity of a blind pleural needle biopsy in making a diagnosis of cancer in patients with a suspected MPE is similar to that of thoracentesis (44%–52%).[107–109] However, the sensitivity of a needle biopsy is diminished (17%–37%)[108,109] in patients in whom an initial thoracentesis was negative. Thus, pleural biopsy is not nearly as useful in establishing a diagnosis in patients with cancer as it is in patients with a more diffuse pleural process such as tuberculosis.

Thoracoscopy has consistently shown to have a sensitivity of 95% in making the diagnosis of cancer in patients with a suspected MPE.[110–112] The sensitivity of thoracoscopy remains 90% in patients in whom initial tests such as fluid aspiration or needle biopsy have been nondiagnostic.[112,113] However, confirmation of the diagnosis of cancer may not be necessary in patients with a history of cancer. Recurrent cancer was found to be the cause of a pleural effusion in 86% and 100% of patients with a history of cancer in two studies.[112,114]

If the effusion is due to a cancer that is responsive to chemotherapy, such as lymphoma or SCLC, the recommended treatment is systemic therapy alone.[115,116] No data is available on how often this approach results in resolution of the effusion, but presumably the response rates are similar to the response rates for other manifestations of these types of cancer. Some authors have also recommended that a pleural effusion in women with hormone-responsive breast cancer also be treated initially with hormone therapy.[106] However, no data is available examining the efficacy of such an approach, and most often an MPE in women with breast cancer is treated with pleural drainage and sclerotherapy.

For the vast majority of patients with an MPE, palliation involves pleural drainage as well as a local therapy to prevent fluid reaccumulation. A wide variety of agents have been instilled into the pleural cavity in order to cause adhesions between the visceral and parietal pleura, thus obliterating the pleural space.[116] This approach requires that the lung is able to fully expand and come in contact with the chest wall. Few studies have documented the incidence of failure of the lung to re-expand. Two studies involving >100 patients found this was the case in 18% and 35% of all patients.[117,118] It has been suggested that earlier referral of patients for sclerotherapy may decrease this incidence,[118] but data to substantiate this is not available. Treatment options for patients who do not have full lung expansion are discussed later in this chapter.

Thoracentesis alone rarely provides durable palliation in

TABLE 29–4. TYPE OF CANCER CAUSING MALIGNANT PLEURAL EFFUSION

CANCER TYPE	%
Lung	35
Breast	23
Lymphoma	10
Unknown primary	12
Gynecologic	6
Gastrointestinal	5
Genitourinary	2
Other	7

Data from a review of 811 patients with a malignant pleural effusion.
From Hausheer FH, Yarbro JW. Diagnosis and treatment of malignant pleural effusion. Semin Oncol. 1985; 12:54–75.[106]

patients with an MPE and should be used primarily in patients who are expected to survive for only several weeks. In one study, an attempt was made to manage 94 patients with thoracentesis alone. The median time to fluid recurrence was found to be 4 days, and at 1 month, 97% had developed a recurrent effusion.[119] Other smaller studies have found that the effusion recurred in all patients after thoracentesis alone.[120,121]

Chest tube drainage alone has been reported to be effective in an average of 39% of patients.[119,121–125] However, most of these studies involve only small numbers of patients (100 total), the range of reported effectiveness is wide (0-86%), and none has clearly defined the criteria and timepoint used to measure response.

A large number of studies of various sclerotherapy agents have been published, as well as several extensive reviews.[106,115,116] However, interpretation of this data is difficult. Many of these studies involved only small numbers of patients and did not define the criteria or timepoint used for assessment of response. Furthermore, patient selection is poorly delineated in most of these reports. Presumably, sclerotherapy was not attempted in most patients in whom the lung did not expand up against the chest wall, although only a few studies have explicitly stated this.[126–128] The results from studies explicitly stating this are not perceptibly different from the others. Therefore, the following paragraphs are restricted to studies with at least 20 patients that provide an objective assessment of the efficacy of a variety of common pleural sclerotherapy agents by CXR at 1 month. A complete response is defined as the absence of any fluid reaccumulation on CXR, whereas a partial response is defined as a reaccumulation of some fluid that is not sufficient either to cause symptoms or to warrant an intervention. Interpretation of response data at later times[126,128–133] is difficult because of patient dropout, which may be more likely to involve those patients with a poor result.

The results of studies reporting objective response criteria by CXR at 1 month in patients with an MPE treated with several common sclerotherapy agents are reported in Table 29–5. The best results are reported with the use of talc, with a 75% complete response and a 90% overall response at 1 month. Most commonly, talc has been insufflated during thoracoscopy, but equal results have been reported using a slurry of talc administered via a chest tube.[134,135] Although talc itself is inexpensive (<$10 per dose), the cost of hospitalization and thoracoscopy is substantial.[115,116]

The side effects associated with talc are mild and primarily involve a brief period of fever or pain. Although the studies reported in Table 29–5 provide little information on the incidence of these symptoms, in one review fever was reported in 16% of patients and pain in 7%.[116] The variability in the reported incidence of these symptoms may be related to the definition of fever and the subjective assessment of what constitutes significant pain. When a fever does occur, it is generally seen within 12 hours and lasts 1 to 3 days.[136] Empyema has occasionally been reported, with an incidence of 0 to 3%.[136] Anecdotal cases of pneumonitis and adult respiratory distress syndrome have been reported following instillation of talc.[129] However, these have been rare and may be related to the use of larger doses (10 g) of talc than is used today (2.5–5 g).[136]

Pleurodesis with talc has been shown not to have significant long-term detrimental effects. In a 22- to 35-year follow-up study of 114 patients, pulmonary function was found not to be altered.[137] In this study, as well as another long-term follow-up study (14–40 years) of 210 patients, no cases of mesothelioma were encountered.[137,138] Talc currently marketed in the United States is asbestos free. However, such long-term issues are not important in patients being treated for an MPE.

Tetracycline was a popular agent for sclerotherapy until its manufacture was discontinued in 1992. Despite its former popularity, tetracycline was only moderately effective, with an objective response rate of approximately 60% at 1 month. Doxycycline has been explored as an alternative to talc. It appears to be as effective as talc, if not slightly better. However, this data is limited to a few small studies, and in some instances, multiple instillations of doxycycline are necessary in order to achieve these results.

Bleomycin, an antineoplastic agent, has been used as a sclerotherapy agent for >20 years and has been shown to be moderately effective. On rare occasions, it has been associated with a sepsis-like syndrome.[139] A major limitation of bleomycin is the cost (~$1200 per dose).[115,116] Furthermore, approximately 45% of the dose is systemically absorbed, although side effects such as myelosuppression or hair loss are seen only rarely.[116] The benefit of bleomycin appears to be related to its ability to cause pleural inflammation rather than an antineoplastic effect.

A number of other chemotherapy drugs have been instilled into the pleural space of patients with an MPE. These include cisplatin, doxorubicin, etoposide, 5-fluorouracil, mitomycin C, and interferon. In one review, the reported response rates were relatively low, ranging from 0 to 66%, but definition of the criteria and timepoints for assessing response usually were not provided.[116] Numerous side effects were encountered, and these agents are now used only rarely.[116] Quinacrine, *Corynebacterium*, and radioactive isotopes have been investigated, but they are only of historic interest now.[106,116] Although response rates of 60% to 80% for these agents have been reported, this data involves small trials with vague endpoints.[106,116]

Although randomized studies comparing sclerotherapy agents have been reported, most have involved <50 patients total, giving them poor statistical power.[140] The studies involving ≥50 evaluable patients with clearly defined endpoints are shown in Table 29–6. The data from these studies is too limited to allow any definite conclusions to be drawn about the superiority of any particular agent. A large Cancer and Leukemia Group B trial (CALGB 9334) involving >400 patients completed accrual in 1999, and preliminary data suggests no major difference between the arms, which compared talc administered via a chest tube with talc administered via thoracoscopy. A three-arm trial conducted by the Eastern Cooperative Oncology Group, comparing bleomycin with doxycycline and talc slurry was closed prematurely.

Surgical pleurectomy is highly effective. Two reports involving 50 and 106 patients found 2% recurrences at 1 month.[134,135] However, the operative mortality in these studies was found to be 10% and 18%, with a 23% incidence of major complications.[141,142] Because of this, open surgical pleurectomy or decortication is currently used rarely.

Approximately 20% of patients in the studies listed in

TABLE 29–5. OBJECTIVE RESPONSE[a] TO COMMON PLEURAL SCLEROTHERAPY AGENTS IN PATIENTS WITH A MALIGNANT PLEURAL EFFUSION

STUDY	N[b]	AGENT	% DEAD AT 1 mo	MST (mo)	% WITH FEVER	% WITH PAIN	CR AT 1 mo (%)	CR+PR AT 1 mo (%)
Viallat et al[131]	327	Talc	9	6	10	—	86	90
Sanchez-Armengol et al[117]	119	Talc	—	4	—	—	69	87
Kennedy et al[134]	47	Talc[c]	19	—	63	34	—	81
Jacobi et al[135]	33	Talc[c]	8	—	—	—	—	94
Hartman et al[130]	33	Talc	15	—	—	—	—	97
Danby et al[157]	23	Talc	4	11	—	—	71	88
Aelony et al[152]	21	Talc	16	4	—	—	—	86
Fentiman et al[158]	20	Talc	20	—	—	—	—	90
Average (talc)					?	?	75	89
Sherman et al[132]	75	Tetra[d]	23	—	12	~30	—	73
Martinez-Moragón et al[159]	31	Tetra[d]	—	15	0	32	52	81
Ruckdeschel et al[126]	27	Tetra	15	3	7	17	—	33
Parker et al[160]	20	Tetra	—	—	—	—	—	48
Average (tetracycline)					10	26		59
Patz et al[145]	29	Doxy[e]	46	—	0	20	34	79
Pulsiripunya et al[161]	27	Doxy	—	—	—	60	89	100
Heffner et al[133]	23	Doxy[f]	15	—	4	33	—	65
Seaton et al[127]	21	Doxy	43	—	—	—	81	95
Average (doxycycline)					2	38	68	85
Martinez-Moragón et al[159]	31	Bleo	—	11	19	22	45	84
Patz et al[145]	29	Bleo[d]	44	—	13	11	41	72
Ruckdeschel et al[126]	28	Bleo	17	3	9	9	—	64
Ostrowski[129]	25	Bleo[g]	—	—	12	28	48	72
Average (bleomycin)					13	18	45	73
Average for all			21	7				

Inclusion criteria: Studies of ≥20 evaluable patients undergoing pleural sclerosis with selected agents and reporting objective (CXR) findings at 1 month.
[a]OR, defined as either a CR or a PR.
[b]Evaluable patients, meaning patients alive at 1 mo with a CXR.
[c]Delivered as a slurry through a chest tube.
[d]1500 mg.
[e]Through pigtail catheter
[f]Multiple instillations in many patients.
[g]Various doses.
Bleo, bleomycin, 60 units; CR, complete response (no fluid reaccumulation on CXR at 1 month); CXR, chest radiograph; Doxy, doxycycline, 500 mg; PR, partial response (fluid accumulation on CXR at 1 mo that is not symptomatic and does not warrant intervention); Talc, talc powder, 2–5 g administered via thoracosacopy; Tetra, tetracycline, 1000 mg; ?, unknown.

Table 29–5 died within 1 month of treatment (range, 4%–46%). The wide range undoubtedly reflects differences in selection criteria in this population of patients who generally have end stage cancer, and this range probably has nothing to do with the type of treatment used for the MPE.

Nevertheless, the median survival in patients with an MPE is approximately 7 months. The survival may be slightly better in patients with breast cancer compared with other cancer types.[117] There is conflicting data about whether a low pleural fluid pH is associated with a poorer prognosis

TABLE 29–6. RANDOMIZED COMPARISONS OF TREATMENTS FOR MALIGNANT PLEURAL EFFUSION

STUDY	n EVALUABLE	AGENTS		CR AT 1 mo (%)		
		Arm 1	Arm 2	Arm 1	Arm 2	P
Groth et al[162]	95	VATS/mitoxantrone[a]	VATS	71	64	NS
Masuno et al[163]	76	Adriamycin/LC9018[b]	Adriamycin	32	18	.006
Ruckdeschel et al[126]	85	Tetracycline	Bleomycin	33	64	.021
Martinez-Moragón et al[128]	62	Tetracycline	Bleomycin	52	45	NS
Patz et al[145]	58	Doxycycline	Bleomycin	34	41	NS

Inclusion criteria: Randomized studies of ≥50 evaluable patients with a malignant pleural effusion.
[a]Mitoxantrone is a cytostatic agent.
[b]LC9018 is a biologic response modifier (lyophilized lactobacillus casei YIT9018).
CR, complete response, defined as no reaccumulation of fluid; NS, not significant; VATS, video-assisted thoracic surgery (thoracoscopy).

in patients with an MPE.[143,144] The palliative benefits of treatment of an MPE must be balanced against the morbidity and mortality associated with any therapy. Clearly, there is a large group of patients who can derive significant benefit from definitive treatment of an MPE, and treatment of this condition seems justified as long as patients with an extremely limited life expectancy are excluded.

For those patients in whom the lung is able to fully re-expand after drainage of an MPE, sclerotherapy to prevent fluid reaccumulation is of major palliative benefit. Talc appears to have the greatest efficacy. Talc insufflation at the time of thoracoscopy may shorten the hospital stay for these patients with limited life expectancy, but it involves the expense and risk of an operative procedure. The use of small-bore pigtail catheters and perhaps even outpatient management may have an impact on the treatment of this disease.[127,145-147] Good results have been reported in 100 patients who underwent outpatient placement of an in-dwelling pleural catheter as the definitive management of an MPE.[147]

Several options are available for patients in whom full expansion of the lung against the chest wall is not achieved. Several authors have reported that talc sclerotherapy in these patients (in conjunction with thoracoscopic lysis of adhesions) carries a 50% success rate.[117,131] These studies provide no details about the number of patients involved or the definition of success, but presumably symptoms are relieved to the point where no further interventions are needed. It is likely that the patients selected for this procedure had apposition of the lung and chest wall in a major portion of the hemithorax.

The second option, which can be used regardless of the degree of lung expansion, is a pleuroperitoneal shunt. A small (2 mL) pump chamber must be actively compressed because fluid must move against the pressure gradient. This requires a cooperative patient whose rate of fluid accumulation is not extremely rapid. Several studies have reported good results in 71% to 100% of patients (142 patients total).[118,148-151] Shunt occlusion was seen in 10% to 25% of patients.[118,148-151]

A third method of treating an MPE in which the lung does not re-expand involves placement of a pigtail catheter through a long skin tunnel. Fluid can be aspirated with a large syringe every 1 to 2 days by the patient, a family member, or a visiting nurse. The incidence of catheter infection is low, even after several months, and symptom relief has been found to be good.[146]

EDITORS' COMMENTS

It is crucial to realistically assess whether the appropriate goal of treatment for a particular patient should be a potential cure or palliation. Although many advances have been made in curative treatments for lung cancer, the fact remains that most patients will die of this disease. An honest assessment of the chance of cure and a patient's expected median survival time is important. Often, both the patient and the physician want to believe that the chance of survival is better than what the data indicates.

The fact that no curative therapy is available for a patient does not mean that nothing can be done. In reality, palliation remains the area in which physicians can make the greatest difference. A wide variety of palliative treatments are available, including surgery, chemotherapy, and various forms of RT. In some instances (eg, brain metastases or large airway obstruction), therapy can not only relieve symptoms but also prolong survival. Most often, however, the benefit of palliative therapy is in improving the patient's quality of life. In addition, many cancer patients attest that one of the most important factors affecting their quality of life is their physician's attitude toward them. A treating physician who is compassionate, gentle, and strong enough to face the facts together with the patient can provide enormous palliation, even without providing treatment.

A substantial amount of data is available regarding the outcomes of various palliative treatments. However, the impact of this data seems to be limited because palliative treatment regimens often appear to be derived from curative strategies rather than tailored to suit the needs of incurable patients. The issues leading to the design of

DATA SUMMARY: MALIGNANT PLEURAL EFFUSION			
	AMOUNT	**QUALITY**	**CONSISTENCY**
The sensitivity of cytology in confirming the malignant nature of a pleural effusion is 55%	Mod	High	High
In patients with a history of cancer, pleural effusion is due to cancer recurrence in 90%	Mod	Poor	High
Re-expansion of the lung is possible in 70% of patients	Mod	Mod	Mod
Chest tube drainage alone is of palliative benefit in 40% of patients	High	Poor	Poor
Talc results in a complete response (CR) in 90% of patients in whom lung re-expansion is possible	High	Mod	High
Doxycycline results in a CR in 85% of patients	High	Mod	Mod
Bleomycin results in a CR in 75% of patients	High	Mod	High
The median survival of patients with an MPE is 7 months	High	Mod	Poor

Type of data rated: Plain text: descriptive statement   *Italics: controlled comparison*   **Bold: randomized comparison**
CR, complete response.

curative regimens may not be germane in a palliative setting. For example, when patient survival is short, a reluctance to treat with large radiation fractions because of concern about late toxicity is probably not warranted. Limiting the patient's treatment time relative to the length of their survival is probably a more important concern. Certainly, individual judgment is important in choosing appropriate therapy, and this is probably even more true in the case of palliative treatments. However, the data indicates that the rate and duration of palliation of a wide variety of symptoms is equivalent in shorter and simpler treatment regimens compared with more complex regimens. It is surprising that this is not more widely recognized.

A variety of treatments are available for specific symptoms such as airway obstruction or MPE. These treatments can be accomplished quickly and result in major palliation in the majority of patients. Which of these treatments is best is not clear. For airway obstruction, the modality chosen should be individualized and based on patient characteristics. An MPE that is symptomatic should be treated definitively, rather than with repeated thoracentesis, unless the patient is clearly likely to survive only for a few weeks. Too often, such palliative treatment is withheld for a long time because of pessimism about the ability to offer a benefit to patients with a terminal illness.

References

1. Zimm S, Wampler GL, Stablein D, et al. Intracerebral metastases in solid-tumor patients: natural history and results of treatment. Cancer. 1981;48:384–394.
2. Newman SJ, Hansen HH. Frequency, diagnosis, and treatment of brain metastases in 247 consecutive patients with bronchogenic carcinoma. Cancer. 1974;33:492.
3. Richards P, McKissock W. Intracranial metastases. BMJ. 1963;1:15–18.
4. Stoier M. Metastatic tumors of the brain. Acta Neurol Scand. 1965;41:262–268.
5. Borgelt B, Gelber R, Kramer S, et al. The palliation of brain metastases: final results of the first two studies by the Radiation Therapy Oncology Group. Int J Radiat Oncol Biol Phys. 1980;6:1–9.
6. Kurtz JM, Gelber R, Brady LW, et al. The palliation of brain metastases in a favorable patient population: a randomized clinical trial by the Radiation Therapy Oncology Group. Int J Radiat Oncol Biol Phys. 1981;7:891–895.
7. Priestman TJ, Dunn J, Brada M, et al. Final results of the Royal College of Radiologists' trial comparing two different radiotherapy schedules in the treatment of cerebral metastases. Clin Oncol. 1996;8:308–315.
8. Komarnicky LT, Phillips TL, Martz K, et al. A randomized phase III protocol for the evaluation of misonidazole combined with radiation in the treatment of patients with brain metastases (RTOG-7916). Int J Radiat Oncol Biol Phys. 1991;20:53–58.
9. Epstein BE, Scott CB, Sause WT, et al. Improved survival duration in patients with unresected solitary brain metastasis using accelerated hyperfractionated radiation therapy at total doses of 54.4 Gray and greater. Cancer. 1993;71:1362–1367.
10. Haie-Meder C, Pellae-Cosset B, Laplanche A, et al. Results of a randomized clinical trial comparing two radiation schedules in the palliative treatment of brain metastases. Radiother Oncol. 1993;26:111–116.
11. Gaspar L, Scott C, Rotman M, et al. Recursive partitioning analysis (RPA) of prognostic factors in three Radiation Therapy Oncology Group (RTOG) brain metastases trials. Int J Radiat Oncol Biol Phys. 1997;37:745–751.
12. Vecht CJ, Hovestadt A, Verbiest HBC, et al. Dose-effect relationship of dexamethasone on Karnofsky performance in metastatic brain tumors: a randomized study of doses of 4, 8, and 16 mg per day. Neurology. 1994;44:675–680.
13. Ryan GF, Ball DL, Smith JG. Treatment of brain metastases from primary lung cancer. Int J Radiat Oncol Biol Phys. 1995;31:273–278.
14. Chang D-B, Yang P-C, Luh K-T, et al. Late survival of non-small cell lung cancer patients with brain metastases: influence of treatment. Chest. 1992;101:1293–1297.
15. Weissman DE, Janjan NA, Erickson B, et al. Twice-daily tapering dexamethasone treatment during cranial radiation for newly diagnosed brain metastases. J Neurooncol. 1991;11:235–239.
16. Cohen N, Strauss G, Lew R, et al. Should prophylactic anticonvulsants be administered to patients with newly diagnosed cerebral metastases? A retrospective analysis. J Clin Oncol. 1988;6:1621–1624.
17. Cairncross JG, Kim J-H, Posner JB. Radiation therapy for brain metastases. Ann Neurol. 1980;7:529–541.
18. Murray KJ, Scott C, Greenberg HM, et al. A randomized phase III study of accelerated hyperfractionation versus standard in patients with unresected brain metastases: a report of the Radiation Therapy Oncology Group (RTOG) 9104. Int J Radiat Oncol Biol Phys. 1997;39:571–574.
19. Diener-West M, Dobbins TW, Phillips TL, et al. Identification of an optimal subgroup for treatment evaluation of patients with brain metastases using RTOG study 7916. Int J Radiat Oncol Biol Phys. 1989;16:669–673.
20. Arriagada R, Le Chevalier T, Borie F, et al. Prophylactic cranial irradiation for patients with small-cell lung cancer in complete remission. J Natl Cancer Inst. 1995;87:183–190.
21. Crossen JR, Garwood D, Glatstein E, et al. Neurobehavioral sequelae of cranial irradiation in adults: a review of radiation-induced encephalopathy. J Clin Oncol. 1994;12:627–642.
22. DeAngelis LM, Mandell LR, Thaler HT, et al. The role of postoperative radiotherapy after resection of single brain metastases. Neurosurgery. 1989;24:798–805.
23. Kelly K, Bunn PA Jr. Is it time to reevaluate our approach to the treatment of brain metastases in patients with non–small cell lung cancer? Lung Cancer. 1998;20:85–91.
24. Ellis R, Gregor A. The treatment of brain metastases from lung cancer. Lung Cancer. 1998;20:81–84.
25. Gilbert RW, Kim JH, Posner JB. Epidural spinal cord compression from metastatic tumor: diagnosis and treatment. Ann Neurol. 1978;3:40–51.
26. Byrne TN. Spinal cord compression from epidural metastases. N Engl J Med. 1992;327:614–619.
27. Bach F, Agerlin N, Sorensen JB. Metastatic spinal cord compression secondary to lung cancer. J Clin Oncol. 1992;10:1781–1787.
28. Pedersen AG, Bach F, Melgaard B. Frequency, diagnosis, and prognosis of spinal cord compression in small bronchogenic carcinoma: a review of 817 consecutive patients. Cancer. 1985;55:1818–1822.
29. Stark RJ, Henson RA, Evans SJ. Spinal metastases: a retrospective survey from a general hospital. Brain. 1982;105:189–213.
30. Portenoy RK, Galer BS, Salaman O, et al. Identification of epidural neoplasm: radiography and bone scintigraphy in the symptomatic and asymptomatic spine. Cancer. 1989;64:2207–2213.
31. Smoker WR, Godersky JC, Knutzon RK, et al. The role of MR imaging in evaluating metastatic spinal disease. AJR Am J Roentgenol. 1987;149:1241–1248.
32. Carmody RF, Yang PJ, Seeley GW, et al. Spinal cord compression due to metastatic disease: diagnosis with MR imaging versus myelography. Radiology. 1989;173:225–229.
33. Weissman DE. Glucocorticoid treatment for brain metastases and epidural spinal cord compression: a review. J Clin Oncol. 1988;6:543–551.
34. Greenberg HS, Kim JH, Posner JB. Epidural spinal cord compression from metastatic tumor: results with a new treatment protocol. Ann Neurol. 1980;8:361–366.
35. Sundaresan N, Bains M, McCormack P. Surgical treatment of spinal cord compression in patients with lung cancer. Neurosurgery. 1985;16:350–356.
36. Young RF, Post EM, King GA. Treatment of spinal epidural metastases: randomized prospective comparison of laminectomy and radiotherapy. J Neurosurg. 1980;53:741–748.
37. Price P, Hoskin PJ, Easton D, et al. Prospective randomised trial of single and multifraction radiotherapy schedules in the treatment of painful bony metastases. Radiother Oncol. 1986;6:247–255.

38. Nielsen OS, Bentzen XM, Sandberg E, et al. Randomized trial of single dose vs. fractionated palliative radiotherapy of bone metastases. Radiother Oncol. 1998;47:233–240.
39. Hoskin PJ, Prince P, Easton D, et al. A prospective randomised trial of 4 Gy or 8 Gy single doses in the treatment of metastatic bone pain. Int J Radiat Oncol Biol Phys. 1992;23:74–78.
40. Tong D, Gillick L, Hendrickson FR. The palliation of symptomatic osseous metastases: final results of the study by the Radiation Therapy Oncology Group. Cancer. 1982;50:893–899.
41. Niewald M, Tkocz H-J, Abel U, et al. Rapid course radiation therapy versus more standard treatment in a randomized trial for bone metastasis. Int J Radiat Oncol Biol Phys. 1996;36:1085–1089.
42. Jeremic B, Shibamoto Y, Acimovic L, et al. A randomized trial of three single-dose radiation therapy regimens in the treatment of metastatic bone pain. Int J Radiat Oncol Biol Phys. 1998;42:161–167.
43. Gaze MN, Kelly CG, Kerr GR, et al. Pain relief and quality of life following radiation therapy for bone metastases: a randomised trial of two fractionation schedules. Radiother Oncol. 1997;45:109–116.
44. Mithal NP, Needham PR, Hoskin PJ. Retreatment with radiotherapy for painful bone metastases. Int J Radiat Oncol Biol Phys. 1994;29:1011–1014.
45. Rasmusson B, Vejborg I, Jensen AB, et al. Irradiation of bone metastases in breast cancer patients: a randomized study with 1 year follow-up. Radiother Oncol. 1995;34:179–184.
46. Poulter CA, Cosmatos D, Rubin P, et al. A report of RTOG 82-06: a phase III study of whether the addition of single dose hemibody irradiation to standard fractionated local field irradiation is more effective than local field irradiation alone in the treatment of symptomatic osseous metastases. Int J Radiat Oncol Biol Phys. 1992;23:207–214.
47. Bleehen NM, Girling DJ, for the MRC Lung Cancer Working Party. Inoperable non–small-cell lung cancer (NSCLC): a Medical Research Council randomised trial of palliative radiotherapy with two fractions or ten fractions: report to the Medical Research Council by its Lung Cancer Working Party. Br J Cancer. 1991;63:265–270.
48. Bleehen NM, Girling DJ, Machin D, et al. A Medical Research Council (MRC) randomised trial of palliative radiotherapy with two fractions or a single fraction in patients with inoperable non–small-cell lung cancer (NSCLC) and poor performance status. Br J Cancer. 1992;65:934–941.
49. Simpson JR, Francis ME, Perez-Tamayo R, et al. Palliative radiotherapy for inoperable carcinoma of the lung: final report of a RTOG multi-institutional trial. Int J Radiat Oncol Biol Phys. 1985;11:751–758.
50. Macbeth FR, Bolger JJ, Hopwood P, et al. Randomized trial of palliative two-fraction versus more intensive 13-fraction radiotherapy for patients with inoperable non–small cell lung cancer and good performance status. Medical Research Council Lung Cancer Working Party. Clin Oncol. 1996;8:167–175.
51. Rees GJG, Devrell CE, Barley VL, et al. Palliative radiotherapy for lung cancer: two versus five fractions. Clin Oncol. 1997;9:90–95.
52. Roswit B, Patno ME, Rapp R, et al. The survival of patients with inoperable lung cancer: a large-scale randomized study of radiation therapy versus placebo. Radiology. 1968;90:688–697.
53. Durrant KR, Berry RJ, Ellis F, et al. Comparison of treatment policies in inoperable bronchial carcinoma. Lancet. (April 10) 1971;1:715–719.
54. Johnson DH, Einhorn LH, Bartolucci A, et al. Thoracic radiotherapy does not prolong survival in patients with locally advanced, unresectable non–small cell lung cancer. Ann Intern Med. 1990;113:33–38.
55. Carroll M, Morgan SA, Yarnold JR, et al. Prospective evaluation of a watch policy in patients with inoperable non–small cell lung cancer. Eur J Cancer Clin Oncol. 1986;22:1353–1356.
56. Collins TM, Ash DV, Close HJ, et al. An evaluation of the palliative role of radiotherapy in inoperable carcinoma of the bronchus. Clin Radiol. 1988;39:284–286.
57. Speiser BL, Spratling L. Remote afterloading brachytherapy for the local control of endobronchial carcinoma. Int J Radiat Oncol Biol Phys. 1993;25:579–587.
58. Cavaliere S, Venuta F, Foccoli P, et al. Endoscopic treatment of malignant airway obstructions in 2,008 patients. Chest. 1996;110:1536–1542.
59. Ornadel D, Duchesne G, Wall P, et al. Defining the roles of high dose rate endobronchial brachytherapy and laser resection for recurrent bronchial malignancy. Lung Cancer. 1997;16:203–213.
60. Trédaniel J, Hennequin C, Zalcman G, et al. Prolonged survival after high-dose rate endobronchial radiation for malignant airway obstruction. Chest. 1994;105:767–772.
61. Fernandez C, Rosell R, Abad-Esteve A, et al. Quality of life during chemotherapy in non–small cell lung cancer patients. Acta Oncol. 1989;28:29–33.
62. Ofiara L, Roman T, Schwartzman K, et al. Local determinants of response to endobronchial high-dose rate brachytherapy in bronchogenic carcinoma. Chest. 1997;112:946–953.
63. Mehta MP, Shahabi S, Jarjour NN, et al. Endobronchial irradiation for malignant airway obstruction. Int J Radiat Oncol Biol Phys. 1989;17:847–851.
64. Osoba D, Rusthoven JJ, Turnbull KA, et al. Combination chemotherapy with bleomycin, etoposide, and cisplatin in metastatic non–small-cell lung cancer. J Clin Oncol. 1985;3:1478–1485.
65. Ellis PA, Smith IE, Hardy JR, et al. Symptom relief with MVP (mitomycin C, vinblastine and cisplatin) chemotherapy in advanced non–small-cell lung cancer. Br J Cancer. 1995;71:366–370.
66. Crino L, Scagliotti G, Marangolo M, et al. Cisplatin-gemcitabine combination in advanced non–small-cell lung cancer: a phase II study. J Clin Oncol. 1997;15:297–303.
67. Mehta M, Petereit D, Chosy L, et al. Sequential comparison of low dose rate and hyperfractionated high dose rate endobronchial radiation for malignant airway occlusion. Int J Radiat Oncol Biol Phys. 1992;23:133–139.
68. Burt PA, O'Driscoll BR, Notley HM, et al. Intraluminal irradiation for the palliation of lung cancer with the high dose rate micro-Selectron. Thorax. 1990;45:765–768.
69. Schray MF, McDougall JC, Martinez A, et al. Management of malignant airway compromise with laser and low dose rate brachytherapy: the Mayo Clinic experience. Chest. 1988;93:264–269.
70. Hetzel MR, Nixon C, Edmondstone WM, et al. Laser therapy in 100 tracheobronchial tumours. Thorax. 1985;40:341–345.
71. Marasso A, Gallo E, Massaglia GM, et al. Cryosurgery in bronchoscopic treatment of tracheobronchial stenosis. Chest. 1993;103:472–474.
72. Slawson RG, Scott RM. Radiation therapy in bronchogenic carcinoma. Radiology. 1979;132:175–176.
73. Montebello JF, Aron BS, Manatunga AK, et al. The reirradiation of recurrent bronchogenic carcinoma with external beam irradiation. Am J Clin Oncol. 1993;16:482–488.
74. Jackson MA, Ball DL. Palliative retreatment of locally recurrent lung cancer after radical radiotherapy. Med J Aust. 1987;147:391–394.
75. Green N, Melbye RW. Lung cancer: retreatment of local recurrence after definitive irradiation. Cancer. 1982;49:865–868.
76. Gressen EL, Werner-Wasik M, Cohn J, et al. Thoracic reirradiation for symptomatic relief after prior radiotherapeutic management for lung cancer. Am J Clin Oncol. 2000;23:160–165.
77. Mathisen DJ, Grillo HC. Endoscopic relief of malignant airway obstruction. Ann Thorac Surg. 1989;48:469–475.
78. Mathur PN, Wolf KM, Busk MF, et al. Fiberoptic bronchoscopic cryotherapy in the management of tracheobronchial obstruction. Chest. 1996;110:718–723.
79. Dumon JF, Shapshay S, Bourcereau J, et al. Principles for safety in application of neodymium-YAG laser in bronchology. Chest. 1984;86:163–168.
80. Personne C, Colchen A, Leroy M, et al. Indications and technique for endoscopic laser resections in bronchology: a critical analysis based upon 2,284 resections. J Thorac Cardiovasc Surg. 1986;91:710–715.
81. Brutinel WM, Cortese DA, McDougall JC, et al. A two-year experience with the neodymium-YAG laser in endobronchial obstruction. Chest. 1987;91:159–165.
82. Hauck RW, Lembeck RM, Emslander HP, et al. Implantation of Accuflex and Strecker stents in malignant bronchial stenoses by flexible bronchoscopy. Chest. 1997;112:134–144.
83. Wilson GE, Walshaw MJ, Hind CRK. Treatment of large airway obstruction in lung cancer using expandable metal stents inserted under direct vision via the fiberoptic bronchoscope. Thorax. 1996;51:248–252.
84. Monnier P, Mudry A, Stanzel F, et al. The use of the covered

wallstent for the palliative treatment of inoperable tracheobronchial cancers: a prospective, multicenter study. Chest. 1996;110:1161–1168.

85. Lam S, Müller NL, Miller RR, et al. Predicting the response of obstructive endobronchial tumors to photodynamic therapy. Cancer. 1986;58:2298–2306.

86. Hayata Y. Photoradiation. Chest. 1986;89:332S.

87. McCaughan JS Jr, Williams TE. Photodynamic therapy for endobronchial malignant disease: a prospective fourteen-year study. J Thorac Cardiovasc Surg. 1997;114:940–947.

88. Homasson JP, Renault P, Angebault M, et al. Bronchoscopic cryotherapy for airway strictures caused by tumors. Chest. 1986;90:159–164.

89. Walsh DA, Maiwand MO, Nath AR, et al. Bronchoscopic cryotherapy for advanced bronchial carcinoma. Thorax. 1990;45:509–513.

90. Maiwand MO. Cryotherapy for advanced carcinoma of the trachea and bronchi. BMJ. 1986;293:181–182.

91. Maiwand MO. The role of cryosurgery in palliation of tracheobronchial carcinoma. Eur J Cardio-Thorac Surg. 1999;15:764–768.

92. Hernandez P, Gursahaney A, Roman T, et al. High dose rate brachytherapy for the local control of endobronchial carcinoma following external irradiation. Thorax. 1996;51:354–358.

93. Huber R, Fischer R, Hautmann H, et al. Palliative endobronchial brachytherapy for central lung tumors: a prospective, randomized comparison of two fractionation schedules. Chest. 1995;107:463–470.

94. Taulelle M, Chauvet B, Vincent P, et al. High dose rate endobronchial brachytherapy: results and complications in 189 patients. Eur Respir J. 1998;11:162–168.

95. Speiser BL, Spratling L. Radiation bronchitis and stenosis secondary to high dose rate endobronchial irradiation. Int J Radiat Oncol Biol Phys. 1993;25:589–597.

96. Gollins SW, Ryder WDJ, Burt PA, et al. Massive haemoptysis death and other morbidity associated with high dose rate intraluminal radiotherapy for carcinoma of the bronchus. Radiother Oncol. 1996;39:105–116.

97. Khanavkar B, Stern P, Alberti W, et al. Complications associated with brachytherapy alone or with laser in lung cancer. Chest. 1991;99:1062–1065.

98. Bedwinek J, Petty A, Bruton C, et al. The use of high dose rate endobronchial brachytherapy to palliate symptomatic endobronchial recurrence of previously irradiated bronchogenic carcinoma. Int J Radiat Oncol Biol Phys. 1991;22:23–30.

99. Sutedja G, Baris G, Schaake-Koning C, et al. High dose rate brachytherapy in patients with local recurrences after radiotherapy of non–small cell lung cancer. Int J Radiat Oncol Biol Phys. 1992;24:551–553.

100. Mehta MP. Endobronchial radiotherapy for lung cancer. In: Pass HI, Mitchell JB, Johnson DH, et al, eds. Lung Cancer: Principles and Practice. Philadelphia, Pa: Lippincott-Raven; 1996:741–750.

101. Miller RR, McGregor DH. Hemorrhage from carcinoma of the lung. Cancer. 1980;46:200–205.

102. Mantravadi RVP, Gates JO, Crawford JN, et al. Unresectable non–oat cell carcinoma of the lung: definitive radiation therapy. Radiology. 1989;172:851–855.

103. Chetty KG, Moran EM, Sassoon CSH, et al. Effect of radiation therapy on bronchial obstruction due to bronchogenic carcinoma. Chest. 1989;95:582–584.

104. Majid OA, Lee S, Khushalani S, et al. The response of atelectasis from lung cancer to radiation therapy. Int J Radiat Oncol Biol Phys. 1986;12:231–232.

105. Chella A, Ambrogi MC, Ribechini A, et al. Combined Nd-YAG laser/HDR brachytherapy versus Nd-YAG laser only in malignant central airway involvement: a prospective randomized study. Lung Cancer. 2000;27:169–175.

106. Hausheer FH, Yarbro JW. Diagnosis and treatment of malignant pleural effusion. Semin Oncol. 1985;12:54–75.

107. Salyer WR, Eggleston JC, Erozan YS. Efficacy of pleural needle biopsy and pleural fluid cytopathology in the diagnosis of malignant neoplasm involving the pleura. Chest. 1975;67:536–539.

108. Winkelmann M, Pfitzer P. Blind pleural biopsy in combination with cytology of pleural effusions. Acta Cytol. 1981;25:373–376.

109. Prakash UBS, Reiman HM. Comparison of needle biopsy with cytologic analysis for the evaluation of pleural effusion: analysis of 414 cases. Mayo Clin Proc. 1985;60:158–164.

110. Weissberg D, Kaufman M. Diagnostic and therapeutic pleuroscopy: experience with 127 patients. Chest. 1980;78:732–735.

111. Boutin C, Cargnino P, Viallat JR. Thoracoscopy in the early diagnosis of malignant pleural effusions. Endoscopy. 1980;12:155–160.

112. Bal S, Hasan SS. Thoracoscopic management of malignant pleural effusion. Int Surg. 1993;78:324–327.

113. Ohri SK, Oswal SK, Townsend ER, et al. Early and late outcome after diagnostic thoracoscopy and talc pleurodesis. Ann Thorac Surg. 1992;53:1038–1041.

114. Yim APC, Chung SS, Lee TW, et al. Thoracoscopic management of malignant pleural effusions. Chest. 1996;109:1234–1238.

115. Belani CP, Pajeau TS, Bennett CL. Treating malignant pleural effusions cost consciously. Chest. 1998;113:78S–85S.

116. Walker-Renard PB, Vaughan LM, Sahn SA. Chemical pleurodesis for malignant pleural effusions. Ann Intern Med. 1994;120:56–64.

117. Sanchez-Armengol A, Rodriguez-Panadero F. Survival and talc pleurodesis in metastatic pleural carcinoma, revisited: report of 125 cases. Chest. 1993;104:1482–1485.

118. Petrou M, Kaplan D, Goldstraw P. Management of recurrent malignant pleural effusions: the complementary role of talc pleurodesis and pleuroperitoneal shunting. Cancer. 1995;75:801–805.

119. Anderson CB, Philpott GW, Ferguson TB. The treatment of malignant pleural effusions. Cancer. 1974;33:916–922.

120. Sarma P, Moore MR. Approach to the management of pleural effusion in malignancy. South Med J. 1978;71:133–136.

121. Lambert CJ, Shah HH, Urschel HC Jr, et al. The treatment of malignant pleural effusions by closed trocar tube drainage. Ann Thorac Surg. 1967;3:1–5.

122. Zaloznik AJ, Oswald SG, Langin M. Intrapleural tetracycline in malignant pleural effusions: a randomized study. Cancer. 1983;51:752–755.

123. Sørensen PG, Svendsen TL, Enk B. Treatment of malignant pleural effusion with drainage, with and without instillation of talc. Eur J Respir Dis. 1984;65:131–135.

124. Izbicki R, Weyhing BT III, Baker L, et al. Pleural effusion in cancer patients: a prospective randomized study of pleural drainage with the addition of radioactive phosphorus to the pleural space vs. pleural drainage alone. Cancer. 1975;36:1511–1518.

125. O'Neill W, Spurr C, Muss H, et al. A prospective study of chest tube drainage and tetracycline (TCN) sclerosis versus chest tube drainage alone in the treatment of malignant pleural effusion [abstract]. Proc ASCO. 1980; p 349.

126. Ruckdeschel JC, Moores D, Lee JY, et al. Intrapleural therapy for malignant pleural effusions: a randomized comparison of bleomycin and tetracycline. Chest. 1991;100:1528–1535.

127. Seaton KG, Patz EF Jr, Goodman PC. Palliative treatment of malignant pleural effusions: value of small-bore catheter thoracostomy and doxycycline sclerotherapy. AJR Am J Roentgenol. 1995;164:589–591.

128. Martinez-Moragón E, Aparicio J, Rogado MC, et al. Pleurodesis in malignant pleural effusions: a randomized study of tetracycline versus bleomycin. Eur Respir J. 1997;10:2380–2383.

129. Ostrowski MJ. Intracavitary therapy with bleomycin for the treatment of malignant pleural effusions. J Surg Oncol. 1989;1(suppl):7–13.

130. Hartman DL, Gaither JM, Kesler KA, et al. Comparison of insufflated talc under thoracoscopic guidance with standard tetracycline and bleomycin pleurodesis for control of malignant pleural effusions. J Thorac Cardiovasc Surg. 1993;105:743–748.

131. Viallat J-R, Rey F, Astoul P, et al. Thoracoscopic talc poudrage pleurodesis for malignant effusions: a review of 360 cases. Chest. 1996;110:1387–1393.

132. Sherman S, Grady, KJ, Seidman JC. Clinical experience with tetracycline pleurodesis of malignant pleural effusions. South Med J. 1987;80:716–719.

133. Heffner JE, Standerfer RJ, Torstveit J, et al. Clinical efficacy of doxycycline for pleurodesis. Chest. 1994;105:1743–1747.

134. Kennedy L, Rusch VW, Strange C, et al. Pleurodesis using talc slurry. Chest. 1994;106:342–346.

135. Jacobi CA, Wenger FA, Schmitz-Rixen T, et al. Talc pleurodesis in recurrent pleural effusions. Langenbecks Arch Surg. 1998;383:156–159.

136. Kennedy L, Sahn SA. Talc pleurodesis for the treatment of pneumothorax and pleural effusion. Chest. 1994;106:1215–1222.

137. Lange P, Mortensen J, Groth S. Lung function 22-35 years after

treatment of idiopathic spontaneous pneumothorax with talc poudrage or simple drainage. Thorax. 1988;43:559–561.

138. Chappell AG, for the Research Committee of the British Thoracic Association and the Medical Research Council Pneumoconiosis Unit. A survey of the long-term effects of talc and kaolin pleurodesis. Br J Dis Chest. 1979;73:285–288.

139. Weiss RB, Bruno S. Hypersensitivity reactions to cancer chemotherapeutic agents. Ann Intern Med. 1981;94:66–72.

140. Reed CE. Management of the malignant pleural effusion. In: Pass HI, Mitchell JB, Johnson DH, et al, eds. Lung Cancer: Principles and Practice. Philadelphia, Pa: Lippincott-Raven; 1996:643–654.

141. Jensik R, Cagle JE Jr, Milloy F, et al. Pleurectomy in the treatment of pleural effusion due to metastatic malignancy. J Thorac Cardiovasc Surg. 1963;46:322–330.

142. Martini N, Bains MS, Beattie EJ. Indications for pleurectomy in malignant effusion. Cancer. 1975;35:734–738.

143. Heffner JE, Nietert PJ, Barberi C. Pleural fluid pH as a predictor of survival for patients with malignant pleural effusions. Chest. 2000;117:79–86.

144. Burrows CM, Mathews C, Colt HG. Predicting survival in patients with recurrent symptomatic malignant pleural effusions: an assessment of the prognostic values of physiologic, morphologic, and quality of life measures of extent of disease. Chest. 2000;117:73–78.

145. Patz EF Jr, McAdams HP, Erasmus JJ, et al. Sclerotherapy for malignant pleural effusions: a prospective randomized trial of bleomycin vs doxycycline with small-bore catheter drainage. Chest. 1998;113:1305–1311.

146. Parker LA, Jaffe TA, Little K. Outpatient management of intrathoracic fluid collections with small bore catheters [abstract]. AJR Am J Roentgenol. 1999;172(suppl):29.

147. Putnam JB Jr, Walsh GL, Swisher SG, et al. Outpatient management of malignant pleural effusion by a chronic indwelling pleural catheter. Ann Thorac Surg. 2000;69:369–375.

148. Tsang V, Fernando HC, Goldstraw P. Pleuroperitoneal shunt for recurrent malignant pleural effusions. Thorax. 1990;45:369–372.

149. Ponn RB, Blancaflor J, D'Agostino RS, et al. Pleuroperitoneal shunting for intractable pleural effusions. Ann Thorac Surg. 1991;51:605–609.

150. Lee KA, Harvey JC, Reich H, et al. Management of malignant pleural effusions with pleuroperitoneal shunting. J Am Coll Surg. 1994;178:586–588.

151. Little AG, Ferguson MK, Golomb HM, et al. Pleuroperitoneal shunting for malignant pleural effusions. Cancer. 1986;58:2740–2743.

152. Aelony Y, King RR, Boutin C. Thoracoscopic talc poudrage in malignant pleural effusions: effective pleurodesis despite low pleural pH. Chest. 1998;113:1007–1012.

153. Cavaliere S, Foccoli P, Farina PL. Nd:YAG laser bronchoscopy: a five-year experience with 1,396 applications in 1,000 patients. Chest. 1988;94:15–21.

154. Gollins SW, Burt PA, Barber PV, et al. High dose rate intraluminal radiotherapy for carcinoma of the bronchus: outcome of treatment of 406 patients. Radiother Oncol. 1994;33:31–40.

155. Aygun C, Weiner S, Scariato A, et al. Treatment of non–small cell lung cancer with external beam radiotherapy and high dose rate brachytherapy. Int J Radiat Oncol Biol Phys. 1992;23:127–132.

156. Kabarowski R, Maczko M, Skrzypczynska E, et al. Endobronchial BRT HDR in NSCLC: valuation of early clinical results of particular fractions—preliminary report. Lung Cancer. 1998;21(suppl 1):S56.

157. Danby CA, Adebonojo SA, Moritz DM. Video-assisted talc pleurodesis for malignant pleural effusions utilizing local anesthesia and IV sedation. Chest. 1998;113:739–742.

158. Fentiman IS, Rubens RD, Hayward JL. Control of pleural effusions in patients with breast cancer: a randomized trial. Cancer. 1983;52:737–739.

159. Martinez-Moragón E, Aparicio J, Sanchis J, et al. Malignant pleural effusion: prognostic factors for survival and response to chemical pleurodesis in a series of 120 cases. Respiration. 1998;65:108–113.

160. Parker LA, Charnock GC, Delany DJ. Small bore catheter drainage and sclerotherapy for malignant pleural effusions. Cancer. 1989;64:1218–1221.

161. Pulsiripunya C, Youngchaiyud P, Pushpakom R, et al. The efficacy of doxycycline as a pleural sclerosing agent in malignant pleural effusion: a prospective study. Respirology. 1996;1:69–72.

162. Groth G, Gatzemeier U, Häubingen K, et al. Intrapleural palliative treatment of malignant pleural effusions with mitoxantrone versus placebo (pleural tube alone). Ann Oncol. 1991;2:213–215.

163. Masuno T, Kishimoto S, Ogura T, et al. A comparative trial of LC9018 plus doxorubicin and doxorubicin alone for the treatment of malignant pleural effusion secondary to lung cancer. Cancer. 1991;68:1495–1500.

164. Macha HN, Koch K, Stadler M, et al. New technique for treating occlusive and stenosing tumours of the trachea and main bronchi: endobronchial irradiation by high-dose iridium-192 combined with laser canalisation. Thorax. 1987;42:511–515.

SATELLITE NODULES AND MULTIPLE PRIMARY CANCERS

Frank C. Detterbeck, David R. Jones,
and William K. Funkhouser, Jr.

DEFINITIONS

Occasionally, patients are encountered who have more than one focus of lung cancer within the pulmonary parenchyma. The presentation may be metachronous, in which case the two foci of cancer are temporally separated, often by many years. Alternatively, patients may be seen with two foci presenting synchronously. These may involve tumors within the same lobe or within the same lung, and patients may also present with bilateral lung cancers. The tumors may have similar or different histologic types. The second cancer may be discovered because of symptoms or may be found incidentally either during evaluation of the first cancer or during follow-up.

A classification system for multiple foci of cancer should ideally predict the biologic behavior of the cancers and thereby determine the optimal treatment. Three different theoretical situations can be defined in which the tumors are likely to exhibit markedly different behaviors and require different treatment approaches. First, a tumor may involve multiple foci that represent a form of local intrapulmonary spread without systemic hematogenous dissemination. Second, two primary lung cancers may develop that are completely independent of one another. Finally, more than one focus of cancer within the lung parenchyma may be a manifestation of hematogenous systemic spread of a primary lung cancer (or of a nonpulmonary malignancy).

Independent development of multiple primary lung cancers (MPLC) and hematogenous dissemination of a single primary lung cancer certainly do occur. A reasonable amount of evidence also suggests that local intralobar spread of pulmonary malignancies can also occur (as will be discussed). This chapter analyzes data related to satellite nodules and MPLC (occurring in either a synchronous or a metachronous fashion). Pulmonary metastases from a primary lung cancer are discussed in Chapter 23.

A set of definitions for satellite nodules, multiple primary lung cancers, and pulmonary metastases is proposed in Table 30–1. These definitions should classify a patient appropriately about 80% of the time, with the possible exception of patients with synchronous tumors of the same histologic type (as discussed later in the section Validity of Classification). Available reports do not necessarily use these definitions, however. For example, most authors do not clearly define what they mean by satellite nodules. Most reports of MPLC have used the definition proposed by Martini and Melamed[1] in 1975, albeit with minor modifications. The definition of MPLC in Table 30–1 is also similar to the definition proposed by Martini and Melamed, with the exception that the minimum time interval between cancers of the same histologic type is increased to at least 4 years. The ability to perform molecular genetic characterization of tumors may provide another method of defining "histologically" distinct tumors in the future.

Some studies have excluded patients with bronchioloalveolar carcinoma (BAC), but others have not. These tumors exhibit a strong propensity to be multifocal and to develop widespread pulmonary metastases without extrathoracic metastases (see Chapter 27). Such tumors should be excluded from studies of satellite nodules. It seems best to exclude BAC from studies of multiple primary cancers as well, although including them may be reasonable if they represent a tumor of different histologic type. However, it is difficult to retrospectively exclude BAC from the reported data in the studies that have included these tumors. Fortunately, BAC represents a relatively small percentage (<10%) of the tumors in most studies.

TABLE 30–1. DEFINITION OF SATELLITE NODULES, MULTIPLE PRIMARY LUNG CANCERS, AND PULMONARY METASTASES

SATELLITE NODULES

Satellite Nodules From Primary Tumor

Same histology
and same lobe as primary cancer
and no systemic metastases

MULTIPLE PRIMARY LUNG CANCERS

Same Histology, Anatomically Separated

Cancers in different lobes
and no N2,3 involvement
and no systemic metastases
or

Same Histology, Temporally Separated

≥4-year interval between cancers
and no systemic metastases from either cancer
or

Different Histology

Different histologic type
or different molecular genetic characteristics
or arising separately from foci of carcinoma in situ

HEMATOGENOUSLY SPREAD PULMONARY METASTASES

Same Histology and Multiple Systemic Metastases
or

Same Histology, in Different Lobes

and presence of N2,3 involvement,
or <2-year interval

SATELLITE NODULES

The term *satellite nodule* has been used to denote a synchronous secondary tumor nodule of identical histology to the main tumor. Histologic confirmation of the secondary nodule requires a tissue biopsy; hence, the reports of satellite nodules involve patients who underwent resection, with few exceptions. Some authors have used the term *ipsilateral pulmonary metastases* to describe such cases. Most authors have included both patients with satellite nodules occurring in the same lobe as the primary tumor and

patients with satellite nodules occurring in a different (ipsilateral) lobe.

This section examines the characteristics and outcomes of patients with a secondary tumor nodule or nodules occurring in the same lobe, which will be called *same-lobe satellite nodule* (SLSN). The focus in this section is on studies in which at least 80% of patients had SLSN because little data is available that involves these patients exclusively. Studies in which the majority of patients had BAC are excluded.[2,3]

A summary of the larger set of studies that have included both SLSN and secondary lesions occurring in different lobes is shown in Table 30–2. The occurrence of such satellite nodules is surprisingly common, being found consistently in approximately 7% of patients who have undergone resection. Adenocarcinoma has generally been the most common tumor type, and approximately half of patients have been N0. Even though more than half of the patients have had SLSN, the average 5-year survival for this larger group of patients is only 19%.

Studies reporting primarily (≥80%) on patients with SLSN are shown in Table 30–3. Once again, adenocarcinoma is generally reported as the most common cell type. Although studies in which most of the patients have BAC have been excluded,[2,3] most studies have not specifically reported on the proportion of patients who had BAC. The one study that specifically mentioned a low incidence of BAC also included relatively few patients with adenocarcinoma.[4] Approximately half of the patients have been N0, with the remainder split relatively evenly between N1 and N2.

The overall 5-year survival for patients with SLSN is relatively good (35%). Although the data is limited, the 5-year survival of patients with SLSN who were N0 is approximately 60%. This suggests better survival for the patients with SLSN compared with patients with a secondary cancer nodule in a different lobe. The survival of this latter group of patients has been reported specifically in four studies.[5–8] The largest of these reported a 5-year survival of 23% in 38 patients.[8] The 5-year survival was found to be 0% and 20% in two studies reporting on <10 patients each.[5,6] The fourth study included 21 patients and found a

TABLE 30–2. CHARACTERISTICS OF PATIENTS WITH IPSILATERAL SECONDARY PULMONARY LESIONS

| STUDY | N | Incid[a] | % OF ALL PATIENTS | | | | | | 5-y SURVIVAL (%) | |
			SLSN	BAC	Adeno	N0	N1	N2	All	N0
Naruke et al[55]	146	8	61	?	—	—	—	—	13	—
Okada[8]	89	10	57	0	80	36	19	37	(27)[b]	45
Deslauriers et al[4]	84	8	81	5	25	51	37	12	22	54
Watanabe et al[56]	49	7	—	?	—	—	—	—	14	—
Shimizu et al[6]	42	5	88	?	67	46	18	36	26	44
Yoshino et al[57]	42	8	—	?	74	40	21	36	(26)[b]	—
Fukuse et al[7]	41	4	49	?	66	44	10	44	26	26
Average[c]		7	67		62	43	21	33	20	42

Inclusion criteria: Studies from 1980 to 2000 reporting on ≥20 patients with ipsilateral secondary pulmonary lesions, excluding studies with ≥50% patients with BAC.
[a]Percentage of patients with satellite nodules relative to all patients who underwent resection at that institution during the study period.
[b]Estimated.
[c]Excluding the values in parentheses.
Adeno, adenocarcinoma; BAC, bronchioloalveolar carcinoma; Incid, incidence; SLSN, same-lobe satellite nodules.

TABLE 30–3. CHARACTERISTICS OF PATIENTS WITH SATELLITE NODULES IN THE SAME LOBE (SLSN)

| STUDY | N | % OF ALL PATIENTS | | | | | 5-y SURVIVAL %) | |
		BAC	Adeno	N0	N1	N2	All	N0
Deslauriers et al[4a]	68	5	25	51	37	12	22	54
Okada[8]	51	0	—	35	23	38	30	68
Yano et al[5]	39	—	62	26	31	44	37	70
Shimizu et al[6b]	37	—	67	46	18	36	42	—
Fukuse et al[7]	20	—	—	—	—	—	37	—
Average				**40**	**27**	**33**	**34**	**64**

Inclusion criteria: Studies from 1980 to 2000 reporting on ≥20 patients, in which ≥80% have SLSN, excluding studies with ≥50% of patients with BAC.
[a]Includes 19% different lobe secondary tumors.
[b]Includes 12% different lobe primary tumors.
Adeno, adenocarcinoma; BAC, bronchioloalveolar carcinoma.

3-year survival of 21%, with an estimated 5-year survival of <10%.[7] Each of these studies reported poorer survival in patients with secondary cancers in a lobe different from that in patients with SLSN, although the difference in one of these was small.[8] Furthermore, multivariate analysis in one of these studies found that the localization of a secondary cancer nodule to a different lobe was an independent predictor of poor survival. Only two studies have suggested no difference in survival. However, one of these included mostly patients with BAC,[3] and the other included many patients with pleural metastases and patients who did not undergo resection.[9] One review of this topic also concluded that patients with secondary cancer nodules occurring in a different lobe have poorer survival than patients with SLSN.[10]

Despite the relatively good survival of resected patients with SLSN, the survival of patients with a satellite nodule is worse than that of patients without a satellite nodule. This is most clearly shown in the study by Deslauriers et al,[4] which compared patients with and without satellite nodules, stage for stage (Fig. 30–1). In this study, the stage of tumor was classified independent of the satellite nodule.

Another somewhat smaller study found only a slight trend to poorer survival in N0 patients with a satellite nodule than in patients without a satellite nodule when stage was assessed independent of the satellite lesion.[5] A multivariate analysis of the larger study found that the presence of satellite nodules was an independent predictor of poorer survival (hazard ratio, 1.6; $P = 0.001$).[4]

The relatively good survival of patients with SLSN suggests that a local mechanism of spread is occurring, as opposed to diffuse hematogenous seeding. Theoretically, local spread could occur by an airborne mechanism, via lymphatic channels, or through the pulmonary arterial circulation. Spread through the pulmonary venous circulation is likely to be systemic.

Some limited data suggests that spread through the pulmonary arterial circulation may account for SLSN. All studies that have examined the relative location of the primary tumor and the satellite nodule have found that in two-thirds of patients the satellite nodules are either adjacent to or *distal* to the primary tumor.[4,11,12] Spread via lymphatic channels seems less likely, considering that approximately 50% of the patients have no lymph node

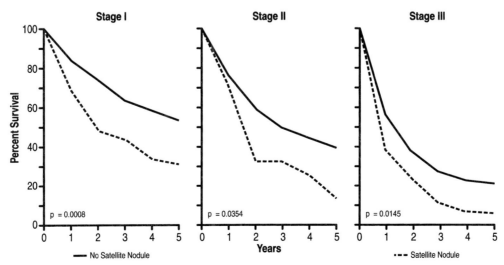

FIGURE 30–1. Survival of resected patients by stage according to the presence of satellite nodules. (From Deslauriers J, Brisson J, Cartier R, et al. Carcinoma of the lung: evaluation of satellite nodules as a factor influencing prognosis after resection. J Thorac Cardiovasc Surg. 1989;97:504–512.[4])

involvement, even though most patients have large primary tumors.[4,11] In addition, most studies have been careful to exclude patients who have satellite nodules associated with intrapulmonary lymphatics or lymph nodes. Finally, there is no data to support airborne metastases, except in the case of BAC. Perhaps future studies will provide more information about the mechanism of spread by examining the relationship of pulmonary arterial, venous, and lymphatic invasion to SLSN, as well as more careful studies of the anatomic relationship of primary tumors and satellite nodules.

MULTIPLE PRIMARY LUNG CANCERS

Incidence

A large number of reports have been published on patients with MPLC (Table 30–4). Overall, such patients account for approximately 6% of patients with lung cancer. There appears to be little difference between surgical series (involving resected patients) and general series (involving patients entered in a registry). This is not surprising because there are few patients who are not treated surgically who survive long enough to develop a second lung cancer. Approximately 30% of the multiple lung cancers are synchronous.

Because of differing lengths of follow-up, the relative number of all patients with lung cancer who develop MPLC does not provide an estimate of the risk of developing a new primary lung cancer. To assess this, the incidence of metachronous cancers developing during a known period of follow-up must be assessed. Several studies have examined this and have consistently found the incidence to be between 0.5% and 4% per patient per year of follow-up.[13–23] The average incidence in these studies is 1.6% per patient per year. Several of these studies have focused specifically on patients whose first cancer was stage I and have reported similar results.[14–16,18–20]

The incidence of second primary lung cancers does not appear to decrease with time. In fact, the rate was found to be 1% per patient per year during the first 5 years after the initial cancer was diagnosed, but increased to 2% per patient per year between 5 and 10 years after diagnosis in the careful long-term study of 907 patients with T1N0 disease reported by Thomas and Rubinstein.[14] A higher incidence of MPLC during late follow-up was also suggested by another study of patients who survived ≥10 years after a first lung cancer was diagnosed.[24] Sixteen percent of these patients were found to develop a new lung primary. These results suggest that follow-up of patients who have had lung cancer should continue indefinitely.

Reports have suggested that the incidence of new primary lung cancer is much higher in patients who originally had a central tumor.[25–31] On average, 9% of patients with a central tumor were found to have either a synchronous or a metachronous second primary lung cancer. The incidence of a second primary lung cancer in these studies has consistently ranged between 8% and 15% with only one exception (2%).[27] Although these crude rates do not allow an estimation of the risk of a new primary lung cancer per patient per year, the fact that the crude rates for central tumors are consistently reported to be higher than the crude rates for multiple lung cancers in general suggests that patients with central tumors may be more prone to developing a new primary lung cancer. It is also interesting to note that squamous cell carcinomas, which are more likely

TABLE 30–4. INCIDENCE OF MULTIPLE PRIMARY LUNG CANCERS[a]

STUDY	STUDY SIZE[b]	N[c]	STUDY TYPE	% BAC	% SYNCHRONOUS	CRUDE RATE[d] (%)
van Bodegom et al[36]	1540	153	All	0	42	9.9
Deschamps et al[32]	9611	117	All	19	38	1.2
Adebonojo et al[37]	1325	68	All	0	29	5.1
Mathisen et al[38]	—	90	Surgical	9	11	—
van Bodegom et al[36]	498	77	Surgical	0	—	15.0
Ribet and Dambron[17]	1980	75	Surgical	—	32	3.8
Martini et al[16e]	598	69	Surgical	—	24[f]	10.0[f]
Antakli et al[13]	1572	65	Surgical	—	40	4.1
Okada et al[33]	908	57	Surgical	0	49	6.3
Verhagen et al[40]	1287	55	Surgical	—	27	4.3
Adebonojo et al[37]	576	52	Surgical	0	29	9.0
Wu et al[39]	3815	30	Surgical	—	33	0.8
Ferguson et al[34g]	>2100	28	?	0	(100)[g]	(<1.3)[g]
Van Meerbeeck et al[18h]	534	23	Surgical	4	(0)[h]	(4.3)[h]
Average[i]					33	6.3

Inclusion criteria: Studies from 1980 to 2000 of >20 patients with multiple primary lung cancers, excluding earlier overlapping reports from the same institution.
[a]All studies used the definition of multiple primary cancer suggested by Martini and Melamed,[1] except as indicated.
[b]Total number of patients in study.
[c]Number of patients with multiple primary lung cancers.
[d]Percentage of all patients who had a secondary primary lung cancer.
[e]Unclear definition.
[f]Excluding patients with previous lung cancer, before beginning of study.
[g]Patients with synchronous cancers only.
[h]Patients with metachronous cancers only.
[i]Excluding values in parentheses.
BAC, bronchioloalveolar carcinoma; Surgical, series of patients undergoing resection.

TABLE 30–5. CHARACTERISTICS OF SYNCHRONOUS MULTIPLE PRIMARY LUNG CANCERS

STUDY	N	% INCIDENTAL[a]	% BAC	% SAME HISTOLOGY	% IPSILATERAL	% SAME LOBE
van Bodegom et al[36]	64	—	0	81	—	0
Deschamps et al[32]	36	42	18	33	86	—
Rosengart et al[35]	33	—	8	48	76	36
Ferguson et al[34]	28	18	0	68	39	0
Okada et al[33]	28	39	0	43	75	—
Antakli et al[13]	26	19	—	—	46	15
Ribet and Dambron[17]	24	—	—	58	38	—
Average		**30**		**55**	**60**	

Inclusion criteria: Studies from 1980 to 2000 of ≥20 patients with synchronous multiple primary lung cancers.
[a]Percentage discovered incidentally at the time of resection.
BAC, bronchioloalveolar carcinoma.

to involve the central airways, account for approximately 70% of all MPLC in almost all reports.

Synchronous Primary Lung Cancers

Approximately one-third of MPLC present as synchronous cancers, and approximately one-third of these synchronous primary lung cancers are found incidentally at the time of thoracotomy (Table 30–5). It is not surprising, therefore, that approximately two-thirds of synchronous primary lung cancers have been found on the same side. Studies that included a high proportion of incidental second primary lung cancers reported that approximately 75% of synchronous primary lung cancers were ipsilateral.[32,33] Other studies have found ipsilateral tumors to occur in approximately 40% of patients.[13,17,34]

The number of patients with synchronous tumors of the same histologic type varies considerably among studies. Reports in which most tumors were of the same histologic type found that the majority of cases involved bilateral tumors. This may represent a reluctance by the authors to classify tumors of the same histologic type as multiple primaries if they are unilateral. Two studies have reported a relatively high incidence of synchronous primary lung cancers occurring within the same lobe.[13,35] It is not clear whether these tumors were of different histologic types. It may be that at least some of these tumors would be more appropriately classified as satellite nodules if they were of the same histologic type.

The most common histologic type among synchronous MPLC has been squamous cell carcinoma (Table 30–6). The two studies in Table 30–6 with a high proportion of incidentally discovered tumors have both reported a more balanced distribution of squamous cell carcinoma and adenocarcinoma.[32,33]

The majority of synchronous MPLC have been early stage tumors (Table 30–6). When stage is reported as the poorer stage of the two cancers, stage I disease is found in approximately 50% of patients. It might be expected that series reporting primarily on patients who underwent resection would consist mostly of early stage tumors, but this is not consistently the case. At least 30% of patients are found to be stage III or IV, even in series involving primarily resected patients.

The ability to resect both cancers in patients with synchronous MPLCs has been reported to be high (Table 30–7). This likely represents a bias, with resected patients being more likely to be reported. In patients who are not resected, it is probably difficult to clearly establish histologically that the patients have synchronous MPLC. Although approximately 80% of tumors are able to be resected, approximately 30% of these resections involve a segmentectomy or a wedge resection.

The 5-year survival of patients with synchronous MPLC has been disappointingly low (see Table 30–7; Fig. 30–2). Although not many reports have included survival data, the data that is available generally indicates that most of these patients will not be 5-year survivors. Even among patients in whom each tumor was pathologically stage I, the sur-

TABLE 30–6. HISTOLOGIC TYPE AND STAGE OF SYNCHRONOUS MULTIPLE PRIMARY LUNG CANCERS[a]

STUDY	N	Squam	Adeno	Other	SCLC	I	II	IIIa	IIIb-IV
van Bodegom et al[36]	64	70	20	9	2	28	9	——63——	
Deschamps et al[32b]	36	36	35	28	1	67	19	11	—
Rosengart et al[35b]	33	63	24	11	2	58	15	15	12
Ferguson et al[34]	28	68	18	12	2	38	19	42	0
Okada et al[33b]	28	46	43	5	2	39	18	18	25
Ribet and Dambron[17]	24	67	21	2	10	54	25	21	0
Average		**58**	**27**	**11**	**3**	**47**	**18**	**21**	**9**

Inclusion criteria: Studies from 1980 to 2000 of ≥20 patients with synchronous multiple primary lung cancers.
[a]Values shown are percentages. Histologic types are calculated per tumor (each cancer is counted separately). Stage is reported per patient by counting only the higher stage of the two tumors.
[b]Surgical series with ≥90% of patients having been resected.
Adeno, adenocarcinoma; SCLC, small cell lung cancer; Squam, squamous cell carcinoma.

TABLE 30–7. SURVIVAL OF PATIENTS WITH SYNCHRONOUS MULTIPLE PRIMARY LUNG CANCERS

STUDY	N	% INCIDENTAL[a]	% RESECTED	% LIMITED[b] RESECTION	OPERATIVE MORTALITY (%)	5-y SURVIVAL (%)		
						All	Resected	pI
van Bodegom et al[36]	64	—	50	34	—	—	—	24[c]
Deschamps et al[32d]	36	42	100	21	6	—	16	—
Rosengart et al[35d]	33	—	91	33	—	44	—	—
Ferguson et al[34]	28	18	68	47	0	0	0	0
Okada et al[33d]	28	39	96	7	0	70	—	79[c]
Antakli et al[13]	26	19	92	42	—	5	12	—
Ribet and Dambron[17]	24	—	63	40	4	—	—	—
Average		30	80	32	3			

Inclusion criteria: Studies from 1980 to 2000 of ≥20 patients with synchronous multiple primary lung cancers.
[a]Percentage found incidentally at time of resection.
[b]Percentage of resected patients who underwent wedge resection or segmentectomy.
[c]Stage I and II.
[d]Surgical series with ≥90% of patients having been resected.
pI, pathologic stage I patients.

vival has been low in two series.[34,36] Only one series has reported good survival.[33] In this series, few patients underwent a limited resection, and the second cancer was found incidentally at the time of resection in a high proportion of patients.[33] The cause of death has been reported to be recurrent cancer in approximately 75% of patients.[17,32,37] This was relatively evenly split between local and distant recurrences in the one study reporting this data, which included 40% of patients who underwent a limited resection.[17]

Metachronous Multiple Primary Lung Cancers

A number of reports of metachronous MPLC have been published between 1980 and 2000. Most included patients seen in the 1970s and 1980s, although a few investigators have reported on patients seen in the 1960s and 1970s,[32,38,39] and others have focused primarily on more recently treated patients.[18,33,37] Characteristics of these patients are shown in Table 30–8. The average interval between the first and second primary lung cancer is 48 months. A surprising amount of variation is seen, with intervals ranging from 18 to 79 months. It is not clear why this is the case. A shorter interval tends to be reported when the definition of multiple primaries does not include a minimum time interval for patients with tumors of the same histologic type,[18,32,37] but this is not consistent.[13] The discrepancy may possibly be related to the average follow-up, although this is not reported in most studies. The differences do not appear to be related to possible epidemiologic differences among tumors diagnosed in Europe, North America, or Asia.

Less than half of metachronous lung cancers occur on the same side as the original lung cancer. This is not surprising when one considers that the original lung cancer was invariably treated by resection, with the result that less lung tissue remains on the ipsilateral side as a potential site for a second primary. Considering that most lung cancers are somewhat more likely to occur in the upper lobes, the finding that two-thirds of second primary lung cancers occur on the opposite side seems appropriate.[13,35,37,39,40] In contrast, a greater proportion of synchronous primary lung cancers occur on the same side. Because most reported series are of resected patients, this finding may be the result of a greater likelihood that ipsilateral

DATA SUMMARY: SYNCHRONOUS FOCI OF LUNG CANCER	AMOUNT	QUALITY	CONSISTENCY
Approximately 7% of tumors have satellite nodules	High	Mod	High
Same-lobe satellite nodules (SLSN) are most commonly seen with adenocarcinoma	Mod	High	Mod
The 5-year survival of stage I patients with SLSN is 60%	Mod	High	High
Approximately one-third of multiple primary lung cancers (MPLC) are synchronous	High	High	High
Approximately 30% of synchronous MPLC are discovered incidentally at thoracotomy	High	Mod	Mod
60% of synchronous MPLC are squamous cell carcinomas	High	High	Mod
50% of synchronous MPLC are of the same histologic type	High	High	Mod
The 5-year survival of resected patients with synchronous MPLC is 10%-20%	High	Mod	Mod

Type of data rated: Plain text: descriptive statement   *Italics: controlled comparison*   **Bold: randomized comparison**

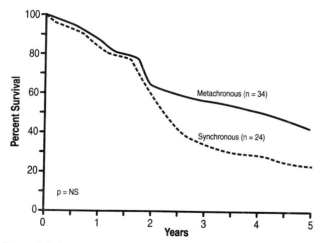

FIGURE 30–2. Survival of 24 patients with synchronous primary lung cancers whose most advanced cancer was stage pI, compared with 34 patients with metachronous primary lung cancers whose second cancer was stage pI (from the day of resection of the *second* cancer). (From Deschamps C, Pairolero PC, Trastek VF, et al. Multiple primary lung cancers: results of surgical treatment. J Thorac Cardiovasc Surg. 1990;99:769–778.[32])

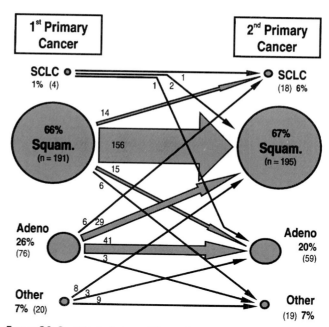

FIGURE 30–3. Histologic type of first and second primary lung cancer in 291 patients with metachronous multiple primary lung cancers. **Inclusion criteria:** Studies from 1980 to 2000 including >20 patients with metachronous cancers and reporting individual histologic types (includes 2% patients with bronchioloalveolar carcinoma). (Data from references 17, 32, 33, 36, 37, 40.)

Adeno, adenocarcinoma; SCLC, small cell lung cancer; Squam, squamous cell carcinoma.

synchronous primary tumors will be resected. Such a bias due to technical surgical issues probably does not occur in reports of metachronous tumors. In most instances, a second resection should be better tolerated if it is ipsilateral rather than contralateral to the first resection.

The histology of the metachronous second primary lung cancer is the same as that of the first lung cancer in two-thirds of patients (see Table 30–8). The survival rate of patients with tumors of the same histologic type has consistently been found to be no different from that of patients with tumors of different histologic types,[32,35,37,38,40] suggesting that same-histology metachronous tumors are *not* metastases. A more likely explanation is that the same factors that induced the development of the first lung cancer may predispose to the development of a second, similar tumor (of the same histologic type, yet occurring independently). This is supported by a molecular genetic analysis of seven patients with metachronous MPLC of similar

histology in whom the primary and secondary cancers were found to have different p53 mutations in all patients.[41]

Approximately two-thirds of metachronous primary lung cancers are squamous cell carcinomas (Fig. 30–3). The consistency of this finding among published reports strongly suggests that this histologic subtype may be more predisposed to the development of multiple primary cancers. This is also supported by the observation that patients with central tumors may be more likely to develop MPLC. A bias due to technical factors in surgical series is not likely to be involved. Technical factors would predispose

TABLE 30–8. CHARACTERISTICS OF METACHRONOUS MULTIPLE PRIMARY LUNG CANCERS

STUDY	N	% BAC	INTERVAL[a] (mo)	% SAME HISTOLOGY	% IPSILATERAL
van Bodegom et al[36]	89	0	79[b]	73	—
Mathisen et al[38]	80	9	46	—	—
Rosengart et al[35]	78	12	48	65	33
Ribet and Dambron[17]	51	—	70	82	39
Deschamps et al[32]	44	16	24[c]	70	—
Verhagen et al[40]	40	—	71	70	48
Antakli et al[13]	39	0	55[c]	—	33
Adebonojo et al[37]	37	0	24[c]	54	27
Okada et al[33]	29	0	49	63	—
Van Meerbeeck et al[18 c]	23	4	18[c]	48	26
Wu et al[39]	20	—	48[b]	70	40
Average			**48**	**66**	**35**

Inclusion criteria: Studies from 1980 to 2000 of ≥20 patients with metachronous second primary lung cancers.
[a]Interval between first and second lung cancer in months. All studies required a minimum of 2 years for cancers of the same histologic type unless otherwise stated.
[b]Minimum of 3 years required if of same histologic type.
[c]No minimum time between cancers required if of same histologic type.
BAC, bronchioloalveolar carcinoma.

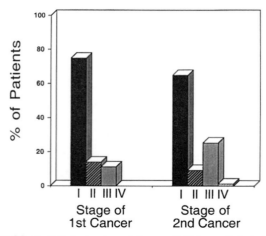

FIGURE 30–4. Pathologic stage (when available) or clinical stage of metachronous multiple primary lung cancers. Data shown is the average of percentages reported in studies from 1980 to 2000 of ≥20 patients (total of 368 patients). (Data from references 17, 32, 33, 35–37, 40.)

to the inclusion of more peripheral tumors, which are more likely to be adenocarcinomas.

The stages of the first and second lung cancer are shown in Figure 30–4. The overwhelming predominance of stage I among first primary lung cancers is explained by the fact that few patients with stage II or IIIa disease survive long enough to manifest a second primary lung cancer. However, the vast majority of second primary cancers are also stage I. This is seen even in reports including *all patients* who developed a metachronous tumor, whether the second primary cancer was resected or not.[17,35,36] The most likely explanation for this finding is that patients received close follow-up after their first lung cancer, leading to diagnosis of the second lung cancer at an early stage. In fact, approximately 80% of second primary lung cancers were discovered by a routine follow-up chest radiograph (CXR) in studies reporting this data (Table 30–9). Most studies, however, have not provided sufficient information regarding

the frequency of follow-up to allow a more detailed correlation.

Approximately two-thirds of patients are able to undergo resection of a second primary lung cancer. Most of those who do not undergo resection are thought to have inadequate pulmonary reserve. The survival of resected patients is shown in Table 30–9 (see Fig. 30–2). The average 5-year survival of 36% is disappointingly low. Even among patients who have stage I tumors, a 5-year survival of <50% has been found by all investigators. The hypothesis that the poor survival is related to a high proportion of limited resections is not borne out by the findings in Table 30–9 or by a direct comparison of survival after lobectomy versus survival after limited resection.[37] The poor survival also cannot be accounted for by a tenuous pulmonary status following a second resection because approximately 60% of patients die of recurrent disease, and only a minority of patients die of respiratory failure.[32,37,40] Thus, the relatively poor prognosis for patients with resected metachronous MPLC appears to be related to the biology of the cancer itself.

Third Primary Lung Cancers

Third primary lung cancers have been reported sporadically in most of the major series.[13,16,17,32,33,35,37,38,40,42] Sixty-five patients with a third primary lung cancer have been reported between 1980 and 2000, out of 663 patients with MPLC. One study has even reported three patients with four and five MPLC.[13]

The data is too limited to draw any firm conclusions. Fifty-four percent of the third primaries had a metachronous presentation.[13,16,17,32,38,40,42] The three primary lung cancers were all of the same cell type in approximately one-third of the patients when this data was reported.[17,32,40,42] Approximately 60% of the third primary lung cancers were able to be resected.[17,32,40,42] The resection of the third primary lung cancer involved a limited resection in slightly

TABLE 30–9. OUTCOME OF TREATMENT IN PATIENTS WITH METACHRONOUS MULTIPLE PRIMARY LUNG CANCERS

STUDY	N (ALL)	% INCIDENTAL[a]	% RESECTED	% LIMITED[b]	OPERATIVE MORTALITY (%)	5-y SURVIVAL (%) All	Resected	pI
von Bodegom et al[36]	89	—	51	16	9	—	20	20[c]
Mathisen et al[38]	80	80	(100)[d]	(61)[e]	8[e]	33	—	—
Rosengart et al[35]	78	—	73	37	2	23	38	38
Ribet and Dambron[17]	51	63	33	35	11	—	58	—
Deschamps et al[32]	44	86	(100)[d]	43	5	—	34	41
Verhagen et al[40]	40	90	83	18	15	18	—	27[c]
Antakli et al[13]	39	—	54	49	—	8	23	—
Adebonojo et al[37]	37	100	97	22	6	—	37	39
Okada et al[33]	29	—	(100)[d]	—	0	—	33	50[c]
Wu et al[39]	20	55	(100)[d]	30	—	—	42	—
Average[f]		**79**	**65**	**33**	**7**		**36**	

Inclusion criteria: Studies from 1980 to 2000 of ≥20 patients with metachronous second primary lung cancers reporting survival data.
[a] Asymptomatic or found by routine follow-up chest radiograph.
[b] Percentage of resected patients who underwent wedge resection or segmentectomy.
[c] Both stage I and II.
[d] Included only patients undergoing resection.
[e] Includes patients with synchronous multiple primary cancers (11%).
[f] Excluding values in parentheses.
pI, pathologic stage I patients.

more than half of the patients in those series reporting this data.[17,32,38] Of 23 resected patients for whom survival data is available, 5 were reported to be alive at 5 years (22% absolute 5-year survival).[32,38,42] Although it is difficult to suppress the suspicion that a third lung tumor represents a metastasis when the histology is the same as one of the previous cancers, the survival figures are more suggestive of a new primary cancer than a metastasis.

VALIDITY OF CLASSIFICATION

Multiple foci of cancer are classified in this chapter as satellite lesions, synchronous or metachronous multiple primary lung cancers, and pulmonary metastases. It is reasonable to question whether these theoretical scenarios really exist (particularly the concept of satellite nodules) or actually occur with some regularity in clinical practice (particularly MPLC). If the concepts are valid and occur frequently enough to be clinically relevant, then being able to differentiate among the groups prospectively is important. At the very least, it is important to know which clinical scenarios are associated with a great deal of uncertainty.

Data from several lines of reasoning argues that the concept of satellite nodules caused by a local mechanism of pulmonary spread is indeed valid. The incidence of SLSN is much higher than the estimated incidence of both isolated pulmonary metastases in the same lobe and synchronous MPLC in the same lobe. The histologic types reported for SLSN are different from those for MPLC. Furthermore, the survival of patients with SLSN is different from that of patients with pulmonary metastases or synchronous MPLC. On the other hand, a limited study (n = 4) using flow cytometry to distinguish tumors has yielded some conflicting data and has suggested that local field cancerization may lead to the development of multiple primary cancers in close proximity to one another.[43] Much more data, however, supports the concept of satellite nodules of cancer spread by a local mechanism.

An estimate of the incidence of SLSN, MPLC, and pulmonary metastases in several different clinical scenarios is shown in Table 30–10. These estimated incidences must be viewed as rough approximations because the data used is not direct, but involves an extrapolation from various types of staging and follow-up studies. When data from several studies is combined, there is an inherent danger that the patient groups in the studies may have been dissimilar, making the combined results invalid. Nevertheless, the results in Table 30–10 provide the best estimate available of the incidence of SLSN, MPLC, and pulmonary metastases in patients with multiple foci of cancer. The results indicate that, overall, each of these three mechanisms occurs frequently enough to be clinically relevant.

The ability to prospectively distinguish SLSN from MPLC or pulmonary metastases is not a major issue. The data in Table 30–10 suggests that the incidence of SLSN is 10 times the incidence of a hematogenously spread pulmonary metastasis in the same lobe and is also much higher than the chance of a synchronous primary cancer of the same histologic type. Most important, the good survival data in published studies of SLSN indicates that a favorable patient population has, in fact, been identified. Classification of only patients with satellite nodules *in the same lobe* in the group postulated to have local intrapulmonary spread not only has the advantage of being easy to apply prospectively but also selects only those patients with a distinctly favorable prognosis.

Multiple primary cancers are easily defined when cancers of different histologic types are involved. This situation accounts for approximately 40% of MPLC. Classification of cancers involving the same histologic type, on the other hand, is problematic. The presence of a precursor lesion in association with an invasive carcinoma (such as invasive squamous cell carcinoma together with carcinoma in situ) implies a local origin and makes metastasis unlikely.[44] There is no data on how often tumors of the same histologic type are classified as MPLC on the basis of associated carcinoma in situ, but personal experience indicates that this occurs in only a small minority of patients.

For metachronous tumors of the same histologic type, an interval of >2 years between the diagnosis of the first and second cancers makes the chance that a second focus of cancer represents a new primary only slightly higher than the estimated chance of metastasis from the original cancer. If the interval is >4 years, the incidence of a new primary cancer of the same histologic type is about five times as likely as a metastasis. It makes little difference whether the original tumor involved mediastinal lymph

DATA SUMMARY: METACHRONOUS MULTIPLE PRIMARY LUNG CANCERS	AMOUNT	QUALITY	CONSISTENCY
The risk of a second primary lung cancer is 2% per patient per year	High	High	High
The average interval between metachronous multiple primary lung cancers (MPLC) is 48 months	High	High	Mod
Two-thirds of metachronous MPLC are of the same histologic type	High	High	Mod
Two-thirds of metachronous MPLC are squamous cell carcinomas	High	Mod	High
Two-thirds of metachronous MPLC can be resected	High	High	Mod
The 5-year survival of resected patients with metachronous MPLC is 36%	High	High	Mod

Type of data rated: Plain text: descriptive statement   *Italics: controlled comparison*   **Bold: randomized comparison**

TABLE 30–10. ESTIMATED INCIDENCE OF SATELLITE NODULES, MULTIPLE PRIMARY LUNG CANCERS, AND PULMONARY METASTASES FOR VARIOUS CLINICAL SCENARIOS INVOLVING MULTIPLE FOCI OF LUNG CANCER IN STAGE cI,III PATIENTS[a]

CLINICAL SCENARIO	ESTIMATED INCIDENCE[b]		
	SLSN[c]	MPLC[d]	Pulm Met[e]
Synchronous Satellite Nodule	5%	—	0.5%
Same histology, same lobe No metastases, any N status			
Synchronous Second Primary Cancer	—	1%	0.5%
Same histology, different lobe No metastases, no N2,3 involvement			
Isolated Pulmonary Metastasis	—	—	2%
Synchronous Same histology, different lobe No metastases, but positive N2,3 nodes			
Metachronous Second Primary Cancer[g]	—	3%	2%[f]
>2-y interval Same histology, different lobe No metastases, any N status			
Metachronous Second Primary Cancer[g]	—	3%	0.5%[h]
>4-y interval Same histology, different lobe No metastases, any N status			
Second Primary Cancer, Different Histology	—	2.5%	—
Synchronous or metachronous Different histology, any lobe			

[a]As defined in Table 30–1.
[b]Rounded to nearest 0.5%.
[c]From data in Table 30–2.
[d]From data in Tables 30–4, 30–5, 30–8.
[e]From data in Chapter 6 and assumptions noted below.
[f]2.2% for stage I,II of first cancer, 2.0% for stage III of first cancer.
[g]Assuming first cancer resected.
[h]0.6% for stage I,II of first cancer, 0.4% for stage III of first cancer.
Assumptions: The organ distribution of distant metastases at the time of recurrence is assumed to be the same as that in patients with distant metastases at the time of presentation. The rate of recurrence in patients with stage I,II NSCLC is estimated to be 40% (see Chapters 11 and 12), 55% of which occur within 2 years and 85% within 4 years.[16,58] The rate of distant recurrences in patients with stage III NSCLC is assumed to be 80% (see Chapter 17), 75% of which occur within 2 years and 95% within 4 years.[55,56] Metastases are assumed to be evenly distributed among five lobes.
MPLC, multiple primary lung cancers; NSCLC, non–small cell lung cancer; Pulm met, pulmonary metastases; SLSN, same-lobe satellite nodule.

nodes. Although the chance of a recurrence is much higher in stage III non–small cell lung cancer (NSCLC), these recurrences generally present sooner. The available data suggests that the chance of a recurrence becoming apparent *after* 2 years and *after* 4 years is similar whether the original tumor was stage I or III.

These speculations regarding the relative frequency of MPLC and pulmonary metastases suggest that an interval of >4 years is necessary before one can confidently classify a second tumor of the same histologic type as a second primary lung cancer. This is corroborated by the finding

that patients who had a long time interval between tumors have significantly better survival.[35,40] However, most reports have required a minimum of only 2 years for metachronous MPLC of similar histology. The average survival of 36% in such (resected) patients would argue that these studies did not include a large proportion of patients who actually had pulmonary metastases from their original cancer. Furthermore, the survival of patients with metachronous MPLC of the same histologic type has consistently been found to be the same as that for patients with metachronous MPLC of different histologic types.[32,35,37,38,40] This also argues that most patients with MPLC of the same histologic type did not have a metastasis. In addition, genetic analysis in a limited number of such patients (n = 7) suggests that the first and second cancers were different tumors in all cases, despite intervals of <4 years in most of these patients.[41]

The most difficult scenario is that of a patient with two synchronous foci of cancer of the same histologic type located in different lobes. The estimates in Table 30–10 indicate that even in cI,II patients, the incidence of isolated pulmonary metastases is nearly as high as the reported incidence of synchronous MPLC of the same histologic type. The survival data is varied, with some studies reporting practically no long-term survivors,[13,32,34] whereas others have reported intermediate[35,36] or even good survival.[33] This discrepancy may result from classifying varying numbers of patients with pulmonary metastases as having synchronous MPLC. At any rate, reliable classification of patients with two synchronous foci of cancer of the same histologic type is difficult at best. Molecular genetic analysis of such tumors may greatly aid appropriate classification.

PROSPECTIVE APPROACH TO PATIENTS

The most important task is to formulate an approach to patients with multiple foci of lung cancer that can be used prospectively. This is hampered by the fact that all the available studies are retrospective and have rarely included a clear description of the patients' clinical presentation. Furthermore, the data is limited and provides only a partial understanding of the biology of multiple foci of lung cancer. Nevertheless, a prospective approach to these patients is needed.

In the following paragraphs, a prospective approach is formulated for patients with cI-III NSCLC in whom a second focus of cancer is not only identified radiographically but is also proved to be malignant by cytologic studies. Patients with disseminated disease (extrathoracic metastases) are excluded. In addition, the 30% of patients with synchronous MPLC in whom the second cancer was found incidentally at thoracotomy (see Table 30–5) are excluded for obvious reasons. Patients with BAC should also be considered separately. Finally, it must be emphasized that the majority (57%-86%) of additional nodules seen radiographically in patients with cI,III NSCLC are benign lesions.[9,45] Therefore, the considerations noted in the following discussion are relevant only when a histologic diagnosis of MPLC has been made.

Among patients who present with a synchronous second focus of cancer, those with a same-lobe satellite nodule can be expected to have a favorable outcome after resection (see Table 30–3). Because of this, there is little reason to perform any additional preoperative staging investigations (eg, mediastinoscopy, computed tomography of the head, bone scan) in patients with a second nodule in the same lobe as the primary tumor, other than what is dictated by the patient's clinical status and the primary tumor. In fact, there is probably little reason to attempt to definitively diagnose the second lesion preoperatively because a resection should be carried out in patients with cI,II tumors with a second radiographic nodule in the same lobe regardless of the diagnosis.

Treating patients with a synchronous second focus of lung cancer in a different lobe is more problematic. Patients with cancers of different histologic types clearly have two distinct primary tumors. However, one must be cautious in accepting this diagnosis based on cytology alone because the accuracy of determining cell type by cytologic studies is only 60% to 80% (see Table 4–12).[46–49] A histologic or core needle diagnosis should probably be obtained, especially if there is evidence of mediastinal lymph node involvement, because this increases the chance of an isolated pulmonary metastasis. Even when the diagnosis of a synchronous second primary cancer of different histologic type is secure, careful staging with distant organ scanning and mediastinoscopy should be carried out because the survival of patients with synchronous MPLC is poor, even in patients who have cancers of different histologic types.[32]

Patients with a synchronous second cancer of similar histologic type present a conundrum. These patients should undergo an extensive search for mediastinal involvement or distant metastases. Genetic marker analysis may be useful in distinguishing between MPLC and a metastasis. In the absence of distant metastases, lymph node involvement, or evidence that the second focus of cancer is a metastasis, resection is reasonable, although the reported survival is generally poor.

A careful search for sites of recurrence should be conducted in patients who present with a nodule that is suspected to be a metachronous second primary lung cancer. This is particularly important if the histologic type is the same as the primary cancer and if the interval between cancers has been <4 years. A new cancer appearing in <2 years should be assumed to be a metastasis unless it is clearly of a different histologic type. Most cancers appearing between 2 and 4 years after the first primary lung cancer are probably MPLC, although a fair amount of doubt about this exists until the interval has been >4 years. Resection of an early stage second primary lung cancer should be undertaken, although the prognosis is not as good as that for an early stage single primary lung cancer.

CHEMOPREVENTION

The ability to prevent the development of a new lung cancer would be of great benefit, especially in patients who have had a previous lung cancer. A randomized trial of chemoprevention to prevent MPLC has been carried out using a high dose of vitamin A.[15] This study randomized

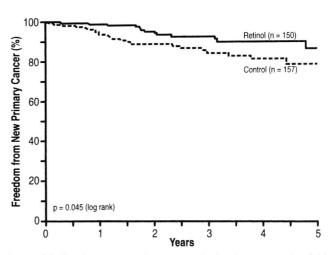

FIGURE 30–5. Time to new primary tumor in the chemoprevention field (lung, head and neck, or bladder cancers) among 307 resected patients with pI non–small cell lung cancer randomized to daily retinol versus observation. (From Pastorino U, Infante M, Maiolo M, et al. Adjuvant treatment of stage I lung cancer with high-dose vitamin A. J Surg Oncol. 1993;11:1216–1222. Copyright © 1993 Wiley-Liss, Inc. Reprinted by permission of Wiley-Liss, Inc., a division of John Wiley & Sons, Inc.[15])

307 patients with resected stage I NSCLC to observation only or to treatment with 300 000 IU of retinol palmitate each day for 2 years. Most patients treated with vitamin A experienced mild side effects, but compliance was >80%, and only 3% of patients discontinued treatment because of toxicity. After a mean follow-up period of 46 months, a statistically significant reduction in the rate of new smoking-induced primary cancers (lung, head and neck, and bladder) was found in the patients randomized to receive vitamin A (Figure 30–5). At 5 years, the rate of new smoking-induced cancers was 11% for the vitamin A arm versus 20% for the observation arm ($P = 0.045$), with most (80%) of the new cancers being new primary lung cancers.[15] These results are strengthened by a similar study in patients with head and neck cancer, which found a statistically significant reduction in the rate of second cancers in patients randomized to treatment with 13-cis-retinoic acid, a synthetic derivative of vitamin A.[50] A larger randomized trial of similar design (1486 stage I NSCLC patients, National Cancer Institute #91-0001) has recently completed accrual, but no data is available yet. Another trial in Europe (Euroscan) involving either vitamin A or N-acetylcysteine in 2573 patients with a history of either lung or head and neck cancer has also completed accrual, and results will be available soon.[51]

Three other randomized chemoprevention trials (total of 69 518 patients) investigating the risk of lung cancer have shown no benefit, but have used different drugs and targeted a different population.[52–54] Three trials have investigated the effect of β-carotene, either alone,[54] in combination with vitamin E,[52] or in combination with low dose vitamin A (25 000 IU).[53] All three trials have analyzed the incidence of primary lung cancer, either in smokers age 50 to 69 years,[52,53] or in male physicians, 50% of whom had never smoked.[54] The two trials involving smokers found that β-carotene *increased* the risk of lung cancer (relative risk 1.18, $P = 0.01$; and relative risk 1.28, $P = 0.02$), as well as the risk of cardiovascular deaths (relative risk 1.11, P not given; and relative risk 1.26, $P = $ NS).[52,53] The third trial found no significant difference in either of these endpoints.[54] Because the trial using low dose vitamin A combined this with β-carotene, it does not allow any conclusions to be drawn about the effect of vitamin A on the incidence of a first primary lung cancer.[53] Therefore, none of these three trials diminishes the credibility of the study discussed in the previous paragraph, which demonstrated a reduction in the risk of a *second primary* lung cancer with *high dose vitamin A.*[15]

EDITORS' COMMENTS

The area of multiple primary lung cancers and satellite nodules is marked by a fair amount of confusion, stemming in part from vague and inconsistently used definitions. When the data is viewed as a whole, however, several conclusions can be drawn with a reasonable amount of confidence. Many questions remain, but it is likely that more consistent classification and the use of molecular genetic analysis will result in a much better understanding in the near future.

Evidence from a number of avenues strongly suggests that satellite lesions within the same lobe are not manifestations of hematogenous or lymphatic spread, although the exact mechanism by which these satellite nodules occur remains to be elucidated. It is clear that the prognosis is good for these patients. Radiographic evidence of a synchronous second focus of cancer in a different lobe should not necessarily be assumed to be a sign of hematogenous dissemination and a diagnosis should be pursued aggressively. However, if a second focus of cancer is documented, the prognosis is relatively poor.

It is quite likely that many patients with a second focus of cancer of the same histologic type actually have a metastasis, despite being classified as having either synchronous MPLC or metachronous MPLC with a short interval (<4 years) between tumors. Even though it is tempting to be optimistic about the chance of cure of two apparently early stage cancers, the possibility that the second focus of cancer represents a metastasis must be considered. The prognosis may not be as favorable as the patient and the physician would like to believe.

Many questions remain regarding the classification of additional foci of lung cancer, and there is much opportunity for progress through further research. The ability to "fingerprint" tumors by molecular genetic analysis may alter our understanding in the future. As the treatment of primary lung cancer improves, an understanding of how to approach patients with a suspected second primary lung cancer will become more important.

References

1. Martini N, Melamed MR. Multiple primary lung cancers. J Thorac Cardiovasc Surg. 1975;70:606–612.
2. Suzuki K, Nagai K, Yoshida J, et al. The prognosis of resected lung carcinoma associated with atypical adenomatous hyperplasia: a comparison of the prognosis of well-differentiated adenocarcinoma associated with atypical adenomatous hyperplasia and intrapulmonary metastasis. Cancer. 1997;79:1521–1526.
3. Nakajima J, Furuse A, Oka T, et al. Excellent survival in a subgroup of patients with intrapulmonary metastasis of lung cancer. Ann Thorac Surg. 1996;61:158–163.
4. Deslauriers J, Brisson J, Cartier R, et al. Carcinoma of the lung: evaluation of satellite nodules as a factor influencing prognosis after resection. J Thorac Cardiovasc Surg. 1989;97:504–512.
5. Yano M, Arai T, Inagaki K, et al. Intrapulmonary satellite nodule of lung cancer as a T factor. Chest. 1998;114:1305–1308.
6. Shimizu N, Ando A, Date H, et al. Prognosis of undetected intrapulmonary metastases in resected lung cancer. Cancer. 1993;71:3868–3872.
7. Fukuse T, Hirata T, Tanaka F, et al. Prognosis of ipsilateral intrapulmonary metastases in resected non–small cell lung cancer. Eur J Cardiothorac Surg. 1997;12:218–223.
8. Okada M, Tsubota N, Yoshimura M, et al. Evaluation of TMN classification for lung carcinoma with ipsilateral intrapulmonary metastasis. Ann Thorac Surg. 1999;68:326–331.
9. Kunitoh H, Eguchi K, Yamada K, et al. Intrapulmonary sublesions detected before surgery in patients with lung cancer. Cancer. 1992;70:1876–1879.
10. Urschel JD, Urschel DM, Anderson TM, et al. Prognostic implications of pulmonary satellite nodules: are the 1997 staging revisions appropriate? Lung Cancer. 1998;21:83–87.
11. Shimizu J, Watanabe Y, Oda M, et al. Results of surgical treatment of stage I lung cancer. Nippon Geka Gakkai Zasshi (J Jpn Surg Soc). 1993;94:505–510.
12. Naruke T, Yamasaki S. The results of surgical treatment of lung cancer with intrapulmonary metastasis [in Japanese]. Chiryougaku. 1989;23:193–197.
13. Antakli T, Schaefer RF, Rutherford JE, et al. Second primary lung cancer. Ann Thorac Surg. 1995;59:863–867.
14. Thomas PA Jr, Rubinstein L. Malignant disease appearing late after operation for T1N0 non-small-cell lung cancer. J Thorac Cardiovasc Surg. 1993;106:1053–1058.
15. Pastorino U, Infante M, Maioli M, et al. Adjuvant treatment of stage I lung cancer with high-dose vitamin A. J Surg Oncol. 1993;11:1216–1222.
16. Martini N, Bains MS, Burt ME, et al. Incidence of local recurrence and second primary tumors in resected stage I lung cancer. J Thorac Cardiovasc Surg. 1995;109:120–129.
17. Ribet M, Dambron P. Multiple primary lung cancers. Eur J Cardiothorac Surg. 1995;9:231–236.
18. Van Meerbeeck J, Weyler J, Thibaut A, et al. Second primary lung cancer in Flanders: frequency, clinical presentation, treatment and prognosis. Lung Cancer. 1996;15:281–295.
19. Ginsberg, RJ, Rubinstein LV, for the Lung Cancer Study Group. Randomized trial of lobectomy versus limited resection for T1 N0 non–small cell lung cancer. Ann Thorac Surg. 1995;60:615–623.
20. Pairolero PC, Williams DE, Bergstralh EJ, et al. Postsurgical Stage I bronchogenic carcinoma: morbid implications of recurrent disease. Ann Thorac Surg. 1984;38:331–338.
21. Levi F, Randimbison L, Te V-C, et al. Second primary cancers in patients with lung carcinoma. Cancer. 1999;86:186–190.
22. Tockman MS, Mulshine JL, Piantadosi S, et al. Prospective detection of preclinical lung cancer: results from two studies of hnRNP overexpression. Clin Cancer Res. 1997;3:2237–2348.
23. Saito Y, Sato M, Sagawa M, et al. Multicentricity in resected occult bronchogenic squamous cell carcinomas. Ann Thorac Surg. 1994;57:1200–1205.
24. Temeck BK, Flehinger BJ, Martini N. A retrospective analysis of 10 year survivors from carcinoma of the lung. Cancer. 1984;53:1405–1408.
25. Weisel RD, Cooper JD, Delarue NC, et al. Sleeve lobectomy for carcinoma of the lung. J Thorac Cardiovasc Surg. 1979;78:839–849.
26. Deslauriers J, Gaulin P, Beaulieu M, et al. Long-term clinical and functional results of sleeve lobectomy for primary lung cancer. J Thorac Cardiovasc Surg. 1986;92:871–879.
27. Watanabe Y, Shimizu J, Oda M, et al. Results in 104 patients undergoing bronchoplastic procedures for bronchial lesions. Ann Thorac Surg. 1990;50:607–614.
28. Van Schil PEY, de la Riviere AB, Knaepen PJ, et al. Second primary lung cancer after bronchial sleeve resection: treatment and results in eleven patients. J Thorac Cardiovasc Surg. 1992;104:1451–1455.

29. Watanabe Y, Shimizu J, Oda M, et al. Early hilar lung cancer: its clinical aspect. J Surg Oncol. 1991;48:75–80.

30. Huidekoper HJ, van Ginneken PJJ. Sleeve resection. Respiration. 1985;47:303–308.

31. Murakami S, Watanabe Y, Saitoh H, et al. Treatment of multiple primary squamous cell carcinomas of the lung. Ann Thorac Surg. 1995;60:964–969.

32. Deschamps C, Pairolero PC, Trastek VF, et al. Multiple primary lung cancers: results of surgical treatment. J Thorac Cardiovasc Surg. 1990;99:769–778.

33. Okada M, Tsubota N, Yoshimura M, et al. Operative approach for multiple primary lung carcinomas. J Thorac Cardiovasc Surg. 1998;115:836–840.

34. Ferguson MK, DeMeester TR, DesLauriers J, et al. Diagnosis and management of synchronous lung cancers. J Thorac Cardiovasc Surg. 1985;89:378–385.

35. Rosengart TK, Martini N, Ghosn P, et al. Multiple primary lung carcinomas: prognosis and treatment. Ann Thorac Surg. 1991;52:273–279.

36. van Bodegom PC, Wagenaar SS, Corrin B, et al. Second primary lung cancer: importance of long term follow up. Thorax. 1989;44:788–793.

37. Adebonojo SA, Moritz DM, Danby CA. The results of modern surgical therapy for multiple primary lung cancers. Chest. 1997;112:693–701.

38. Mathisen DJ, Jensik RJ, Faber LP, et al. Survival following resection for second and third primary lung cancers. J Thorac Cardiovasc Surg. 1984;88:502–510.

39. Wu S, Lynn Z, Xu C, et al. Multiple primary lung cancers. Chest. 1987;92:892–896.

40. Verhagen AFTM, Tavilla G, van de Wal HJCM, et al. Multiple primary lung cancers. Thorac Cardiovasc Surgeon. 1994;42:40–44.

41. Mitsudomi T, Yatabe Y, Koshikawa T, et al. Mutations of the p53 tumor suppressor gene as clonal marker for multiple primary lung cancers. J Thorac Cardiovasc Surg. 1997;114:354–360.

42. Carey FA, Donnelly SC, Walker WS, et al. Synchronous primary lung cancers: prevalence in surgical material and clinical implications. Thorax. 1993;48:344–346.

43. Ichinose Y, Hara N, Ohta M. Synchronous lung cancers defined by deoxyribonucleic acid flow cytometry. J Thorac Cardiovasc Surg. 1991;102:418–424.

44. Auerbach O, Gere JB, Forman JB, et al. Changes in the bronchial epithelium in relation to smoking and cancer of the lung. N Engl J Med. 1957;256:97–104.

45. Keogan MT, Tung KT, Kaplan DK, et al. The significance of pulmonary nodules detected on CT staging for lung cancer. Clin Radiol. 1993;48:94–96.

46. Jolly PC, Hutchinson CH, Detterbeck F, et al. Routine computed tomographic scans, selective mediastinoscopy, and other factors in evaluation of lung cancer. J Thorac Cardiovasc Surg. 1991;102:266–271.

47. Payne CR, Hadfield JW, Stovin PG, et al. Diagnostic accuracy of cytology and biopsy in primary bronchial carcinoma. J Clin Pathol. 1981; 34:773–778.

48. Truong LD, Underwood RD, Greenberg SD, et al. Diagnosis and typing of lung carcinomas by cytopathologic methods: a review of 108 cases. Acta Cytol. 1985;29:379–384.

49. Cataluna. JJS, Perpiná M, Greses JV, et al. Cell type accuracy of bronchial biopsy specimens in primary lung cancer. Chest. 1996;109:1199–1203.

50. Hong WK, Lippman SM, Itri LM, et al. Prevention of second primary tumors with isotretinoin in squamous-cell carcinoma of the head and neck. N Engl J Med. 1990;323:795–801.

51. de Vries N, van Zandwijk N, Pastorino U, et al. The Euroscan study. Br J Cancer. 1991;64:985–989.

52. Heinonen OP, Albanes D, et al, for the Alpha-Tocopherol, Beta Carotene Cancer Prevention Study Group. The effect of vitamin E and beta carotene on the incidence of lung cancer and other cancers in male smokers. N Engl J Med. 1994;330:1029–1035.

53. Omenn GS, Goodman GE, Thornquist MD, et al. Effects of a combination of beta carotene and vitamin A on lung cancer and cardiovascular disease. N Engl J Med. 1996;334:1150–1155.

54. Hennekens CH, Buring JE, Manson JE, et al. Lack of effect of long-term supplementation with beta carotene on the incidence of malignant neoplasms and cardiovascular disease. N Engl J Med. 1996;334:1145–1149.

55. Naruke T, Tomoyuki G, Tsuchiya R, et al. Prognosis and survival in resected lung carcinoma based on the new international staging system. J Thorac Cardiovasc Surg. 1988;96:440–447.

56. Watanabe Y, Shimizu J, Oda M, et al. Proposals regarding some deficiencies in the new international staging system for non-small cell lung cancer. Jpn J Clin Oncol. 1991;21:160–168.

57. Yoshino I, Nakanishi R, Osaki T, et al. Postoperative prognosis in patients with non-small cell lung cancer with synchronous ipsilateral intrapulmonary metastasis. Ann Thorac Surg. 1997;64:809–813.

58. Cangemi A, Volpino P, D'Andrea N, et al. Local and/or distant recurrences in T1-2/N0-1 non-small cell lung cancer. Eur J Cardiothorac Surg. 1995;9:473–478.

PULMONARY METASTASES FROM EXTRAPULMONARY CANCER

John D. Sadoff and Frank C. Detterbeck

The lung is a common site of metastatic involvement from cancers originating elsewhere in the body. In fact, pulmonary and liver metastases together account for the majority of metastases in patients with disseminated cancer. In autopsy studies of patients with extrathoracic primary cancers, 20% to 50% had pulmonary metastases.[1,2] Surgical treatment of isolated pulmonary metastases is currently considered to be the standard of care in many situations. Indeed, resection is possible in the majority (>50%) of patients with pulmonary metastases from several types of tumors that preferentially metastasize to the lungs, such as sarcomas, germ cell tumors, and pediatric malignant tumors.[3]

This chapter focuses on the surgical treatment of isolated pulmonary metastases from extrathoracic cancers. The outcome of surgical treatment and prognostic factors associated with better survival are discussed. The indications for surgical resection are examined, as are issues associated with the selection of patients for surgical resection of pulmonary metastases. Issues associated with pulmonary metastases from a primary lung cancer are discussed in Chapter 23, and malignant pleural involvement is discussed in Chapter 29.

HISTORICAL PERSPECTIVE

The recorded history of pulmonary metastasectomy dates back to 1855 when Sedillot et al[4] first reported a pulmonary resection for metastatic disease. However, this involved direct spread to the pulmonary parenchyma from a primary chest wall tumor and not a discrete pulmonary metastasis. In 1882, Weinlechner[5] resected a discrete pulmonary metastasis that was discovered during resection of a chest wall sarcoma. In 1939, Barney and Churchill[6] performed a planned resection of a preoperatively recognized solitary metastasis from a renal adenocarcinoma. In fact, this patient lived another 23 years, and this case received considerable publicity.

In the 1970s, two authors provided clear evidence that resection of multiple bilateral metastases could be accomplished with minimal morbidity and mortality and could result in extended survival.[7,8] Martini et al[7] reported no perioperative mortality, very low morbidity, and an overall 5-year survival of 27% in 39 patients with testicular cancer who underwent a planned resection of isolated pulmonary metastases. Similarly, in an analysis of 60 patients who underwent resection of pulmonary metastases for "cure," Morton et al[8] reported a 2-year survival rate of 94% in patients with a tumor doubling time of >40 days, although the rate was only 6% if the tumor doubling time was <40 days. Each of these reports significantly influenced the attitude toward surgical treatment of metastatic cancer at the time. In fact, many of the policies regarding metastasectomy proposed by these authors are still followed today.

DIAGNOSIS OF ISOLATED PULMONARY NODULES

Diagnosis of the nature of a pulmonary nodule in patients with extrathoracic malignancies can be considered in several contexts. The focus of this chapter is on patients with a recent history of cancer in whom the primary tumor is controlled but who are found to have an isolated pulmonary nodule or nodules (ie, no extrathoracic metastases). Patients with an uncontrolled primary tumor or multiple sites of extrathoracic metastases raise entirely different diagnostic issues that are beyond the scope of this chapter. Furthermore, the focus of this chapter is on pulmonary nodules

TABLE 31–1. PROPORTION OF TYPES OF PRIMARY CANCER IN PATIENTS UNDERGOING RESECTION OF PULMONARY METASTASES

STUDY[a]	N	SARCOMA (%)	TERATOMA (%)	OTHER (%)[b]	COLON (%)	BREAST (%)	GU (%)	MELANOMA (%)	GYN (%)
Pastorino et al[23]	5206	43	(5)[c]	13	14	9	8	6	2
Vogt-Moykopf et al[63]	729	27	(3)[c]	24	12	11	15	3	5
Robert et al[73]	276	46	32	5	7	1	6	2	1
Marincola et al[56]	217	35	———32———		8	6	8	6	5
Girard et al[78]	186	29	———25———		11	17	9	4	5
Venn et al[72]	118	38	37	————————————25————————————					
Average		**36**	———**28**———		**10**	**9**	**9**	**4**	**4**

Inclusion criteria: Studies from 1980 to 2000 with ≥100 patients.
[a]Germ cell and Wilms' tumors are often not included in these studies because of the role of preoperative chemotherapy followed by surgery.
[b]Includes head and neck.
[c]Includes only extragonadal teratomas.
GU, genitourinary; Gyn, gynecologic.

that are at least moderately suspicious for metastases. For example, patients with clear stigmata of infectious processes are excluded. Also excluded are patients in whom the risk of pulmonary metastases is considered low, either because of a long time interval (>5 or 10 years) since the prior cancer was treated or because the type of cancer (eg, skin or superficial bladder cancer) makes a metastasis unlikely. Finally, patients in whom the risk of primary lung cancer is minimal (eg, lifelong nonsmokers, patients <45 years of age) represent a special group for which the following probabilities may not apply.

The task in patients with a pulmonary nodule and a recent history of cancer is to assess the likelihood that the nodule represents a metastasis versus a new primary lung cancer. A chronic benign process is usually already excluded because a normal chest radiograph (CXR) was likely obtained in the vast majority of patients at the time of diagnosis of the previous cancer. An infectious cause is also unlikely in the absence of clinical signs or symptoms. An important factor influencing the chance that a nodule is a metastasis is the site of origin of the prior cancer. Table 31–1 lists the types of primary cancers most frequently involved in patients who are considered for resection of pulmonary metastases.

Usually histologic confirmation of the nature of a pulmonary nodule is eventually necessary. In clinical practice, however, some decisions must be made on the basis of a presumptive diagnosis. For example, a decision must be made whether to pursue a separate diagnostic procedure (transthoracic needle biopsy or thoracoscopic wedge resection) or to undertake an operative procedure that is both diagnostic and therapeutic. Such a procedure might involve a wedge excision via sternotomy if metastasis is likely or a lobectomy through a thoracotomy if primary lung cancer is likely. The presumptive diagnosis may also dictate whether specific preoperative tests, such as pulmonary function testing or mediastinoscopy, are appropriate.

In some clinical contexts, the likelihood of a particular diagnosis is so high (≥80%) that an initial treatment approach may be confidently planned without a histologic diagnosis, whereas in other instances it is prudent to obtain a definitive diagnosis first. A tissue diagnosis is usually not necessary when multiple lesions are present in a patient with a history of cancer. Virtually all patients (99%) were

found to have metastases in one study that analyzed 146 such patients in whom a definitive diagnosis was eventually established (either by biopsy or by follow-up).[9] The chance that a *solitary* nodule is a metastasis varies according to the histologic type of the primary tumor, as shown in Figure 31–1. A solitary nodule is highly likely to be a metastasis in patients with a prior sarcoma, many of whom are relatively young. The chance that a nodule is a metastasis is also high in melanoma patients. A history of an adenocarcinoma from various sites results in an approximately 50% chance that a nodule is a metastasis. The likelihood of metastasis is low in patients with a prior squamous cell cancer, as well as in those with prostate cancer.

The reports from which the data shown in Figure 31–1 is taken focused explicitly on patients with a solitary pulmonary nodule and a history of cancer. Nevertheless, some characteristics of these studies should be noted to understand the limitations in generalizing the results. Although not explicitly stated, most of the patients were presumably

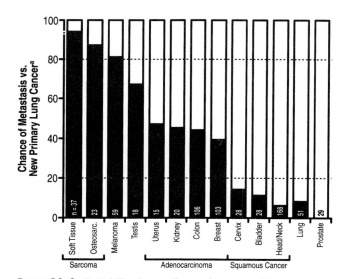

FIGURE 31–1. Probability that a solitary pulmonary nodule is a metastasis in patients with a history of cancer according to cancer type. Inclusion criteria: studies reporting data on ≥15 patients with a solitary pulmonary nodule and a history of a specific type of cancer. [a]Benign diagnoses excluded. (Data from references 10, 69, and 116.)

free of cancer at other sites (or at least more accessible sites) because the patients were subjected to a thoracotomy to establish the diagnosis. Because the studies were carried out primarily in the 1970s, the detection of a solitary pulmonary nodule was probably based primarily on chest radiograph and linear tomography rather than on computed tomography (CT) scans. The higher resolution of CT can certainly lead to the detection of additional small lesions (≤5 mm) that are difficult to characterize further. The implications of such small lesions were *not* addressed in the studies included in Figure 31–1. Furthermore, the data in this figure primarily addresses the risk of a metastasis versus a new primary lung cancer. Although the studies included some patients with benign nodules, it is not clear whether a significant proportion of patients with benign disease was excluded. In studies providing this information, approximately 18% of patients (range, 5%-32%) with a pulmonary nodule and a history of cancer were found to have benign disease.[10–13]

Factors other than the number of lesions and the type of prior cancer must also be taken into account, of course, but are probably of lesser importance. Although the clinical context (ie, interval from diagnosis of previous cancer, risk of primary lung cancer, and so on) is certainly important, it is probably not a major factor if patients with a high or low likelihood of metastases are excluded (eg, >5–10 year interval, young nonsmoker). Furthermore, although much attention has been directed toward the radiographic characteristics of a nodule, they seem to be of only minor importance in establishing a presumptive diagnosis.

The classic picture of pulmonary metastases consists of multiple lesions that are smooth and well circumscribed.[13–15] In addition, most metastatic nodules tend to be peripheral (82%-92%) and in the lung bases (75%), which probably reflects the location of the smaller capillaries and the majority of pulmonary blood flow.[2,14,16–18] The size of a lesion is not helpful in distinguishing a metastasis from a primary lung cancer.[2,19] Most metastatic nodules are <5 mm in size,[2] but larger lesions (>2.5 cm) are actually more likely to be metastases.[13,20] Growth rate characteristics vary significantly among different cell types, from patient to patient, and even from metastasis to metastasis, and there is no way to correlate growth rate accurately with diagnosis.[21] Even in combination, none of these characteristics (growth rate, size, or location) is sufficiently diagnostic to be helpful.[2] To state it differently, radiologic characteristics are usually not particularly useful in differentiating benign and malignant lesions because both benign and malignant lesions are generally small and peripheral.

A few rare radiographic findings may occasionally be of diagnostic value. Less than 4% of all metastatic nodules to the lung undergo cavitation,[16,18] whereas this process is commonly seen in infectious processes.[14] When cavitation of metastatic nodules does occur, it usually is seen following radiation or chemotherapy and in metastatic squamous cell carcinomas.[14,16] Calcifications are usually associated with benign disease but may be seen in metastatic osteosarcoma or any metastatic nodule following radiation or chemotherapy.[14–16,22]

Specific Diagnostic Issues

Pulmonary hilar or mediastinal lymph node involvement from metastatic extrapulmonary cancers is rare but can occur either with or without pulmonary parenchymal involvement. In data from the International Registry of Lung Metastases, 5% of all patients who underwent resection exhibited nodal involvement (11% of germ cell, 8% of melanoma, 6% of epithelial carcinoma, and 2% of sarcoma patients).[23] The prognosis for these patients appears to be poor (median survival, ≤6 months), even when the nodes are completely resected.[24,25] Therefore, mediastinoscopy is strongly recommended if mediastinal lymph node involvement is suspected. Lymph node enlargement (>1 cm on CT scan) implied a 67% chance of malignant involvement in one study of 30 such patients with pulmonary metastases.[26]

Cytologically proven endobronchial metastases are rare, occurring in only 2% to 5% of isolated pulmonary metastases in one study, and most commonly involve breast, colon, and renal cell carcinomas.[27] Patients with endobronchial metastases are usually symptomatic (75%) and have atelectasis due to obstruction (primarily involving the upper lobes).[27–29] The diagnosis of an endobronchial metastasis can be made by bronchoscopy in most cases.[27] Evidence of endobronchial metastases as the first presenting symptom of metastases is extremely rare and usually indicates an advanced stage of disease (involving bone, brain, and pleural metastases in 87% of patients) and a poor prognosis (with a mean survival of only 13 months despite surgical therapy).[27] Therefore, identification of an endobronchial metastasis usually implies that the goal of treatment is palliation.[27]

Unilateral, prominent interstitial markings on CT may signify lymphangitic spread, which is secondary tumor deposition in pulmonary lymph channels after initial hematogenous spread to the pulmonary capillaries.[30] However, the CT appearance is not diagnostic and can easily be confused with lymphedema or pneumonia. A clinical diagnosis can often be made from the constellation of symptoms, physical examination, and radiographic studies. If necessary, a transbronchial biopsy usually provides definitive confirmation. Lymphangitic cancer typically involves an adenocarcinoma,[31] especially breast, gastric, colon, prostate, and pancreatic carcinoma.[14] When this type of pulmonary involvement is clinically apparent, the disease is usually widespread[14] and carries a poor prognosis (median survival, 3–6 months).[32] In autopsy studies, lymphangitic pulmonary involvement is relatively frequent, being seen in 24% to 79% of patients with pulmonary metastases.[16,31]

In patients with a germ cell tumor (testicular cancer, embryonal cancer, and teratoma), persistence of pulmonary masses may occasionally be seen after treatment with chemotherapy.[14,33] On resection, 50% to 90% of these lesions are found to be necrotic-fibrotic tissue, scar, or a mature, benign teratoma.[14,33–37] Although recurrent disease is unlikely if the serum tumor markers (α-fetoprotein and β-human chorionic gonadotropin) are negative, viable cancer cells may be present despite low levels of these markers.[34,37,38] Resection of persistent lesions in patients with germ cell tumors is usually indicated because no test currently exists to prove the benign nature of these lesions[33,37,39] and because residual benign teratomas may grow over time or dedifferentiate into malignant disease.[37,40]

Plain chest radiographs identify an average of only about 50% of pulmonary metastases (Table 31–2).[20,41,42] Standard CT reveals approximately 70% of the isolated metastases

TABLE 31–2. DIAGNOSTIC EFFICACY OF PLAIN RADIOGRAPHS AND STANDARD AND SPIRAL COMPUTED TOMOGRAPHY IN THE DIAGNOSIS OF PULMONARY METASTASES COMPARED WITH OPERATIVE EXPLORATION AND PATHOLOGIC EXAMINATION

RADIOLOGIC STUDY	RESOLUTION[c]	% DETECTED OF ALL NODULES[a]		% DETECTED OF ALL METASTASES[b]	
		Average	Range	Average	Range
Plain CXR	6–10 mm[41]	42	21–59[20,42,104]	48	36–56[2,20,104]
Standard CT	3–6 mm[48]	69	61–78[13,20,42,104]	71	58–84[20,30,42,104]
Spiral CT[d]	2–4 mm[29,48,105]	?	?	?	?

Inclusion criteria: Studies from 1978 to 2000 with ≥25 patients that provided histologic confirmation of the diagnosis of pulmonary nodules.
[a]Percentage of nodules seen radiographically compared with number of nodules found at thoracotomy (both benign and malignant nodules).
[b]Percentage of all metastases seen radiographically compared with the total number found at thoracotomy.
[c]Smallest size of a nodule that can be reliably seen, given the usual density.
[d]Spiral CT may identify 20% more lesions than conventional CT, but this is not confirmed.[46,47]
CT, computed tomography; CXR, chest radiograph.

that are eventually identified at operation.[20,29,41,43,44] CT is also more sensitive for associated factors such as the presence of enlarged lymph nodes, a pleural or pericardial effusion, or interstitial markings that imply lymphangitic spread.[29,41] CT is much more sensitive for pulmonary metastases than plain CXR (73% versus 27%) but is less specific (58% versus 90%) (see Table 31–2).[20,29,41,45,46] Limited data has suggested that spiral CT may be superior to conventional CT in terms of early detection of pulmonary lesions.[47] It is estimated that the resolution of spiral CT is in the order of 1 to 3 mm, given optimal collimation and interpolation algorithms,[48] and that it may reveal up to 20% more lesions than does conventional CT.[46,47]

Preoperative radiographic work-up of patients with suspected pulmonary metastases using a combination of plain films and conventional CT is reported to be accurate 61% of the time, with 25% underestimating and 14% overestimating the extent of isolated pulmonary metastases.[23] However, when only patients who had bilateral explorations are analyzed, prospective radiologic work-up (including both plain CXR and CT scan) is much less accurate (Fig. 31–2).[23] The peripheral nature and small size of many pulmonary metastases, combined with a propensity to mimic benign lesions, make these metastases difficult to diagnose on any radiograph.[2,29] The essential clinical questions are

whether preoperative radiographic studies can predict that lesions are resectable and whether they are sufficiently reliable to justify a unilateral approach to solitary lesions. These issues are addressed in the section on treatment.

TREATMENT

Goal of Treatment

The goal of treatment in patients with pulmonary metastases is cure, which implies that all known disease must be effectively treated. Definitive treatment of pulmonary metastases usually involves surgical resection because there is no curative role for radiation of pulmonary metastases, and effective chemotherapy is not available except for a few tumor types. Patients with an uncontrolled primary tumor and patients with other extrathoracic sites of disease are not candidates for resection of pulmonary metastases because cure is not possible if extrathoracic disease remains. As a result, it has become widely accepted that several essential requirements must be met for a patient to be considered a candidate for surgical resection of pulmonary metastases: (1) the primary tumor is controlled, (2) no other extrathoracic metastases exist, (3) all the intrathoracic disease can be completely resected, and (4) the patient is fit to tolerate an operation.[23,43,49–59] An exception to this tenet is the patient with colon cancer with a hepatic and a pulmonary metastasis in whom a resection of both can be accomplished because this can result in reasonable long-term survival (average 5-year survival of 20% in one review).[60]

There is no role for surgical resection of pulmonary metastases as a palliative treatment. Patients with pulmonary metastases are almost always asymptomatic because most lesions are peripheral. Symptoms usually imply situations that are not amenable to resection because of an extensive pulmonary tumor burden or local (pleural, endobronchial, or mediastinal) invasion,[61] although occasionally an extended resection can be accomplished and can result in reasonable long-term survival.[62] Furthermore, it is generally assumed that noncurative surgical resection of pulmonary metastases does not result in a palliative prolongation of survival, although this issue has not been studied in a controlled fashion. However, certain chemosensitive tumors such as germ cell cancers, lymphoma, and high-grade

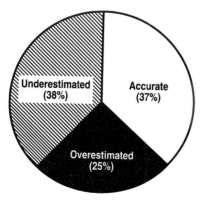

FIGURE 31–2. Accuracy of preoperative radiologic assessment of the number of pulmonary metastases among 1134 patients undergoing a bilateral exploration. (From Pastorino U, for The International Registry of Lung Metastases. Long-term results of lung metastasectomy: prognostic analyses based on 5206 cases. J Thorac Cardiovasc Surg. 1997;113:37–49.[23])

DATA SUMMARY: DIAGNOSTIC ISSUES IN PATIENTS WITH SUSPECTED PULMONARY METASTASIS

	AMOUNT	QUALITY	CONSISTENCY
In patients with a history of cancer who present with multiple pulmonary nodules, the chance of metastasis is 95%	Mod	Mod	High
In patients with a solitary pulmonary nodule and a history of sarcoma or melanoma, the chance of metastasis is >80%	Mod	Mod	Mod
In patients with a solitary pulmonary nodule and a history of an adenocarcinoma, the chance of metastasis is 50%	Mod	Mod	Mod
In patients with a solitary pulmonary nodule and a history of squamous cell cancer, the chance of metastasis is 10%	Mod	Mod	Mod
Nodal involvement occurs in 5% of patients with pulmonary metastases	Mod	High	High
Endobronchial metastases are usually seen in the context of widespread disease	Mod	Mod	High
Conventional computed tomography scans demonstrate approximately 70% of the metastases that are found at thoracotomy	High	High	Mod
The number of metastases actually present is either overestimated or underestimated in one-fourth to one-third of the patients (each) by preoperative radiographic studies	Mod	High	Mod

Type of data rated: Plain text: descriptive statement   *Italics: controlled comparison*   **Bold: randomized comparison**

---

sarcomas may be an exception. In these instances, some authors have suggested that surgical tumor reduction may improve the response to chemotherapy.[63]

Results

The primary outcome measure that has been studied is long-term survival. Five-year survival is usually taken to be synonymous with cure, although occasionally recurrences are seen after this time. Overall, approximately one-third of patients who undergo "curative" resection of isolated pulmonary metastases are found to be 5-year survivors.[23] A fair amount of variation exists in reported survival rates among different primary tumor types, although there is surprisingly little variation among different studies of a single tumor type (Table 31–3).

The fairly good survival of patients who undergo a complete resection of pulmonary metastases stands in sharp contrast to the survival of patients who are not resected. Although there are no randomized or matched controlled studies, there can be little doubt that there are few, if any, long-term survivors of nonsurgical therapy for cancer that is metastatic to the lungs. In a study of 89 untreated patients with pulmonary metastases, all were dead within 2 years.[64] With the exception of germ cell tumors (and, arguably, some sarcomas), there is currently no curative nonsurgical therapy for isolated pulmonary metastases,[59] and the available data demonstrates that untreated pulmonary metastases are invariably fatal.[64–67]

Technical Surgical Issues

A wedge resection results in adequate excision of pulmonary metastases and has the added advantage of preservation of pulmonary parenchyma. There is no difference in survival between patients undergoing wedge resection and those undergoing lobectomy or pneumonectomy as long as a complete resection is undertaken.[51,68–70] Local recurrences at excision sites are rare and are no more frequent after wedge resection than after a lobectomy.[71,72] Furthermore, the incidence of nodal involvement is rare (5%), which argues that larger resections are unnecessary. The majority of pulmonary metastases (60%-80%) are peripheral and are currently treated by wedge resection. In 20% of patients, a more central tumor necessitates a lobectomy, and in 5%, a pneumonectomy is required to achieve a complete resection.[50,51,63,66,70,72–76]

No clear data exists regarding what constitutes an adequate margin when a wedge resection is performed. Little recorded data is available regarding the size of the margins obtained, and local recurrence rates differ widely among studies, probably because of differences in how local recurrence is defined. Simple enucleation of metastases was attempted in the past but was abandoned because it resulted

TABLE 31–3. OVERALL 5-YEAR SURVIVAL FOR PATIENTS WITH ISOLATED PULMONARY METASTASES AFTER RESECTION

	5-y SURVIVAL (%)	
CANCER TYPE	Range	Average
Germ cell[23,37,38,72,107]	68-90	80
Gynecologic[56,108]	50-56	53
Head and neck[50,56,80]	40-41	44
Renal[50,56,63,76,109]	39-53	43
Colon[50,63,90–92,110,111]	30-52	38
Sarcoma[23,50,56,63,72,74,88,101,106]	20-50	34
Breast[50,58,63,103,112,113]	27-38	34
Melanoma[11,23,50,56,66,85,89,96,114,115]	5-31	16

Inclusion criteria: Studies from 1980 to 2000 with ≥20 patients with isolated pulmonary metastases from a specific tumor type.

in high rates of locoregional recurrence.[63] A margin of 0.5 cm was recommended together with a negative cytologic touch preparation in one review, but no data was presented.[53] Another study reported only one local recurrence at the site of a previously excised pulmonary metastasis among 112 wedge resections but did not provide data on the size of the margins.[72] A $\geq$ 1 cm margin was obtained in 99 patients undergoing a video-assisted thoracic surgery (VATS) wedge resection with curative intent; only 3% of all patients developed a local recurrence after a mean follow-up of 37 months.[71] In another study, a margin of at least 1 cm was obtained, yet a high recurrence rate was noted.[77] However, this study did not distinguish between a recurrence at the site of a previous resection and pulmonary recurrences elsewhere in the lung. In fact, 73% of the recurrences in this study were either in the opposite lung or in both lungs, suggesting that the tumor biology was the issue rather than the size of the margin. Furthermore, adjacent occult "microfoci" of cancer were found in some of the patients and were associated with a higher rate of pulmonary recurrence (93% versus 31%).[77]

Preoperative radiographic assessment (usually with CT) allows prediction of resectability in the vast majority of patients. In patients selected for metastasectomy (whose disease was presumably judged preoperatively to be resectable), a complete resection is achieved in an average of 86% of patients (range, 78%-99%).[23,37,65,75,76,78–80] This is the case even though additional lesions are often found at surgical exploration that were not apparent radiographically (see Table 31–2, Fig. 31–2).

Bilateral exposure for pulmonary metastasectomy can be achieved via a number of types of incisions, including sternotomy, bilateral anterior thoracotomy with transverse sternotomy ("clamshell incision"), and separate bilateral thoracotomies. A sternotomy is associated with less pain and generally provides adequate exposure to allow careful palpation of both lungs and the performance of wedge resections of peripheral nodules. A unilateral thoracotomy is usually reserved for patients with unilateral disease that is either central or far posterior, making resection via sternotomy difficult. Some surgeons have advocated a VATS approach.[71,81] This approach requires that the lung containing the metastasis be handled in an atraumatic manner and the specimen retrieved in a protective bag to avoid recurrences at the port access sites.[71,82] There is no data as yet regarding whether the VATS approach yields acceptable long-term survival results. The gold standard is still an open procedure with manual palpation.

An important issue underlying the selection of an optimal surgical approach is whether palpation of both lungs is essential to find all identifiable disease. A retrospective study involving 65 sarcoma patients compared median sternotomy to unilateral thoracotomy and found that bilateral palpation (via sternotomy) identified additional metastases in 40% of patients who were previously thought to have unilateral disease on the basis of CT or linear tomography.[12] Data regarding the ability of standard CT scanning to demonstrate all pulmonary metastases also suggests that without palpation, metastases will be missed in approximately 25% of patients (see Table 31–2).[30,42] Spiral CT techniques may identify more pulmonary metastatic lesions than conventional CT does, but the data

concerning this modality is preliminary.[46,47] How well spiral CT correlates with palpation in identifying metastases has not been studied.

The more important issue—when one considers the possibility of subsequent resection of additional nodules that become apparent later—is whether survival is affected if only radiographically demonstrable disease is resected at an initial operation (without palpation) rather than resection of all disease that can be identified at thoracotomy. There is ample data indicating that recurrent pulmonary metastases are subsequently found in approximately 50% of patients, despite careful palpation of the lungs.[23] Furthermore, the survival of patients (undoubtedly carefully selected) who have undergone second or even third resections is no different from that of patients who have undergone only one resection.[3,23,83] A retrospective study that compared patients with radiographically unilateral disease who underwent sternotomy with those who underwent unilateral thoracotomy also found no survival difference between these groups.[12] If other studies can corroborate similar survival of patients undergoing bilateral palpation versus patients undergoing resection of only radiographically visible lesions *and* subsequent resection of eventual recurrences, VATS resection of pulmonary metastases may be warranted provided that a complete resection can be accomplished via VATS. A large randomized study addressing this question was initiated in 1999 (Cancer and Leukemia Group B [CALGB] 39804).

PROGNOSTIC FACTORS
Complete Resection

The prognostic factor with the greatest impact is complete resection of all known tumor (Fig. 31–3). Numerous authors have reported good survival when all disease is resected, regardless of the number of resected metastases.[8,23,24,51,52,55,56,65,67,72–74,78,84–87] Patients who undergo complete resection have consistently been found to have markedly better survival than patients whose disease is unresectable.[23,49,50,65–67,70,72,79,87–89]

Relatively few reports provide survival data on the actual outcome of patients who undergo an incomplete resection, but it is apparent that incomplete resection results in far worse survival (see Fig. 31–3).[52,70,75,78,79,85,86] In the International Registry, a 5-year survival of 13% was found in these patients,[23] and Vogt-Moykopf et al[63] reported a 17% 5-year survival in 176 patients who underwent incomplete resection. Some authors have suggested that long-term survival after incomplete resection is related primarily to the effect of chemotherapy in patients with germ cell tumors.[63] Other studies have reported that patients who undergo incomplete resection have a prognosis equivalent to that of nonoperative therapy and that almost all such patients die within 2 years.[24,67,74,75,79,87] It is plausible that there may be a slight difference between patients with a microscopically positive margin (R_1) and those with gross tumor left behind (R_2), but no data is available to assess this point.

Histology

There is no doubt that the type of cancer involved has a significant impact on the chance of survival in patients

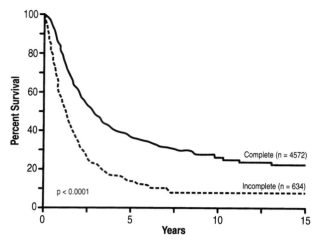

Figure 31-3. Survival after lung metastasectomy: complete resection versus incomplete resection. (From Pastorino U, for The International Registry of Lung Metastases. Long-term results of lung metastasectomy: prognostic analyses based on 5206 cases. J Thorac Cardiovasc Surg. 1997;113:37–49.[23])

undergoing resection of isolated pulmonary metastases. This is seen clearly in the results shown in Table 31–3. The data from the International Registry of Lung Metastases involving 4501 patients who underwent complete resection is also consistent with these results (Fig. 31–4).[23] The tumor type carries independent prognostic significance because the differences were still apparent when adjusted for other factors (age, sex, disease-free interval [DFI], number of lesions) using multivariate analysis in this study (Fig. 31–5). Analysis of these results indicates that three different groups can be distinguished on the basis of long-term prognosis. It is clear that the patients with the best prognosis are those with Wilms' tumors and germ cell tumors. Melanoma involving the lung carries the worst prognosis, whereas a large variety of other cancer types have fairly similar 5-year survival rates clustered between 35% and 55%.[23]

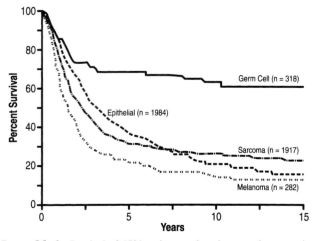

Figure 31-4. Survival of 4501 patients undergoing complete resection, according to the four major primary tumor types: germ cell, sarcoma, epithelial carcinoma, and melanoma. (From Pastorino U, for The International Registry of Lung Metastases. Long-term results of lung metastasectomy: prognostic analyses based on 5206 cases. J Thorac Cardiovasc Surg. 1997;113:37–49.[23])

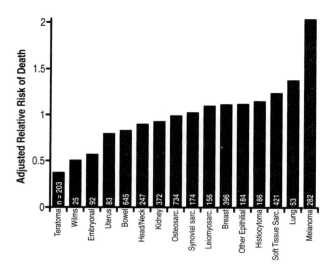

Figure 31-5. Relative risk of death among various types of cancer in completely resected patients when adjusted for the influence of other prognostic factors (number of lesions, disease-free interval, age, sex). Sarc, sarcoma. (Data from Pastorino U, for The International Registry of Lung Metastases. Long-term results of lung metastasectomy: prognostic analyses based on 5206 cases. J Thorac Cardiovasc Surg. 1997;113:37–49.[23])

Number of Preoperative Lesions

The number of metastases is an important prognostic factor. Because of the discrepancy between what is seen radiographically and what is found at surgery, it is important to distinguish between the number of nodules seen preoperatively and the number of metastases found pathologically in the resected specimens. There is ample evidence that the fewer the number of metastases present, the better the postresection survival.[52,76,85,90–93] Many studies have reported that the 5-year survival of patients with only one metastasis identified at surgery was markedly better than that of patients who were found to have multiple metastases (average, 47% versus 17%; range, 35%-53% versus 8%-26%).[85,90–93] The International Registry study[23] found that the 5-year survival of patients with one metastasis was better than that of patients with two to three metastases, who, in turn, survive longer than patients with four or more metastases (Fig. 31–6). However, at 15 years there was no difference among patients with more than one metastasis, and only those with a solitary metastasis exhibited better survival. When outcomes in the Registry data were corrected for the influence of other prognostic factors, independent prognostic significance was associated primarily with the presence of only one pulmonary metastasis, whereas the number of metastases greater than one had little importance (Fig. 31–7).[23]

It does not appear that there is a threshold number of metastases found *intraoperatively* above which resection becomes futile. In the past, some surgeons limited their resections to ≤ four lesions because it was felt that a number greater than this made the patient's disease unresectable.[8] One study suggested that patients with more than six metastases found intraoperatively were likely to be unresectable,[86] but reported that the 5-year survival of such patients was 20% (compared with nearly 40% in patients with six or fewer metastases). The International Registry

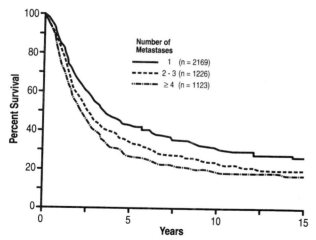

FIGURE 31–6. Survival of 4518 patients undergoing complete resection, according to the number of pathologically proven metastases: single lesions, two to three lesions, and four or more lesions. (From Pastorino U, for The International Registry of Lung Metastases. Long-term results of lung metastasectomy: prognostic analyses based on 5206 cases. J Thorac Cardiovasc Surg. 1997;113:37–49.[23])

found a 5-year survival of 26% in patients with four or more lesions who underwent complete resection.[23] Another study involving 44 patients (with various cancer types) who underwent resection of eight or more metastases found no significant survival difference compared with 412 patients with less than eight nodules (5-year survivals of 28% and 34%, respectively).[65] The survival rates in these studies in patients in whom multiple metastases were resected are high enough to justify the procedure. Thus, there appears to be no reason to abort a metastasectomy operation no matter how many metastases are found intraoperatively as long as a complete resection can be accomplished and the patient can tolerate the procedure. Anecdotally, up to 117 metastases have been resected (in multiple operations) in a

patient with soft tissue sarcoma with no further recurrences 6½ years after the last resection.[65]

The important clinical question is whether patients in whom resection is not warranted can be identified *preoperatively*. Patients with a single pulmonary nodule (identified preoperatively) have been shown to have better survival than patients with multiple nodules seen preoperatively.[24,91] Most of the studies that have analyzed the influence of the number of nodules on survival have involved patients with sarcomas; the thresholds chosen in these studies have been ≤3, 4, or 5 nodules. These studies have found an average 5-year survival of 34% (range, 15%-47%) among patients with ≤4 nodules (or sometimes ≤3 or 5 nodules), whereas the average 5-year survival was 2% (range, 0%-8%) among patients with ≥ 4 preoperatively identified nodules.[67,84,94,95] Therefore, patients with a sarcoma who have > four nodules seen radiographically that are suspected to represent metastatic disease are extremely unlikely to benefit from metastasectomy.

Disease-Free Interval

The *DFI* is defined as the time from the start of therapy for the primary tumor to the diagnosis of metastases. Using this classification, a tumor in which pulmonary metastases are often present at the time of diagnosis of the primary (such as testicular cancer) will have a short average DFI. Therefore, when analyses involve all types of patients, the effect of DFI is confounded by its association with particular types of cancer. The International Registry's study of patients with all types of cancer found a better prognosis as the DFI became longer, although the difference in survival at 5 years was minimal unless the DFI was ≥36 months (Fig. 31–8).[23] Many studies have also reported that a longer DFI confers better overall 5-year survival,[23–25,52,59,67,68,85,86,90] but a number of other authors have found that when all visible tumor could be resected, the DFI alone was not predictive of survival.[8,50,56–58,73,84,96]

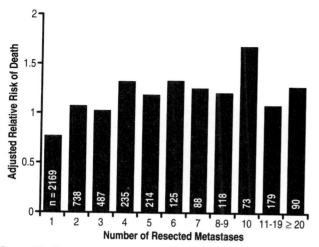

FIGURE 31–7. Relative risk of death according to number of metastases in completely resected patients when adjusted for the influence of other prognostic factors (cancer type, disease-free interval, age, sex). (Data from Pastorino U, for The International Registry of Lung Metastases. Long-term results of lung metastasectomy: prognostic analyses based on 5206 cases. J Thorac Cardiovasc Surg. 1997;113:37–49.[23])

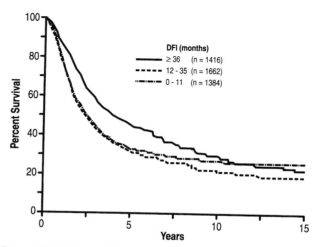

FIGURE 31–8. Survival of 4462 patients undergoing complete resection, according to the disease-free interval (DFI): 0 to 11 months, 12 to 35 months, and 36 or more months. (From Pastorino U, for The International Registry of Lung Metastases. Long-term results of lung metastasectomy: prognostic analyses based on 5206 cases. J Thorac Cardiovasc Surg. 1997;113:37–49.[23])

The variable results may be due to the confounding influence of other factors such as the type of cancer or the number of lesions. The studies that have examined DFI among patients with the same cancer type have generally found that the DFI has prognostic value,[24,50,58,63,75,79,88] with few exceptions.[89,91] When corrected for other prognostic factors, the International Registry data indicated a progressively higher risk of death as the DFI became shorter. However, patients with synchronous metastases had somewhat better survival, an unexplained and seemingly inconsistent finding (Fig. 31–9).[23] It is reasonable to conclude that, in general, the longer the period from treatment of the primary lesion to diagnosis of a metastasis, the better the prognosis, although other variables must be taken into account. However, there does not appear to be a DFI that makes resection futile.

Tumor Doubling Time

Tumor doubling time (TDT) refers to the time it takes for the volume of a metastasis to double and represents a crude assessment of the biologic aggressiveness of a cancer. In general, patients with a TDT ≤20 days have a worse prognosis than do those with a TDT >20 days.[52,64] In patients with a sarcoma, Casson et al[84] found that a TDT ≥40 days conferred almost double the median survival when compared with doubling times <40 days. In patients with melanoma, the TDT has been found to be an independent prognostic factor.[89] However, TDT has been difficult to use in actual practice. Obviously, the TDT is closely associated with the type of primary cancer involved and requires that the tumor be observed for a time before resection is undertaken. Furthermore, it is difficult to predict prognosis based on this measurement alone, especially in light of possible concomitant therapies that may alter tumor cell biology.[94] In addition, different nodules from the same tumor can grow at different rates, thus making estimation of TDT difficult in many situations.[52,64]

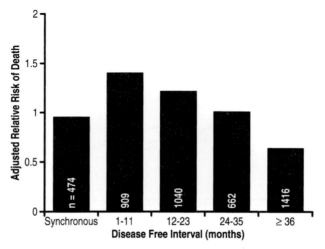

Figure 31–9. Relative risk of death according to the disease-free interval in completely resected patients when adjusted for the influence of other prognostic factors (cancer type, number of lesions, age, sex). (Data from Pastorino U, for The International Registry of Lung Metastases. Long-term results of lung metastasectomy: prognostic analyses based on 5206 cases. J Thorac Cardiovasc Surg. 1997;113:37–49.[23])

Other Factors (Bilaterality, Age, Gender, and Size)

Intuitively, one would think that unilateral disease would be less aggressive and have better overall survival than bilateral disease. However, several studies have found that patients with bilateral metastases do not have a worse prognosis, as long as a complete resection is achieved.[23,25,52,60,63,76,88] These studies provide an indirect argument for routine palpation of *both* lungs whenever possible.

It does not appear that age or sex influences overall prognosis as an independent factor. Men and women have roughly an equal chance of developing pulmonary metastases,[23,52] although certain types of cancer occur primarily in a specific gender. One study showed that women with metastatic pulmonary disease die faster than men,[73] but this observation is likely due to the fact that only men develop teratomas, which carry a much better long-term prognosis.[73] Younger patients (<40 years old) undergoing surgery tend to have better outcomes than do older patients,[74] but once again, younger patients are much more likely to have germ cell tumors, which carry a better prognosis. Overall, age and sex should not be considered as prognostic factors.[68]

Larger pulmonary metastases have been reported to portend poorer survival in patients who have undergone resection.[50,59,68,73] However, it is not clear whether this is due to the size of the tumor per se or whether the larger size decreases the ability to achieve a complete resection because invasion of the chest wall or mediastinum may have occurred. In addition, germ cell tumors may confound the analysis because they are usually small and have a high 5-year survival (see Table 31–3). Overall, no specific size criteria have emerged that have a defined prognostic value in determining patient selection or prognosis.[65]

Multivariate Analysis

It is clear that many of the prognostic factors examined are interrelated, and examination of each factor individually makes it difficult in many instances to draw definite conclusions. Unfortunately, many of the available studies have not included enough patients to make multivariate analysis practical. By far the largest cohort of patients analyzed in this manner comes from the International Registry.[23] Among 4572 patients who underwent complete resection of a pulmonary metastasis, the DFI, number of metastases, and histologic cell type were significant prognostic factors both alone and in combination. Specifically, a DFI ≥36 months and a single metastasis (as defined postoperatively by pathologic examination) were statistically significant, independent positive prognostic factors. Teratomas and germ cell tumors carried a statistically significant better prognosis as independent factors, and Wilms' tumors also had a similar better prognosis, although this was not quite statistically significant, probably because of the small numbers of these patients. Melanoma was found to be a significant independent negative prognostic factor. Carcinomas of the bowel and soft tissue sarcomas were found to have a relative risk similar to that in the majority of other tumor types, although from a statistical viewpoint, the risk

DATA SUMMARY: TREATMENT OF PULMONARY METASTASES

	AMOUNT	QUALITY	CONSISTENCY
A complete resection (R_0) is achieved in 85% of those patients selected for surgery	Mod	Mod	High
Incomplete resection results in very poor (10%) long-term survival	Mod	High	High
Survival after complete resection of pulmonary metastases by wedge resection or lobectomy is equivalent	Mod	Poor	High
Additional lesions are missed in 25% of the patients if the lungs are not palpated	High	High	Mod
The 5-year survival after metastasectomy in patients with a germ cell tumor is 80%	High	High	Mod
The 5-year survival after metastasectomy in patients with a sarcoma or a carcinoma is 35%-50%	High	High	High
The 5-year survival after metastasectomy in patients with melanoma is 20%	High	High	High
The 5-year survival after metastasectomy in patients with sarcoma who have ≥4-5 nodules identified *preoperatively* is poor (≤10%)	High	High	High
The 5-year survival after metastasectomy in patients who have ≥4-5 metastases found *intraoperatively* is 25% if a complete resection is achieved	Mod	High	High
Survival after metastasectomy is progressively better in patients who had a progressively longer disease-free interval	High	Mod	Poor

Type of data rated: Plain text: descriptive statement   *Italics: controlled comparison*   **Bold: randomized comparison**

of death for certain tumor types was found to be either slightly reduced (bowel) or slightly increased (sarcomas). The clinical significance of this finding in these two tumor types is questionable.

In summary, the key prognostic factor is whether or not a complete resection is achieved (see Fig. 31–3). Among completely resected patients, the cancer type, number of lesions, and the DFI have independent prognostic value. The International Registry has the broadest predictive power because of the number of patients involved.[23] Other large studies (≥200 patients) using multivariate analysis have been in general agreement with the conclusions of the International Registry, finding that histology (germ cell versus sarcomas or carcinomas versus melanoma), the number of metastases (1 versus >1), and the DFI (>30 versus <30 months) significantly affect prognosis.[73,74]

PATIENT SELECTION

It is widely accepted that a pulmonary metastasectomy is contraindicated if the patient will not be rendered disease free by the resection, because the goal of metastasectomy is cure.[23,43,50–53,55–57,63,90] Cure requires that there be no extrathoracic sites of cancer and that all the disease in the chest can be completely resected. However, despite meeting these essential requirements, some patients are not considered candidates for surgery because the chance that they will derive a survival benefit is extremely low. Such patient selection involves the use of preoperative patient characteristics that have prognostic value to estimate the chance of long-term survival. Of course, deciding what threshold of

survival probability is high enough to justify resection is a matter of individual judgment.

From the data presented previously, it is clear that the major prognostic factors are the type of cancer (germ cell versus most carcinomas and sarcomas versus melanoma), the number of lesions (1 versus >1), and the DFI (≥36 months versus <36 months). This assumes that the pulmonary metastases are judged to be completely resectable and that there is no extrathoracic disease. The International Registry data suggested definition of four prognostic groups, based on these factors.[23] These are shown in Table 31–4, together with the observed 5-year survival rates. Because the Registry included such a large number of

TABLE 31–4. SURVIVAL OF 4673 RESECTED PATIENTS WITH CARCINOMA, SARCOMA, AND MELANOMA METASTASES TO THE LUNG, DIVIDED INTO PROGNOSTIC GROUPS (GERM CELL TUMORS ARE EXCLUDED)

GROUP	DEFINITION	5-y SURVIVAL (%)
Group I	Resectable, single metastasis, DFI ≥36 mo	51
Group II	Resectable, *either* multiple metastases *or* DFI <36 mo	37
Group III	Resectable, multiple metastases *and* DFI <36 mo	24
Group IV	Unresectable	13

DFI, disease-free interval (between treatment of primary tumor and appearance of metastasis).

Data from Pastorino U, for the International Registry of Drug Metastases. Long-term results of lung metastasectomy: prognostic analyses based on 5206 cases. J Thorac Cardiovasc Surg. 1997;113:37–49.[23]

patients, it represents the best available assessment of how to select patients for resection.[23] However, it is important to note that this model excluded patients with germ cell tumors and Wilms' tumors. Furthermore, it is also important to note that the number of lesions in the International Registry's prognostic model refers to the number of *metastases resected* rather than to the number of nodules seen *preoperatively*. Finally, the reported 13% 5-year survival in patients whose disease is "unresectable" should not be used to justify surgery in patients whose disease is *thought preoperatively to be unresectable*. Although disease in these patients was found to be unresectable, all patients underwent surgery and, therefore, their disease was presumably thought prospectively to be resectable.

From a practical standpoint, patients with germ cell tumors should usually undergo pulmonary metastasectomy even in the face of multiple nodules and a short DFI provided that the lesions are resectable. Although a solid survival estimate for such patients is not available, it is likely that the 5-year survival is high enough (probably at least 10%-20%) to justify resection. This approach also appears to be advocated by the authors of the analysis of the International Registry, as evidenced by the fact that patients with germ cell cancers were excluded from the prognostic grouping.[23]

Conversely, the survival of patients with isolated pulmonary metastases from melanoma is so poor (15% at 5 years for all patients)[23,85] that it is difficult to justify metastasectomy when there are multiple nodules or the DFI is short. The reported survival of approximately 15% at 5 years after metastasectomy involves single metastases in the vast majority of patients,[23,85] and in fact only 10% of all patients with pulmonary metastases from melanoma are able to undergo a complete resection.[66,85] The survival of patients with multiple nodules appearing after a short interval is likely to be <10% despite pulmonary metastasectomy. However, it must be conceded that this survival rate is an estimate and is not based on solid data.

For most types of cancers (any non–germ cell and non-melanoma malignancy), the decision about when to undertake a metastasectomy is more difficult. Clearly those patients with solitary nodules (defined at resection) and a DFI ≥36 months can be expected to have a good chance of long-term survival. In the International Registry analysis, the 5-year survival of this group was 51%.[23] The survival of patients with both multiple (resected) nodules and a DFI <36 months is 24%,[23] making the outlook less favorable, although resection may still be warranted. In such instances, the balance may be tipped one way or another by a number of subjective factors, such as assessment of the likelihood of a complete resection or the medical fitness of the patient. Other factors that will probably influence the decision include the number of nodules seen preoperatively, just how short the DFI is, and the type of cancer (gynecologic and renal carcinomas have a marginally better prognosis than does breast cancer).

RECURRENT PULMONARY METASTASES

Recurrent disease can be expected in more than 50% of patients who undergo surgical resection of pulmonary me-

tastases.[23,79] This implies that other metastatic foci were already present at the time of the first resection because it is assumed that the primary tumor site is controlled. The recurrence rate is highest in patients with melanoma (64%) and sarcoma (64%) compared with epithelial tumors (46%) or germ cell tumors (26%).[23] The prognosis for patients with recurrent melanoma is poor because 73% of the recurrences involve extrathoracic sites, whereas in the case of sarcomas, only 34% of recurrences are extrathoracic. Extrathoracic recurrences account for 56% of recurrence of epithelial cancers and 46% of germ cell cancers.[23]

The 5-year survival after a second or even a third resection in these patients has been reported by several studies to be 37% (range, 25%-48%, measured from the time of the most recent resection).[23,50,51,59,83,87] In fact, the long-term survival after repeat metastasectomy is no different from that in patients undergoing metastasectomy in general.[50,51,75,79,83,87,97] In the International Registry, 40% of all patients with recurrences were able to undergo a second metastasectomy.[23] The rate was much higher for patients with sarcoma (53%) and germ cell tumors (40%) than for those with epithelial cancers (28%) or melanoma (16%).[23]

Obviously, the patients undergoing repeat metastasectomy are carefully selected. However, the good survival of these patients provides strong encouragement that this approach is worthwhile. The same basic prerequisites must be met—that is, no extrathoracic cancer is present and all the disease in the chest can be completely resected.[51] One multivariate analysis of prognostic factors for repeat metastasectomy found that a DFI of ≥18 months (between pulmonary metastasectomy procedures), as well as younger age, was associated with better survival.[87] In the absence of other studies, it seems reasonable to use the same selection criteria for a repeat resection as those suggested for patients being considered for a first metastasectomy.

OTHER TREATMENT ISSUES

Diagnostic Delay

In patients being considered for resection of isolated pulmonary metastases (with no extrathoracic sites of disease), it must be assumed that seeding of the lung with foci of cancer occurred before resection of the primary tumor. The discovery of a subsequent pulmonary nodule raises an obvious concern that there may be many more foci of cancer that cannot yet be seen radiographically. An argument can be made to delay resection for 2 to 3 months to see whether more nodules become apparent when the decision to pursue surgical resection would be different for one as opposed to multiple nodules.[50,63] However, some physicians argue that this action subjects the patient to a risk of further spread of tumor cells originating from the pulmonary metastasis.[98]

No prospective studies addressing the value of a "diagnostic delay" period have been reported, and no retrospective studies have examined how often additional nodules are discovered at the end of such an observation interval. One retrospective study found that the same number of patients developed additional subsequent metastases after resection regardless of the interval between detection of the first pulmonary metastasis and metastasectomy.[50] Furthermore, there was no difference in the proportion of patients in whom a second metastasis appeared within 6 months of operation regardless of how long the patients waited before operation.[50]

Five-year survival has been retrospectively examined relative to a diagnostic delay period in two studies.[50,99] The first study found no difference in 5-year survival among several groups of patients with an interval between diagnosis and resection ranging from ≤ 2 weeks to ≥ 3 months (Fig. 31–10).[50] The other study found better survival ($P = 0.05$) in patients with metastatic colorectal carcinoma resected within 1 month compared with patients who underwent resection more than 1 month after isolated pulmonary metastases were first detected.[99] Therefore, although the data is limited, there appears to be no obvious benefit to delaying resection once a metastasis has been discovered.

Adjuvant Chemotherapy

It is reasonable to consider whether postoperative "adjuvant" therapy after pulmonary metastasectomy has a role in decreasing the recurrence rate, which is approximately 50% after resection alone. There is little data addressing this question, in part because the issue must be addressed separately for each tumor type. However, it stands to reason that as a general principle, there is no point in considering this approach unless a chemotherapy regimen is available that has at least a moderate amount of activity in the tumor type in question. Although there are no guidelines regarding what constitutes an acceptable minimal response rate in this context, it is reasonable to conclude that adjuvant therapy currently has no role in tumors for which effective systemic therapy is lacking, such as melanoma and renal and gynecologic cancers (for which reported response rates are $\leq 20\%$).

In the case of pulmonary metastases from sarcomas, the use of perioperative chemotherapy is controversial, and there are no prospective randomized studies comparing surgery alone with combination therapy.[74,100] When chemo-

therapy is used, two cycles are frequently given preoperatively, with the argument that this allows assessment of the response. Additional cycles of postresection chemotherapy can then be limited to only those patients who have demonstrated a response.[87] However, no prospective trials have addressed the use of preoperative chemotherapy, and no prospective or retrospective studies have examined the combination of surgery and postoperative chemotherapy.[74] One study of 24 patients found that the response to preoperative chemotherapy did not predict survival after resection.[101] Until solid data is available, decisions regarding postoperative or preoperative therapy in patients with pulmonary metastases from a sarcoma must be based on intuition and individual judgment.

Germ cell tumors are responsive to chemotherapy, and 70% to 80% of patients with pulmonary metastases demonstrate a complete response after three or four cycles of chemotherapy.[35] As discussed in Specific Diagnostic Issues, in the 20% to 30% of patients who have evidence of residual metastatic disease following chemotherapy, resection is indicated if feasible.[14,33–36] If residual carcinoma is found, postoperative chemotherapy can be administered, but a favorable outcome can be expected with or without postoperative chemotherapy.[35] Although the prognosis is worse if the residual tumor mass is larger than 3 cm, adjuvant radiotherapy or repeat surgical intervention has resulted in $\geq 90\%$ 5-year survival.[102]

Only one retrospective study of 63 patients with breast cancer metastatic to only the lungs has reported on the use of systemic chemotherapy or hormonal therapy following pulmonary metastasectomy and has compared this to systemic chemotherapy or hormonal therapy alone (without metastasectomy).[103] These patients were carefully matched with respect to age, stage of disease, DFI, type of initial therapy for the primary breast cancer, initial stage of the primary breast cancer, and whether the pulmonary metastases were single or multiple. The patients who underwent surgical resection were found to have better 5-year survival than the matched patients who received chemotherapy and/or hormonal therapy alone (36% versus 11%, $P = 0.02$).[103] However, this study does not permit assessment of metastasectomy with adjuvant therapy versus metastasectomy alone.

EDITORS' COMMENTS

Although many patients with a recurrence of cancer present with widespread metastases, those individuals who are found to have only pulmonary metastases should be strongly considered for metastasectomy. The success of this approach in these patients lends strong support to the concepts of oligometastases (limited number of metastatic deposits) and a limited ability of circulating tumor cells to establish a nidus for growth and develop into a clinically apparent metastasis.

The key prerequisite is to leave no tumor behind following metastasectomy. This requires that the primary site be controlled, that there are no other sites of metastases, and that the disease in the chest can be completely resected. In addition, many relative prognostic factors must be taken into account in selecting patients appropriately, including histology, the number of metastases suspected preopera-

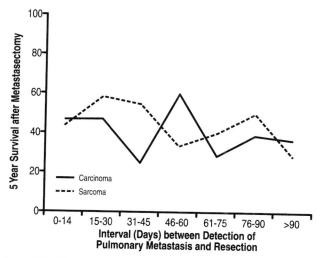

FIGURE 31–10. Effect of interval between first detection of a pulmonary metastasis and metastasectomy. (From Mountain CF, McMurtrey MJ, Hermes KE. Surgery for pulmonary metastasis: a 20-year experience. Ann Thorac Surg. 1984;38:323–330.[50])

DATA SUMMARY: ADDITIONAL SELECTION AND TREATMENT ISSUES

	AMOUNT	QUALITY	CONSISTENCY
Recurrent disease occurs in 50% of patients after pulmonary metastasectomy	Mod	Mod	Mod
Approximately 40% of patients with recurrence are candidates for repeat metastasectomy	Mod	Mod	Mod
Repeat metastasectomy in (selected) patients who develop recurrent pulmonary metastases results in survival equivalent to that of patients undergoing a first metastasectomy	Mod	Mod	High
Resection of only those patients who do not develop additional lesions during a 2–3 month diagnostic delay period does not result in better survival	Mod	Mod	High
Adjuvant chemotherapy following metastasectomy in chemoresponsive tumors does not improve survival	*Poor*	*Mod*	—

Type of data rated: Plain text: descriptive statement   *Italics: controlled comparison*   **Bold: randomized comparison**

tively, and the interval between control of the primary and the appearance of a metastasis. Following the assessment that a complete resection can be achieved, the histologic type of cancer is the next most important determinant of prognosis after metastasectomy. Patients with germ cell tumors have such a good prognosis with metastasectomy that this procedure should be undertaken in practically all cases, regardless of other relative prognostic factors. Patients with melanoma have a poor prognosis, and resection of metastases should probably be reserved for those patients in whom other prognostic factors are favorable.

In patients with sarcoma or carcinoma and isolated pulmonary metastases, other prognostic factors play a large role in patient selection. The number of nodules seen *preoperatively* that are suspected of being a metastasis is of major importance. In the case of sarcoma, the data is clear that those patients with four or more lesions have such a poor outcome that metastasectomy is probably not justified. There is little data in other tumor types, but it is likely that the outcomes are similar. This is different from the number of metastases found *intraoperatively*. In this situation, although there is a difference in survival between patients with only one versus those with more than one metastasis, the actual number of metastatic deposits in those with multiple (>1) foci has little prognostic influence, as long as a complete resection can be achieved. A longer disease-free interval is also associated with a better prognosis, especially if the interval is more than 3 years.

The gold standard is still an operation that allows the lungs to be carefully palpated. It is clear that more metastases are found by palpation of the lung than are found by conventional imaging studies. Although spiral CT may represent a significant advance in the detection of small lesions, an assessment of the accuracy of this technique is not yet available. Therefore thoracoscopic resection of radiographically detected lesions without palpation should be regarded as a suboptimal procedure. The best test of microscopic foci of cancer, however, may be continued follow-up and repeat resection if additional lesions become apparent. Although a diagnostic delay period of 2 to 3 months before metastasectomy is not useful, detection of additional lesions on longer postoperative follow up with repeat resection does allow salvage of a substantial number of these patients.

References

1. Abrams HL, Spiro R, Goldstein N. Metastases in carcinoma: analysis of 1000 autopsied cases. Cancer. 1950;3:74.
2. Crow J, Slavin G, Kreel L. Pulmonary metastasis: a pathologic and radiologic study. Cancer. 1981;47:2595–2602.
3. Pastorino U, Gasparini M, Tavecchio L, et al. The contribution of salvage surgery to the management of childhood osteosarcoma. J Clin Oncol. 1991;9:1357–1362.
4. Merkle NM, Meyer G, Bülzebruck H. Operative Behandlung von Lungenmatastasen. In: Schildberg FW, ed. Chirurgische Behandlung von Tumormetastasen. Melsungen: Bibliomed; 1987:191–206.
5. Weinlechner. Lungenchirurgie. Wien Med Wochenschr. 1882;20–21.
6. Barney JD, Churchill EJ. Adenocarcinoma of the kidney with metastases to the lung. J Urol. 1939;42:269–276.
7. Martini N, McCormack PM, Bains MS. Indications for surgery for intrathoracic metastases in testicular carcinoma. Semin Oncol. 1979;6:99–103.
8. Morton DL, Joseph WL, Ketcham AS, et al. Surgical resection and adjunctive immunotherapy for selected patients with multiple pulmonary metastases. Ann Surg. 1973;178:360–366.
9. Patz EF, Fidler J, Knelson M, et al. Significance of percutaneous needle biopsy in patients with multiple pulmonary nodules and a single known primary malignancy. Chest. 1995;107:601–604.
10. Casey JJ, Stempel BG, Scanlon EF, et al. The solitary pulmonary nodule in the patient with breast cancer. Surgery. 1984;96:801–805.
11. Pogrebniak HW, Stovroff M, Roth JA, et al. Resection of pulmonary metastases from malignant melanoma: results of a 16-year experience. Ann Thorac Surg. 1988;46:20–23.
12. Roth JA, Pass HI, Wesley MN, et al. Comparison of median sternotomy and thoracotomy for resection of pulmonary metastases in patients with adult soft tissue sarcomas. Ann Thorac Surg. 1986;42:134–138.
13. Gross BH, Glazer GM, Bookstein FL. Multiple pulmonary nodules detected by computed tomography: diagnostic implications. J Comput Assist Tomogr. 1985;9:880–885.
14. Libshitz HI, North LB. Pulmonary metastases. Radiol Clin North Am. 1982;20:437–451.
15. Hirakata K, Nakata H, Nakagawa T. CT of pulmonary metastases with pathological correlation. Semin Ultrasound CT MR. 1995;16:379–394.
16. Hirakata K, Nakata H, Haratake J. Appearance of pulmonary metastases on high resolution CT scans: comparison with histopathological findings from autopsy specimens. AJR Am J Roentgenol. 1993;161:7–43.
17. Snyder BJ, Pugatch RD. Imaging characteristics of metastatic disease to the chest. Chest Surg Clin North Am. 1998;8:29–48.

18. Coppage L, Shaw C, McBride-Curtis A. Metastatic disease to the chest in patients with extra-thoracic malignancy. J Thorac Imaging. 1987;2:24–37.
19. Toomes H, Delphendahl A, Manke H-G, et al. The coin lesion of the lung: a review of 955 resected coin lesions. Cancer. 1983;51:534–537.
20. Chang AE, Schaner EG, Conkle DM, et al. Evaluation of computed tomography in the detection of pulmonary metastases: a prospective study. Cancer. 1979;43:913–916.
21. Ladanyi M, Cha C, Lewis R, et al. MDM2 gene amplification in metastatic osteosarcoma. Cancer Res. 1993;53:16–18.
22. Chai J, Patz E. CT of the lung: patterns of calcification and other high attenuation abnormalities. AJR Am J Roentgenol. 1994;162:1063–1066.
23. Pastorino U, for The International Registry of Lung Metastases. Long-term results of lung metastasectomy: prognostic analyses based on 5206 cases. J Thorac Cardiovasc Surg. 1997;113:37–49.
24. Takita H, Edgerton F, Karakousis C, et al. Surgical management of metastases to the lung. Surg Gynecol Obstet. 1981;152:191–194.
25. Putnam JB Jr, Roth JA, Wesley MN, et al. Analysis of prognostic factors in patients undergoing resection of pulmonary metastases from soft tissue sarcomas. J Thorac Cardiovasc Surg. 1984;87:260–267.
26. Glazer GM, Orringer MB, Gross BH, et al. The mediastinum in non–small cell lung cancer: CT-surgical correlation. AJR Am J Roentgenol. 1984;142:1101–1105.
27. Heitmiller RF, Marasco WJ, Hruban RH, et al. Endobronchial metastasis. J Thorac Cardiovasc Surg. 1993;106:537–542.
28. Braman SS, Whitcomb ME. Endobronchial metastases. Arch Intern Med. 1975;135:543–547.
29. Davis S. CT evaluation for pulmonary metastases in patients with extra-thoracic malignancy. Radiology. 1991;180:1–12.
30. Ren H, Hruban RH, Kuhlman JE, et al. Computed tomography of inflated fixed lungs: the beaded septum sign of pulmonary metastases. J Comput Assist Tomogr. 1989;13:411–416.
31. Janower ML, Blennerhassett JB. Lymphangitic spread of metastatic cancer to the lung. Radiology. 1971;101:267–273.
32. Sadoff F, Grossman J, Weiner N. Lymphangitic pulmonary metastases secondary to breast cancer with normal chest x-rays and abnormal perfusion lung scans. Oncology. 1975;31:164–171.
33. Cagini L, Nicholson AG, Horwich A, et al. Thoracic metastasectomy for germ cell tumors: long term survival and prognostic factors. Ann Oncol. 1998;9:1185–1191.
34. Murphy BR, Breeden ES, Donohue JP, et al. Surgical salvage of chemorefractory germ cell tumors. J Clin Oncol. 1993;11:324.
35. Einhorn LH, Williams SD, Mandelbaum I, et al. Surgical resection in disseminated testicular cancer following chemotherapeutic cytoreduction. Cancer. 1981;48:904.
36. Libshitz HI, Jing BS, Wallace S, et al. Sterilized metastases: a diagnostic and therapeutic dilemma. AJR Am J Roentgenol. 1983;140:15–19.
37. Liu D, Abolhoda A, Burt ME, et al. Pulmonary metastasectomy for testicular germ cell tumors: a 28-year experience. Ann Thorac Surg. 1998;66:1709–1714.
38. The International Germ Cell Cancer Collaborative Group. International Germ Cell Consensus Classification: a prognostic factor–based system for metastatic germ cell cancers. J Clin Oncol. 1997;15:594.
39. Anyanwu E, Krysa S, Buelzebruck H, et al. Pulmonary metastasectomy as secondary treatment for testicular tumors. Ann Thorac Surg. 1994;57:1222–1228.
40. Logothetis CJ, Samuels ML, Trindade A, et al. The growing teratoma syndrome. Cancer. 1982;50:1629–1635.
41. Dinkel E, Mundinger A, Schopp D, et al. Diagnostic imaging in metastatic lung disease. Lung. 1990;168(suppl):1129–1136.
42. Peuchot M, Libshitz HI. Pulmonary metastatic disease: radiologic-surgical correlation. Radiology. 1987;164:719–722.
43. Todd TR. The surgical treatment of pulmonary metastases. Chest. 1997;112:287S–290S.
44. Goldstraw P. The surgical treatment of pulmonary metastases. Helv Chir Acta. 1989;56:791–797.
45. Pelotti P, Ciminari R, Bacci G, et al. Usefulness of stratigraphy and computerized tomography in the initial staging of osteosarcoma of the extremities: retrospective study of 217 cases. Minerva Med. 1988;79:41–44.
46. Collie DA, Wright AR, Williams JR, et al. Comparison of spiral-acquisition computed tomography and conventional computed tomography in the assessment of pulmonary metastatic disease. Br J Radiol. 1994;67:436–444.
47. Remy-Jardin M, Remy J, Giraud F, et al. Pulmonary nodules: detection with thick-section spiral CT versus conventional CT. Radiology. 1993;187:513–520.
48. Paranjpe DV, Bergin CJ. Spiral CT of the lungs: optimal technique and resolution compared with conventional CT. AJR Am J Roentgenol. 1994;162:561–567.
49. McCormack P. Surgical treatment of pulmonary metastases: Memorial Hospital experience. In: Weiss L, Gilbert HA, eds. Pulmonary Metastasis. Boston, Mass: GK Hall; 1978:19.
50. Mountain CF, McMurtrey MJ, Hermes KE. Surgery for pulmonary metastasis: a 20-year experience. Ann Thorac Surg. 1984;38:323–330.
51. McCormack PM. Surgery for pulmonary metastases. In: Cohen AM, Winawer SJ, eds. Cancer of the Colon, Rectum and Anus. New York, NY: McGraw-Hill; 1995:857–861.
52. Putnam JB Jr, Roth JA. Prognostic indicators in patients with pulmonary metastases. Semin Surg Oncol. 1990;6:291–296.
53. Dresler CM, Goldberg M. Surgical management of lung metastases: selection factors and results. Oncology. 1996;10:649–655.
54. Harvey JC, Lee K, Beattie EJ. Surgical management of pulmonary metastases. Chest Surg Clin North Am. 1994;4:55–66.
55. Todd TR. Pulmonary metastasectomy: current indications for removing lung metastases. Chest. 1993;103:401S.
56. Marincola FM, Mark JB. Selection factors resulting in improved survival after surgical resection of tumors metastatic to the lungs. Arch Surg. 1990;125:1387–1393.
57. Takita H, Merrin C, Didolkar MS. The surgical management of multiple lung metastases. Ann Thorac Surg. 1977;24:359–364.
58. Wright JO, Brandt B, Ehrenhaft JL. Results of pulmonary resection for metastatic lesions. J Thorac Cardiovasc Surg. 1982;83:94–99.
59. Ishida T, Kaneko S, Yokohama H, et al. Metastatic lung tumors and extended indications for surgery. Int Surg. 1992;77:173–177.
60. McCormack PM, Ginsberg RJ. Current management of colorectal metastases to lung. Chest Surg Clin North Am. 1998;8:119–129.
61. Martini N, McCormack PM. Evolution of the surgical management of pulmonary metastases. Chest Surg Clin North Am. 1998;8:13–27.
62. Putnam JB Jr, Suell DM, Natarajan G, et al. Extended resection of pulmonary metastases: is the risk justified? Ann Thorac Surg. 1993;55:1440–1446.
63. Vogt-Moykopf I, Krysa S, Bulzebruck H, et al. Surgery for pulmonary metastases: the Heidelberg experience. Chest Surg Clin North Am. 1994;4:85–112.
64. Joseph WL, Morton DL, Adkins PC. Prognostic significance of tumor doubling time in evaluating operability in pulmonary metastatic disease. J Thorac Cardiovasc Surg. 1971;61:23–32.
65. Girard P, Baldeyrou P, Le Chevalier T, et al. Surgical resection of pulmonary metastases: up to what number? Am J Respir Crit Care Med. 1994;149:469–476.
66. Tafra L, Dale PS, Wanek LA, et al. Resection and adjuvant immunotherapy for melanoma metastatic to the lung and thorax. J Thorac Cardiovasc Surg. 1995;110:119–129.
67. Jablons D, Steinberg SM, Roth J, et al. Metastasectomy for soft tissue sarcoma: further evidence for efficacy and prognostic indicators. J Thorac Cardiovasc Surg. 1989;97:695–705.
68. van de Wal HJ, Verhagen A, Lecluyse A, et al. Surgery of pulmonary metastases. Thorac Cardiovasc Surg. 1986;34:153.
69. Cahan WC, Castro EB, Hajdu SI. The significance of a solitary lung shadow in patients with colon carcinoma. Cancer. 1974;33:414–421.
70. Koong HN, Pastorino U, for the International Registry of Lung Metastases, Ginsberg RJ. Is there a role for pneumonectomy in pulmonary metastases? Ann Thorac Surg. 1999;68:2039–2043.
71. Lin JC, Wiechmann RJ, Szwerc MF, et al. Diagnostic and therapeutic video-assisted thoracic surgery resection of pulmonary metastases. Surgery. 1999;126:636–642.
72. Venn GE, Sarin S, Goldstraw P. Survival following pulmonary metastasectomy. Eur J Cardiothorac Surg. 1989;3:105–109.
73. Robert JH, Ambrogi V, Mermillod B, et al. Factors influencing long-term survival after lung metastasectomy. Ann Thorac Surg. 1997;63:777–784.
74. van Geel AN, Pastorino U, Jauch KW, et al. Surgical treatment of lung metastases. Cancer. 1996;77:675–682.
75. Verazin GT, Warneke JA, Driscoll DL, et al. Resection of lung metastases from soft-tissue sarcomas: a multivariate analysis. Arch Surg. 1992;127:1407–1411.
76. Friedel G, Hürtgen M, Penzenstadler M, et al. Resection of pulmo-

nary metastases from renal cell carcinoma. Anticancer Res. 1999;19:1593–1596.

77. Gundry SR, Coran AG, Lemmer J, et al. The influence of tumor microfoci on recurrence and survival following pulmonary resection of metastatic osteogenic sarcoma. Ann Thorac Surg. 1984;38:473–478.

78. Girard P, Baldeyrou P, LeChevalier T, et al. Surgery for pulmonary metastases: who are the 10-year survivors? Cancer. 1994;74:2791–2797.

79. Gadd MA, Casper ES, Woodruff JM, et al. Development and treatment of pulmonary metastases in adult patients with extremity soft tissue sarcoma. Ann Surg. 1993;218:705–712.

80. Liu D, Labow DM, Dang N, et al. Pulmonary metastasectomy for head and neck cancers. Ann Surg Oncol. 1999;6:572–578.

81. Dowling RD, Keenan RJ, Ferson PF, et al. Video-assisted thoracoscopic resection of pulmonary metastases. Ann Thorac Surg. 1993;56:772.

82. Downey RJ, McCormack P, for The Video-Assisted Thoracic Surgery Study Group, et al. Dissemination of malignant tumors after video-assisted thoracic surgery: a report of twenty-one cases. J Thorac Cardiovasc Surg. 1996;111:954–960.

83. Casson AG, Putnam JB, Natarajan G, et al. Efficacy of pulmonary metastasectomy for recurrent soft tissue sarcoma. J Surg Oncol. 1991;47:1–4.

84. Casson AG, Putnam JB, Natarajan G, et al. Five-year survival after pulmonary metastasectomy for adult soft tissue sarcoma. Cancer. 1992;69:662–668.

85. Harpole DH Jr, Johnson CM, Wolfe WG, et al. Analysis of 945 cases of pulmonary metastatic melanoma. J Thorac Cardiovasc Surg. 1992;103:743–750.

86. Vogt-Moykopf I, Bülzebruck H, Merkle NM. Results of surgical treatment of pulmonary metastases. Eur J Cardiothorac Surg. 1988;2:224–232.

87. Pogrebniak HW, Roth JA, Steinberg SM, et al. Reoperative pulmonary resection in patients with metastatic soft tissue sarcoma. Ann Thorac Surg. 1991;52:197–203.

88. Billingsley KG, Burt ME, Jara E, et al. Pulmonary metastases from soft tissue sarcoma: analysis of patterns of disease and postmetastasis survival. Ann Surg. 1999;229:602–612.

89. Ollila DW, Stern SL, Morton DL. Tumor doubling time: a selection factor for pulmonary resection of metastatic melanoma. J Surg Oncol. 1998;69:206–211.

90. Mansel JK, Zinsmeister AR, Pairolero PC, et al. Pulmonary resection of metastatic colorectal adenocarcinoma: a ten year experience. Chest. 1986;89:109–112.

91. Girard P, Ducreux M, Baldeyrou P, et al. Surgery for lung metastases from colorectal cancer: analysis of prognostic factors. J Clin Oncol. 1996;14:2047–2053.

92. Okumura S, Kondo H, Tsuboi M, et al. Pulmonary resection for metastatic colorectal cancer: experiences with 159 patients. J Thorac Cardiovasc Surg. 1996;112:867–874.

93. Goya T, Miyazawa N, Kondo H, et al. Surgical resection of pulmonary metastases from colorectal cancer: ten year follow-up. Cancer. 1989;64:1418–1421.

94. Roth JA, Putnam JB Jr, Wesley MN, et al. Differing determinants of prognosis following resection of pulmonary metastases from osteogenic and soft tissue sarcoma patients. Cancer. 1985;55:1361–1366.

95. Meyer WH, Schell MJ, Jumar PM, et al. Thoracotomy for pulmonary metastatic osteosarcoma: an analysis of prognostic indicators of survival. Cancer. 1987;59:374–379.

96. Gorenstein LA, Putnam Jr JB, Natarajan G, et al. Improved survival after resection of pulmonary metastases from malignant melanoma. Ann Thorac Surg. 1991;52:204–210.

97. Potter DA, Kinsella T, Glatstein E, et al. High grade soft tissue sarcomas of the extremities. Cancer. 1986;58:190–195.

98. Valente M, Pastorino U. Secondary lung cancer resection with curative intent: causes of success and failure and prognostic factors. Tumori. 1982;68:337–340.

99. van Halteren H, van Geel AN, Hart AAM, et al. Pulmonary resection for metastases of colorectal origin. Chest. 1995;107:1526–1531.

100. Belli L, Scholl S, Livartowski A, et al. Resection of pulmonary metastases in osteosarcoma: a retrospective analysis of 44 patients. Cancer. 1989;63:2546–2550.

101. Lanza LA, Putnam JB Jr, Benjamin RS, et al. Response to chemotherapy does not predict survival after resection of sarcomatous pulmonary metastases. Ann Thorac Surg. 1991;51:219–224.

102. Puc H, Hellan R, Mazumdar M, et al. Management of residual mass in advanced seminoma: results and recommendations from the Memorial Sloan-Kettering Cancer Center. J Clin Oncol. 1996;14:454.

103. Staren ED, Salerno C, Rongione A, et al. Pulmonary resection for metastatic breast cancer. Arch Surg. 1992;127:1282–1284.

104. Schaner EG, Chang AE, Doppman JL, et al. Comparison of computed and conventional whole lung tomography in detecting pulmonary nodules: a prospective radiologic-pathologic study. AJR Am J Roentgenol. 1978;131:51–54.

105. Coakley FV, Cohen MD, Waters DJ, et al. Detection of pulmonary metastases with pathological correlation: effect of breathing on the accuracy of spiral CT. Pediatr Radiol. 1997;27:576–579.

106. Carter SR, Grimer RJ, Sneath RS, et al. Results of thoracotomy in osteogenic sarcoma with pulmonary metastases. Thorax. 1991;46:727–731.

107. Daugaard G, Hansen HH, Rorth M. Treatment of malignant germ cell tumors. Ann Oncol. 1990;1:195–202.

108. Seki M, Nakagawa K, Tsuchiya S, et al. Surgical treatment of pulmonary metastases from uterine cervical cancer: operation method by lung tumor size. J Thorac Cardiovasc Surg. 1992;104:876–881.

109. Cerfolio RJ, Allen MS, Deschamps C, et al. Pulmonary resection of metastatic renal cell carcinoma. Ann Thorac Surg. 1994;57:339–344.

110. McCormack PM, Burt ME, Bains MS, et al. Lung resection for colorectal metastases: ten year results. Arch Surg. 1992;127:1403–1406.

111. Regnard JF, Grunenwald D, Spaggiari L, et al. Surgical treatment of hepatic and pulmonary metastases from colorectal cancers. Ann Thorac Surg. 1998;66:214–219.

112. Friedel G, Linder A, Toomes H. The significance of prognostic factors for the resection of pulmonary metastases of breast cancer. Thorac Cardiovasc Surg. 1994;42:71–75.

113. McDonald ML, Deschamps C, Ilstrup DM, et al. Pulmonary resection for metastatic breast cancer. Ann Thorac Surg. 1994;58:1599–1602.

114. Wong JH, Euhus DM, Morton DL. Surgical resection for metastatic melanoma to the lung. Arch Surg. 1988;23:1091–1095.

115. Karp NS, Boyd A, DePan HJ, et al. Thoracotomy for metastatic malignant melanoma of the lung. Surgery. 1990;107:256–261.

116. Cahan WG, Shaw JP, Castro EL. Benign solitary lung lesions in patients with cancer. Ann Surg. 1978;187:241–244.

INDEX

Note: Page numbers in *italics* refer to illustrations; page numbers in **boldface** refer to data summaries; page numbers followed by t refer to tables.

A

ISBN 0-7216-9192-7

90038

9 780721 691923

WMD 200418